To my loving wife, Brenda. The years have been kind to her; and she has been even kinder to me.

Contributors

D. Greg Anderson, MD
Assistant Professor
Department of Orthopaedic Surgery
University of Virginia
Assistant Professor
Department of Orthopaedic Surgery
University of Virginia Medical Center
Charlottesville, Virginia
Trauma

Mark R. Brinker, MD
Clinical Professor of Orthopaedic Surgery
Tulane University School of Medicine
New Orleans, Louisiana
Clinical Professor of Orthopaedic Surgery
Texas Tech University
Health Sciences Center School of Medicine
Lubbock, Texas
Director of Acute and Reconstructive Trauma
Texas Orthopedic Hospital
Fondren Orthopedic Group, LLP
Houston, Texas
Basic Sciences

David B. Carmack, MD, Major, USAF, MC
Chief
AF C-STARS Orthopaedic Trauma Surgery
Department of Orthopaedic Surgery
R Adams Cowley Shock Trauma Center
Baltimore, Maryland
Trauma

Anikar Chhabra, MD
Resident
Department of Orthopaedic Surgery
University of Virginia,
Charlottesville, Virginia
Sports Medicine

Brian J. Cole, MD, MBA
Associate Professor
Department of Orthopaedics and Anatomy (Conjoint)
Rush Medical College
Director
Rush Cartilage Restoration Center
Rush Presbyterian St. Luke's Medical Center
Chicago, Illinois
Sports Medicine

Deborah A. Frassica, MD
Assistant Professor of Radiation Oncology
Department of Radiation Oncology and Molecular Radiation Sciences
Johns Hopkins University
Baltimore, Maryland
Orthopaedic Pathology

Frank J. Frassica, MD
Robert A. Robinson Professor and Chairman of Orthopaedic Surgery
Department of Orthopaedic Surgery
Professor of Oncology
Sidney Kimmel Comprehensive Cancer Center
Johns Hopkins University
Department Director
Department of Orthopaedic Surgery
Johns Hopkins Hospital
Baltimore, Maryland
Orthopaedic Pathology

Frank A. Gottschalk, MD, FRCS Ed, FCS(SA) Orth
Professor
Department of Orthopaedic Surgery
University of Texas Southwestern Medical Center at Dallas
Attending
Department of Orthopaedic Surgery
Zale Lipshy University Hospital
Attending
Department of Orthopaedic Surgery
Parkland Health & Hospital System
Dallas, Texas
Rehabilitation: Gait, Amputations, Prosthetics, Orthotics

Richard F. Howard, DO
Assistant Clinical Professor
Department of Orthopedic Surgery
Saint Louis University
Chief of Surgery
Des Peres Hospital
Program Director
Des Peres Hospital Orthopedic Surgery Program
St. Louis, Missouri
Hand and Microsurgery

Kerry G. Jepsen, MD, Major, USAF, MC, FS
Department of Orthopedics and Podiatry
Landstuhl Regional Medical Center
Germany
Principles of Practice and Statistics

Leonid I. Katolik, MD
Chief Resident
Department of Orthopaedic Surgery
Rush University School of Medicine
Chief Resident
Department of Orthopaedic Surgery
Rush Presbyterian St. Luke's Medical Center
Chicago, Illinois
Fellow in Hand and Microvascular Surgery
Department of Orthopaedic Surgery
Division of Hand and Microvascular Surgery
University of Washington Combined Program
Seattle, Washington
Sports Medicine

William C. Lauerman, MD
Professor
Deparment of Orthopaedic Surgery
Georgetown University Hospital
Washington, D.C.
Spine

C. Michael LeCroy, MD
Director
Orthopaedic Trauma Service
Mission Hospitals and Clinics
Asheville, North Carolina
Trauma

Brian R. McCall, MD
Chief Resident
Department of Orthopaedic Surgery
Georgetown University Hospital
Washington, D.C.
Spine

Edward F. McCarthy, MD
Professor of Pathology and Orthopaedics
Johns Hopkins Hospital
Baltimore, Maryland
Orthopaedic Pathology

Edward J. McPherson, MD, FACS
Associate Professor of Orthopaedic Surgery
Department of Orthopaedics
University of Southern California
Associate Professor of Orthopaedic Surgery
USC University Hospital
Los Angeles, California
Adult Reconstruction

Todd A. Milbrandt, MD, MS
Chief Resident
Department of Orthopaedics
University of Virginia
Charlottesville, Virginia
Pediatric Orthopaedics
Trauma

Brian Mullis, MD
Resident
Department of Orthopaedic Surgery
University of North Carolina at Chapel Hill
Resident
Department of Orthopaedic Surgery
UNC Hospitals
Chapel Hill, North Carolina
Trauma

Daniel P. O'Connor, PhD
President
Joe W. King Orthopedic Institute
Houston, Texas
Basic Sciences

Raymond Pavlovich, Jr., MD
Fellow
Department of Sports Medicine
Rush St. Luke's Presbyterian Hospital
Chicago, Illinois
Sports Medicine

Kevin D. Plancher, MD, MS
Associate Clinical Professor
Department of Orthopaedics
Albert Einstein College of Medicine
Attending
Department of Orthopaedics
Beth Israel North
New York, New York
Attending
Department of Orthopaedics
The Stamford Hospital
Stamford, Connecticut
Attending
Department of Orthopaedics
Westchester Square Hospital
Bronx, New York
Principles of Practice and Statistics

E. Greer Richardson, MD
Professor
Co-Director
Foot and Ankle Fellowship
Department of Orthopaedic Surgery
University of Tennessee Campbell Clinic
President
Medical Staff
Baptist Memorial Hospital
Consulting Staff
Methodist Hospitals
Memphis, Tennessee
Disorders of the Foot and Ankle

LtCol Damian M. Rispoli, MD
Assistant Professor
Department of Surgery
Uniformed Services University School of Medicine
Bethesda, Maryland
Director of Orthopaedic Education
Department of Orthopaedics
Malcolm Grow Medical Center
Andrews AFB, Maryland
Principles of Practice and Statistics

Franklin D. Shuler, MD, PhD
Assistant Professor
Department of Orthopaedic Surgery and Rehabilitation
Division of Orthopaedic Trauma
Vanderbilt University
Nashville, Tennessee
Anatomy

Daniel J. Sucato, MD, MS
Assistant Professor
Department of Orthopaedic Surgery
University of Texas at Southwestern Medical Center
Orthopaedic Surgeon
Department of Orthopaedic Surgery
Texas Scottish Rite Hospital
Dallas, Texas
Pediatric Orthopaedics

Preface

> Look beneath the surface; let not the several quality of a thing nor its worth escape thee.
>
> Marcus Aurelius (121-180); Meditations vi 3.

It is my distinct pleasure to introduce the Fourth Edition of the popular textbook *Review of Orthopaedics,* a book more familiar to some residents than their "significant other." I have been blessed with an extremely positive response from residents all over the world to both this book and the *Colorado Orthopaedic Review Course* that it fostered. It is a special treat for me to have so many of you personally thank me for what **we** have put together. For that I am tremendously grateful and offer my heartfelt thanks.

I would be remiss, however, if I did not emphasize that small two-letter word—**we**. After the first edition, I made the transition from author to editor. There is no way that I could do justice to a review of anything but Sports Medicine at this point in my career. Perhaps this is a product of further sub-specialization in Orthopaedics, or perhaps it is a reflection of the never-ending explosion of knowledge in our specialty. Regardless, I owe a special debt of gratitude to the authors of *Review of Orthopaedics.* They have done a fabulous job! We all recognize that some multiple-edition texts offer little more than a new cover.

By the way, I was very pleased that we moved on from the salmon color of the third edition—fortunately, the old refrain that you can't judge a book by its cover held true. This edition is a complete renovation—we brought back the trauma tables (and included pediatric trauma), we invited several new authors who have extensively revised outdated chapters, we made new tables, included new illustrations, added new material, and (thankfully) changed the cover. Basically, **we** made sure that this edition will prepare **you** for In-Training Examinations, Board Examinations, Recertification, *and* your daily practice of Orthopaedic Surgery.

Mark D. Miller, MD

Contents

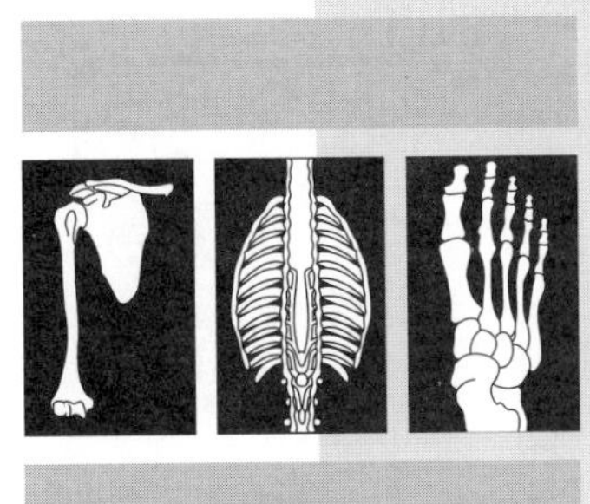

1

Basic Sciences

MARK R. BRINKER
DANIEL P. O'CONNOR

SECTION 1

Bone

I. Histology of Bone

A. Types—Normal bone is lamellar and can be cortical or cancellous. Immature and pathologic bone is woven, is more random with more osteocytes than lamellar bone, has increased turnover, and is weaker and more flexible than lamellar bone. Lamellar bone is stress oriented; woven bone is not stress oriented.

1. Cortical Bone (Compact Bone) (Fig. 1-1; Table 1-1)—Makes up 80% of the skeleton; composed of tightly packed osteons or haversian systems connected by haversian (or Volkmann's) canals containing arterioles, venules, capillaries, nerves, and possibly lymphatic channels. Interstitial lamellae lie between the osteons. Fibrils frequently connect lamellae but do not cross cement lines (where bone resorption has stopped and new bone formation has begun). Cement lines define the outer border of an osteon. Intraosseous circulation (canals and canaliculi [cell processes of osteocytes]) provides nutrition. Cortical bone has a slow turnover rate, a relatively high Young's modulus (*E*), and a higher resistance to torsion and bending than cancellous bone.
2. Cancellous Bone (Spongy or Trabecular Bone) (see Fig. 1-1)—Less dense and undergoes more remodeling according to lines of stress (Wolff's law). It has a higher turnover rate, has a smaller Young's modulus, and is more elastic than ortical bone.

B. Cellular Biology

1. Osteoblasts—Form bone. Derived from undifferentiated mesenchymal cells. These cells have

Table 1-1. TYPES OF BONES

MICROSCOPIC APPEARANCE	SUBTYPES	CHARACTERISTICS	EXAMPLES
Lamellar	Cortical	Structure is oriented along lines of stress Strong	Femoral shaft
	Cancellous	More elastic than cortical bone	Distal femoral metaphysis
Woven	Immature	Not stress oriented	Embryonic skeleton Fracture callus
	Pathologic	Random organization Increased turnover Weak Flexible	Osteogenic sarcoma Fibrous dysplasia

Modified from Brinker, M.R., and Miller, M.D.: Fundamentals of Orthopaedics. Philadelphia, WB Saunders, 1999, p.1.

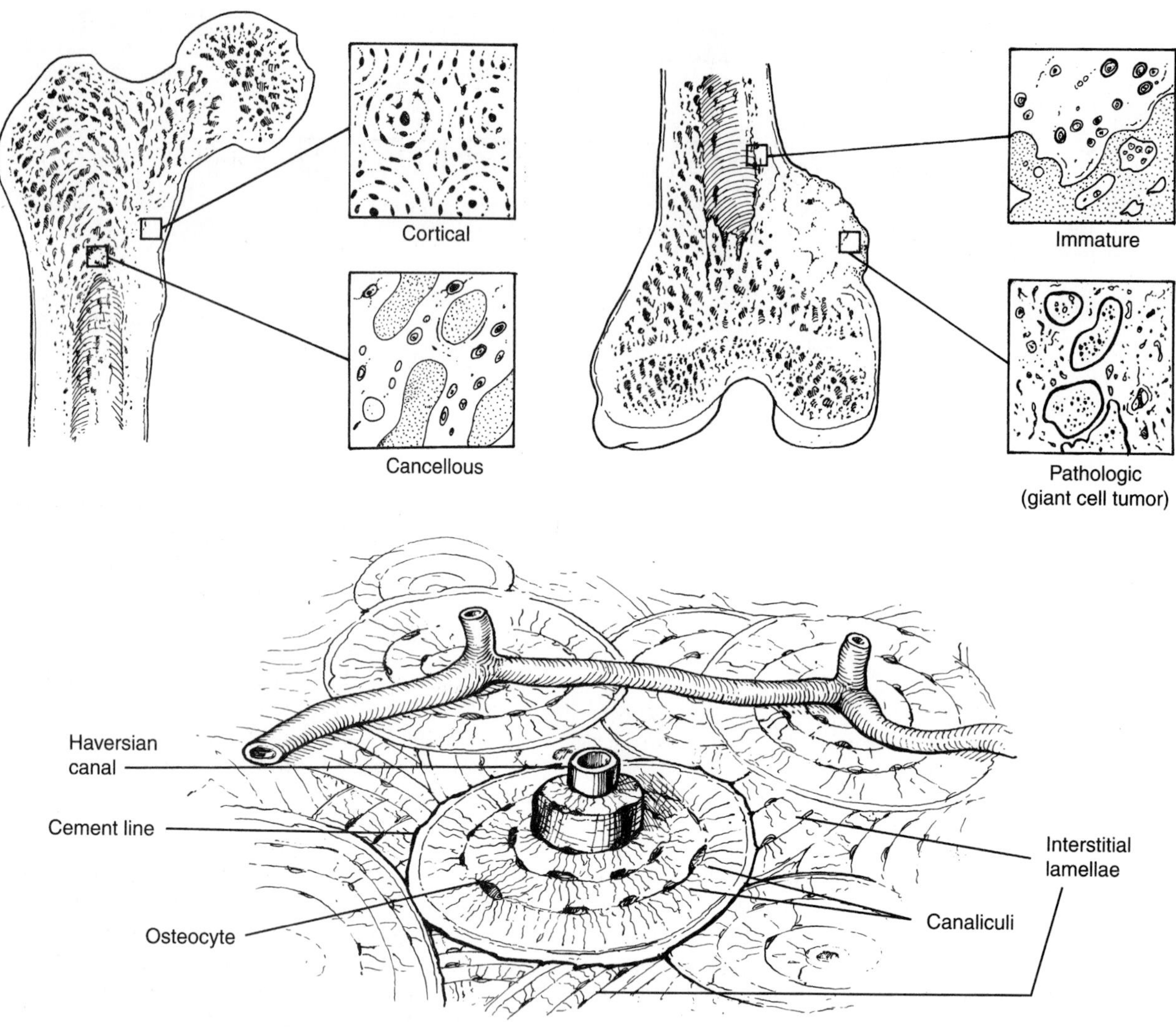

FIGURE 1-1 ■ Types of bone. *Cortical* bone consists of tightly packed osteons. *Cancellous* bone consists of a meshwork of trabeculae. In *immature* bone, there is unmineralized osteoid lining the immature trabeculae. In *pathologic bone,* atypical osteoblasts and architectural disorganization are seen. (From Brinker, M.R., and Miller, M.D.: Fundamentals of Orthopaedics. Philadelphia, WB Saunders, 1999, p. 2.)

more endoplasmic reticulum, Golgi apparatus, and mitochondria than other cells (for synthesis and secretion of matrix). More differentiated, metabolically active cells line bone surfaces and less active cells in "resting regions" or entrapped cells maintain the ionic milieu of bone. Disruption of the lining cell layer activates these cells. Osteoblast differentiation in vivo is effected by the interleukins, platelet-derived growth factor (PDGF), and insulin-derived growth factor (IDGF). **Osteoblasts respond to parathyroid hormone (PTH)**, produce alkaline phosphatase, produce type I collagen, and produce osteocalcin (stimulated by 1,25-dihydroxyvitamin D). Osteoblasts have receptor-effector interactions for (1) PTH; (2) 1,25-dihydroxyvitamin D; (3) glucocorticoids; (4) prostaglandins; and (5) estrogen (Table 1-2). Certain antiseptic agents are toxic to cultured osteoblasts (including hydrogen peroxide and povidone-iodine [Betadine] solution and scrub). Bacitracin is believed to be less toxic.

2. Osteocytes (see Fig. 1-1)—Maintain bone. Make up 90% of the cells in the mature skeleton; are former osteoblasts trapped in newly formed matrix (which they help preserve). Osteocytes have a high nucleus/cytoplasm ratio with long interconnecting cytoplasmic processes. Not as active in matrix production as osteoblasts. Important for control of extracellular calcium and phosphorus concentration.

Table 1-2. BONE CELL TYPES, RECEPTOR TYPES, AND EFFECTS

CELL TYPE	RECEPTOR	EFFECT
Osteoblast	PTH	Releases a secondary messenger (exact mechanism unknown) to stimulate osteoclastic activity. Activates adenylate cyclase.
	1–25 Vitamin D_3	Stimulates matrix and alkaline phosphatase synthesis and production of bone-specific proteins (such as osteocalcin).
	Glucocorticoids	Inhibits the synthesis of DNA, production of collagen, and synthesis of osteoblastic proteins.
	Prostaglandins	Activates adenylate cyclase and stimulates resorption of bone.
	Estrogen	Anabolic (bone production) and anticatabolic (prevents bone resorption) effect on bone. Increases the levels of mRNA for alkaline phosphatase and inhibits the activation of adenylate cyclase.
Osteoclast	Calcitonin	Inhibits the function of osteoclasts (inhibits bone resorption).

PTH, Parathyroid hormone.

Directly stimulated by calcitonin and inhibited by PTH.

3. Osteoclasts—Resorb bone. Multinucleated, irregularly shaped giant cells originate from hematopoietic tissues (**monocyte progenitors** form giant cells by fusion). Possess a ruffled ("brush") border (plasma membrane enfoldings that increase surface area; are important in bone resorption) and a surrounding clear zone. Bone resorption occurs in depressions (Howship's lacunae); bone formation and resorption are linked ("coupled"), but resorption occurs more rapidly. **Osteoblasts (and tumor cells) express the RANK ligand (RANK L), which is a molecule that binds to receptors on osteoclasts, thus increasing bone resorption**; this mechanism is inhibited by osteoprotegerin binding to RANK L and preventing interaction with osteoclasts. **Osteoclasts synthesize tartrate-resistant acid phosphate.** Osteoclasts bind to bone surfaces via cell attachment (anchoring) proteins (**integrins**), which effectively seals the space below the osteoclast. Osteoclasts produce hydrogen ions (via carbonic anhydrase), which lowers the pH and increases the solubility of hydroxyapatite crystals, and the organic matrix is then removed by proteolytic digestion. Patients deficient in carbonic anhydrase cannot resorb bone by this mechanism. **Osteoclasts have specific receptors for calcitonin** to allow them to regulate bone resorption directly (see Table 1-2). **Osteoclasts are responsible for the bone resorption seen in multiple myeloma and metastatic bone disease. Interleukin-1 (IL-1) is a potent stimulator of osteoclastic bone resorption and has been found in the membranes sur-rounding loose total joint implants. IL-10 suppresses osteoclast formation. Bisphosphonates inhibit osteoclast resorption of bone (by preventing the osteoclast from forming the ruffled border necessary for expression of acid hydrolases) and reduce the incidence of skeletal events in patients with multiple myeloma.**
4. Osteoprogenitor Cells—Become osteoblasts. Line haversian canals, endosteum, and periosteum, awaiting the stimulus to differentiate into osteoblasts.
5. Lining Cells—Narrow, flattened cells that form an "envelope around bone."

C. Matrix—Composed of organic components (40%) and inorganic components (60%) (Table 1-3).
   1. Organic Components—40% of the dry weight of bone.
      a. Collagen—Primarily type I collagen ("bone" contains the word "one"; remember bone is primarily type I collagen). **Hole zones** (gaps) exist within the collagen fibril between the **ends** of molecules. **Pores** exist between the **sides** of parallel molecules. Mineral deposition (calcification) occurs within the hole zones and pores (Fig. 1-2). Cross-linking decreases collagen solubility and increases its tensile strength.
      b. Proteoglycans.
      c. Matrix Proteins (Noncollagenous)—**Osteocalcin** is inhibited by PTH and stimulated by 1,25-dihydroxyvitamin D. **Osteocalcin levels can be measured in the serum or urine as a marker of bone turnover**; elevated in Paget's disease, renal osteodystrophy, and hyperparathyroidism.
      d. Growth Factors and Cytokines.
   2. Inorganic (Mineral) Components—60% of the dry weight of bone.
      a. Calcium Hydroxyapatite [$Ca_{10}(PO_4)_6(OH)_2$].
      b. Osteocalcium Phosphate (Brushite).

D. Bone Remodeling
   1. General
      a. Wolff's Law—Bone remodels in response to mechanical stress. Increasing mechanical stress leads to significant bone gain. Removing external mechanical stresses can lead to significant bone loss, which is reversible (to varying degrees) upon remobilization.

Table 1-3. COMPONENTS OF BONE MATRIX

	FUNCTION	COMPOSED OF	TYPES	NOTES
Organic Matrix				
Collagen	Provides tensile strength.	Primarily type I collagen.		90% of organic matrix. Structure: triple helix of two α_1 and one α_2 chains, quarter-staggered to produce a fibril.
Proteoglycans	Partly responsible for compressive strength.	Glycosaminoglycan (GAG)-protein complexes (see Section 2: Joints).		Inhibit mineralization.
Matrix Proteins (noncollagenous)	Promote mineralization and bone formation.		Osteocalcin (bone γ-carboxyglutamic acid–containing protein [bone Gla protein]).	Attracts osteoclasts; direct regulation of bone density; most abundant noncollagenous matrix protein (10-20% of total).
			Osteonectin (SPARC).	Secreted by platelets and osteoblasts; postulated to have role in regulating Ca or organizing mineral in matrix.
			Osteopontin.	Cell-binding protein, similar to an integrin.
Growth Factors and Cytokines	Aid in bone cell differentiation, activiation, growth, and turnover.		Transforming growth factor-beta (TGF-β). Insulin-like growth factor (IGF). Interleukins (IL-1, IL-6). Bone morphogenetic proteins ($BMP_{1\text{-}6}$).	Present in small amounts in bone matrix (for more information, see Table 1-9)
Inorganic Matrix				
Calcium Hydroxyapatite [$Ca_{10}(PO_4)_6(OH)_2$]	Provides compressive strength.			Makes up most of the inorganic matrix; primary mineralization in collagen gaps (holes and pores), secondary mineralization on periphery.
Osteocalcium Phosphate (Brushite)				Makes up the remaining inorganic matrix.

b. Piezoelectric Charges—Bone remodels in response to electrical charges. The compression side of bone is electronegative, stimulating osteoblasts (formation); the tension side of bone is electropositive, stimulating osteoclasts (resorption). Both cortical and cancellous bone are continuously remodeled throughout life by osteoclastic and osteoblastic activity (Fig. 1-3).

c. Hueter-Volkmann Law—Remodeling occurs in small packets of cells known as **basic multicellular units (BMUs)**, modulated by systemic hormones and local cytokines. The **Hueter-Volkmann law** suggests that mechanical factors can influence longitudinal growth, bone remodeling, and fracture repair; compressive forces inhibit growth and tensile forces stimulate growth; this may play a role in the progression of scoliosis and Blount's disease.

2. Cortical Bone—Remodels by osteoclastic tunneling (cutting cones) (Fig. 1-4), followed by layering of osteoblasts and successive deposition of layers of lamellae (after the cement line has been laid down) until the tunnel size has narrowed to the diameter of the osteonal central canal. The head of the cutting cone is made up of osteoclasts, which bore holes through hard cortical bone. Behind the osteoclast front are capillaries, followed by osteoblasts that lay down osteoid to fill the resorption cavity.
3. Cancellous Bone—Remodels by osteoclastic resorption, followed by osteoblasts laying down new bone.

E. Bone Circulation

1. Anatomy—As an organ, bone receives 5-10% of the cardiac output. Long bones receive blood from three sources: (1) nutrient artery system; (2) metaphyseal-epiphyseal system; and (3) periosteal system. Bones with a tenuous blood supply include the scaphoid, talus, femoral head, and odontoid.

a. Nutrient Artery System—Nutrient arteries branch from the major systemic arteries,

MINERAL ACCRETION: ***BIOLOGICAL CONSIDERATIONS***
HETEROGENEITY WITHIN A COLLAGEN FIBRIL

PROGRESSIVELY INCREASING MINERAL MASS DUE TO:

1. **INCREASED NUMBER OF NEW MINERAL PHASE PARTICLES (NUCLEATION)**
   a. **HETEROGENEOUS NUCLEATION BY MATRIX IN COLLAGEN HOLES (? PORES)**
   b. **2° CRYSTAL INDUCED NUCLEATION IN HOLES AND PORES**
2. **INITIAL GROWTH OF PARTICLES TO ~ 400Å x 15–30Å x 50–75Å**

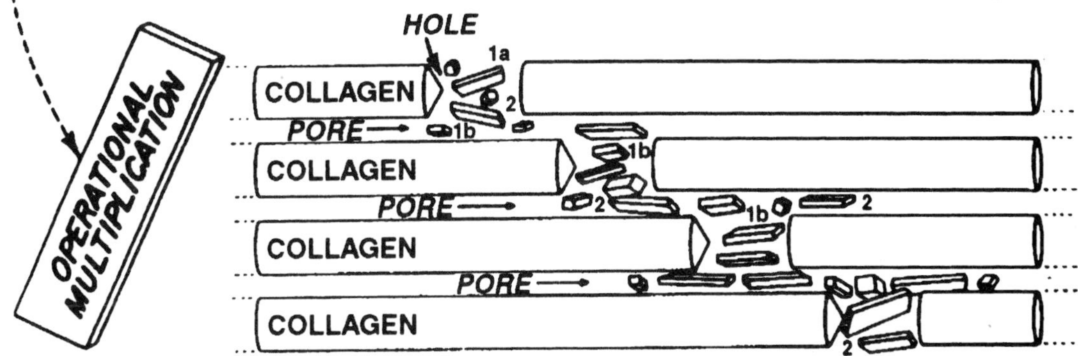

FIGURE 1-2 ■ Mineral accretion. (From Simon, S.R., ed.: Orthopaedic Basic Science, 2nd ed., p. 139. Rosemont, IL, American Academy of Orthopaedic Surgeons, 1994.)

enter the diaphyseal cortex (outer and inner tables) through the nutrient foramen, and then enter the medullary canal, branching into ascending and descending small arteries (Fig. 1-5). These branch into arterioles in the endosteal cortex and supply at least the inner two thirds of mature diaphyseal cortex via vessels in the haversian system (Figs. 1-6, 1-7). The nutrient artery system is **high pressure**.

b. Metaphyseal-Epiphyseal System—Arises from the periarticular vascular plexus (e.g., geniculate arteries).

c. Periosteal System—Composed primarily of capillaries that supply the outer one third (at most) of the mature diaphyseal cortex. The periosteal system is **low pressure**.

2. Physiology

   a. Direction of Flow (Fig. 1-8)—Arterial flow in mature bone is centrifugal (inside to outside), a result of the net effect of the high-pressure nutrient arterial system (endosteal system) and the low-pressure periosteal system. In a completely displaced fracture with disruption of the endosteal (nutrient) system, the pressure gradient reverses, the periosteal system pressure predominates, and blood flow is centripetal (outside to inside). Arterial flow in immature developing bone is centripetal because the periosteum is highly vascularized and is the predominant component of bone blood flow. Venous flow in mature bone is centripetal; cortical capillaries drain to venous sinusoids, which drain in turn to the emissary venous system.

   b. Fluid Compartments of Bone

Extravascular	65%
Haversian	6%
Lacunar	6%
RBCs	3%
Other	20%

   c. Physiologic States' Effect on Bone Blood Flow

   (1) Hypoxia—increases flow
   (2) Hypercapnia—increases flow
   (3) Sympathectomy—increases flow

3. Fracture Healing—**Bone blood flow is the major determinant of fracture healing.** Bone blood flow delivers nutrients to the site of bony injury. The **initial response** is **decreased bone blood flow** after vascular disruption at the fracture site. **Within hours to days, bone blood flow increases** (as part of the **regional acceleratory phenomenon), peaks at approximately 2 weeks, and returns to normal between 3 and 5 months.**

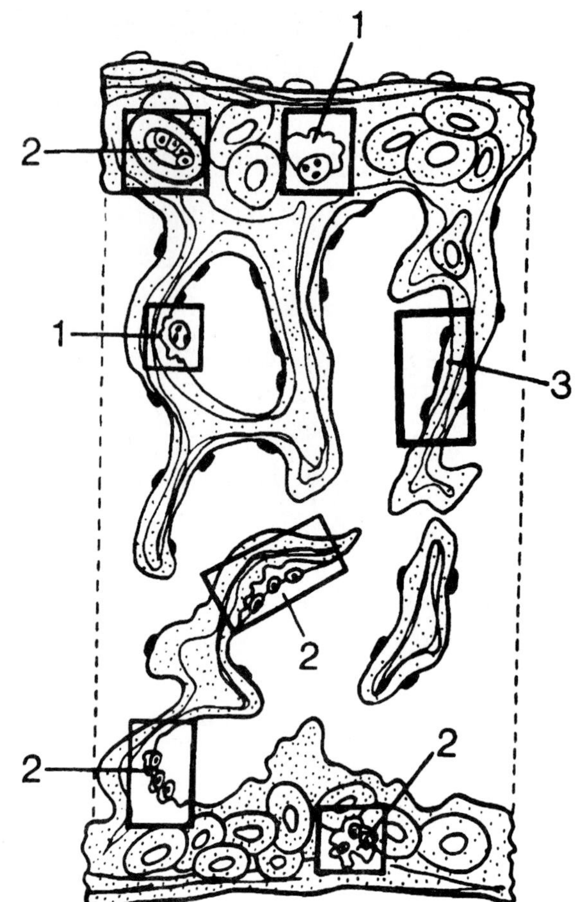

FIGURE 1-3 ■ Bone remodeling. *1,* Bone resorbed by osteoclastic activity in the cortex and trabeculae. *2,* Osteoblasts form new bone at the site of prior bone resorption. *3,* Osteoblasts become incorporated into bone as osteocytes. (From Simon, S.R., ed.: Orthopaedic Basic Science, 2nd ed., p. 141. Rosemont, IL, American Academy of Orthopaedic Surgeons, 1994.)

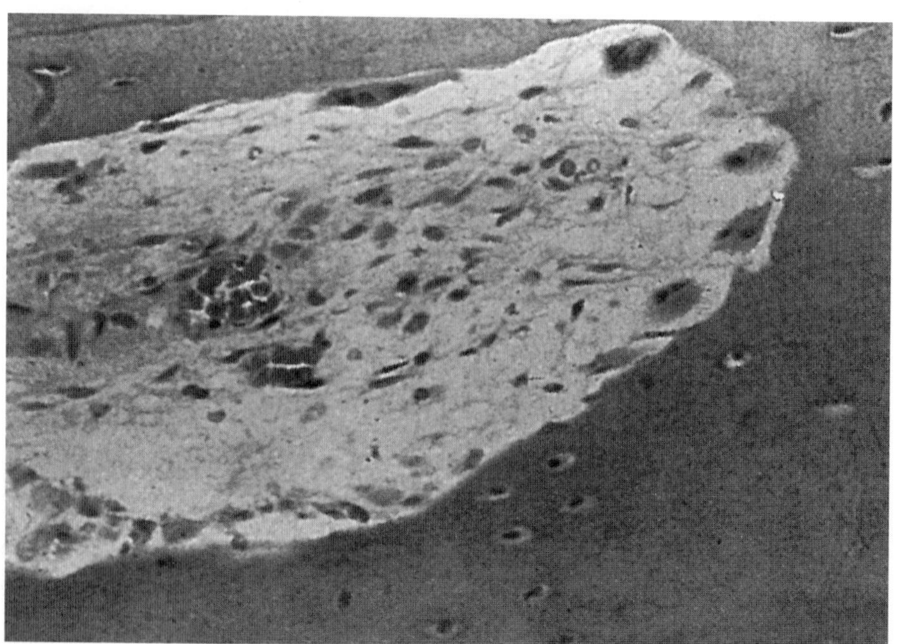

FIGURE 1-4 ■ Mechanism of cortical bone remodeling via cutting cones. (From Simon, S.R., ed.: Orthopaedic Basic Science, 2nd ed., p. 142. Rosemont, IL, American Academy of Orthopaedic Surgeons, 1994.)

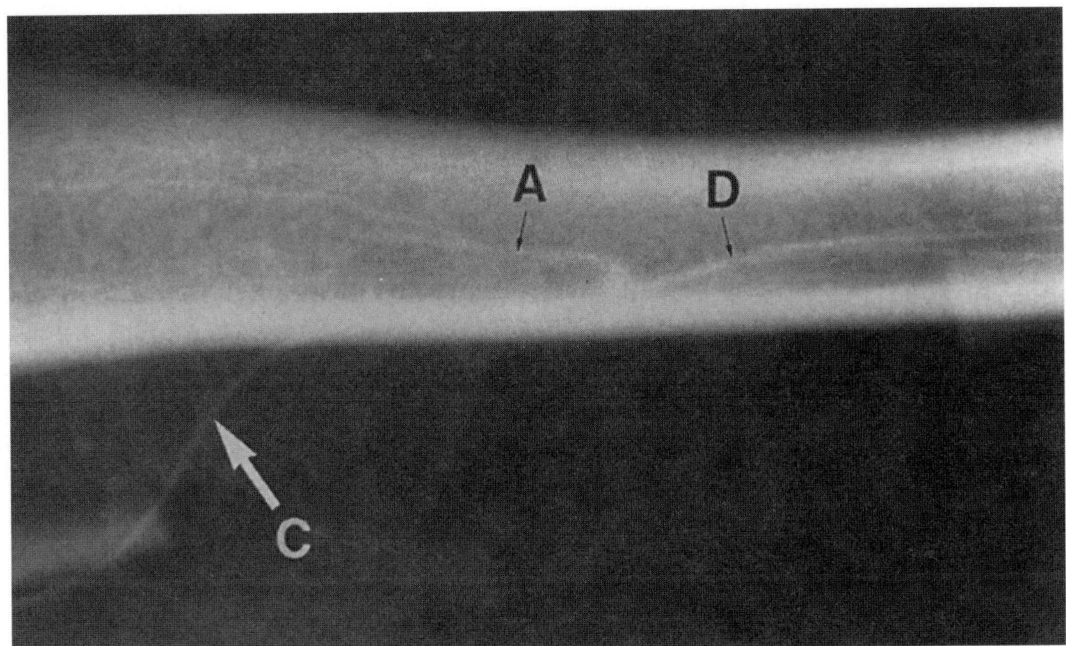

FIGURE 1-5 ■ Intraoperative arteriogram (canine tibia) demonstrating ascending (*A*) and descending (*D*) branches of the nutrient artery. *C*, Cannula. (From Brinker, M.R., Lipton, H.L., Cook, S.D., and Hyman, A.L.: Pharmacological regulation of the circulation of bone. J. Bone Joint Surg. [Am.] 72:964–975, 1990.)

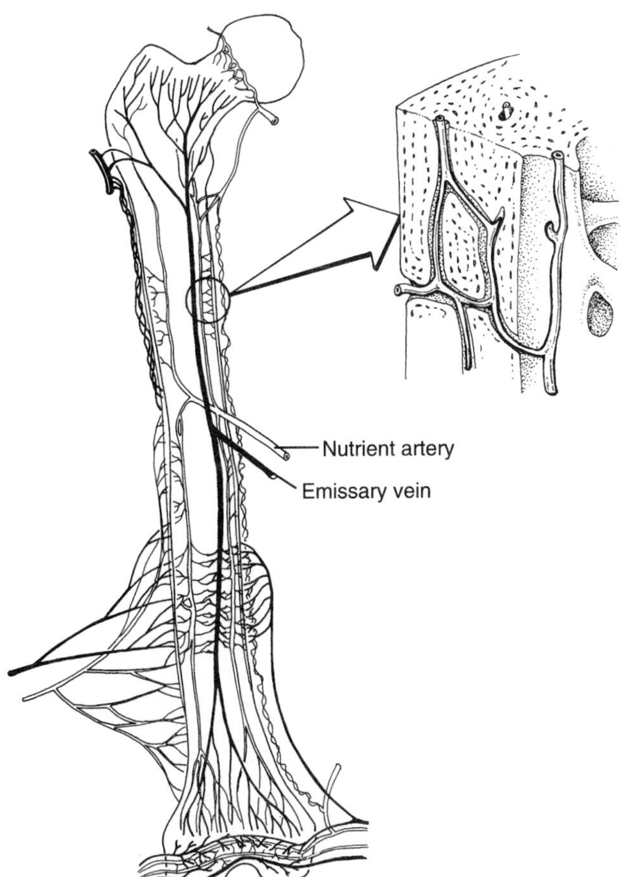

FIGURE 1-6 ■ Blood supply to bone. (From Brinker, M.R., and Miller, M.D.: Fundamentals of Orthopaedics. Philadelphia, WB Saunders, 1999, p. 4.)

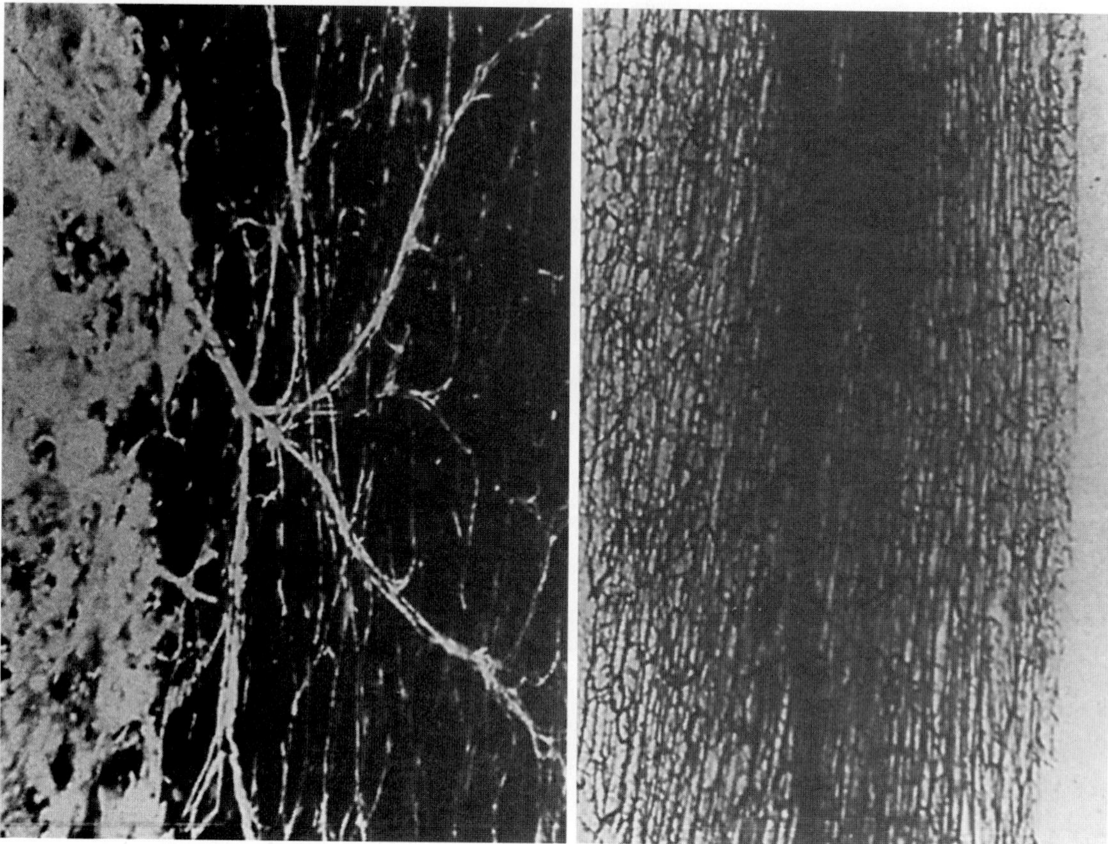

FIGURE 1-7 ■ Vasculature of cortical bone. (From Simon, S.R., ed.: Orthopaedic Basic Science, 2nd ed., p. 131. Rosemont, IL, American Academy of Orthopaedic Surgeons, 1994.)

The major advantage of unreamed intramedullary (IM) nails is preservation of the endosteal blood supply. Loose-fitting nails spare cortical perfusion and allow more rapid reperfusion compared with canal-filling nails. Reaming devascularizes the inner 50-80% of cortex; this is associated with the greatest delay in revascularization of the endosteal blood supply.

4. Regulation—Bone blood flow is under the control of metabolic, humoral, and autonomic inputs. The arterial system of bone has great potential for vasoconstriction (from the resting state) and much less potential for vasodilation. The vessels within bone possess a variety of vasoactive receptors (β-adrenergic, muscarinic, thromboxane/prostaglandin) that may be useful in the future for pharmacologic treatment of bone diseases related to aberrant circulation (e.g., osteonecrosis [ON], fracture nonunions).

F. Tissues Surrounding Bone

1. Periosteum—Connective tissue membrane that covers bone. It is more highly developed in children because of its role in the deposition of cortical bone, which is responsible for growth in bone diameter. The inner layer of periosteum, or cambium, is loose, is more vascular, and contains cells that are capable of becoming osteoblasts (to form bone); these cells are responsible for enlarging the diameter of bone during growth and forming periosteal callus during fracture healing; the outer, fibrous layer is less cellular and is contiguous with joint capsules.
2. Bone Marrow—Source of progenitor cells; controls the inner diameter of bone.
   a. Red Marrow—Hematopoietic (40% water, 40% fat, 20% protein). Red marrow slowly changes to yellow marrow with age, first in the appendicular skeleton and later in the axial skeleton.
   b. Yellow Marrow—Inactive (15% water, 80% fat, 5% protein).

G. Types of Bone Formation (Table 1-4)

1. **Enchondral Bone Formation/Mineralization**
   a. General Comments—Undifferentiated cells secrete cartilaginous matrix and differentiate into chondrocytes. The matrix mineralizes and is invaded by vascular buds that bring osteoprogenitor cells. Osteoclasts resorb calcified cartilage, and osteoblasts form bone. **Remember: Bone replaces the cartilage model; cartilage is not converted to bone. Examples of enchondral bone formation include (1) embryonic long**

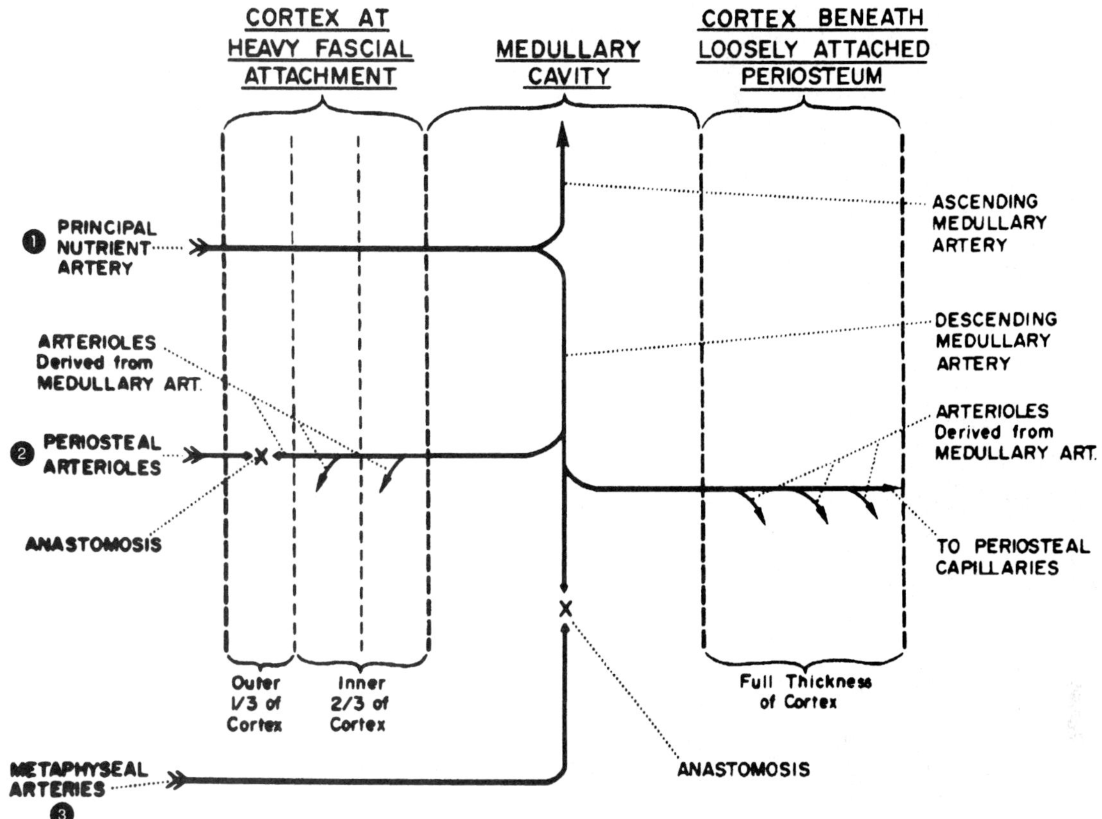

FIGURE 1-8 ■ Major components of the afferent vascular system of long bone. Components 1, 2, and 3 constitute the total nutrient supply to the diaphysis. Arrows indicate the direction of blood flow. (From Rhinelander, F.W.: Circulation in bone. In Bourne, G., ed.: The Biochemistry and Physiology of Bone, 2nd ed., vol. 2. Orlando, FL, Academic Press, 1972.)

Table 1-4. TYPES OF BONE FORMATION

TYPE OF OSSIFICATION	MECHANISM	EXAMPLES OF NORMAL MECHANISMS	EXAMPLES OF DISEASES WITH ABNORMAL OSSIFICATION
Enchondral	Bone replaces a cartilage model	1) Embryonic long bone formation 2) Longitudinal growth (physis) 3) Fracture callus 4) The type of bone formed with the use of demineralized bone matrix	Achondroplasia
Intramembranous	Aggregates of undifferentiated mesenchymal cells differentiate into osteoblasts, which form bone	1) Embryonic flat bone formation 2) Bone formation during distraction osteogenesis 3) Blastema bone	Cleidocranial dysostosis
Appositional	Osteoblasts lay down new bone on existing bone	1) Periosteal bone enlargement (width) 2) The bone formation phase of bone remodeling	Paget's disease Infantile hyperostosis (Caffey's disease) Melorheostosis

bone formation, (2) longitudinal growth (physis), (3) fracture callus, and (4) the bone formed with the use of demineralized bone matrix.

b. Embryonic Long Bone Formation (Figs. 1-9, 1-10)—Formed from mesenchymal anlage, usually at 6 weeks in utero. Enchondral bone formation is responsible for the development of embryonic long bones. Vascular buds invade the mesenchymal model, bringing in osteoprogenitor cells that differentiate into osteoblasts and form the primary centers of ossification at approximately 8 weeks. The cartilage model grows through appositional (width) and interstitial (length) growth. The marrow is formed by resorption of the central portion of the cartilage anlage by invasion of myeloid precursor cells brought in by the capillary buds. Secondary centers of ossification develop at the bone ends, forming epiphyseal centers of ossification (growth plates), which are responsible for longitudinal growth of immature bones. During this developmental stage, there is a

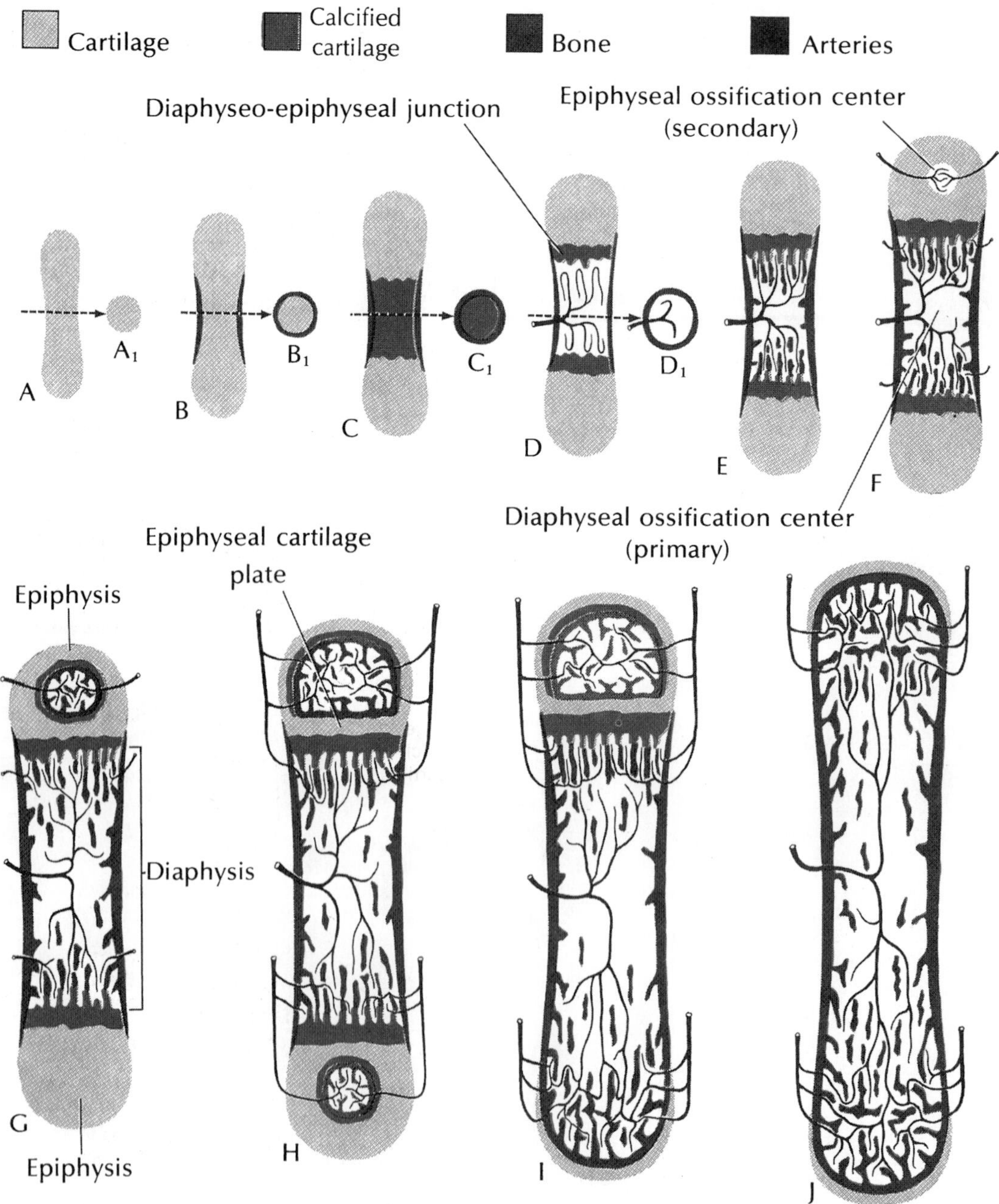

FIGURE 1-9 ■ Enchondral ossification of long bones. Note that phases *F-J* often occur after birth. (From Moore, K.L.: The Developing Human, p. 346. Philadelphia, WB Saunders, 1982.)

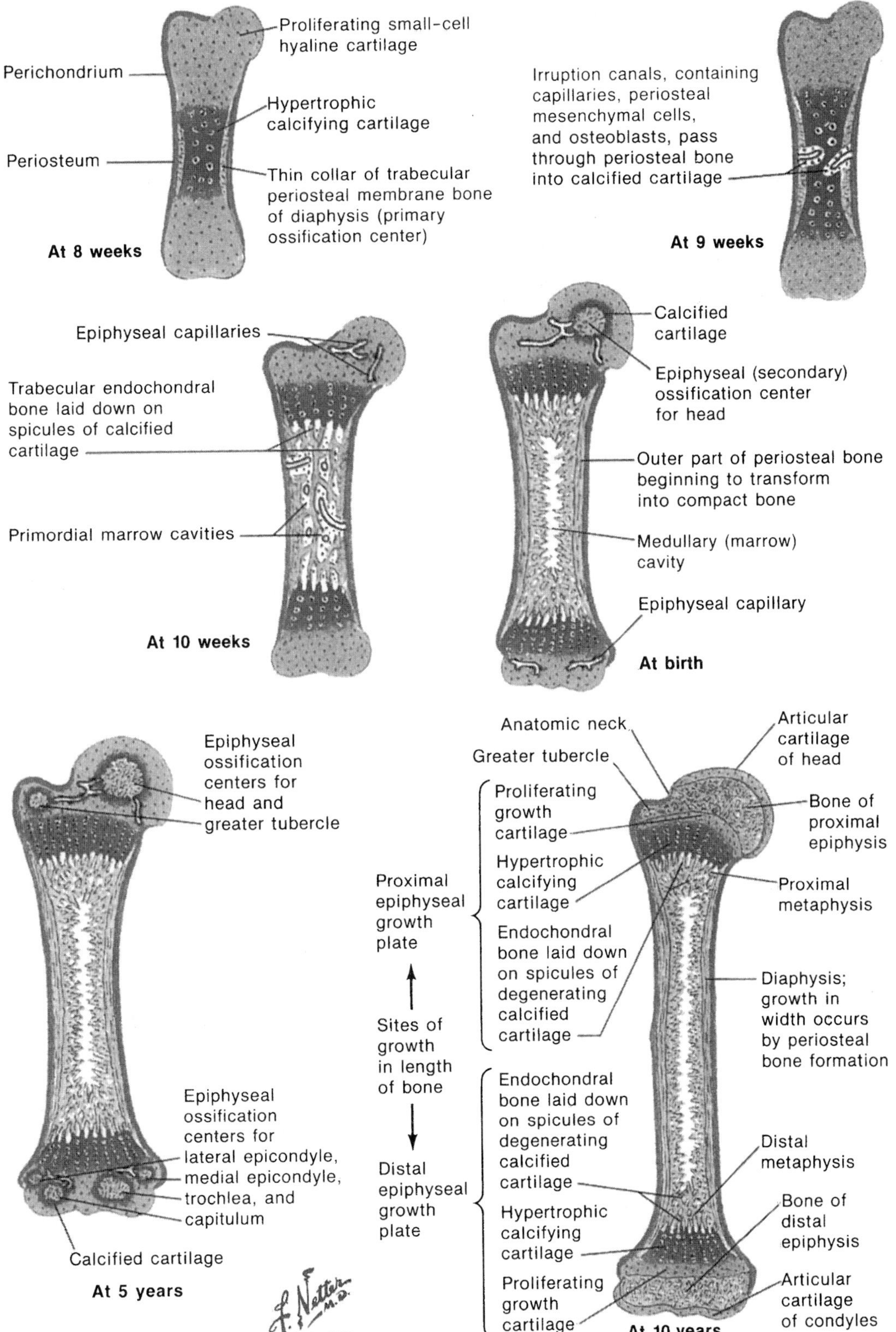

FIGURE 1-10 ■ Development of a typical long bone: Formation of the growth plate and secondary centers of ossification. (From the Ciba Collection of Medical Illustrations, vol. 8, part I, p. 136, 1987. Illustrated by Frank H. Netter. Reprinted by permission.)

rich arterial supply composed of an epiphyseal artery (which terminates in the proliferative zone), metaphyseal arteries, nutrient arteries, and perichondrial arteries (Fig. 1-11).

c. Physis—Two growth plates exist in immature long bones: (1) **horizontal** (the physis); and (2) **spherical** (allows growth of the epiphysis). The spherical growth plate has the same arrangement as the physis but is less organized. Acromegaly and spondyloepiphyseal dysplasia affect the physis; multiple epiphyseal dysplasia affects the epiphysis. Physeal cartilage zones are based on growth (see Fig. 1-11) and function (Figs. 1-12, 1-13).

(1) Reserve Zone—Cells store lipids, glycogen, and proteoglycan aggregates for later growth and matrix production. Decreased oxygen tension occurs in this zone. **Lysosomal storage diseases (Gaucher's)** and other diseases can affect this zone.

(2) Proliferative Zone—Longitudinal growth occurs with stacking of chondrocytes (the top cell is the dividing "mother" cell). There is increased oxygen tension and increased proteoglycans in the surrounding matrix, which inhibits calcification. This zone functions in cellular proliferation and matrix production. Defects in this zone (chondrocyte proliferation and column formation) are seen in **achondroplasia** (see Fig. 1-13) (does not affect intramembranous bone [width]).

(3) Hypertrophic Zone—Sometimes subdivided into three zones: **maturation, degeneration,** and **provisional calcification**. Normal mineralization of matrix occurs in the lower hypertrophic zone. In the hypertrophic zone, chondrocytes increase five times in size, accumulate calcium in their mitochondria, and then die (releasing calcium from matrix vesicles). **The rate of chondrocyte maturation**

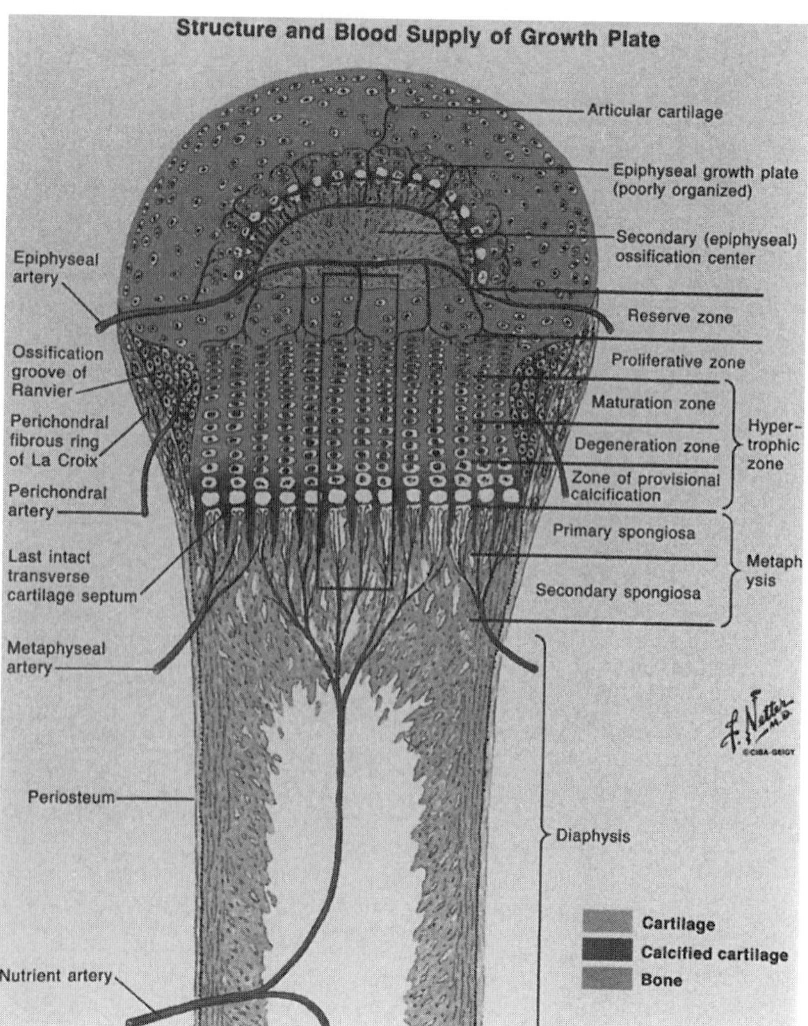

FIGURE 1-11 ■ Structure and blood supply of a typical growth plate. (From the Ciba Collection of Medical Illustrations, vol. 8, part I, p. 166, 1987. Illustrated by Frank H. Netter. Reprinted by permission.)

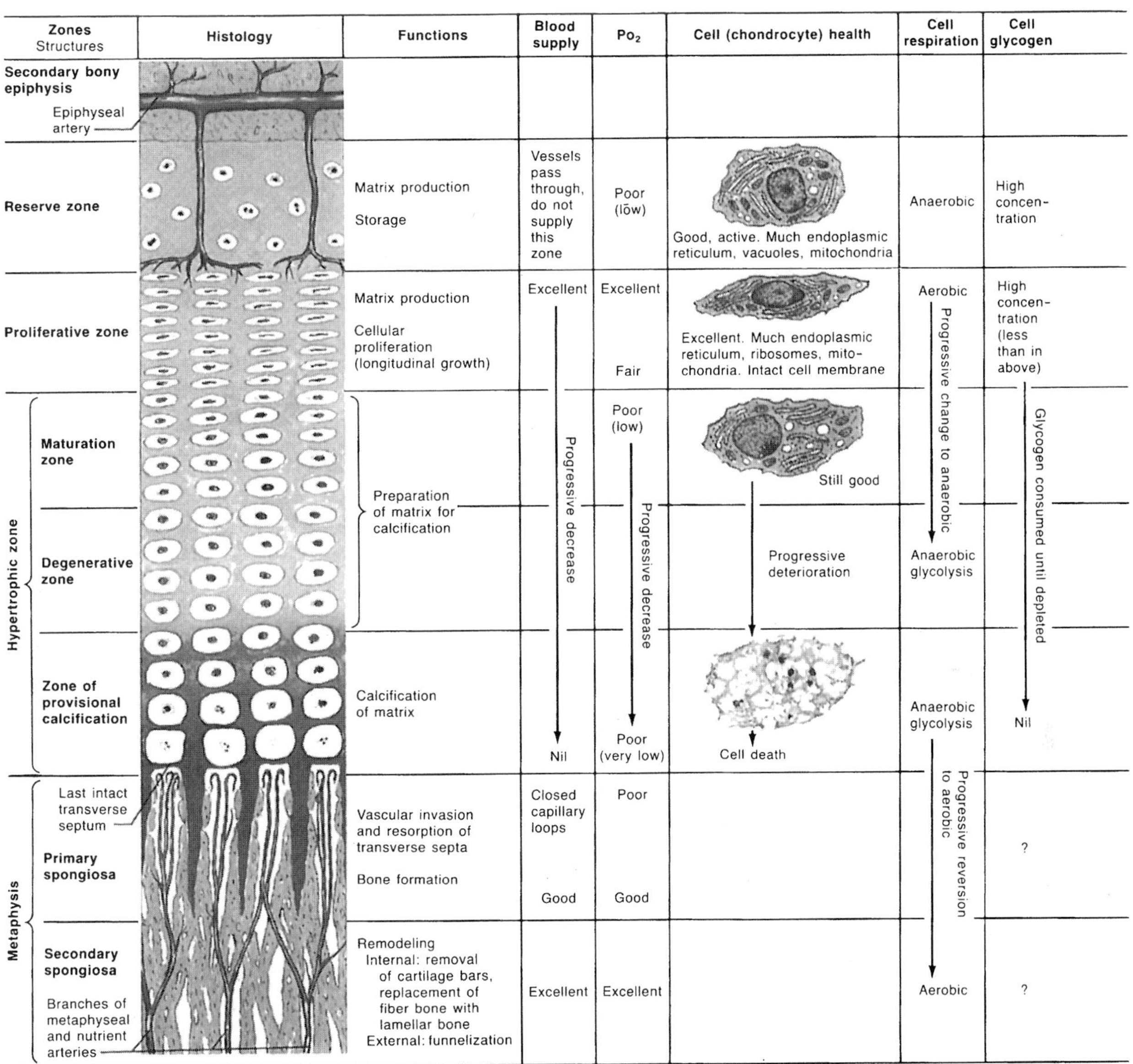

Zones Structures	Histology	Functions	Blood supply	Po_2	Cell (chondrocyte) health	Cell respiration	Cell glycogen
Secondary bony epiphysis Epiphyseal artery							
Reserve zone		Matrix production Storage	Vessels pass through, do not supply this zone	Poor (lōw)	Good, active. Much endoplasmic reticulum, vacuoles, mitochondria	Anaerobic	High concentration
Proliferative zone		Matrix production Cellular proliferation (longitudinal growth)	Excellent	Excellent Fair	Excellent. Much endoplasmic reticulum, ribosomes, mitochondria. Intact cell membrane	Aerobic	High concentration (less than in above)
Hypertrophic zone: Maturation zone		Preparation of matrix for calcification	Progressive decrease	Poor (low)	Still good	Progressive change to anaerobic	Glycogen consumed until depleted
Hypertrophic zone: Degenerative zone				Progressive decrease	Progressive deterioration	Anaerobic glycolysis	
Hypertrophic zone: Zone of provisional calcification		Calcification of matrix	Nil	Poor (very low)	Cell death	Anaerobic glycolysis	Nil
Metaphysis: Last intact transverse septum Primary spongiosa		Vascular invasion and resorption of transverse septa Bone formation	Closed capillary loops Good	Poor Good		Progressive reversion to aerobic	?
Metaphysis: Secondary spongiosa Branches of metaphyseal and nutrient arteries		Remodeling Internal: removal of cartilage bars, replacement of fiber bone with lamellar bone External: funnelization	Excellent	Excellent		Aerobic	?

FIGURE 1-12 ■ Zonal structure, function, and physiology of the growth plate. (From the Ciba Collection of Medical Illustrations, vol. 8, part I, p. 164, 1987. Illustrated by Frank H. Netter. Reprinted by permission.)

Zones Structures	Histology	Functions	Exemplary diseases	Defect (if known)
Secondary bony epiphysis Epiphyseal artery	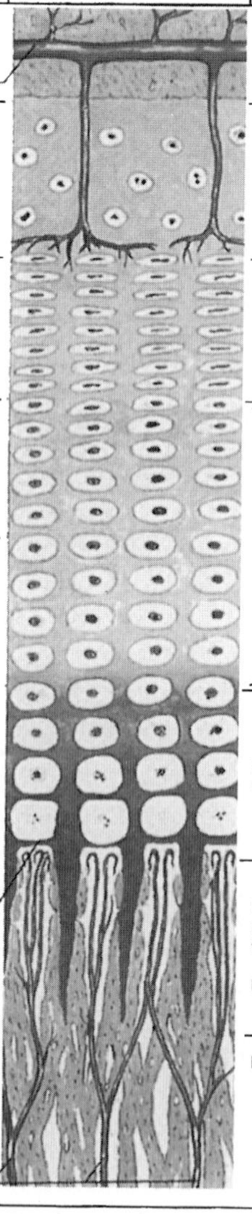			
Reserve zone		Matrix production Storage	Diastrophic dwarfism (also, defects in other zones)	Defective type II collagen synthesis
			Pseudoachondroplasia (also, defects in other zones)	Defective processing and transport of proteoglycans
			Kneist syndrome (also, defects in other zones)	Defective processing of proteoglycans
Proliferative zone		Matrix production Cellular proliferation (longitudinal growth)	Gigantism	Increased cell proliferation (growth hormone increased)
			Achondroplasia	Deficiency of cell proliferation
			Hypochondroplasia	Less severe deficiency of cell proliferation
			Malnutrition, irradiation injury, glucocorticoid excess	Decreased cell proliferation and/or matrix synthesis
Hypertrophic zone: **Maturation zone**; **Degenerative zone**		Preparation of matrix for calcification	Mucopolysaccharidosis (Morquio's syndrome, Hurler's syndrome)	Deficiencies of specific lysosomal acid hydrolases, with lysosomal storage of mucopolysaccharides
Hypertrophic zone: **Zone of provisional calcification**		Calcification of matrix	Rickets, osteomalacia (also, defects in metaphysis)	Insufficiency of Ca^{++} and/or P for normal calcification of matrix
Metaphysis: Last intact transverse septum; **Primary spongiosa**		Vascular invasion and resorption of transverse septa	Metaphyseal chondrodysplasia (Jansen and Schmid types)	Extension of hypertrophic cells into metaphysis
		Bone formation	Acute hematogenous osteomyelitis	Flourishing of bacteria due to sluggish circulation, low PO_2, reticuloendothelial deficiency
Metaphysis: **Secondary spongiosa**; Branches of metaphyseal and nutrient arteries		Remodeling Internal: removal of cartilage bars, replacement of fiber bone with lamellar bone	Osteopetrosis	Abnormality of osteoclasts (internal remodeling)
			Osteogenesis imperfecta	Abnormality of osteoblasts and collagen synthesis
			Scurvy	Inadequate collagen formation
		External: funnelization	Metaphyseal dysplasia (Pyle disease)	Abnormality of funnelization (external remodeling)

FIGURE 1-13 ■ Zonal structure and pathologic defects of cellular metabolism. (From the Ciba Collection of Medical Illustrations, vol. 8, part I, p. 165, 1987. Illustrated by Frank H. Netter. Reprinted by permission.)

is regulated by systemic hormones and local growth factors (parathyroid-related peptide inhibits chondrocyte maturation; Indian hedgehog is produced by growth plate chondrocytes and regulates the expression of parathyroid-related peptide). Osteoblasts migrate from sinusoidal vessels and use cartilage as a scaffolding for bone formation. Low oxygen tension and decreased proteoglycan aggregates aid this process. **This zone widens in rickets** (see Fig. 1-13), where little or no provisional calcification occurs. **Enchondromas** also originate in this zone. **Mucopolysaccharidic diseases** (see Fig. 1-13) also affect this zone, leading to chondrocyte degeneration (swollen, abnormal chondrocytes). Physeal fractures were classically believed to occur through the provisional calcification zone (within the hypertrophic zone), but probably traverse several zones depending on the type of loading (Fig. 1-14). **The hypertrophic zone is believed to be involved in slipped capital femoral epiphysis (SCFE), except SCFE associated with renal failure, in which the slippage occurs through the metaphyseal spongiosa.**

d. Metaphysis—Adjacent to the physis, the metaphysis expands with skeletal growth. Osteoblasts from osteoprogenitor cells align on cartilage bars produced by physeal expansion. Primary spongiosa (calcified cartilage bars) mineralizes to form woven bone and remodels to form secondary spongiosa and a "cutback zone" at the metaphysis. Cortical bone is made by remodeling of physeal (enchondral) and intramembranous bone in response to stress along the periphery of the growing long bones.

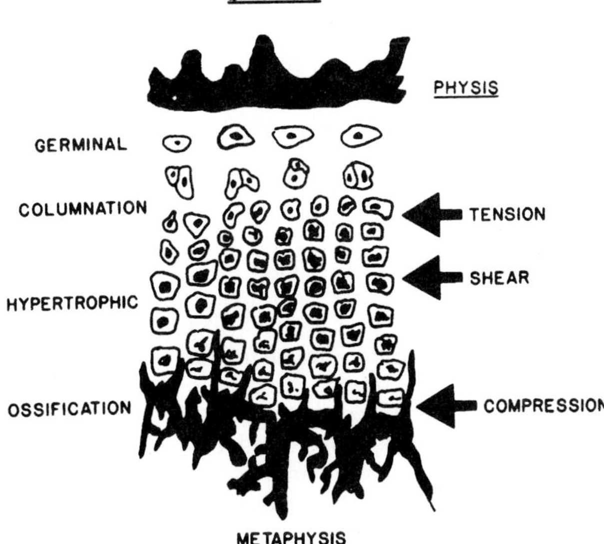

FIGURE 1-14 ■ Histologic zone of failure varies with the type of loading applied to a specimen. (From Moen, C.T., and Pelker, R.R.: Biomechanical and histological correlations in growth plate failure. J. Pediatr. Orthop. 4:180–184, 1984.)

e. Periphery of the Physis—Composed of two elements.
   (1) Groove of Ranvier—Supplies chondrocytes to the periphery of the growth plate for lateral growth (width).
   (2) Perichondrial Ring of LaCroix—Dense fibrous tissue that is the primary limiting membrane that anchors and supports the periphery of the physis.

f. Mineralization—Consists of seeding of collagen hole zones with calcium hydroxyapatite crystals through branching and accretion (crystal growth).

g. Effect of Hormones and Growth Factors on the Growth Plate—Several hormones and growth factors have both direct and indirect effects on the developing growth plate. Some factors are produced and act within the growth plate (paracrine or autocrine), and others are produced at a site distant from the growth plate (endocrine). The actions of hormones and growth factors are via their effect on chondrocytes and matrix mineralization (summarized in Fig. 1-15 and Table 1-5).

2. **Intramembranous Ossification**—Occurs without a cartilage model. Undifferentiated mesenchymal cells aggregate into layers (or membrane). These cells differentiate into osteoblasts and deposit organic matrix that mineralizes to form bone. **Examples of intramembranous bone formation include (1) embryonic flat bone formation (pelvis, clavicle, vault of skull), (2) bone formation during distraction osteogenesis, and (3) blastema bone (occurs in young children with amputations).**

3. Appositional Ossification—Osteoblasts align themselves on the existing bone surface and lay down new bone. **Examples of appositional ossification include (1) periosteal bone enlargement (width) and (2) the bone formation phase of bone remodeling.**

II. Bone Injury and Repair

A. **Fracture Repair**—A continuum proceeding from **inflammation** through **repair** (soft callus followed by hard callus) and ending in **remodeling**. Fracture healing may be influenced by a variety of biologic and mechanical factors (Table 1-6). **The most important factor in fracture healing is blood supply (bone blood flow).** Head injury can increase the osteogenic response to fracture. **Nicotine from smoking increases the time to**

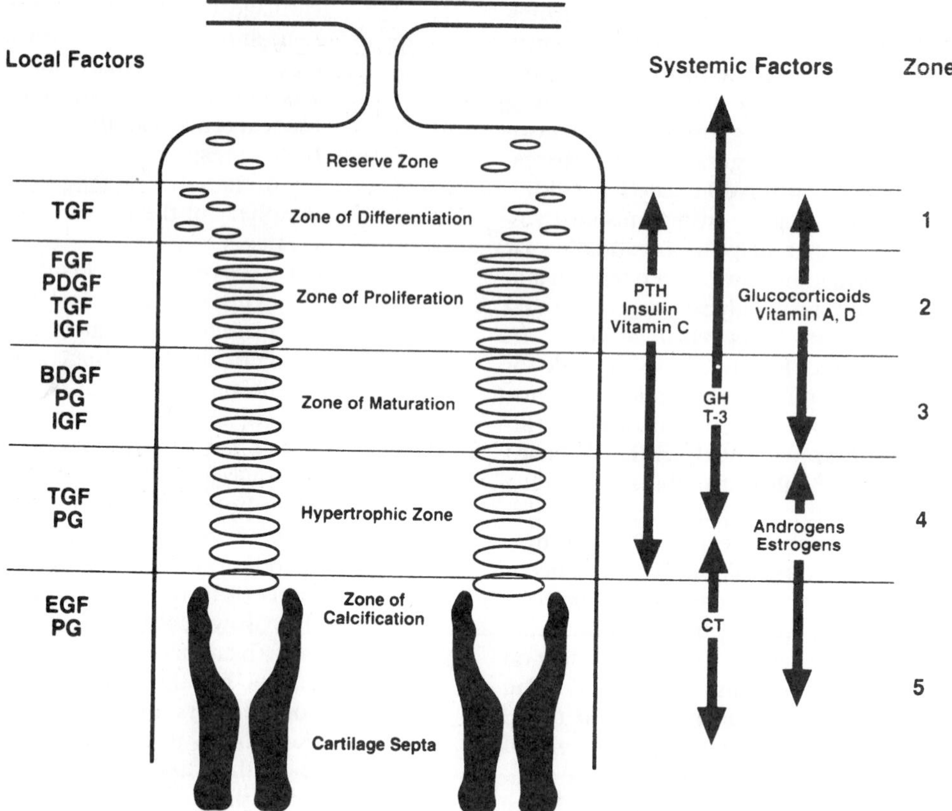

FIGURE 1-15 ■ Growth plate, demonstrating the proposed sites of action of hormones, growth factors, and vitamins. (From Simon, S.R., ed.: Orthopaedic Basic Science, 2nd ed., p. 197. Rosemont, IL, American Academy of Orthopaedic Surgeons, 1994.)

fracture healing, increases the risk of nonunion (particularly in the tibia), and decreases the strength of the fracture callus. Smoking also increases the risk of pseudarthrosis after lumbar fusion by up to 500%. Nonsteroidal anti-inflammatory drugs (NSAIDs) have an adverse effect on fracture healing and healing of lumbar spinal fusions.

1. Stages of Fracture Repair
   a. Inflammation—Bleeding from the fracture site and surrounding soft tissues creates a hematoma, which provides a source of hematopoietic cells capable of secreting growth factors. Subsequently, fibroblasts, mesenchymal cells, and osteoprogenitor cells are present at the fracture site, and granulation tissue forms around the fracture ends. Osteoblasts, from surrounding osteogenic precursor cells, fibroblasts, or both, proliferate.
   b. Repair—Primary callus response occurs within 2 weeks. If the bone ends are not in continuity, **bridging (soft) callus** occurs. The soft callus is replaced later, via the process of enchondral ossification, by **woven bone (hard callus)**. Another type of callus, **medullary callus**, supplements the bridging callus, although it forms more slowly and occurs later (Fig. 1-16). During fracture callus formation in an unstable fracture, type II collagen is expressed early, followed by type I collagen. Fracture healing varies with the method of treatment (Table 1-7). The amount of callus formation is inversely proportional to the extent of immobilization of the fracture. Primary cortical healing, which resembles normal remodeling, occurs with rigid immobilization and anatomic (or near-anatomic) reduction. With closed treatment, "enchondral healing" with periosteal bridging callus occurs. With rigidly fixed fractures (compression plate), direct osteonal or primary bone healing occurs without visible callus. The initial histologic change observed in hypertrophic nonunions treated with plate stabilization is fibrocartilage mineralization.
   c. Remodeling—This process begins during the middle of the repair phase and continues long after the fracture has clinically healed (up to 7 years). Remodeling allows the bone to assume its normal configuration

Table 1-5. EFFECTS OF HORMONES AND GROWTH FACTORS ON THE GROWTH PLATE

HORMONE/ FACTOR	SYSTEMIC/LOCAL DERIVATION	BIOLOGIC EFFECT *Proliferation*	*Macro-Molecule Biosynthesis*	*Maturation Degradation*	*Matrix Calcification*	ZONE PRIMARILY AFFECTED
Thyroxine	Systemic (thyroid)	+ (T_3 with IGF-I)	0	+ (T_3 alone)	0	Proliferative zone and upper hypertrophic zone
Parathyroid	Systemic (Parathyroid)	+	+ +(Proteoglycan)	0	0	Entire growth plate
Calcitonin	Systemic (thyroid)	0	0	+	+	Hypertrophic zone and metaphysis
Excess corticosteroids	Systemic (adrenals)	–	–	–	0	Entire growth plate
Growth hormone	Systemic (pituitary)	+ (through IGF-I locally)	+ (Slight)	0	0	Proliferative zone
Somatomedins	Systemic Local paracrine (liver, chondrocytes)	+	+ (Slight)	0	0	Proliferative zone
Insulin	Systemic (pancreas)	+ (through IGF-I receptor)	0	0	0	Proliferative zone
1,25-$(OH)_2D_3$	Systemic (liver, kidney)	0	0	+ (Indirect effect serum [Ca] x [PO])		Hypertrophic zone
24,25-$(OH)_2D_3$	Systemic (liver, kidney)	+	+ (Collagen II)	0	0	Proliferative zone and hypertrophic zone
Vitamin A	Systemic (diet)	0	0	–	0	Hypertrophic zone
Vitamin C	Systemic (diet)	0	+ (Collagen)	0	+ (Matrix vesicles)	Proliferative zone and hypertrophic zone
EGF	Local paracrine (endothelial cells)	+	– (Collagen)	0	0	Metaphysis
FGF	Local paracrine (endothelial cells)	+	0	0	0	Proliferative zone
PDGF	Local paracrine (platelets)	+	+ (Noncollagenous proteins)	0	0	Proliferative zone
TGF-β	Local paracrine (platelets, chondrocytes)	±	±	0	0	Proliferative zone and hypertrophic zone
BDGF	Local paracrine (bone matrix)	0	+ (Collagen)	0	0	Upper hypertrophic zone
IL-I	Local paracrine (inflammatory cells, synoviocytes)	0	–	+ + Activates tissue metalloproteinases	0	Entire growth plate
Prostaglandin	Local autocrine	±	+ (Proteoglycan) – (Collagen and alkaline phosphatase)	0	Bone resorption with osteoclasts	Hypertrophic zone and metaphysis

+, Increase stimulation; 0, no known effect; –, inhibitory; ±, depending on the local hormonal milieu.

EGF, epidermal growth factor; FGF, fibroblast growth factor; PDGF, platelet-derived growth factor; TGF-β, transforming growth factor-beta; BDGF, bone-derived growth factor; IL-1, interleukin-1; IGF-I, insulin-like growth factor I.

From Simon, S.R.: Orthopaedic Basic Science, 2nd ed., p. 196. Rosemont, IL, American Academy of Orthopaedic Surgeons, 1994; reprinted by permission.

Table 1-6. BIOLOGIC AND MECHANICAL FACTORS INFLUENCING FRACTURE HEALING

BIOLOGIC FACTORS	MECHANICAL FACTORS
Patient age	Soft-tissue attachments to bone
Comorbid medical conditions	Stability (extent of immobilization)
Functional level	Anatomic location
Nutritional status	Level of energy imparted
Nerve function	Extent of bone loss
Vascular injury	
Hormones	
Growth factors	
Health of the soft-tissue envelope	
Sterility (in open fractures)	
Cigarette smoke	
Local pathologic conditions	
Level of energy imparted	
Type of bone affected	
Extent of bone loss	

Table 1-7. TYPE OF FRACTURE HEALING BASED ON TYPE OF STABILIZATION

TYPE OF STABILIZATION	PREDOMINANT TYPE OF HEALING
Cast (closed treatment)	Periosteal bridging callus and interfragmentary enchondral ossification
Compression plate	Primary cortical healing (cutting cone–type remodeling)
Intramedullary nail	Early: periosteal bridging callus; enchondral ossification Late: medullary callus
External fixator	Dependent on extent of rigidity Less rigid: periosteal bridging callus More rigid: primary cortical healing
Inadequate immobilization with adequate blood supply	Hypertrophic nonunion (failed enchondral ossification); type II collagen predominates
Inadequate immobilization without adequate blood supply	Atrophic nonunion
Inadequate reduction with displacement at the fracture site	Oligotrophic nonunion

and shape based on the stresses to which it is exposed (Wolff's law). Throughout the process, woven bone formed during the repair phase is replaced with lamellar bone. Fracture healing is complete when there is repopulation of the marrow space.

2. Biochemistry of Fracture Healing—Four biochemical steps of fracture healing have been described (Table 1-8).
3. Growth Factors of Bone (Table 1-9)
4. Endocrine Effects on Fracture Healing (Table 1-10)
5. Ultrasound and Fracture Healing—Clinical studies show that low-intensity pulsed ultrasound accelerates fracture healing and increases the mechanical strength of callus, including torque and stiffness. The postulated mechanism of action is that the cells responsible for fracture healing respond favorably to the mechanical energy transmitted by the ultrasound signal.
6. Effect of Radiation on Bone—High-dose irradiation causes long-term changes within the haversian system and also decreases cellularity.

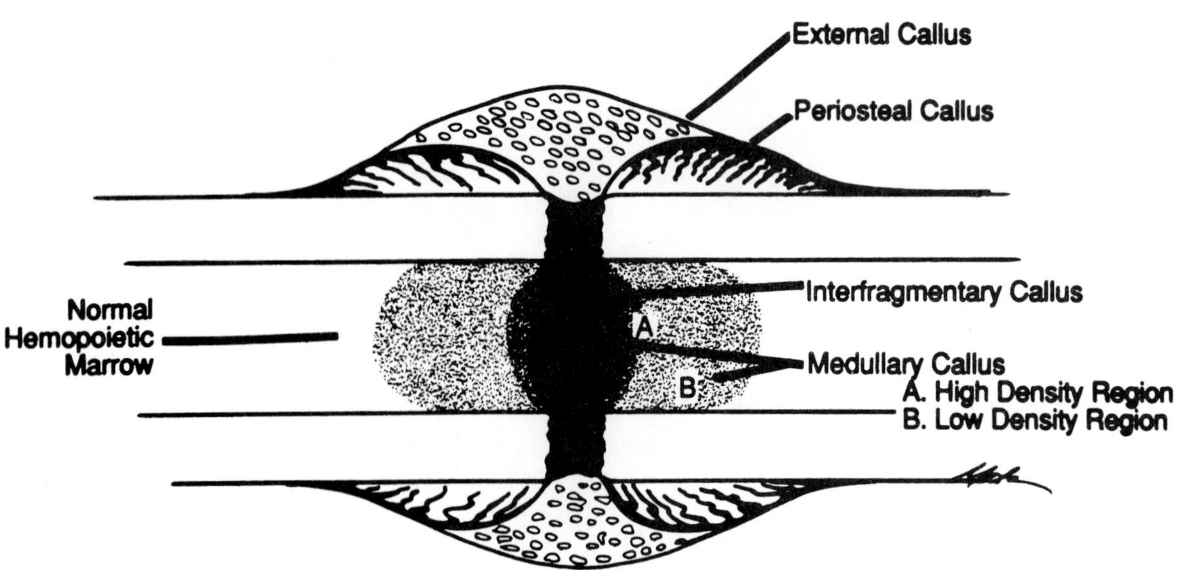

FIGURE 1-16 ■ Histology of typical fracture healing. (From Brighton, C.T., and Hunt, R.M.: Early histological and ultrastructural changes in medullary fracture callus. J. Bone Joint Surg. [Am.] 73:832–847, 1991.)

Table 1-8. BIOCHEMICAL STEPS OF FRACTURE HEALING

STEP	COLLAGEN TYPE
Mesenchymal	I, II, (III, V)
Chondroid	II, IX
Chondroid-osteoid	I, II, X
Osteogenic	I

Table 1-10. ENDOCRINE EFFECTS ON FRACTURE HEALING

HORMONE	EFFECT	MECHANISM
Cortisone	–	Decreased callus proliferation
Calcitonin	+?	Unknown
TH/PTH	+	Bone remodeling
Growth hormone	+	Increased callus volume

TH/PTH, thyroid hormone/parathyroid hormone.

Immediate postoperative irradiation adversely affects the incorporation of anterior spinal interbody strut grafts (delaying radiation for 3 weeks eliminates these effects). High-dose irradiation (90 kGy—the dose needed for viral inactivation) of allograft bone significantly reduces its structural integrity.

7. Electricity and Fracture Healing
   a. Definitions
      (1) Stress-Generated Potentials—Serve as signals that modulate cellular activity. Piezoelectric effect and streaming potentials are examples of stress-generated potentials.
      (2) Piezoelectric Effect—Charges in tissues are displaced secondary to mechanical forces.
      (3) Streaming Potentials—Occur when electrically charged fluid is forced over a tissue (cell membrane) with a fixed charge.
      (4) Transmembrane Potentials—Generated by cellular metabolism.
   b. Fracture Healing—Electrical properties of cartilage and bone depend on their charged molecules. Devices intended to stimulate fracture repair by altering a variety of cellular activities have been introduced.
   c. Types of Electrical Stimulation
      (1) Direct Current (DC)—Stimulates an inflammatory-like response (stage I).
      (2) Alternating Current (AC)—"Capacity coupled generators." Affects cyclic adenosine monophosphate (cAMP), collagen synthesis, and calcification during the repair stage.
      (3) Pulsed Electromagnetic Fields (PEMFs)—Initiate calcification of fibrocartilage (cannot induce calcification of fibrous tissue).
8. Pathologic Fracture—Results through areas of weakened bone from tumor, infection, or metabolic bone disease. The factors most predictive of the risk of pathologic fracture are pain, anatomic location, and the pattern of bony destruction (scoring system of Mirels). **The anatomic site with the highest risk of pathologic fracture is the subtrochanteric femur.**

B. Bone Grafting—Bone grafts have four important properties (Table 1-11).
   1. Graft Properties
      a. Osteoconductive Matrix—Acts as a scaffold or framework into which bone growth occurs.
      b. Osteoinductive Factors—Growth factors such as bone morphogenetic protein (BMP) and transforming growth factor beta (TGF-β) that signal local factors to stimulate bone formation.

Table 1-9. GROWTH FACTORS OF BONE

GROWTH FACTOR	ACTION	NOTES
Bone Morphogenetic Protein (BMP)	Osteoinductive; stimulates bone formation. Induces metaplasia of mesenchymal cells into osteoblasts.	Target cells of BMP are the undifferentiated perivascular mesenchymal cells.
Transforming Growth Factor-Beta (TGF-β)	Induces mesenchymal cells to produce type II collagen and proteoglycans. Induces osteoblasts to synthesize collagen.	Found in fracture hematomas; believed to **regulate cartilage and bone formation in fracture callus**. Coating porous implants with TGF-β enhances bone ingrowth.
Insulin-Like Growth Factor II (IGF-II)	Stimulates type I collagen, cellular proliferation, cartilage matrix synthesis, and bone formation.	
Platelet-Derived Growth Factor (PDGF)	Attracts inflammatory cells to the fracture site (chemotactic).	Released from platelets.

Table 1-11. TYPES OF BONE GRAFTS AND BONE GRAFT PROPERTIES

GRAFT	OSTEOCONDUCTION	OSTEOINDUCTION	OSTEOGENIC CELLS	STRUCTURAL INTEGRITY	OTHER PROPERTIES
Autograft					
Cancellous	Excellent	Good	Excellent	Poor	Rapid incorporation
Cortical	Fair	Fair	Fair	Excellent	Slow incorporation
Allograft	Fair	Fair	None	Good	**Fresh** has the highest immunogenicity **Freeze-dried** is the least immunogenic but has the least structural integrity (weakest) **Fresh frozen** preserves BMP
Ceramics	Fair	None	None	Fair	
Demineralized bone matrix	Fair	Good	None	Poor	
Bone marrow	Poor	Poor	Good	Poor	

BMP, bone morphogenic protein.
Modified from Brinker, M.R., and Miller, M.D.: Fundamentals of Orthopaedics. Philadelphia, WB Saunders, 1999. p. 7.

c. Osteogenic Cells—Include primitive mesenchymal cells, osteoblasts, and osteocytes.
d. Structural Integrity

2. Overview of Bone Grafts—Commonly, autografts (from same person) or allografts (from another person). Cancellous bone is commonly used for grafting nonunions or cavitary defects because it is quickly remodeled and incorporated (via creeping substitution). Cortical bone is slower to turn over than cancellous bone and is used for structural defects.
   a. Osteoarticular (osteochondral) allograft use is increasing in frequency for tumor surgery; they are immunogenic (cartilage is vulnerable to inflammatory mediators of immune response [cytotoxicity from antibodies and lymphocytes]); articular cartilage preserved with glycerol or dimethyl sulfoxide (DMSO); **cryogenically preserved grafts leave few viable chondrocytes**. Tissue-matched (sygeneic) osteochondral grafts produce minimal immunogenic effect and incorporate well.
   b. Vascularized bone grafts, though technically difficult, allow more rapid union and cell preservation; best for irradiated tissues or large tissue defects (may be donor site morbidity [i.e., fibula]).
   c. Nonvascular bone grafts are more common than vascularized grafts.
   d. Allograft bone
      (1) Types
         (a) Fresh—Increased immunogenicity.
         (b) Fresh Frozen—Less immunogenic than fresh. BMP preserved.
         (c) Freeze-Dried (Lyophilized)—Loses structural integrity and depletes BMP, **least immunogenic, purely osteoconductive, and lowest likelihood of viral transmission**, commonly known as "croutons."
         (d) Bone Matrix Gelatin (BMG—digested Source of BMP)—**Demineralized bone matrix (Grafton) is osteoconductive and osteoinductive.**
      (2) Antigenicity—Bone allografts are composite materials and therefore possess a spectrum of potential antigens. The primary mechanism of rejection is cellular, as opposed to humoral. Bone marrow cells of allograft incite the greatest immunogenic response. Class I and II cellular antigens contained within allograft are recognized by T-lymphocytes in the host. Cellular components that contribute to antigenicity include those of marrow origin, endothelium, and retinacular activating cells. Both the cellular components and the extracellular matrix elicit an antigenic response, with the former eliciting a relatively greater response. Type I collagen (organic matrix) stimulates both cell-mediated and humoral responses. The noncollagenous portion of the matrix (proteoglycans, osteopontin, osteocalcin, and other glycoproteins) also stimulates an immunogenic response. **Hydroxyapatite has not been shown to elicit an immune response. Allograft incorporation is related to cellularity and Major Histocompatibility Complex incompatibility between host tissue and allogenic tissue.**

(e) Five Stages of Graft Healing (Urist) (Table 1-12)

3. **Specific Bone Graft Types**
   a. Cortical Bone Grafts—Slower incorporation through remodeling of existing haversian systems via resorption (weakens the graft), followed by deposition of new bone (restoring strength). Resorption confined to osteon borders; interstitial lamellae are preserved. Used for structural defects.
   b. Cancellous Grafts—Revascularize and incorporate quickly; osteoblasts lay down new bone on old trabeculae, which are later remodeled ("creeping substitution"). Allografts must be harvested with sterile technique, and donors must be screened for potential transmissible diseases. The major factors influencing bone graft incorporation are shown in Figure 1-17.
   c. Synthetic Bone Grafts—Composed of silicon, calcium, or aluminum.
      (1) Silicate-Based Grafts—Incorporate the element silicon (Si) as silicate (silicon dioxide).
         a. Bioactive Glasses
         b. Glass-Ionomer Cement
      (2) Calcium Phosphate-Based Grafts—Capable of osseoconduction and osseointegration. **These materials biodegrade at a very slow rate.** Many are prepared as ceramics (heated apatite crystals fuse into crystals [sintered]).
         (a) Tricalcium Phosphate
         (b) Hydroxyapatite (e.g., Collagraft Bone Graft Matrix [Zimmer, Inc., Warsaw, IN]); purified bovine dermal fibrillar collagen plus ceramic hydroxyapatite granules and tricalcium phosphate granules.
      (3) Calcium Sulfate—Osteoconductive (e.g., OsteoSet [Wright Medical Technology, Inc., Arlington, TN]).
      (4) Calcium Carbonate (chemically unaltered marine coral)—Is resorbed and replaced by bone (osteoconductive) (e.g., Biocora [Inoteb, France]).
      (5) Coralline Hydroxyapatite—Calcium carbonate skeleton is converted to calcium phosphate via a thermoexchange process (e.g., Interpore 200 and 500 [Interpore Orthopaedics, Irvine, CA]).
      (6) Other Materials
         a. Aluminum Oxide—Alumina ceramic bonds to bone in response to stress and strain between implant and bone.
         b. Hard Tissue—Replacement polymer.

Table 1-12. STAGES OF GRAFT HEALING

STAGE	ACTIVITY
1-Inflammation	Chemotaxis stimulated by necrotic debris
2-Osteoblast differentiation	From precursors
3-Osteoinduction	Osteoblast and osteoclast function
4-Osteoconduction	New bone forming over scaffold
5-Remodeling	Process continues for years

C. Distraction Osteogenesis (Fig. 1-18)
   1. Definition—The use of distraction to stimulate formation of bone.
   2. Clinical Applications
      a. Limb lengthening
      b. Hypertrophic nonunions
      c. Deformity correction (via differential lengthening)
      d. Segmental bone loss (via bone transport)
   3. Biology
      a. Under optimal stable conditions, **bone forms via intramembranous ossification**.
      b. In an unstable environment, bone forms via enchondral ossification; in an extremely unstable environment, pseudoarthrosis may occur.
      c. Histologic Phases
         (1) Latency phase (5-7 days).
         (2) Distraction phase (1 mm per day, approximately 1 inch per month).
         (3) Consolidation phase (typically twice as long as the distraction phase).
   4. Conditions that Promote Optimal Bone Formation During Distraction Osteogenesis
      a. Low-energy corticotomy/osteotomy.
      b. Minimal soft-tissue stripping at the corticotomy site (preserves blood supply).
      c. Stable external fixation to eliminate torsion, shear, and bending moments.
      d. Latency period (no lengthening) of 5-7 days.
      e. Distraction at 0.25 mm 3-4 times per day (0.75-1.0 mm per day).
      f. Neutral fixation interval (no distraction) during consolidation.
      g. Normal physiologic use of the extremity, including weight bearing.

D. Heterotopic Ossification (HO)—Ectopic bone forms in the soft tissues, most commonly in response to an injury or a surgical dissection.
   1. Myositis ossificans (MO) is a specific form of HO when the ossification occurs in muscle.
   2. Patients with traumatic brain injuries are particularly prone to HO; recurrence after resection is likely if neurologic compromise is severe. **Timing of surgery for HO after traumatic brain injury depends on the time since injury (usually 3-6 months is**

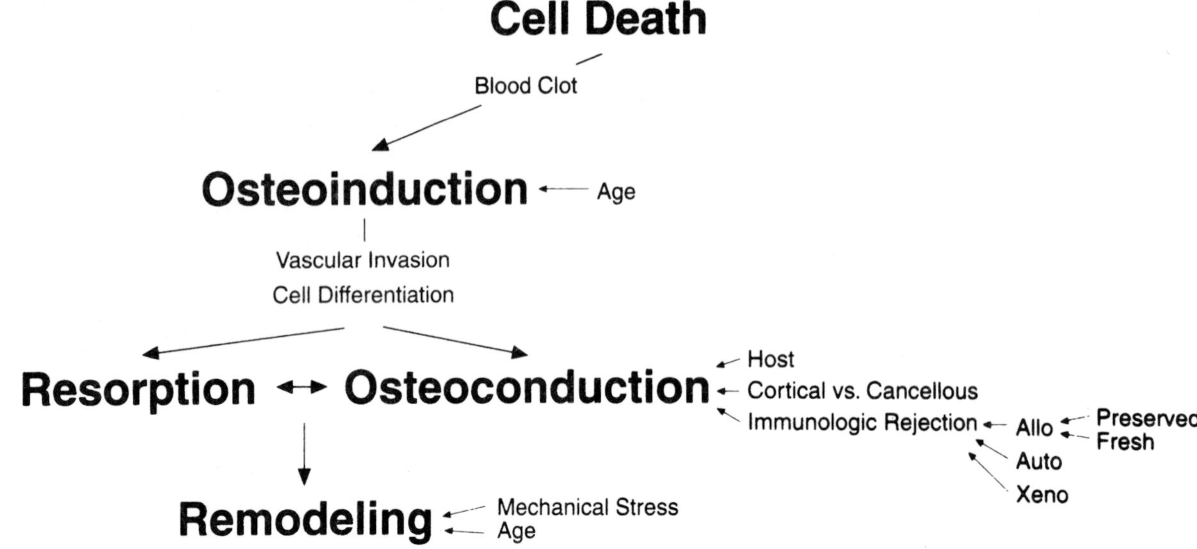

FIGURE 1-17 ■ Major factors influencing bone graft incorporation. (From Simon, S.R., ed.: Orthopaedic Basic Science, 2nd ed., p. 284. Rosemont, IL, American Academy of Orthopaedic Surgeons, 1994.)

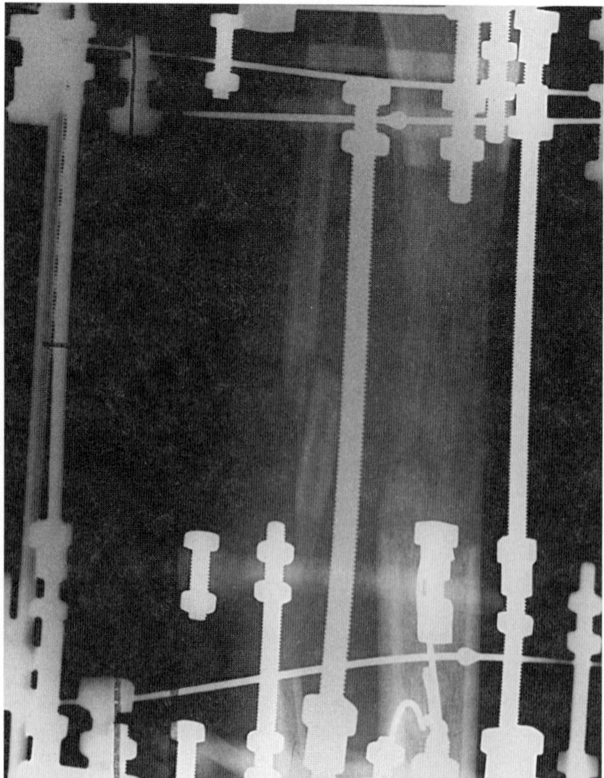

FIGURE 1-18 ■ Radiograph of a patient who has undergone bone transport for a large distal tibial segmental defect. This AP radiograph of the proximal tibia shows early regeneration of distraction osteogenesis; bone formation is via intramembranous ossification.

adequate; there is usually no need to wait longer than 6 months) and evidence of bone maturation on plain radiographs (sharp demarcation and a trabecular pattern).

3. When resecting HO after total hip arthroplasty (THA) (should be delayed for ≥6 months after THA), adjuvant radiation therapy is useful to prevent HO recurrence; **irradiation (optimal therapy is a single postoperative dose of 700 rad) prevents proliferation and differentiation of primordial mesenchymal cells into osteoprogenitor cells that can form osteoblastic tissue.**
4. **Preoperative radiation helps to prevent the formation of HO following THA in patients who are at high risk.** The incidence of HO after THA in patients with Paget's disease is high (approximately 50%).
5. Oral diphosphonate inhibits mineralization of osteoid but does not prevent the formation of osteoid matrix; when oral diphosphonate therapy is discontinued, mineralization with formation of HO may occur.

III. Conditions of Bone Mineralization, Bone Mineral Density, and Bone Viability

A. Normal Bone Metabolism

1. Calcium—Bone serves as a reservoir for more than 99% of the body's calcium. Calcium is also important in muscle and nerve function, clotting mechanisms, and many other areas. Plasma calcium (<1% of total body calcium) is about equally free and bound (usually to albumin). It is absorbed in the duodenum by active transport (requiring adenosine triphosphate [ATP] and calcium-binding protein and

regulated by 1,25-$(OH)_2$-vitamin D_3) and by passive diffusion in the jejunum. The kidney reabsorbs 98% of calcium (60% in the proximal tubule). **The primary homeostatic regulators of serum calcium are PTH and 1,25-$(OH)_2$-vitamin D_3.** The dietary requirement of **elemental calcium** is approximately 600 mg/day for children, about 1300 mg/day for adolescents and young adults (growth spurt [ages 10-25 years]), and 750 mg/day for adult men and women (ages 25-65 years). Pregnant women require 1500 mg/day, and **lactating women require 2000 mg/day. Postmenopausal women and patients with a healing long bone fracture require 1500 mg/day.** Most people have a positive calcium balance during their first three decades of life and a negative balance after the fourth decade. About 400 mg of calcium is released from bone daily. Calcium may be excreted in stool.

2. Phosphate—In addition to being a key component of bone mineral, phosphate is also important in enzyme systems and molecular interactions (metabolite and buffer). Approximately 85% of the body's phosphate stores are in bone. Plasma phosphate is mostly unbound and is reabsorbed by the kidney (proximal tubule). Dietary intake of phosphate is usually adequate (requirement = 1000-1500 mg/day). Phosphate may be excreted in urine.
3. Parathyroid Hormone (PTH)—An 84-amino-acid peptide synthesized in and secreted from the chief cells of the (four) parathyroid glands. PTH helps regulate plasma calcium. PTH directly activates osteoblasts and modulates renal phosphate filtration. Decreased calcium levels in the extracellular fluid stimulates β_2 receptors to release PTH, which acts at the intestine, kidney, and bone (see Table 1-11). PTH may affect bone loss in the elderly. **PTH-related protein and its receptor have been implicated in metaphyseal dysplasia.**
4. Vitamin D—Naturally occurring steroid activated by UV irradiation from sunlight or utilized from dietary intake (Fig. 1-19). It is hydroxylated to 25-(OH)-vitamin D_3 in the liver and is hydroxylated a second time in the kidney. Conversion to the 1,25-$(OH)_2$-vitamin D_3 form activates the hormone, whereas

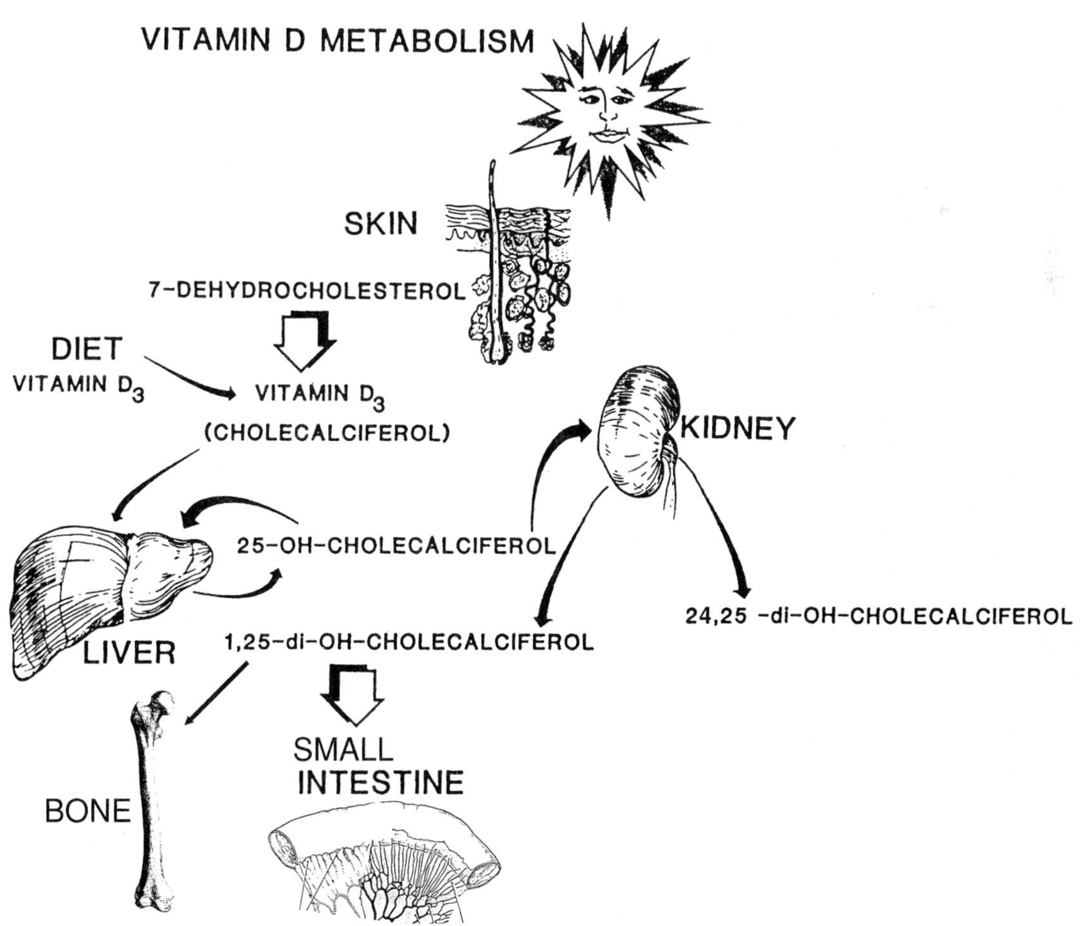

FIGURE 1-19 ■ Vitamin D metabolism. (Modified from Orthopaedic Science Syllabus, p. 11. Park Ridge, IL, American Academy of Orthopaedic Surgeons, 1986.)

conversion to the 24,25-$(OH)_2$-vitamin D_3 form inactivates it (Fig. 1-20). The active form works at the intestine, kidney, and bone (Table 1-13). Phenytoin (Dilantin) causes impaired metabolism of vitamin D.

5. Calcitonin—A 32-amino-acid peptide hormone produced by the clear cells in the parafollicles of the **thyroid gland**; has a limited role in calcium regulation. Increased extracellular calcium levels causes secretion of calcitonin, controlled by a β_2 receptor. **Calcitonin inhibits osteoclastic bone resorption (osteoclasts have calcitonin receptors; decreases osteoclast number and activity) and decreases serum calcium.** May also have a role in fracture healing and reducing vertebral compression fractures in high-turnover osteoporosis.
6. Other Hormones Affecting Bone Metabolism
   a. Estrogen—**Prevents bone loss by inhibiting bone resorption** (a decrease in urinary pyridoline cross-links is observed). **However, because bone formation and resorption are coupled, estrogen therapy also decreases bone formation (see the following discussion on bone loss).** Supplementation is helpful in postmenopausal women only if started within 5-10 years after onset of menopause; the risk of endometrial cancer for patients taking estrogen is reduced when combined with cyclic progestin therapy. **Recent studies suggest a higher risk of heart disease and breast cancer with certain hormone replacement therapy regimens; other post menopausal pharmacologic interventions (alendronate, raloxifene) should therefore be strongly considered to slow bone loss in patients at lower risk.**
   b. Corticosteroids—**Increase bone loss** (decrease gut absorption of calcium by decreasing binding proteins; decrease bone formation [cancellous more affected than cortical bone] by inhibiting collagen synthesis and inhibiting osteoblast productivity; they do not affect mineralization). Alternate-day therapy may reduce effects.
   c. Thyroid Hormones—Affect bone resorption more than bone formation, **leading to osteoporosis** (large [thyroid-suppressive] doses of thyroxine can lead to osteoporosis). **Regulates skeletal growth at the physis** by stimulating chondrocyte growth, type X collagen synthesis, and alkaline phosphatase activity.
   d. Growth Hormone—**Causes a positive calcium balance** by increasing gut absorption of calcium more than it increases urinary excretion. Insulin and somatomedins participate in this effect.
   e. Growth Factors—TGF-β, PDGF, and mono/lymphokines have a role in bone and cartilage repair (discussed elsewhere in this chapter).
7. Interaction—Calcium and phosphate metabolism are affected by an elaborate interplay of hormones and even the levels of the metabolites themselves. Feedback mechanisms play an important role in the regulation of plasma levels of calcium and phosphate. It is now believed that peak bone mass usually occurs between 16 and 25 years of age and is greater in men and African Americans. After this peak, bone loss occurs at a rate of 0.3-0.5% per year (2-3% per year for untreated women during the sixth through tenth years after menopause).
8. Bone Loss—Occurs at the onset of menopause, when there is both accelerated bone formation and resorption. **Markers of bone resorption include urinary hydroxyproline and pyridoline cross-links (when there is bone resorption, both of these are elevated). Serum alkaline phosphatase is a marker for bone formation (elevated when bone formation is increased). Estrogen therapy for osteoporosis in high-risk patients results in a decrease in urinary pyridoline (decreased bone resorption) and a decrease in serum alkaline phosphatase (decreased bone formation); estrogen also increases bone density of the femoral neck and thereby reduces the rate of hip fracture.**

B. Conditions of Bone Mineralization—Include hypercalcemic disorders, hypocalcemic disorders, and hypophosphatasia (Tables 1-14, 1-15, and 1-16).

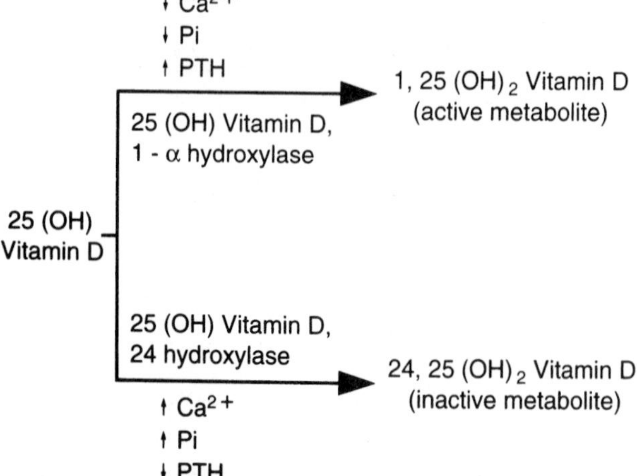

FIGURE 1-20 ■ Vitamin D metabolism in the renal tubular cell. (From Simon, S.R., ed.: Orthopaedic Basic Science, 2nd ed., p. 165. Rosemont, IL, American Academy of Orthopaedic Surgeons, 1994.)

Table 1-13. REGULATION OF CALCIUM AND PHOSPHATE METABOLISM

PARAMETER	PARATHYROID HORMONE (PTH) (PEPTIDE)	1,25-$(OH)_2$ D (STEROID)	CALCITONIN (PEPTIDE)
Origin	Chief cells of parathyroid glands	Proximal tubule of kidney	Parafolicular cells of thyroid gland
Factors stimulating production	Decreases serum Ca^{2+}	Elevated PTH Decreased serum Ca^{2+} Decreased serum P_i	Elevated serum Ca^{2+}
Factors inhibiting production	Elevated serum Ca^{2+} Elevated 1,25 $(OH)_2$ D	Decreased PTH Elevated serum Ca^{2+} Elevated serum P_i	Decreased serum Ca^{2+}
Effect on end-organs for hormone action			
Intestine	No direct effect Acts indirectly on bowel by stimulating production of 1,25-$(OH)_2$ D in kidney	Strongly stimulates intestinal absorption of Ca^{2+} and P_i	?
Kidney	Stimulates 25-(OH)D-1α-OH_{ase} in mitochondria of proximal tubular cells to convert 25-(OH) D to 1,25-$(OH)_2$ D Increases fractional resorption of filtered Ca^{2+} Promotes urinary excretion of P_i	?	?
Bone	Stimulates osteoclastic resorption of bone Stimulates recruitment of preosteoclasts	Strongly stimulates osteoclastic resorption of bone	Inhibits osteoclastic resorption of bone ? Role in normal human physiology
Net effect on Ca^{2+} and P_i concentrations in extracellular fluid and serum	Increased serum Ca^{2+} Decreased serum P_i	Increased serum Ca^{2+} Increased serum P_i	Decreased serum Ca^{2+} (transient)

1,25-$(OH)_2$ D, 1,25-dihyroxyvitamin D; PTH, parathyroid hormone; 25-(OH)D, 25-hydroxyvitamin D.
Adapted from an original figure by Frank H. Netter. From The Ciba Collection of Medical illustrations, vol. 8, part I, p. 179. Copyright by Ciba-Geigy Corporation.

Table 1-14. OVERVIEW OF CLINICAL AND RADIOGRAPHIC ASPECTS OF METABOLIC BONE DISEASES

DISEASE	ETIOLOGY	CLINICAL FINDINGS	RADIOGRAPHIC FINDINGS
Hypercalcemia			
Hyperparathyroidism	PTH overproduction—adenoma	Kidney stone, hyperreflexia	Osteopenia, osteitis fibrosa cystica
Familial syndromes	PTH overproduction—MEN/renal	Endocrine/renal abnormalities	Osteopenia
Hypocalcemia			
Hypoparathyroidism	PTH underproduction-idiopathic	Neuromuscular irritability, eye	Calcified basal ganglia
PHP/Albright's	PTH receptor abnormality	Short MC/MT, obesity	Brachydactyly, exostosis
Renal osteodystrophy	CRF—↓ phosphate excretion	Renal abnormalities	"Rugger jersey" spine
Rickets (osteomalacia)			
Vit. D—deficient	↓ Vit. D diet; malabsorption	Bone deformities, hypotonia	"Rachitic rosary," wide growth plates, fxs
Vit. D—dependent (types I and II)	(see Table 1-15)	Total baldness	Poor mineralization
Vit. D—resistant (hypophosphatemic)	↓Renal tubular phosphate resorption	Bone deformities, hypotonia	Poor mineralization
Hypophosphatasia	↓Alkaline phosphatase	Bone deformities, hypotonia	Poor mineralization
Osteopenia			
Osteoporosis	↓Estrogen—↓ bone mass	Kyphosis, fxs	Compression vertebral fxs, hip fxs
Scurvy	Vit. C deficiency—defective collagen	Fatigue, bleeding, effusions	Thin cortices, corner sign
Osteodense			
Paget's disease	Osteoclastic abn.—↑ bone turnover	Deformities, pain, CHF, fxs	Coarse trabeculae, "picture frame" vertebrate
Osteopetrosis	Osteoclastic abn.—unclear	Hepatosplenomegaly, anemia	Bone within bone

↓, decreased; ↑, increased; Def., defective; abn., abnormality; PTH, parathyroid hormone; MC, metacarpal; MT, metatarsal; CRF, chronic renal failure; CHF, congestive heart failure; fxs, fractures; PHP, pseudohypoparathyroidism; MEN, multiple endocrine neoplasia.

Table 1-15. LABORATORY FINDINGS AND CLINICAL DATA REGARDING PATIENTS WITH THE VARIOUS METABOLIC BONE DISEASES

DISORDER	SERUM Ca	SERUM PHOS	ALK PHOS	PTH	25(OH) VIT D	1,25-$(OH)_2$ VIT D	URINARY CALCIUM	OTHER FINDINGS/ POSSIBLE FINDINGS	TREATMENT	COMMENTS
Primary hyperparathyroidism	↑	N or ↓	N or ↑	↑	N	N or ↑	↑	Active turnover seen on bone biopsy with peritrabecular fibrosis	Surgical excision of parathyroid edema Treat hypercalcemia (see text)	Most commonly due to parathyroid adenoma Because PTH stimulates conversion of the inactive form to the active form [1,25 (OH_2) Vit D] in the kidney, ↑ production of PTH leads to ↑ levels of 1,25 $(OH)_2$ Vit D
Malignancy with bony metastases	↑	N or ↑	N or ↑	N or ↓	N	N or ↓	↑	**Brown tumors** Destructive lesions in bone	Treat cancer and hypercalcemia (see text)	↑ Calcium levels may lead to ↓PTH production via feedback mechanism. ↓1,25 $(OH)_2$ Vit D levels are due to ↓ PTH (which is responsible for conversion of the inactive to the active form of Vit D in the kidney). Multiple myeloma will display an abnormal urinary and serum protein electrophoresis
Hyperthyroidism	↑	N	N	N or ↓	N	N	↑	↑Free thyroxin index ↓thyroid-stimulating hormone Tachycardia, tremors		↑ Calcium levels due to ↑ bone turnover (hypermetabolic state)
Vitamin D intoxication	↑	N or ↑	N or ↑	N or ↓	↑↑↑	N	↑			History of excessive Vit D intake Dietary vitamin D is converted to 25 (OH) Vit D in the liver This results in very high concentrations of 25 (OH) Vit D that cross-react with intestinal Vit D receptors to ↑ resorption of calcium to cause hypercalcemia
Hypoparathyroidism	↓	↑	N	↓	N	↓	↓	Basal ganglia calcification Hypocalcemia findings		↓ PTH production most commonly follows surgical ablation of the thyroid (with the parathyroid) gland ↓PTH leads to ↓ serum calcium and ↑ serum phosphate (due to ↓ urinary excretion of phosphate)

Pseudohypo-parathyroidism	↓	↑	N	N or ↑	N	↓	↓	Hypocalcemic findings		Because PTH stimulates conversion from the inactive to the active form of Vit D (in the kidney), 1,25 $(OH)_2$ Vit D is also ↓ PTH has no effect at the target cells (in the kidney, bone and intestine) due to a PTH receptor abnormality. This leads to a ↓ in the active form of Vit D. Therefore serum calcium levels are ↓ due to: 1) the lack of effect of PTH on bone 2) ↓ levels of 1,25 $(OH)_2$ Vit D
Renal osteodystrophy (high-turnover bone disease of renal disease [secondary hyperparathyroidism])	↓ (or N)	↑↑↑	↑	↑↑↑	N	↓	–	Findings of secondary hyperparathyroidism "Rugger jersey" spine Osteitis fibrosa Amyloidosis	1) Correct underlying renal abnormality 2) Maintain normal serum phosphorous and calcium 3) Dietary phosphate restriction 4) Phosphate binding antacid (calcium carbonate) 5) Administration of the active form of Vit D—1, 25 $(OH)_2$ Vit D (calcitriol)	↓ Renal phosphorous excretion leads to hyperphosphatemia Phosphorous retention leads to ↓ serum calcium and ↑↑↑ PTH (which can lead to secondary hyperparathyroidism) Elevated BUN and creatinine Associated with long-term hemodialysis
Renal osteodystrophy (low-turnover bone disease of renal disease [aluminum toxicity])	↑ (or N)	N or ↑	↑	N (or mildly elevat-ed)	N	↓	—	"Rugger jersey" spine Osteitis fibrosa Amyloidosis Osteomalacia may be seen		PTH levels are ↓ because of: 1) Frequent episodes of hypercalcemia 2) Direct inhibitory effect of aluminum on PTH **No Secondary hyperparathyroidism is present** Elevated BUN and creatinine Associated with long-term hemodialysis
Nutritional rickets—vitamin D deficiency	↓ or N	↓	↑	↑	↓	↓	↓	Osteomalacia, hypotonia Muscle weakness, tetany Bowing deformities of the long bones Rachitic rosary	Oral administration of Vit D (1500–5000 IU/day)	With ↓ vitamin D intake, intestinal calcium and phosphate absorption are reduced leading to hypocalcemia. ↓ Serum calcium stimulates ↑PTH (secondary hyperparathyroidism) that leads to bone resorption and to ↑ serum calcium (toward or to normal levels)

(Continued)

Table 1-15. LABORATORY FINDINGS AND CLINICAL DATA REGARDING PATIENTS WITH THE VARIOUS METABOLIC BONE DISEASES—CONT'D

DISORDER	SERUM CA	SERUM PHOS	ALK PHOS	PTH	25(OH) VIT D	1,25-$(OH)_2$ VIT D	URINARY CALCIUM	OTHER FINDINGS/ POSSIBLE FINDINGS	TREATMENT	COMMENTS
										Sources of vitamin D include: 1) Sunlight 2) Fish liver foods 3) Fortified milk
Nutritional rickets—calcium deficiency	↓ or N	↓	↑	↑	N	↑ (or N)	↓	Similar clinical findings as vitamin D deficiency	Oral administration of calcium (700 mg/day)	Hypocalcemia leads to secondary hyperparathyroidism. ↑ PTH leads to enhanced renal conversion of 25 (OH) Vit D to 1,25 $(OH)_2$ Vit D
Nutritional rickets—phosphate deficiency	N	↓	↑	N	N	↑↑↑	N	No changes of secondary hyperparathyroidism are seen	Oral supplementation of phosphate	Neither secondary hyperparathyroidism nor Vit D deficiency is present ↓ Serum phosphate leads to ↑ renal production of 1,25 $(OH)_2$ Vit D
Hereditary vitamin D—dependent rickets type I ("pseudo-vitamin D deficiency")	↓	↓	↑	↑	N (or ↑)	↓↓↓	↓	Osteomalacia Clinical findings similar (but more severe) than nutritional rickets—vitamin D deficiency	Oral administration of physiologic doses (1–2 μg/day) of 1,25 $(OH)_2$ Vit D	There is a defect in renal 25 (OH) Vit D 1 α hydroxylase. This enzymatic defect inhibits conversion from the inactive form [25(OH) Vit D] to the active form [1,25 $(OH)_2$ Vit D] of vitamin D in the kidney
Hereditary vitamin D—dependent rickets type II ("hereditary	↓	↓	↑	↑	N (or ↑)	↑↑↑	↓	Osteomalacia Alopecia Clinical findings similar (but more severe) than	Long-term (3-6 months) daily administration of high-dose vitamin D	There is an intracellular receptor defect for 1,25 $(OH)_2$ Vit D Patients with this disorder have the highest

resistance to 1,25 $(OH)_2$ Vit D")							nutritional rickets—vitamin D deficiency	analogue [1,25 $(OH)_2$ Vit D or 1 α (OH) Vit D] plus 3 g/day of elemental calcium	1,25 $(OH)_2$ Vit D levels observed in humans; this ↑↑↑ level of 1,25 $(OH)_2$ Vit D distinguishes hereditary vitamin D–dependent rickets type II from type I (the level of 1,25 $(OH)_2$ Vit D is ↓↓↓)
Hypophosphatemic rickets (vitamin D—resistant rickets) ("phosphate diabetes") (Albright's syndrome is an example of a hypophosphatemic syndrome)	N	↓↓↓	↑	N	N	N	N	Osteomalacia No changes of secondary hyperparathyroidism Classic triad: 1) Hypophosphatemia 2) Lower limb deformities 3) Stunted growth rate	Oral administration of elemental phosphate (1–3 g/day) plus high-dose vitamin D (20,000–70,000 IU/day). Vitamin D administration is needed to counterbalance the hypocalcemic effect of phosphate administration, which otherwise could lead to severe secondary hyperparathyroidism	There is an inborn error in phosphate transport (probably located in the proximal nephron). This leads to failure of reabsorption of phosphate in the kidney and "spilling" of phosphate (phosphate diabetes) in the urine While the absolute levels of 1,25 $(OH)_2$ Vit D are normal, they are inappropriately low considering the degree of phosphaturia [production of 1, 25 $(OH)_2$ Vit D is normally stimulated by ↓ serum phosphorous (see Table 1-11)] **This is the most commonly encountered form of rickets**
Hypophosphatasia	↑	↑	↓↓↓	N	N	N	↑	Osteomalacia Early loss of teeth	There is no established medical therapy	There is an inborn error in the tissue-nonspecific (kidney, bone, liver) isoenzyme of alkaline phosphatase Elevated urinary phosphoethanolamine is diagnostic

Table 1-16. DIFFERENTIAL DIAGNOSIS OF THE METABOLIC BONE DISEASES BASED ON BLOOD CHEMISTRIES

↑CALCIUM	↓CALCIUM	NORMAL CALCIUM	↑PHOSPHORUS	↓PHOSPHORUS	NORMAL PHOSPHORUS
Primary hyperparathyroidism Hyperthyroidism Vitamin D intoxication Malignancy without bony metastasis Malignancy with bony metastasis Multiple myeloma Lymphoma Sarcoidosis Milk-alkali syndrome Severe generalized immobilization Multiple endocrine neoplasias Addison's disease Steroid administration Peptic ulcer disease Hypophosphatasia	Hypoparathyroidism Pseudohypoparathyroidism Renal osteodystrophy (high-turnover bone disease) Nutritional rickets—vitamin D deficiency Nurtitional rickets—calcium deficiency Hereditary vitamin D–dependent rickets (types I and II)	Osteoporosis Pseudohypoparathyroidism Nutritional rickets—vitamin D deficiency Nutritional rickets—calcium deficiency Nutritional rickets—phosphate deficiency Hypophosphatemic rickets	Malignancy with bony metastasis Multiple myeloma Lymphoma Vitamin D intoxication Hypoparthyroidism Pseudohypoparathyroidism Renal osteodystrophy Hypophosphatasia Sarcoidosis Milk-alkali syndrome Severe generalized immobilization	Primary hyperparathyroidism Malignancy without bony metastasis Nutritional rickets—vitamin D deficiency Nutritional rickets—calcium deficiency Nutritional rickets—phosphate deficiency Hereditary vitamin D–dependent rickets (types I and II) Hypophosphatemic rickets	Osteoporosis Primary hyperparathyroidism Malignancy with bony metastasis Multiple myeloma Lymphoma Hyperthyroidism Vitamin D intoxication Renal osteodystrophy (*only* low-turnover bone disease) Sarcoidosis Milk-alkali syndrome Severe generalized immobilization
Primary hyperparathyroidism Pseudohypoparathyroidism Renal osteodystrophy Nutritional rickets—vitamin D deficiency Nutritional rickets—calcium deficiency Hereditary vitamin D—dependent rickets (types I and II)	Malignancy with bony metastasis Malignancy without bony metastasis Multiple myeloma Lymphoma Hyperthyroidism Vitamin D intoxication Hypoparathyroidism Sarcoidosis Milk-alkali sydrome Severe generalized immobilization	Osteoporosis Malignancy with bony metastasis Multiple myeloma Lymphoma Vitamin D intoxication Pseudohypoparathyroidism Renal osteodystrophy (*only* low-turnover bone disease) Nutritional rickets—phosphate deficiency Hypophosphatemic rickets Hypophosphatasia Sarcoidosis Hyperthyroidism Milk-alkali syndrome Severe generalized immobilization	Primary hyperparathyroidism Nutritional rickets—calcium deficiency Nutritional rickets—phosphate deficiency Hereditary vitamin D–dependent rickets type II Sarcoidosis	Malignancy with bony metastasis Malignancy without bony metastasis Multiple myeloma Lymphoma Hypoparathyroidism Pseudohypoparathyroidism Renal osteodystrophy Nutritional rickets—vitamin D deficiency Hereditary vitamin D–dependent rickets type I	Osteoporosis Primary hyperparathyroidism Malignancy with bony metastasis Multiple myeloma Lymphoma Hyperthyroidism Vitamin D intoxication Nutritional rickets—calcium deficiency Hypophosphatemic rickets Hypophosphatasia

1. Hypercalcemia—Can present as polyuria, **polydipsia**, kidney stones, excessive bony resorption ± fibrotic tissue replacement (osteitis fibrosa cystica), central nervous system (CNS) effects (confusion, stupor, weakness), and gastrointestinal (GI) effects (constipation). Can also cause **anorexia, nausea, vomiting, dehydration, and muscle weakness**.
   a. Primary Hyperparathyroidism—Caused by overproduction of PTH, usually as a result of a parathyroid adenoma (which generally affects only one parathyroid gland). Excessive PTH causes a net **increase in plasma calcium** and a **decrease in plasma phosphate** (due to enhanced urinary excretion). It results in **increased osteoclastic resorption** and failure of repair attempts (poor mineralization due to low phosphate). Diagnosis is based on signs and symptoms of hypercalcemia (described earlier) and characteristic laboratory results (increased serum calcium, PTH, urinary phosphate; decreased serum phosphate). Bony changes include osteopenia, osteitis fibrosa cystica (fibrous replacement of marrow), **"brown tumors"** (Fig. 1-21) (increased giant cells, extravasation of red blood cells [RBCs], hemosiderin staining, fibrous tissue hemosiderin), and chondrocalcinosis. Radiographs may demonstrate deformed, osteopenic bones, fractures, "shaggy" trabeculae, areas of radiolucency (phalanges, distal clavicle, skull), **destructive metaphyseal lesions**, and calcification of the soft tissues. Histologic changes include osteoblasts and osteoclasts active on both sides of trabeculae (as seen in Paget's disease), areas of destruction, and wide osteoid seams. Surgical parathyroidectomy is curative.
   b. Other Causes of Hypercalcemia
      (1) Familial Syndromes—Hypercalcemia can result from pituitary adenomas associated with multiple endocrine neoplasia (MEN) types I and II and from familial hypocalciuric hypercalcemia (which is caused by poor renal clearance of calcium).
      (2) Other Disorders—Include malignancy (most common), PTH-related protein secretion (lung carcinoma), lytic bone metastases and lesions (such as multiple myeloma), hyperthyroidism, vitamin D intoxication, prolonged immobilization, Addison's disease, steroid administration, peptic ulcer disease (milk alkali syndrome), kidney disease, sarcoidosis, and hypophosphatasia. Hypercalcemia related to malignancy can be life-threatening (and is commonly associated with muscle weakness). Initial treatment should include hydration with normal saline (reverses dehydration). Hypercalcemia of malignancy can occur in the absence of extensive bone metastasis; hypercalcemia of malignancy most commonly results from the release of systemic growth factors and cytokines that stimulate osteoclastic bone resorption (at bony sites not involved in the tumor process).
   c. Treatment of Hypercalcemia
      (1) Hydration (saline diuresis)
      (2) Loop diuretics
      (3) Dialysis (for severe cases)

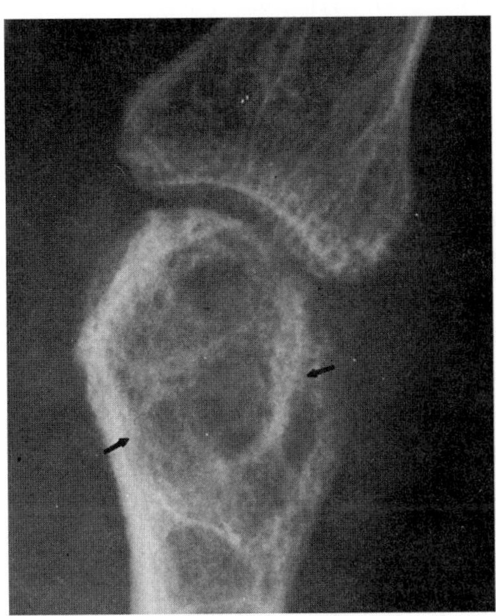

A

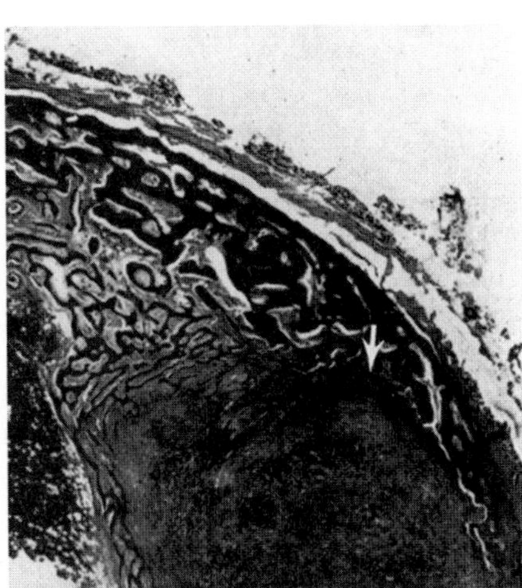

B

FIGURE 1-21 ■ Brown tumor of hyperparathyroidism. *A*, Radiographic changes of brown tumors in the metacarpal head of a patient with hyperparathyroidism. *B*, The photomicrograph shows giant cells within the tumor; rarefied bone with fibrous replacement is also observed. (From Resnick, D. and Niwayama, G.: Diagnosis of Bone and Joint Disorders. Philadelphia, W.B. Saunders, 1981, p. 1826.)

(4) Mobilization (prevents further bone resorption)
(5) Specific drug therapy (bisphosphonates, mithramycin, calcitonin, and gallium nitrate)

2. Hypocalcemia—(Fig. 1-22) Low-plasma calcium can result from low PTH or vitamin D_3. Hypocalcemia leads to increased neuromuscular irritability (tetany, seizures, Chvostek's sign), cataracts, fungal infections of the nails, EKG changes (prolonged QT interval), and other signs and symptoms.
   a. Hypoparathyroidism—Decreased PTH decreases plasma calcium and increases plasma phosphate (urinary excretion not enhanced because of lack of PTH). Common findings include fungal nail infections, hair loss, and blotchy skin (pigment loss; vitiligo). Skull radiographs may show basal ganglia calcification. **Iatrogenic hypoparathyroidism most commonly follows thyroidectomy.**
   b. Pseudohypoparathyroidism (PHP)—A rare genetic disorder caused by a lack of effect of PTH at the target cells. PTH level is normal or even high, but PTH action at the cellular level is blocked by an abnormality at the receptor, by the cAMP system, or by a lack of required cofactors (e.g., Mg^{2+}). **Albright hereditary osteodystrophy**, a form of PHP, is associated with short first, fourth, and fifth metacarpals and metatarsals, brachydactyly, exostoses, obesity, and diminished intelligence. Pseudopseudohypoparathyroidism (pseudo-PHP) is a normocalcemic disorder that is phenotypically similar to PHP. However, in pseudo-PHP there is a normal response to PTH.
   c. Renal Osteodystrophy (Fig. 1-23)—A spectrum of disorders of bone mineral metabolism in patients with chronic renal disease. Renal disease impairs excretion of certain endogenous and exogenous substances and compromises mineral homeostasis, which leads to abnormalities of bone mineral metabolism. Renal bone diseases are subdivided into high-turnover disease and low-turnover disease.
      (1) High-Turnover Renal Bone Disease—Chronically elevated serum PTH leading to **secondary hyperparathyroidism** (hyperplasia of the chief cells of the parathyroid gland). Factors contributing to sustained increased secretion of PTH (and ultimately hyperplasia of the chief cells of the parathyroid gland [secondary hyperparathyroidism]) include the following:
         (a) Diminished Renal Phosphorous Excretion—Chronic renal failure leads to an inability to excrete phosphate. Phosphorous retention promotes PTH secretion by three mechanisms: (1) hyperphosphatemia leads to lowered serum calcium directly and thereby stimulates PTH; (2) phosphorous impairs renal 1 α-hydroxylase activity, therefore impairing production of 1,25-$(OH)_2$-vitamin D_3; (3) phosphorous retention may directly increase the synthesis of PTH. Increased secretion of PTH can lead to secondary hyperparathyroidism.
         (b) Hypocalcemia
         (c) Impaired renal calcitriol
         (d) Alterations in the control of PTH gene transcription secretion
         (e) Skeletal resistance to the actions of PTH

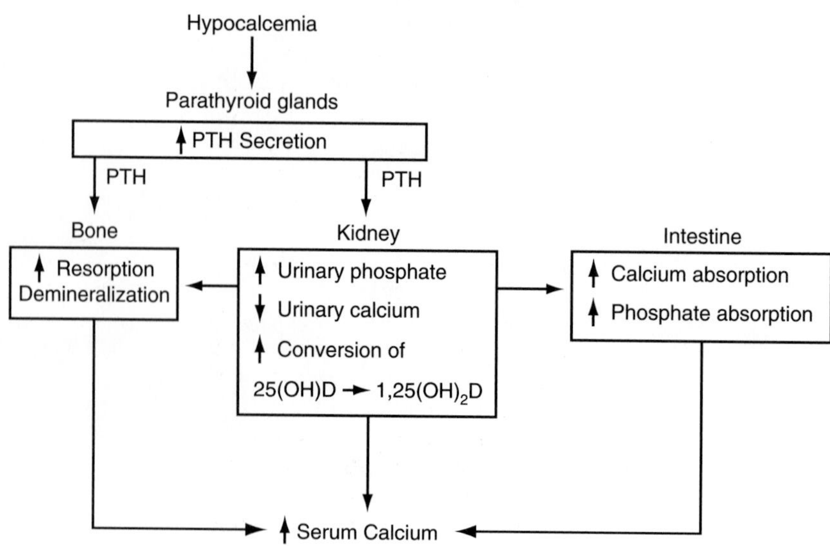

FIGURE 1-22 ■ Body's reaction to hypocalcemia with the consequent resorption of bone. (From Favus, M.J., ed.: Primer on Metabolic Bone Diseases and Disorders of Mineral Metabolism, 3rd ed. Philadelphia, Lippincott-Raven, 1996, p. 302.)

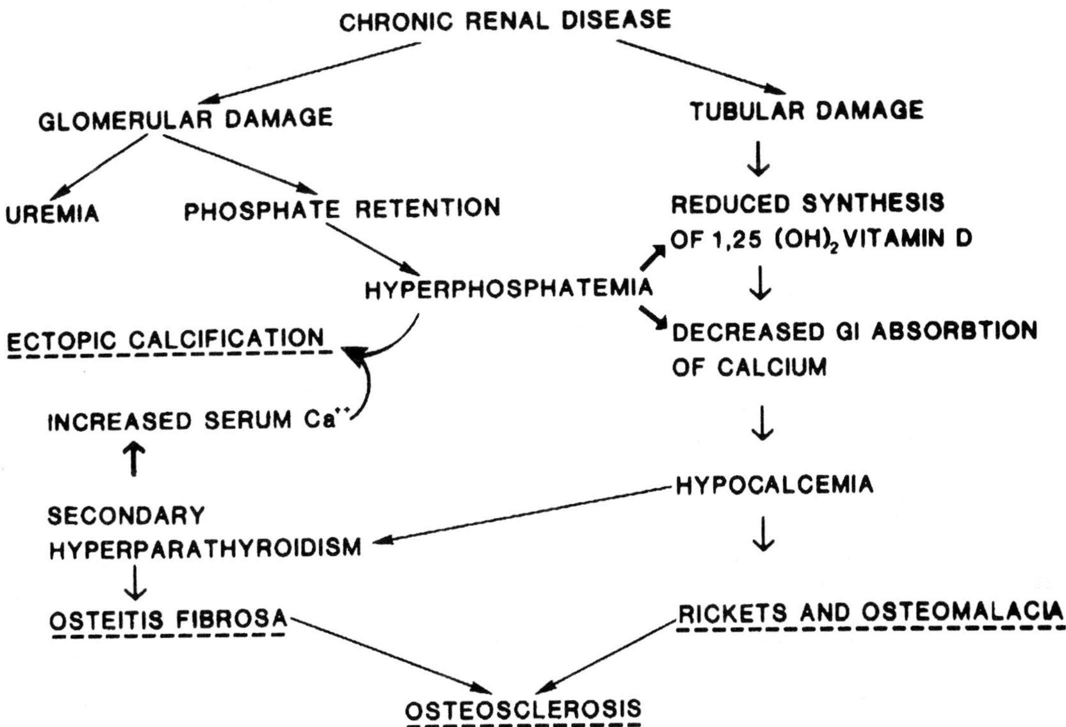

FIGURE 1-23 ■ Pathogenesis of bone changes in renal osteodystrophy. (From Simon, S.R., ed.: Orthopaedic Basic Science, 2nd ed., p. 171. Rosemont, IL, American Academy of Orthopaedic Surgeons, 1994.)

(2) Low-Turnover Renal Bone Disease (Adynamic Lesion of Bone and Osteomalacia)—**These patients do not have secondary hyperparathyroidism**; serum PTH is normal or mildly elevated. Bone formation and turnover are reduced. Excess deposition of aluminum into bone (aluminum toxicity) negatively affects bone mineral metabolism:

(a) Impairs differentiation of precursor cells to osteoblasts
(b) Impairs proliferation of osteoblasts
(c) Impairs PTH release from the parathyroid gland
(d) Disrupts the mineralization process. Depending on the severity of involvement, the low-turnover lesion may represent an adynamic lesion or osteomalacia.
(e) Adynamic lesion—Accounts for the majority of cases of low-turnover bone disease in patients with chronic renal failure.
(f) Osteomalacia—In addition to slowed bone formation and turnover, there is a defect in the mineralization of newly formed bone.

In renal osteodystrophy, radiographs may demonstrate a "rugger jersey" spine, like that in childhood osteopetrosis, and soft-tissue calcification. **An additional complication of chronic dialysis is the accumulation of beta-2 microglobulin, which leads to amyloidosis. Amyloidosis may be associated with carpal tunnel syndrome, arthropathy, and pathologic fractures.** The material in amyloidosis stains pink with Congo red. Laboratory tests in renal osteodystrophy show an abnormal glomerular filtration rate (GFR); increased alkaline phosphatase, blood urea nitrogen (BUN), and creatinine; and decreased venous bicarbonate. Treatment should be directed at relieving the urologic obstruction or kidney disease.

d. Rickets (Osteomalacia in Adults)—**Failure of mineralization** leading to changes in the physis in the zone of provisional calcification (increased width and disorientation) and bone (cortical thinning, bowing).

The causes of rickets and osteomalacia are summarized in Table 1-17.

(1) Nutritional Rickets (see Table 1-15)

(a) Vitamin D Deficiency Rickets—Rare after addition of vitamin D to milk; but still seen in Asian immigrants, patients with dietary peculiarities, premature infants, and those with malabsorption (sprue) or chronic parenteral nutrition. Decreased intestinal absorption of calcium and phosphate leads to secondary hyperparathyroidism (PTH continues to be produced because of low plasma calcium). **Laboratory studies** show **low normal calcium** (maintained by high PTH), **low phosphate** (excreted because of the effect of PTH), **increased PTH**, and **low levels of vitamin D**. Enlargement of the costochondral junction (**"rachitic rosary"**), bony deformities (**bowing of the knees**, "codfish" vertebrae), retarded bone growth (defect in the hypertrophic zone with widened osteoid seams and physeal cupping), muscle hypotonia, dental disease, pathologic fractures (Looser's zones [pseudofracture on the compression side of bone]), **milkman's fracture** ([pseudofracture in adults] Fig. 1-24), a waddling gait, and other problems may result. Affected children are commonly below the fifth percentile for height. Treatment with vitamin D (5000 IU daily) resolves most deformities. Characteristic radiographic changes seen in rickets include physeal widening, physeal cupping, and coxa vara.

(b) Calcium Deficiency Rickets (Fig. 1-25)

(c) Phosphate Deficiency Rickets

(2) Hereditary Vitamin D-Dependent Rickets Type I and type II—Rare disorders with features similar to vitamin D deficiency (nutritional) rickets, except **may be worse** and patients may have total baldness.

(a) Vitamin D-Dependent Rickets Type I—**Defect in renal 25-(OH)-vitamin D 1 α-hydroxylase**, inhibiting conversion of the inactive form of vitamin D to the active form of vitamin D. The inheritance pattern is autosomal recessive (AR). The gene responsible is on chromosome 12q14.

Table 1-17. CAUSES OF RICKETS AND OSTEOMALACIA

Nutritional Deficiency
Vitamin D deficiency
Dietary chelators (rare) of calcium
Phytates
Oxalates (spinach)
Phosphorus deficiency (unusual)
Antacid (aluminium-containing) abuse leading to severe dietary phosphate binding
Gastrointestinal Absorption Defects
Postgastrectomy (rare today)
Biliary disease (interference with absorption of fat-soluble vitamin D)
Enteric absorption defects
Short bowel syndrome
Rapid-transit (gluten-sensitive enteropathy) syndromes
Inflammatory bowel disease
Crohn's disease
Celiac disease
Renal Tubular Defects (Renal Phosphate Leak)
X-linked dominant hypophosphatemic vitamin D-resistant rickets (VDRR) or osteomalacia
Classic Albright's syndrome or Fanconi's syndrome type I
Fanconi's syndrome type II
Phosphaturia and glycosuria
Fanconi's syndrome type III
Phosphaturia, glycosuria, aminoaciduria
Vitamin D—dependent rickets (or osteomalacia) type I (a genetic or acquired deficiency of renal tubular 25-hydroxyvitamin D 1-alpha hydroxylase enzyme that prevents conversion of 25-hydroxy-vitamin D to the active polar metabolite 1,25-dihydroxy-vitamin D)
Vitamin D-dependent rickets (or osteomalacia) type II (this entity represents enteric end-organ insensitivity to 1,25-dihydroxy-vitamin D and is probably caused by an abnormality in the 1,25- dihydroxy-vitamin D nuclear receptor)
Renal tubular acidosis
Acquired—associated with many systemic diseases
Genetic
Debre-De Toni-Fanconi syndrome
Lignac-Fanconi syndrome (cysteinosis)
Lowe's syndrome
Renal Osteodystrophy Miscellaneous Causes
Soft-tissue tumors secreting putative factors
Fibrous dysplasia
Neurofibromatosis
Other soft-tissue and vascular mesenchymal tumors
Anticonvulsant medication (induction of the hepatic P450 microsomal enzyme system by some anticonvulsants—phenytoin, Phenobarbital, mysoline—causes increased degradation of vitamin D metabolites)
Heavy metal intoxication
Hypophosphatasia
High-dose diphosphonates
Sodium fluoride

Adapted from Simon, S.R.: Orthopaedic Basic Science, 2nd ed., p. 169. Rosemont, IL, American Academy of Orthopaedic Surgeons, 1994.

(b) Vitamin D-Dependent Rickets Type II—**Defect in an intracellular receptor for 1,25-$(OH)_2$-vitamin D_3.**

(3) Familial Hypophosphatemic Rickets (Vitamin D-Resistant Rickets; also known as "Phosphate Diabetes")—**Most commonly encountered form of**

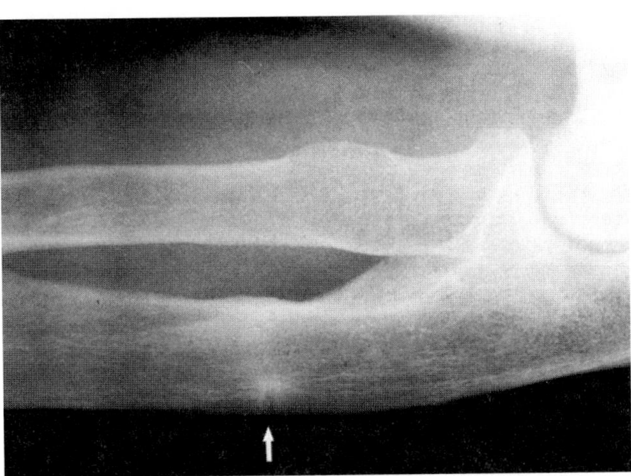

FIGURE 1-24 ■ Pseudofracture (*arrow*) in an adult patient with X-linked hypophosphatemic osteomalacia occurring in characteristic location in proximal ulna. Note bowing of ulna. (From Pitt, M.J., et al.: Crit. Rev. Radiol. Sci. 10:145, 1977.)

rickets. X-linked dominant disorder that is a result of impaired renal tubular reabsorption of phosphate. Affected patients have a normal GFR and an impaired vitamin D_3 response. Phosphate replacement (1-3 g daily) with high-dose vitamin D_3 can correct the effects of the disorder, which are similar to those of the other forms of rickets.

3. Hypophosphatasia (Fig. 1-26)—AR disorder caused by an inborn error in the tissue-nonspecific isoenzyme of alkaline phosphatase that leads to **low levels of alkaline phosphatase**, which is required for the synthesis of inorganic phosphate, important in bone matrix formation. **Features are similar to those of rickets,** and treatment may include phosphate therapy. **Increased urinary phosphoethanolamine is diagnostic.**

C. Conditions of Bone Mineral Density—Bone mass is regulated by the relative rates of deposition and withdrawal (Fig. 1-27).

1. Osteopenia
   a. Osteoporosis—Age-related **decrease in bone mass** usually associated with loss of estrogen in postmenopausal women (Fig. 1-28). **The World Health Organization defines osteoporosis as a lumbar (L2-4) density level 2.5 standard deviations below the peak bone mass of a 25-year-old individual.** Osteoporosis is responsible for more than 1 million fractures per year (vertebral body most common). The lifetime risk of fracture in white women after 50 years of age is approximately 75%; the risk of hip fracture is 15-20%. **Osteoporosis is a quantitative, not a qualitative, defect in bone; mineralization of bone remains normal.**

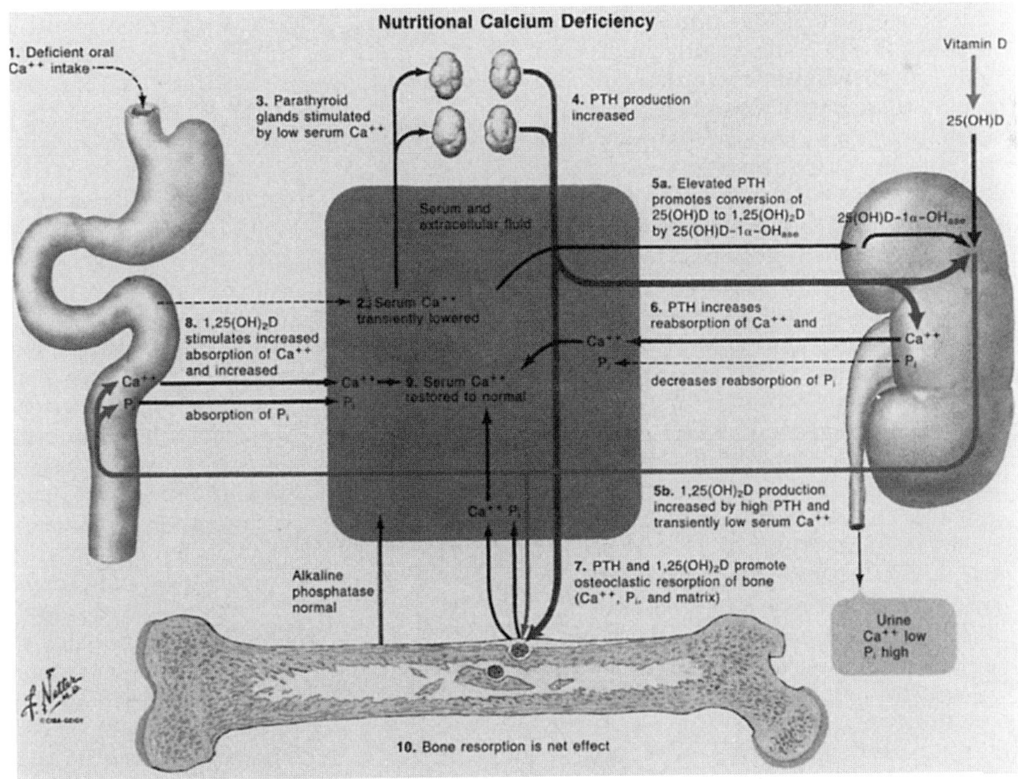

FIGURE 1-25 ■ Nutritional calcium deficiency. (From the Ciba Collection of Medical Illustrations, vol. 8, part I, p. 184, 1987. Illustrated by Frank H. Netter. Reprinted by permission.)

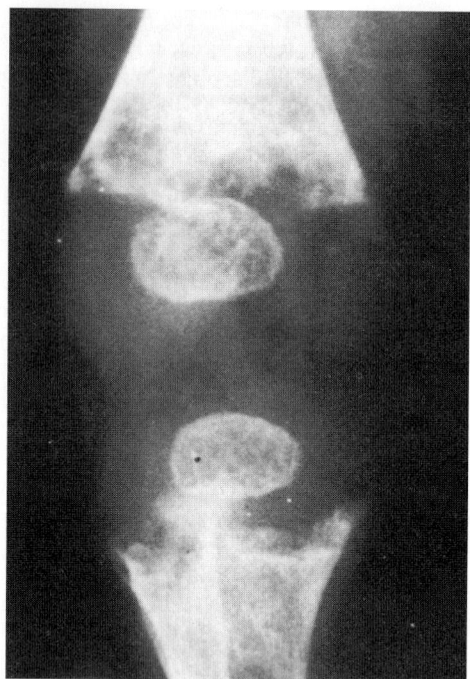

FIGURE 1-26 ■ Hypophosphatasia. Deossification is present adjacent to the growth plates. Characteristic radiolucent areas extend from the growth plates into the metaphysis. (From Resnick, D., and Niwayama, G.: Diagnosis of Bone and Joint Disorders. Philadelphia, W.B. Saunders, 1981, p. 1710.)

Sedentary, thin **Caucasian women of northern European descent** (fair skin and hair), particularly **smokers,** heavy **drinkers,** and patients on **phenytoin [Dilantin] (impairs vitamin D metabolism),** with low-calcium and low-vitamin D diets who **breast-fed their infants,** are at greatest risk. **A history of two osteoporotic vertebral compression fractures is the strongest predictor of subsequent vertebral fracture in postmenopausal women; positive family history and premature menopause also increase the risk. Cancellous bone is most markedly affected**. Clinical features include kyphosis and vertebral fractures (compression fractures of T11–L1 [creating an anterior wedge-shaped defect or resulting in a centrally depressed "codfish" vertebrae]), hip fractures, and distal radius fractures. Two types of osteoporosis have been characterized: type I (postmenopausal) and type II (age related).

(1) Type I Osteoporosis (Postmenopausal)—Affects trabecular bone primarily; vertebral and distal radius fractures are common.

(2) Type II Osteoporosis (Age Related)—Seen in patients older than 75 years; affects both trabecular and cortical bone; is related to poor calcium absorption; hip and pelvic fractures are common. Laboratory studies, including urinary calcium and hydroxyproline and serum alkaline phosphatase, are helpful for evaluating osteopenic conditions; **these studies are usually unremarkable in osteoporosis**; but hyperthyroidism (reversible osteoporosis), hyperparathyroidism, Cushing's syndrome, hematologic disorders, and malignancy should be ruled out. **Plain radiographs are usually not helpful unless bone loss is >30%.** Special studies used for the work-up of osteoporosis include single-photon (appendicular) and double-photon (axial) absorptiometry, quantitative computed tomography (CT), and dual-energy x-ray absorptiometry (DEXA). **DEXA is most accurate and emits less radiation.** Biopsy (after tetracycline labeling) may be used to evaluate the severity of osteoporosis and to identify osteomalacia. Histologic changes: thinning trabeculae, decreased osteon size, and enlarged haversian and marrow spaces. Physical activity, calcium supplements (more effective in type II [age-related] osteoporosis), **estrogen-progesterone therapy (in type I [postmenopausal] osteoporosis; works best when initiated within 6 years of menopause),** and fluoride (inhibits bone resorption, but bone is more brittle) have a role in the treatment of osteoporosis. Bisphosphonates bind to bone resorption surfaces and inhibit osteoclastic membrane ruffling without destroying the cells. Other drugs, such as intramuscular calcitonin, may also be helpful but are expensive and may cause hypersensitivity reactions. The future of bone augmentation with PTH, growth factors, prostaglandin inhibitors, and other therapies remains to be determined. **An overview of recommended treatments for osteoporosis is shown in Figure 1-29.** The best prophylaxis for at-risk patients comprises: (1) diet with adequate calcium intake; (2) weight-bearing exercise program; and (3) estrogen therapy evaluation at menopause.

(3) Idiopathic Transient Osteoporosis of the Hip—Uncommon; diagnosis of exclusion; most common during the third trimester of pregnancy but can also occur in men. Presents with groin pain, limited range of motion (ROM), and localized osteopenia (without a history of trauma). Treatment includes

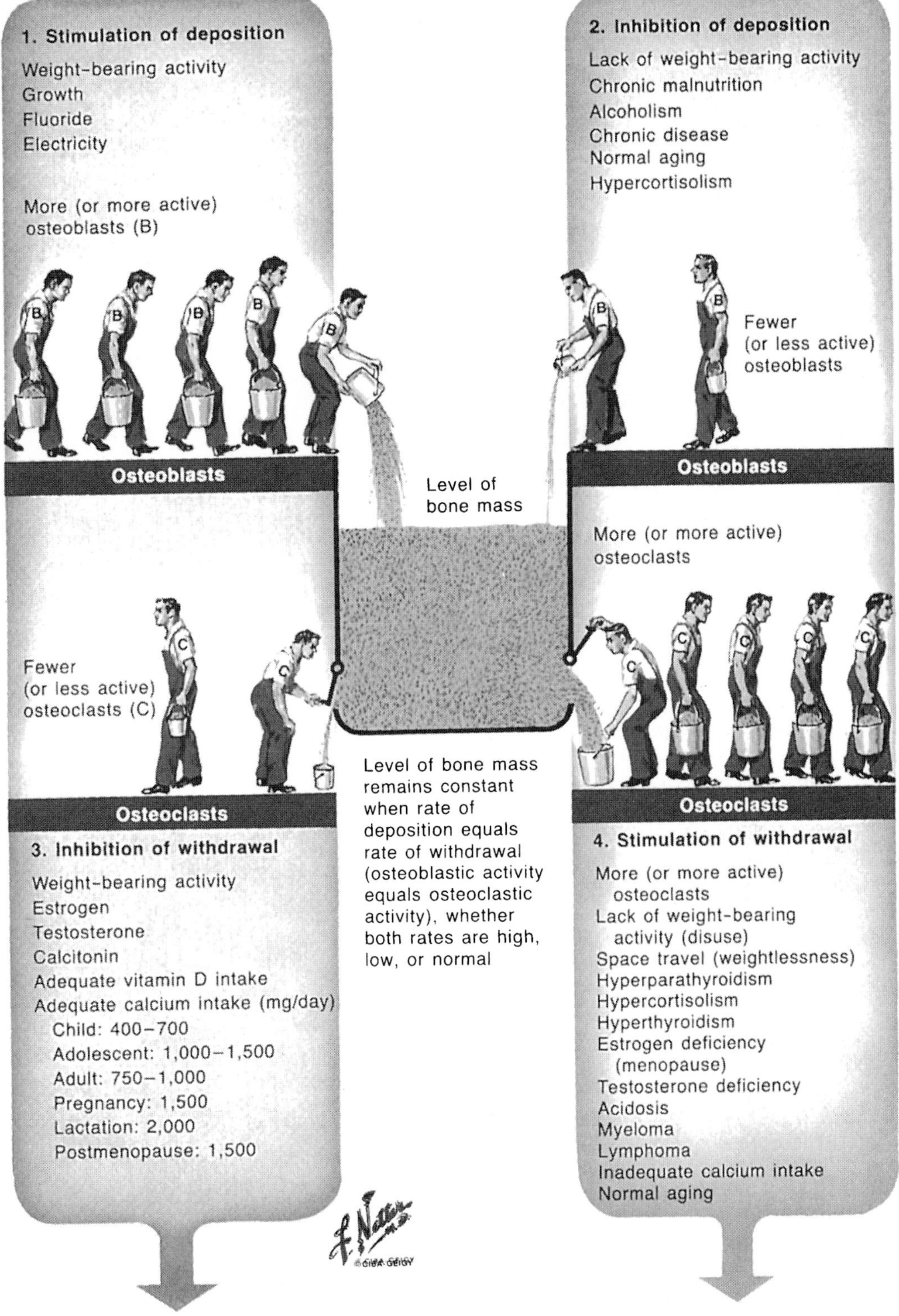

FIGURE 1-27 ■ Four mechanisms of bone mass regulation. (From the Ciba Collection of Medical Illustrations, vol. 8, part I, p. 181, 1987. Illustrated by Frank H. Netter. Reprinted by permission.)

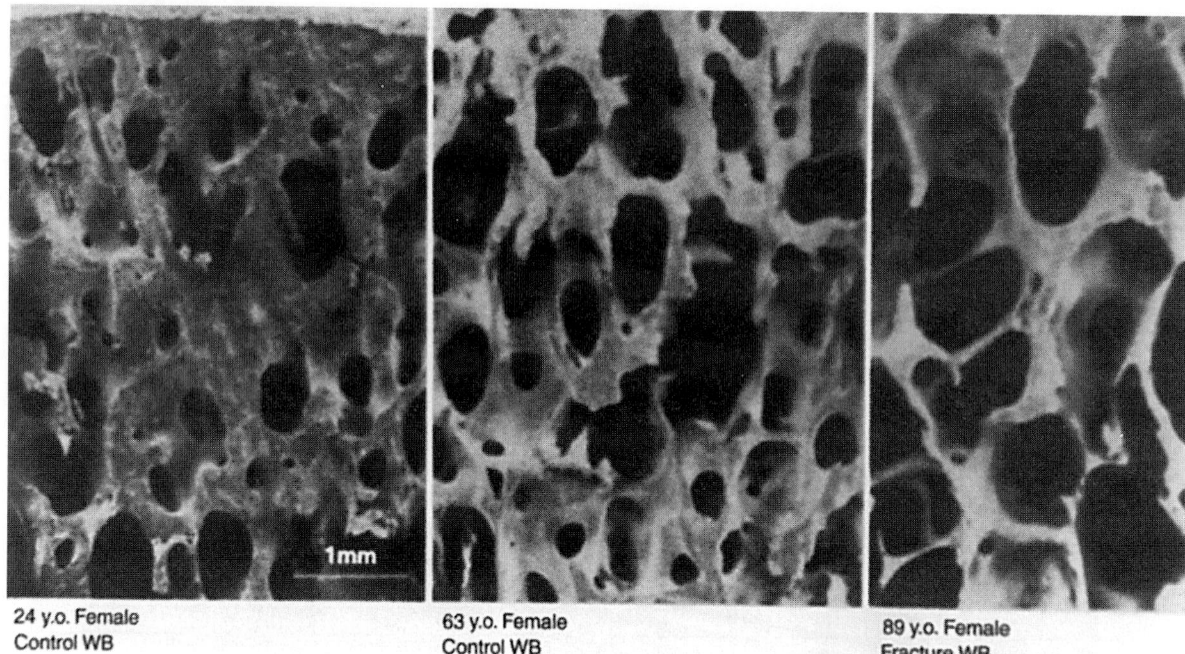

FIGURE 1-28 ■ Age-related changes in density and architecture of human trabecular bone from the lumbar spine. (Reprinted from Keaveney, T.M., and Hayes, W.C.: Mechanical properties of cortical and trabecular bone. Bone 7:285–344, 1993, by permission from Elsevier Science.)

limited weight bearing and analgesics. The disease is generally self-limited and tends to resolve spontaneously after 6-8 months (distinguishes it from osteonecrosis, in which the symptoms are progressive and do not resolve spontaneously). Stress fractures may occur.

(4) Bone Loss Related to Spinal Cord Injury—With paraplegia and quadraplegia, bone mineral loss occurs throughout the skeleton (except the skull) for approximately 16 months and levels off at two thirds of the original bone mass (high risk of fracture). Bone loss occurs to the greatest extent in the lower extremities.

b. Osteomalacia—Discussed with rickets. **Defect in mineralization** results in a large amount of **unmineralized osteoid (qualitative defect).** Osteomalacia is caused by vitamin D–deficient diets, GI disorders, renal osteodystrophy, and certain drugs (aluminum-containing phosphate-binding antacids [aluminum deposition in bone prevents mineralization], and phenytoin). **Like osteoporosis, osteomalacia is also associated with chronic alcoholism**. It is commonly associated with Looser's zones (microscopic stress fractures), other fractures, biconcave vertebral bodies, and a trefoil pelvis seen on plain radiographs. Biopsy (transiliac) is required for diagnosis (histologically, widened osteoid seams are seen). Femoral neck fractures are common in patients with osteomalacia. Treatment usually includes large doses of vitamin D. Osteoporosis and osteomalacia are compared in Figure 1-30.

c. Scurvy—**Vitamin C (ascorbic acid) deficiency produces a decrease in chondroitin sulfate synthesis, which leads to defective collagen growth and repair and impaired intracellular**

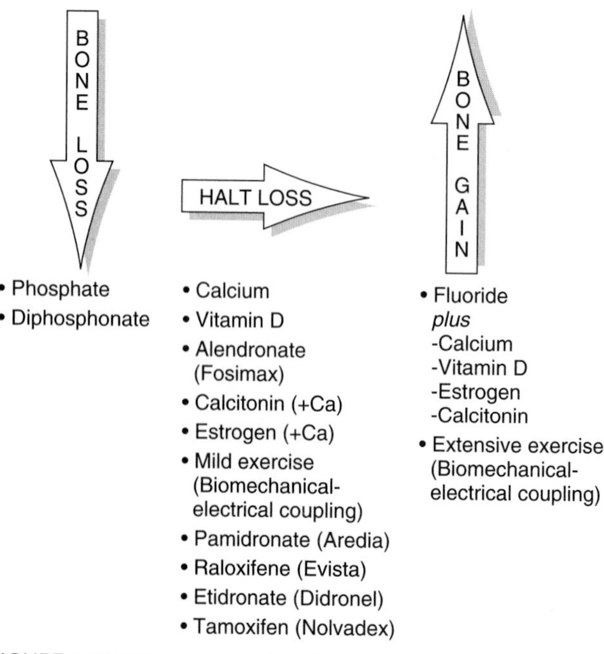

FIGURE 1-29 ■ Treatment options for osteoporosis. (From Simon, S.R., ed.: Orthopaedic Basic Science, 2nd ed., p. 174. Rosemont, IL, American Academy of Orthopaedic Surgeons, 1994.)

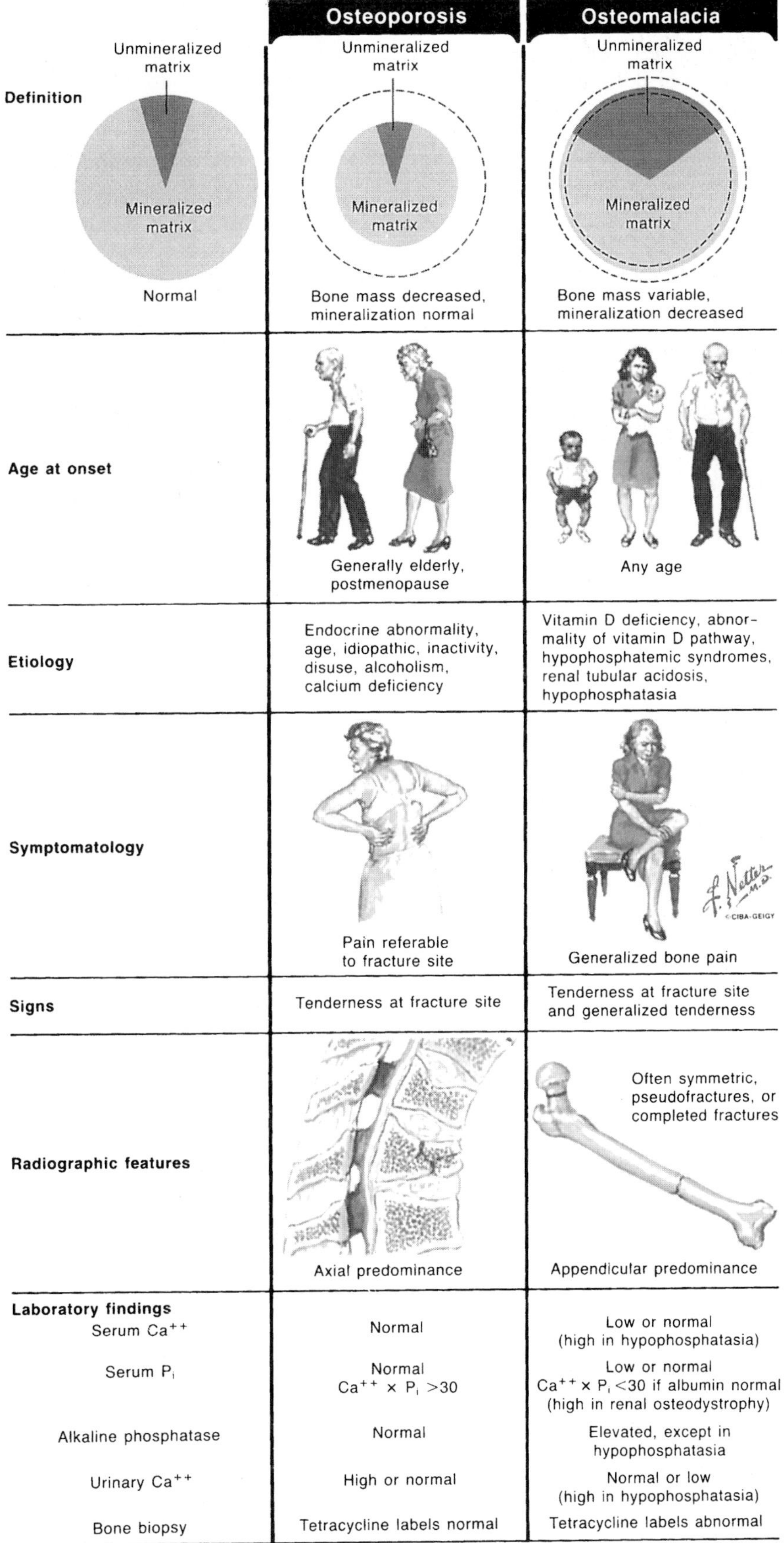

Comparison of Osteoporosis and Osteomalacia
Osteoporosis
Osteomalacia
Definition
Unmineralized matrix
Mineralized matrix
Normal
Unmineralized matrix
Mineralized matrix
Bone mass decreased, mineralization normal
Unmineralized matrix
Mineralized matrix
Bone mass variable, mineralization decreased
Age at onset
Generally elderly, postmenopause
Any age
Etiology
Endocrine abnormality, age, idiopathic, inactivity, disuse, alcoholism, calcium deficiency
Vitamin D deficiency, abnormality of vitamin D pathway, hypophosphatemic syndromes, renal tubular acidosis, hypophosphatasia
Symptomatology
Pain referable to fracture site
Generalized bone pain
F. Netter M.D.
© CIBA-GEIGY
Signs
Tenderness at fracture site
Tenderness at fracture site and generalized tenderness
Radiographic features
Axial predominance
Often symmetric, pseudofractures, or completed fractures
Appendicular predominance
Laboratory findings
Serum Ca++
Normal
Low or normal (high in hypophosphatasia)
Serum Pi
Normal Ca++ × Pi >30
Low or normal Ca++ × Pi <30 if albumin normal (high in renal osteodystrophy)
Alkaline phosphatase
Normal
Elevated, except in hypophosphatasia
Urinary Ca++
High or normal
Normal or low (high in hypophosphatasia)
Bone biopsy
Tetracycline labels normal
Tetracycline labels abnormal

FIGURE 1-30 ■ Osteoporosis versus osteomalacia. (From the Ciba Collection of Medical Illustrations, vol. 8, part I, p. 228, 1987. Illustrated by Frank H. Netter. Reprinted by permission.)

hydroxylation of collagen peptides. Clinical features include fatigue, gum bleeding, ecchymosis, joint effusions, and iron deficiency. Radiographic changes may include thin cortices and trabeculae and metaphyseal clefts (corner sign). Laboratory studies are normal. Histologic changes include replacement of primary trabeculae with granulation tissue, areas of hemorrhage, and widening of the zone of provisional calcification in the physis. **The greatest effect on bone formation occurs in the metaphysis.**

d. Marrow Packing Disorders—Myeloma, leukemia, and other disorders can cause osteopenia (see Chapter 8, Orthopaedic Pathology).

e. Osteogeneis Imperfecta (see Chapter 2, Pediatric Orthopaedics)—**Caused by abnormal collagen synthesis (failure of normal collagen cross-linking). Abnormality is primarily due to a mutation in the genes responsible for the metabolism and synthesis of type I collagen.**

2. Increased Osteodensity

a. Osteopetrosis (Marble Bone Disease)—A group of bone disorders that leads to increased sclerosis and obliteration of the medullary canal due to **decreased osteoclast (and chondroclast) function** (there is failure of bone resorption). The number of osteoclasts may be increased, decreased, or normal. The disorder may result from an abnormality of the immune system (thymic defect). Histologically, osteoclasts lack the normal ruffled border and clear zone. Marrow spaces fill with **necrotic calcified cartilage**, and cartilage may be trapped within osteoid. Empty lacunae and plugging of haversian canals are also seen. The most severe infantile AR ("malignant") form leads to a "bone within a bone" appearance on radiographs, hepatosplenomegaly, and aplastic anemia and can lead to death during infancy. Bone marrow transplantation (of osteoclast precursors) can be life-saving during childhood. High doses of calcitriol ± steroids may also be helpful. The autosomal dominant (AD) "tarda" (benign) form **(Albers-Schönberg disease)** demonstrates generalized osteosclerosis (including the typical **"rugger jersey" spine**), usually without other anomalies (Figs. 1-31, 1-32). Pathologic fractures through abnormal (brittle) bone are common.

b. Osteopoikilosis ("Spotted Bone Disease")—Islands of deep cortical bone appear within the medullary cavity and the cancellous bone of the long bones (especially in the hands and feet). These areas are usually

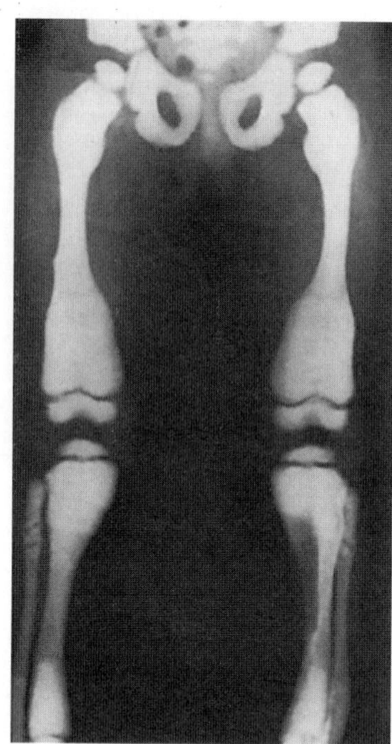

FIGURE 1-31 ■ Typical "marble bone" appearance of osteopetrosis. (From Tachdijian, M.O.: Pediatric Orthopaedics, 2nd ed., p. 795. Philadelphia: WB Saunders, 1990.)

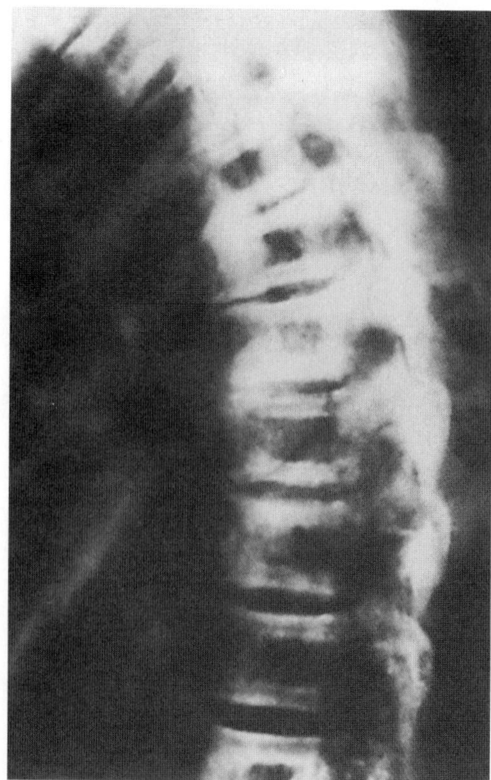

FIGURE 1-32 ■ Typical "rugger jersey" spine seen in osteopetrosis. (From Tachdijian, M.O.: Pediatric Orthopaedics, 2nd ed., p. 797. Philadelphia, WB Saunders, 1990.)

asymptomatic, and there is no known incidence of malignant degeneration.

3. Paget's Disease—**Elevated serum alkaline phosphatase and urinary hydroxyproline; virus-like inclusion bodies observed in osteoclasts.** Can display both decreased and increased osteodensity (depending on the phase of the disease). See Chapter 8, Orthopaedic Pathology.
   a. Active Phase
      (1) Lytic Phase—Intense osteoclastic bone resorption
      (2) Mixed Phase
      (3) Sclerotic Phase—Osteoblastic bone formation predominates
   b. Inactive Phase

D. Conditions of Bone Viability
   1. Osteonecrosis—Death of bony tissue (usually adjacent to a joint surface) from causes other than infection. It is usually caused by loss of blood supply due to trauma or another etiology (e.g., after a slipped capital femoral epiphysis). **Recent studies suggest that idiopathic ON of the femoral head and Legg-Calvé-Perthes disease occur in patients with coagulation abnormalities** [deficiency of antithrombin factors protein C and protein S and increased levels of lipoprotein (a)]. ON commonly affects the hip joint, leading to eventual collapse and flattening of the femoral head, most frequently in the anterolateral region. The condition is associated with steroid and heavy alcohol use; also associated with blood dyscrasias (e.g., sickle cell disease), dysbaric (caisson disease), excessive radiation therapy, and Gaucher's disease.
      a. Etiology—Theories regarding the etiology of ON vary (Fig. 1-33). It may be related to

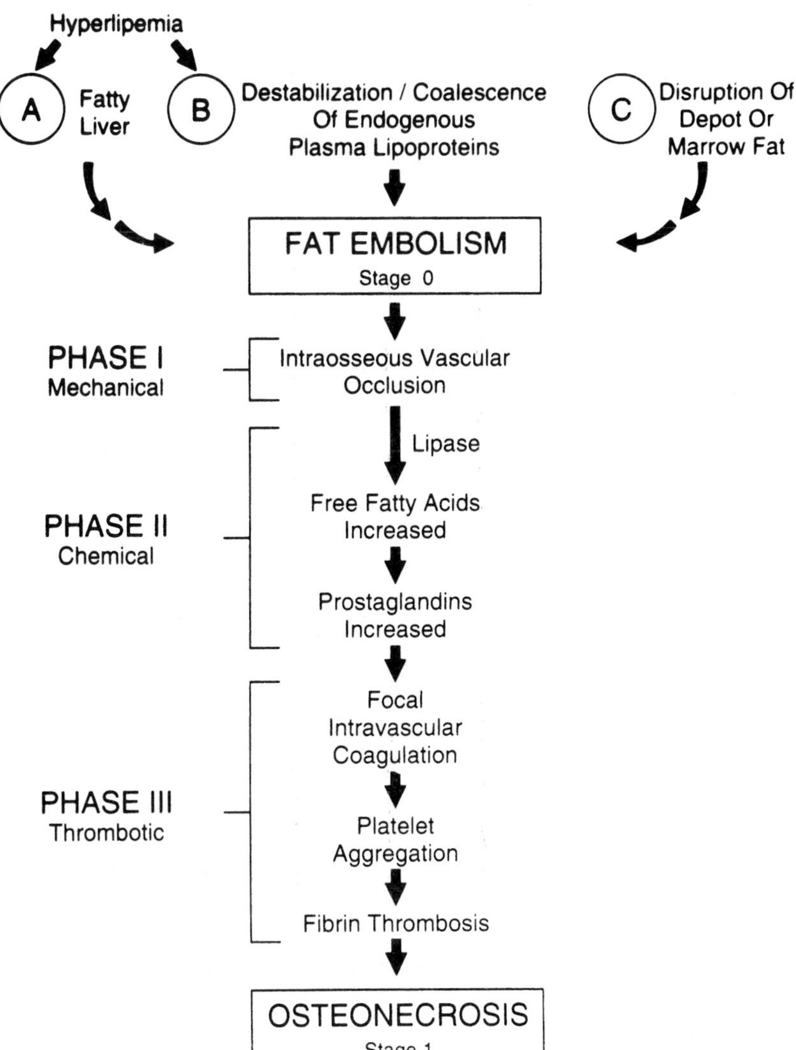

FIGURE 1-33 ■ Possible mechanisms of intraosseous fat embolism leading to focal intravascular coagulation and osteonecrosis. (From Jones, J.P., Jr.: Fat embolism and osteonecrosis. Orthop. Clin. North Am. 16:595–633, 1985.)

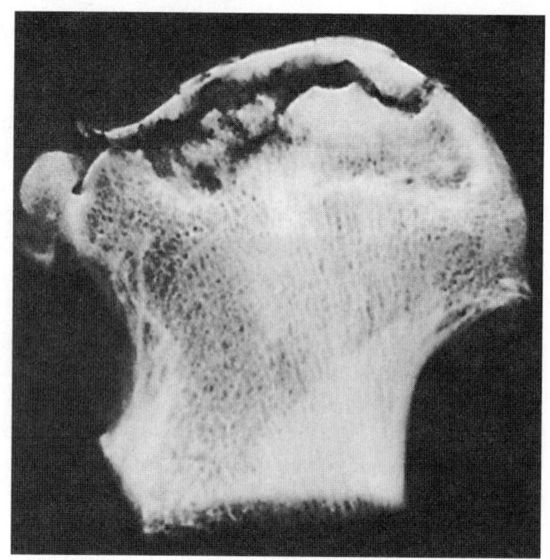

FIGURE 1-34 ■ Fine-grain radiograph demonstrating space between the articular surface and subchondral bone: "Crescent sign" of osteonecrosis. (From Steinberg, M.E.: The Hip and Its Disorders, p. 630. Philadelphia, WB Saunders, 1991.)

enlargement of space-occupying marrow fat cells, which leads to ischemia of adjacent tissues. Vascular insults and other factors may also be significant. Idiopathic ON (Chandler's disease) is diagnosed when no other cause can be identified. Idiopathic, alcohol, and dysbaric ON are associated with multiple insults. ON may arise secondary to an underlying hemoglobinopathy (such as sickle cell disease) or a marrow disorder (such as hemochromatosis). Cyclosporine has reduced the incidence of ON of the femoral head in renal transplant patients.

b. Pathologic Changes—Grossly necrotic bone, fibrous tissue, and subchondral collapse may be seen (Figs. 1-34, 1-35). Histologically, early changes involve autolysis of osteocytes (14-21 days) and necrotic marrow, followed by (1) inflammation with invasion of buds of primitive mesenchymal tissue and capillaries; (2) later, **new woven bone is laid down on top of dead trabecular bone;** and (3) this stage is followed by resorption of dead trabeculae and remodeling via **"creeping substitution."** The bone is weakest during resorption and remodeling, and **collapse (crescent sign, seen on radiographs)** and fragmentation can occur.

c. Evaluation—Careful history taking (risk factors) and physical examination (e.g., decreased ROM, limp) should precede additional studies. Evaluation of other joints (especially the contralateral hip) is important in order to identify the disease process early. The process is bilateral in the hip in 50% of cases of idiopathic ON and up to 80% of steroid-induced ON. Magnetic resonance imaging (MRI)

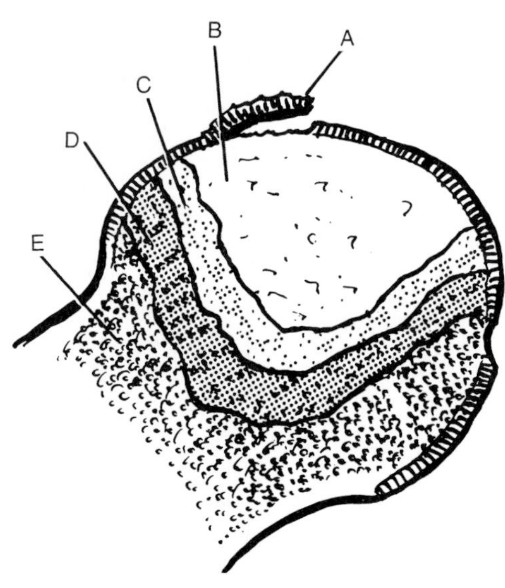

FIGURE 1-35 ■ Pathology of avascular necrosis. *A*, Articular cartilage. *B*, Necrotic bone. *C*, Reactive fibrous tissue. *D*, Hypertrophic bone. *E*, Normal trabeculae. (From Steinberg, M.E.: The Hip and Its Disorders, p. 630. Philadelphia, WB Saunders, 1991.)

(earliest positive study; highest sensitivity and specificity) and bone scanning are helpful for making an early diagnosis. Femoral head pressure measurement is possible but invasive. Pressure >30 mm Hg or increased by >10 mm Hg with injection of 5 mL of saline (stress test) is considered abnormal (but these values have varied widely from one investigation to another).

d. Treatment—Replacement arthroplasty of the hip is associated with increased loosening. Nontraumatic ON of the distal femoral condyle and proximal humerus may improve spontaneously without surgery. The precise role of core decompression remains unresolved, but results are best for early hip disease (Ficat stage I).

2. Osteochondroses—Can occur at traction apophyses in children and may or may not be associated with trauma, inflammation of the joint capsule, or vascular insult/secondary thrombosis. The pathology is similar to that described for ON in the adult. Table 1-18 shows the common osteochondroses. Most are discussed separately in the chapters covering the respective sites of disease.

Table 1-18. COMMON OSTEOCHONDROSES

DISORDER	SITE	AGE (YEARS)
Van Neck's disease	Ischipubic synchrondrosis	4-11
Legg-Calvé-Perthes disease	Femoral head	4-8
Osgood-Schlatter disease	Tibial tuberosity	11-15
Sinding-Larsen-Johansson syndrome	Inferior patella	10-14
Blount's disease (infant)	Proximal tibial epiphysis	1-3
Blount's disease (adolescent)	Proximal tibial epiphysis	8-15
Sever's disease	Calcaneus	9-11
Köhler's disease	Tarsal navicular	3-7
Freiberg's infarction	Metatarsal head	13-18
Scheuermann's disease	Discovertebral junction	13-17
Panner's disease	Capitellum of humerus	5-10
Thiemann's disease	Phalanges of hand	11-19
Kienböck's disease	Carpal lunate	20-40

SECTION 2

Joints

I. Articular Tissues

A. Cartilage—Types: **growth plate (physeal) cartilage** (previously discussed); **fibrocartilage** at tendon and ligament insertion into bone (and healing articular cartilage); **elastic cartilage** in tissues such as the trachea; **fibroelastic cartilage** makes up menisci; and **articular cartilage**, the focus of this section, which is critical to joint function. Articular cartilage decreases friction and distributes loads and is classically described as avascular, aneural, and alymphatic. Chondrocytes receive nutrients and oxygen from synovial fluid via diffusion through the cartilage matrix. The pH of cartilage is 7.4; changes in pH can disrupt cartilage structure. **Unlike mature articular cartilage, immature articular cartilage has a stem cell population.** Animal models (rabbit knee) suggest that autologous osteochondral progenitor cells can be isolated (from bone marrow) and grown in vitro, apparently without losing their ability to differentiate into cartilage or bone. They therefore may be clinically useful for repairing articular cartilage defects (and subchondral bone). Animal models (rabbit) also suggest that TGF-β can induce chondrogenesis in periosteal explants cultured in agarose gel.

1. Articular Cartilage Composition
   a. Water (65-80% of wet weight)—Shifts in and out of cartilage to allow deformation of cartilage surface in response to stress. Water is not distributed homogeneously (65% in deep zone, 80% at surface). Water content increases (90%) in osteoarthritis (Table 1-19). Water is also responsible for nutrition and lubrication. Increased water content leads to increased permeability, decreased strength, and decreased Young's modulus of elasticity.
   b. Collagen (10-20% of wet weight; >50% of dry weight) (Fig. 1-36)—Type II collagen accounts for approximately 90-95% of the total collagen content of articular cartilage and provides a cartilaginous framework and **tensile strength.** Increased amounts of glycine, proline, hydroxyproline, and hydrogen bonding are responsible for its unique characteristics. Hydroxyproline is unique to collagen and can be measured in the urine to assess bone turnover. Small amounts of types V, VI, IX, X, and XI collagen are present in the matrix of articular cartilage. An overview of all collagen types is shown in Table 1-20. Collagen type VI is a minor component of normal articular cartilage, but its content increases significantly in early osteoarthritis. **Collagen type X is produced only by hypertrophic chondrocytes during enchondral ossification (growth plate, fracture callus, HO formation, calcifying cartilaginous tumors) and is associated with calcification of cartilage; a genetic defect in type X collagen is responsible for Schmid's metaphyseal chondrodysplasia (affects the hypertrophic physeal zone). Collagen type XI is an adhesive holding the collagen lattice together.**

Table 1-19. BIOCHEMICAL CHANGES OF ARTICULAR CARTILAGE

	AGING	OSTEOARTHRITIS (OA)
Water content (hydration; permeability)	↓	↑
Collagen	Content remains relatively unchanged	Becomes disorderly (breakdown of matrix framework) Content ↓ in severe OA Relative concentration ↑ (due to loss of proteoglycans)
Proteoglycan content (concentration)	↓ (also the length of the protein core and GAG chains decreases)	↓
Proteoglycan synthesis		↑
Proteoglycan degradation	↓	↑↑↑
Chondroitin sulfate concentration (includes both chondroitin 4 and 6–sulfate)	↓	↑
Chondroitin 4–sulfate concentration	↓	↑
Keratin sulfate concentration	↑	↓
Chondrocyte size	↑	
Chondrocyte number	↓	
Modulus of elasticity	↑	↓

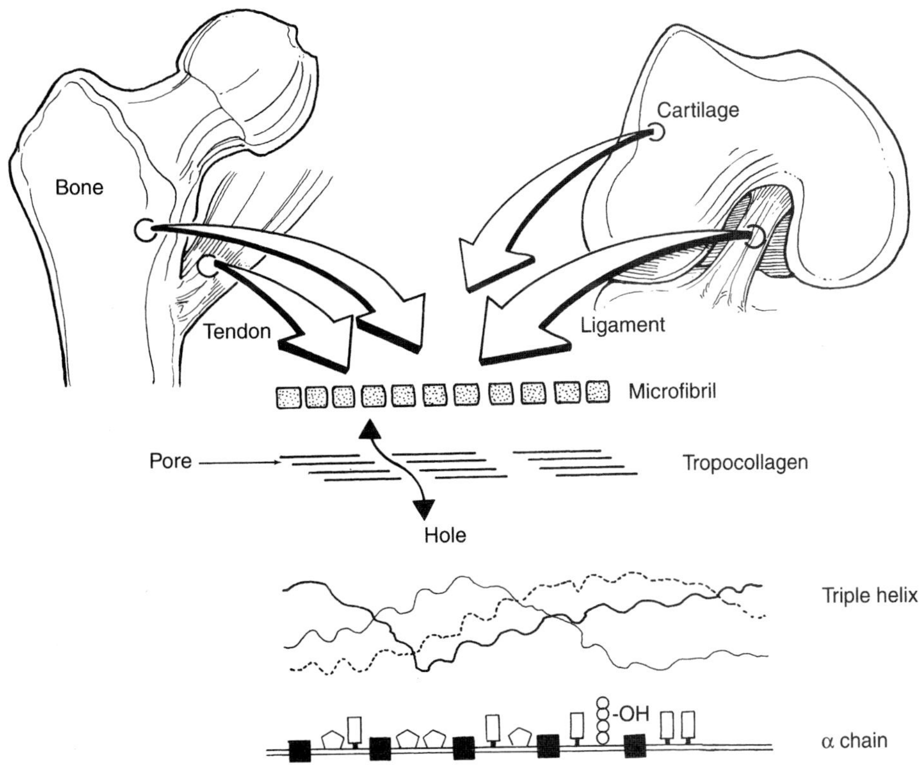

FIGURE 1-36 ■ Microstructure of collagen. Collagen is composed of microfibrils that are quarter-staggered arrangements of tropocollagen. Note hole and pore regions for mineral deposition (for calcification). Tropocollagen, in turn, is made up of a triple helix of α chains of polypeptides. (From Brinker, M.R., and Miller, M.D.: Fundamentals of Orthopaedics. Philadelphia, WB Saunders, 1999, p. 3.)

Table 1-20. TYPES OF COLLAGEN

TYPE	LOCATION
I	Bone Tendon Meniscus Annulus of intervertebral disc Skin
II	Articular cartilage Nucleus pulposus of intervertebral disc
III	Skin Blood vessels
IV	Basement membrane (basal lamina)
V	Articular cartilage (in small amounts)
VI	Articular cartilage (in small amounts) Tethers the chondrocyte to its pericellular matrix
VII	Basement membrane (epithelial)
VIII	Basement membrane (epithelial)
IX	Articular cartilage (in small amounts)
X	Hypertrophic cartilage Associated with calcification of cartilage (matrix mineralization)
XI	Articular cartilage (in small amounts) (acts as an adhesive)
XII	Tendon
XIII	Endothelial cells

c. Proteoglycans (10-15% of wet weight)—Protein polysaccharides provide **compressive strength**. Proteoglycans are produced by chondrocytes, are secreted into the extracellular matrix, and are composed of subunits known as **glycosaminoglycans** (GAGs, disaccharide polymers). **These GAGs include two subtypes of chondroitin sulfate (the most prevalent GAG in cartilage) and keratin sulfate. The concentration of chondroitin-4-sulfate decreases with age, that of chondroitin-6-sulfate remains essentially constant, and that of keratin sulfate increases with age.** GAGs are bound to a protein core by **sugar bonds** to form a proteoglycan aggrecan molecule. **Link proteins** stabilize these aggrecan molecules to hyaluronic acid to form a proteoglycan aggregate. Proteoglycans have a half-life of 3 months, produce cartilage's porous structure, and trap and hold water **(regulate and retain fluid in the matrix)**. Figure 1-37 illustrates a proteoglycan aggregate and an aggrecan molecule.

d. Chondrocytes (5% of wet weight)—Active in protein synthesis, possess a double effusion

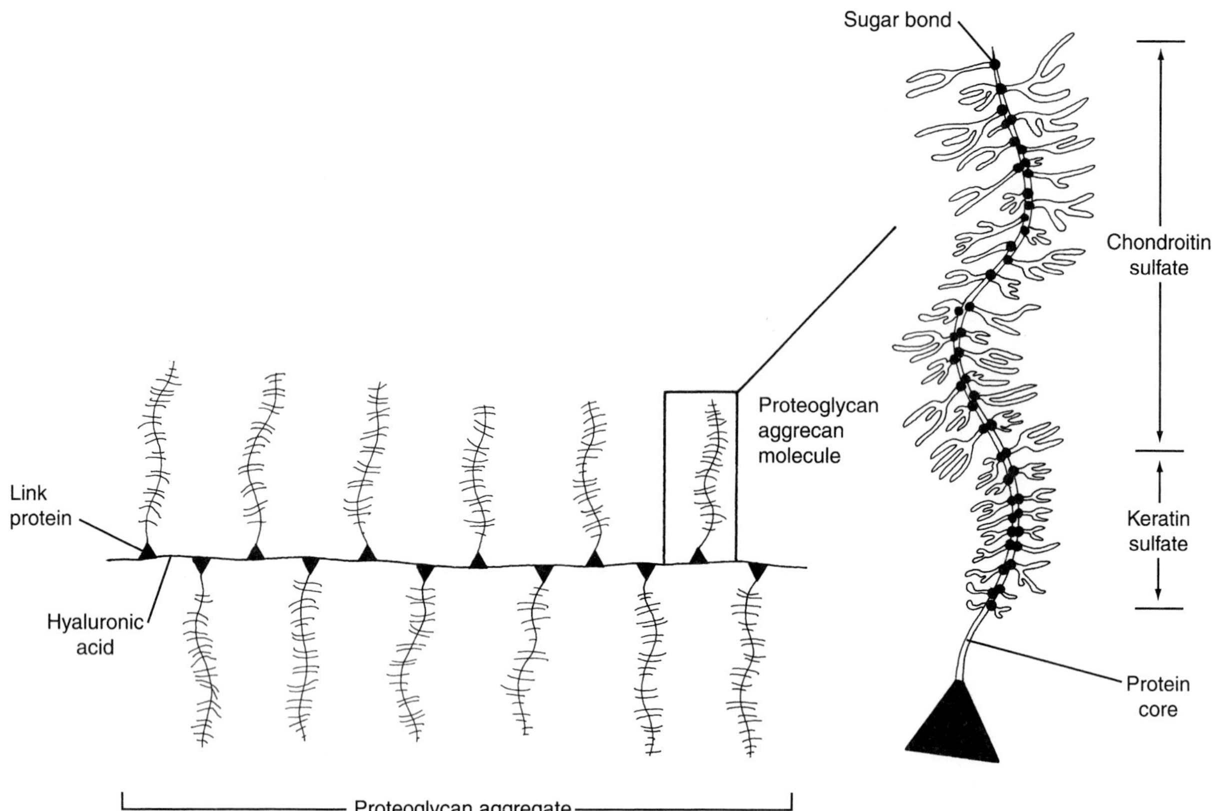

FIGURE 1-37 ■ Proteoglycan aggregate and aggrecan molecule. (From Brinker, M.R., and Miller, M.D.: Fundamentals of Orthopaedics. Philadelphia, WB Saunders, 1999, p. 9.)

barrier; produce collagen, proteoglycans, and some enzymes for cartilage metabolism; least active in the calcified zone. Deeper cartilage zones have chondrocytes with decreased rough endoplasmic reticulum (RER) and increased intraplasmic filaments (degenerative products). Chondroblasts, derived from undifferentiated mesenchymal cells (stimulated by motion), are later trapped in lacunae to become chondrocytes.

e. Other Matrix Components
   (1) Adhesives (fibronectin, chondronectin, anchorin CII)—Involved in interactions between chondrocytes and fibrils. Fibronectin may be associated with osteoarthritis.
   (2) Lipids—Unknown function.

2. Articular Cartilage Layers—The various layers of articular cartilage are described in Table 1-21 and are illustrated in Figure 1-38. **The tangential zone has a high concentration of collagen fibers** arranged at right angles to each other (parallel to the articular surface). The calcified zone forms a transitional region of intermediate stiffness between articular cartilage and subchondral bone. The superficial zone has the greatest tensile stiffness. The deeper zones have increased chondrocyte volume; collagen fibers are oriented perpendicular to the joint surface.
3. Articular Cartilage Metabolism
   a. Collagen Synthesis—Figure 1-39 shows the events and sites involved in collagen synthesis.

Table 1-21. ARTICULAR CARTILAGE LAYERS

LAYER	WIDTH (μM)	CHARACTERISTIC	ORIENTATION	FUNCTION
Gliding zone (superficial)	40	↓ Metabolic activity	Tangential	vs. Shear
Transitional zone (middle)	500	↑ Metabolic activity	Oblique	vs.Compression
Radial zone (deep)	1000	↑ Collagen size	Vertical	vs.Compression
Tidemark	5	Undulating barrier	Tangential	vs. Shear
Calcified zone	300	Hydroxyapatite crystals		Anchor

↑, increased; ↓, decreased.

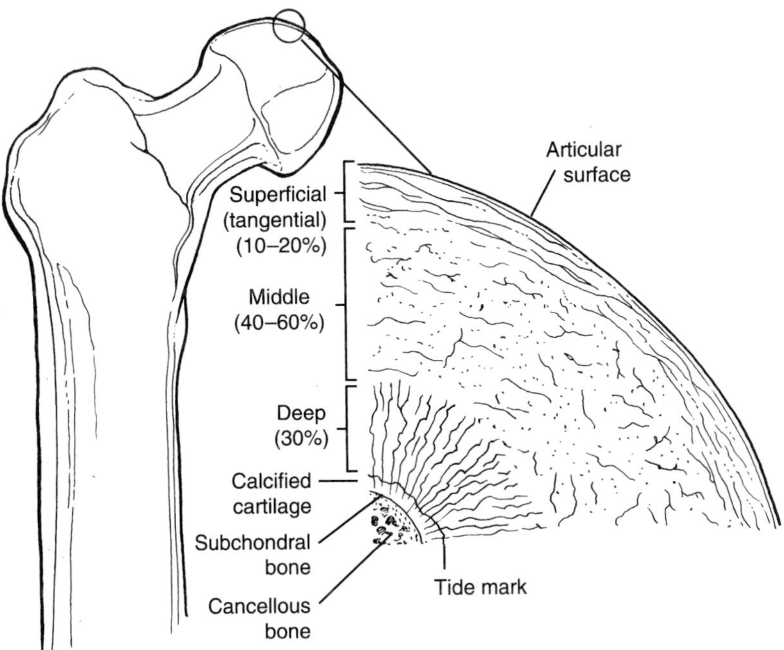

FIGURE 1-38 ■ Articular cartilage layers. (From Brinker, M.R., and Miller, M.D.: Fundamentals of Orthopaedics. Philadelphia, WB Saunders, 1999, p. 9.)

b. Collagen Catabolism—Little is known of the exact mechanism. Enzymatic processes have been proposed that involve metalloproteinase collagenase cleaving the triple helix. Mechanical factors may also play a role.
c. Proteoglycan Synthesis (Fig. 1-40)—A series of molecular events beginning with proteoglycan gene expression and transcription of messenger RNA and concluding with proteoglycan aggregate formation in the extracellular matrix.
d. Proteoglycan Catabolism (Fig. 1-41)

4. Articular Cartilage Growth Factors—Regulate cartilage synthesis; may have a role in osteoarthritis.
   a. PDGF—May affect healing of cartilage lacerations (and perhaps osteoarthritis).
   b. TGF-β—**Stimulates proteoglycan synthesis while suppressing synthesis of**

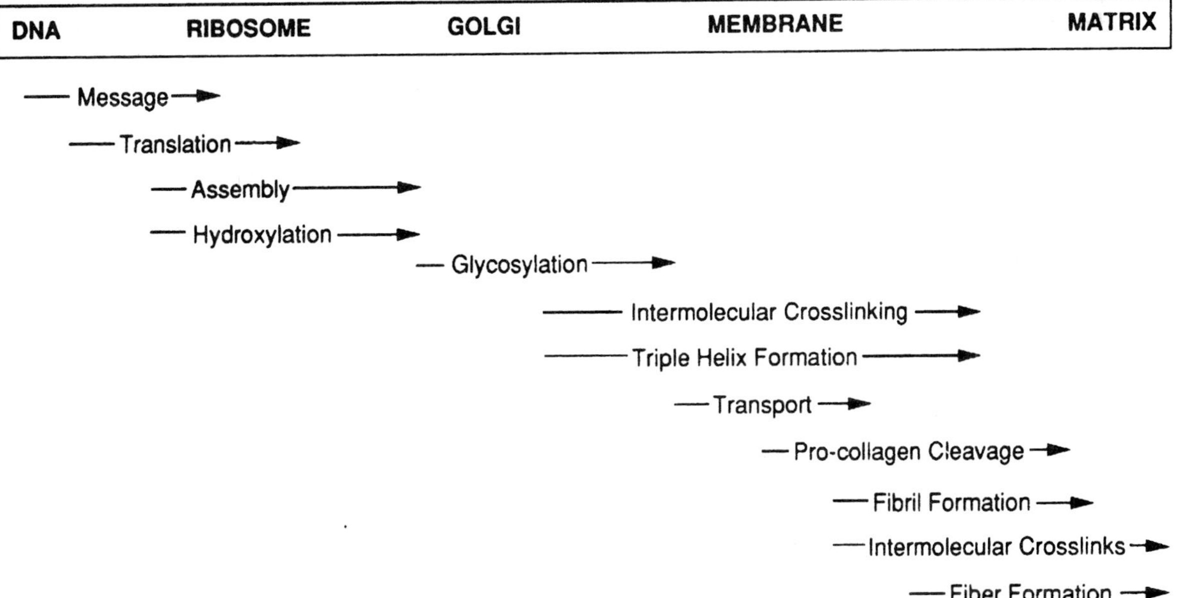

FIGURE 1-39 ■ Collagen synthesis is accomplished at various intracellular sites. (From Mankin, H.J., and Brandt, K.D.: Biochemistry and metabolism of articular cartilage in osteoarthritis. In Moskowitz, R.W., Howell, D.S., Goldberg, V.M., et al., eds.: Osteoarthritis: Diagnosis and Medical/Surgical Management, 2nd ed., p. 124. Philadelphia, WB Saunders, 1992.)

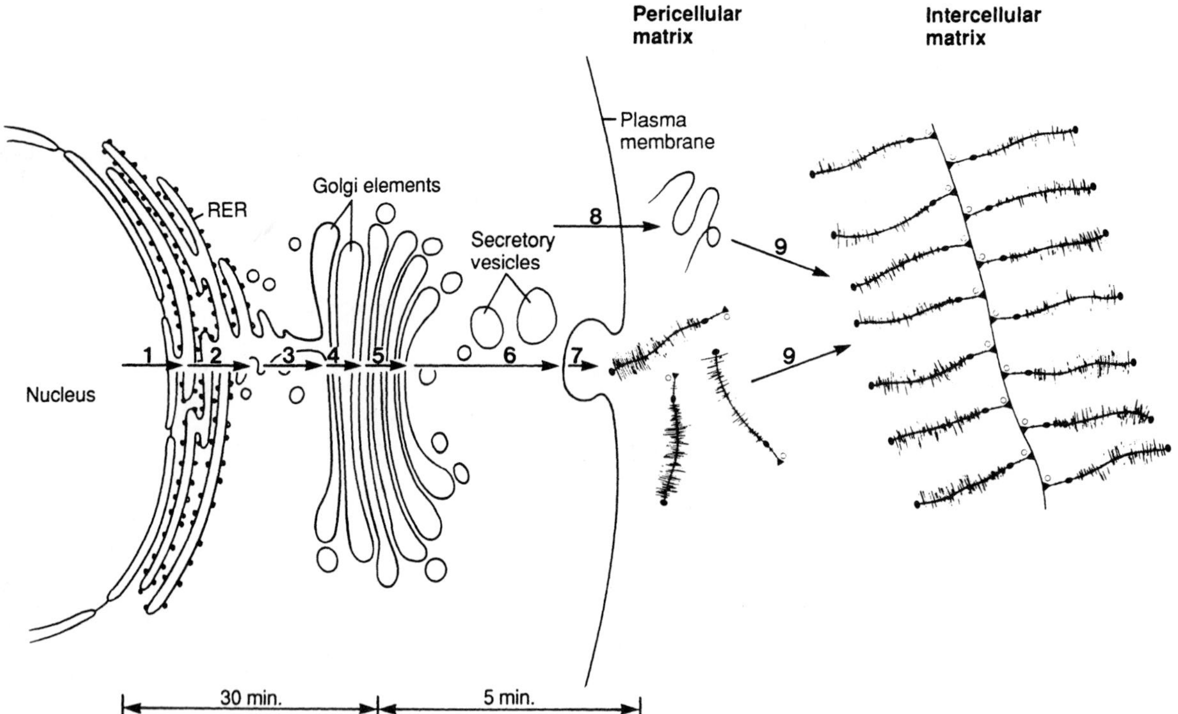

FIGURE 1-40 ■ Synthesis and secretion of proteoglycan aggrecan molecules and link protein by a chondrocyte. *1,* Transcription of aggrecan and link protein genes to mRNA. *2,* Translation of mRNA to form protein core. *3,* Transportation. *4, 5, cis* and medial *trans* Golgi compartments, respectively, where glycosaminoglycan chains are added to the protein core. *6,* Transportation to the secretory vesicles. *7,* Release into the extracellular matrix. *8, 9,* Hyaluronate from the plasma membrane binds with the aggrecan and link proteins to form aggregates in the extracellular matrix. RER, rough endoplasmic reticulum. (From Simon, S.R., ed.: Orthopaedic Basic Science, 2nd ed., p. 13. Rosemont, IL, American Academy of Orthopaedic Surgeons, 1994.)

type II collagen. Stimulates the formation of plasminogen activator inhibitor-1 and tissue inhibitor of metalloproteinase (TIMP), which prevent the degradative action of plasmin and stromelysin.

c. Fibroblast Growth Factor (Basic) (b-FGF)—Stimulates DNA synthesis in adult articular chondrocytes; may affect cartilage repair.

d. Insulin-Like Growth Factor-I (IGF-I)—Previously known as somatomedin C. Stimulates DNA and cartilage matrix synthesis in adult articular cartilage and immature cartilage of the growth plate.

5. Lubrication and Wear Mechanisms of Articular Cartilage (Figs. 1-42 to 1-44)

a. General Comments—The primary mechanism responsible for lubrication of articular cartilage (low coefficient of friction) during dynamic function is **elastohydrodynamic lubrication.** The coefficient of friction for human joints (such as the knee and hip) varies from 0.002-0.04. Factors decreasing the coefficient of friction of articular cartilage include fluid film formation, elastic deformation of articular cartilage, synovial fluid, and efflux of fluid from the cartilage. An example of a factor that increases the coefficient of friction is fibrillation of articular cartilage. Almost all joints, during ROM, undergo both rolling and sliding (for more information, see Section 8, Biomaterials and Biomechanics).

b. Specific Types of Lubrication (see Figs. 1-42 and 1-43)

(1) **Elastohydrodynamic Lubrication—The predominant mechanism during dynamic joint function.** Deformation of articular surfaces and thin films of joint lubricants separate the surfaces (the coefficient of friction is primarily a function of lubricant properties, not the surfaces). Coefficient of friction is generally low.

(2) **Boundary Lubrication** (Slippery Surfaces)—The bearing surface is largely nondeformable, and therefore the lubricant only partially separates the surfaces.

(3) **Boosted Lubrication** (Fluid Entrapment)—Describes the concentration of lubricating fluid in pools trapped by regions of bearing surfaces that are making contact. The coefficient of friction is generally higher for boosted than elastohydrodynamic lubrication.

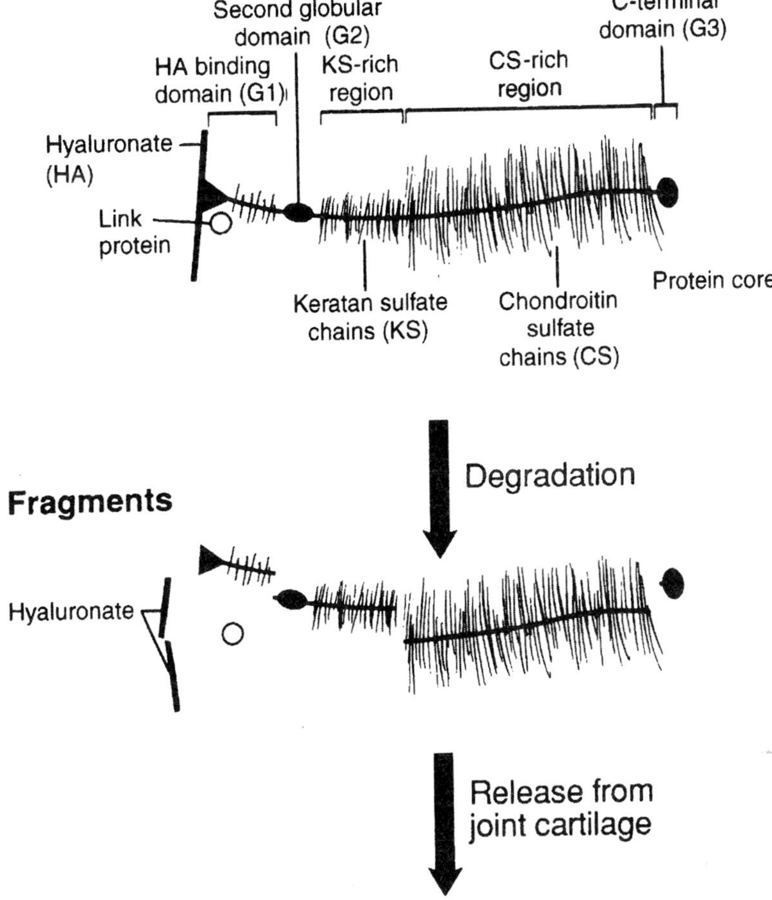

FIGURE 1-41 ■ Proteoglycan degradation in articular cartilage. Cleavage of the G1 and G2 domains make the fragments nonaggregating. (Modified from Simon, S.R., ed.: Orthopaedic Basic Science, 2nd ed., p. 14. Rosemont, IL, American Academy of Orthopaedic Surgeons, 1994.)

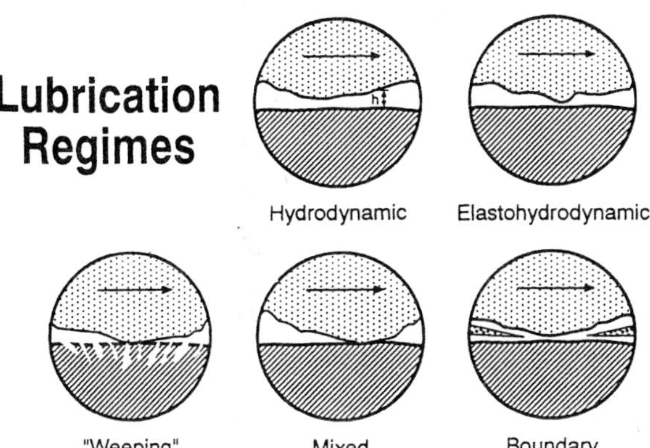

FIGURE 1-42 ■ Types of lubrication. (From Simon, S.R., ed.: Orthopaedic Basic Science, 2nd ed., p. 465. Rosemont, IL, American Academy of Orthopaedic Surgeons, 1994.)

(4) **Hydrodynamic Lubrication**—Fluid separates the surfaces under load.

(5) **Weeping Lubrication**—Fluid shifts to loaded areas.

6. Articular Cartilage Aging (and Other Special Circumstances) (see Table 1-19)—With aging, chondrocytes become larger, acquire increased lysosomal enzymes and no longer reproduce (so cartilage becomes relatively **hypocellular**). **Cartilage increases stiffness and decreases solubility with aging.** Also, cartilage proteoglycans decrease in mass and size (decreased length of the chondroitin sulfate chains) and change in proportion (decreased concentration of chondroitin sulfate and **increased concentration of keratin sulfate**). Protein content increases with aging and **water content decreases;** these changes decrease cartilage elasticity. Moderate joint impact (without a fracture) decreases proteoglycan concentration and increases tissue hydration.

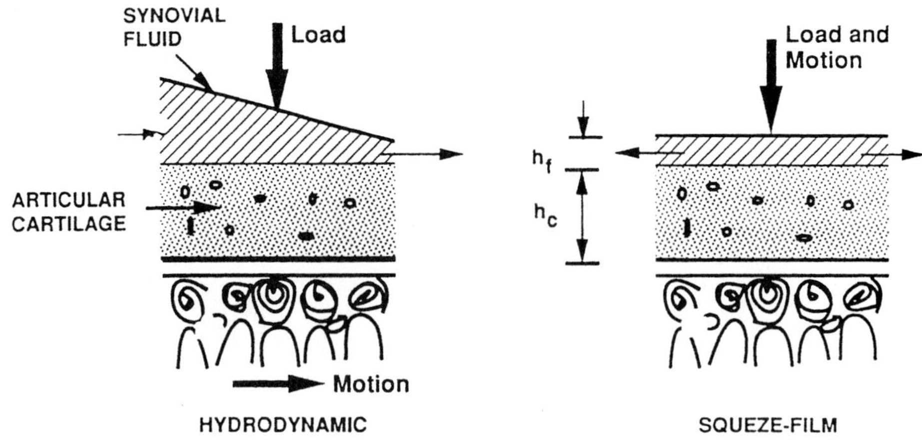

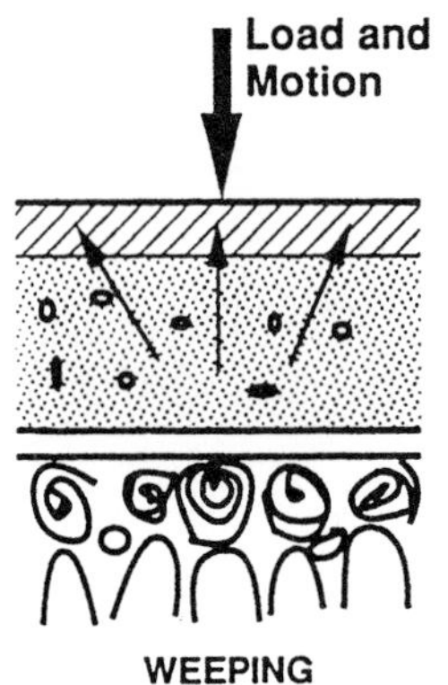

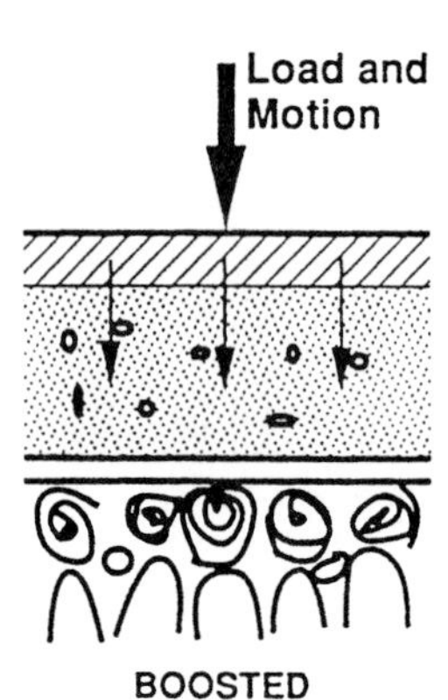

FIGURE 1-43 ■ Fluid film lubrication models include Hydrodynamic, Squeeze-Film, Weeping, and Boosted. (From Mow, V.C., and Soslowsky, L.J.: Friction, lubrication, and wear of diarthrodial joints. In Basic Orthopaedic Biomechanics, Mow, V.C., and Hayes, W.C., eds., pp. 245–292. New York, Raven Press, 1991.)

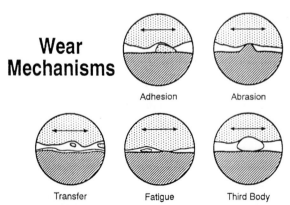

7. Articular Cartilage Healing—**Deep lacerations** extending below the tidemark that penetrate the underlying subchondral bone may heal with fibrocartilage. **The fibrocartilage is produced by undifferentiated marrow mesenchymal stem cells** that differentiate into cells capable of producing fibrocartilage (this is the theory behind abrasion chondroplasty); an abundance of type I collagen is typical at 1 year following injury. Remember, fibrocartilage is not as durable as hyaline cartilage. Blunt trauma may induce changes in cartilage similar to those seen with osteoarthritis. **Superficial articular cartilage lacerations** that do not cross the tidemark cause chondrocytes to proliferate but **do not heal because cartilage is avascular**. Continuous passive motion is believed to benefit cartilage healing; joint immobilization leads to atrophy or cartilage degeneration. In animal models, 4 weeks of joint disuse (knee immobilization) decreases the ratio of proteoglycan to collagen, which returns to normal after 8 weeks of joint mobilization. Joint instability (transection of the anterior cruciate ligament [ACL]) initially decreases the ratio of proteoglycan to collagen (at 4 weeks), but later (12 weeks) elevates the ratio of proteoglycan to collagen and increases hydration. Joint instability markedly decreases hyaluronan, whereas joint disuse does not.

B. Synovium—Synovium mediates the nutrient exchange between blood and joint (synovial) fluid. Synovial tissue is composed of vascularized connective tissue that lacks a basement membrane. Two cell types are present: **type A**, important in **phagocytosis**; and **type B (fibroblast-like cells)**,

Wear Mechanisms

Adhesion

Abrasion

Transfer

Fatigue

Third Body

FIGURE 1-44 ■ Wear mechanisms. (From Simon, S.R., ed.: Orthopaedic Basic Science, 2nd ed., p. 466. Rosemont, IL, American Academy of Orthopaedic Surgeons, 1994.)

which produce synovial fluid (broth). Other undifferentiated cells have a reparative role. A third type of cell, type C, may exist as an intermediate cell type. **Synovial fluid** consists of hyaluronic acid, lubricin (a lubricating glycoprotein), proteinase, collagenases, and prostaglandins. Synovial fluid is an ultrafiltrate (dialysate) of blood plasma added to fluid produced by the synovial membrane; it contains no RBCs, clotting factors, or hemoglobin. It **lubricates articular cartilage and provides nourishment through diffusion. Synovial fluid exhibits non-newtonian flow characteristics** (the viscosity coefficient μ is not a constant; the fluid is not linearly viscous); its **viscosity increases as the shear rate decreases. Lubricin, a glycoprotein,** is the key lubricating component. **Hyaluronan molecules** in the knee become entangled and behave like an elastic solid during high-strain activities (running, jumping). Analysis of synovial fluid in disease processes is important and is discussed later in this section under arthroses.

C. Meniscus—Deepens the articular surface of a variety of synovial joints (acromioclavicular [AC], sternoclavicular [SC], glenohumeral, hip, knee), broadening the contact area and distributing the load such as on the tibial plateau. Meniscus is more elastic and less permeable than articular cartilage. The meniscus of the knee is the focus of this section. **Three years after total meniscectomy of the knee, 20% of patients have significant arthritic lesions and 70% have radiographic changes; all experience arthrosis by 20 years. The severity of degenerative changes is proportional to the amount of meniscus excised.**

1. Anatomy (Knee Meniscus)—Triangular semilunar structure. Peripheral border is attached to the joint capsule. Medial meniscus is semicircular; lateral meniscus is circular.
2. Histology—Meniscus is composed of **fibroelastic cartilage** (Fig. 1-45), with an interlacing network of collagen fibers, proteoglycans, glycoproteins, and cellular elements (Table 1-22).

Table 1-22. HISTOLOGIC FEATURES OF MENISCUS

EXTRACELLULAR MATRIX
- Collagen—**primarily type I collagen** (55-65% of dry weight)
- Also types II, III, V, and VI (5-10% of dry weight)
  - ***Superficial layer***—mesh-like fibers oriented primarily radially
  - ***Surface layer***—(deep to superficial layer) irregularly aligned collagen bundles
  - ***Middle layer***—(deep) parallel circumferential fibers
- Elastin (0.6% of dry weight)
- Proteoglycans, Glycoproteins } (1-3% of dry weight)
- Adhesive glycoproteins (fibronectin, thrombospondin)

CELLULAR COMPONENTS—Synthesize and maintain extracellular matrix
—anaerobic metabolism (few mitochondria)

- Chondrocytes, Fibroblasts } **Fibrochondrocytes:**
  - *Fusiform cells*
    - Found in superficial layer
    - Resemble fibroblasts and chondrocytes
    - Found in lacunae
    - Contain abundant endoplasmic reticulum (ER) and Golgi
  - *Ovoid cells*
    - Found in surface and middle layer
    - Contain abundant ER and Golgi

3. Innervation and Blood Supply (Knee Meniscus)—The peripheral two thirds is innervated by type I and type II nerve endings (concentrated in the anterior and posterior horns; few fibers are found in the meniscal body). **Blood supply is from the geniculate arteries.** Vessels branch circumferentially to form a plexus supplying the **peripheral 25% of the meniscus;** the remaining meniscus receives nutrition via diffusion. Peripheral meniscal tears in the vascularized region ("red zone") can heal via fibrovascular scar formation; more central

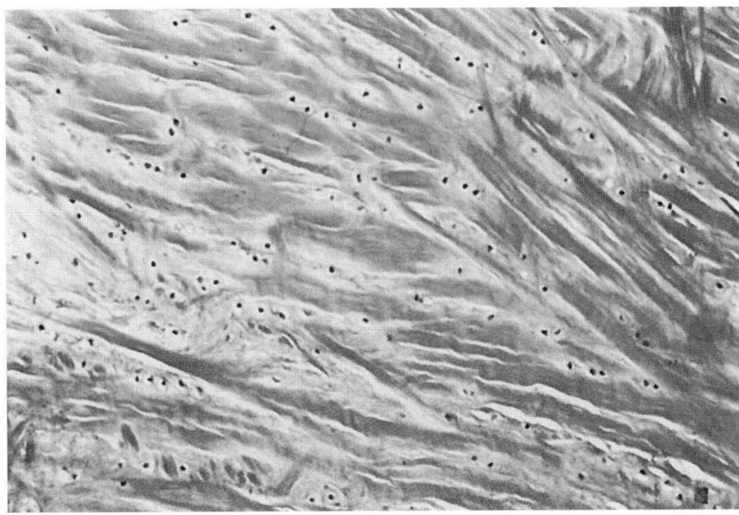

FIGURE 1-45 ■ Histology of menisci.

tears in the avascular region ("white zone") cannot. **The cell responsible for meniscal healing is the fibrochondrocyte. Peripheral meniscal tears with a rim width <4 mm have the best healing characteristics.**

II. Arthroses

A. Introduction—Arthroses may be classified into four basic groups based on their common characteristics (Table 1-23).

1. **Noninflammatory Arthritides**—Include osteoarthritis, neuropathic arthropathy, acute rheumatic fever, and a variety of other entities (ON, osteochondritis dissecans, osteochondromatosis).
2. **Inflammatory Arthritides**—Include many rheumatologic disorders: rheumatoid arthritis, systemic lupus erythematosus, the spondyloarthropathies, and crystalline arthropathies. These disorders may be associated with a human leukocyte antigen (HLA) complex region.
3. **Infectious Arthritides**—Include pyogenic arthritis, tuberculous arthritis, fungal arthritis, and Lyme disease.
4. **Hemorrhagic Arthritides**—Include hemophilic arthropathy, sickle cell joint destruction, and pigmented villonodular synovitis.

B. Joint Fluid Analysis (Table 1-24)

1. Noninflammatory Arthritides—200 white blood cells (WBCs) with 25% polymorphonuclear neutrophil leukocytes (PMNs); glucose and protein equal serum values; normal viscosity (high), straw color, firm mucin clot.
2. Inflammatory Arthritides—2000-75,000 WBCs with up to 50% PMNs; moderately decreased glucose (25 mg/dL lower than serum glucose); low viscosity, yellow-green, friable mucin clot. Synovial fluid complement is decreased in rheumatoid arthritis and normal in ankylosing spondylitis.
3. Infectious Arthritides—More than 80,000 WBCs with more than 75% PMNs, a positive Gram stain (also positive cultures later), low glucose (25 mg/dL lower than serum glucose), opaque fluid, increased synovial lactate.

C. Noninflammatory Arthritides

1. Osteoarthritis (Degenerative Joint Disease) (see Table 1-23)—**Most common form** of arthritis, but little is known about this disease.

Table 1-23. COMPARISON OF COMMON ARTHRITIDES

ARTHRITIS	AGE	SEX	SYM?	JOINTS	PHYSICAL EXAM
Noninflammatory					
Osteoarthritis	Old	M > F	Asym	Hip, knee, CMC	↓ ROM, crepitus
Neuropathic	Old	M > F	Asym	Foot, ankle, LE	Effusion, unstable
ARF	Child	M = F	Asym	Mig; lg joints	Red tender joint, rash
Ochronosis	Adult	M = F	Asym	Lg joints/spine	↓ ROM, locking
Inflammatory					
Rheumatoid	Young	F > M	Sym	Hands, feet	Ulnar dev, claw toes
SLE	Young	F > M	Sym	PIP, MCP, knee	Red swollen joint, rash
JRA	Child	F > M	Sym	Knee, multiple	Swollen joint, normal color
Relapsing polychondritis	Old	M = F	Sym	All joints	Eye, ear involved
Spondylorthropathies					
AS	Young	M > F	Sym	SI, spine, hip	Rigid spine, "chin on chest"
Reiter's syndrome	Young	M > F	Asym	Wt-bearing	Urethral D/C, conjunctivitis
Psoriatic	Young	M = F	Asym	DIP, small joints	Rash, sausage digit, pitting
Entereopathic	Young	M > F	Asym	Wt-bearing	Synovitis, GI manifestations
Crystal Deposition Disease					
Gout	Young	M > F	Asym	Great toe, LE	Tophi, red, swollen
Chondrocalcinosis	Old	M = F	Asym	Knee, LE	Acute swelling
Infectious					
Pyogenic	Any	M = F	Asym	Any joint	Red, hot, swollen
Tuberculous	Old	M > F	Asym	Spine, LE	Indolent, swelling
Lyme disease	Young	M = F	Asym	Any joint	Acute effusion
Fungal	Any	M > F	Asym	Any joint	Indolent
Hemorrhagic					
Hemophilia	Young	M	Asym	Knee, UE (elbow, shoulder)	↓ ROM, swelling
Sickle cell	Young	M = F	Asym	Hip, any bone	Pain, ↓ ROM
PVNS	Young	M = F	Asym	Knee, LE	Pain, synovitis

ARF, acute rheumatic fever; SLE, systemic lupus erythematosus; JRA, juvenile rheumatoid arthritis; AS, ankylosing spondylitis; PVNS, pigmented villonodular synovitis; Asym, asymmetric; Sym, symmetric; CMC, carpometacarpal; LE, lower extremity; Mig, migratory; Lg, large; PIP, proximal interphalangeal; MCP, metacarpophalangeal; SI, sacroiliac; DIP, distal interphalangeal; UE, upper extremity; ↓ROM, decreased range of motion; D/C, discharge; GI, gastrointestinal; ASO, antistreptolysin O; ESR, erythrocyte sedimentation rate; CRP, C-reactive protein; RF, rheumatoid factor; ANA, antinuclear antibody; alk. Phos, alkaline phosphatase; CPK, creatine phosphokinase; HLA, human leukocyte antigen; Birefr., birefringent; WBC, white blood cells; PPD, purified protein derivative; AFB, acid fast bacilli; ELISA, enzyme linked immunosorbent assay; PTT, partial thromboplastin time; resorp., resorption; arth, arthritis; MT, metatarsal; DIP, distal interphalangeal; Art, articular; fibrocart, fibrocartilage; Eryth. marg., erythema marginatum; Pericard., pericardial; Pulm, pulmonary; Eryth., erythema; ECM, erythema chronicum migrans; Neuro., neurologic; NSAID, nonsteroidal anti-inflammatory drug; TJA, total joint arthroplasty; TX, treat/treatment; reconstr. surg., reconstructive surgery; RA, rheumatoid arthritis; ASA, acetylsalicylic acid; PT, physical therapy; I&D, incise and drain; IV, intravenous; 5-FU, 5-flucytosine.

Table 1-23. COMPARISON OF COMMON ARTHRITIDES—CONT'D

LAB TESTS	RADIOGRAPHY	SYSTEMIC	TREATMENT
Nonspecific	Asym. narrowing, eburnation, cysts, osteophytes	None	NSAID, arthrodesis, osteotomy, TJA
For underlying disease	Destruction/heterotopic bone	None	Brace, TJA contraindicated
ASO titer	Usually normal	Eryth. marg. nodules, carditis	Symptomatic
Urine homogentisic acid	Destruction, disc calcification	Spondylosis	Supportive
ESR, CRP, RF	Sym. narrow, periart. resorp.	Pericard. & pulm. disease	Pyramid Tx. synovitis, reconstr. surg.
ANA	Less destruction	Cardiac, renal, pancytopenia	Drug therapy like RA
RF/ANA	Juxta-art. late, osteopenia	Iridocyclitis, rash	ASA; 75% remission
ESR	Normal	Ear, cardiac	Supportive, dapsone?
ESR, alk; phos., CPK, HLA-B27	SI arth., bamboo spine	Uveitis	PT, NSAID, osteotomy
ESR, WBC, HLA-B27	MT head erosion, periostis	Urethritis, conjunctivitis, ulcer	PT, NSAID, sulfa?
ESR, HLA-B27	DIP—pencil in cup	Rash, conjunctivitis	Drug therapy as for RA
ESR, HLA-B27	Normal	Eryth. nodosum, pyoderma	Tx bowel disease, symptomatic
Uric acid; – Birefr. crystals	Soft tissue swell, erosions	Tophi, renal stones	Colchicine, indomethacin
+ Birefr. rod-shaped crystals	Art, fibrocart. calcified	Ochronosis, hyperparathyroidism, hypothyroidism	Symptomatic, avoid surgery
WBC, ESR, bacteria	Joint narrowing (late)	Fever, chills, infection	I&D, IV antibiotics
PPD, AFB, cultures	Both sides, cysts	Lung, multiorgan	Antibiotics ± I&D
Culture, ELISA	Usually normal	ECM rash, neuro., cardiac	Penicillin, tetracycline
Special studies/cultures	Minimal changes	Immunocompromised	5-FU, amphotericin
PTT, factor VIII	Squared-off patella	Soft tissue bleeding	Support, synovectomy, TJA (unless + inhibitor)
Sickle prep.	Osteonecrosis	Infarcts, osteonecrosis	
Aspirate, biopsy	Juxtacortical erosion	None	Surgical excision

a. Etiology—On a cellular level, osteoarthritis (OA) may be a result of a failed attempt of chondrocytes to repair damaged cartilage. Osteoarthritic cartilage is characterized by **increased water content** (in contrast to the decreased water content seen with aging) (see Table 1-19), **alterations in proteoglycans** (shorter chains and increased chondroitin/keratin sulfate ratio), **collagen abnormalities** (disrupted by collagenase), and **binding of proteoglycans to hyaluronic acid** (caused by proteolytic enzymes from increased prostaglandin E [PGE] and decreased link proteins). Cathepsins B and D levels and **metalloproteinases** (collagenase, gelatinase, stromelysin) **increase in OA cartilage. IL-1** enhances enzyme synthesis and may have a **catabolic effect** leading to cartilage degeneration; GAGs and polysulfuric acid may have a protective effect. **Biochemical changes seen in articular cartilage with aging and osteoarthritis are compared in Table 1-19.** Figure 1-46 shows the enzymatic cascade involved in articular cartilage degradation. Cartilage degeneration is encouraged by shear stress and is prevented with normal compressive forces. Excessive stresses and inadequate chondrocyte response lead to degeneration. Genetic predisposition may be important in OA. **Postmenopausal arthritis of the medial clavicle** seen on the dominant extremity side in elderly women is not

Table 1-24. JOINT FLUID ANALYSIS

TYPES OF ARTHRITIS	WHITE BLOOD CELLS (/mm³)	POLYMORPHONUCLEAR LEUKOCYTES (%)	OTHER CHARACTERISTICS
Noninflammatory	200	25	Joint aspirate glucose and protein equal to serum values
Inflammatory	2000-75,000	50	↓ Joint aspirate glucose
Infectious	>80,000	>75	Thick cloudy fluid + Gram's stain + Cultures ↓ Joint aspirate glucose, ↑ joint aspirate protein

From Brinker, M.R., and Miller, M.D.: Fundamentals of Orthopaedics. Philadelphia, WB Saunders, 1999, p. 26.

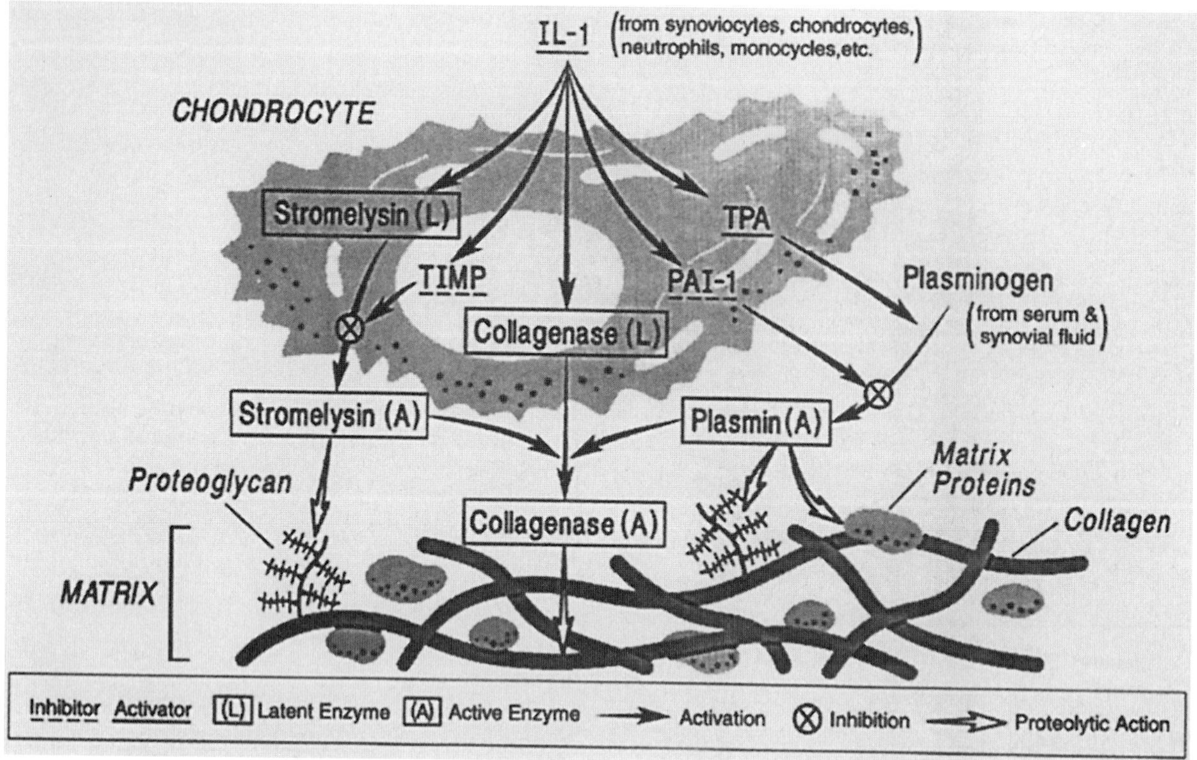

FIGURE 1-46 ■ Enzyme cascade of interleukin-1-stimulated degradation of articular cartilage. (From Simon, S.R., ed.: Orthopaedic Basic Science, 2nd ed., p. 40. Rosemont, IL, American Academy of Orthopaedic Surgeons, 1994.)

associated with any systemic arthritis; treatment is with NSAIDs. **Rapidly destructive OA** occurs most commonly in the hip and may mimic septic arthritis, rheumatoid arthritis, seronegative arthritis, neuropathic arthritis, or ON. In the hip, the femoral head may be so flattened that appears to have been "sheared off."

b. General Characteristics—OA can be primary (intrinsic defect) or secondary (trauma, infection, congenital). Changes that occur in OA begin with deterioration and loss of the bearing surface, followed by osteophyte development and osteochondral junction breakdown. Later, cartilage disintegration and subchondral microfractures expose the bony surface. **Subchondral cysts** (which arise secondary to microfracture and may contain an amorphous gelatinous material) and **osteophytes,** which are part of this process, along with **"joint space narrowing"** and eburnation of bone are demonstrated on radiographs. Microscopic changes include loss of superficial chondrocytes, **chondrocyte cloning** (>1 chondrocyte per lacuna), replication and breakdown of the tidemark, fissuring, cartilage destruction with eburnation of subchondral "pagetoid" bone, and other changes (Figs. 1-47, 1-48). Physical examination findings include decreased ROM and crepitus. **The knee is the most common joint affected in OA.** Treatment begins with supportive measures (e.g., activity modification, cane) and includes NSAIDs (misoprostol [Cytotec] may lower GI complications via a prostaglandin effect). Surgical procedures ranging from arthroscopic débridement to total joint arthroplasties (TJAs) may be useful in advanced cases that are resistant to nonoperative treatment.

c. Radiographic Characteristics—Osteophytes, "joint space" narrowing, subchondral cysts (from microfractures/bone repair) on both sides of the joint, and subchondral sclerosis are typical. Tomograms or CT scans are best at showing these OA-related changes.
   (1) Hand—Distal interphalangeal (DIP), proximal interphalangeal (PIP), and carpometacarpal (CMC) joints
   (2) Hip—Superolateral involvement
   (3) Knee—Asymmetric involvement

2. Neuropathic Arthropathy (Charcot Joint Disease) (see Table 1-23 and Fig. 1-49)—An extreme form of OA caused by disturbed sensory innervation. Causes include diabetes (foot), tabes dorsalis (lower extremity), **syringomyelia (the most common cause of upper-extremity neuropathic arthropathy** [most common in the shoulder and

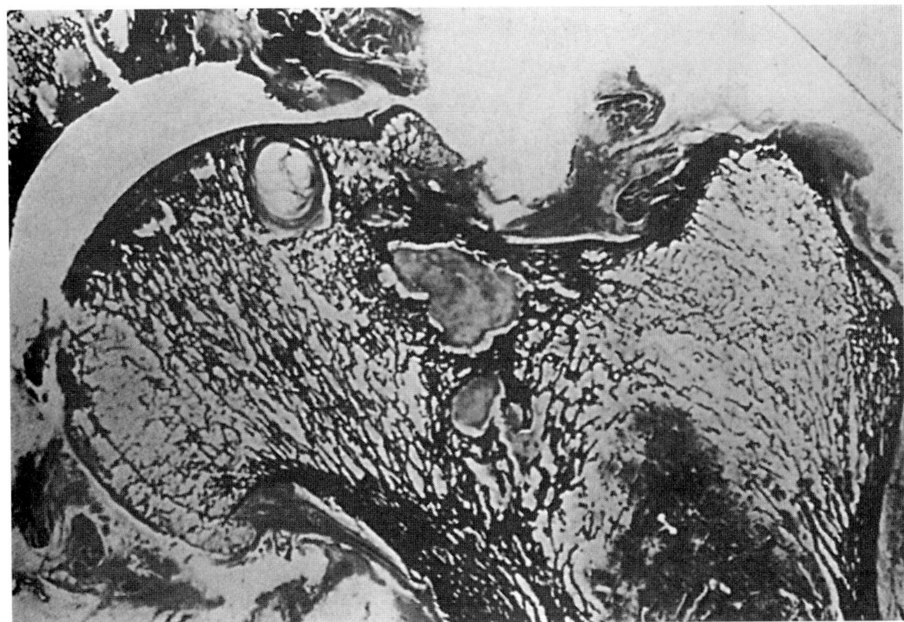

FIGURE 1-47 ■ Macro section of an osteoarthric human femoral head demonstrating subarticular cysts, sclerotic bone formation, and an inferior femoral head osteophyte. (From Simon, S.R., ed.: Orthopaedic Basic Science, 2nd ed., p. 35. Rosemont, IL, American Academy of Orthopaedic Surgeons, 1994.)

elbow]), Hansen's disease (the second most common cause of upper-extremity neuropathic arthropathy), myelomeningocele (ankle and foot), congenital insensitivity to pain (ankle and foot), and other neurologic problems (such as spinal cord injury). A Charcot joint develops in 25% of patients with syringomyelia (80% involve the upper extremity). Typically seen in an older patient with an unstable, painless, swollen joint, who may experience a hemarthrosis. Radiographs show advanced (severe) destructive changes on both sides of the joint, scattered "chunks" of bone embedded in fibrous tissue, joint distention by fluid, and heterotopic ossification. **It may be very difficult to differentiate Charcot's arthropathy and osteomyelitis based on physical examination and plain radiographs.** Symptoms common to the two conditions include swelling, warmth, erythema, minimal pain, and a variable WBC count and erythrocyte sedimentation rate (ESR); both are common in diabetic patients. **Technetium bone scan may look similar ("hot") for**

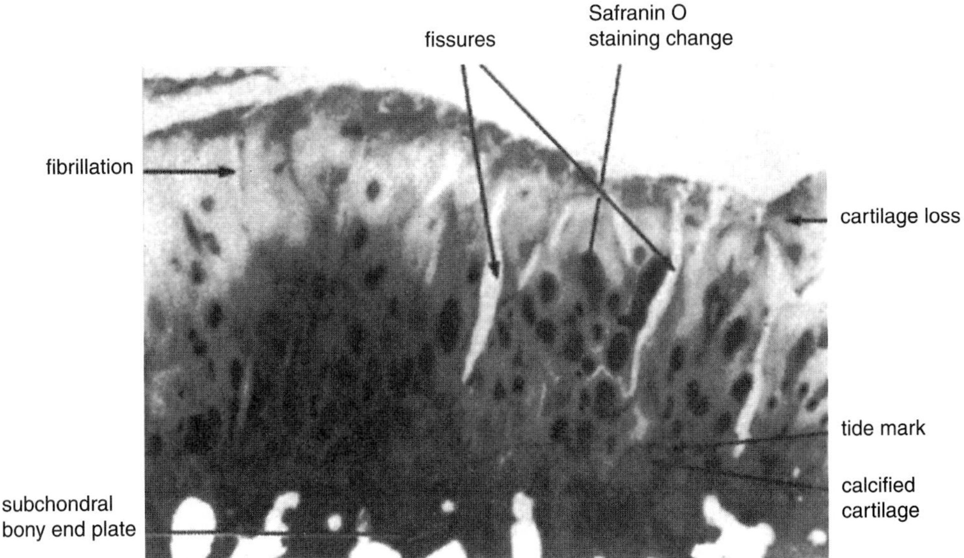

FIGURE 1-48 ■ Low-power micrograph of osteoarthritis demonstrating fibrillation, fissures, and cartilage loss. (From Simon, S.R., ed.: Orthopaedic Basic Science, 2nd ed., p. 34. Rosemont, IL, American Academy of Orthopaedic Surgeons, 1994.)

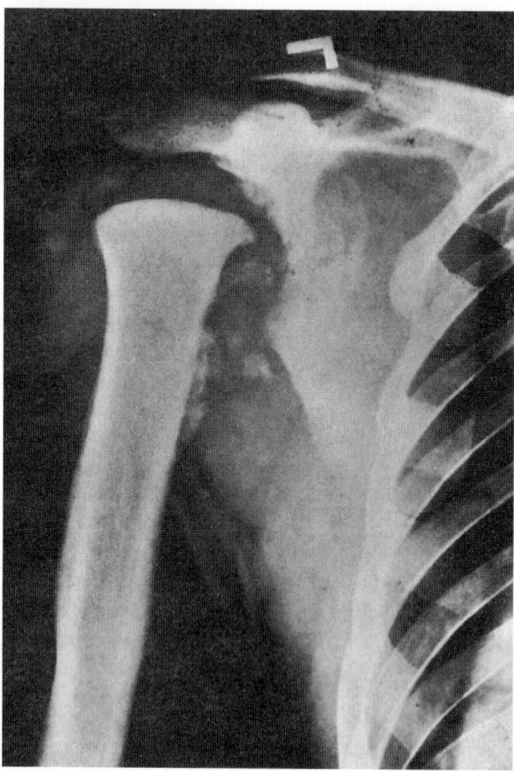

FIGURE 1-49 ■ AP radiograph of a shoulder showing severe destructive changes characteristic of neuropathic arthropathy. (From Weissman, B.N.W., and Sledge, C.B.: Orthopedic Radiology. Philadelphia, WB Saunders, 1986, p. 238.)

both osteomyelitis and Charcot's arthropathy; indium leukocyte scan will be "hot" (positive) for osteomyelitis and "cold" (negative) for Charcot's arthropathy. Treatment of Charcot's arthropathy is focused on limitation of activity and appropriate bracing or casting **(involved-side skin temperature similar to the uninvolved side is the best indicator for discontinuing a total contact cast)**. A Charcot joint is usually a contraindication for total joint arthroplasty and the use of other orthopaedic hardware.

3. Acute Rheumatic Fever (see Table 1-23) (Sometimes Included in the Inflammatory Group)—Formerly the most common cause of childhood arthritis, acute rheumatic fever is rarely seen since the advent of antibiotics. Arthritis and arthralgias can follow **untreated group A β-hemolytic strep infections** and can present with acute onset of red, tender, extremely painful joint effusions. Systemic manifestations include carditis, erythema marginatum (painless macules with red margins usually on the abdomen but never on the face), subcutaneous nodules (extensor surfaces of the upper extremities), and chorea. The arthritis is **migratory** and typically involves **multiple large joints**. Diagnosis is based on the **Jones' criteria** (preceding strep infection with two major criteria [carditis, polyarthritis, chorea, erythema marginatum, subcutaneous nodules] or one major and two minor criteria [fever, arthralgia, prior rheumatic fever, elevated ESR, prolonged PR interval on EKG]). **Antistreptolysin O titers are elevated in 80% of affected patients.** Treatment includes penicillin and salicylates.
4. Ochronosis (see Table 1-23)—Degenerative arthritis resulting from **alkaptonuria**, a rare inborn defect of the **homogentisic acid oxidase enzyme system** (tyrosine and phenylalanine catabolism). **Excess homogentisic acid is deposited in the joints** and then polymerizes (turns black), leading to early degenerative changes (can also be deposited in other tissues such as the heart valves).These patients may also experience **black urine. Ochronotic spondylitis** (Fig. 1-50), which usually occurs during the fourth decade of life, includes progressive degenerative changes and **disc space narrowing and calcification (Table 1-25)**.
5. Secondary Pulmonary Hypertrophic Osteoarthropathy—A clinical diagnosis. Involves a lung tumor mass, joint pain and stiffness, periostitis of the long bones, and clubbing of the fingers.

D. Inflammatory Arthritides—Tables 1-26 and 1-27 show an overview of commonly confused laboratory findings in inflammatory arthritic conditions. Generally, inflammatory arthritides produce radiographic evidence of destruction on both sides of a joint.

1. Rheumatoid Arthritis (RA) (see Table 1-23)—The most common form of inflammatory arthritis, RA affects 3% of women and 1% of men. Required diagnostic criteria, developed by the American Rheumatism Association, are morning stiffness, swelling, nodules, positive laboratory tests, and radiographic findings.
   a. Etiology—Unclear, but probably related to a cell-mediated immune response (T cell) that incites an inflammatory response initially against soft tissues and later against cartilage (chondrolysis) and bone (periarticular bone resorption). **Mononuclear cells are the primary cellular mediator of tissue destruction in RA**. RA may be associated with an infectious etiology or an HLA locus **(HLA-DR4 and HLA-DW4)**. Lymphokines, cytokines (particularly IL-1 and tumor necrosis factor-α), and other inflammatory mediators initiate a destructive cascade that leads to joint destruction. RA cartilage is sensitive to PMN degradation and IL-1 effects (phospholipase A_2, PGE_2, and plasminogen activators). **Class II molecules** are involved in antigen-T-lymphocyte interaction.

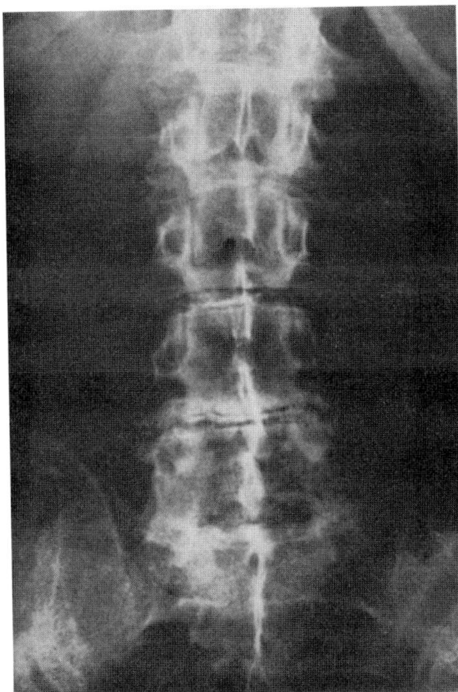
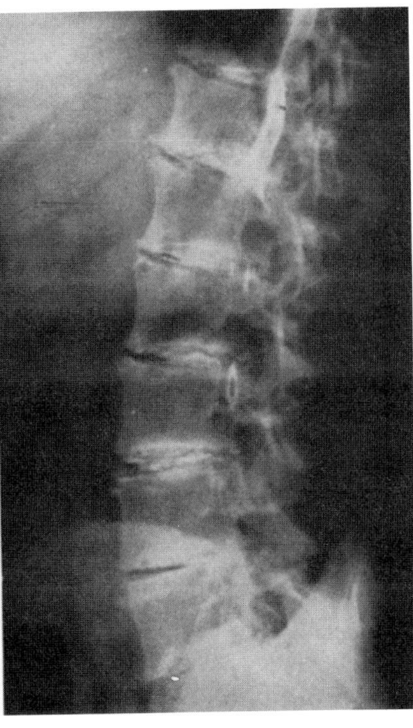

FIGURE 1-50 ■ Ochronosis. Irregular calcification and narrowing of the intervertebral discs are present. Radiolucent streaks, evident anteriorly between the vertebral bodies, are not uncommon. There is only minimal lipping of the vertebral bodies. (Courtesy of Samuel Fisher, M.D.)

Table 1-25. COMPARATIVE BONY CHANGES OF THE SPINE IN THE ARTHRITIDES

DISORDER	BONY CHANGE	RADIOGRAPHIC APPEARANCE
Ochronosis	Syndesmophytes (ossification of the annulus fibrosis of the intervertebral disc)	Vertical syndesmophytes extending from the body of one vertebra to the adjacent vertebra
Ankylosing Spondylitis	Syndesmophytes	Similar to above
Reiter's Syndrome and Psoriatic Spondylitis	Ossification of the connective tissues adjacent to the spine	Area of ossification is separated from the margin of the vertebral body and/or the intervertebral disc
Disseminated Idiopathic Skeletal Hyperostosis	Ossification of the connective tissues adjacent to the spine, the anterior longitudinal ligament, and the intervertebral disc	Undulating osseous extension along the anterior portion of the spine

Table 1-26. COMMONLY CONFUSED LABORATORY FINDINGS IN INFLAMMATORY ARTHRITIC CONDITIONS

FINDING	MAY BE POSITIVE FOR	USUALLY NEGATIVE FOR
Rheumatoid factor (RF)	Rheumatoid arthritis Sjögren's syndrome Sarcoid Systemic lupus erythematosus	Ankylosing spondylitis Gout Psoriatic arthritis Reiter's syndrome
HLA-B27*	Ankylosing spondylitis Reiter's syndrome Psoriatic arthritis Enteropathic arthritis	
Antinuclear antibody (ANA)	Systemic lupus-erythematosus Sjögren's syndrome Scleroderma	

*Approximately 6% of all whites are HLA-B27-positive.

Modified from Brinker, M.R., and Miller, M.D.: Fundamentals of Orthopaedics, Philadelphia, WB Saunders, 1999, p. 27.

Table 1-27. ASSOCIATIONS BETWEEN HUMAN LEUKOCYTE ANTIGEN ALLELES AND SUSCEPTIBILITY TO SOME RHEUMATIC DISEASES

DISEASE	HLA MARKER	FREQUENCY (%) IN PATIENTS (WHITES)	FREQUENCY (%) IN CONTROLS (WHITES)	RELATIVE RISK
Ankylosing spondylitis	B27	90	9	87
Reiter's syndrome	B27	79	9	37
Psoriatic arthritis	B27	48	9	10
Inflammatory bowel disease with spondylitis	B27	52	9	10
Adult rheumatoid arthritis	DR4	70	30	6
Polyarticular juvenile rheumatoid arthritis	DR4	75	30	7
Pauciarticular juvenile rheumatoid arthritis	DR8	30	5	5
	DR5	50	20	4.5
	DR2.1	55	20	4
Systemic lupus erythematosus	DR2	46	22	3.5
	DR3	50	25	3
Sjögren's syndrome	DR3	70	25	6

From Nepom, B.S., and Nepom, G.T.: Immunogenetics and the rheumatic diseases. In McCarty, D.J., ed.: Arthritis and Allied Conditions: A Textbook of Rheumatology, 12th ed. Philadelphia, Lea & Febiger, 1993.

b. General Characteristics—Usually an insidious onset of morning stiffness and polyarthritis. Most commonly the hands (ulnar deviation and subluxation of the metacarpophalangeals [MCPs]) and the feet (metatarsophalangeals [MTPs], claw toes, and hallux valgus) are affected early, but also common in the knees, elbows, shoulders, ankles, and cervical spine. **Subcutaneous nodules**, which are strongly associated with positive serum rheumatoid factor (RF), are seen in 20% of RA patients (over their lifetime). Synovium and soft tissues are affected first; only later are joints significantly involved. Pannus ingrowth denudes articular cartilage and leads to chondrocyte death. **Laboratory findings** include **elevated ESR and C-reactive protein** and **a positive RF titer (immunoglobulin M, IgM)** in approximately 80% of patients. Joint fluid assays can also demonstrate RF, decreased complement levels, and other helpful findings. **Systemic manifestations** can include rheumatoid vasculitis, pericarditis, and pulmonary disease (pleurisy, nodules, fibrosis). Popliteal cysts in rheumatoid patients (confirmed by ultrasonography) can mimic thrombophlebitis. Felty's syndrome is RA with splenomegaly and leukopenia. Still's disease is acute-onset of arthritis with fever, rash, and splenomegaly. Sjögren's syndrome is an autoimmune exocrinopathy often associated with RA; symptoms include **decreased salivary and lacrimal gland secretion** (keratoconjunctivitis sicca complex) and lymphoid proliferation.

c. Treatment—**RA treatment** goals: control synovitis and pain, maintain joint function, and prevent deformities. A multidisciplinary approach is necessary, involving therapeutic drugs, physical therapy, and sometimes surgery. The "pyramid" approach to RA drug therapy is to begin with NSAIDs and slowly progress to antimalarials, remittive agents (methotrexate, sulfasalazine, gold, and penicillamine), steroids, cytotoxic drugs, and finally experimental drugs. The pyramidal approach has been challenged recently in favor of a more aggressive approach (beginning with remittive agents). Surgery includes synovectomy (only if aggressive drug therapy fails), soft-tissue realignments (usually not favored because the deformity progresses), and various reconstructive procedures (increased risk of infection after TJA). If done early, chemical and radiation synovectomy can be successful. **Operative synovectomy** (open or arthroscropic), especially in the knee, **decreases the pain and swelling associated with the synovitis but does not prevent radiographic progression or the future need for total knee arthroplasty (TKA) nor does it improve joint ROM.** After all forms of synovectomy, the synovium initially regenerates normally, but degenerates to rheumatoid synovial tissue over time. Evaluation of the cervical spine with preoperative radiographs is important.

d. Radiographic Characteristics (Fig. 1-51)—Include **periarticular erosions** and **osteopenia.** Areas commonly affected are the hand (MCPs, PIPs, and carpal bones),

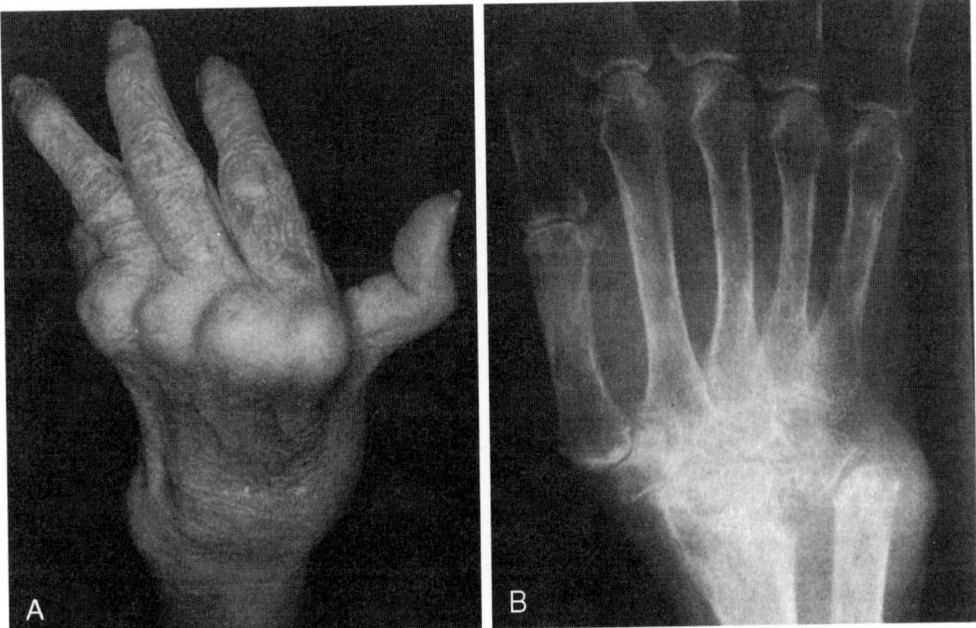

FIGURE 1-51 ■ *A,* Clinical photograph of the hand of a patient with advanced rheumatoid arthritis. Note ulnar drift of the metacarpophalangeal (MCP) joints caused by the ulnar shift of the extensor tendons, dislocations of the MCP joints, and thumb deformities. *B,* AP radiograph of the hand and wrist of a patient with rheumatoid arthritis. Note severe erosive destruction of the distal radioulnar joint and diffuse osteopenia. (From Bogumil, G.P.: The hand. In Wiesel, S.W., and Delahay, J.N: Essentials of Orthopaedic Surgery, 2nd ed. Philadelphia, WB Saunders, 1997, p. 263.)

wrist, and C-spine. All three knee compartments may show osteoporosis and erosions. **Protrusio acetabuli** (medial displacement of the acetabulum beyond the radiographic teardrop with medial migration of the femoral head into the pelvis) is common in RA, as well as ankylosing spondylitis, Paget's disease, metabolic bone diseases, Marfan's syndrome, Otto's pelvis, and other conditions.

2. Systemic Lupus Erythematosus (SLE) (see Tables 1-23, 1-26, and 1-27)—Chronic inflammatory disease of unknown origin usually affecting women (especially African Americans). Probably immune-complex related. Manifestations include **fever, butterfly malar rash**, pancytopenia, pericarditis, nephritis, and polyarthritis. **Joint involvement is the most common feature**, affecting more than 75% of SLE patients. Arthritis typically presents as acute, red, tender swelling of the PIPs, MCPs, carpus, knees and other joints. **SLE is typically not as destructive as RA.** Treatment for SLE arthritis usually includes the same medications described for RA. Mortality in SLE is usually related to renal disease. Differential diagnosis of SLE includes polymyositis and dermatomyositis, which also present with symmetric weakness ± a characteristic "heliotropic" rash of the upper eyelids. SLE patients are typically positive for antinuclear antibody (ANA) and HLA-DR3 and may be positive for RF.
3. Polymyalgia Rheumatica—Common among the elderly. Aching and stiffness of the shoulder and pelvic girdle, associated with malaise, headaches, and anorexia, are common symptoms. Physical examination is usually unremarkable. Laboratory studies show a **markedly elevated ESR**, anemia, increased alkaline phosphatase, and increased immune complexes. Usually treated symptomatically, with steroid use for refractory cases. **May be associated with temporal arteritis**, which requires a biopsy for definitive diagnosis and requires timely treatment with high-dose steroids (if left untreated, may rapidly result in total blindness).
4. Juvenile Rheumatoid Arthritis (JRA) (see Tables 1-23 and 1-27)—Also discussed in Chapter 2, Pediatric Orthopaedics. Three major types of JRA are recognized: systemic (20% of JRA patients), polyarticular (50%), and pauciarticular (30%). **Seronegative** denotes RF-negative, **seropositive** denotes RF-positive; the incidence of seropositive JRA is estimated to be <15% and is associated with a higher incidence of chronic, active, and progressive disease. **Pauciarticular** denotes ≤4 joints are involved, **polyarticular** denotes ≥5 joints are involved. **Early-onset** denotes onset of disease before the teens, **late-onset** denotes

onset of disease as a teenager or later. **Seronegative polyarticular JRA** is characterized by >5 joints being involved and is more frequent in girls. **Seropositive polyarticular JRA** also involves >5 joints, is more frequent in girls, exhibits a **positive RF** and **destructive degenerative joint disease (DJD),** and **frequently develops into adult RA. Early-onset pauciarticular JRA** involves ≤4 joints, is more frequent in girls, and is associated with **iridiocyclitis** in 50% of cases (particularly those with a positive ANA). **Late-onset pauciarticular JRA** involves ≤4 joints and is seen in **boys** more commonly than girls. JRA may also be associated with an HLA locus (HLA-DR2, HLA-DR4, HLA-DR5, HLA-DR8, and HLA-B27 in boys). Treatment of JRA includes high-dose aspirin, only occasionally gold or remittive agents (refractory polyarticular), and frequent ophthalmologic examinations (with a slit lamp) for asymptomatic ocular involvement. **The most common joint affected in JRA is the knee**, followed by the finger/wrist, ankle, and hip and C-spine.

5. Relapsing Polychondritis (see Table 1-23)—Rare disorder associated with episodic **inflammation, diffuse self-limited arthritis**, and progressive cartilage destruction ± systemic vasculitis. The disorder typically involves the **ears (thickening of the auricle)**; also seen are inflammatory eye disorders, tracheal involvement, hearing disorders, and sometimes cardiac involvement. It may be an autoimmune disorder (type II collagen affected). Treatment is supportive, although dapsone may have a role in the future.
6. Spondyloarthropathies/Enthesopathies (Occur at Ligament Insertions into Bone)—Characterized by a **positive HLA-B27** (sixth chromosome, D locus) and a **negative RF** titer.
   a. Ankylosing Spondylitis (AS) (see Tables 1-23, 1-26, and 1-27)—Bilateral sacroiliitis ± acute anterior uveitis in an HLA-B27–positive man is diagnostic. There is insidious onset of back pain (and associated morning stiffness) and hip pain during the third to fourth decade of life. AS progresses for approximately 20 years **(progressive spinal flexion deformities)**. Radiographic changes (Fig. 1-52, Table 1-25) in the spine include **squaring of the vertebrae, vertical syndesmophytes**, obliteration of sacroiliac (SI) joints, and "whiskering" of the enthesis. Ascending ankylosis of the spine usually begins in the thoracolumbar (TL) spine, often causing the entire spine to become rigid. Spinal manifestations include the "chin on chest" deformity (which may require corrective osteotomy of the cervicothoracic junction), **difficult cervical spine fractures (associated with epidural hemorrhage [high mortality rate]) that are best diagnosed via CT scan (75% rate of neurologic involvement)**, and severe kyphotic deformities (corrected via a posterior-closing wedge osteotomy). Spondylodiscitis may develop in the late stage. Lower spinal deformities with hip flexion deformities and pain (plus **morning stiffness**) are often helped with bilateral total hip arthroplasty (THA). Associated protrusio acetabuli requires special THA techniques. The need for prophylaxis for heterotopic bone formation has been questioned in patients with AS undergoing routine primary, noncemented THA. Initial treatment with physical therapy (PT) and NSAIDs (phenylbutazone is best but can cause bone marrow depression). AS is often associated with heart disease and pulmonary fibrosis. Other extraskeletal manifestations include iritis, aortitis, colitis, arachnoiditis, amyloidosis, and sarcoidosis. Pulmonary involvement (restriction of chest excursion [<2 cm]), hip involvement, and young age at onset are prognostic of poor outcomes.

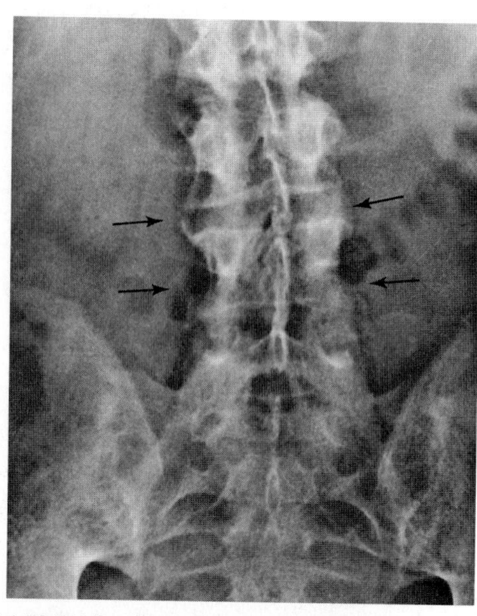

FIGURE 1-52 ■ AP radiograph of the lumbar spine and sacroiliac joints demonstrating marginal syndesmophytes *(arrows)* typical in ankylosing spondylitis. Note bilateral involvement of the sacroiliac joints. (From Bullough, P.G., and Vigorita, V.J.: Atlas of Orthopaedic Pathology. Philadelphia, Gower Medical Publishing, 1984, p. 8.11, by permission from Mosby.)

   b. Reiter's Syndrome (see Tables 1-23, 1-25, 1-26, and 1-27); (Fig. 1-53)—Classic presentation is a young man with the triad of **conjunctivitis, urethritis, and oligoarticular arthritis** ("can't see, pee, or bend the knee"). Painless **oral ulcers, penile lesions,**

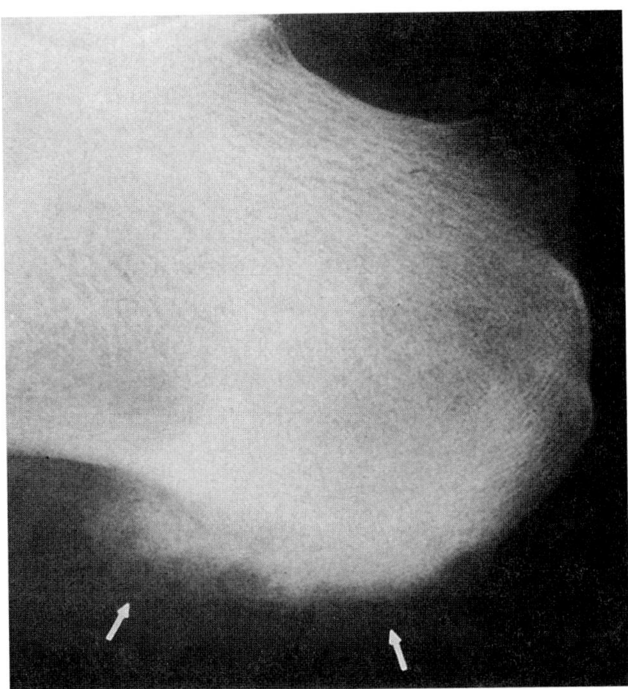

FIGURE 1-53 ■ Lateral radiograph of the calcaneus of a patient with Reiter's syndrome shows fluffy perosteal calcifications *(arrows)*.

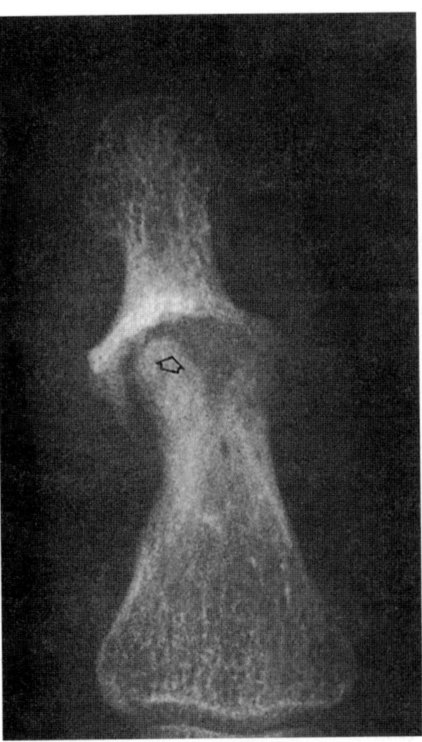

FIGURE 1-54 ■ AP radiograph of the distal interphalangeal joint of the foot in a patient with psoriatic arthritis shows the classic "pencil and cup" deformity.

and **pustular lesions** on the extremities, **palms** and **soles (keratoderma blennorrhagicum)** and plantar heel pain are common. The arthritis usually causes sudden asymmetric swelling and pain in weight-bearing joints. Recurrence is common and can lead to metatarsal (MT) head erosion and calcaneal periostitis. Approximately **80-90% of patients with Reiter's syndrome are HLA-B27 positive**, and 60% with chronic disease have **sacroiliitis**. Treatment includes NSAIDs, PT, and possibly sulfa drugs in the future.

c. Psoriatic Arthropathy (see Tables 1-23, 1-25, 1-26, and 1-27)—Affects approximately 5-10% of patients with psoriasis. Many HLA loci may be involved, but HLA-B27 is found in 50% of patients with psoriatic arthritis. Many forms exist; most patients have the oligoarticular form, which (asymmetrically) affects the small joints of the hands and feet. **Nail pitting** (also fragmentation and discoloration), **"sausage" digits, and "pencil in cup" deformity (with DIP involvement)** are characteristic (Fig. 1-54). Treatment is similar to that for RA.

d. Enteropathic Arthritis (see Tables 1-23, 1-26, and 1-27)—Approximately 10-20% of Crohn's disease and ulcerative colitis patients experience peripheral joint arthritis, and 5% or more experience axial disease. This nondeforming arthritis occurs more commonly in large, weight-bearing joints. It usually presents as an acute monarticular synovitis that may precede any bowel symptoms. Enteropathic arthritis is HLA-B27 positive in approximately half of all affected persons and is associated with AS in 10-15% of cases.

7. Crystal Deposition Disease

a. Gout (see Table 1-23 and Fig. 1-55)—Disorder of nucleic acid metabolism causing hyperuricemia, which leads to monosodium urate (MSU) crystal deposition in joints. Crystals activate inflammatory mediators (proteases, chemotactic factors, prostaglandins, leukotriene B4, and free oxygen radicals). The inflammatory mediators are **inhibited by colchicine**. The crystals also activate platelets, IL-1, and the complement system. **Phagocytosis is inhibited by phenylbutazone and indomethacin (Indocin).** Local polypeptides may inhibit the crystal inflammatory response via a glycoprotein "coating." Recurrent arthritis attacks, especially in men 40-60 years of age (usually in the lower extremity, **especially the great toe [podagra]**), crystal deposition as **tophi** (ear helix, eyelid, olecranon, Achilles; usually seen in the chronic form), and renal disease/stones (2% Ca^{2+} versus normal 0.2%) are characteristic. The kidneys are

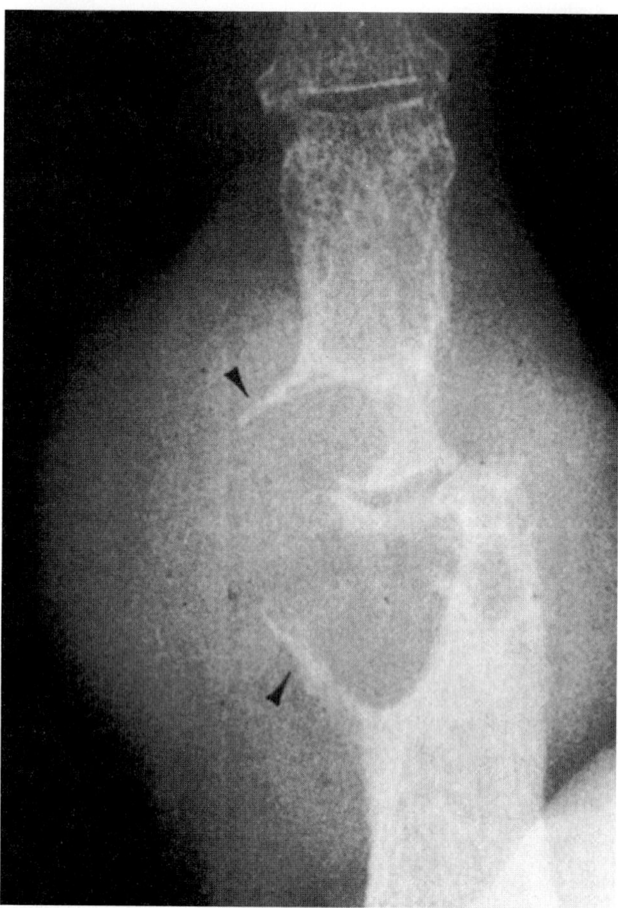

FIGURE 1-55 ■ AP radiograph of the proximal interphalangeal joint of a finger in a patient with gout. Note the soft-tissue swelling and "punched out" periarticular erosions and sclerotic overhangings bordering the joint *(arrows)*. (From Resnick, D., and Niwayama, G.: Diagnosis of Bone and Joint Disorders. Philadelphia, W.B. Saunders, 1981, p. 1478.)

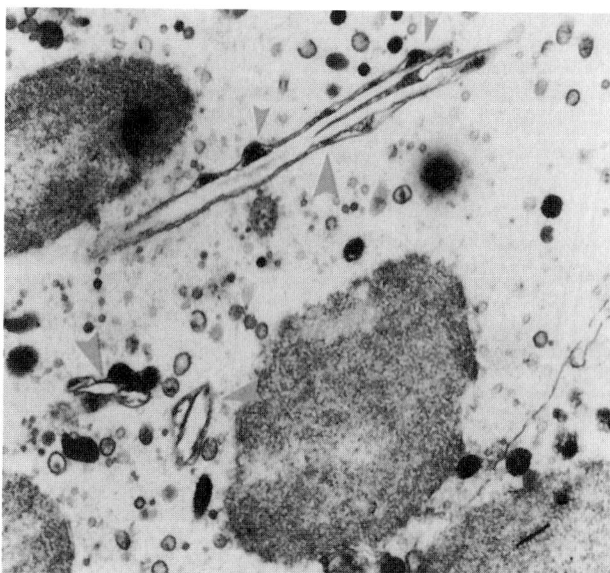

FIGURE 1-56 ■ A neutrophil has phagocytosed a number of MSU crystals *(large arrows)*. Although the crystals have almost completely dissolved, the outlines of the vacuoles remain, one still needle shaped. Lysosomes discharge their contents directly into the phagosomes (*small arrows*). (Magnification, ×22,000; original magnification, ×31,250.) (From Krey, P.R., and Lazaro, D.M.: Analysis of Synovial Fluid. Summit, NJ, Ciba-Geigy, 1992.)

the second most commonly affected organ. **Gout may be precipitated by chemotherapy for myeloproliferative disorders. Radiographs may show soft-tissue changes and "punched-out" periarticular erosions with sclerotic overhanging borders** (see Fig. 1-55). Elevated serum uric acid level is not diagnostic of gout; MSU crystals that are **thin, tapered intracellular crystals that are strongly negatively birefringent** (Fig. 1-56) in joint aspirate are essential for diagnosis. **Initial treatment with indomethacin** (75 mg tid) is indicated, followed by a rheumatology consultation (patients with GI symptoms or a history of peptic ulcer disease should receive intravenous colchicine for acute attacks). **Allopurinol** is used to lower serum uric acid levels in hyperuricemic patients with chronic gout and is given prior to chemotherapy for myeloproliferative disorders. **Allopurinol is a xanthine oxidase inhibitor** (xanthine oxidase is needed for the conversion of hypoxanthine to xanthine, and xanthine to uric acid). Colchicine can be used for **prophylaxis after recurrent attacks**.

b. Chondrocalcinosis (see Table 1-23)—Caused by several disorders, including (1) **calcium pyrophosphate (dihydrate crystal) deposition disease (CPPD—also known as pseudogout)**, (2) ochronosis, (3) hyperparathyroidism, (4) hypothyroidism, and (5) hemochromatosis. **CPPD** (a common cause of chondrocalcinosis) is a disorder of pyrophosphate metabolism that occurs in older patients and occasionally causes acute attacks (usually in the lower extremities, especially the **knee**), which can be mistaken for septic arthritis. **Short, blunt, rhomboid-shaped crystals that are weakly positively birefringent** (Fig. 1-57) are seen in neutrophilic leukocytes in knee aspirate. **Chondrocalcinosis of knee menisci is often related to a previous knee injury.** Radiographs show fine linear calcification in hyaline cartilage and more diffuse calcification of **menisci** (Fig. 1-58) **and other fibrocartilage (triangular fibrocartilage complex**, acetabular labrum). NSAIDs are often helpful. Intra-articular yttrium-90 injections have also been successful in chronic cases.

c. Calcium Hydroxyapatite Crystal Deposition Disease—Also associated with chondrocalcinosis and DJD. It is a **destructive arthropathy** commonly seen in the knee and shoulder. The **"Milwaukee shoulder"** is

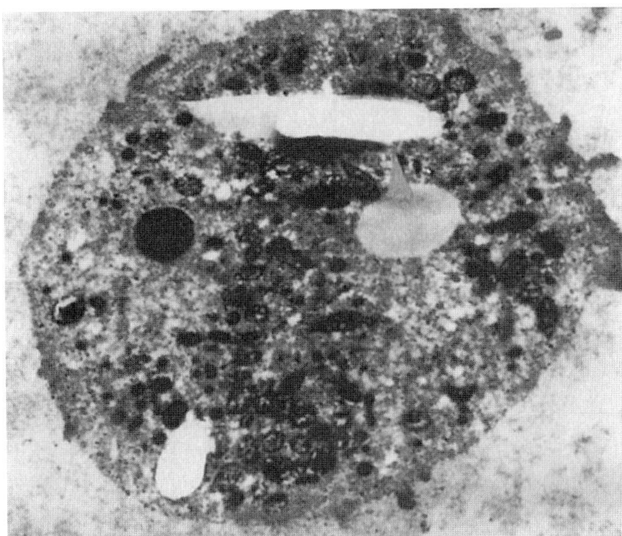

FIGURE 1-57 ■ A synovial fluid leukocyte showing the outline of a phagocytosed CPPD crystal that has dissolved *(arrow)*. (Magnification, ×14,000; original magnification, ×17,000.) (From Krey, P.R., and Lazaro, D.M.: Analysis of Synovial Fluid. Summit, NJ, Ciba-Geigy, 1992.)

basic calcium phosphate deposition in the shoulder along with cuff tear arthropathy. Calcium hydroxyapatite crystals are too small to see with light microscopy; treatment is generally supportive.

d. Birefringence
   (1) Positive—Long axis of crystal parallel to the compensator (of the microscope): the crystal is blue.
   (2) Negative—Long axis of crystal parallel to the compensator: the crystal is yellow. (*Note*: when the crystal's long axis is perpendicular to the compensator, color rules are reversed.)
   (3) Weak—Dull crystal.
   (4) Strong—Bright, shiny crystal.

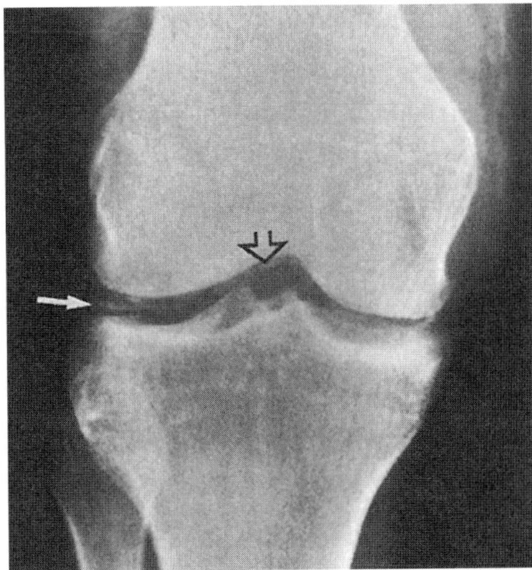

FIGURE 1-58 ■ AP radiograph demonstrating calcium pyrophosphate deposition disease (pseudogout) in the meniscus of the knee. Note calcification within the (fibrocartilage) meniscus *(closed arrow)* and articular involvement with fine linear calcification of hyaline cartilage *(open arrow)*. (From Weissman, B.N.W., and Sledge, C.B.: Orthopaedic Radiology, p. 549. Philadelphia, WB Saunders, 1986).

E. Infectious Arthritides
   1. Pyogenic Arthritis (see Table 1-23)—Results from hematogenous spread or by extension of osteomyelitis. Commonly occurs in children (see Chapter 2, Pediatric Orthopaedics). In adult patients, pyogenic arthritis occurs more commonly in persons who are at risk, including IV drug abusers (especially the SC and SI joints); sexually active young adults (gonococcal infection [intracellular diplococci], especially if seen with skin papules); diabetics (feet and lower extremities); and RA patients. It is also seen after trauma (fight bites, open injuries) or surgery (iatrogenic). Histology may demonstrate synovial hyperplasia, numerous PMNs, and cartilage destruction. Destruction of cartilage can be direct (proteolytic enzymes) or indirect (caused by pressure and lack of nutrition). Treatment includes I&D(s) (irrigation and debridement) and up to several weeks of antibiotics.
   2. Tuberculous Arthritis (see Table 1-23)—Chronic granulomatous infection caused by *Mycobacterium tuberculosis* usually invades joints by **hematogenous spread**. The spine and lower extremities are most often involved, typically in Mexicans and Asians. Approximately 80% of cases are monarticular. Radiographically, tuberculous arthritis causes changes on both sides of the joint. Diagnosis is helped with a **positive purified protein derivative (PPD)**, demonstration of **acid-fast bacilli** and **"rice bodies" (fibrin globules) in the synovial fluid,** positive cultures (may take several weeks), and characteristic radiographs (subchondral osteoporosis, cystic changes, notch-like bony destruction at the joint edge, and joint space narrowing with osteolytic changes on both sides of the joint). Histology may demonstrate **characteristic granulomas with Langhans giant cells** (peripheral nuclei). Treatment includes I&D and long-term antibiotics (isoniazid, rifampin, pyrazinamide, and pyridoxine).
   3. Fungal Arthritis (see Table 1-23)—More common in neonates, **AIDS patients**, and drug users. Pathogens include *Candida albicans*. Potassium hydroxide (KOH) preparations of synovial fluid are helpful because cultures require prolonged incubation. Arthritis can be treated with 5-flucytosine. Blastomycosis, coccal infections, and other fungal infections often require treatment with amphotericin (this treatment is sometimes administered intra-articularly with fewer side effects).
   4. Lyme Disease (see Table 1-23)—Acute, self-limited joint effusions (especially in the shoulder and knee) that recur frequently. Caused by the **spirochete *Borrelia burgdorferi***

(*Borrelia garinii* in Europe), which is transmitted by **tick bites** (*Ioxodes*), endemic in half of the United States. Transmission of *B. burgdorferi* occurs in approximately 10% of bites by infected ticks. Sometimes called the "great mimicker." Systemic signs may include a characteristic "bull's-eye" rash **(erythema chronicum migrans) or** neurologic (Bell's palsy is common) or cardiac symptoms. The disease occurs in three stages: I—rash, II—neurologic symptoms, III—arthritis. **Immune complexes and cryoglobulins accumulate in the synovial fluid** of affected persons. Diagnosis is confirmed by **enzyme-linked immunosorbent assay (ELISA) testing**, which should be sought in endemic areas after a Gram stain and joint cultures of an infectious aspirate show no organisms. **Treatment** is with doxycycline (most effective), amoxicillin, cefuroxime, erythromycin, or ceftriaxone (for carditis).

F. Hemorrhagic Effusions

1. Hemophilic Arthropathy (Table 1-23)—**X-linked recessive disorder, factor VIII deficiency** (hemophilia A—classic) or factor IX deficiency (hemophilia B—Christmas disease) associated with repeated hemarthrosis due to minor trauma, leading to synovitis, cartilage destruction (enzymatic processes), and joint deformity. Disease severity related to the degree of factor deficiency (mild, 5-25% levels; moderate, 1-5% levels; severe, 0-1% levels). Repeated episodes of hemarthrosis lead to replacement of the normal joint capsule with dense scar tissue. **The knee is most commonly involved**, followed by the elbow, ankle, shoulder, and spine. Joint swelling, decreased ROM, and pain are characteristic. **A joint aspirate should be obtained to rule out a concomitant infection.** Radiographs later in the disease process may demonstrate variable changes to the patella (**"squared off" patella = Jordan's sign** [also seen in JRA]), widening of the intercondylar notch, and enlarged femoral condyles that appear to "fall off" the tibia (Fig. 1-59). Ultrasonography can be used to diagnose and follow intramuscular bleeding episodes. **Iliacus hematomas can cause femoral nerve palsies.** Management includes correction of factor levels, splints, compressive dressings, bracing, and analgesics. Occasionally, steroids are helpful. Surgical management

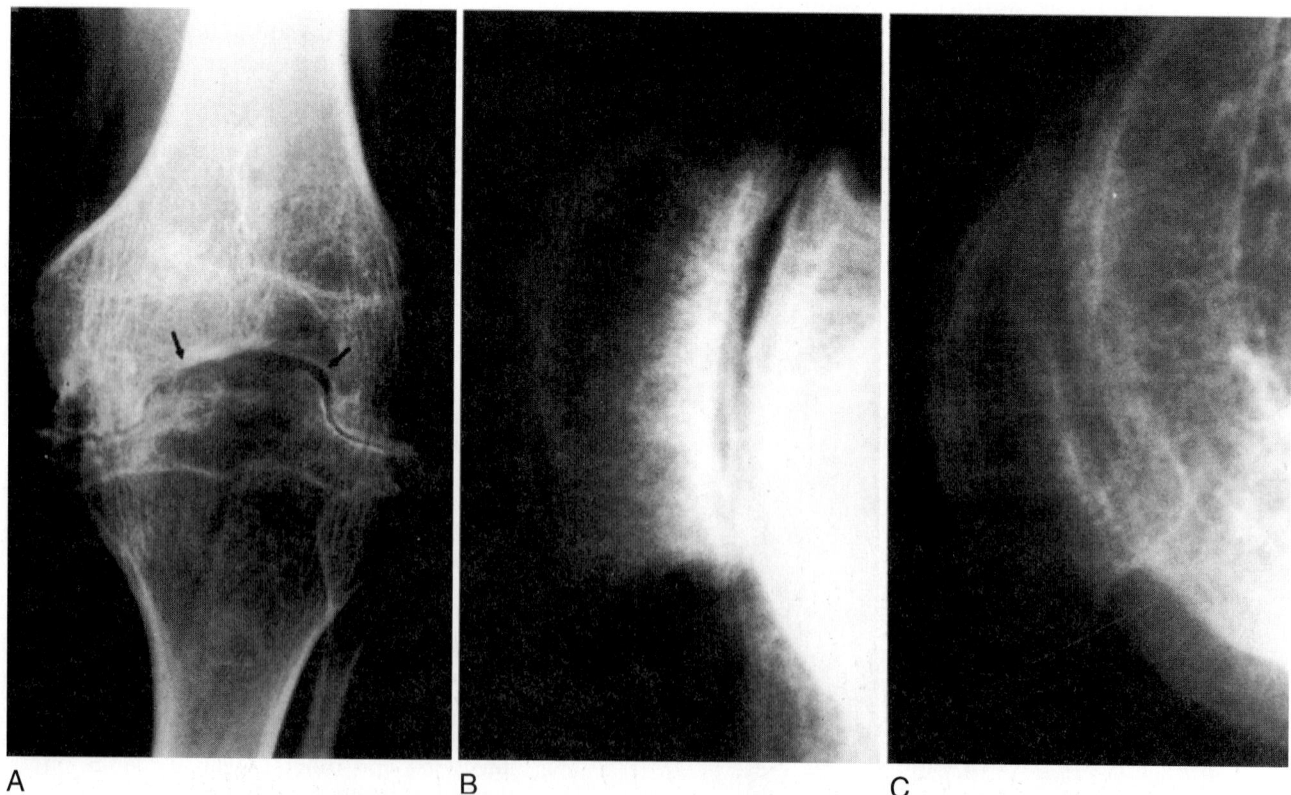

FIGURE 1-59 ■ Radiographic changes of hemophilia. *A*, AP radiograph of the knee shows enlargement and ballooning of the distal femur, flattening of the distal femoral condyles, marked joint space narrowing, and severe widening of the intercondylar notch. *B* and *C* show the variable radiographic changes that can occur in the patella with *B* appearing "squared off" (Jordan's sign) and *C* appearing elongated and thinned. (From Resnick, D., and Niwayama, G.: Diagnosis of Bone and Joint Disorders. Philadelphia, W.B. Saunders, 1981, p. 2025.)

includes synovectomy (for recurrent hemarthroses and synovial hypertrophy refractory to conservative treatment), TJA (for end-stage arthropathy), or arthrodesis (especially for the ankle). **Synovectomy** has been shown to reduce the incidence of recurrent hemarthroses (less pain and swelling). **Synoviorthesis** (destruction of synovial tissue by intra-articular injection of a radioactive agent) with colloidal ^{32}P chromic phosphate may be useful for the treatment of chronic hemophilic synovitis that is resistant to conventional treatment. **Factor levels** should be maintained near 100% during the first postoperative week and at 50-75% during the second week. There is a high incidence of HIV positivity in hemophiliacs (up to 90%). **The presence of an inhibitor that represents an IgG antibody to the clotting factor protein (that causes the patient to have no response to factor replacement therapy) is a relative contraindication to any elective surgical procedure.** Inhibitor is present in 5-25% of patients and can develop at any time. New monoclonal recombinant factor VIII products are prone to induce inhibitors. When an inhibitor to factor VIII develops, other strategies to provide hemostasis must be used.

2. Sickle Cell Disease—Hemoglobin SS is found in 1% of African Americans and leads to local infarction due to capillary stasis. Bony infarcts and ischemic necrosis may occur in multiple bones in sickle cell disease (thalassemia does not produce infarcts or ischemic necrosis). Dactylitis with metacarpal/metatarsal periosteal new bone formation may also be seen. Osteomyelitis is not uncommon in patients with sickle cell disease (***Salmonella* is the most characteristic organism, and *Staphylococcus* is the most common**); *Salmonella* spread can come from a gallbladder infection. The ESR is usually falsely low. ON (especially of the femoral head, which leads to joint destruction and may require THA) is common in sickle cell patients. Results of TJA are poor owing to ongoing negative bone remodeling.
3. Pigmented Villonodular Synovitis (PVNS) (see Table 1-23) (Fig. 1-60)—Synovial disease often affecting young adults with **exuberant**

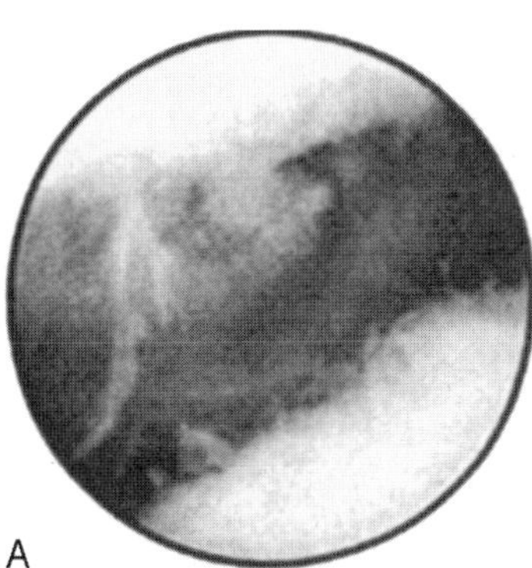

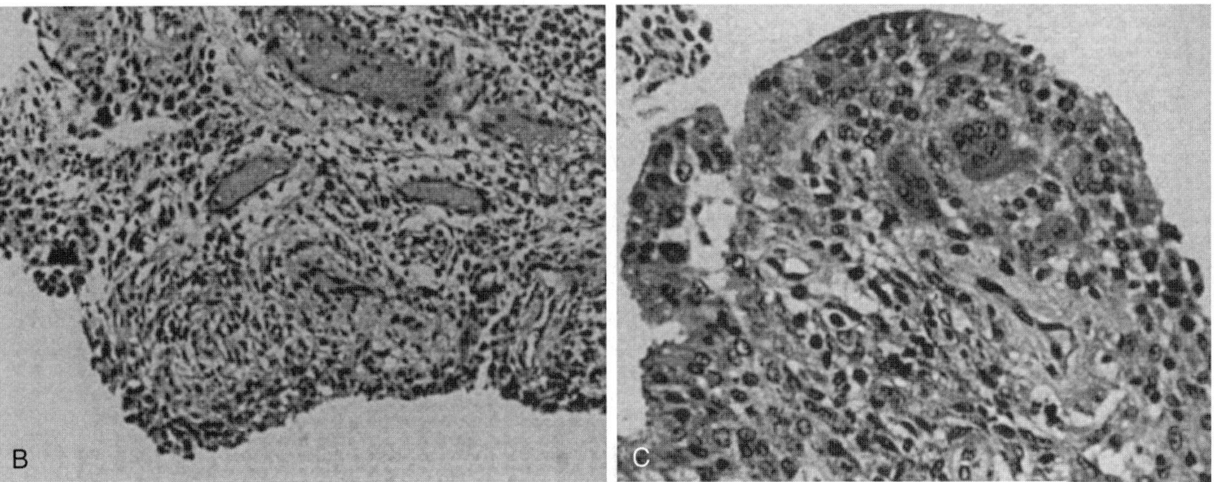

FIGURE 1-60 ■ Localized pigmented villonodular synovitis. *A,* Arthroscopic view localized to the medial knee joint. *B,* Histologic picture shows vascular channels, giant cells, and blood pigments (hematoxylin and eosin stain, ×100). *C,* Giant cells in synovial villus (hematoxylin and eosin stain, ×400).

proliferation of villi and nodules. The synovium is frequently rust-colored or brown because of extensive **hemosiderin deposits.** Pain, swelling, synovitis, and a **rust-colored or bloody effusion** are common. **The knee is the most frequent site of PVNS**, with occasional involvement of the hip and ankle. Radiographs show well-defined juxtacortical erosions with sclerotic margins. Histologic features include pigmented synovial histiocytes, foam cells (lipid-laden histiocytes), and multinucleated giant cells. Treatment is surgical excision **(total synovectomy)** of the affected synovium. Microscopic residual disease may be treated with intra-articular dysprosium (a radioisotope).

SECTION 3

Neuromuscular and Connective Tissues

I. Skeletal Muscle and Athletics

A. Noncontractile Elements (Fig. 1-61)

1. Muscle Body—**Epimysium** surrounds individual muscle bundles; **perimysium** surrounds muscle fascicles; and **endomysium** surrounds individual fibers.
2. Myotendon Junction—**The weak link in the muscle, often the site of tears**, especially with eccentric contractions. Sarcolemma filaments interdigitate with the basement membrane (type IV collagen) and tendon tissue (type I collagen). Involution of muscle cells in this region gives maximum surface area for attachment. Linking proteins and specialized membrane proteins are also present.
3. Sarcoplasmic Reticulum—Stores calcium in intracellular membrane-bound channels, including T-tubules (which go to each myofibril) and cisternae (small storage areas) (Fig. 1-62).

B. Contractile Elements (see Fig. 1-61)—Derived from myoblasts. Each muscle is composed of several muscle **fascicles**, which in turn contain muscle **fibers** (the basic unit of contraction); fibers are composed of **myofibrils** (1-3 μm in diameter and 1-2 cm long); a myofibril is a collection of **sarcomeres**. A muscle fiber is an elongated cell. Fibers are usually parallel, but can run oblique to one another (e.g., bipennate muscle). Muscle fiber architecture is specific for the required function.

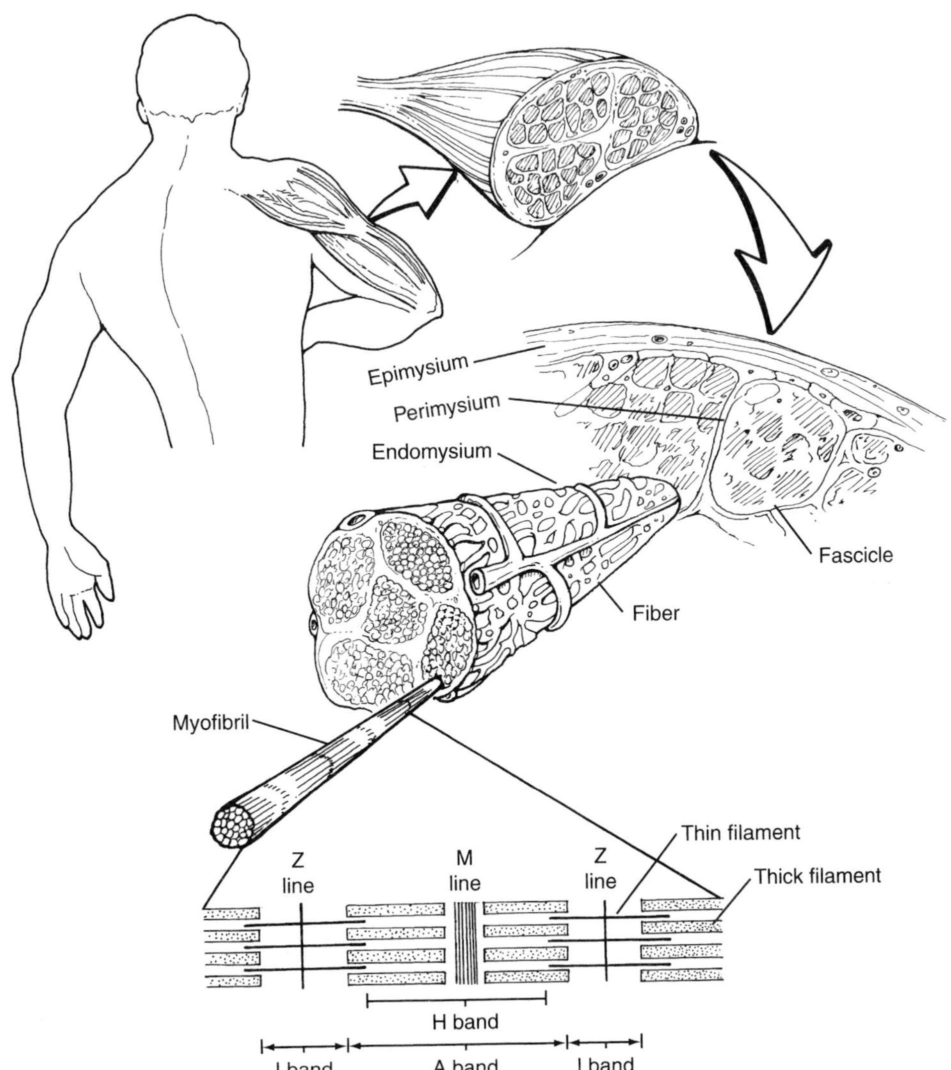

FIGURE 1-61 ■ Skeletal muscle architecture. (From Brinker, M.R., and Miller, M.D.: Fundamentals of Orthopaedics. Philadelphia, WB Saunders, 1999, p. 10.)

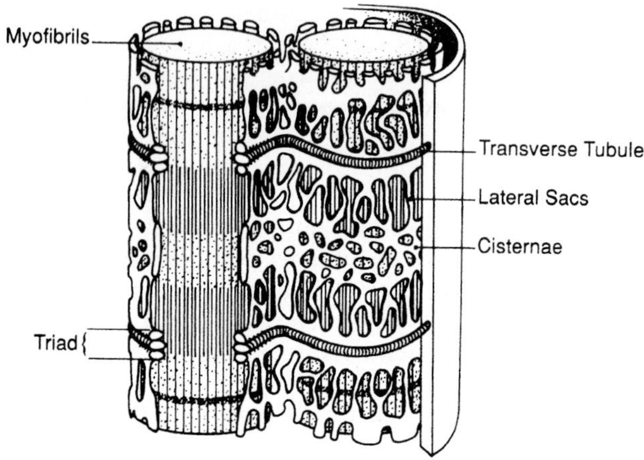

FIGURE 1-62 ■ Sarcoplasmic reticulum. Action potentials travel down the transverse tubules, causing calcium release from the outer vesicles. (From Simon, S.R., ed.: Orthopaedic Basic Science, 2nd ed., p. 94. Rosemont, IL, American Academy of Orthopaedic Surgeons, 1994.)

Table 1-28. SARCOMERE

A band	Contains actin and myosin
I band	Contains actin only
H band	Contains myosin only
M line	Interconnecting site of the thick filaments
Z line	Anchors the thin filaments

From Brinker, M.R., and Miller, M.D.: Fundementals of Orthopaedics. Philadelphia, WB Saunders, 1999, p. 11.

1. Sarcomere—Composed of thick (**myosin**) and thin (**actin**) filaments intricately arranged to allow the fibers to slide past each other. The sarcomere is arranged into bands and lines (see Fig. 1-61) (Table 1-28). The **H band** contains only thick (myosin) filaments, and the **I band is composed solely of thin (actin) filaments**. Thin filaments are attached to the **Z line** and extend across I bands, partially into the A band. Each sarcomere is bounded by two adjacent Z lines.

C. Action—Stimulus for a muscle contraction originates in the cell body of a nerve and is carried toward the neuromuscular junction via an electrical impulse that is propagated down the entire length of the axon (from the spinal cord to skeletal muscle). Once the impulse reaches the **motor endplate** (a specialized synapse formed between muscle and nerve) (Fig. 1-63), acetylcholine (stored in presynaptic vesicles) is released. Acetylcholine then diffuses across the **synaptic cleft** (50 nm) to bind a specific receptor on the muscle membrane (myasthenia gravis is a shortage of acetylcholine receptors; botulinum A injections reduce spasticity by blocking acetylcholine release at the end plate). Acetylcholine binding triggers depolarization of the sarcoplasmic reticulum, which releases calcium into the muscle cytoplasm.

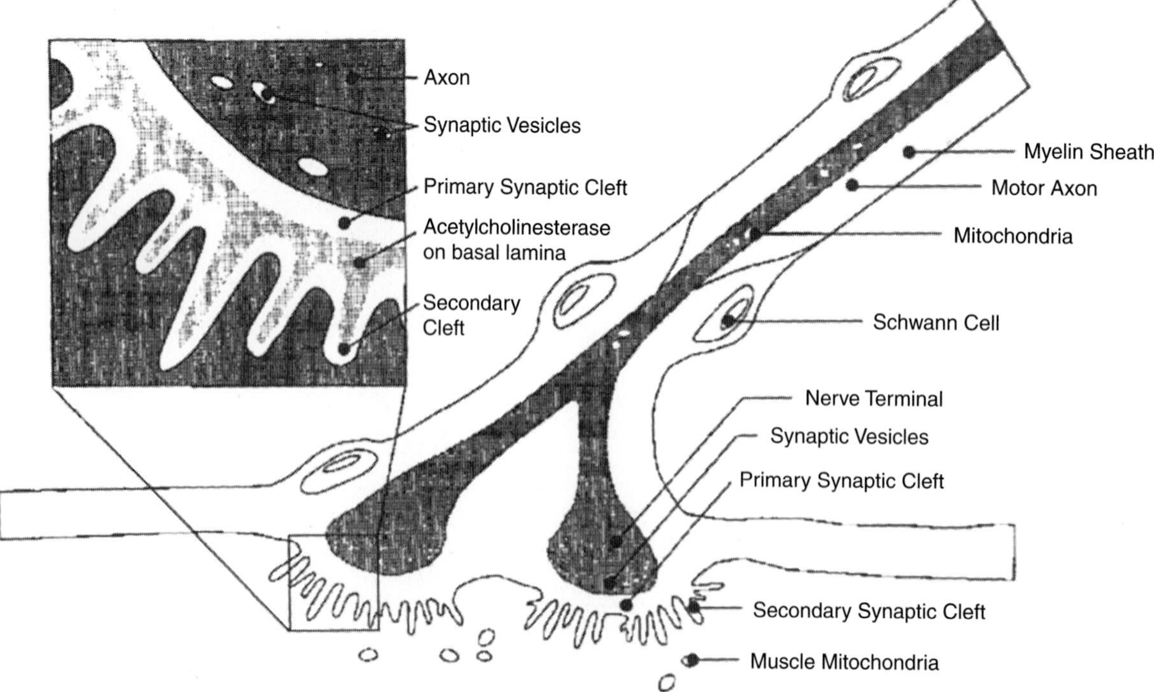

FIGURE 1-63 ■ Motor endplate. (From Simon, S.R., ed.: Orthopaedic Basic Science, 2nd ed., p. 93. Rosemont, IL, American Academy of Orthopaedic Surgeons, 1994.)

Calcium binds to troponin (on the thin filaments), causing them to change the position of tropomycin (also on the thin filaments) and exposing the actin filament. Actin-myosin cross-bridges form; and with the breakdown of ATP, the thick and thin filaments slide past one another, contracting the muscle. Table 1-29 shows the effects of some commonly used agents that affect impulse transmission.

D. Types of Muscle Contractions—Table 1-30

E. Types of Muscle Fibers—Include slow twitch (type I) and fast twitch (type II); fibers are a part of a motor unit (a motor unit is a motorneuron and the muscle fibers it innervates). Table 1-31 shows the characteristics of type I and type II muscle fibers.

1. Slow Twitch (ST) (Type I; Oxidative ["Red"]) Fibers—**Aerobic** and therefore have **more mitochondria**, enzymes, and triglycerides (energy source) than type II fibers. They have low concentrations of glycogen and glycolytic enzymes (ATPase). Remember **"slow red ox"**—type I are slower, more vascular [red], and undergo aerobic oxidation. Type I fibers perform **endurance activities** and are the first lost without rehabilitation.
2. Fast Twitch (FT) (Type II; Glycolytic ["White"]) Fibers—Anaerobic; contract more quickly and have larger and stronger motor units (increased ATPase) than ST fibers, but are consequently less efficient. Type II fibers develop a large amount of force per cross-sectional area, with high contraction speeds and quick relaxation times. Type II fibers are well suited for high-intensity, short-duration activities (sprinting) and fatigue rapidly. Type II fibers have low intramuscular triglycerine stores. Type IIA and IIB fibers are associated with sprinting (adenosine triphosphate—creatine phosphate system); subtypes of type II fibers are based on myosin heavy chains.

F. Energetics—Three energy systems generate muscle activity, depending on the duration and intensity of the muscular activity required (Fig. 1-64).

1. **Adenosine Triphosphate—Creatine Phosphate (ATP-CP) System (also known as the Phosphagen System).** Meets the metabolic requirements for intense muscle activities that last up to 20 seconds, such as **sprinting a 100-200-meter dash**. Converts stored carbohydrates from within the muscle fiber itself to energy. **Does not use oxygen and does not produce lactate**; it is therefore an alactive anaerobic activity. Energy is derived from the high-energy phosphate bonds during hydrolysis:

   $$\text{ATP} \rightarrow \text{ADP} + \text{P} + \text{Energy}$$

   $$\text{ADP} \rightarrow \text{AMP} + \text{P} + \text{Energy}$$

2. **Lactic Anaerobic System (also known as Lactic Acid Metabolism)** (Fig. 1-65)—Meets the metabolic requirements for intense muscle activities that last for 20-120 seconds, such as a **400 meter sprint**. Involves hydrolysis of one glucose molecule to ultimately produce lactic acid plus energy converting two molecules of adenosine diphosphate (ADP) to two molecules of ATP.
3. **Aerobic System** (Figs. 1-65 and 1-66)—When oxygen is available, the aerobic system replenishes ATP through oxidative phosphorylation and the Krebs cycle; uses glucose or fatty acids to produce ATP. Meets the metabolic requirements for **episodes of longer duration and lower-intensity muscle activities**.

G. Athletes and Training—The distribution of FT versus ST fibers is genetically determined; however, specific training can selectively improve these fibers. **Endurance athletes typically have a higher percentage of ST fibers**, whereas athletes participating in "strength"-type sports (and sprinters) have more FT fibers. **Training for endurance sports** consists of decreased tension and increased repetitions, which increases the efficiency of the ST fibers and increases the number of mitochondria, capillary density, and oxidative capacity; this type of training also improves blood lipid profiles. **Training for strength** consists of

Table 1-29. AGENTS THAT AFFECT NEUROMUSCULAR IMPULSE TRANSMISSION

AGENT	SITE OF ACTION	MECHANISM	EFFECT
Nondepolarizing drugs (curare, pancuronium, vecuronium)	Neuromuscular junction	Competitively binds to acetylcholine receptor to block impulse transmission	Paralytic agent (long term)
Depolarizing drugs (succinylcholine)	Neuromuscular junction	Binds to acetylcholine receptor to cause temporary depolarization of muscle membrane	Paralytic agent (short term)
Anticholinesterases (neostigmine, edrophonium)	Autonomic ganglia	Prevents breakdown of acetylcholine to enhance its effect	Reverses effect of nondepolarizing drugs; muscarinic effects (bronchospasm, bronchorrhea, bradycardia)

Table 1-30. TYPES OF MUSCLE CONTRACTIONS

TYPE OF MUSCLE CONTRACTION	DEFINITION	EXAMPLE	PHASES
Isotonic	**Muscle tension is constant through the range of motion.** Muscle length changes through the range of motion. This is a measure of dynamic strength.	Biceps curls using free weights.	**Concentric Contration**—The muscle shortens during the contraction. Tension within the muscle is proportional to the externally applied load. An example of an isotonic concentric contraction is the "curl" (elbow moving toward increasing flexion) portion of a biceps curl. **Eccentric Contraction**—The muscle lengthens during the contraction (internal force is less than external force). **Eccentric contractions have the greatest potential for high muscle tension and muscle injury.** An example of an isotonic eccentric contraction is "the negative" (elbow moving toward increasing extension) portion of a biceps curl.
Isometric	Muscle tension is generated but the length of the muscle remains unchanged. This is a measure of static strength.	Pushing against an immovable object (such as a wall).	
Isokinetic	Muscle tension is generated as the muscle maximally contracts at a constant velocity over a full range of motion. Isokinetic exercises are best for maximizing strength and are a measure of dynamic strength.	Isokinetic exercises require special equipment, such as a Cybex machine.	Concentric Eccentric

increased tension and decreased repetitions, which increases the number of myofibrils/fibers and induces **hypertrophy (increased cross-sectional area) of FT (type II) fibers**; a well-conditioned muscle may be able to fire more than 90% of its fibers simultaneously. Both types of training slow the lactate response to exercise. The cross-sectional area of skeletal muscle reliably predicts the potential for contractile force. **Isokinetic exercises produce more strength gains than do isometric exercises.** Isotonic exercises produce a uniform strength increase throughout joint ROM. **Plyometric ("bounding") exercises** consist of a muscle stretch followed immediately by a rapid contraction. The stretch stores elastic energy, which increases the force of the concentric muscle contraction. **Plyometrics are the most efficient method of conditioning for improvement in power. Closed chain exercise** is loading an extremity with the most distal segment stabilized or not moving; this allows muscular co-contraction around a joint, which minimizes joint shear (e.g., placing less stress on the ACL). Oxygen consumption (VO_2) is an important consideration when training athletes. **Aerobic conditioning (cardiorespiratory fitness)** in a healthy adult is recommended at 3-5 days per week for 20-60 minutes per session (training at 60-90% of maximum

Table 1-31. CHARACTERISTICS OF HUMAN SKELETAL MUSCLE FIBER TYPES

CHARACTERISTIC	TYPE I	TYPE IIA	TYPE IIB
Other names	Red, slow twitch (ST) Slow oxidative (SO)	White, fast twitch (FT) Fast oxidative glycolytic (FOG)	Fast glycolytic (FG)
Speed of contraction	Slow	Fast	Fast
Strength of contraction	Low	High	High
Fatigability	Fatigue-resistant	Fatigable	Most fatigable
Aerobic capacity	High	Medium	Low
Anaerobic capacity	Low	Medium	High
Motor unit size	Small	Larger	Largest
Capillary density	High	High	Low

From Simon, S.R.: Orthopaedic Basic Science, 2nd ed., p. 100. Rosemont, IL, American Academy of Orthopaedic Surgeons, 1994.

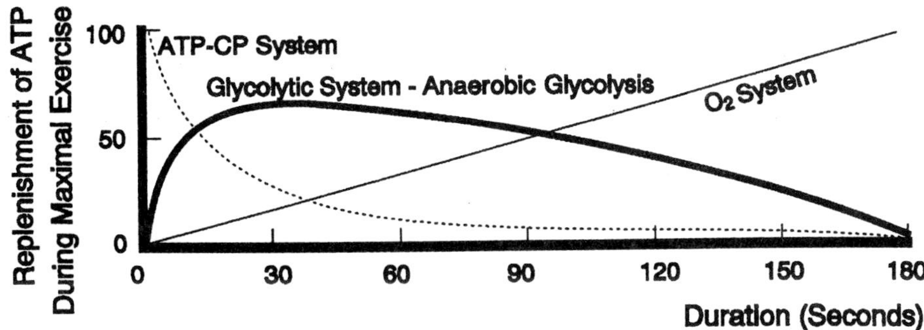

FIGURE 1-64 ■ Energy sources for muscle activity. (From Simon, S.R., ed.: Orthopaedic Basic Science, 2nd ed., p. 102. Rosemont, IL, American Academy of Orthopaedic Surgeons, 1994.)

heart rate). Long-distance runs increase aerobic capacity and endurance but decrease flexibility and optimum explosive strength. Aerobic conditioning has proved effective in lowering the incidence of back injury in workers and in helping the elderly to remain ambulatory. A significant decline in aerobic fitness ("detraining") occurs after just 2 weeks of no training. **Weight reduction** with fluid and food restriction (wrestlers, boxers, and jockeys trying to "make weight") is associated with reduced cardiac output, increased heart rate, smaller stroke volumes, lower oxygen consumption, decreased renal blood flow, and electrolyte loss. **Anabolic (androgenic) steroids** cause increased muscle strength (due to increased protein synthesis and an increase in aggressive behavior that promotes increased weight training), increased body weight, testicular atrophy, irreversible deepening of the female voice, reduction in testosterone and gonadotropic hormones, growth retardation, oligospermia, azoospermia, gynecomastia, hypertension, striae, cystic acne, alopecia (irreversible), liver tumors, increased low-density lipoprotein (LDL), decreased high-density lipoprotein (HDL), and abnormal liver isoenzymes lactate dehydrogenase (LDH). Anabolic steroids do not increase aerobic power or capacity for muscular exercise, but have been shown to be more effective than corticosteroids for long-term muscle strength recovery after contusion injury. Athletes who use pure testosterone extract to enhance performance have both anabolic and androgenic effects. The anabolic effects include muscle development, increased muscle mass, and erythropoiesis. Doping control (drug testing) for anabolic steroids is tested by the International Olympic Committee using urine sampling. Abuse of the **growth hormone somatotropin** among adults causes selective hypertrophy of type I muscle fibers, which produces atrophy of type II fibers, leading to muscle hypertrophy with weakness and fatigue. A syncopal episode in a young athlete suggests a serious underlying cardiac abnormality (and a risk of sudden death); a timely medical evaluation is mandatory before returning to athletics. The most common cause of **sudden death** in young athletes is hypertrophic obstructive cardiomyopathy. Abdominal injuries in athletes most commonly affect the kidney. Wrap-around polycarbonate glasses should be worn to protect the eyes in racquet sports. **Carbohydrate loading** involves increasing carbohydrates 3 days prior to an event (e.g., marathon) and decreasing physical activity. The best **fluid replacement** regimen for a competitive athlete is to replace enough water to maintain prepractice weight and maintain a

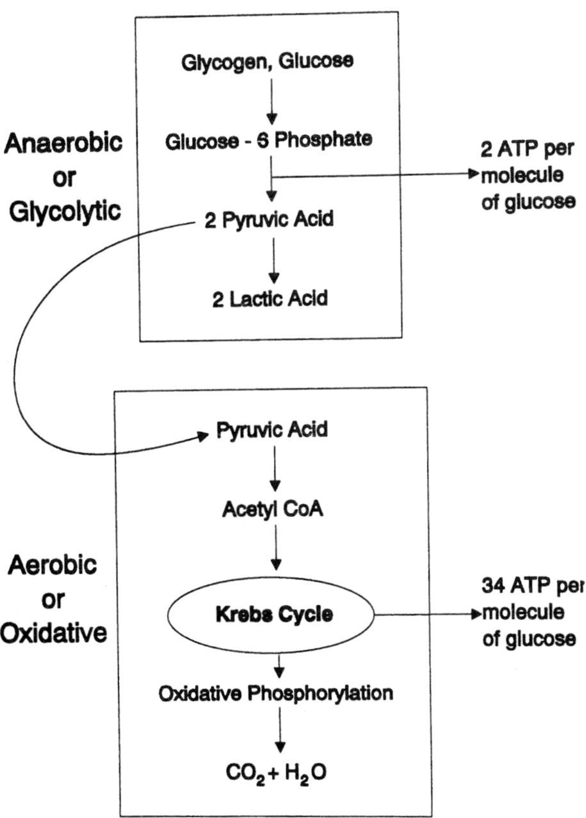

FIGURE 1-65 ■ ATP production via anaerobic and aerobic breakdown of carbohydrates: Glycolysis and anaerobic metabolism occur in the cytoplasm; oxidative phosphorylation occurs in the mitochondria. (From Simon, S.R., ed.: Orthopaedic Basic Science, 2nd ed., p. 104. Rosemont, IL, American Academy of Orthopaedic Surgeons, 1994.)

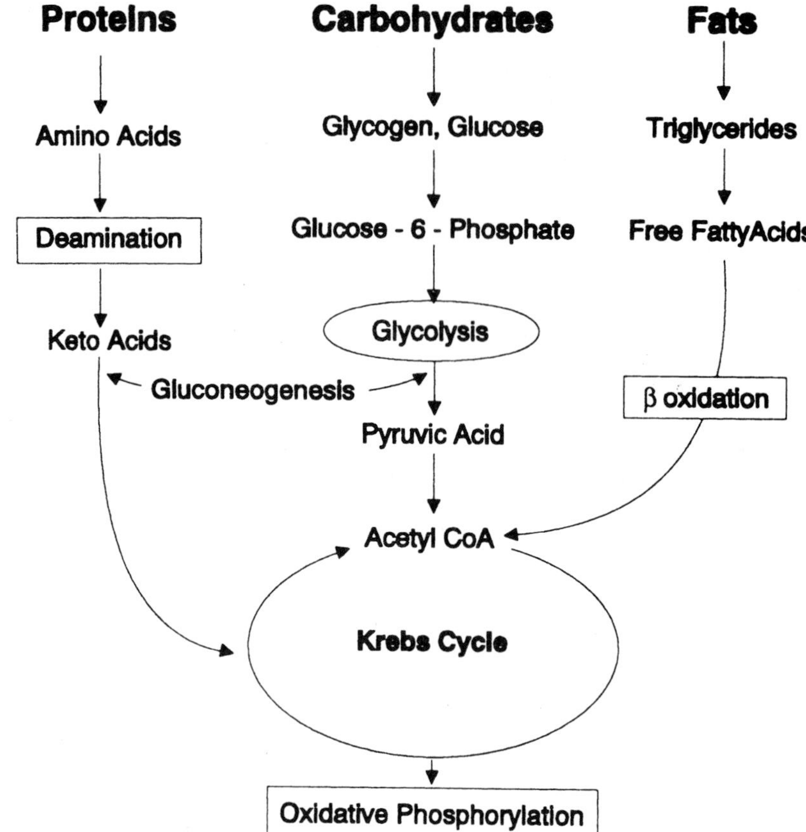

FIGURE 1-66 ■ Aerobic system for ATP (energy) production of skeletal muscle. (From Simon, S.R., ed.: Orthopaedic Basic Science, 2nd ed., p. 103. Rosemont, IL, American Academy of Orthopaedic Surgeons, 1994.)

normal diet. Fluid carbohydrate and electrolyte replacement is most effective when the osmolality of the replacement fluid is <10% (glucose polymers minimize osmolality); fluid absorption by the gut is enhanced by solutions of low osmolality. **Creatine supplements** are used by some athletes to attempt to enhance performance. The physiological basis for this is that creatine is converted to phosphocreatine, which acts as an energy reservoir for ATP in muscle. Recent studies have shown that **creatine supplementation can increase the amount of work that is produced in the first few maximum-effort anaerobic trials but does not increase peak force production**. Treatment of **heat cramps** includes passive stretching, cooling, and fluid/electrolyte replacement.

H. Female Athletes—The "female athlete triad" is **amenorrhea, osteoporosis,** and **anorexia**. Amenorrhea results from a decrease in the percentage of body fat, increased training, hormonal changes, competitive running before menarche, and changes in the hypothalamic-pituitary axis. Exercise-induced secondary amenorrhea leads to premature bone demineralization. Female athletes with stress fracture and a history of amenorrhea should undergo bone mineral density testing (using DEXA) to assess for bone loss. Initial management includes increasing weight, decreasing exercise, and possibly administration of cyclic estrogens or progesterones.

I. Muscle Injury—Most **muscle strains** (the most common sports injury) occur at the myotendinous junction in muscles that cross two joints (hamstring, gastrocnemius) and have increased type II fibers. Initially there is inflammation and later fibrosis. **Muscle tears occur most commonly at the myotendinous junction, often during a rapid (high-velocity) eccentric contraction; eccentric contractions develop the highest forces observed in skeletal muscle.** Muscle tears typically heal with dense scarring. Surgical repair of clean lacerations in the midbelly of skeletal muscle usually results in minimal regeneration of muscle fibers distally, scar formation at the laceration, and recovery of about one half of muscle strength. Muscle activation (via stretching) allows twice the energy absorption prior to failure; "bouncing" types of stretching are deleterious. **Muscle soreness** may result from eccentric muscle contractions and may be associated with changes in the I band of the sarcomere. Denervation causes muscle atrophy and increased sensitivity to acetylcholine, causing spontaneous fibrillations at 2-4 weeks after damage to the motor axon. Spasticity is related to increased muscle reactivity to stretch. Muscle strength gains during the first 10 days of rehabilitation are due to improved neural firing patterns. Later strength gains are due to increases in ROM, muscle fiber size, muscle repair, and tendon repair. Trunk extensors are stronger than trunk flexors.

J. Immobilization—Changes the number of sarcomeres at the musculotendinous junction and accelerates granulation tissue response in the injured muscle. Immobilization in lengthened positions decreases contractures and maintains strength. Atrophy can result from disuse or altered nervous system recruitment. Electrical stimulation can help offset these effects.

II. Nervous System

A. Organization

1. CNS—Patients may continue to improve up to 6 months after a **stroke** and up to 18 months after **traumatic brain injury**. The most common mechanism of **spinal cord injury** in adults is motor vehicle accidents. **Neurogenic shock** (a state of vasodilation presenting with paradoxical hypotension and bradycardia) following cervical or upper thoracic spinal cord injury occurs because the descending sympathetic pathways are disrupted. **Spinal cord injury patients seeking treatment <8 hours after injury have the best chance for optimizing their neurologic outcome if given methylprednisolone: <3 hours from injury = an initial bolus of 30 mg/kg followed by an infusion of 5.4 mg/kg/hr for 24 hours; between 3 and 8 hours from injury = an initial bolus of 30 mg/kg followed by an infusion of 5.4 mg/kg/hr for 48 hours.** This regimen is associated with improved root function at the level of the injury, although improvement of spinal cord function may or may not occur. **The regimen is not indicated for nerve root deficits, brachial plexus deficits, or gunshot wounds. Concussion** (Table 1-32) is a jarring injury to the brain that results in disturbance (to some degree) of cerebral function. Grade I injuries (mild): an athlete may return to play when asymptomatic. Grade II injuries (moderate): characterized by retrograde amnesia (persists for several minutes after injury) despite resolution of confusion and disorientation; a first-time grade II concussion allows return to play after a week without symptoms. Long periods without play (months) are required for a third-time grade I concussion, a second grade II concussion, or a first-time grade III (severe) concussion. Folic acid, as a dietary supplement, can decrease the chance of having a child with myelomeningocele.

2. Peripheral Nervous System (PNS) (Fig. 1-67)
   a. Nerves—Bundles of axons enclosed in a connective tissue sheath
   b. Nerve fiber—Axon plus surrounding Schwann cell sheath
      (1) Myelinated Fibers—An axon 1-2 μm in diameter is considered myelinated. Each myelinated axon is associated with one Schwann cell. Conduction velocity is faster than in unmyelinated fibers.
      (2) Unmyelinated fibers—One Schwann cell surrounds several axons. Conduction velocity is relatively slow.
      (3) Nerve Fibers
         (a) Afferents—Transmit information from sensory receptors to the CNS.
            1. Somatic Afferents—Originate in receptors in muscle, skin, and the sensory organs of the head (vision, hearing, taste, smell).
            2. Visceral Afferents—Originate in viscera.
         (b) Efferents—Transmit information from the CNS to the periphery. Motor efferents innervate skeletal muscle fibers.
            1. Somatic Efferents—Innervate skin, skeletal muscle, and joints.
            2. Autonomic Efferents (Splanchnics)—Innervate viscera.

B. Histology and Signal Generation

1. Neuron (Fig. 1-67)—Composed of four regions: cell body, axon, dendrites, and presynaptic terminal.

Table 1-32. CONCUSSION

SEVERITY	CHARACTERISTICS	TREATMENT
Grade I (mild)	No loss of consciousness No retrograde amnesia	Return to play as soon as asymptomatic (Long-term suspension of play for a third-time grade I concussion)
Grade II (moderate)	Loss of consciousness <5 minutes Retrograde amnesia (there is always some permanent loss of memory regarding the injury itself) Confusion and disorientation resolve rapidly	*First episode*—Return to play after asymptomatic for 1 week *Repeat episode*—Long-term suspension of play
Grade III (severe)	Prolonged unconsciousness Permanent retrograde amnesia Confusion and disorientation persist	Long-term suspension of play

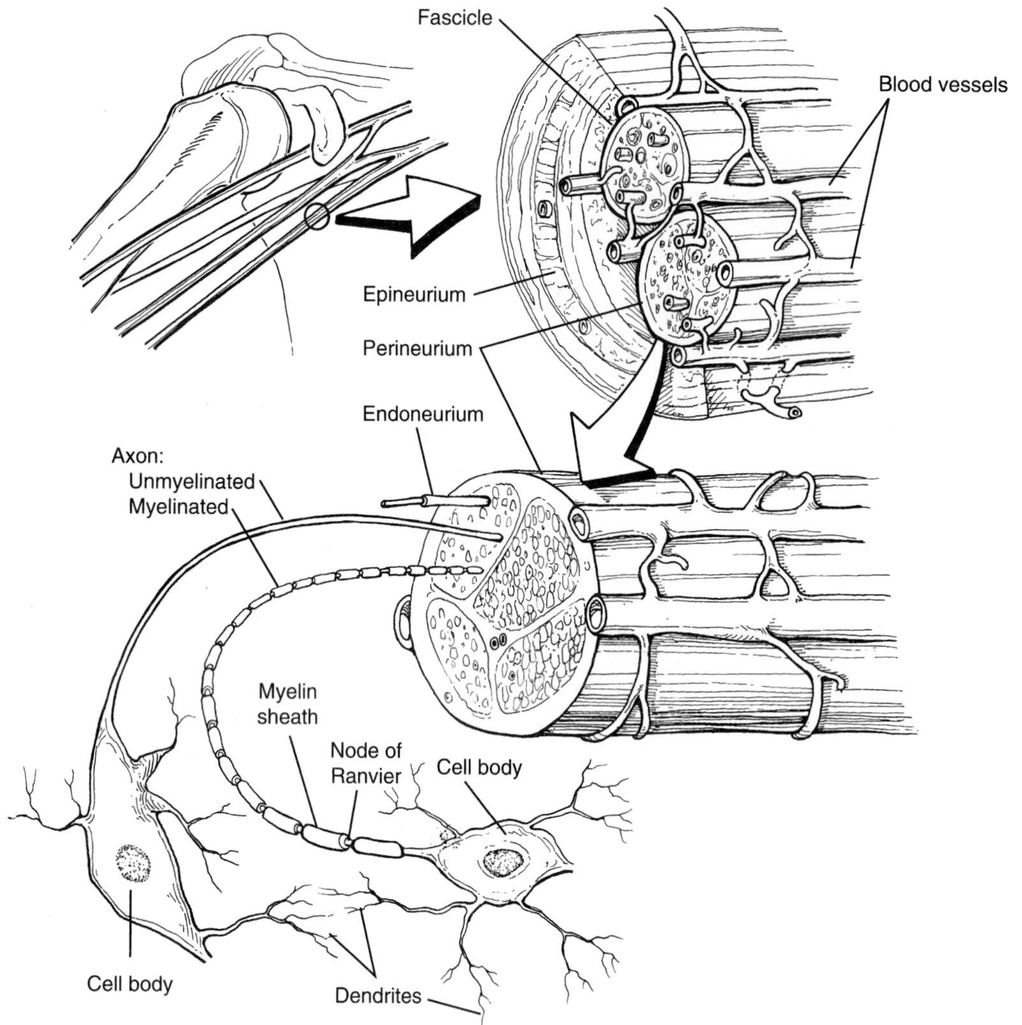

FIGURE 1-67 ■ Nerve architecture. (From Brinker, M.R., and Miller, M.D.: Fundamentals of Orthopaedics. Philadelphia, WB Saunders, 1999, p. 13.)

a. Cell Body—The metabolic center; accounts for <10% of neuron size; gives rise to a single axon.
b. Axon—Primary conducting vehicle of the neuron; conveys electrical signals (over long distances) via action potentials.
c. Dendrites—Thin processes branching from the cell body; receive input (synaptic) from surrounding nerve cells.
d. Presynaptic Terminals—Transmit information from one neuron to another (to the cell body or dendrites of the "receiving" neuron).

2. Glial Cells (Fig. 1-68)—Three basic types have been described: Schwann cells, oligodendrocytes, and astrocytes.
   a. Schwann cells—**Responsible for myelinating peripheral nerve axons** (forms an elongated double-membrane structure). Loss of the myelin sheath (demyelination) disrupts conduction of action potentials along the axon. Myelin is 70% lipid and 30% protein.
   b. Oligodendrocytes—Only in the CNS; form myelin.
   c. Astrocytes—Most common of the glial cells. Only in the CNS. Astrocytes have many functions but serve primarily as a supporting structure of the brain.
3. Resting and Action Potentials
   a. Resting Potential—Results from unequal distribution of ions on either side of the neuronal cell membrane (lipid bilayer). The four most plentiful ions about the cell membrane are Na^+, K^+, Cl^-, and a group of other organic ions (A^-). Resting potential of a neuron is −50 to −80 mV (cell inside is negative relative to outside) (Fig. 1-69).
   b. Action Potential—Transmits signals rapidly via electrical impulses to other neurons or effector organs (e.g., muscle). Depolarization

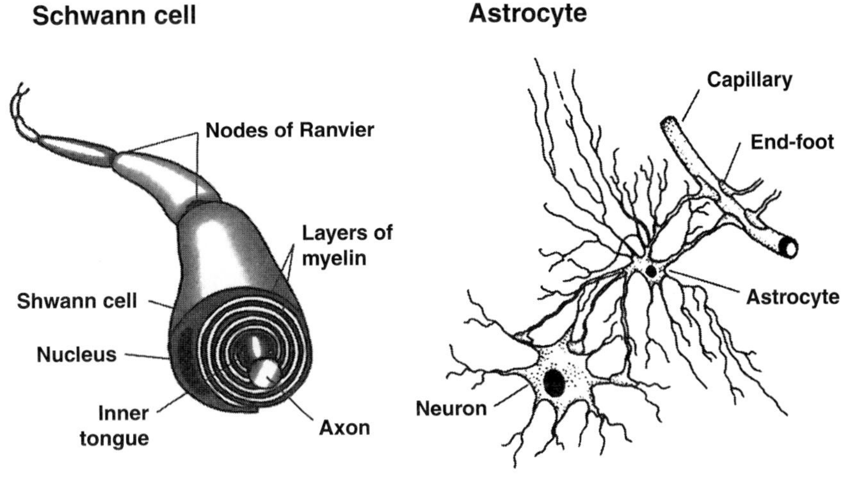

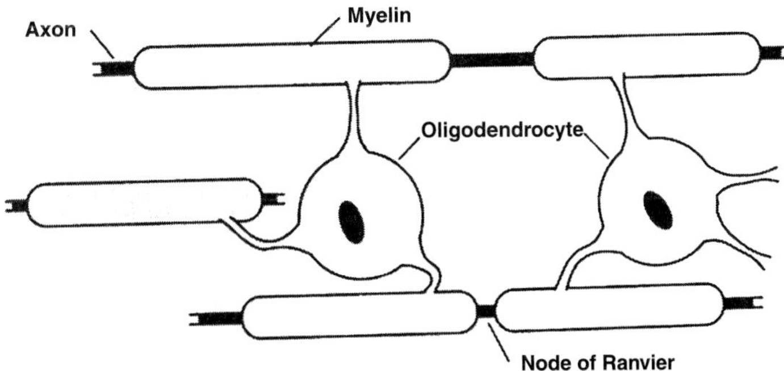

FIGURE 1-68 ■ Glial cells include the Schwann cell, astrocytes, and oligodendrocytes. (From Simon, S.R., ed.: Orthopaedic Basic Science, 2nd ed., p. 320. Rosemont, IL, American Academy of Orthopaedic Surgeons, 1994.)

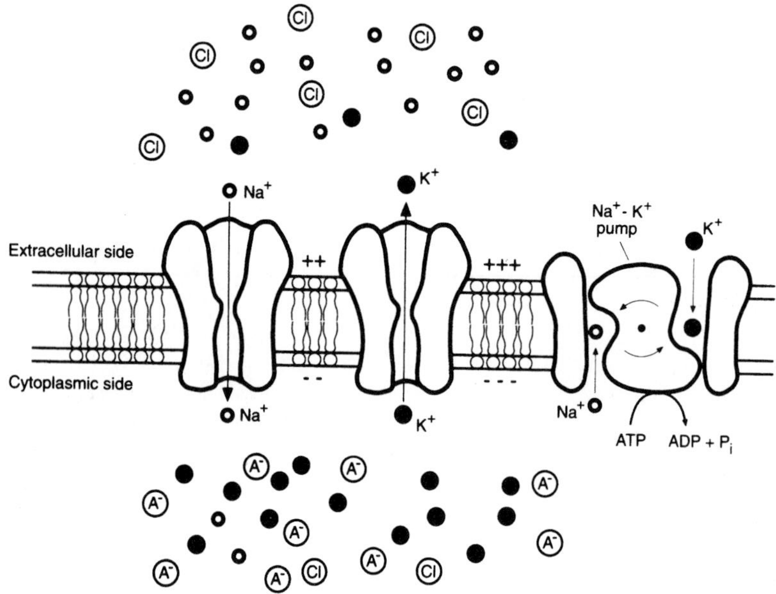

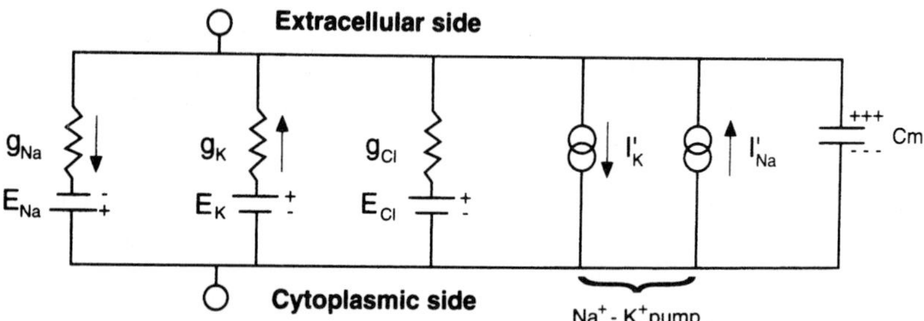

FIGURE 1-69 ■ Electrolyte transport across cell walls. *Top,* Passive fluxes of Na^+ and K^+ into and out of the cell are balanced by the energy-dependent sodium-potassium pump. *Bottom,* Electrical circuit model of a neuron at rest. (From Simon, S.R., ed.: Orthopaedic Basic Science, 2nd ed., p. 332. Rosemont, IL, American Academy of Orthopaedic Surgeons, 1994.)

and the action potential result from an increase in cell membrane permeability to Na^+ in response to a stimulus. This process is related to the three types of gated ion channels (Fig. 1-70): voltage-gated channels, mechanical gated channels, and chemical-transmitter gated channels. Action potentials propagate via both passive current flow and active membrane changes (Fig. 1-71).

C. Sensory System—**Sensory receptors** (located peripherally) receive messages from the environment and other parts of the body and transmit them to the CNS. The four attributes of a stimulus are quality, intensity, duration, and location. Sensory receptor types include photoreceptors (vision), mechanoreceptors (hearing, balance, mechanical stimuli), thermoreceptors (temperature), chemoreceptors (taste, smell), and nociceptors (pain). Neurogenic pain (and inflammatory) mediators are identifiable within the dorsal root ganglion of the lumbar spine. The pain associated with an osteoid osteoma comes from prostaglandins secreted by the tumor itself.

1. Somatosensory System—Conveys three modalities: mechanical, pain, and thermal. Each of these is mediated by a specific type of sensory receptor (Table 1-33). Somatosensory input from each of these three modalities is transmitted to the spinal cord (or brainstem) via the **dorsal root ganglion** (see Fig. 1-72).

D. Motor System—Organized into four areas: spinal cord, brainstem, motor cortex, and premotor cortical areas (basal ganglia and cerebellum).

1. Spinal Cord (Fig. 1-72)
   a. White Matter (peripheral)—Ascending and descending fiber tracts; myelinated and unmyelinated axons.
   b. Gray Matter (central)—Contains neuronal cell bodies, glial cells, dendrites, and axons (myelinated and unmyelinated); contains three types of neurons.
      (1) Motoneurons (α and γ)—Axons exit via ventral roots.
      (2) Interneurons—Axons remain in the spinal cord.
      (3) Tract Cells—Axons ascend to supraspinal centers.
   c. Spinal Cord Reflexes (Table 1-34)—A reflex is a "stereotyped response" to a specific sensory stimulus. **A reflex pathway involves a sensory organ (receptor), an interneuron, and a motoneuron.**
      (1) Monosynaptic Reflex—Only one synapse is involved between receptor and effector.
      (2) Polysynaptic Reflex—Involves one or more interneurons. **Most human reflexes are polysynaptic.**
2. Motor Unit—Composed of an α-motoneuron and the muscle fibers it innervates. Four types exist, based on physiologic demands (Table 1-35): type S (slow, fatigue resistant); type FR (fast, fatigue resistant); type FI (fast, fatigue intermediate); and type FF (fast fatigue).
3. Upper and Lower Motoneurons
   a. Upper Motoneurons—Located in the descending pathways of the cortex, brainstem, and spinal cord.
   b. Lower Motoneurons—Located in the ventral gray matter of the spinal cord.
   c. Motoneuron Lesions—Table 1-36 **shows findings associated with upper and lower motoneuron lesions. Spasticity**

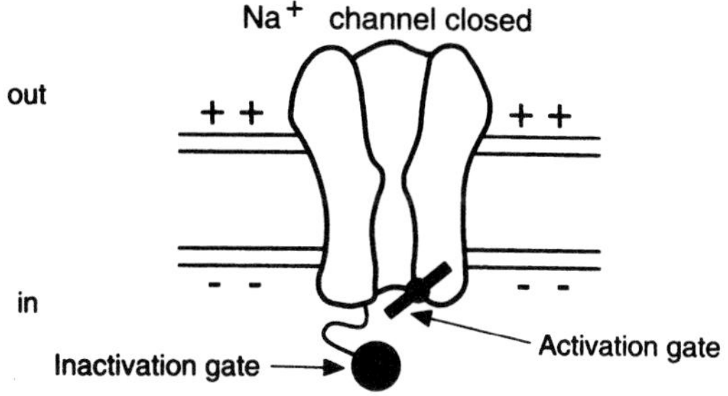

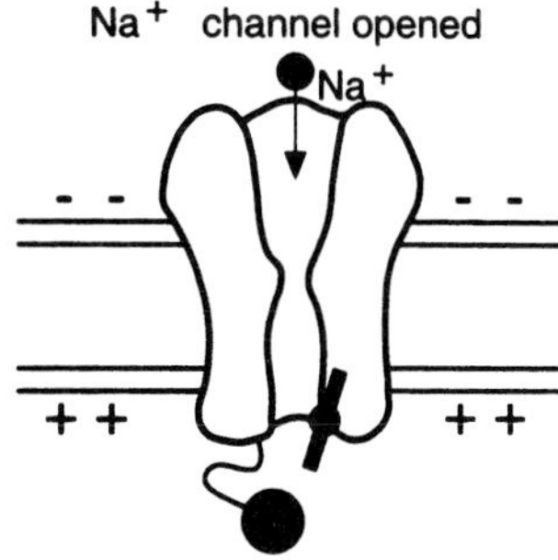

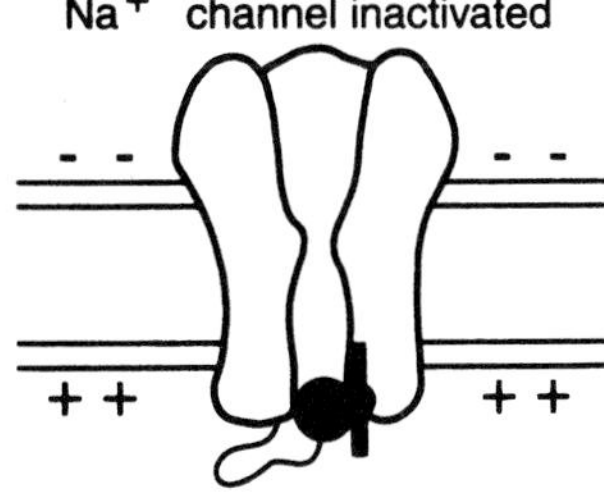

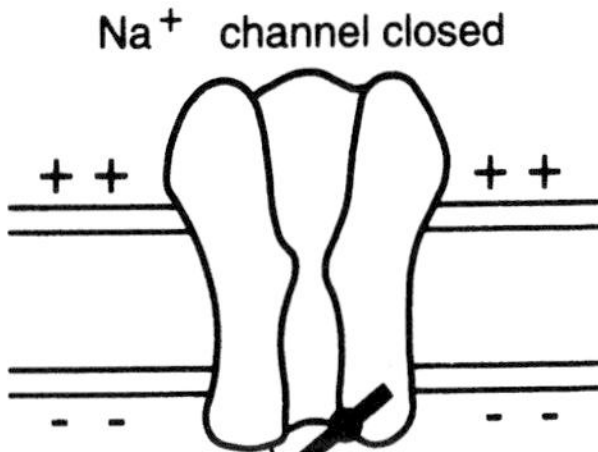

FIGURE 1-70 ■ Gated sodium channel response during an action potential. *Top to bottom:* rest, depolarization, maintenance of depolarization, repolarization. (From Kandel, E.R., Schwartz, J.H., and Jessel, T.M.: Principles of Neural Science, 3rd ed., p. 14. Norwalk, CT, Appleton & Lange, 1991.)

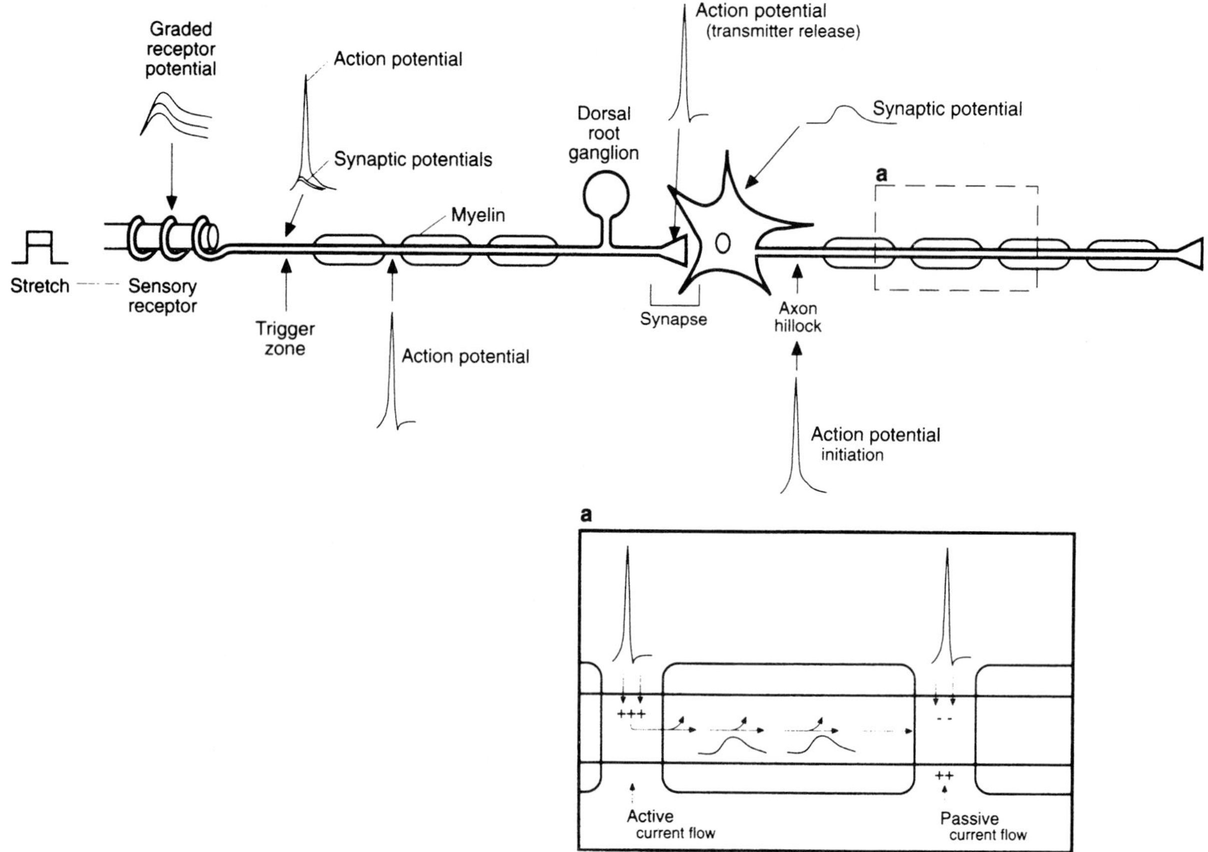

FIGURE 1-71 ■ Action potential is propagated to the terminal region, where it triggers the release of transmitter, which initiates a synaptic potential in the motoneuron. Action potential propagation results from the spread of local passive depolarizing currents between the nodes of Ranvier (*inset*). At the nodes, voltage-gated channels open, producing an action potential. (From Simon, S.R., ed.: Orthopaedic Basic Science, 2nd ed., p. 337. Rosemont, IL, American Academy of Orthopaedic Surgeons, 1994.)

Table 1-33. RECEPTOR TYPES

RECEPTOR TYPE	FIBER TYPE	QUALITY
Nociceptors		
Mechanical	Aδ	Sharp, pricking pain
Thermal and mechanothermal	Aγ	Sharp, pricking pain
Thermal and mechanothermal	C	Slow, burning pain
Polymodal	C	Slow, burning pain
Cutaneous and subcutaneous mechanoreceptors		
Meissner's corpuscle	Aβ	Touch
Pacini's corpuscle	Aβ	Flutter
Ruffini's corpuscle	Aβ	Vibration
Merkel's receptor	Aβ	Steady skin indentation
Hair-guard, hair-tylotrich	Aβ	Steady skin indentation
Hair down	Aβ	Flutter
Muscle and skeletal mechanoreceptors		
Muscle spindle primary	Aα	Limb proprioception
Muscle spindle secondary	Aβ	Limb proprioception
Golgi tendon organ	Aα	Limb proprioception
Joint capsule mechanoreceptor	Aβ	Limb proprioception

From Kandel, E.R., Schwartz, J.H., and Jessel, T.M., eds.: Principles of Neural Science, 3rd ed., p. 342. Norwalk, CT, Appleton & Lange, 1991.

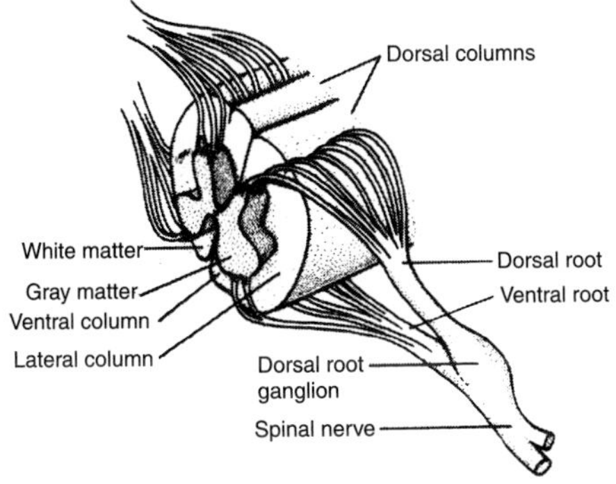

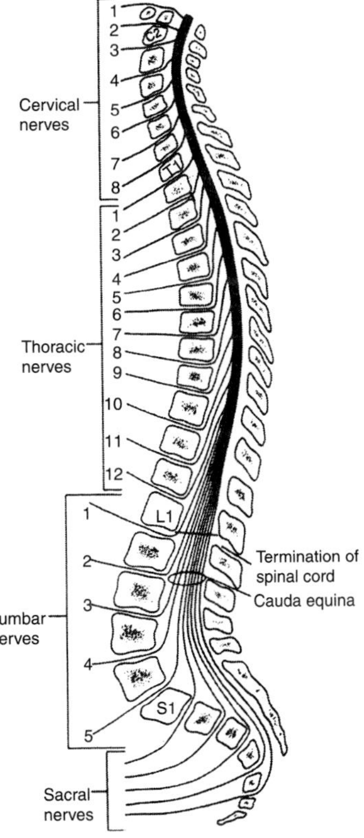

FIGURE 1-72 ■ Spinal cord anatomy. *Left,* Each spinal nerve has a dorsal (sensory) and a ventral (motor) root. Dorsal roots are branches from dorsal root ganglia cells; ventral roots are motor axons from cells in the ventral horn. *Right,* Note that the spinal cord terminates at the L1 vertebra. The dorsal and ventral roots of the lumbar and sacral nerves are collectively called the cauda equina. (From Kandel, E.R., Schwartz, J.H., and Jessel, T.M.: Principles of Neural Science, 3rd ed., pp. 285–286. Norwalk, CT, Appleton & Lange, 1991.)

is common in patients with an **upper motoneuron lesion**.

E. Peripheral Nerve
   1. Morphology (see Fig. 1-67)—The peripheral nerve is a highly organized structure composed of nerve fibers, blood vessels, and connective tissues. Axons, coated with a fibrous tissue called **endoneurium**, group into nerve bundles called **fascicles**, which are covered with connective tissue called **perineurium**. Peripheral nerves are composed of one (mono), a few (oligo), or several (poly) fascicles and surrounding areolar connective tissue **(epineurium)** enclosed within an epineural sheath.
   2. Nerve Fibers (Axons) (2-25 μm in diameter)—Three types of nerve fibers are shown in Table 1-37.
   3. Conduction—As has been previously discussed, myelinated axons conduct action potentials rapidly, facilitated by **nodes of Ranvier** (gaps between Schwann cells).
   4. Blood Supply
      a. Extrinsic—Vessels run in loose connective tissue surrounding the nerve trunk.
      b. Intrinsic—Vascular plexuses in the epineurium, perineurium, and endoneurium (with interconnections between these three plexuses).

F. Injury to the Nervous System—**Peripheral nerve injury** leads to death of the distal axons and **wallerian degeneration** (of myelin), which extends distal to the somatosensory receptor. Proximal axonal budding occurs (after a 1-month delay) and leads to regeneration at the rate of about

Table 1-34. SUMMARY OF SPINAL REFLEXES

SEGMENTAL REFLEX	RECEPTOR ORGAN	AFFERENT FIBER
Phasic stretch reflex	Muscle spindle (primary endings)	Type Ia (large myelinated)
Tonic stretch reflex	Muscle spindle (secondary endings)	Type II (intermediate myelinated)
Clasp-knife response	Muscle spindle (secondary endings)	Type II (intermediate myelinated)
Flexion withdrawal reflex	Nociceptors (free nerve endings), touch and pressure receptors	Flexor-reflex afferents: small unmyelinated cutaneous afferents (A-delta, C and muscle afferents, group III)
Autogenic inhibition	Golgi tendon organ	Type 1b (large myelinated)

From Simon, S.R.: Orthopaedic Basic Science, 2nd ed., p. 350. Rosemont, IL, American Academy of Orthopaedic Surgeons, 1994.

Table 1-35. GENERAL CHARACTERISTICS OF MOTOR UNIT TYPES

PARAMETER	MOTOR UNIT TYPES		
	FF	*FR*	*S*
Muscle unit physiology[a]			
Contraction time	Fastest	Slightly slower	Slowest
Sag	Present	Present	Absent
Maximum tension	Largest	Smaller	Smallest
Fatigue index	<0.25	<0.75-1.00	0.7-1.0
Muscle unit anatomy[b]			
Innervation ratio	2.9	2.1	1.0
Fiber cross-sectional area	1.3	0.98	1.0
Specific tension	1.4	1.2	1.0
Muscle unit metabolism			
Fiber type	FG	FOG	SO
Myosin heavy chain	IIB	IIA	I
Glycogen	High	High	Low
Hexokinase	Low	Intermediate	High
Glycolytic enzymes	High	High	Low
Oxidative enzymes	Low	High	High
Cytochrome c	Low	High	High
Capillary supply	Sparse	Rich	Very rich
Motoneuron			
Cell body size	Largest	Slightly smaller	Smallest
Conduction velocity	Fastest	Slightly slower	Slowest
After-hyperpolarization duration	Shortest	Slightly shorter	Longest
Input resistance	Lowest	Slightly higher	Highest

FF, fast fatigable; FR, fast fatigue-resistant; S, fatigue-resistant; FG, fast glycolytic; FOG, fast oxidative glycolytic; SO, slow oxidative.
[a]Data relative to the FF unit.
[b]Data relative to the slow unit.
From Simon, S.R.: Orthopaedic Basic Science, 2nd ed., p. 344. Rosemont, IL, American Academy of Orthopaedic Surgeons, 1994; reprinted by permission.

1 mm/day (possibly 3-5 mm/day in children). Nerve regeneration is influenced by contact guidance (attraction to the basal lamina of the Schwann cell), neurotrophism (factors enhancing growth), and neurotropism (preferential attraction toward nerves rather than other tissues). **Pain is the first modality to return. Nerve injury may be characterized as one of three types (Table 1-38).** Mechanical deformation of a compressed peripheral nerve is greatest in superficial regions and in zones between compressed and uncompressed segments. **Nerve stretching** can also affect function: 8% elongation diminishes a nerve's microcirculation; 15% elongation disrupts axons. **"Stingers"** (or "burners") refer to neuropraxia from a brachial plexus stretch injury, seen most commonly in football players; time for recovery is variable as are residual sequela (e.g., permanent muscle atrophy). Neurologic studies electromyography [EMG], nerve conduction studies [NCS] may be useful to document injury extent in patients with muscle atrophy or motor weakness. Cortical evoked potential testing is the most sensitive method of predicting neural compression. In a patient with an injury of the brachial plexus, a **positive histamine response** implies that there is an intact reflex arc (afferent nerve,

Table 1-36. FINDINGS IN UPPER AND LOWER MOTONEURON LESIONS

FINDINGS	UPPER MOTONEURON LESIONS	LOWER MOTONEURON LESIONS
Strength	Decreased	Decreased
Tone	Increased	Decreased
Deep tendon reflexes	Increased	Decreased
Superficial tendon reflexes	Decreased	Decreased
Babinski's sign	Present	Absent
Clonus	Present	Absent
Fasciculations	Absent	Present
Atrophy	Absent	Present

From Simon, S.R.: Orthopaedic Basic Science, 2nd ed., p. 354. Rosemont, IL, American Academy of Orthopaedic Surgeons, 1994.

Table 1-37. TYPES OF NERVE FIBERS

TYPE	DIAMETER (μM)	MYELINATION	SPEED	EXAMPLES
A	10-20	Heavy	Fast	Touch
B	<3	Intermediate	Medium	ANS
C	<1.3	None	Slow	Pain

ANS, autonomic nervous system.

Table 1-38. TYPES OF NERVE INJURIES

INJURY	PATHOPHYSIOLOGY	PROGNOSIS
Neuropraxia	Reversible conduction block characterized by local ischemia and selective demyelination of the axon sheath	Good
Axonotmesis	More severe injury with disruption of the axon and myelin sheath but leaving the epineurium intact	Fair
Neurotmesis	Complete nerve division with disruption of the endoneurium	Poor

efferent nerve, intervening cell body or ganglion), indicating that the lesion is proximal to the ganglion (preganglionic). **Cauda equina** syndrome is discussed in Chapter 7, Spine. A double-level cauda equina nerve root compression (even at low pressures) results in a dramatic reduction in impulse conduction and blood flow as compared with a single-level cauda equina compression. The nucleus pulposus induces an inflammatory response when in contact with the nerve roots: the response includes leukotaxis, increased vascular permeability, and decreased nerve conduction velocities.

G. Nerve Repair—Several methods are available. Younger patients have a better chance of recovery than do older patients after an operative repair of a nerve transection. It is critical to properly align nerve ends during surgical repair in order to maximize potential for functional recovery.
   1. Direct Muscular Neurotization—Insert the proximal nerve stump into the affected muscle belly; results in less than normal function, but is indicated in selected cases.
   2. Epineural Repair—Primary repair of the outer connective tissue layer of the nerve at the site of injury after resecting the proximal neuroma and distal glioma. Care is taken to ensure proper rotation and lack of tension on the repair.
   3. Grouped Fascicular Repair—Identical to epineural repair, but with reapproximation of individual fascicles under microscopic control. Used for large nerves, but no significant improvement in results over epineural repair has been demonstrated.

III. Connective Tissues

A. Tendons (Fig. 1-73)—Dense, regularly arranged tissues that attach muscle to bone. Tendons are composed of fascicles (groups of collagen bundles),

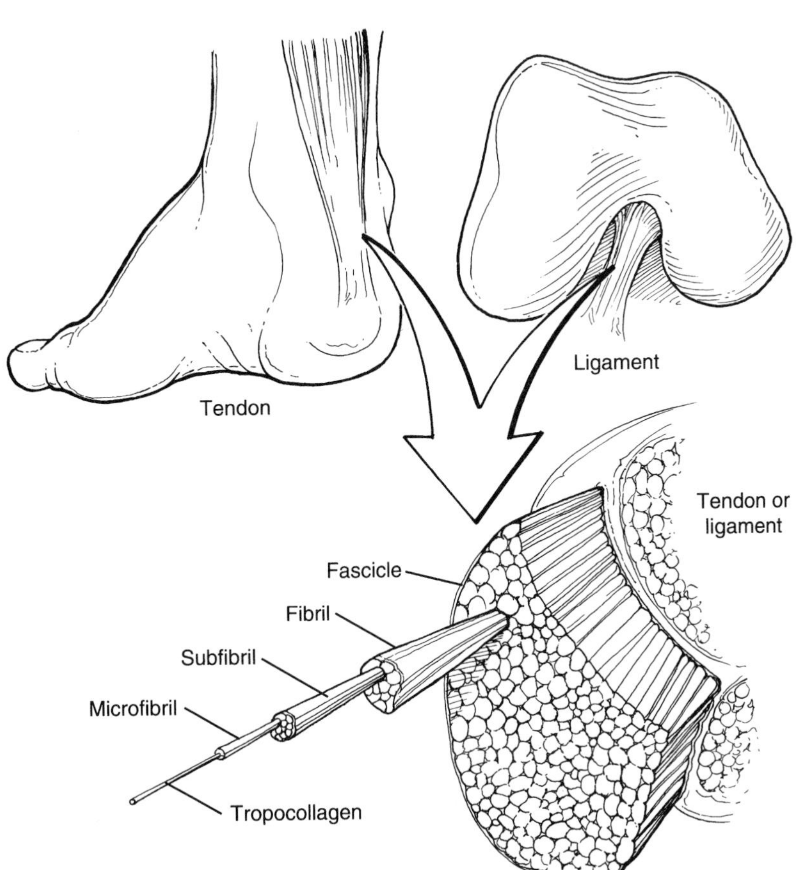

FIGURE 1-73 ■ Tendon and ligament architecture. (From Brinker, M.R., and Miller, M.D.: Fundamentals of Orthopaedics. Philadelphia, WB Saunders, 1999, p. 15.)

separated by **endotenon** and surrounded by **epitenon**. Tendons consist of fibroblasts (predominant cell type) arranged in parallel rows (Fig. 1-74) in fascicles (composed of fibrils) with surrounding loose areolar tissue (peritenon). Fibroblasts produce mostly type I collagen (85% of the dry weight of tendon). **Tendon inserts into bone via four transitional tissues (for force dissipation): tendon, fibrocartilage, mineralized fibrocartilage (Sharpey's fibers), and bone.** Two types of tendons exist: (1) paratenon-covered tendons and (2) sheathed tendons. Paratenon-covered tendons (vascular tendons) have many vessels supplying a rich capillary system (Fig. 1-75). With a sheathed tendon, a mesotenon (vincula) carries a vessel that supplies only one tendon segment; avascular areas receive nutrition via diffusion from vascularized segments (Fig. 1-76). Because of these vascular differences, paratenon-covered tendons heal better. Tendinous structures tend to orient themselves along stress lines. Tendinous healing after injury is initiated by fibroblasts from the epitenon and macrophages that initiate healing and remodeling. Treatment affects the repair process. Tendon healing occurs in large part through intrinsic capabilities. Tendon repairs are **weakest at 7-10 days**; they regain most of their original strength at 21-28 days and achieve **maximum strength at 6 months**. Early mobilization allows

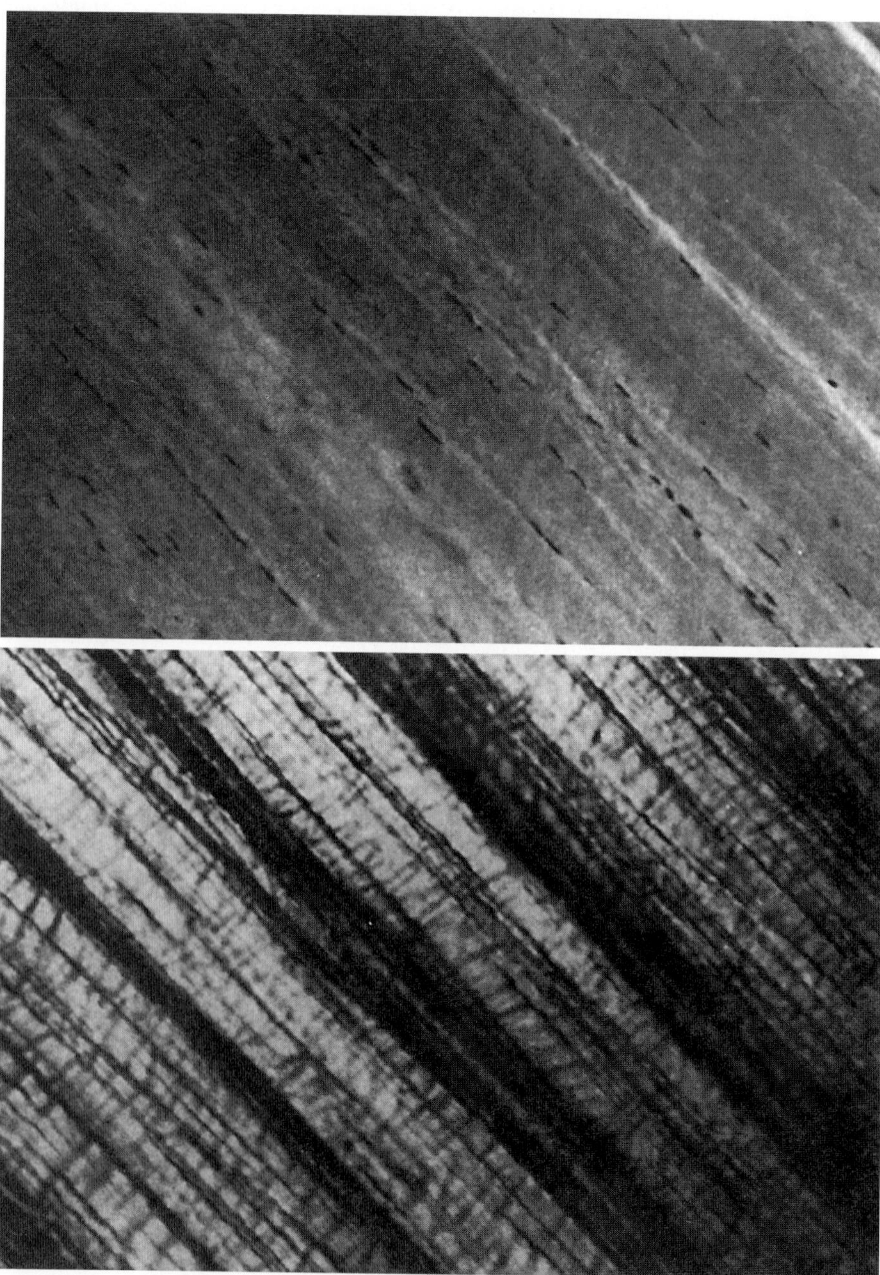

FIGURE 1-74 ■ *Top,* Photomicrograph of a flexor tendon with parallel rows of fibroblasts and collagen bundles. *Bottom,* Polarized light photograph of the same section illustrating parallel, longitudinally arranged collagen bundles. (From Simon, S.R., ed.: Orthopaedic Basic Science, 2nd ed., p. 49. Rosemont, IL, American Academy of Orthopaedic Surgeons, 1994.)

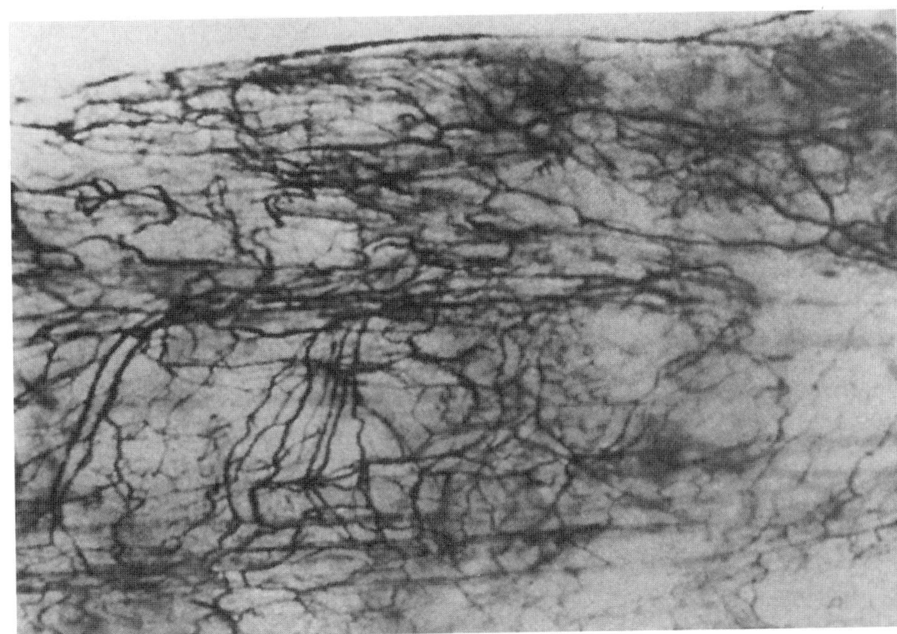

FIGURE 1-75 ■ India ink injection of rabbit calcaneal tendon (Spalteholz technique) demonstrating the vasculature of the paratenon. (From Simon, S.R., ed.: Orthopaedic Basic Science, 2nd ed., p. 50. Rosemont, IL, American Academy of Orthopaedic Surgeons, 1994.)

increased ROM but results in decreased tendon repair strength. Immobilization leads to increased tendon substance strength at the expense of ROM but tends to decrease the strength at the tendon-bone interface. Bony avulsions of tendon insertions heal more rapidly than midsubstance tears. Animal experiments (goats) have demonstrated no significant benefit from the creation of a trough (exposing the tendon to cancellous bone) for a tendon repair as compared with direct repair to cortical bone.

B. Ligaments (see Fig. 1-73)—Composed of type I collagen (70% of the dry weight of ligament), these structures help to stabilize joints. Their ultrastructure is similar to that of tendons, but the fibers are more variable and have a **higher elastin content. Unlike tendons, ligaments have a "uniform microvascularity," which receives its supply at the insertion site.** They also possess mechanoreceptors and free nerve endings that may play a role in stabilizing joints. Collagen sliding plays an important role in changes in ligament length (during growth and contracture). **Ligament insertion into bone** represents a transition from one material to another and can be classified into two types: **indirect insertion** (more common) and **direct insertion**. Indirect insertion: superficial ligament fibers insert at acute angles into the periosteum. Direct insertion: has both superficial and deep fibers; the deep fibers attach to bone at 90-degree angles and the **transition from ligament to bone occurs in four phases: ligament, fibrocartilage, mineralized fibrocartilage, and bone**. Healing (three phases, as in bone) benefits from normal stress and strain across the joint. **Early ligament healing is with type III collagen that is later converted to type I collagen.** Immobilization adversely affects the strength (elastic modulus decreases) of an intact ligament and of a ligament repair. In animal studies (rabbit), medial collateral ligament (MCL) breaking strength was reduced dramatically (66%) after 9 weeks of cast immobilization. The negative effects of immobilization reverse slowly upon remobilization. The mechanical properties of a ligament return toward normal much more rapidly than those of an insertion site. Exercise increases ligaments' mechanical and structural properties. **The most common mechanism of ligament failure is rupture of sequential series of collagen fiber bundles** distributed throughout the body of the ligament and not localized to one specific area. **Ligaments do not plastically deform** ("they break, not bend"). **Midsubstance ligament tears are common in adults; avulsion injuries are more common in children.** Local injection of corticosteroids at the site of an injured ligament is detrimental to the healing process. **Ligamentous avulsion typically occurs between the unmineralized and mineralized fibrocartilage layers.** The fixation site is the most common location for an immediate postoperative failure of a bone-patellar tendon-bone ACL reconstruction. **The major blood supply for the cruciate ligaments is the middle genicular artery.**

C. Intervertebral Discs—Allow spinal motion and stability. Two components: central nucleus pulposus (a hydrated gel with compressibility; high GAG/low collagen) and a surrounding annulus

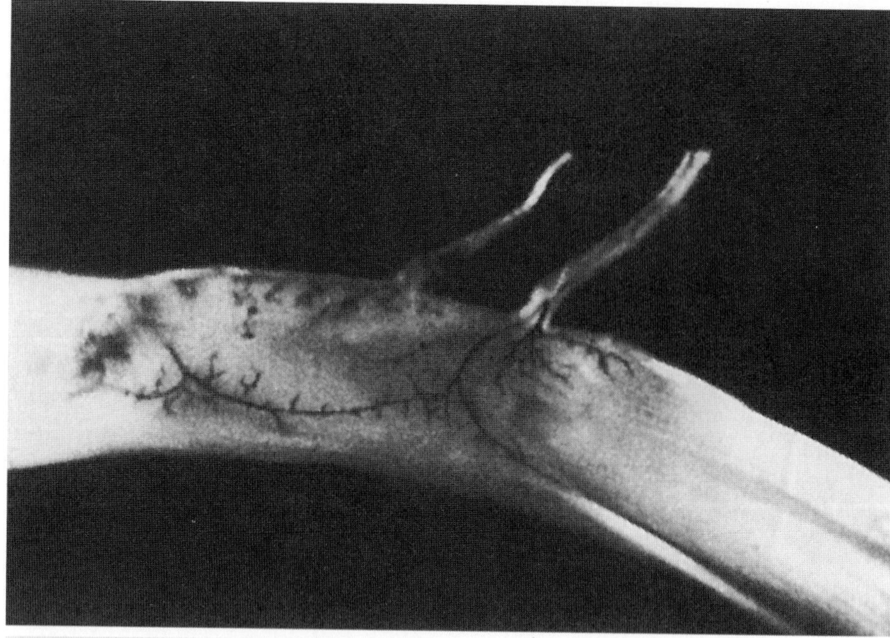

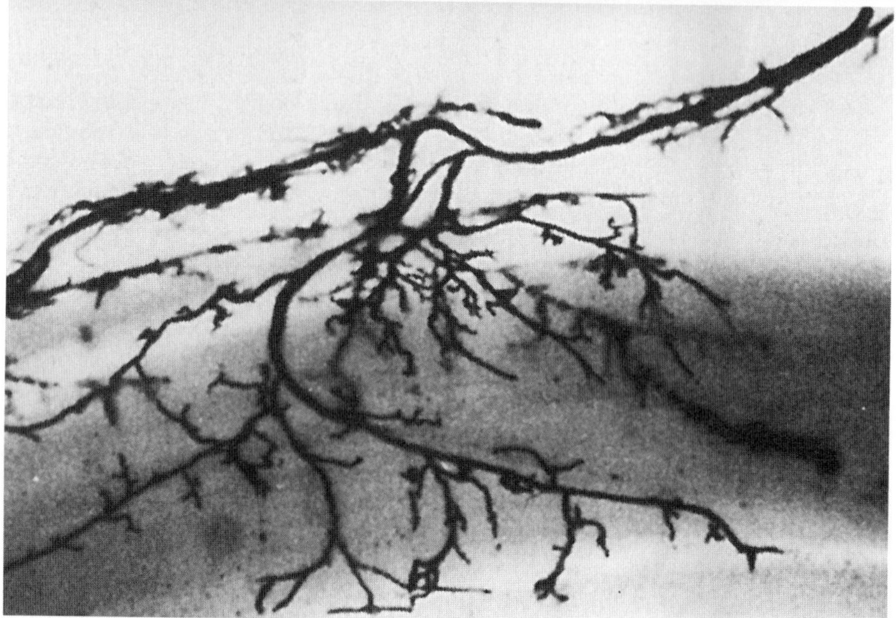

FIGURE 1-76 ■ *Top,* India ink specimens demonstrating the vascular supply of the flexor tendons via vincula. *Bottom,* Close-up of the specimen. (From Simon, S.R., ed.: Orthopaedic Basic Science, 2nd ed., p. 51. Rosemont, IL, American Academy of Orthopaedic Surgeons, 1994.)

fibrosis (extensibility and increased tensile strength; high collagen/low GAG). Composed of water (85%), proteoglycans, and **collagen types I and II** (type I in the annulus fibrosis; type II in the nucleus pulposus). The aging disc shows decreased water content (as a result of a lack of large proteoglycans and aggrecans and decreased proteoglycan concentration; but keratin sulfate concentration increases with age) and increased collagen. The superficial layer of the annulus contains nerve fibers. Various neuropeptides, (believed to be involved in sensory transmission, nociceptive transmission, neurogenic inflammation, and skeletal metabolism) include substance P, calcitonin gene-related peptide, vasoactive intestinal peptide (VIP), and the c-flanking peptide of neuropeptide Y (CPON). Cigarette smoking is a predisposing factor to degenerative disc disease.

D. Soft-Tissue Healing
   1. Four phases of soft-tissue healing have been described.
      a. Hemostasis—Primary platelet plug is formed within 5 minutes of injury. Secondary clotting via the coagulation cascade and fibrin occurs within 10-15 minutes. Fibronectin, a large glycoprotein, binds fibrin to cells and acts as a chemotactic factor. Platelets release factors that activate the next phase of healing.

b. Inflammation—Involves débridement of injured/necrotic tissue via macrophages and occurs within the first week. It has three stages: (1) activation (immediate); (2) amplification (48-72 hours); and (3) débridement (using bacteria, phagocytosis, and matrix [biochemical] means). Prostaglandins help to mediate the inflammatory response.
c. Organogenesis—Occurs at 7-21 days and consists of tissue modeling. Mesenchymal precursors differentiate into myofibroblasts. Angiogenesis occurs. Further differentiation leads to the final stage of healing.
d. Remodeling (of Individual Tissue Lines)—Continues for up to 18 months. Realignment and cross-linking of collagen fibers allows increased tensile strength.

2. Growth Factors—Require activation, are redundant, and function through feedback loop mechanisms.
   a. Chemotactic Factors—Attract cells. The factors include prostaglandins (PMNs), prostanoids (PMNs), complement (PMNs and macrophages), PDGF (macrophages and fibroblasts), and angiokines (endothelial cells).
   b. Competence Factors—Activate dormant (G_0) cells. Include PDGF and prostaglandins.
   c. Progression Factors—Allow cell growth. Induce epidermal growth factor, IL-1, and somatomedins.
   d. Inductive Factors—Stimulate differentiation. Include angiokines, bone morphogenic protein, and specific tissue growth factors.
   e. Transforming Factors—Cause dedifferentiation and proliferation.
   f. Permissive Factors—Enhancing factors; include fibronectin and osteonectin.

E. Soft-Tissue Implants
1. Introduction—Usually used around the knee (ACL); implants can be allografts, autografts, and synthetics.
2. Allografts—Have no donor-site morbidity but incite an immune response and may transmit infection **(risk of HIV exposure from a ligament allograft is 1 in 1 million)**. Freeze-drying reduces the immunogenic response, but also decreases strength (deep freezing without drying does not significantly affect strength). If not harvested under sterile conditions, treatment with cold ethylene oxide gas may have adverse effects **(graft failure)**, particularly if >3 M rad irradiation is used in conjunction (2 M rad with ethylene oxide does not appear to significantly decrease the mechanical properties). Allograft ligaments exhibit slower, less predictable histologic recovery than autografts.
3. Synthetic Ligaments—Unlike autografts or allografts, these structures have no initial period of weakness. However, they suffer from wear (debris) and are associated with **sterile joint effusions** having increased levels of neutral proteinases **(collagenase** and gelatinase) and chondrocyte activation factor (IL-1).

F. Miscellaneous—Fibroblastic proliferation in Dupuytren's contracture is associated with PDGF, TGF-β, and epidermal growth factor. A **fibrillin** (a component of the elastic fiber system) metabolism defect has been demonstrated in some patients with adolescent idiopathic scoliosis and fibrillin abnormalities have been demonstrated in most patients with Marfan's syndrome.

SECTION 4

Cellular and Molecular Biology, Immunology, and Genetics of Othopaedics

The fields of molecular biology, immunology, and genetics are rapidly expanding, including advances specific to the field of musculoskeletal science. This section introduces the basic concepts of these fields.

I. Cellular and Molecular Biology

A. Chromosomes—Human chromosomes are located in the nucleus of every cell (46 chromosomes; 23 pairs [22 pairs of autosomes and 1 pair of sex chromosomes]). Each chromosome contains >150,000 **genes**. The genes are regulated so that a relatively small number of genes are expressed for any given cell. Regulation of **gene expression** determines the unique biologic qualities of each cell. Chromosomes contain both DNA and ribonucleic acid (RNA).

B. DNA—All nuclear DNA resides in the 23 chromosome pairs. Located within the chromosome (in the cell nucleus), DNA is responsible for regulating cellular functions via **protein synthesis**. DNA has been classically described as a double helix (double strands) that contains **two sugar molecules** (each strand of DNA represents one sugar molecule), each of which has one of four nitrogenous bases (adenine, guanine, cytosine, thymine) (Fig. 1-77). The nitrogenous bases from one strand are linked to those of the other strand via hydrogen bonds. (In DNA, adenine is always linked to thymine, and guanine is always linked to cytosine.) DNA is important for three cellular processes: (1) DNA replication; (2) transcription of messenger RNA (mRNA); (3) regulation of cell division and the production of mRNA.

C. Nucleotide—The sugar molecule plus one nitrogenous base. The nucleotide sequence in one strand of DNA determines the complimentary nucleotide sequence in the other strand. The genetic message is grouped into three-letter words known as **codons**. The codon specifies one of the possible 20 amino acids that are the building blocks of all proteins (Fig. 1-78).

D. Gene—Portion of DNA that codes for a specific enzyme ("one gene equals one enzyme").

E. Transcription (Fig. 1-79)—To produce a specific protein, the DNA of the gene for that specific protein must be transcribed to an mRNA molecule (via RNA polymerase).

F. Translation (see Fig. 1-79)—Process by which mRNA builds proteins from amino acids.

G. Protein Coding and Regulation—Each **codon** is a sequence of three nucleotides in DNA or RNA that provides the genetic code information for one of the 20 amino acids that are the building blocks of all proteins (Figs. 1-78 and 1-80). Between functional coding sequences are large noncoding sequences known as **regulating DNA**. The **gene promoter** is part of the regulatory DNA and is required for transcription. **Consensus sequences** (named for a specific nucleotide sequence) serve as binding sites for specific proteins involved in gene regulation. **Gene enhancers** are binding sites for proteins (transcription factors) that are involved in the regulation of transcription. Protein coding and regulation are shown in Figure 1-81.

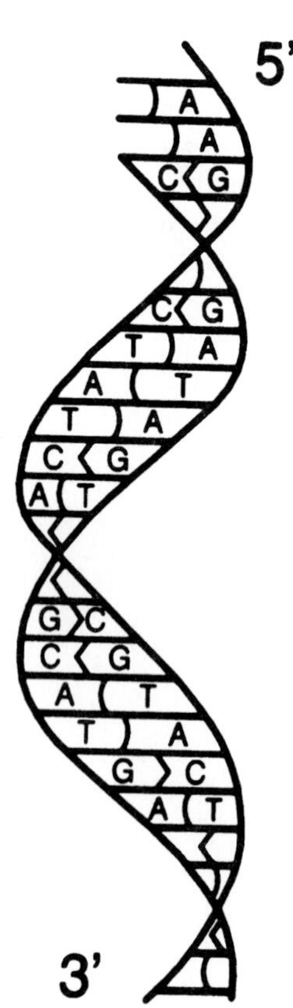

FIGURE 1-77 ■ DNA structure. The two deoxyribose strands are connected by a pair of nucleotides (which form the rung of the ladder) connected by hydrogen bonds. A, adenine; T, thymine; C, cytosine; G, guanine. (From Simon, S.R., ed.: Orthopaedic Basic Science, 2nd ed., p. 221. Rosemont, IL, American Academy of Orthopaedic Surgeons, 1994.)

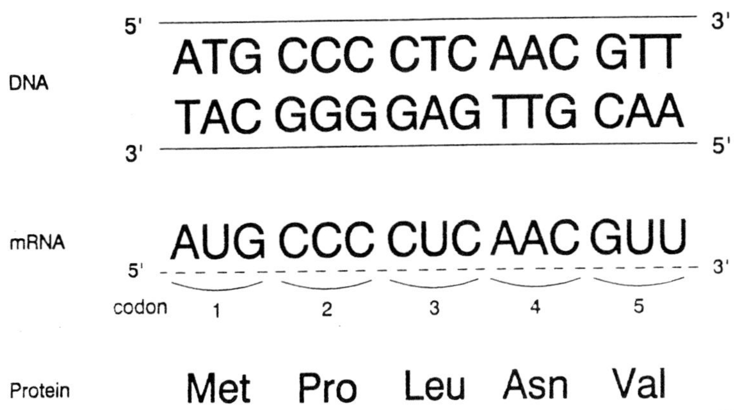

FIGURE 1-78 ■ A genetic message begins as a double-stranded DNA molecule, which serves as the template for messenger RNA. The mRNA, in groups of three nucleotides to a codon, directs the order of amino acids in protein. (From Ross, D.W., ed.: Introduction to Molecular Medicine, 2nd ed., p. 4. New York, Springer-Verlag, 1996.)

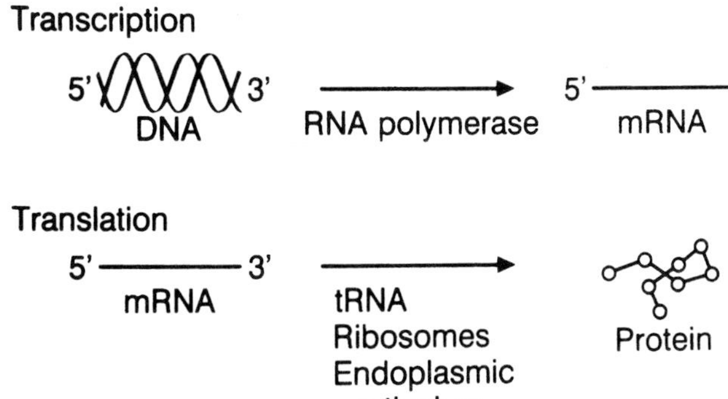

FIGURE 1-79 ■ DNA information is transcribed into RNA in the nucleus. mRNA is then transported to the cytoplasm where translation into proteins occurs in the endoplasmic reticulum. DNA, deoxyribonucleic acid; RNA, ribonucleic acid; mRNA, messenger RNA; tRNA, transfer RNA. (From Simon, S.R., ed.: Orthopaedic Basic Science, 2nd ed., p. 222. Rosemont, IL, American Academy of Orthopaedic Surgeons, 1994.)

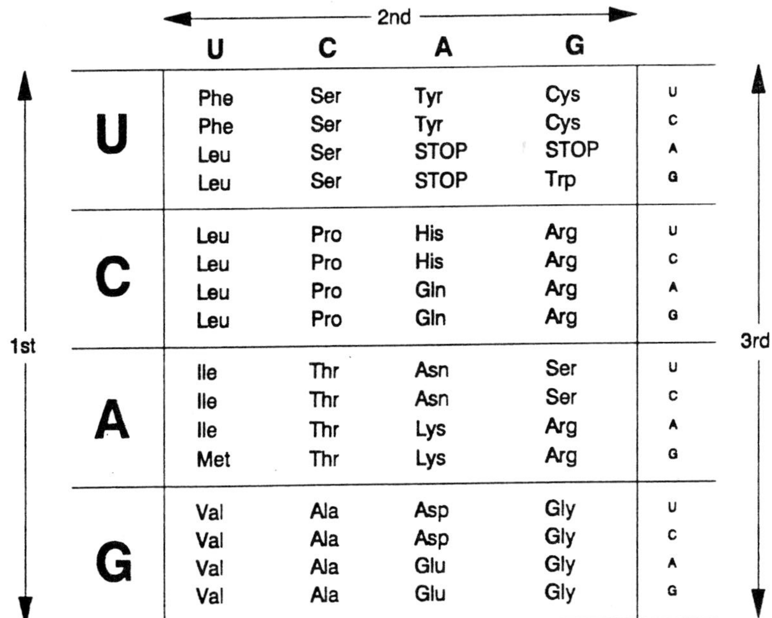

1st	2nd: U	C	A	G	3rd
U	Phe	Ser	Tyr	Cys	U
	Phe	Ser	Tyr	Cys	C
	Leu	Ser	STOP	STOP	A
	Leu	Ser	STOP	Trp	G
C	Leu	Pro	His	Arg	U
	Leu	Pro	His	Arg	C
	Leu	Pro	Gln	Arg	A
	Leu	Pro	Gln	Arg	G
A	Ile	Thr	Asn	Ser	U
	Ile	Thr	Asn	Ser	C
	Ile	Thr	Lys	Arg	A
	Met	Thr	Lys	Arg	G
G	Val	Ala	Asp	Gly	U
	Val	Ala	Asp	Gly	C
	Val	Ala	Glu	Gly	A
	Val	Ala	Glu	Gly	G

FIGURE 1-80 ■ The genetic code for translation of the triplet nucleotide codons of mRNA into amino acids in proteins. (From Ross, D.W., ed.: Introduction to Molecular Medicine, 2nd ed., p. 7. New York, Springer-Verlag, 1996.)

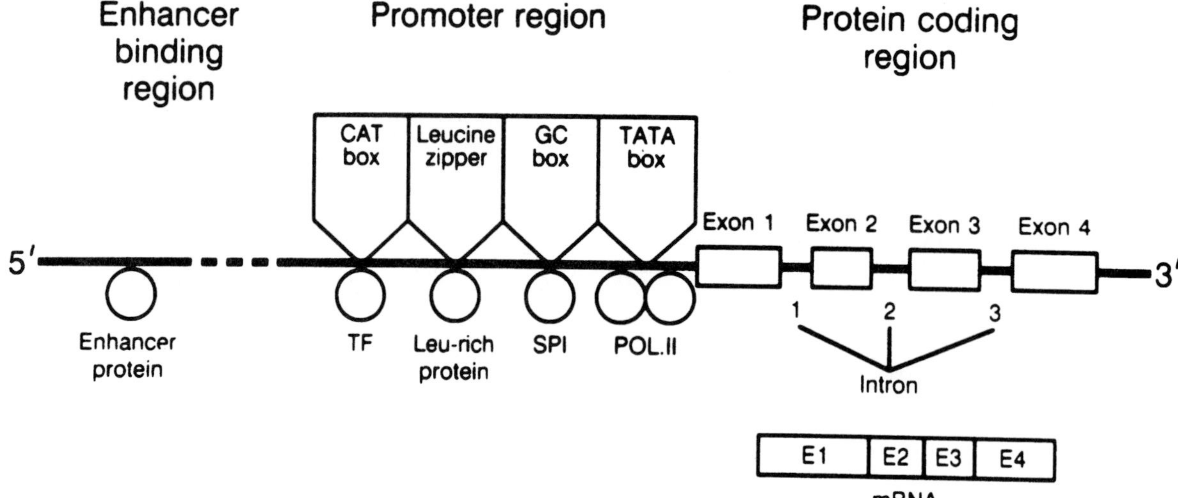

FIGURE 1-81 ■ Protein coding and regulation. mRNA, messenger ribonucleic acid; TF, transcription factor; POL II, RNA polymerase II; SPI, serum promoter. (From Simon, S.R., ed.: Orthopaedic Basic Science, 2nd ed., p. 223. Rosemont, IL, American Academy of Orthopaedic Surgeons, 1994.)

H. Techniques of Study Used to Study Genetic (Inherited) Disorders
   1. Restriction Enzymes—Used to cut DNA at a precise, reproducible cleavage location. Fragments of DNA that have been cleaved this way are called **restriction fragments. Linkage analysis** uses statistical methods to estimate the probability of a genetic trait or disease being associated with various polymorphisms (alternate gene expressions) identified in the restriction fragments.
   2. Agarose Gel Electrophoresis—When exposed to an electrical field, negatively charged DNA suspended in agarose gel moves through the gel toward the positive pole of the field. The gel acts as a "sieve": small DNA fragments move more easily (further in a given time) than large fragments. Agarose gel electrophoresis is commonly used after (and in conjunction with) restriction enzymes.
   3. DNA Ligation—Process of attaching genes removed from human DNA to pieces of nonhuman DNA known as **plasmids** to facilitate the study of specific genes. Two DNA fragments linked via ligation form **recombinant DNA**.
   4. Plasmid Vectors—Used to produce large quantities of a gene to be studied. The gene is ligated into a plasmid (which is then known as a **recombinant plasmid**) and inserted into a bacterium (the vector) using a process called **transformation**. The recombinant plasmid replicates inside the bacterium and thus increases the recombinant DNA (and the gene).
   5. Genomic Screening (Fig. 1-82).
   6. Transgenic Animals (Fig. 1-83)—Used to investigate the function of cloned genes. A transgenic animal is produced by inserting a foreign gene **(transgene)** into a single-cell embryo, which then replicates and carries the transgene to every cell in the body.
   7. Southern Hybridization—Technique used to identify a **particular DNA sequence** in an extract of mixed DNA.
   8. Northern Hybridization—Technique used to identify a particular **RNA sequence** in an extract of mixed RNA.
   9. Polymerase Chain Reaction (PCR) Amplification—**Method used to repetitively synthesize (amplify) a specific DNA sequence** in vitro such that the number of DNA copies doubles each cycle. PCR amplification has gained widespread use and has been employed for the prenatal diagnosis of sickle cell disease and screening DNA for gene mutations.

I. Cloning
   1. Definition—Cloning is the making of identical biological entities.
   2. Types
      a. Therapeutic Cloning—DNA is removed from a patient and inserted into an embryo. Stem cells are then removed from the growing embryo (which then dies) and stimulated so that they differentiate into a specific tissue. The goal of therapeutic cloning is to produce a specific type of tissue or an organ that will be transplanted back into the patient to avoid transplantation of an organ from another person (and thus avoiding organ rejection and the associated complications of immunosuppressive agents).
      b. Reproductive Cloning—DNA is removed from a host and inserted into an embryo. The embryo is then implanted into a healthy womb and allowed to develop. The goal of

Genomic screening

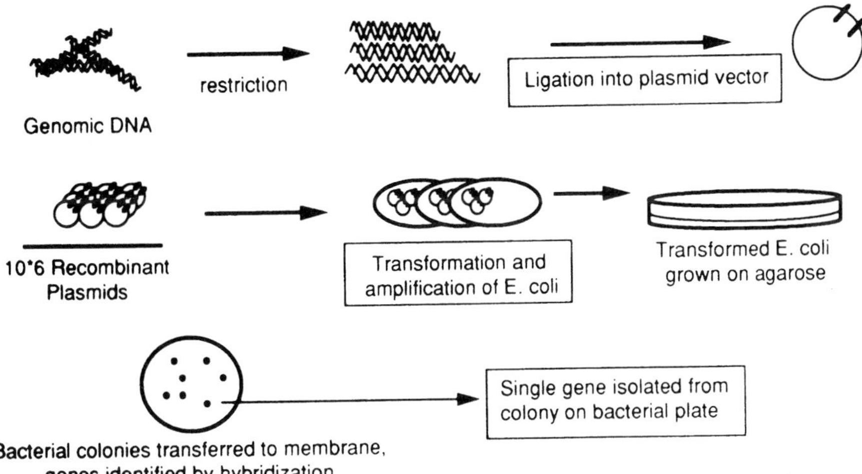

cDNA screening

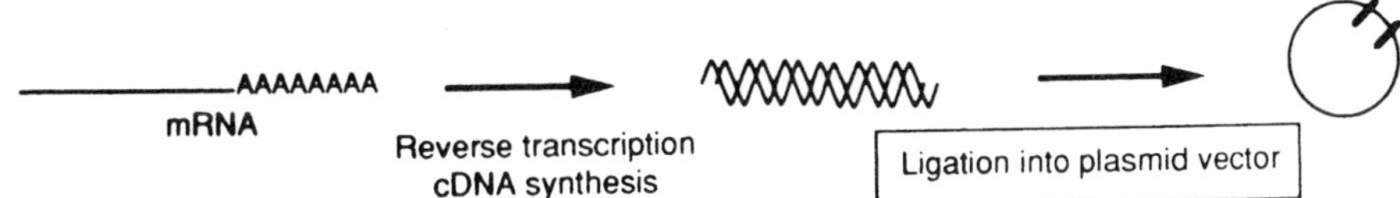

FIGURE 1-82 ■ Genomic library of recombinant plasmids with fragments of all the DNA in the chromosome. The entire genome, restricted into small fragments, is ligated into plasmid vectors restricted by the same enzymes. These recombinant plasmids transform bacteria, which can be screened to isolate specific genes of interest. (From Simon, S.R., ed.: Orthopaedic Basic Science, 2nd ed., p. 227. Rosemont, IL, American Academy of Orthopaedic Surgeons, 1994.)

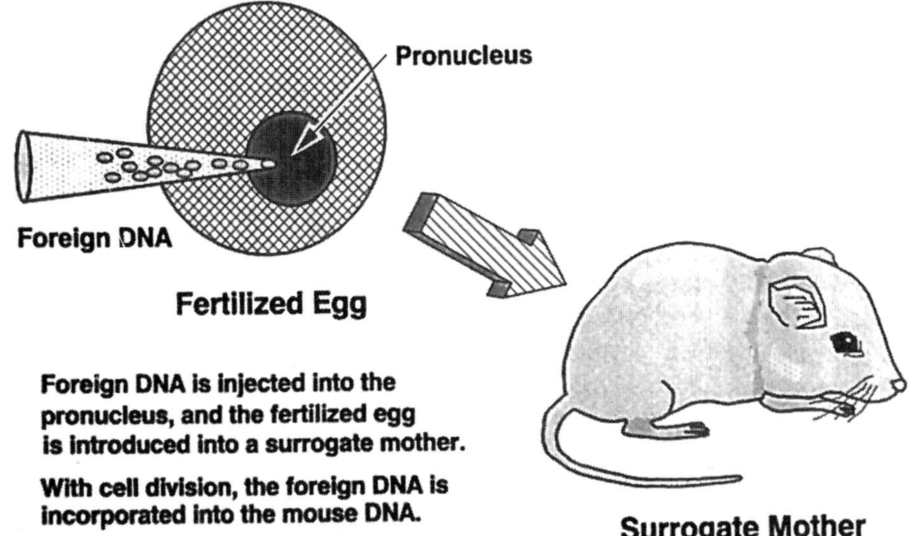

Pronucleus
Foreign DNA
Fertilized Egg
Foreign DNA is injected into the
pronucleus, and the fertilized egg
is introduced into a surrogate mother.
With cell division, the foreign DNA is
incorporated into the mouse DNA.
Offspring have foreign DNA
in every cell.
Surrogate Mother

FIGURE 1-83 ■ Transgenic mice. Recombinant DNA is injected into a fertilized mouse egg. The foreign DNA incorporates into the chromosome with cell division. As the egg develops into an embryo, every cell in the animal contains the foreign DNA. (From Simon, S.R., ed.: Orthopaedic Basic Science, 2nd ed., p. 228. Rosemont, IL, American Academy of Orthopaedic Surgeons, 1994.)

reproductive cloning is to produce an animal that is genetically identical to the host.

c. Embryo Cloning—One or more cells are removed from a fertilized embryo and stimulated to develop in utero. The goal of embryo cloning is to produce several genetically identical animals (such as twins or triplets).

II. Immunology

A. Overview—Immunology is the study of the body's defense mechanisms. Areas of particular relevance to the musculoskeletal system are infection, transplantation, tumors, autoimmune disorders (e.g., RA), and bone remodeling. Two types of immune responses have been described: nonspecific and specific.

B. Nonspecific Immune Response—**Inflammatory reaction** that begins when a foreign antigen is recognized. May arise as a result of a fracture, soft-tissue injury, or foreign body. Histamine is released and results in local vasodilation (exudate) with phagocytic cells that enzymatically digest "offending material." The inflammatory response may be enhanced by activation of the complement system or quieted by anti-inflammatory medication.

C. Specific Immune Response (Fig. 1-84)—Includes **cell-mediated** and **humoral antibody-mediated** immune responses. The cells involved in specific immune responses (B cells and T cells) arise from primitive mesenchymal cells from the bone marrow (Fig. 1-85). B lymphocytes mature in the lymph nodes; T lymphocytes originate in the bone marrow and pass through the thymus during fetal development before moving to the lymph nodes and blood. T cells include helper T cells, suppressor T cells, and killer T cells. **Antigens** evoke an immune response. **Macrophages and monocytes** are responsible for processing antigen so it is able to stimulate lymphocytes. Lymphocytes have the unique ability to mount specific reactions to millions of potential antigens. They do this by rearranging their genes (no other cell can do this) to achieve antigenic diversity and thus produce millions of antibodies.

1. **Cell-mediated immune response** (Fig. 1-86)—Involves T lymphocytes. The protein produced by T cells' gene rearrangement stays fixed to the surface of T cells and acts as a receptor molecule. The T-cell receptor acts indirectly on a foreign antigen (it does not bond directly as is seen with B lymphocytes).
2. **Humoral antibody-mediated immune response** (Fig. 1-87)—Involves B lymphocytes. B lymphocytes differentiate into **plasma cells** to produce immunoglobins against specific antigens. **B lymphocytes are associated with**

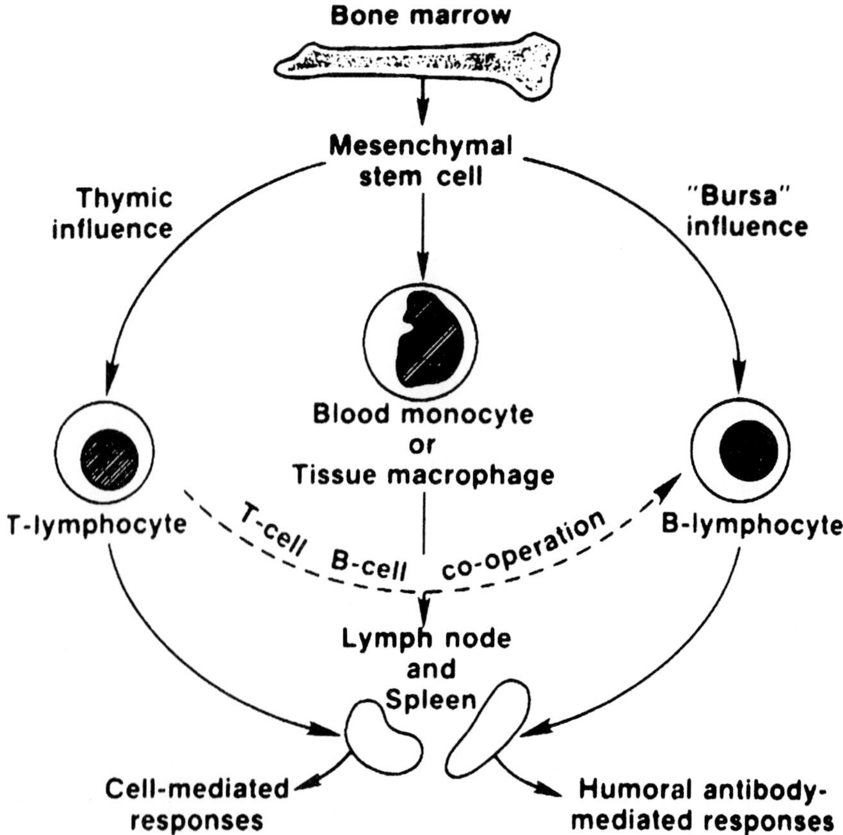

FIGURE 1-84 ■ Bone marrow primitive mesenchymal cells differentiate into B and T lymphocytes and macrophages and cooperate in cell-mediated and humoral responses. (From Friedlander, G.E.: Immunology. In Albright, J.A., and Brand, R.A., eds.: The Scientific Basis of Orthopaedics, 2nd ed., p. 484. Norwalk, CT, Appleton & Lange, 1987.)

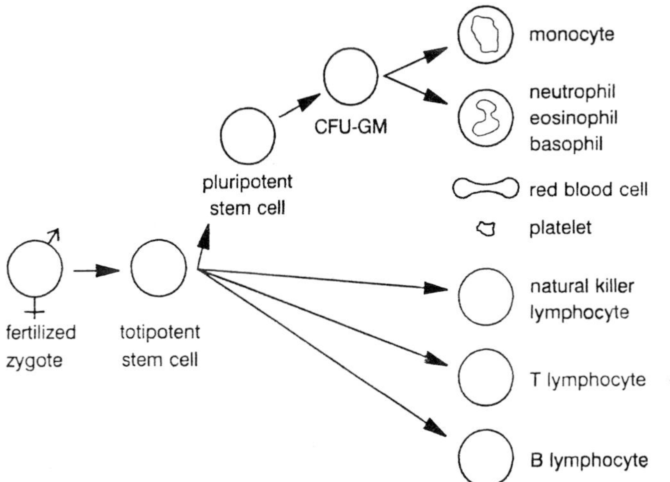

FIGURE 1-85 ■ Stem cells generate all the cell types of the blood and immune systems by a process of proliferation and differentiation in response to growth signals. CFU-GM = colony-forming unit of the granulocyte/monocyte. (From Ross, D.W., ed.: Introduction to Molecular Medicine, 2nd ed., p. 112. New York, Springer-Verlag, 1996.)

immunoglobins and the HLA system, whereas T lymphocytes are not. Immunoglobins are produced by plasma cells in a Y configuration (Fig. 1-88). Five classes of immunoglobulin have been described.
   a. IgA—Mucosal surfaces.
   b. IgM—Produced earliest by fetus; largest; RF is an IgM.
   c. IgG—Most common; arises in response to infection.
   d. IgD—Acts as a receptor.
   e. IgE—Allergic responses.

D. Cytokines—Proteins (or glycoproteins) that are cell products secreted in response to a foreign antigen. They are produced by T cells and regulate inflammatory and immune responses. Cytokines have been described in four broad categories.
   1. Interferons
   2. Growth Factors
   3. Colony-Stimulating Factors
   4. Interleukins

E. Complement System (Fig. 1-89)—A group of 25 proteins that act in a "cascading sequence" to amplify an immune response.

F. Immunogenetics—HLAs contribute to the "specificity of immune recognition" and are associated with a variety of rheumatologic diseases. The HLA gene is located on chromosome 6 (short arm); there are 6 class I loci and 14 class II loci.

G. Transplantation
   1. Allogenic Grafting—Transplantation between nonidentical members of the same species.
   2. Xenografting—Transplantation of tissues across species.
   3. Graft Preparation
      a. Freezing—Cellular response diminished.
      b. Freeze-Drying (Lyophilization)—Cellular response nearly undetectable.

H. Oncology (Fig. 1-90)—Cancer is a disease characterized by abnormal, uncontrolled cell growth, due to damage to the cell's DNA. The molecular approach to cancer seeks to discover the

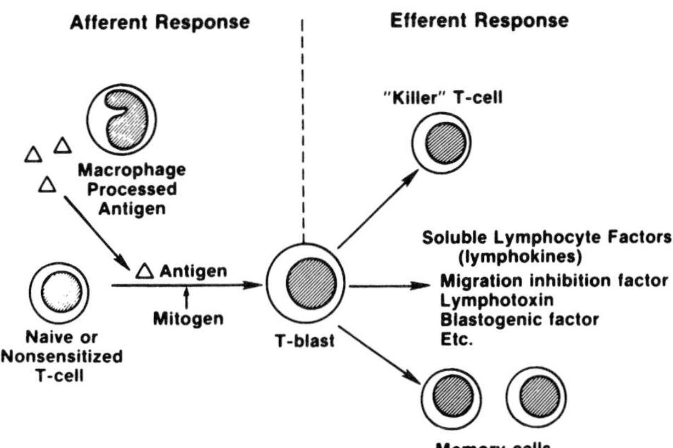

FIGURE 1-86 ■ The cell-mediated immune response. (From Friedlander, G.E.: Immunology. In Albright, J.A., and Brand, R.A., eds.: The Scientific Basis of Orthopaedics, 2nd ed. Norwalk, CT, Appleton & Lange, 1987, p. 493.)

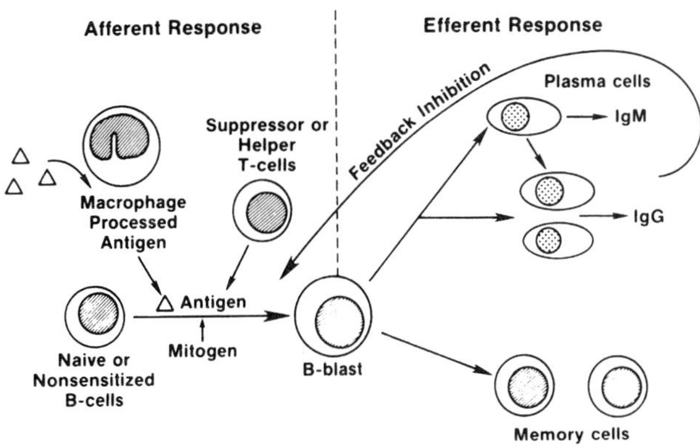

FIGURE 1-87 ■ The humoral antibody response; activation of B cells and immunoglobin production. (From Friedlander, G.E.: Immunology. In Albright, J.A., and Brand, R.A., eds.: The Scientific Basis of Orthopaedics, 2nd ed. Norwalk, CT, Appleton & Lange, 1987, p. 492.)

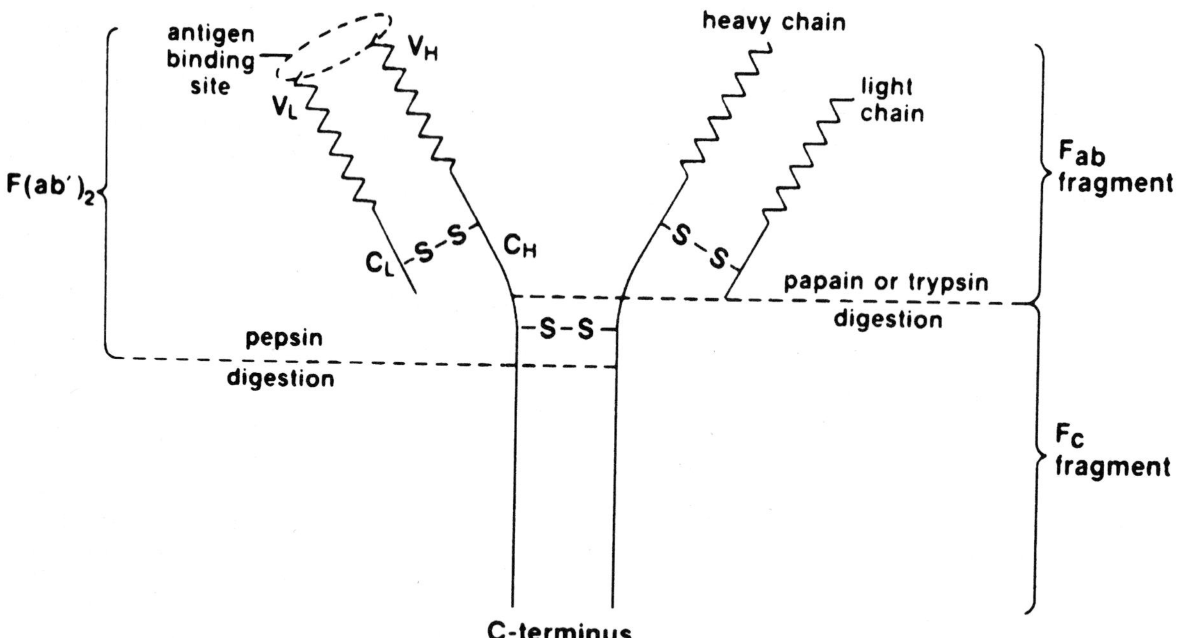

FIGURE 1-88 ■ Basic subunit structure of the immunoglobulin molecule. (From Friedlander, G.E.: Immunology. In Albright J.A., and Brand, R.A., eds.: The Scientific Basis of Orthopaedics, 2nd ed., p. 486. Norwalk, CT, Appleton & Lange, 1987.)

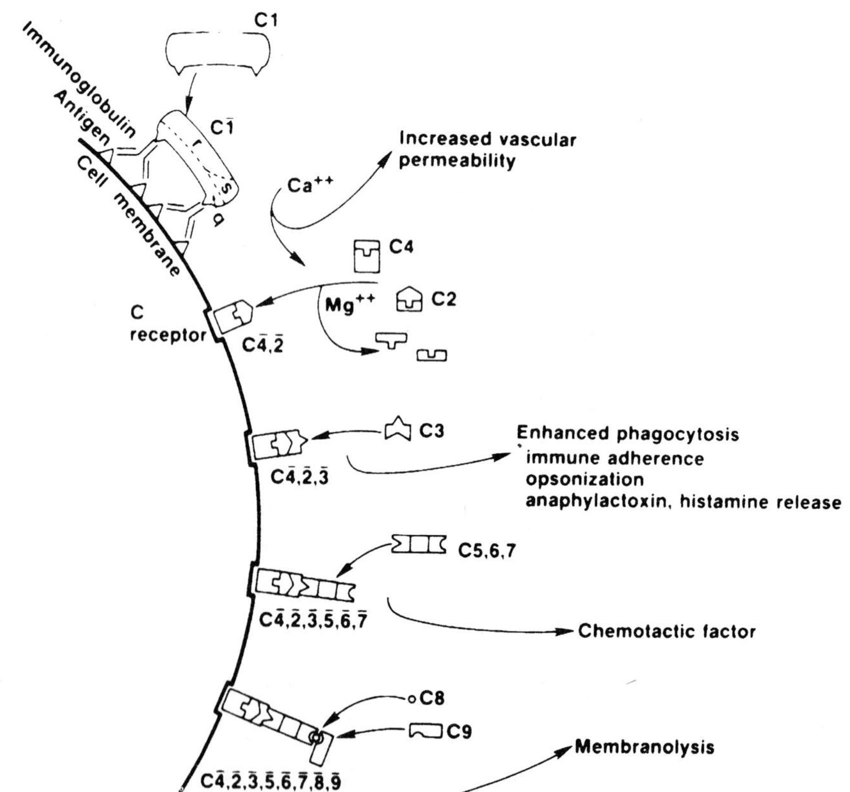

FIGURE 1-89 ■ Complement cascade. (From Friedlander, G.E.: Immunology. In Albright, J.A., and Brand, R.A., eds.: The Scientific Basis of Orthopaedics, 2nd ed., p. 491. Norwalk, CT, Appleton & Lange, 1987.)

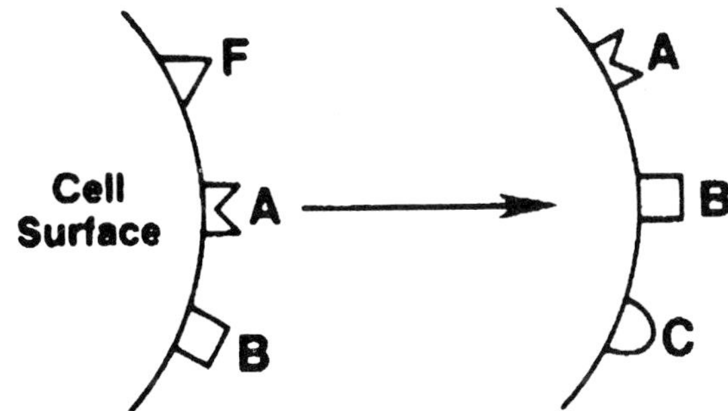

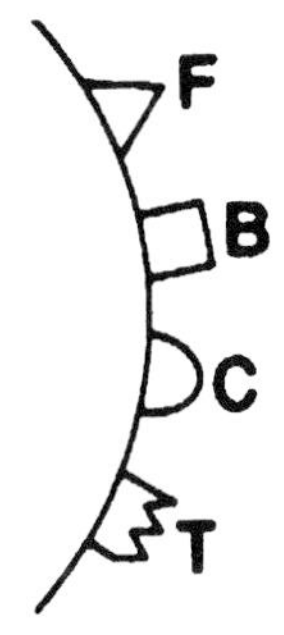

FIGURE 1-90 ■ Tumor cells have cell-surface antigens common to other normal cells reflecting the tissue of origin *(B, C)*. They may also demonstrate antigens normally present only on fetal cells *(F)* and loose antigens common to the cell type of origin *(A)*. In addition, they acquire new tumor-associated antigens *(T)*. (From Friedlander, G.E.: Immunology. In Albright, J.A., and Brand, R.A., eds.: The Scientific Basis of Orthopaedics, 2nd ed., p. 502. Norwalk, CT, Appleton & Lange, 1987.)

mechanisms by which normal cells become cancer cells. Various mechanisms may damage normal cells and result in malignancy: a point mutation in DNA; a gene deletion; or a chromosomal translocation (which results in gene rearrangement).

1. **Oncogenes**—Growth-control genes. Improper expression of an oncogene results in unregulated cell growth as seen in cancer cells.
2. **Anti-Oncogenes (Tumor Suppressor Genes)**—Suppress growth in damaged cells to inhibit tumors.
3. Metastases—The sequence of events for primary tumor cells to metastasize to a distant organ:
   a. Sequence of Events
      (1) Progressive growth of the primary tumor
      (2) Neovascularization of the tumor
      (3) Basement membrane erosion and invasion.
         (a) **Matrix metalloproteinases have the capacity to degrade type IV collagen, which is present in the basement membrane** (see Table 1-20).
         (b) Matrix metalloproteinases are therefore believed to be important for tumor cell metastasis.
      (4) Entry of tumor cells into adjacent blood vessels
      (5) Detachment of cells from the primary tumor
      (6) Embolization of tumor cells into the general circulation
      (7) Attachment of tumor cells at a distant site
      (8) Invasion into vessel walls with migration into surrounding parenchyma
      (9) Progressive tumor growth in the new site
   b. Types of Tumors—**The most common tumors that metastasize to bone, in decreasing order of incidence, are: breast, prostate, lung, kidney, and thyroid.**
4. Miscellaneous—**Flow cytometry and cytofluorometry** are methods used to quantify the amount of DNA in cells. **These techniques are useful for determining the amount of abnormal (aneuploid) DNA in a malignant tumor. P-glycoprotein** is an energy-dependent cell-wall pump that functions to eliminate natural toxins (and some chemotherapeutic agents) from the cytoplasm. P-glycoprotein allows both cancer and normal cells to develop resistance to chemotherapeutic agents.

I. **Miscellaneous Topics Related to Specific Immune-Related Orthopaedic Conditions—Latex allergy** has been reported as an intraoperative complication, particularly in patients with myelomenigocele. Latex allergy in these children is likely due to repetitive mucosal and parenteral latex exposure (e.g., operations, examinations). **Type I hypersensitivity to latex involves IgE antibodies** that are specific for proteins to the sap from the rubber tree (*Hevea brasiliensis*) used to make gloves. Preoperative prophylaxis (cimetidine and diphenyhydramine) decreases the frequency of potentially catastrophic events (anaphylaxis). The development of rheumatoid arthritis is related to a reaction between T cells (helper/inducer) and antigen-presenting cell macrophage.The foreign-body response to particulate biomaterials appears to be initiated by macrophages. Lymphocytes do not appear to be essential for this response. Endosteal bone erosion (osteolysis; aggressive granulomatous lesions) surrounding an uninfected femoral stem following THA is associated with monocytes-macrophages.

III. Genetics

A. Introduction—Although more than 3000 genetic disorders have been identified, very few genes responsible for musculoskeletal diseases and disorders have been identified.

B. Mendelian Inheritance—Mendelian traits are those that follow specific patterns of inheritance controlled by a single gene pair ("monogenic").

A **genetic locus** is a gene's specific position on a chromosome. An **allele** is one of several possible alternative forms of a gene. Because the chromosomes are paired (46 chromosomes; 23 pairs [22 pairs of autosomes and 1 pair of sex chromosomes]) there are two copies (loci) for every gene. An individual is **homozygous** if the two alleles on each of the paired chromosomes are identical; the individual is **heterozygous** if the alleles differ. The term **phenotype** refers to the features exhibited by an individual due to genetic make-up; **genotype** refers to the presence or absence of particular genes, not the associated traits that are expressed. Mendelian traits may be inherited by one of four modes.

1. Autosomal dominant
2. Autosomal recessive
3. X-linked dominant
4. X-linked recessive

A detailed description of these four modes of mendelian inheritance is shown in Table 1-39. The overall incidence of mendelian disorders in humans is approximately 1%. Non-mendelian traits may be inherited via "polygenic" transmission (caused by the action of several genes).

C. Mutations—Genetic disorders arise from alterations (mutations) in the genetic material. Mutations may be passed from generation to generation, following mendelian inheritance, or the mutation may represent a new mutation **(sporadic mutation)** that occurs in the sperm or egg of the parents or in the embryo.

D. Chromosomal Abnormalities—Result from disruptions in the normal arrangement or number of chromosomes. These include:
   1. Aneuploidy—An abnormal number of chromosomes
      a. Triploidy—Three copies of chromosomes (69 chromosomes).
      b. Tetraploids—Four copies of chromosomes (92 chromosomes).
      c. Monosomy—One chromosome of one pair is absent (45 chromosomes).
      d. Trisomy—One chromosome pair has an extra chromosome (47 chromosomes).
   2. Deletion—A section of one chromosome (in a chromosome pair) is absent.

Table 1-39. MENDELIAN INHERITANCE

INHERITANCE PATTERN	DESCRIPTION	PUNNETT SQUARE(S)
Autosomal dominant[*]	Typically represent **structural defects** Heterozygote state (Aa) manifests the condition 50% of the offspring are affected (assuming only one parent is affected) Normal offspring do not transmit the condition There is no gender preference	A a a: Aa aa a: Aa aa
Autosomal recessive[†]	Typically represent **biochemical or enzymatic defects** Homozygote state (aa) manifests the condition Parents are unaffected (they are most commonly heterozygotes) 25% of offsprings are affected (assuming each parent is a heterozygote) There is no gender preference	A a A: AA Aa a: Aa aa
X-linked dominant[‡]	Heterozygotes (X'X or X'Y) manifests the condition Affected females (mating with unaffected males) transmit the X-linked gene to 50% of daughters and 50% of sons	X Y X': X'X X'Y X: XX XY
	Affected males (mating with unaffected females) transmit the X-linked gene to all daughters and no sons	X' Y X: X'X XY X: X'X XY
X-linked recessive[§]	Heterozygote (X'Y) male manifests the condition Heterozygote (X'X) female is unaffected Affected male (mating with a normal female) transmits the X-linked gene to all daughters (who are carriers) and no sons	X' Y X: X'X XY X: X'X XY
	Carrier female (mating with a normal male) transmits the X-linked gene to 50% of daughters (who are carriers) and 50% of sons (who are affected)	X Y X': X'X X'Y X: XX XY

[*] A is the mutant dominant allele.
[†] a is the mutant recessive allele.
[‡] X' is the mutant dominant X allele.
[§] X' is the mutant recessive X allele.

Table 1-40. OVERVIEW OF THE INHERITANCE PATTERNS OF SOME MUSCULOSKELETAL-RELATED DISORDERS

AUTOSOMAL DOMINANT	AUTOSOMAL RECESSIVE	X-LINKED DOMINANT	X-LINKED RECESSIVE
Achondroplasia Spondyloepiphyseal dysplasia (congenita form) Multiple epiphyseal dysplasia Metaphyseal chondrodysplasia (Schmid and Jansen types) Kniest's dysplasia Malignant hyperthermia Marfan's syndrome Ehlers-Danlos syndrome Osteogenesis imperfecta (types I and IV) Osteochondromatosis Polydactyly	Metaphyseal chondrodysplasia (McKusick type) Diastrophic dysplasia Laron's dysplasia Sickle cell anemia Hurler's syndrome Osteogenesis imperfecta (types II and III) Hypophosphatasia Hereditary vitamin D–dependent rickets Homocystinuria	Hypophosphatemic rickets	Spondyloepiphyseal dysplasia (tarda form) Hemophilia Hunter's syndrome Duchenne's muscular dystrophy

3. Duplication—An extra section of one chromosome (in a chromosome pair) is present.
4. Translocation—A portion of one chromosome is exchanged with a portion of another chromosome.
5. Inversion—A broken portion of a chromosome reattaches to the same chromosome in the same location but in a reverse direction.

E. The Genetics of Musculoskeletal Conditions and Conditions Associated with Musculoskeletal Abnormalities—Table 1-40 shows the inheritance pattern of the musculoskeletal (and related) disorders that appear most often on board examinations. Table 1-41 is a comprehensive compilation of the known genetic defects involved in disorders that display musculoskeletal manifestations.

Table 1-41. COMPREHENSIVE COMPILATION OF INHERITANCE PATTERN, DEFECT, AND ASSOCIATED GENE OF MUSCULOSKELETAL-RELATED DISORDERS

	DISORDER	INHERITANCE PATTERN	DEFECT	ASSOCIATED GENE
Dysplasias	Achondroplasia	Autosomal dominant	Defect in the fibroblast growth factor (FGF) receptor 3	FGF receptor 3 gene
	Diastrophic dysplasia	Autosomal recessive	Mutation of a gene coding for a sulfate transport protein	Sulfate-transporter gene (chromosome 5)
	Kniest's dysplasia	Autosomal dominant	Defect in type II collagen	COL 2A1
	Laron's dysplasia (pituitary dwarfism)	Autosomal recessive	Defect in the growth hormone receptor	
	McCune-Albright syndrome (polyostotic fibrous dysplasia, café-au-lait spots, precocious puberty)	Sporadic mutation	Germ line defect in the Gsα protein	Mutation of Gsα subunit of the receptor/adenylate cyclase—coupling G proteins
	Metaphyseal chondrodysplasia (Jansen form)	Autosomal dominant		
	Metaphyseal chondrodysplasia (McKusick form)	Autosomal recessive		
	Metaphyseal chondrodysplasia (Schmid-tarda form)	Autosomal dominant	Defect in type X collagen	COL 10A1
	Multiple epiphyseal dysplasia	Autosomal dominant (most commonly)	Cartilage oligomeric matrix protein	
	Spondyloepiphyseal dysplasia	Autosomal dominant (congenita form) X-Linked recessive (tarda form)	Defect in type II collagen	Linked to X p22.12-p22.31 and COL 2A1

(Continued)

Table 1-41. COMPREHENSIVE COMPILATION OF INHERITANCE PATTERN, DEFECT, AND ASSOCIATED GENE OF MUSCULOSKELETAL-RELATED DISORDERS—CONT'D

	DISORDER	INHERITANCE PATTERN	DEFECT	ASSOCIATED GENE
	Achondrogenesis	Autosomal recessive	Fetal cartilage fails to mature	
	Apert syndrome	Sporadic mutation/ Autosomal dominant		
	Chondrodysplasia punctata (Conradi–Hünerman)	Autosomal dominant		
	Chondrodysplasia punctata (rhizomelic form)	Autosomal recessive	Defect in subcellular organelles (perioxisomes)	
	Cleidocranial dysplasia (dysostosis)	Autosomal dominant		
	Dysplasia epiphysealis hemimelica (Trevor's disease)	??		
	Ellis-van Creveld syndrome (chondroectodermal dysplasia)	Autosomal recessive		
	Fibrodysplasia ossifican progressiva	Sporadic mutation/ Autosomal dominant		
	Geroderma osteodysplastica (Walt Disney dwarfism)	Autosomal recessive		
	Grebe chondrodysplasia	Autosomal recessive		
	Hypochondroplasia	Sporadic mutation/ Autosomal dominant		
	Kabuki make-up syndrome	Sporadic mutation		
	Mesomelic dysplasia (Langer type)	Autosomal recessive		
	Mesomelic dysplasia (Nievergelt type)	Autosomal dominant		
	Mesomelic dysplasia (Reinhardt-Pfeiffer type)	Autosomal dominant		
	Mesomelic dysplasia (Werner type)	Autosomal dominant		
	Metatrophic dysplasia	Autosomal recessive		
	Progressive diaphyseal dysplasia (Camurati-Engelmann disease)	Autosomal dominant		
	Pseudoachondroplastic dysplasia	Autosomal dominant		
	Pycnodysostosis	Autosomal recessive		
	Spondylometaphyseal chondrodysplasia	Autosomal dominant		
	Spondylothoracic dysplasia (Jarcho-Levin syndrome)	Autosomal recessive		
	Thanatophoric dwarfism	Autosomal dominant		
	Tooth-and-nail syndrome	Autosomal dominant		
	Treacher Collins syndrome (mandibulo-facial dysotosis)	Autosomal dominant		
Metabolic bone diseases	Hereditary vitamin D–dependent rickets	Autosomal recessive	(See Table 1-15)	
	Hypophosphatasia	Autosomal recessive	(See Table 1-15)	
	Hypophosphatemic rickets (vitamin D–resistant rickets)	X-linked dominant	(See Table 1-15)	
	Osteogenesis imperfecta	Autosomal dominant (types I and IV) Autosomal recessive (types II and III)	Defect in type I collagen (abnormal cross-linking)	COL 1A1, COL 1A2
	Albright hereditary osteodystrophy (pseudohypoparathyroidism)	Uncertain	Parathyroid hormone has no effect at the target cells (in the kidney, bone, and intestine)	
	Infantile cortical hyperostosis (Caffey's disease)	???		
	Ochronosis (alkaptonuria)	Autosomal recessive	Defect in the homogentisic acid oxidase system	
	Osteopetrosis	Autosomal dominant (mild, tarda form) Autosomal recessive (infantile, malignant form)		
Connective tissue disorders	Marfan's syndrome	Autosomal dominant	Fibrillin abnormalities (some patients also have type I collagen abnormalities)	Fibrillin gene (chromosome 15)

(Continued)

	DISORDER	INHERITANCE PATTERN	DEFECT	ASSOCIATED GENE
Connective tissue disorders *(Continued)*	Ehlers-Danlos syndrome (there are at least 13 varieties)	Autosomal dominant (most common)	Defects in types I and III collagen have been described for some varieties; lysyl oxidase abnormalities	COL 1A2 (for Ehlers-Danlos type VII)
	Homocystinuria	Autosomal recessive	Deficiency of the enzyme cystathionine β-synthase	
Mucopolysaccharidosis	Hunter's syndrome ("gargoylism")	X-linked recessive		
	Hurler's syndrome	Autosomal recessive	Deficiency of the enzyme alpha-L-iduronidase	
	Maroteaux-Lamy syndrome	Autosomal recessive		
	Morquio's syndrome	Autosomal recessive		
	Sanfilippo's syndrome	Autosomal recessive		
	Scheie's syndrome	Autosomal recessive	Deficiency of the enzyme alpha-L-iduronidase	
Muscular dystrophies	Duchenne's muscular dystrophy	X-linked recessive	Defect on the short arm of the X chromosome	Dystrophin gene
	Becker's dystrophy	X-linked recessive		
	Fascioscapulohumeral dystrophy	Autosomal dominant		
	Limb-girdle dystrophy	Autosomal recessive		
	Steinert's disease (myotonic dystrophy)	Autosomal dominant		
Hematologic disorders	Hemophilia (A and B)	X-linked recessive	Hemophilia A-factor VIII deficiency Hemophilia B-factor IX deficiency	
	Sickle cell anemia	Autosomal recessive	Hemoglobin abnormality (hemoglobin S)	
	Gaucher's disease	Autosomal recessive	Deficient activity of the enzyme β-glucosidase (glucocerebrosidase)	
	Hemochromatosis	Autosomal recessive		
	Niemann-Pick disease	Autosomal recessive	Accumulation of sphingomyelin in cellular lysosomes	
	Smith-Lemli-Optiz syndrome	Uncertain		
	Thalassemia	Autosomal recessive	Abnormal production of hemoglobin A	
	von Willebrand's disease	Autosomal dominant		
Chromosomal disorders with musculoskeletal abnormalities	Down syndrome		Trisomy of chromosome 21	
	Angelman's syndrome		Chromosome 15 abnormality	
	Clinodactyly		Associated with many genetic anomalies including trisomy of chromosomes 8 and 21	
	Edward's syndrome		Trisomy of chromosome 18	
	Fragile X syndrome	X-linked trait (does not follow the typical pattern of an X-linked trait)		Xq27-Xq28
	Klinefelter's syndrome (XXY)		Male has an extra X chromosome	
	Langer-Giedion syndrome	Sporadic mutation	Chromosome 8 abnormality	
	Nail-patella syndrome	Autosomal dominant	Chromosome 9 abnormality	
	Patau's syndrome		Trisomy of chromosome 13	
	Turner's syndrome (XO)		Female missing one of the two X chromosomes	
Neurologic disorders	Charcot-Marie-Tooth disease	Autosomal dominant (most common)		
	Congenital insensitivity to pain	Autosomal recessive		
	Dejerine-Sottas disease	Autosomal recessive		
	Friedreich's ataxia	Autosomal recessive		
	Huntington's disease	Autosomal dominant		
	Menkes' syndrome	X-linked recessive	Inability to absorb and use copper	
	Pelizaeus-Merzbacher disease	X-linked recessive	Defect in the gene for proteolipid (a component of myelin)	
	Riley-Day syndrome	Autosomal recessive		
	Spinal muscular atrophy (Werdnig-Hoffman disease and Kugelberg-Welander disease)	Autosomal recessive		

(Continued)

Table 1-41. COMPREHENSIVE COMPILATION OF INHERITANCE PATTERN, DEFECT, AND ASSOCIATED GENE OF MUSCULOSKELETAL-RELATED DISORDERS—CONT'D

	DISORDER	INHERITANCE PATTERN	DEFECT	ASSOCIATED GENE
Neurologic disorders *(Continued)*	Sturge-Weber syndrome	Sporadic mutation		
	Tay-Sachs disease	Autosomal recessive	Deficiency in the enzyme hexosaminidase A	
Diseases associated with neoplasias	Ewing's sarcoma			11;22 chromosomal translocation
	Multiple endocrine neoplasia I (MEN I)	Autosomal dominant		RET
	MEN II	Autosomal dominant		
	MEN III	Autosomal dominant	Chromosome 10 abnormality	
	Neurofibromatosis (von Recklinghausen's disease)	Autosomal dominant		NF1, NF2
Miscellaneous disorders	Malignant hyperthermia	Autosomal dominant		
	Osteochondromatosis	Autosomal dominant		
	Polydactyly	Autosomal dominant (a small number of cases of sporadic gene mutations have been reported)		
	Captodactyly	Autosomal dominant		
	Cerebro-oculo-facio-skeletal syndrome	Autosomal recessive		
	Congential contractural arachnodactyly			Fibrillin gene (chromosome 5)
	Distal arthrogryposis syndrome	Autosomal dominant		
	Dupuytren's contracture	Autosomal dominant (with partial sex-limitation)		
	Fabry's disease	X-linked recessive	Deficiency of alpha-galactosidase A	
	Fanconi's pancytopenia	Autosomal recessive		
	Freeman-Sheldon syndrome (craniocarpotarsal dysplasia; whistling face syndrome)	Autosomal dominant Autosomal recessive		
	GM1 gangliosidosis	Autosomal recessive		
	Hereditary anonychia	Autosomal dominant Autosomal recessive		
	Holt-Oram syndrome	Autosomal dominant		
	Humeroradial synostosis	Autosomal dominant Autosomal recessive		
	Klippel-Feil syndrome		Faulty development of spinal segments along the embryonic neural tube	
	Klippel-Trénaunay-Weber syndrome	Sporadic mutation		
	Krabbe's disease	Autosomal recessive	Deficiency of galactocerebroside β-galactosidase	
	Larsen's syndrome	Autosomal dominant Autosomal recessive		
	Lesch-Nyham disease	X-linked trait	Absence of the enzyme hypoxanthine guanine phosphoribosyl transferase	
	Madelung's deformity	Autosomal dominant		
	Mannosidosis	Autosomal recessive	Deficiency of the enzyme alpha-monosidase	
	Maple syrup urine disease	Autosomal recessive	Defective metabolism of the amino acids leucine, isoleucine, and valine	
	Meckel syndrome (Gruber's syndrome)	Autosomal recessive		
	Mobius' syndrome	Autosomal dominant		
	Mucolipidosis (oligosaccharidosis)	Autosomal recessive	A family of enzyme deficiency diseases	
	Multiple exostoses	Autosomal dominant		
	Multiple pterygium syndrome	Autosomal recessive		
	Noonan's syndrome	Sporadic mutation		
	Oral-facial-digital (OFD) syndrome	OFDI—X-linked dominant OFDII (Mohr's syndrome)—autosomal recessive		

(Continued)

	DISORDER	INHERITANCE PATTERN	DEFECT	ASSOCIATED GENE
Miscellaneous disorders *(Continued)*	Osler-Weber-Rendu syndrome (hereditary hemorrhagic telangiectasia)	Autosomal dominant		
	Pfeiffer's syndrome (acrocephalosyndactyly)	Sporadic mutation/ autosomal dominant		
	Phenylketonuria	Autosomal recessive	Enzyme deficiency characterized by the inability to convert phenylalanine to tyrosine due to a chromosome 12 abnormality	
	Phytanic acid storage disease	Autosomal recessive		
	Progeria (Hutchinson-Gilford progeria syndrome)	Autosomal dominant		
	Proteus syndrome	Autosomal dominant		
	Prune-belly syndrome	Uncertain	Localized mesodermal defect	
	Radioulnar synostosis	Autosomal dominant		
	Rett's syndrome	Sporadic mutation/ X-linked dominant		
	Roberts' syndrome (pseudothalidomide syndrome)	Sporadic mutation/ autosomal recessive		
	Russell-Silver syndrome	Sporadic mutation (possibly X-linked)		
	Saethre-Chotzen syndrome	Autosomal dominant		
	Sandhoff's disease	Autosomal recessive	Enzyme deficiency of hexosaminidase A and B	
	Schwartz-Jampel syndrome	Autosomal recessive		
	Seckel's syndrome (bird-headed dwarfism)	Autosomal recessive		
	Stickler's syndrome (hereditary progressive arthroopthalmopathy)	Autosomal dominant	Collagen abnormality	
	TAR syndrome (thrombocytopenia–aplasia of radius syndrome)	Autosomal recessive		
	Tarsal coalition	Autosomal dominant		
	Trichorrhinophalangeal syndrome	Autosomal dominant		
	Urea cycle defects	Argininemia—autosomal recessive Argininosuccinic aciduria—autosomal recessive Carbamyl phosphate synthetase deficiency—autosomal recessive Citrullinemia—autosomal recessive Ornathine transcarbamylase deficiency—X-linked	A group of enzyme disorders characterized by high levels of ammonia in the blood and tissues	
	VATER association	Sporadic mutation		
	Werner's syndrome	Autosomal recessive		
	Zygodactyly	Autosomal dominant		

SECTION 5

Orthapaedic Infections and Microbiology

I. Musculoskeletal Infections

The following is an overview. Specific infections unique to particular orthopaedic areas are detailed in the chapters that follow. In general, the following initial treatment regimen recommendations are based on the presumed type of infection as determined by clinical findings and symptoms. Definitive treatment should be based on final culture results, when available. Glycocalyx is an exopolysaccharide coating that envelops bacteria. Bacterial adherence to biologic implants is promoted by an inflammatory tissue interface and inhibited by a noninflammatory tissue interface.

A. Soft-Tissue Infections—Table 1-42.
   1. Bite injuries—Table 1-43.

B. Bone Infections—Osteomyelitis is an infection of bone and bone marrow that may be caused by direct inoculation of an open traumatic wound or by blood-borne organisms (hematogenous). **It is not possible to determine the microscopic organism causing chronic osteomyelitis based on the clinical picture and patient age; thus a specific microbiologic diagnosis via deep cultures is essential (organisms isolated from sinus tract drainage typically do not accurately reflect the organisms present deep within the wound and within bone).**
   1. Acute Hematogenous Osteomyelitis—Bone and bone marrow infection caused by blood-borne organisms, commonly in children (boys more often than girls). In children, the infection is most common in the metaphysis or epiphysis of the long bones, more commonly in the lower extremity than the upper extremity. Radiographic changes of acute hematogenous osteomyelitis include soft-tissue swelling (early), bone demineralization (10-14 days), and **sequestra** (dead bone with surrounding granulation tissue) and **involucrum** (periosteal new bone) later. Pain, loss of function of the involved extremity, and a soft-tissue abscess may be present. Patients commonly show an elevated WBC count and an elevated ESR; blood cultures may be positive. **C-reactive protein is the most sensitive monitor of the course of infection in children with acute hematogenous osteomyelitis.** Nuclear medicine studies may be helpful in equivocal cases. **MRI shows changes in bone and bone marrow before plain films.** Empiric therapy should be started after cultures have been obtained, either by aspiration or surgical drainage when indicated. The indications for operative intervention include (1) drainage of an abscess, (2) débridement of infected tissues to prevent further destruction, and (3) refractory cases that show no improvement following nonoperative treatment. The treatment of acute osteomyelitis may be summarized as follows: (1) identify the organisms, (2) select appropriate antibiotics, (3) deliver antibiotics to the infected site, and (4) halt tissue destruction. Before definitive cultures become available, empiric therapy is based on the patient's age and/or special circumstances.
      a. **Newborn (up to 4 Months of Age)**—The most common organisms include *S. aureus*, gram-negative bacilli, and group B streptococcus. Primary empiric therapy includes nafcillin or oxacillin plus a third-generation cephalosporin. Alternative antibiotic therapy includes vancomycin plus a third-generation cephalosporin. Newborns with hematogenous osteomyelitis may be afebrile, and the best predictors of the osteomyelitis are local signs in the extremity, including warmth. Almost 70% of newborn patients with hematogenous osteomyelitis have positive blood cultures.
      b. **Children 4 Years of Age or Older**—The most common organisms are *S. aureus*, group A Strep, and coliforms (uncommon). The empiric treatment of choice is nafcillin or oxacillin; alternative regimens include vancomycin or clindamycin. When the Gram stain shows gram-negative organisms, a third-generation cephalosporin should be added. **With recent immunization programs, *H. influenzae* bone infections causing hematogenous osteomyelitis have almost been completely eliminated.**
      c. **Adults 21 Years of Age or Older—The most common organism is *S. aureus*,** but a wide variety of other organisms have been isolated. Initial empiric therapy includes nafcillin or oxacillin or cefazolin; vancomycin can be used as an alternative initial therapy.
      d. Sickle Cell Anemia—*Salmonella* is a characteristic organism. The primary treatment is with one of the fluoroquinolones (only in adults); alternative treatment is with a third-generation cephalosporin.
      e. Hemodialysis Patients and IV Drug Abusers—*S. aureus*, *S. epidermidis*, and *Pseudomonas aeruginosa* are common organisms. The treatment of choice is one of the penicillinase resistant synthetic penicillins (PRSPs) plus ciprofloxacin; an alternative treatment is vancomycin with ciprofloxacin.

2. Acute Osteomyelitis (After Open Fracture or Open Reduction with Internal Fixation)—Clinical findings may be similar to acute hematogenous osteomyelitis. Treatment includes radical irrigation and débridement with removal of orthopaedic hardware as necessary. Open wounds may require rotational or free flaps. The most common offending organisms are *S. aureus*, *P. aeruginosa*, and coliforms. Empiric therapy prior to definitive cultures is nafcillin with ciprofloxacin; alternative therapy is vancomycin with a third-generation cephalosporin. Patients with acute osteomyelitis and vascular insufficiency and those who are immunocompromised generally show a polymicrobic picture.
3. Chronic Osteomyelitis—May arise as a result of an inappropriately treated acute osteomyelitis, trauma, or soft-tissue spread, especially in the Cierney type C elderly host (Table 1-44), the immunosuppressed, diabetics, and IV drug abusers. Chronic osteomyelitis may be classified anatomically (Fig. 1-91). Skin and soft tissues are often involved and the sinus tract may occasionally develop squamous cell carcinoma. Periods of quiescence (of the infection) are often followed by acute exacerbations. Nuclear medicine studies are often helpful for determining the activity of the disease. **Operative sampling of deep specimens from multiple foci is the most accurate means of identifying the pathologic organisms.** A combination of IV antibiotics (based on deep cultures), surgical débridement **(complete removal of compromised bone and soft tissue, and retained hardware is the most important factor in eliminating infection). It is almost impossible to eliminate implant-associated infection without removing the implant because organisms grow in a glycocalyx [biofilm] that shields them from antibodies and antibiotics**. Following sterilization of the affected area, bone grafting and soft-tissue coverage is often required. Unfortunately, amputations are still required in certain cases. *S. aureus*, Enterobacteriaceae, and *P. aeruginosa* are the most frequent offending organisms. **Treatment is based on deep cultures and sensitivity testing: empiric therapy is not indicated in chronic osteomyelitis.**
4. Subacute Osteomyelitis—Usually discovered radiologically in a patient with a painful limp and no systemic (and often no local) signs or symptoms. Subacute osteomyelitis may arise secondary to a partially treated acute osteomyelitis, or it occasionally develops in a fracture hematoma. Unlike acute osteomyelitis, the WBC count and blood cultures are frequently normal. ESR, bone cultures, and radiographs are often useful. Subacute osteomyelitis most commonly affects the femur and tibia; and unlike acute osteomyelitis, it can cross the physis, even in older children. Radiographic changes include **Brodie's abscess** (a localized radiolucency usually seen in the metaphyses of long bones). It is sometimes difficult to differentiate from Ewing's sarcoma. Treatment of Brodie's abscess in the metaphysis includes surgical curettage. When localized to the epiphysis only, other lesions (e.g., chondroblastoma) must be ruled out. **Epiphyseal osteomyelitis is caused almost exclusively by *S. aureus*.** Epiphyseal osteomyelitis requires surgical drainage only if pus is present, otherwise 48 hours of IV antibiotics followed by 6 weeks of oral antibiotics is curative.
5. Chronic Sclerosing Osteomyelitis—An unusual infection that primarily involves diaphyseal bones of adolescents. Typified by intense proliferation of the periosteum leading to bony deposition, it may be caused by anaerobic organisms. Insidious onset, dense progressive sclerosis on radiographs, and localized pain and tenderness are common. Malignancy must be ruled out.
6. Chronic Multifocal Osteomyelitis—Caused by an infectious agent, it appears in children without systemic symptoms. Normal laboratory values, except for an elevated ESR, are common. Radiographs demonstrate multiple metaphyseal lytic lesions, especially in the medial clavicle, distal tibia, and distal femur. Usually resolves spontaneously, requiring only symptomatic treatment.
7. Osteomyelitis with Unusual Organisms—Several unusual organisms occur in certain clinical settings (Table 1-45). Radiographs show characteristic features in syphilis (*Treponema pallidum*) (radiolucency in the metaphysis from granulation tissue) and tuberculosis (joint destruction on both sides of a joint). Histology can also be helpful (e.g., tuberculosis with granulomas).

C. Joint Infections

1. Septic Arthritis—Commonly follows hematogenous spread or extension of metaphyseal osteomyelitis in children. Can also arise as a complication of a diagnostic or therapeutic procedure. Most cases involve infants (hip) and children. **The metaphysis of the proximal femur, proximal humerus, radial neck, and distal fibula are within their respective joint capsules; metaphyseal osteomyelitis can rupture into the joint in these areas. The most common site at which septic arthritis follows acute osteomyelitis is the proximal femur/hip.** RA (tuberculosis most characteristic, *S. aureus* most common) and IV drug abuse (*Pseudomonas* most characteristic) predispose adults to septic arthritis. Surgical drainage or daily aspiration is the mainstay of treatment. Open (or arthroscopic)

Table 1-42. SOFT-TISSUE INFECTIONS

TYPE	AFFECTED TISSUES	CLINICAL FINDINGS	ORGANISMS	TREATMENT
Cellulitis	Subcutaneous; generally deeper and with less distinct margins than erysipelas	Erythema; tenderness; warmth; lymphangitis; lymphadenopathy	Group A strep (most common) *S. aureus* (less common)	Initial antibiotic treatment is penicillinase-resistant synthetic penicillins (PRSPs [nafcillin or oxacillin]) Alternate therapies: erythromycin, first-generation cephalosporins, amoxicillin/clavulanate (Augmentin), azithromycin, and clarithromycin
Erysipelas	Superficial; progressively enlarging, well-demarcated, red, raised, painful plaque	Similar to cellulitis but more superficial and well-demarcated	In diabetics: group A strep, *S. aureus,* Enterobacteriaceae, and clostridia	Same as cellulitis Second- or third-generation cephalosporin or amoxicillin for early and mild cases Severe cases may require imipenem (Primaxin), meropenem, or trovafloxacin Diabetics may require surgical débridement to rule out necrotizing fasciitis and obtain definitive cultures Septic patients should receive x-ray examinations to rule out gas in the soft tissues
Necrotizing fasciitis	Muscle fasica	Aggressive, life-threatening; may be associated with an underlying vascular disease (particularly diabetes) Commonly occurs after surgery, trauma, or streptococcal skin infection	Many acute cases involve several organisms Group A strep is the most common Clostridia or polymicrobial infections (aerobic plus anaerobic) are also seen	Requires emergent extensive surgical débridement (involving the entire length of the overlying cellulitis) and IV antibiotics Initial antibiotic treatments penicillin G for strep or clostridia; imipenem cilastatin or meropenem for polymicrobial infections Alternative therapies include ceftriax-one or erythromycin
Gas gangrene	Muscle; commonly in grossly contaminated traumatic wounds, particularly those that are closed primarily	Progressive severe pain, edema (distant from the wound), foul-smelling serosanguineous discharge, high fever, chills, tachycardia, confusion Clinical findings consistent with toxemia Radiographs typically show widespread gas in the soft tissues (facilitates rapid spread of the infection)	Classically caused by *Clostridium perfringens* or *Clostridium specticum* or other histotoxic *Clostridium* species These gram-positive anaerobic spore-forming rods produce exotoxins that cause necrosis of fat and muscle, and thrombosis of local vessels	Surgical (radical) débridement with fasciotomies is the primary treatment Hyperbaric oxygen may be a useful adjuvant therapy, although its effectiveness remains inconclusive Initial antibiotic treatment is clindamycin plus penicillin G Alternative therapies include ceftriaxone or erythromycin

Toxic Shock Syndrome (TSS): Staphylococcal	Remember, TSS is a form of toxemia, not a septicemia In orthopaedics, TSS is secondary to colonization of surgical or traumatic wounds (even after minor trauma) TSS can be associated with tampon use via colonization of the vagina with toxin-producing *S. aureus*	Fever, hypotension, erythematous macular rash with a serous exudate (gram-positive cocci are present) The infected wound may look benign and may be misleading with regard to the seriousness of the underlying condition	Caused by toxins produced by *Staphylococcus aureus*	Irrigation and débridement and IV antibiotics Initial antibiotic treatment is a PRSP (nafcillin or oxacillin) Alternative therapies include first-generation cephalosporins Patients may also require emergent fluid resuscitation
Toxic Shock Syndrome (TSS): Streptococcal	Remember, toxemia not septicemia Commonly associated with erysipelas or necrotizing fasciitis	Similar to *staph* TSS	Toxins from Group A, B, C, or G *Streptococcus pyogenes*	Initial antibiotic treatment is clindamycin plus penicillin G Alternative therapies include erythromycin, or ceftriaxone and clindamycin
Surgical wound infection	Varies		Most commonly, *S. aureus,* but Group A strep and Enterobacteriaceae are not uncommon Recently, the incidence of *Staphalococcus epidermidis* wound infections has been increasing Methacillin-resistant *Staphylococcus aureus* (MRSA) species infections are also increasing Vancomycin-methacillin-resistant *S. aureus* (VMRSA) has also been reported	MRSA species are best treated with vancomycin (alternatives to vancomycin for MRSA include teicoplanin, trimethoprim [Bactrim] plus sulfamethoxazole, doxycycline, minocycline, fusidic acid, fosfomycin, rifampin, and novobiocin) VMRSA is currently treated with quinupristin/dalfopristin
Marine injuries	Varies	History of fishing (or other marine activity) injury with signs of infection Culture specimens at 30°C (86°F); cultures may take several weeks to grow on culture media	Marine injuries involve organisms that can cause indolent infections *Vibrio vulnificus* is most likely the organism in infected wounds that were exposed to brackish water or shellfish; can cause a devastating infection Consider atypical mycobacteria (e.g., *Mycobacterium marinum*) for injuries with indolent low-grade infection	*V. vulnificus* is best treated with ceftazidime (doxycycline for penicillin allergy or in addition to ceftazidime); cefotaxime or ciprofloxacin are alternatives *M. marinum* is best treated with clarithromycin or minocycline or doxycycline or trimethoprim/ sulfamethoxazole or rifampin plus ethambutol

Table 1-43. BITE INJURIES

SOURCE OF BITE	ORGANISM(S)	PRIMARY ANTIMICROBIAL (OR DRUG) REGIMEN
Human	*Strep. viridans* (100%) *Bacteroides* *Staph. epidermidis* *Corynebacterium* *Staph. aureus* *Peptostreptococcus* *Eikenella*	Early treatment (not yet infected): amoxicillin/clavulanate (Augmentin) With signs of infection: ampicillin/sulbactam (Unasyn) or cefoxitin or ticarillin/clavulanate (Timentin) or piperacillin-tazobactam Patients with penicillin allergy: clindamycin plus either ciprofloxacin or trimethoprim/sulfamethoxazole *Eikenella* is resistent to clindamycin, nafcillin/oxacillin, metronidazole, and ± to first-generation cephalosporins and erythromycin; susceptible to fluoroquinolones and trimethoprim/sulfamethoxazole; treat with cefoxitin or ampicillin
Dog	*Staph. aureus* *Pasteurella multocida* *Bacteroides* *Fusobacterium* *Capnocytophaga*	Amoxicillin/clavulanate (Augmentin) Consider antirabies treatment
Cat	*Pasteurella multocida* *Staph. aureus* Possibly tularemia	Amoxicillin/clavulanate or cefuroxime axetil or doxycycline
Rat	*Strep. moniliformis*	Amoxicillin/clavulanate or doxycycline Antirabies treatment *not* indicated
Pig	Polymicrobic (aerobes and anerobes)	Amoxicillin/clavulanate
Skunk, raccoon, bat	Varies	Amoxicillin/clavulanate or doxycycline Antirabies treatment is indicated
Pit viper (snake)	*Pseudomonas* Enterobacteriaceae *Staph. epidermidis* *Clostridium*	Antivenin therapy ceftriaxone tetanus prophylaxis
Brown recluse spider	—	Dapsone
Catfish sting	Toxins (may become secondarily infected)	Amoxicillin/clavulanate

Adapted from Gilbert, D.N., Moellering, R.C., and Sande, M.A. The Sanford Guide to Antimicrobial Therapy, p. 36. Hyde Park, VT, Antimicrobial Therapy, Inc., 2002.

drainage is required for septic hip joints. SI joint sepsis is unusual and is best diagnosed by physical examination (flexion abduction external rotation [FABER] most specific), ESR, bone scan, CT scan, and aspiration. A pannus (similar to that of inflammatory arthritis) can be seen in tuberculosis infections. Late sequelae of septic arthritis include soft-tissue contractures that can sometimes be treated with soft-tissue procedures (such as a quadricepsplasty). Empiric therapy before availability of definitive cultures is based on the patient age and/or special circumstances.

a. **Newborn (up to 3 Months of Age)—The most common organisms include**

Table 1-44. INFECTED HOST TYPES

TYPE	DESCRIPTION	RISK
A	Normal immune response; nonsmoker	Minimal
B	Local or mild systemic deficiency; smoker	Moderate
C	Major nutritional or systemic disorder	High

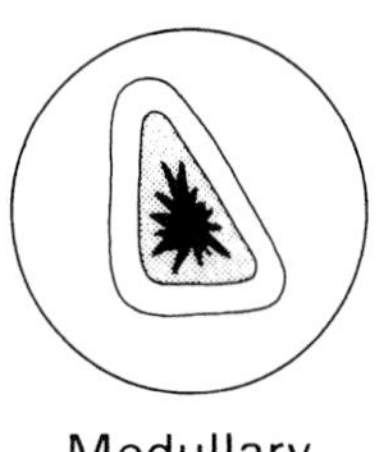

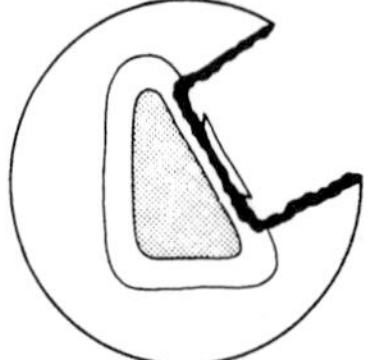

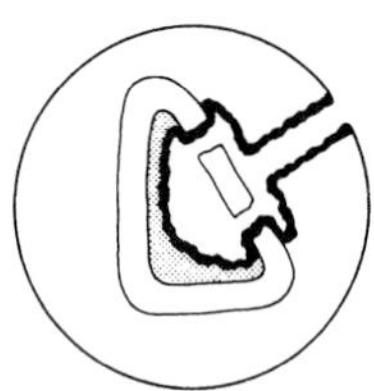

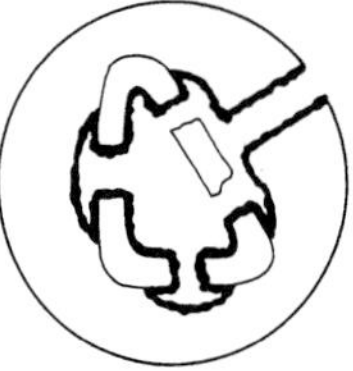

FIGURE 1-91 ■ Cierney's anatomic classification of adult chronic osteomyelitis. (From Cierney, G., III: Chronic osteomyelitis: Results of treatment. Instr. Course Lect. 39:495, 1990.)

Table 1-45. UNUSUAL ORGANISMS THAT MAY BE FOUND IN OSTEOMYELITIS

ORGANISM	RISK FACTOR(S)	SYMPTOMS/SIGNS/FINDINGS	TREATMENT
Serratia marcescens	IV drug abuse	Axial skeleton	Cotrimoxazole
Pseudomonas aeruginosa	IV drug abuse	Nonspecific	Aminoglycoside
Brucella (G–)	Meat handling	Flat bones	Tetracycline/Septra
Salmonella	Sickle cell disease	Asymptomatic	Ampicillin
Anaerobes	Skin contamination	Tissue culture	Clindamycin/cephalosporin
Fungi	Skin contamination	Special study	Amphotericin B
Treponema pallidum	Sexual contact	Nontender swelling	Penicillin
Mycobacteria	TB/leprosy/fishermen	PPD/granuloma/culture at 30°C	PAS, isoniazid

TB, tuberculosis; PPD, purified protein derivative; PAS, *p*-aminosalicylic acid; G–, gram negative.

***S. aureus* and group B strep; less common organisms include** Enterobacteriaceae and *N. gonorrhoeae*. Adjacent bony involvement is seen in almost 70% of patients. Blood cultures are commonly positive. Initial treatment is with a PRSP plus a third-generation cephalosporin. Alternative treatment is with a PRSP plus an antipseudomonal aminoglycosidic (APAG) antibiotic. If the organism is methicillin resistant *s. aureus* (MRSA), use vancomycin (instead of a PRSP) with an APAG.

b. **Children (3 Months to 14 Years of Age)**—The most common organisms are as follows: *S. aureus*, *Streptococcus pyogenes*, *Streptococcus pneumoniae*, *H. influenzae* **(incidence of *H. influenzae* septic arthritis has markedly decreased with vaccination programs)**, and gram-negative bacilli. Initial treatment is with a PRSP plus a third-generation cephalosporin; alternative treatment is with vancomycin plus a third-generation cephalosporin.

c. **Acute Monoarticular Septic Arthritis in Sexually Active Adults**—The most common organisms include *N. gonorrhoeae*, *S. aureus*, streptococci, and aerobic gram-negative bacilli (uncommon). Empiric drug therapy when the Gram stain is negative is ceftriaxone or cefotaxime or ceftizoxime; when the Gram stain shows gram-positive cocci in clusters, the treatment is nafcillin or oxacillin.

d. **Acute Monoarticular Septic Arthritis in Adults Who are Not Sexually Active**—The most common organisms are *S. aureus*, streptococci, and gram-negative bacilli. Antibiotic treatment is a PRSP plus a third-generation cephalosporin or a PRSP plus ciprofloxacin.

e. **Chronic Monoarticular Septic Arthritis**—The most common organisms are *Brucella*, *Nocardia*, *Mycobacteria*, and fungi.

f. **Polyarticular Septic Arthritis**—The most common organisms are gonococci, *Borrelia burgdorferi*, acute rheumatic fever, or viruses.

2. Septic Bursitis—Most commonly caused by an *S. aureus* infection. Treatment is with a PRSP.
3. Infected Total Joint Arthroplasty—Covered in Chapter 4, Adult Reconstruction, but bears some mention here. Perioperative IV antibiotics are the most effective method for decreasing its incidence, although good operative technique, laminar flow (avoiding obstruction between the air source and the operative wound), and special "space suits" also have a role. The ESR is the most sensitive indicator of infection, but it is nonspecific. Culture of the hip aspirate is sensitive and specific. C-reactive protein may also be helpful. Preoperative skin ulcerations are associated with an increased risk for infecting a TKA. **Acute infections (within 2-3 weeks of arthroplasty) can usually be treated with prosthesis salvage, exchanging only polyethylene components (provided the metallic components are stable).** Synovectomy for an acute TKA infection is also beneficial. **Delayed or chronic TJA infections require implant (and cement) removal.** A staged-exchange arthroplasty may be performed later, depending on the virulence of the organism. ***S. epidermidis* is the most common pathogen in infection associated with an implant or other foreign body (including allograft)**; the next most frequent pathogens are *S. aureus* and group B streptococcus. Polymicrobial organisms may form an overlying glycocalyx, making infection control difficult without removing the prosthesis and vigorous débridement. However, according to Cierney, the host is more important than the organism in terms of risk (see Table 1-44). Use of antibiotic-impregnated cement in revision arthroplasties and antibiotic spacers/beads in infected total joints may be helpful. Reimplantation after thorough débridement and use of polymethylmethacrylate (PMMA) with antibiotics has been successful at variable intervals. Some advocate frozen sections at the time of reimplantation

to ensure that local tissues have fewer than 5-10 PMNs per high-power field. The most accurate test for infection of a TJA is a tissue culture. Routine aspiration of all hip joints prior to revision THA results in a high incidence of false-positive cultures; preoperative aspiration of the knee joint prior to revision TKA appears to be a useful study to rule out infection. Most patients who have undergone total joint replacement do not need prophylactic antibiotics when undergoing dental surgery. The most common organism infecting a TJA after a dental procedure is **peptostreptococcus.**

4. Clenched Fist to the Mouth Lacerations—Lacerations overlying the joints of a hand that has struck another person's mouth ("fight bite") should be considered a penetrating joint injury. These wounds should be operatively explored, and the patient should be treated with IV antibiotics.

D. Other Infections

1. Tetanus—**A potentially lethal neuroparalytic disease caused by an exotoxin of *Clostridium tetani*.** Prophylaxis requires classifying the patient's wound (tetanus prone or nontetanus prone) and a complete history of the patient's immunizations. Tetanus-prone wounds: are greater than 6 hours old; have an irregular configuration; have a depth greater than 1 cm, or are the result of a projectile injury, crush injury, burn, or frostbite; have devitalized tissue; and are grossly contaminated. Patients with tetanus-prone wounds who have an unknown tetanus status or have received <3 immunizations require tetanus and diphtheria toxoids and tetanus immune globulin (human). Fully immunized patients with tetanus-prone wounds do not require immune globulin, but tetanus toxoid should be administered if the wound is severe or >24 hours old, or the patient has not received a booster within the past 5 years. The only type of patient with a nontetanus-prone wound who requires any treatment is one with an unknown immunization history or a history of <3 doses of tetanus immunization; these patients require tetanus toxoid. The treatment of established tetanus is primarily to control the patient's muscle spasms with diazepam. Initial antibiotic therapy includes penicillin G or doxycycline; alternative antibiotic therapy includes metronidazole.

2. Rabies—**An acute infection characterized by irritation of the CNS that may be followed by paralysis and death. The organism involved in rabies is a neurotropic virus that may be present in the saliva of rabid animals.** In dog or cat bites, healthy animals should be observed for 10 days; there is no need to start antirabies treatment. If the animal begins to experience symptoms, the patient should receive human rabies immune globulin with human diploid cell vaccine or rabies vaccine absorbed (inactivated). For bites from dogs and cats suspected or known to be rabid, vaccination of the patient should occur immediately. Bites from skunks, raccoons, bats, foxes, and most carnivores should be considered rabid, and the patient should be immunized immediately. Animal bites that rarely require antirabies treatment include: mice, rats, chipmunks, gerbils, guinea pigs, hamsters, squirrels, rabbits, and rodents.

3. Puncture Wounds of the Foot—**The most characteristic organism from the puncture of a nail through the sole of a tennis shoe is *Pseudomonas aeruginosa*** (unless the host is immunocompromised or diabetic). *Pseudomonas infections* (gram-negative rod) require aggressive débridement and appropriate antibiotics (often require a two-antibiotic regimen). The initial antibiotic regimen for an established infection should include ceftazidime or cefepime; alternative initial antibiotic regimen might include ciprofloxacin (except in children), imipenem cilastatin, or a third-generation cephalosporin. The prophylactic antibiotic treatment for a recent (hours) puncture through the sole of a tennis shoe (without infection) remains controversial. **Osteomyelitis develops in 1-2% of children who sustain a puncture wound through the sole of a tennis shoe.**

4. Diabetic Foot Infections
   a. Limited in Extent (No Osteomyelitis, No Previous History of Foot Infection)—The most common organism is aerobic gram-positive cocci. The antibiotic regimen of choice is clindamycin or a first-generation cephalosporin. Débridement of soft tissues is performed as clinically indicated.
   b. Chronic, Recurrent, Limb-Threatening Diabetic Foot—These infections can be life-threatening and, generally, **cultures show a polymicrobial picture** (including aerobic cocci, aerobic bacilli, and anaerobes). **In early cases or relatively milder cases** of chronic recurrent limb-threatening diabetic foot, the initial antibiotic regimen can include ampicillin/sulbactam (Unasyn), piperacillin-tazobactam, ticarcillin/clavulanate (Timentin), or clindamycin plus one of the following: ceftriaxone/cefotaxime, ciprofloxacin, levofloxacin, or aztreonam. In cases of **severe chronic recurrent limb-threatening diabetic foot** or when the patient is septic, the antibiotic regimen of choice includes vancomycin plus one of the following: imipenem/cilastatin (Primaxin), meropenem, or trovafloxacin. Cultures from diabetic foot ulcers are unreliable. **Rapid surgical intervention with irrigation and débridement is essential.** Surgical débridement

helps differentiate diabetic foot from necrotizing fasciitis or gas gangrene.

5. Paronychia—Infection/inflammation of the paronychial fold on the side of the nail.
   a. Nail Biting and Manicuring—The most common organism is *S. aureus*; anaerobes are also common. The initial antibiotic treatment includes clindamycin; erythromycin is an alternative initial antibiotic treatment.
   b. Dentist, Anesthesiologist, Wrestlers (Those Who Are in Contact with the Oral Mucosa of Others)—The most common organism is herpes simplex (herpetic whitlow). Commonly presents with vesicles containing clear fluid. Gram's stain and routine cultures are negative. The treatment of choice is acyclovir; there is no need to débride the vesicles.
   c. Dishwashers or Others Who Engage in Activities that Involve Prolonged Immersion in Water—The most common organism is *Candida*, and the treatment is topical clotrimazole.
6. Fungal Infections—Fungi are multicellular organisms with mycelia (branches) inducing a tissue hypersensitivity reaction, causing chronic granuloma, abscess, and necrosis. Surgical treatment and **amphotericin B** administration are often required. Oral ketoconazole is effective for some limited infections.
7. Human Immunodeficiency Virus (HIV) Infection—Incidence is high in the homosexual male population and is becoming increasingly common in heterosexual patients. Additionally, a large portion of the hemophiliac population is affected. HIV primarily affects the lymphocyte and macrophage cell lines and **decreases the number of T helper cells (formerly known as T4 lymphocytes, now known as CD4 cells). The diagnosis of AIDS requires an HIV-positive test plus one of the following two scenarios: (1) one of the opportunistic infections (such as pneumocystis) or (2) a CD4 count of less than 200 (normal CD4 count = 700-1200).** HIV has increased the importance of blood and body fluid handling precautions during trauma management and surgery. The risk of seroconversion from a contaminated needle stick is 0.3% (increases if the exposure involves a larger amount of blood); the risk of seroconversion from mucous membrane exposure is 0.09%. The risk of HIV transmission via a large, frozen bone allograft is 1 in 1 million; **donor screening is the most important factor in preventing viral transmission. Blood donated for transfusion that tests negative for the HIV antibody may transmit HIV to the recipient because there is a delay (in the donor) between infection with HIV and development of a detectable antibody**. The risk of transmission of HIV via a blood transfusion is 1 in 440,000 to 1 in 600,000 per unit transfused. HIV positivity is not a contraindication to performing required surgical procedures. HIV-positive patients, even if asymptomatic, with traumatic orthopaedic injuries (especially open fractures) or undergoing certain orthopaedic surgical procedures appear to be at increased risk for wound infections and nonwound-related complications (e.g., urinary tract infection, pneumonia). Patients with HIV can develop secondary rheumatologic conditions such as Reiter's syndrome. Fetal AIDS is transmitted across the placenta; affected children typically have a box-like forehead, wide eyes, a small head, and growth failure.
8. Hepatitis—Three types are commonly recognized.
   a. Hepatitis A—Common in areas with poor sanitation and public health concerns. Not a major problem regarding surgical transmission.
   b. Hepatitis B—Approximately 200,000 people are infected with the hepatitis B virus each year, and there are more than 1 million carriers. Screening and vaccination has reduced the risk of transmission for health care workers. Immune globulin is administered after exposure in nonvaccinated persons. Neither the vaccine nor immune globulin administration has been documented as causing HIV transmission.
   c. Hepatitis C (Non-A, Non-B)—The offending virus has been identified (hepatitis C virus). It is the **most common transfusion-associated hepatitis and is also related to IV drug abuse. PCR is the most sensitive method for early detection of infection**.
9. Lyme Disease—Discussed in Section 2 under arthroses. A new Lyme disease vaccine, LYMErix (Recombinant OspA), is available for persons 15-70 years of age.
10. **Cat Scratch Fever (Cat scratch Disease)**—Infection of the lymphatic system by ***Bartonella hensela***. The disease is transmitted via a wound inflicted by a cat. The patient experiences an erythmatous, painful lymphadenitis. Treatment is with azithromycin; alternative treatment is supportive only (resolves in 2-6 months) using needle aspiration of suppurative lymph nodes to relieve pain. **Do not perform incision and drainage on the lesions.**
11. Allograft Infection—May involve up to 20% of allografts; requires aggressive measures to control.
12. Meningococcemia—Can develop in patients with multiple infarcts, such as those with **electrical burns**.
13. Marjolin's Ulcer—Squamous cell carcinoma that develops in patients with chronic drainage from sinus tracts; seen in untreated chronic osteomyelitis.

14. Nutritional Status and Infection—Good nutrition decreases the incidence of postoperative infection. Malnutrition is common after multiple trauma.
15. Postsplenectomy Patients—Susceptible to streptococcal infections and respond poorly to them.
16. Infections of the Spine (Discussed in Chapter 7, Spine)
    a. Discitis—Children experience back pain and may have difficulty walking or sitting. Radiographs may appear normal; bone scans and MRI may show early changes. The initial treatment is immobilization and antibiotics. A biopsy is indicated if initial treatment fails.
    b. Vertebral Osteomyelitis—Activity-related pain of insidious onset is the most common symptom. Neurologic signs are uncommon until late in the disease progression. Weight loss and chills are common. The lumbar spine is the most common site; diabetics are particularly prone. Both a bone scan and MRI are usually diagnostic. Recommended treatment is immobilization and antibiotics. Surgery (I&D and immediate spinal arthrodesis) is indicated if (1) nonoperative treatment fails or (2) vertebral collapse with a neurologic deficit occurs.
    c. Epidural Abscess—Onset of symptoms may be rapid. There is often a history of recent trauma. There is generally markedly limited ROM of the lumbar spine and a positive straight leg raising test (indicating associated inflammation of the dura or nerve root sleeves). Bone scans are typically negative. MRI and contrast CT are excellent for imaging an epidural abscess. Antibiotics are generally ineffective, so surgical drainage is necessary.
    d. Postoperative Spinal Infections—Early diagnosis is difficult; clinical findings are often vague, and there are no excellent diagnostic tests. Following spinal surgery, both the ESR and C-reactive protein peak at 2-3 days and may remain elevated for as long as 2 weeks. Fever spikes and a rising ESR indicate infection (don't forget the blood cultures). Treatment is IV antibiotics, operative débridement, and retention of spinal implants.
    e. Other Spinal Infections
        1. Pyogenic infections
        2. Tuberculous spondylitis
        3. Coccidioidomycosis spondylitis

II. Antibiotics

A. Introduction—Antibiotics in orthopaedics may be used in a variety of ways.
   1. Prophylactic Treatment—Used to prevent postoperative sepsis (for clean surgical cases, administer 1 hour preoperatively and continue for 24 hours postoperatively). Perioperative use of first-generation cephalosporins is efficacious in cases requiring hardware. **Using a shorter course of prophylactic antibiotics decreases the likelihood that bacteria will develop resistance.**
   2. Initial Care After an Open Traumatic Wound—Type I and II open fractures require a first-generation cephalosporin (some authors have recently suggested the addition of an aminoglycoside or the use of a second-generation cephalosporin); type IIIA open fractures require a first-generation cephalosporin plus an aminoglycoside; penicillin is added for grossly contaminated (type IIIB) open fractures.
   3. Treatment of Established Infections—Overall, *S. aureus* remains the leading cause of osteomyelitis and nongonococcal septic arthritis. In general, the virulence of *S. epidermidis* infections is closely related to orthopaedic hardware. **Clindamycin achieves the highest antibiotic concentrations in bone** (nearly equals serum concentrations after IV administration) **and is bacteriostatic**. To prevent the development of vancomycin-resistant strains, vancomycin should not be used in patients with a blood culture of coagulase-negative *S. aureus* that is not methicillin resistant.

B. Antibiotic-Resistant Bacteria—Two types of antibiotic resistance exist.
   1. Intrinsic Resistance—Inherent features of a cell that prevent antibiotics from acting on the cell (such as the absence of a metabolic pathway or enzyme).
   2. Acquired Resistance—A new resistant strain emerges from a population that was previously sensitive (acquired resistance is mediated by plasmids [extrachromosomal genetic elements] and transopsons).

C. Spectrum of Antimicrobial Agents (Table 1-46)
D. Antibiotic Indications and Side Effects (Table 1-47)
E. Mechanism of Action of Antibiotics (Table 1-48)
F. Other Forms of Antibiotic Delivery
   1. Antibiotic Beads or Spacers—PMMA impregnated with antibiotics (usually an aminoglycoside); useful when treating infected TJA or osteomyelitis with bony defects. Antibiotic powder is mixed with cement powder; the antibiotic used is guided by the microorganism, and dosage depends on the selected antibiotic and type of PMMA. Antibiotics that have been used with PMMA for infection are tobramycin, gentamicin, cefazolin (Ancef) and other cephalosporins, oxacillin, cloxacillin, methicillin, lincomycin, clindamycin, colistin, fucidin, neomycin, kanamycin, and ampicillin. Chloramphenicol and tetracycline appear to be inactivated during polymerization. Antibiotics elute from PMMA beads with an exponential decline over a 2-week period and cease to be

Table 1-46. OVERVIEW OF ANTIMICROBIAL AGENTS

Penicillins

Natural
Penicillin G
Penicillin-VK
Penicillinase Resistant (PRSP)
Methicillin (Staphcillin, Celbenin)
Nafcillin (Unipen, Nafcil)
Oxacillin (Prostaphlin, Bactocill)
Cloxacillin (Tegopen, Cloxapen)
Dicloxacillin (Dynapen, Pathocil)
Flucloxacillin (Floxapen, Ladropen, Staphcil)
Aminopenicillins
Ampicillin (Omnipen, Polycillin)
Amoxacillin (Amoxil)
Bacampicillin (Spectrobid)
Amoxicillin/clavulanate (Augmentin)
Ampicillin/sulbactam (Unasyn)
Antipseudomonal Agents
Indanyl carbenicillin (Geocillin)
Ticarcillin (Ticar)
Ticarcillin/clavulanate (Timentin)
Mezlocillin (Mezlin)
Piperacillin (Pipracil)
Piperacillin/tazobactam (Zosyn)

Cephalosporins

First Generation
Cephalothin (Keflin, Seffin)
Cefazolin (Ancef, Kefzol)
Cephapirin (Cefadyl)
Cephradine (Velosef)
Cephalexin (Keflex, Keftab)
Cefadroxil (Duricef, Ultracef)
Second Generation
Cefaclor (Ceclor)
Cefamandole (Mandol)
Cefoxitin (Mefoxin)
Cefuroxime (Zinacef, Kefurox)
Cefuroxime axetil (Ceftin)
Cefmetazole (Zefazone)
Cefotetan (Cefotan)
Cefprozil (Cefzil)
Cefonicid (Monocid)
Loracarbef (Lorabid)
Ceftibuten (Cedax)
Third Generation
Cefetamet pivoxil (R. 15-8075)
Cefoperazone (Cefobid)
Cefoperazone (Claforan)
Ceftizoxime (Cefizox)
Ceftriaxone (Rocephin, Nitrocephin)
Ceftazidime (Fortaz, Tazicef, Tazidime)
Cefixime (Suprax)
Cefpodoxime proxetil (Vantin)
Fourth Generation
Cefpirome (HR 810)
Cefepime (Maxipime)

Carbapenems

Ertapenem (Invanz)
Imipenem + cilastatin (Primaxin)
Meropenem (Merrem)

Monobactams

Aztreonam (Azactam)

Aminoglycosides

Amikacin (Amikin)
Gentamicin (Garamycin)
Kanamycin (Kantrex)
Neomycin
Netilmicin (Netromycin)
Tobramycin (Nebcin)

Fluoroquinolones

Norfloxacin (Noroxin)
Ciprofloxacin (Cipro)
Ofloxacin (Floxin)
Enoxacin (Penetrex)
Gatifloxacin (Tequin)
Grepafloxacin (Raxar)
Lomefloxacin (Maxaquin)
Moxifloxacin (Avelox)
Pefloxacin
Levofloxacin (Levaquin)
Sparfloxacin (Zagam)
Trovafloxacin (Trovan)

Macrolides

Azithromycin (Zithromax)
Clarithromycin (Biaxin)
Dirithromycin (Dynabac)
Erythromycin

Other Antibacterial Agents

Chloramphenicol (Chloromycetin)
Clindamycin (Cleocin)
Vancomycin (Vancocin, Vancoled)
Teicoplanin (Targocid)
Doxycycline (Vibramycin)
Minocycline (Minocin)
Tetracycline (Terramycin)
Polymyxin B (Aerosporin)
Fusidic acid (Fucidin)
Fosfomycin (Monurol)
Sulfisoxazole (Gantrisin)
Trimethoprim/sulfamethoxazole (Bactrim, Septra)
Metronidazole (Flagyl)

Antifungal Agents

Amphotericin B (Fungizone)
Fluconazole (Diflucan)
Flucytosine (Ancobon)
Ketaconazole (Nizoral)
Itraconazole (Sporanox)

Antimycobacterial Agents

Isoniazid [INH (Nydrazid)]
Rifampin (Rifadin)
Ethambutol (Myambutol)
Streptomycin
Pyrazinamide
Ethionamide
Cycloserine (Seromycin)
Amikacin (Amikin)
Capreomycin (Capastat)
Thioacetazone
Rifabutin (Mycobutin)

Antiparasitic Agents

Albendazole (Zentel)
Atovaquone (Mepron)
Dapsone
Ivermectin (Stromectol)
Mefloquine (Lariam)
Pentamidine (Pentam 300)
Pyrimethamine (Daraprim)
Praziquantel (Biltricide)
Quinine

Antiviral Agents

Abacavir (Ziagen)
Acyclovir (Zovirax)
Amantadine (Symmetrel)
Amprenvir (Agenerase)
Cidofovir (Vistide)
Delavirdine (Rescriptor)
Didanosine (Videx)
Efavirenz (Sustiva)
Famciclovir (Famvir)
Foscarnet (Foscavir)
Ganciclovir (Cytovene)
Indinavir (Crixivan)
Lamivudine (Epivir, Epivir-HBV)
Lopinavir/ritonavir (Kaletra)
Nelfinavir (Viracept)
Nevirapine (Viramune)
Oseltamivir (Tamiflu)
Ribavirin (Virazole)
Rimantadine (Flumadine)
Ritonavir (Norvir)
Saquinavir (Invirase, Fortovase)
Stavudine (Zerit)
Valacyclovir (Valtrex)
Zalcitabine (Hivid)
Zidovudine [AZT (Retrovir)]

Adapted from Gilbert, D.N., Moellering, R.C., and Sande, M.A. The Sanford Guide to Antimicrobial Therapy, 32nd ed., pp. 58–78. Hyde Park, VT, Antimicrobial Therapy, Inc., 2002.

Table 1-47. ANTIBIOTIC INDICATIONS AND SIDE EFFECTS

ANTIBIOTICS	ORGANISMS	COMPLICATIONS/OTHER
Aminoglycosides	G–, PM	Auditory (most common) and vestibular toxicity are caused by destruction of the cochlear and vestibular sensory cells from drug accumulation in the perilymph and endolymph; renal toxicity; neuromuscular blockade
Amphotericin	Fungi	Nephrotoxic
Azactam	G–, no anaerobes	
Carbenicillin/ticarcillin/ piperacillin	Better against G–	Bleeding diathesis (carbenicillin)
Cephalosporins		
First generation	Prophylaxis (surgical)	Cephazolin is the drug of choice
Second generation	Some G+/G–	
Third generation	G–, fewer G+	Hemolytic anemia (bleeding diathesis [moxalactam])
Chloramphenicol	*H. influenzae*, anaerobes	Bone marrow aplasia
Ciprofloxacin	G–, methicillin-resistant *S. aureus*	Tendon ruptures; cartilage erosion in children; antacids reduce absorption of cipro; theophylline increases serum concentrations of cipro
Clindamycin	G+, anaerobes	Pseudomembranous enterocolitis
Erythromycin	G+ (PCN allergy)	Ototoxic
Imipenem	G+, some G–	Resistances, seizure
Methicillin/oxacillin/nafcillin	Penicillinase-resistant	Same as penicillin; nephritis (methicillin); subcut. skin slough (nafcillin)
Penicillin	Strep, G+	Hypersensitivity/resistance; hemolytic
Polymyxin/nystatin	GU	Nephrotoxic
Sulfonamides	GU	Hemolytic anemia
Tetracycline	G+ (PCN allergy)	Stains teeth/bone (up to age 8)
Vancomycin	Methicillin-resistance *S. aureus*, *C. difficile*	Ototoxic; erythema with rapid IV delivery

G+, gram positive; G–, gram negative; GU, genitourinary; PM, polymicrobial; PCN, penicillin; subcut., subcutaneous.

present locally in significant levels by 6-8 weeks. Much higher local tissue concentrations of antibiotic can be achieved than with systemic administration, but does not seem to cause problems in doses typically used. (Extremely high local concentrations of antibiotics can decrease cellular replication or even result in cell death.) Increased surface area of PMMA (e.g., with oval beads) enhances antibiotic elution. Beads are inserted only after thorough débridement. Because PMMA may cause a foreign body reaction, the beads should always be removed. Antibiotic powder in doses of 2 g per 40 g of powdered PMMA (simplex P) does not appreciably affect the compressive strength of PMMA. Much higher

Table 1-48. MECHANISM OF ACTION OF ANTIBIOTICS

CLASS OF ANTIBIOTIC	EXAMPLES	MECHANISM OF ACTION
Beta-lactam antibiotics	Penicillin Cephalosporins	Inhibits bacterial peptidoglycan synthesis (the mechanism is via binding to the penicillin-binding proteins on the surface of the bacterial cell membrane)
Aminoglycosides	Gentamicin Tobramycin	Inhibits protein synthesis (the mechanism is via binding to cytoplasmic ribosomal RNA)
Clindamycin and macrolides	Clindamycin Erythromycin Clarithromycin Azithromycin	Inhibit the dissociation of peptidyl-tRNA from ribosomes during translocation (the mechanism is via binding to 50S-ribosomal subunits)
Tetracyclines		Inhibit protein synthesis (on 70S- and 80S-ribosomes)
Glycopeptides	Vancomycin Teicoplanin	Interfere with the insertion of glycan subunits into the cell wall
Rifampin		Inhibits RNA synthesis in bacteria
Quinolones	Ciprofloxacin Levofloxacin Ofloxacin	Inhibit DNA gyrase

concentrations (4-5 g of antibiotic powder per 40 g of PMMA) significantly reduces the compressive strength (important in cemented joint arthroplasties). Antibiotic impregnated cement spacers help prevent soft-tissue contracture after removing an infected TKA.

2. Osmotic Pump—Delivers high concentrations of antibiotics locally. Used mainly for osteomyelitis.
3. Home IV Therapy—Cost-effective alternative for long-term IV antibiotics; facilitated by a Hickman or Broviac indwelling catheter.
4. Immersion Solution—Contaminated bone from an open fracture may be sterilized (100% effective) by immersion in chlorhexidine gluconate scrub and an antibiotic solution.

SECTION 6

Perioperative Problems

I. Pulmonary Problems

A. General Considerations—Pulmonary function tests and blood gas measurements are often helpful for evaluating baseline status. Thoracic and abdominal surgery can significantly affect these values.

B. Blood Gas Evaluation—The following simple working formula is useful for evaluating blood gases:

$$\mathbf{pO_2 = 7\ (FiO_2) - pCO_2}$$

where pO_2 is the anticipated or normal pO_2 given FiO_2 in a normal person, FiO_2 is the percentage of inspired oxygen, and pCO_2 is the value obtained by the blood gas assay.

Example. A 63-year-old-man has acute onset of shortness of breath 12 hours after a THA. Assume that a blood gas assay obtained 15 minutes after placing the patient on 60% oxygen (FiO_2 = 60) reveals the following **observed values**:

$$pO_2 = 120$$

$$pCO_2 = 60$$

$$pO_2 = 7\ (60) - pCO_2 = 420 - pCO_2$$

With a pCO_2 of 60, the anticipated (or normal) pO_2 would be

$$pO_2 = 420 - 60 = 360$$

Therefore, with 60% oxygen and a pCO_2 of 60, expected pO_2 = 360 if all were normal. The observed pO_2 (120) indicates an obvious problem with pulmonary status. To quantify the extent of the problem, calculate the **Aa gradient**:

Aa gradient = (anticipated or normal pO_2 [for a given FiO_2]) – (observed pO_2)

Continuing with the example:

Aa gradient = (360) – (120) = 240

Finally, the **percent physiologic shunt** is calculated.

Percent physiologic shunt = Aa gradient/20

Continuing with the example:

Percent physiologic shunt = 240/20 = 12%

C. Thromboembolism—Common in orthopaedic patients, especially those with procedures about the hip. Risk increases with a history of thromboembolism, obesity, malignancy, aging, congestive heart failure (CHF), birth control pill use, varicose veins, smoking, use of general anesthetics (in contrast with continuous epidural anesthesia), increased blood viscosity, immobilization, paralysis, and pregnancy.

1. Deep Venous Thrombosis (DVT)—Clinical suspicion is often more helpful than physical examination (pain, swelling, Homan's sign) for DVT. Useful studies include **venography (the "gold standard")**, which is 97% accurate (70% for iliac veins), 125I-labeled fibrinogen (operative site artifact causes false positives), impedance plethysmography (poor sensitivity), duplex ultrasonography (B-mode)—90% accurate for DVT proximal to the trifurcation vessels, and Doppler imaging (immediate bedside tool, often best first study). Prophylaxis is the most important factor in decreasing morbidity and mortality; common methods are listed in Table 1-49. Because DVT is relatively uncommon after elective spinal surgery, only mechanical prophylaxis (such as compression stockings) is recommended. **The anticoagulation effects of warfarin (Coumadin) are via inhibition of hepatic enzymes, vitamin K epoxide, and perhaps vitamin K reductase. This inhibition results in decreased carboxylation of the vitamin K–dependent proteins: factors II (prothrombin), VII (the first to be affected), IX, and X. Warfarin does not act by directly binding vitamin K or the clotting factors but by inhibiting posttranslational modification of vitamin K–dependent clotting factors. The anticoagulation effects of warfarin can be reversed with vitamin K or more rapidly with fresh frozen plasma.** Rifampin **and phenobarbital** are antagonists to warfarin. The diagnosis of DVT postoperatively requires initiation of heparin therapy (followed by later conversion to long-term [3 months] warfarin therapy). **Low-dose warfarin given to a patient with a DVT acts by interfering with the metabolism of factors II (prothrombin), VII, IX, and X.** Treatment is recommended for all thigh DVTs; however, treatment of DVTs occurring below the popliteal fossa is controversial. **Preoperative identification of a DVT in a patient with lower-extremity or pelvic trauma is an indication for placement of a vena cava filter. Virchow's triad** of factors involved in venous thrombosis are venous stasis, hypercoagulability, and intimal injury. Thromboembolism formation is summarized in Figure 1-92.
2. Pulmonary Embolism—Pulmonary embolism (PE) should be suspected in postoperative patients with acute onset of pleuritic pain, **tachypnea (90%)**, and tachycardia (60%).

Table 1-49. THROMBOEMBOLISM PROPHYLAXIS

METHOD	EFFECT	ADVANTAGES	DISADVANTAGES
Heparin			
Intravenous	Coagulation cascade—antithrombin III inhibitor	Reversible, effective	Control, embolization
Subcutaneous	Antithrombin III inhibitor	Reversible	No effect in extremity surgery
Coumadin*	Coagulation cascade—vitamin K–dependent clotting factors	Most effective, oral	3-5 days to full effect, control
Aspirin	Inhibits platelet aggregation; inhibits thromboxane–AZ Synthesis	Easy, no monitoring	Limited efficacy
Dextran	Dilutional	Effective	Fluid overload, bleeding
Pneumatic compression (and foot pumps)	Mechanical	Inexpensive, no bleeding	Bulky
Enoxaparin (Lovenox), a low-molecular-weight heparin	Inhibits clotting—forms complexes between antithrombin III and factors IIa and Xa	Fixed dose, no monitoring, improved bioavailability	Bleeding

*See text for details.

Initial work-up includes an EKG (right bundle branch block [RBBB], right axis deviation [RAD] in 25%; may also show ST depression or T wave inversion in lead III), a chest radiograph (hyperlucency rare), and arterial blood gases (ABGs) (normal PO_2 does not exclude PE). Nuclear medicine ventilation-perfusion (V/Q) scan may be helpful, but pulmonary angiography (the "gold standard") is required to make the diagnosis if there is any question. Once PE is diagnosed, heparin therapy (continuous IV infusion) is initiated and monitored by the partial

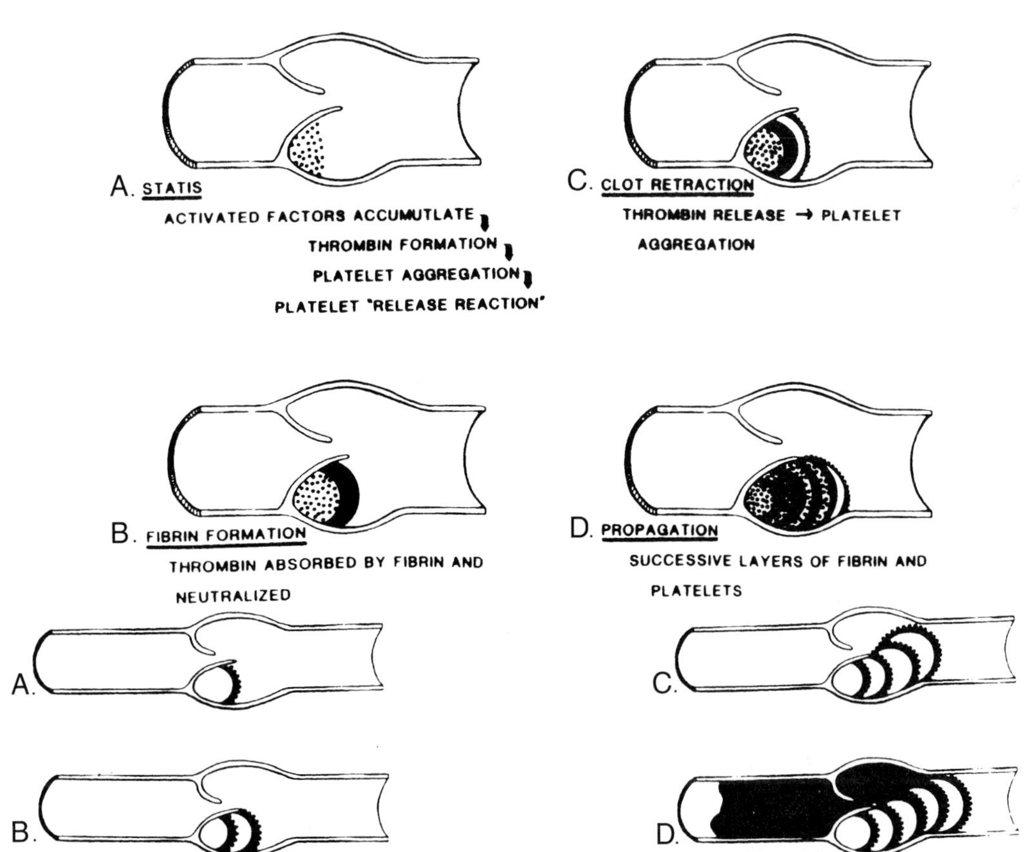

FIGURE 1-92 ■ Venous thromboembolus formation. (From Simon, S.R., ed.: Orthopaedic Basic Science, 2nd ed., p. 492. Rosemont, IL, American Academy of Orthopaedic Surgeons, 1994.)

thromboplastin time (PTT). More aggressive therapy (thrombolytic agents, vena cava filter, or other surgical measures) is required in select cases. Seven to ten days of heparin therapy is followed by 3 months of oral warfarin (monitored by the prothrombin time [PT]). Approximately 700,000 people in the United States have an asymptomatic PE each year, of which 200,000 are fatal. The most important factor for survival is early diagnosis with prompt therapy initiation. The incidence of DVT and fatal PE in unprotected patients is summarized in Table 1-50.

3. Coagulation (Fig. 1-93)—A cascade of enzymatic reactions, beginning with prothrombin-converting activity and concluding with **fibrin** clot formation (as fibrinogen is converted to fibrin). Two interconnecting pathways have been described.
   a. Intrinsic Pathway—Monitored by PTT. Activated when factor XII contacts the collagen of damaged vessels.
   b. Extrinsic Pathway—Monitored by PT. Activated by thromboplastin release into the circulation after cellular injury.
   c. The **bleeding time test measures platelet function**. The **fibrinolytic system** is responsible for dissolving clots. Plasminogen is converted to plasmin (with the help of tissue activators, factor XIIa, and thrombin); plasmin dissolves fibrin clot.

D. Adult Respiratory Distress Syndrome (ARDS)—Acute respiratory failure secondary to pulmonary edema after such events as trauma, shock, or infection. Causes of ARDS include pulmonary infection, sepsis, fat embolism, microembolism, aspiration, fluid overload, atelectasis, oxygen toxicity, pulmonary contusion, and head injury. Complement system activation leads to further progression. Signs include tachypnea, dyspnea, hypoxemia, and decreased lung compliance. **The clinical diagnosis of ARDS after a long-bone fracture is best made using ABGs.** Normal supportive care is often unsuccessful; a 50% mortality rate is not uncommon. Ventilation with PEEP is important; steroids have not been proven to be efficacious. Early stabilization of long-bone fractures (particularly the femur) decreases the risk of pulmonary complications.

E. Fat Embolism (Fig. 1-94)—Usually seen 24-72 hours after trauma (3-4% of patients with long-bone fractures); fatal in 10-15% of cases. **Early skeletal stabilization decreases the incidence of clinically significant fat embolism** and is key in prevention. **Onset may be heralded by hypoxemia (PO_2 < 60 mm Hg), CNS depression, petechiae** (axillae, conjunctivae, palate), tachypnea, pulmonary edema, tachycardia, mental status changes, and confusion. May be caused by bone marrow fat **(mechanical theory)**, chylomicron changes as a result of stress **(metabolic theory)**, or both. Metabolism to free fatty acids, initiation of the clotting cascade, pulmonary capillary leakage, bronchoconstriction, and alveolar collapse result in a **ventilation-perfusion deficit** (hypoxemia) consistent with ARDS. Treatment includes mechanical ventilation with **high levels of positive end expiratory pressure (PEEP)**. Steroids do not appear to have a prophylactic role. Over-reaming the femoral canal can decrease the incidence of fat embolism (embolization of marrow contents) during TKA. **Reamers that have a wider driver shaft increase the risk of fat emboli during femoral reaming.**

F. Pneumonia—Aspiration pneumonia can occur in patients with decreased mentation, supine positioning, and decreased GI motility. Simple measures (raising the head of the bed, using antacids and metoclopramide [Reglan]) can be preventative. Treated by appropriate IV antibiotics and pulmonary toilet.

G. Pulmonary Complications of Orthopaedic Disorders—Scoliosis of significant magnitude can cause pulmonary dysfunction. Spontaneous pneumothorax is common in patients with Marfan's syndrome.

Table 1-50. FREQUENCY OF DEEP VEIN THROMBOSIS AND FATAL PULMONARY EMBOLISM (DIAGNOSED BY VENOGRAPHY)

	FREQUENCY (%)	
UNPROTECTED PATIENTS	*DVT*	*Fatal PE*
Elective hip arthroplasty	70	2
Elective knee arthroplasty	80	1
Open meniscectomy	20	?
Hip fracture	60	3.5
Spinal fracture with paralysis	100	~1
Polytrauma patients	35	?
Pelvic/acetabular fracture	20	?

From Simon, S.R.: Orthopaedic Basic Science, 2nd ed., p. 489. Rosemont, IL, American Academy or Orthopaedic Surgeons, 1994.

II. Other Medical Problems (Nonpulmonary)

A. Nutrition—Adequate nutrition should be ensured prior to elective surgery. Malnutrition may be present in 50% of patients on a surgical ward. Several indicators exist (e.g., anergy panels, albumin levels, transferrin level); **arm muscle circumference measurement is the best indicator of nutritional status**. Wound dehiscence and infection, pneumonia, and sepsis can result from poor nutrition. Lack of enteral feeding can lead to **atrophy of the intestinal mucosae, leading in turn to bacterial translocation**. Nutritional requirements are significantly elevated as a result of stress. Full enteral or parenteral nutrition (nitrogen 200 mg/kg per day) should be provided for patients who cannot tolerate normal intake. Early elemental feeding through a jejunostomy tube can decrease complications in the

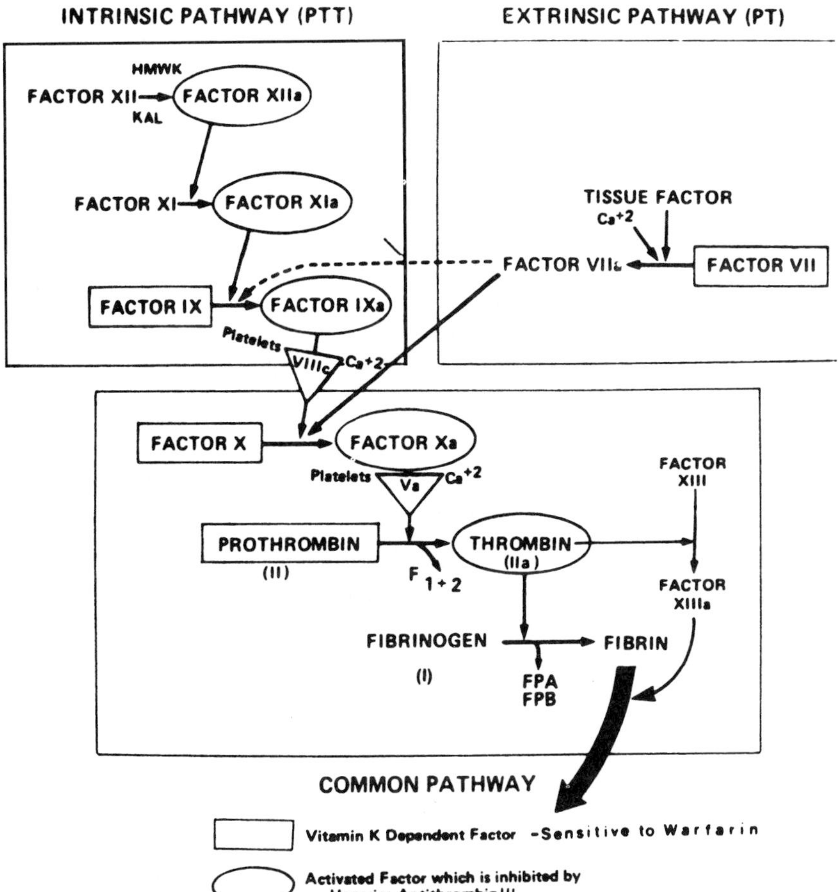

FIGURE 1-93 ■ Coagulation cascade. (From Stead, R.B.: Regulation of hemostasis. In Goldhaber, S.Z., ed.: Pulmonary Embolism and Deep Venous Thromboembolism, p. 32. Philadelphia, WB Saunders, 1985.)

multiple trauma patient. **Enteral protein supplements have proved effective in patients at risk of developing multiple organ system failure.** The metabolic changes of starvation and stress are compared in Table 1-51.

B. Myocardial Infarction (MI)—Acute chest pain, radiation, and EKG changes are classic and warrant monitoring in an appropriate critical care environment where cardiac enzymes and the EKG can be monitored on a continuing basis. Risk factors of MI include increased age, smoking, elevated cholesterol, hypertension, aortic stenosis, a history of coronary artery disease, and a variety of other factors.

C. GI Complications—Can range from ileus (treated with nasogastric suction [NG tube] and antacids) to upper GI bleeding. Postoperative ileus is common in diabetics with neuropathy. Upper GI bleeding is more likely in patients with a history of ulcers, NSAID use, and smoking. Treatment includes lavage, antacids, and H_2-blockers. Vasopressin (left gastric artery) may be required for more serious cases. Ogilvie's syndrome, which includes cecal distention, can follow total joint replacement surgery. If the cecum is >10 cm on an abdominal flat plate radiograph, it must be decompressed (usually can be done colonoscopically).

D. Decubitus Ulcers—Associated with advanced age, critical illness, and neurologic impairment. Common sites include the sacrum, heels, and buttocks, which may be a source of infection and increased morbidity. Prevention with constant changing of position, special mattresses, and treatment of systemic illness and malnutrition is essential. Once established, débridement and sometimes soft-tissue flaps are required for treatment.

E. Urinary Tract Infection (UTI)—Most common nosocomial infection (6-8%). Causes increased risk for joint sepsis after TJA (but may not be from direct seeding). Established UTIs should be adequately treated preoperatively. Perioperative catheterization (removed 24 hours postoperatively) may reduce the rate of postoperative UTI.

F. Prostatic Hypertrophy—Causes postoperative urinary retention. If the history, physical examination (prostate), and urine flow studies (<17 mL/sec peak flow rate) are suggestive, urologic referral should be accomplished preoperatively.

G. Acute Tubular Necrosis—Can cause renal failure in trauma patients. Alkalization of urine is

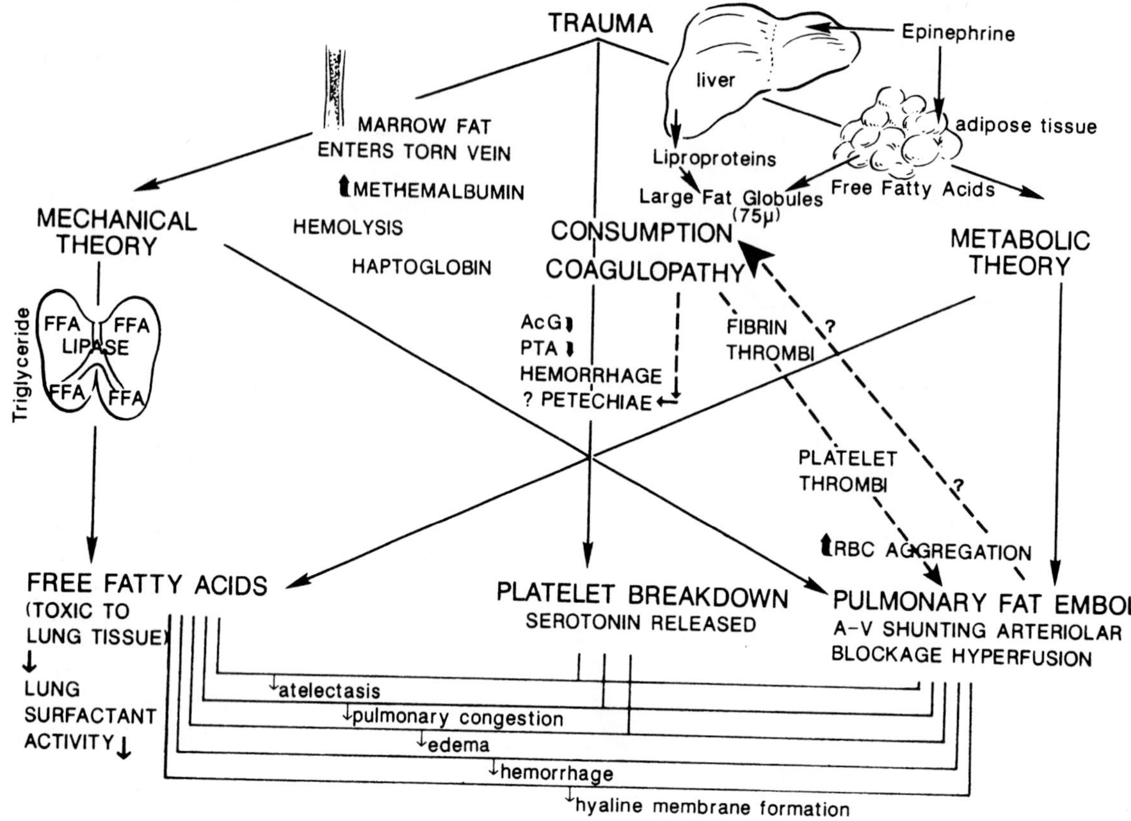

FIGURE 1-94 ■ Pathological events of fat embolism syndrome. (From Simon, S.R., ed.: Orthopaedic Basic Science, 2nd ed., p. 502. Rosemont, IL, American Academy of Orthopaedic Surgeons, 1994.)

important during the early treatment of this disorder.

H. Genitourinary (GU) Injury—NSAIDs can affect the kidney, and appropriate screening laboratory tests are required at regular intervals. Retrograde urethrogram best evaluates lower GU injuries with displaced anterior pelvic fractures.

I. Shock—Capillary blood flow is insufficient for the perfusion of vital tissues and organs. There are four types of shock.

1. Hypovolemic Shock—"Volume loss": decreased cardiac output (CO), increased peripheral vascular resistance (PVR), venous constriction. The most reliable early clinical finding is tachycardia; a drop in systolic blood pressure is a late finding.
2. Cardiogenic Shock—"Ineffective pumping": decreased CO, increased PVR, venous dilation.
3. Vasogenic Shock (PE or pericardial tamponade)—Arteriolar constriction, venous dilation.

Table 1-51. METABOLIC CHANGES OF STARVATION AND STRESS

METABOLIC ACTIVITY	STARVATION		STRESS	
	Early	*Late*	*Hypermetabolism*	*Multisystem*
Energy expenditure	↓	↓↓	↑↑	Organ failure
Mediator activation	None	None	++	++
Metabolic responsiveness	Intact	Intact	Abnormal	Abnormal
Primary fuel	CHO	KB	"Mixed" (no KB)	"Mixed" (no KB)
Hepatic gluconeogenesis	↓	↓	↑	↑ or ↓
Hepatic protein synthesis	↓	↓	↑	↑ or ↓
Whole-body protein catabolism	Sl. ↑	Sl. ↑	↑↑	↑↑↑
Urinary nitrogen excretion	Sl. ↑	Sl. ↑	↑↑	↑↑↑
Malnutrition	Slow	Slow	Rapid	Rapid

CHO, carbohydrate; Sl., slight; KB, ketone bodies.

Adapted from Simon, S.R.: Orthopaedic Basic Science, 2nd ed., p. 510. Rosemont, IL, American Academy of Orthopaedic Surgeons, 1994.

4. Neurogenic Shock/Septic Shock—"Blood pooling": arteriolar, capillary, and venous dilation.

J. Compartment Syndrome—Covered in detail in Chapter 10, Adult Trauma: Upper Extremity, Lower Extremity, and Pelvis. This subject matter is always tested heavily. Questions regarding the foot and thigh appear frequently.

K. Frostbite

1. Superficial—Treat with general rewarming of the entire body plus immersion of the hands or feet in a warm water bath (104°F, 40.0°C) for 15-30 minutes. Splinting, tetanus prophylaxis, analgesics, and antibiotics may also be indicated. Severe swelling may occur upon rewarming; monitor for compartment syndromes.
2. Deep—Débridement is often necessary.

L. **Wound Healing—Adequate healing following surgery is promoted by:**

1. **Transcutaneous oxygen tension >30 mm Hg**
2. **Ischemic index (such as the ankle/brachial systolic index) ≥0.45**
3. Albumin >3.0 g/dL
4. Total lymphocyte count of 1500/mm^3

M. **Anemia**—Physiologic effects include increased heart rate, increased cardiac output, increased coronary blood flow demand, decreased peripheral resistance, and decreased blood viscosity.

III. Intraoperative Considerations

A. Anesthesia—Regional anesthesia may (there is disagreement in the literature) allow quicker recovery, decreased blood loss, and fewer postoperative complications, including reduced blood loss and incidence of DVT/PE in THA patients. Controlled hypotension during surgery helps with blood loss and is a widely accepted technique, especially with THA and spinal arthrodesis (nitroprusside, nitroglycerin, and isoflurane are all effective). Patient positioning on a kneeling frame for spinal surgery decreases (1) intra-abdominal pressure, (2) pressure on the inferior vena cava, (3) pressure on the vertebral venous system, and (4) blood loss. Transient intraoperative decreases in blood pressure (BP) with PMMA insertion are well known. The use of the fiberoptic bronchoscope during surgery has benefited RA patients and others with C-spine abnormalities. The use of local anesthetics for arthroscopy has also gained popularity. **Malignant hyperthermia**, an autosomal dominant, hypermetabolic disorder of skeletal muscle, can be triggered by the use of various anesthetics (especially halothane and succinylcholine) in susceptible patients (e.g., neuromuscular disorders). The disorder involves impaired function of the sarcoplasmic reticulum and calcium homeostasis. Patients with Duchenne's muscular dystrophy, arthrogryposis, and osteogenesis imperfecta are especially at risk. Cell membrane defects affect calcium transport, leading to muscle rigidity and hypermetabolism. Masseter muscle spasm, increased temperature, rigidity, and acidosis are the hallmarks of the disease. Early diagnosis and treatment with **dantrolene sodium (blocks calcium release by stabilizing the sarcoplasmic reticulum while permitting uptake of calcium and thus decreasing the intracellular concentration of calcium)**, balancing of electrolytes, increasing urinary output, respiratory support, and cooling are essential. The **most accurate method for diagnosing malignant hyperthermia is muscle biopsy** (in vitro muscle fiber testing).

B. Spinal Cord Monitoring—Usually involves testing the posterior column, but monitoring of other areas is under investigation. Electrical monitoring includes the use of somatosensory cortical evoked potentials (SCEPs) to record summed input from stimulation of peripheral areas. Somatosensory spinal evoked potentials (SSEPs) are more invasive but can be more sensitive. Preoperative recordings are compared with readings (especially latency and amplitude) at critical times during the procedure. The (Stagnara) wake-up test is still the standard for monitoring and relies on the lightening of anesthesia and the patient moving selected extremities upon command.

C. Tourniquet—Can injure the nerves and muscles directly underneath the tourniquet; electromyography (EMG) abnormalities may occur in 70% of patients after routine surgery using a tourniquet. Careful application, wide cuffs, lower pressures (200 mm Hg in the upper extremity and 250 Hg mm in the lower extremity [or 100-150 mm Hg above systolic BP for the lower extremity]), and double cuffs help avoid these problems. Equilibrium can be reestablished within 5 minutes after 90 minutes of tourniquet application but requires 15 minutes after the use of a tourniquet for 3 hours.

IV. Other Problems

A. Pain Control—Acute pain implies the presence of potential tissue damage; chronic pain (3-6 months) does not. Nociceptors transduce stimuli through substances, allowing transmission along peripheral nerves (type A and C fibers) to the dorsal column, spinothalamic tract, and thalamus. Modulation is via brainstem centers and endogenous opiates. Postoperative pain control can be targeted at any step. Local prostaglandin inhibitors and long-acting local anesthetics target transduction of pain. Perispinal opiates affect modulation, and systemic opiates affect perception and modulation of pain.

1. Local Anesthetics—Result in a transient and reversible loss of sensation that is confined to a particular area. **Local anesthetics achieve their effect by interfering with nerve conduction.** Specifically, these agents interfere with the rate of rise of the depolarization phase of the action potential; cells fail to depolarize

enough to fire after excitation, and the action potential is blocked. Examples of local anesthetics include:

a. Amides—Lidocaine (Xylocaine), bupivacaine (Marcaine), and others
b. Esters of p-Aminobenzoic Acid—Procain (Novocain), butethamine (Monocaine), and others
c. Esters of Meta-Aminobenzoic Acid—Cyclomethycaine (Surfacaine), metabutoxycaine (Primacaine)
d. Esters of Benzoic Acid—Cocaine, ethyl aminobenzoate (Benzocaine), and others

2. NSAIDs—Produce their anti-inflammatory, antipyretic, analgesic, and antiplatelet effects by inhibiting the synthesis and release of prostaglandins. **These drugs inhibit the enzyme cyclooxygenase (COX).** COX catalyzes the synthesis of cyclic endoperoxides, which are important in the formation of prostaglandins.
   a. COX Inhibitors—Two isoforms of COX have been identified (COX-1 and COX-2). In general, the term NSAID refers to an agent that inhibits both COX-1 and COX-2. Examples of NSAIDs include salicylates, salicylate-like anti-inflammatory agents (such as ibuprofen), salicylate-like antipyretic agents (such as acetaminophen), analgesic combinations and mixtures (such as codeine plus aspirin). Several mechanisms exist by which NSAIDs inhibit COX (aspirin binds with a serine residue of COX, which results in irreversible steric hindrance of the active site; ibuprofen is a reversible competitive inhibitor of COX; indomethacin acts at the lipoxygenase side of the arachidonic metabolism pathway, which results in inhibition of leukotriene inflammatory mediators).
   b. COX-2 Specific Inhibitors—One of the major benefits of COX-2 specific inhibitors is that they do not inhibit the beneficial functions of COX-1 (**maintaining gastric mucosa**, regulating renal blood flow, influencing platelet aggregation). It is therefore believed that COX-2-specific inhibitors will have a tremendous beneficial impact in providing safer treatment for patients with arthritis. Examples of COX-2-specific inhibitors include celecoxib (Celebrex) and rofecoxib (Vioxx).
3. Substance P—A sensory neurotransmitter that plays an important role in pain. Capsaicin (pepper cream—obtained from red pepper) is believed to produce analgesia via neuropeptide depletion in unmyelinated C fibers (and depletion of substance P from the spinal cord, which elevates the threshold to painful stimuli).

B. Transfusion—Because of the possibility of disease transmission, transfusion has become an important issue.
   1. Transfusion Reactions—Include allergic, febrile, and hemolytic reactions
      a. Allergic Reaction—Most common; occurs toward the end of transfusion and usually subsides spontaneously. Symptoms include chills, pruritus, erythema, and urticaria. Pretreatment with diphenhydramine (Benadryl) and hydrocortisone may be appropriate in patients with a history of allergic reactions.
      b. Febrile Reaction—Also common; occurs after the initial 100-300 mL of packed RBCs have been transfused. Chills and fever are caused by antibodies to foreign WBCs. Treatment is to hold the transfusion and give antipyretics, similar to that for an allergic reaction.
      c. Hemolytic Reaction—Less common but most serious. It occurs early in the transfusion with symptoms that include chills, fever, tachycardia, chest tightness, and flank pain. Treatment comprises stopping the transfusion, administering IV fluids, performing appropriate laboratory studies, and monitoring the patient in an intensive care setting.
   2. Transfusion Risks—Include transmission of hepatitis (C [2-3%], B [<1%]), cytomegalovirus (CMV; highest incidence but not clinically important), HTLV-1, and HIV (1 in 400,000-600,000 per unit transfused). Donor deferral for high-risk persons and more effective screening methods are helping to manage these risks.
   3. Alternatives to Homologous (Blood Bank) Blood Transfusion—Table 1-52.

C. Heterotopic Ossification—See the discussion on bone injury and repair in Section 1 and Chapter 4, Adult Reconstruction. Seen most commonly following THA in head-injured patients, and in those with elbow injuries. **Indomethacin** is effective for prophylaxis in patients undergoing THA. Single fraction low-dose radiation therapy is recommended as prophylaxis for THA patients at high risk for HO. **Diphosphonates** do not prevent formation of osteoid matrix; after discontinuation of medication, the matrix calcifies, and therefore diphosphonates are not good for prophylaxis. Etidronate sodium inhibits bone resorption at low doses and bone mineralization at high doses.

D. Corticosteroid Injections—The most common complications of intra-articular or extra-articular injection of corticosteroids are subcutaneous fat atrophy and skin pigment changes.

Table 1-52. ALTERNATIVES TO HOMOLOGOUS (BLOOD BANK) BLOOD TRANSFUSION

TYPE	PROCEDURE	NOTES
Autologous deposition	Requires a hemoglobin level of ~11 (and a hematocrit of 33%) and some lead time Iron supplementation during donation is routine	Allows storage of several units of blood prior to elective procedures with significant blood loss anticipated Significant cardiac disease, such as unstable angina, is a contraindication About 20% of THA patients who donate 2 units of autologous blood require a homologous (from another donor) blood transfusion Significantly reduces hepatitis C risk Autologous blood that tests positive for hepatitis can be reinfused, but requires warning labels and special handling and storage **Autologous donation is not recommended unless the risk of transfusion is greater than 10%**
"Cell saver"	Intraoperative autotransfusion	Usually requires 400 mL of blood loss to recover 1 unit (250 mL) Can be used for only 4 hours at one time
Autotransfusion	Allows postoperative drain recuperation and use	Reinfusion should begin within 6 hours of the beginning of collection to reduce febrile reaction risk
Acute preoperative normovolemic hemodilution	Immediate preoperative storage of autologous blood for intra/postoperative use	Replace withdrawn autologous blood with crystalloid
Pharmacologic intervention	Desmopressin (antidiuretic hormone [ADH] analogue that increases levels of plasma factor VIII) Recombinant erythropoietin (stimulates erythrogenesis) Synthetic erythrocyte substitutes	
Judicious use of blood products	Platelet transfusion for massive bleeding or coagulopathies Fresh frozen plasma is reserved for patients with massive bleeding and significantly abnormal coagulation tests Cryoprecipitate is used for hemophilia (less exposure than factor concentrates) and as a source of fibrinogen for consumptive coagulopathies	Platelet transfusion is based on clinical parameters rather than set platelet thresholds

SECTION 7

Imaging and Special Studies

I. Nuclear Medicine

A. Bone Scan—**Technetium-99m pyrophosphate complexes reflect increased blood flow and metabolism and are absorbed onto the hydroxyapatite crystals of bone in areas of infection, trauma, neoplasia, and so on.** Whole-body views and more detailed (pin-hole) views can be obtained. It is particularly useful for the diagnosis of subtle fractures; avascular necrosis (hypoperfused [diminished blood flow] early, increased uptake during the reparative phase); osteomyelitis (especially when a triple-phase study is performed or in conjunction with a gallium or indium scan); THA and TKA loosening (especially femoral components; a technetium scan can be used in conjunction with a gallium scan to rule out concurrent infection); and patellofemoral overload. Three-phase (or even four-phase) studies may be helpful for evaluating diseases such as reflex sympathetic dystrophy and osteomyelitis. The three phases of a triple-phase bone scan are as follows: ***first phase* (blood flow, immediate)**—displays blood flow through the arterial system; ***second phase* (blood pool, 30 minutes)**—displays equilibrium of tracer throughout the intravascular volume; ***third phase* (delayed, 4 hours)**—displays the sites at which the tracer accumulates. Delayed-phase scans may be negative in pediatric septic arthritis. Triple-phase bone scan is the most reliable test for assessing whether a nondisplaced scaphoid fracture exists. A technetium scan is a useful means of evaluating for osteochondritis dissecans of the talus.

B. Gallium Scan—**Gallium-67 citrate localizes in sites of inflammation and neoplasia, probably because of exudation of labeled serum proteins.** Requires delayed imaging (24-48 hours or more). Frequently used in conjunction with a bone scan—a "double tracer" technique. Gallium is less dependent on vascular flow than technetium and may identify foci that would otherwise be missed. It is difficult to differentiate cellulitis from osteomyelitis on a gallium scan.

C. Indium Scan—**Indium-111–labeled WBCs (leukocytes) accumulate in areas of inflammation and do not collect in areas of neoplasia.** Useful for evaluation of **acute infections** (such as osteomyelitis) and possible TJA infections.

D. Technetium-Labeled WBC Scan—Similar to indium scan.

E. Radiolabeled Monoclonal Antibodies—May have a role in identifying primary malignancies and metastatic disease.

F. Other Studies

1. Bone Mineral Analysis—Single-photon absorptiometry (usually of the distal radius and cortical bone; has limited utility), dual-photon absorptiometry (vertebral bodies and femoral neck). (For further details see the following discussion on measurement of bone density.)
2. DVT/Pulmonary Embolism Scan—Radioactive iodine-labeled fibrinogen accumulates in clot and shows up on scanning; is inaccurate in areas of surgical wounds. Radioisotope lung scans may help in evaluating pulmonary blood flow, but is also limited at present.
3. Single-Photon Emission Computed Tomography (SPECT)—Uses scintigraphy and CT to evaluate overlapping structures. Femoral head ON, patellofemoral syndrome, and healing of spondylolytic defects have been evaluated with SPECT.

II. Arthrography—Table 1-53.

III. Magnetic Resonance Imaging (MRI)

A. Introduction—Excellent study to evaluate soft tissues and bone marrow; MRI is not effective for the evaluation of trabecular bone and cortical bone (because these tissues have virtually no hydrogen nuclei and therefore generate no signal). MRI is frequently used to evaluate ON, neoplasms, infection, and trauma. Allows both axial and sagittal representations. Contraindications: pacemakers, cerebral aneurysm clips, or shrapnel or hardware in certain locations.

B. Basic Principles of MRI (Tables 1-54 and 1-55)—MRI uses radiofrequency (RF) pulses on tissues in a magnetic field and displays images in any desired plane without using ionizing radiation. MRI aligns nuclei that have odd numbers of protons/neutrons (with a normally random spin) parallel to a magnetic field. Most MRI magnets have a strength of 0.5-1.5 tesla (1 tesla = 10,000 gauss). RF pulses deflect these particles' nuclear magnetic moments, resulting in an image. The use of surface coils decreases the signal-to-noise ratio. Body coils are used for large joints, smaller coils are available for other studies. Sequences have been developed to demonstrate the differences in T1 and T2 relaxation between tissues. **T1 images are weighted toward fat; T2 images are weighted toward water.** Typically, T1-weighted images have TR (time to repetition) values <1000, and T2 images have TR values >1000. Water, cerebral spinal fluid (CSF), acute hemorrhage, and soft-tissue tumors appear

Table 1-53. ARTHROGRAPHY

ANATOMIC LOCATION	CONDITIONS	DESCRIPTION
Shoulder		Technique can be single- or double-contrast (better detail)
	Rotator cuff tear	Extravasation of contrast through the tear into the subacromial bursa
	Adhesive capsulitis	Demonstrates diminished joint capsule size and loss of the normal axillary fold May be therapeutic (distends the capsule)
	Recurrent dislocations	May demonstrate a distended capsule or disruption of the glenoid labrum Use with tomograms or CT (computed tomography) to better demonstrate capsular or labral pathology
	Other	Bicipital tendon abnormalities Articular pathology Impingement syndrome
Elbow	Articular cartilage defects/loose bodies Osteochondral fractures	Especially helpful when used with tomography
Wrist	Post-traumatic ligament disruption	Digital subtraction techniques are helpful in this area Communication between compartments is used to determine pathology, but remember that communication is common in asymptomatic patients >40 years Communication at the radio-carpal joint and midcarpal joint, suspect S-L or L-T ligament tear Communication at the radio-carpal joint and distal radio-ulnar joint, suspect a triangular fibrocartilage complex (TFCC) tear
Hip		
Infants and children	"Septic" hip	Obtain aspirate and assess joint damage
	Developmental dysplasia of the hip	Degree of joint incongruity—interposed limbus
	Legg-Calvé-Perthes disease	Severity of deformity
Adolescents and adults	Arthritis	Cartilage destruction and loose bodies
	Osteochondral fractures, chondrolysis, and THA loosening	Digital subtraction arthrography can be useful for suspected loose THAs
Knee	Meniscal tears (except posterior horn of the lateral meniscus) and discoid lateral menisci	Can be useful for screening patients with an equivocal history or findings Evaluation of cruciate ligaments is less accurate than evaluation of the mensici
	Articular cartilage evaluation	
	Loose bodies	Air contrast only is recommended for evaluation of loose bodies
	Pathologic synovial tissue	PVNS, popliteal cysts, synovial chondromatosis, plicas
Ankle	Acutely torn ligaments Chronic osseous and osteocartilaginous abnormalities	
Spine	Facet joints	May be useful combined with therapeutic injections (anesthetics and steroids)

dark on T1 studies and bright on T2 studies. Other tissues remain basically the same intensity on both images. Cortical bone, rapidly flowing blood, and fibrous tissue are all dark; muscle and hyaline cartilage are gray; and fatty tissue, nerves, slowly flowing (venous) blood, and bone marrow are bright. **T1 images best demonstrate anatomic structure (high signal-to-noise ratio)**, whereas T2 images are best for contrasting normal and abnormal tissues. When tendon or ligament tissue is oriented near 55 degrees to the magnetic field, T1-weighted images may appear to have increased signal (brightness), thus creating a false appearance of pathology; this is called the **"magic angle phenomena"** and occurs most commonly in the shoulder, ankle, and knee.

C. Specific Applications of MRI
1. Osteonecrosis—**MRI is the method with the highest sensitivity and specificity for early detection of ON** (detects early marrow necrosis and ingrowth of vascularized mesenchymal tissue). MRI is highly specific (98%) and reliable for estimating the age and extent of disease. T1 images demonstrate diseased marrow as dark. MRI allows direct assessment of overlying cartilage.
2. Infection and Trauma—MRI has excellent sensitivity to increases in free water and demonstrates areas of infection and fresh hemorrhage (dark on T1 and bright on T2 studies). **MRI is an excellent (accurate and sensitive) method of evaluating for occult fractures (particularly in the elderly hip).**

Table 1-54. MAGNETIC RESONANCE IMAGING TERMINOLOGY

TERM	EXPLANATION
T1	Time constant of exponential growth of magnetism; T1 measures how rapidly a tissue gains magnetism (see Table 1-55)
T2	Time constant of exponential decay of signal following an excitation pulse; a tissue with a long T2 (such as water) maintains its signal (is bright on T2-weighted image) (see Table 1-55)
T2	Similar to T2 but includes the effects of magnetic field homogeneity
TR	Time to repetition; the time between successive excitation pulses; short TR is less than 80, long TR is greater than 80
TE	Time to echo; the time that an echo is formed by the refocusing pulse; short TE is less than 1000, long TE is greater than 1000
NEX	Number of excitations; higher NEX results in decreased noise with better images
FOV	Field of view
Spin echo	A commonly used pulse sequence in MRI
FSE	Fast spin echo; a type of pulse sequence
GRE	Gradient-recalled echo; a type of pulse sequence

Table 1-55. MRI SIGNAL INTENSITIES

TISSUE	APPEARANCE ON T1-WEIGHTED IMAGE	APPEARANCE ON T2-WEIGHTED IMAGE
Cortical bone	Dark	Dark
Osteomyelitis	Dark	Bright
Ligaments	Dark	Dark
Fibrocartilage	Dark	Dark
Hyaline cartilage	Gray	Gray
Meniscus	Dark	Dark
Meniscal tear	Bright	Gray
Yellow bone marrow (fatty-appendicular)	Bright	Gray
Red bone marrow (hematopoietic-axial)	Gray	Gray
Marrow edema	Dark	Bright
Fat	Bright	Gray
Normal fluid	Dark	Bright
Abnormal fluid (pus)	Gray	Bright
Acute blood collection	Gray	Dark
Chronic blood collection	Bright	Bright
Muscle	Gray	Gray
Tendon	Dark	Dark
Intervertebral disc (central)	Gray	Bright
Intervertebral disc (peripheral)	Dark	Gray

Modified from Brinker, M.R., and Miller, M.D.: Fundamentals of Orthopaedics. Philadelphia, WB Saunders, 1999, p. 24.

3. Neoplasms—MRI has many applications in the study of primary and metastatic bone tumors. Primary tumors, particularly soft-tissue components (extraosseous and marrow), are well demonstrated on MRI. Although nuclear medicine studies remain the procedure of choice for seeking metastatic foci in bone, MRI has a role in evaluating for skip lesions and spinal metastases. Benign bony tumors are typically bright on T1 images and dark on T2 images. Malignant bony lesions are often bright on T2 images. Differential diagnosis, however, is best made based on plain films.
4. Spine—Disc disease is well demonstrated on T2 images. Degenerated discs lose water content and become dark on T2-weighted studies; extent of herniated discs is also well shown. **Recurrent disc herniation is best diagnosed via MRI scan with gadolinium** and can be differentiated from a scar based on the following characteristics: T1 images show scar, decreased signal; free fragment, increased signal; extruded disc, decreased signal; T2 images show scar, increased signal; free fragment, increased signal; extruded disc, decreased signal. Gadolinium-DPTA diethyltriamine pentaacetic acid (DPTA) can also be used to differentiate scar from disc by enhancing edematous structures in T1 images. MRI is the best (most sensitive) study for diagnosing early discitis (decreased signal on T1 and increased signal on T2). **Recent studies have shown the following regarding MRI findings of the spine in asymptomatic persons:** (1) 28% of subjects more than 40 years of age have an abnormality of the cervical spine on MRI, (2) 20-30% of subjects under 40 years of age show evidence of a lumbar disc herniation on MRI, (3) 93% of subjects more than 60 years of age show evidence of degeneration or bulging of one or more lumbar discs on MRI. Biochemical studies have shown that degenerative disc changes occur as early as the second decade of life.
5. Bone Marrow Changes—Best demonstrated by MRI (but nonspecific). Five groups of disorders have been described and are shown in Table 1-56.
6. Knee MRI—Arthrography with MRI can be accomplished with instillation of saline, creating an iatrogenic effusion. This technique can improve joint definition. Knee derangements are well demonstrated on MRI. ACL rupture is correctly diagnosed in 95% of cases. Meniscal pathology has been classified into four groups of myxoid changes (Lotysch) (Table 1-57). **MRI is the best radiological test to demonstrate a posterior cruciate ligament (PCL)**

Table 1-56. IMAGING BONE MARROW DISORDERS

DISORDER	PATHOLOGY	EXAMPLES	MRI CHANGES
Reconversion	Yellow→red	Anemia, metastasis	↓T1 image
Marrow infiltration		Tumor, infection	↓T1 image
Myeloid depletion		Anemia, chemotherapy	↓T1 image
Marrow edema		Trauma, RSD	↓T1, ↑T2 image
Marrow ischemia		Osteonecrosis	↓T1 image

RSD, reflex sympathetic dystrophy; ↑, increased; ↓, decreased.

rupture (physical examination is probably the best test, overall).

7. Shoulder MRI
   a. Rotator Cuff Tears—Results are improving with use (sensitivity and specificity are about 90%). Grade 0 tears show a normal signal, and grade 1, 2, and 3 tears show an increased signal. The morphology of grade 0 and 1 tears is normal; grade 2 tears show abnormal morphology; and grade 3 tears show discontinuity.
   b. Capsular/Labral Tears—MRI is equal to CT arthrography in the presence of an effusion.
8. MRI Spectroscopy—May help with the measurement of metabolic changes (especially ischemic changes).

IV. Other Imaging Studies

A. Computed Tomography—Continues to be important for evaluating many orthopaedic areas. Hounsfield units are used to identify tissue types (−100 = air, −100 to 0 = fat, 0 = water, 100 = soft tissue, 1000 = bone). **CT demonstrates details of bony anatomy better than any other study.** It also shows herniated nucleus pulposis better than myelography alone and may be helpful in differentiating recurrent disc herniation from scar (like MRI). IV contrast material is taken up in scar but not disc tissue. CT is used frequently in conjunction with contrast (e.g., arthrogram CT, myelogram CT). Sagittal and three-dimensional reconstruction techniques may expand its indications. Cine-CT (and MRI) may be helpful for evaluating many joint disorders. CT digital radiography (CT scanogram) can be used for accurate demonstration of leg-length discrepancy with minimal radiation exposure. CT best demonstrates joint incongruity following closed reduction of a dislocated hip. **CT scanning is useful for measuring the cross-sectional dural area in the work-up of cervical spinal stenosis; spinal stenosis is present if this area is less than 100 mm^2.** CT is also important for evaluating subtalar joint injuries and for diagnosing tarsal coalitions; talocalcaneal tarsal coalitions are also well visualized via axial (Harris) view plain radiographs. Dynamic CT scan is the test of choice for patients with atlantoaxial rotatory subluxation (Grisel's syndrome is spontaneous atlantoaxial subluxation occurring in conjunction with inflammation of the soft tissues of the neck [such as pharyngitis]). CT images can be distorted by metal implants.

B. Ultrasonography—Has been used successfully in several areas of orthopaedics.
   1. Shoulder—May be useful for diagnosing rotator cuff tears.
   2. Hip—Effective in diagnosis and follow-up of developmental hip dysplasia and to identify iliopsoas bursitis in adults.
   3. Knee—Used to assess articular cartilage thickness and identify intra-articular fluid.
   4. Other Areas—Helpful for evaluating: soft-tissue masses, hematoma, tendon rupture, abscesses, foreign body location, intraspinal disorders in infants, and the aorta (in patients at increased risk for aortic dilation or rupture [such as Marfan's syndrome]).
   5. Fractures—May help evaluate progression of fracture healing.

C. Guided Biopsies—Aspiration and core biopsy (using a trephine needle) is helpful in the work-up of musculoskeletal lesions; commonly used in conjunction with CT.

D. Myelography—Still useful for evaluating cervical radiculopathy, subarachnoid cysts, and the failed back syndrome. **It is the procedure of choice for extramedullary intradural pathology.** It can be used in conjunction with other studies, such as CT.

E. Discography—Although its use is controversial, it is helpful for evaluating symptomatic disc degeneration. Reproduction of pain with injection and characteristic changes on discograms help identify pathologic discs. It is commonly used in conjunction with CT.

F. Measurement of Bone Density (Noninvasive Methods)—Several methods are available for

Table 1-57. MRI CHANGES OF MENISCAL PATHOLOGY

GROUP	CHARACTERISTICS
I	Globular areas of hyperintense signal
II	Linear hyperintense signal
III	Linear hyperintense signal that communicates with the meniscal surface (tears)
IV	Vertical longitudinal tear/truncation

Table 1-58. NERVE CONDUCTION STUDY RESULTS

CONDITION	LATENCY	CONDUCTION VELOCITY	EVOKED RESPONSE
Normal study	Normal	Upper extremities: >45 m/sec Lower extremities: >40 m/sec	Biphasic
Axonal neuropathy	Increased	Normal or slightly decreased	Prolonged, ↓ amplitude
Demyelinating neuropathy	Normal	Decreased (10-50%)	Normal or prolonged, with ↓ amplitude
Anterior horn cell disease	Normal	Normal (rarely decreased)	Normal or polyphasic with prolonged duration and ↓ amplitude
Myopathy	Normal	Normal	↓ Amplitude, may be normal
Neuropraxia			
Proximal to lesion	Absent	Absent	Absent
Distal to lesion	Normal	Normal	Normal
Axonotmesis			
Proximal to lesion	Absent	Absent	Absent
Distal to lesion	Absent	Absent	Normal
Neurotmesis			
Proximal to lesion	Absent	Absent	Absent
Distal to lesion	Absent	Absent	Absent

Modified from Jahss, M.H.: Disorders of the Foot. Philadelphia, WB Saunders, 1982.

measuring bone density and assessing the risk of fracture.

1. Single Photon Absorptiometry—Basic principle: the density of the cortical bone is inversely proportional to the quantity of photons passing through it. The radioisotope 125I emits a single-energy beam of photons that passes through bone. A sodium iodide scintillation counter detects the transmitted photons. Where the bone is dense, the photon beam is attenuated and fewer photons pass through to the scintillation counter. Single photon absorptiometry is best used in the appendicular skeleton (radius-diaphysis or distal metaphysis); it is unreliable in the axial skeleton (the depth of the soft tissues alters the beam).
2. Dual-Photon Absorptiometry—Like single-photon absorptiometry, dual-photon absorptiometry is an isotope-based means of measuring bone density. Dual-photon absorptiometry, however, allows for measurement of the axial skeleton and the femoral neck by accounting for the attenuation of the signal caused by the soft tissues overlying the spine and the hip.
3. Quantitative Computed Tomography—Allows preferential measurement of trabecular bone density (the bone that is at greatest risk for early metabolic changes). Involves the simultaneous scanning of phantoms of known density, thus creating a standard calibration curve. Precision is excellent; accuracy is within 5-10%. The radiation dose with this technique is higher than that of DEXA.
4. Dual-Energy X-Ray Absorptiometry— **DEXA is the most reliable method of predicting fracture risk. This method is the most accurate with a lower radiation dose than quantitative CT.**

G. Thermography—Maps body surface temperatures. Thermography has low specificity and is not recommended for clinical evaluation of disorders of the spine.

V. Electrodiagnostic Studies

A. Nerve Conduction Studies—Allow evaluation of peripheral nerves and their sensory and motor responses anywhere along their course. Nerve impulses are stimulated and recorded by surface electrodes, allowing calculation of a conduction velocity. Latency (the time between stimulus onset and the response) and response amplitude are measured. Late responses (F and H) allow evaluation of proximal lesions (impulse travels to the spinal cord and returns). Somatosensory evoked potentials can be used to study brachial plexus injuries and for spinal cord monitoring.

B. Electromyography— EMG uses intramuscular needle electrodes to evaluate muscle units. Most studies are done to evaluate for denervation, which demonstrates fibrillations (earliest sign usually at 4 weeks), sharp waves, and an abnormal recruitment pattern.

C. Interpretation—For peripheral nerve entrapment syndromes, distal motor and sensory latencies >3.5 m/sec, nerve conduction velocities of <50 m/sec, and changes over a distinct interval are considered abnormal (Tables 1-58 and 1-59).

Table 1-59. ELECTROMYOGRAPHIC FINDINGS

CONDITION	INSERTIONAL ACTIVITY	ACTIVITY AT REST	MINIMAL CONTRACTION	INTERFERENCE
Normal study	Normal	Silent	Biphasic and triphasic potentials	Complete
Axonal neuropathy	Increased	Fibrillations and positive sharp waves	Biphasic and triphasic potentials	Incomplete
Demyelinating neuropathy	Normal	Silent (occasional activity)	Biphasic and triphasic potentials	Incomplete
Anterior horn cell disease	Increased	Fibrillations, positive sharp waves, fasciculations	Large polyphasic potentials	Incomplete
Myopathy	Increased	Silent or increased spontaneous activity	Small polyphasic potentials	Early
Neuropraxia	Normal	Silent	None	None
Axonotmesis	Increased	Fibrillations and positive sharp waves	None	None
Neurotmesis	Increased	Fibrillations and positive sharp waves	None	None

Modified from Jahss, M.H.: Disorders of the Foot. Philadelphia, WB Saunders, 1982.

SECTION 8

Biomaterials and Biomechanics

I. Basic Concepts

A. Definitions

1. Biomechanics—Science of the action of forces, internal or external, on the living body.
2. Statics—Study of the action of forces on bodies at rest (in equilibrium).
3. Dynamics—Study of bodies in motion and the related forces. There are three subtypes.
   a. Kinematics—Study of motion (displacement, velocity, and acceleration) without reference to the forces causing the motion.
   b. Kinetics—Relates the effects of forces to the motion of bodies.
   c. Kinesiology—Study of human movement/motion.

B. Principal Quantities

1. Basic Quantities—Described by the International System of Units (SI) or the metric system.
   a. Length—Meter (m)
   b. Mass—Amount of matter (kilogram [kg])
   c. Time—Second (sec)
2. Derived Quantities—Derived from basic quantities.
   a. Velocity—Time rate of change of displacement (m/sec).
   b. Acceleration—Time rate of change of velocity (m/sec^2).
   c. Force—Action causing acceleration of a mass (body) (kg·m/sec^2[N]).

C. Newton's Laws

1. First Law: Inertia—If the net external force acting on a body is zero, the body will remain at rest or move uniformly. Allows static analysis via the equation $\Sigma F = 0$ (the sum of the external forces applied to a body equals zero).
2. Second Law: Acceleration—The acceleration (a) of an object of mass m is directly proportional to the force (F) applied to the object ($F = ma$). Helps in dynamic analysis.
3. Third Law: Reactions—For every action (force) there is an equal and opposite reaction (force). Leads to free body analysis.

D. Scalar and Vector Quantities

1. Scalar Quantities—Have magnitude but no direction. Examples include volume, time, mass, and speed (not velocity).
2. Vector Quantities—Have magnitude and direction. Examples include force and velocity. Vectors have four characteristics: (1) magnitude (length of the vector); (2) direction (head of the vector); (3) point of application (tail of the vector); and (4) line of action (orientation of the vector). Vectors can be added, subtracted, and split into components (resolved) for analysis. The resultant of two vectors follows the principle of "parallelogram of forces."

E. Free Body Analysis—Uses forces, moments, and free body diagrams to analyze the action of forces on bodies. **Know how to solve these problems!**

1. Forces—A push or a pull causing external (acceleration) and internal (strain) effects. Force vectors can be split into their components (usually in the x and y directions) for easier analysis. Some elementary knowledge of trigonometry is helpful ($F_x = F \cos \theta$, $F_y = F \sin \theta$). Also, remember the following simple approximations:

   $\sin 30° = \cos 60° \cong 0.5$

   $\sin 45° = \cos 45° \cong 0.7$

   $\sin 60° = \cos 30° \cong 0.9$

2. Moment (M)—The rotational effect of a force acting at a distance from a specified point on a body. The moment (or "torque") equals the force (F) multiplied by the perpendicular distance from the specified point (moment arm = d): $M = F \times d$. **Mass moment of inertia is resistance of the body (or body segment) to rotation**; it is the product of the body's mass times the square of the distance from a specified point on the body (or body segment): $I = m \times d^2$.
3. Free Body Diagram (FBD)—Sketch of a body (or portions thereof) isolated from all other bodies and showing all forces acting on it. Weights of objects act through the center of gravity (CG). **The CG for the human body is just anterior to S2.**
4. Free Body Analysis—After all forces are represented on the FBD, apply the concept of equilibrium (sum of forces and moments both equal zero: $\Sigma F = 0$ and $\Sigma M = 0$) and solve for unknowns. Assumes no change in motion, no deformation, and no friction. The following steps are used in the analysis.
   a. Identify the system (objective, knowns, assumptions).
   b. Select a coordinate system.
   c. Isolate free bodies—FBD.
   d. Apply Newton's laws ($\Sigma F = 0$; $\Sigma M = 0$).
   e. Solve for unknowns.
5. Example—Calculate the biceps force necessary to hold the weight of the forearm (20 N) with the elbow flexed to 90 degrees; assume the biceps insertion is 5 cm distal to the elbow, and the CG of the forearm is 15 cm distal to the elbow (Fig. 1-95). (*Answer*: 60 N.) Also solve for the joint force (J) (see Fig. 1-95). (*Answer*: –40 N.)

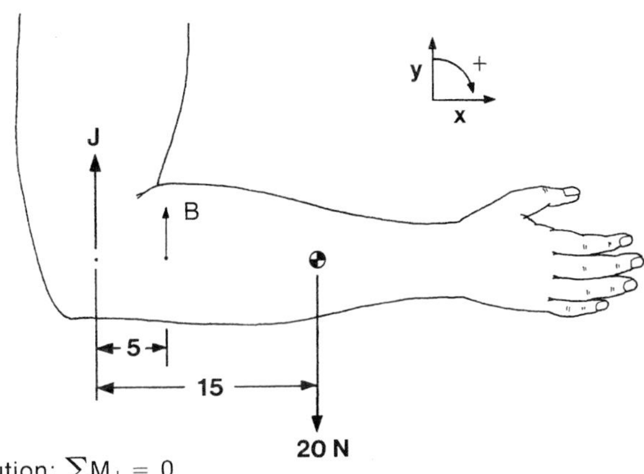

Solution: $\sum M_J = 0$
$-B(.05) \quad 20(.15) = 0$
$.05\ B = 3$
$\underline{B = 60N}$

$\sum F_y = 0$
$+J + B - 20 = 0$
$J = +20 - B$
$\underline{J = -40N}$

FIGURE 1-95 ■ Free body diagram (see text for explanation).

F. Other Important Basic Concepts
   1. Work—The product of a force and the displacement it causes. Work (W) = force (only the vector components parallel to the displacement) × distance. Units: N·m (joules).
   2. Energy—Ability to perform work (also joules). According to the law of conservation of energy, energy is neither created nor destroyed; it is transferred from one condition to another.
      a. Potential Energy—Stored energy; the ability of a body to do work as a result of its position or configuration (strain energy).
      b. Kinetic Energy—Energy of an object due to its motion ($KE = \frac{1}{2}mv^2$).
   3. Friction (f)—Resistance to motion between two bodies when one slides over the other, produced at points of contact. Oriented opposite to the applied force. When the applied force exceeds f, motion begins. Frictional force is proportional to the coefficient of friction and the applied normal (perpendicular) load; f is independent of the area of contact and the shape of the surface.
   4. Piezoelectricity—Electrical charge from deformation of crystalline structures when forces are applied. **Concave (compression) side = electronegative; convex (tension) side = electropositive.**

II. Biomaterials

A. Strength of Materials
   1. Definition—Branch of mechanics that deals with relations between externally applied loads and the resulting internal effects and deformations induced in the body subjected to these loads.
      a. Loads—Forces that act on a body (compression, tension, shear, torsion).
      b. Deformations—Temporary (elastic) or permanent (plastic) change in the shape of a body. Changes in load produce changes in deformation.
   2. Stress—Intensity of internal force: **Stress = force/area**. Used to analyze the internal resistance of a body to a load. Helps in selection of materials. Normal stresses (compressive or tensile) are perpendicular to the surface on which they act. Shear stresses are parallel to the surface on which they act. Stress has the units N/m^2 (pascals [Pa]).
   3. Strain—Relative measure of the deformation (six components) of a body as a result of loading. **Strain = change in length/original length of an object.** It can also be normal or shear. Strain is a proportion and therefore has no units.
   4. Hooke's Law—Basically, stress is proportional to strain up to a limit (the proportional limit).
   5. Young's Modulus (of Elasticity, E)—Measure of the stiffness of a material or its ability to resist deformation: E = stress/strain (in the elastic range of the stress-strain curve, it is the slope). **Modulus of elasticity is the critical factor in load-sharing capacity. A linearly perfect elastic material** has a straight stress-strain curve to the point of failure (the modulus is calculated by dividing the stress at failure (the ultimate stress) by the strain at failure (the ultimate strain).
   6. Stress-Strain Curve—Derived by axially loading a body and plotting stress versus strain (Fig. 1-96).
      a. Yield Point (Proportional Limit)—Transition point from the elastic to the plastic range. Usually 0.2% strain in most metals.
      b. Ultimate Strength—Maximum strength obtained by the material.

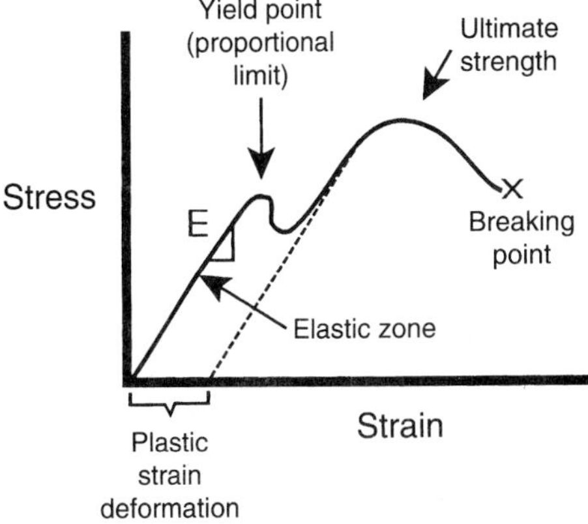

FIGURE 1-96 ■ Stress-strain curve. (Modified from Miller, M.D.: Review of Orthopaedics, 2nd ed. Philadelphia, WB Saunders, 1996, p. 102.)

c. Breaking Point—Point where the material fractures.
d. **Plastic Deformation—Change in length after removing the load (before the breaking point) in the plastic range.**
e. **Strain Energy—The capacity of a material (such as bone) to absorb energy. On a stress-strain curve it is illustrated as the area under the curve.** Total strain energy = recoverable strain energy (resilience) ++ dissipated strain energy. A measure of the toughness (ability to absorb energy before failure) of a material.

B. Materials and Structures
1. Material—Related to a substance or element. Defined by mechanical properties (force, stress, strain) and rheologic properties (elasticity [ability to regain original shape], plasticity [permanent deformation], viscosity [resistance to flow or shear stress], and strength).
   a. **Brittle Materials**—For example, PMMA. Exhibit a linear stress-strain curve up to the point of failure. Brittle materials undergo only **fully recoverable (elastic) deformation** before failure and have little or no capacity to undergo permanent (plastic) deformation before failure.
   b. **Ductile Materials**—For example, metal. Undergo a large amount of plastic deformation prior to failure. Ductility is a measure of post-yield deformation.
   c. **Viscoelastic Materials**—For example, bone and ligaments. **Exhibit stress-strain behavior that is time-rate dependent** (varies with the material); **the materials deformation depends on the load and the rate at which the load is applied. The modulus of a viscoelastic material increases as the strain rate increases. Viscoelastic behavior is a function of the internal friction of a material.**
   d. **Isotropic Materials—Possess the same mechanical properties in all directions (e.g., a golf ball).**
   e. **Anisotropic Materials—Have mechanical properties that vary with the direction of the applied load (e.g., bone).**
   f. Homogeneous Materials—Have a uniform structure or composition throughout.
2. Structure—Related to both the material and the shape of an object and its loading characteristics. A load deformation curve can be constructed similar to a stress-strain curve. The slope of the curve in the elastic range is referred to as the rigidity of the structure. **Bending rigidity of a rectangular structure** is proportional to the base multiplied by the height cubed ($bh^3/12$). **Bending rigidity of a cylinder** is related to the fourth power of the radius. Bending rigidity is **closely related to the area moment of inertia** (*I*, resistance to bending), which is a function of the width and thickness of the structure, and the polar moment of inertia (*J*), which represents the resistance to torsion (twisting). For more information, see the following discussion on intramedullary nails. **Deflection associated with bending** is proportional to the applied force (*F*) divided by the elastic modulus (*E*) of the material being bent multiplied by the area moment of inertia (*I*).

Deflection $\propto F/(E)(I)$

1. Metals—Demonstrate stress-strain curves as discussed earlier. Other important concepts follow.
   a. Fatigue Failure—Occurs with repetitive loading cycles at stress below the ultimate tensile strength. Fatigue failure depends on the magnitude of the stress and number of cycles. If the stress is less than a predetermined amount of stress, called the **endurance limit (the maximum stress under which the material will not fail regardless of how many loading cycles are applied)**, the material may be loaded cyclically an infinite number of times (>106 cycles) without breaking. Above the endurance limit, the fatigue life of a material is expressed by the stress (*S*) versus the number of loading cycles (*n*), or the *S-n* curve.
   b. **Creep (also known as Cold Flow)—Progressive deformation of metals (or other materials [such as polyethylene]) in response to a constant force applied over an extended period.** If sudden stress, followed by constant loading, causes a material to continue to deform, it demonstrates creep. Creep can produce a permanent deformity and may affect mechanical function (such as in a TJA).
   c. Corrosion—Chemical dissolving of metals as may occur in the high-saline environment of the body. Several types of corrosion may occur (Table 1-60); **316L stainless steel is the most likely metal to undergo pitting and crevice corrosion. The risk of galvanic corrosion is highest between 316L stainless steel and cobalt-chromium (Co-Cr) alloy**. Modular components of THA have direct contact between either similar or dissimilar metals (at the modular junctions) and thereby have corrosion products (metal oxides, metal chlorides, and others). Corrosion can be decreased by using similar metals (e.g., with plates and screws of similar metals), with proper design of implants, and with passivation (a thin layer that

Table 1-60 TYPES OF CORROSION

CORROSION	DESCRIPTION
Galvanic	Dissimilar metals[a]; electrochemical destruction
Crevice	Occurs in fatigue cracks with low, O_2 tension
Stress	Occurs in areas with high stress gradients
Fretting	From small movements abrading outside layer
Other	Includes inclusion, intergranular, and others

[a]Metals such as 316L stainless steel and Co-Cr-Mo produce galvanic corrosion.

effectively separates the metal from the solution [e.g., stainless steel coated by chromium oxide]).

d. Types of Metals—Orthopaedic implants are typically made of 316L (L = low carbon) **stainless steel** (iron, chromium, and nickel), "supermetal" alloys **(e.g., cobalt–chromium–molybdenum** [65% Co, 35% Cr, 5% Mo] made with a special forging process), and **titanium alloy** (Ti-6Al-4V). Each possesses a **different stiffness (*E*)** (Fig. 1-97). Problems associated with certain metals include wear, stress shielding (increased in metals with a higher *E*), and ion release (Co-Cr causes macrophage proliferation and synovial degeneration). **Titanium has poor resistance to wear (notch sensitivity)**; particulates may incite a histiocytic response; there is an uncertain association between titanium and neoplasms. Polishing, passivation, and ion implantation improve the fatigue properties of titanium alloy. **Titanium is an extremely biocompatible material; it rapidly forms an adherent oxide coating (self-passivation) that covers its surface (a nonreactive ceramic coating). Another advantage of titanium is its relatively low *E* and high yield strength. Cobalt-chrome alloy generates less metal debris (in THA) than does titanium alloy. Problems with orthoses fabrication: stainless steel is heavy and aluminum has a low endurance limit.**

2. Nonmetals—Include polyethylene, PMMA (bone cement), silicone, and ceramics.
   a. Polyethylene—Ultra-high molecular weight polyethylene (UHMWPE) polymer consists of long carbon chains; used in weight-bearing components of TJAs, such as acetabular cups and tibial trays. These materials have wear characteristics superior to those of high-density polyethylene (HDP); they are tough, ductile, resilient, and resistant to wear and they exhibit low friction. Polyethylenes are viscoelastic and highly susceptible to abrasion. **Wear damage to a UHMWPE articulating surface is most often caused by third-body inclusions. UHMWPE is also thermoplastic and may be altered by temperature or high-dose radiation.** The degradation of polyethylene following gamma irradiation in air is related to free radical formation (which increases susceptibility to oxidation); **gamma irradiation** increases polymer chain cross-links, which greatly **improves wear characteristics but reduces resistance to fatigue and fracture resistance** and decreases elastic modulus, tensile strength, and yield stress. Polyethylenes are weaker than bone in tension and

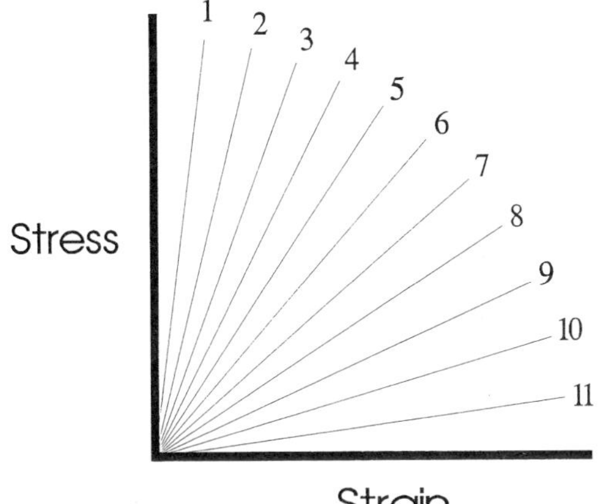

FIGURE 1-97 ■ Comparison of Young's modulus (relative values, not to scale) for various orthopaedic materials.

have a low *E*. Wear debris is associated with a histiocytic osteolytic response. Wear (and the associated osteolytic response) is increased with thinner (<6 mm), flatter, carbon fiber–reinforced polyethylene. Metal backing may help minimize plastic deformation of HDP (and loosening) but decreases its effective thickness (wear). Catastrophic wear of polyethylene tibial inserts is associated with varus knee alignment, thin inserts (<6 mm), flat nonconforming inserts, and heat treatments of the insert. **Polyethylene wear debris is the main factor affecting longevity of THAs.** Fatigue wear is more prevalent in TKA than in THA. **Volumetric wear is most affected by the relative motion between the two surfaces in contact.**

b. Polymethylmethacrylate (PMMA; Bone Cement)—Used for fixation (as a grout, not an adhesive) and load distribution for implants. PMMA reaches its ultimate strength within 24 hours. PMMA can also be used as an internal splint for patients with poor bone stock; it should be thought of as a temporary internal splint until the bone heals (if the bone fails to heal, the PMMA will ultimately fail). **PMMA has poor tensile and shear strength. PMMA is strongest in compression (however, it is not as strong as bone in compression) and has a low *E*.** Reduction in the number of voids (porosity) with insertion (vacuum mixing, centrifugation, good technique) increases cement strength and decreases cracking. **PMMA functions by mechanically interlocking with bone. Insertion can lead to a precipitous drop in blood pressure.** Wear particles can incite a macrophage response that leads to loosening of a prosthesis. **Cement failure is often caused by microfracture and fragmentation of cement.** PMMA may be used to minimize tumor contamination by filling defects in bone created by biopsy or cutterage (this use has not been cleared by the FDA).

c. Silicones—Polymers used for replacement in non–weight-bearing joints. Their poor strength and wear capability are responsible for frequent synovitis with extended use.

d. Ceramics—Broad class of materials that contain metallic and nonmetallic elements bonded ionically in a highly oxidized state; they are good insulators (poor conductors). Include biostable (inert) materials such as Al_2O_3 and bioactive (degradable) substances such as bioglass. **Ceramics are a highly ordered crystalline structure, are typically brittle (no elastic deformation), have a high modulus (*E*), have a high compressive strength, have a low tensile strength, have a low yield strain, and exhibit poor crack resistance characteristics (low fracture toughness [low resistance to fracture]).** Ceramics have the best wear characteristics with polyethylene and a low oxidation rate. **High surface wetability and high surface tension** make them highly conducive to tissue bonding and result in less friction and **diminished wear** ("smooth surface"). Small grain size also allows an ultrasmooth finish and less friction. Calcium phosphates (e.g., hydroxyapatite) may have application as a coating (plasma sprayed) to increase attachment strength and promote bone healing.

e. Other Materials—Polylactic acid (PLA)-coated carbon, which serves as a biodegradable scaffolding, and new polymer composites, some with carbon fiber reinforcement, are still under investigation. Fabrication of these newer devices involves assembling "piles" of carbon fibers impregnated with matrix polymer (polysulfone or polyetherketone). Difficulties with abrasion and impact resistance, radiolucency, and manufacturing are still present.

3. Biomaterials—Possess certain unique characteristics including viscoelasticity (time-dependent stress-strain behavior), creep, and stress relaxation (internal stresses decrease with time). They also are capable of self-adaptation and repair; characteristics change with aging and sampling.

4. Comparison of Common Orthopaedic Materials—Figure 1-97 compares Young's modulus of elasticity (*E*) for various orthopaedic materials.

D. Orthopaedic Structures

1. Bone

a. Mechanical Properties—Bone is a composite of collagen and hydroxyapatite. Collagen has a low *E*, good tensile strength, and poor compressive strength. Calcium apatite is a stiff, brittle material with good compressive strength. The combination is an **anisotropic** material that resists many forces; **bone is strongest in compression, weakest in shear, and intermediate in tension. The mineral content is the main determinant of the elastic modulus of cortical bone.** Cancellous bone is 25% as dense, 10%

as stiff, and 500% as ductile as cortical bone. Cortical bone is excellent in resisting torque; cancellous bone is good in resisting compression and shear. Bone is a dynamic material: able to self-repair; to change with aging (becomes stiffer and less ductile); and to change with prolonged immobilization (becomes weaker). **Material properties of bone decline with aging; to offset the loss in material properties, this amazing organ remodels its geometry to increase the inner and outer cortical diameters, which increases the area moment of inertia and thus decreases bone's bending stresses.** Stress concentration effects occur at defect points within bone or implant-bone interface (stress risers) and reduce the overall loading strength of bone. Stress shielding by implants induces osteoporosis in adjacent bone due to lack of normal physiologic stresses. This commonly occurs under plates and at the femoral calcar in high-riding THAs. A hole that is 20-30% of bone diameter reduces overall strength up to 50%, regardless of whether it is filled with a screw, and does not return to normal until 9-12 months after screw removal. Cortical defects can reduce strength 70% or more (oval defects less than rectangular defects, due to a smaller stress riser).

b. Fracture—Type is based on mechanism of injury.
   (1) **Tension**—By muscle pull, typically transverse, perpendicular to the load and bone axis.
   (2) **Compression**—By axial loading of cancellous bone; results in a crush type of fracture.
   (3) **Shear**—Commonly around joints; the load is parallel to the bone surface, and the fracture is parallel to the load.
   (4) **Bending**—By eccentric loading or direct blows. **The fracture begins on the tension side of the bone and continues transversely/obliquely, eventually bifurcating to produce a butterfly fragment** (with high-velocity bending there will be a comminuted butterfly fracture).
   (5) **Torsion—Creates shear and tensile stresses that most likely result in a spiral fracture.** Because torsional stresses are proportional to the distance from the neutral axis to the periphery of a cylinder, **a long bone under torsion experiences the greatest stresses on the outer (periosteal) surface.**

c. **Comminution—A function of the amount of energy transmitted to bone.**

2. Ligaments and Tendons—Can sustain 5-10% tensile strain before failure (versus 1-4% in bone), commonly from tension rupture of fibers and shear failure between fibers. Most ligaments can undergo plastic strain to the point that function is lost but structure remains in continuity. Soft-tissue implants include stents, ligament augmentation devices, and scaffoldings.
   a. **Tendons**—Strong in tension only; *E* is only 10% that of bone but increases with slower loading; parallel fiber orientation. Tendons demonstrate stress relaxation and creep.
   b. **Ligament Fibers**—Oriented parallel if they resist major joint stress, more randomly if they resist forces from different directions. Stiffness = force/strain, as depicted on a force deformation graph (similar to *E* but does not consider cross-sectional area); the bone-ligament complex is softer (less stiff—decreased *E*). Prolonged immobilization lowers ligament yield point and tensile strength and bone resorbs at the tendon insertion site.
   c. Stents—Internal splint devices: include Proplast Tendon Transfer Stabilizer using synthetic polymers, Goretex prosthetic ligaments, Xenotech (bovine tendon), and polyester implants. These do not allow adequate collagen ingrowth and therefore all eventually fail. Synthetic ligaments produce wear particles that increase levels of proteinases, collagenase, gelatinase, and chondrocyte activation factor.
   d. Ligament Augmentation Devices (LADs)—Such as the Kennedy LAD (polypropylene yarn) and Dacron. LADs do allow some fibrous ingrowth, but their use is limited.
   e. Biodegradable Tissue Scaffoldings—Allow immediate stability and long-term replacement with host tissue. Carbon fiber and PLA-coated carbon fiber devices have been used with limited success (slow ingrowth is improved with PLA coating).

3. Articular Cartilage—The ultimate tensile strength of cartilage is only 5% that of bone, and its *E* is 0.1% that of bone; nevertheless, because of its highly viscoelastic properties, it is well suited for compressive loading. Deformation and shift of water to and from cartilage are largely responsible.

4. Metal Implants
   a. **Screws**—Characterized by pitch (distance between threads), **lead** (distance advanced in one revolution), **root diameter** (minimal/inner diameter $\propto$ tensile strength), and **outer diameter** (determines holding power [pullout strength]). **To maximize pullout strength, a screw should have a large outer diameter, a small root diameter, and a fine pitch.** Pullout strength of a pedicle screw is most affected by the degree of osteoporosis.

b. **Plates**—Strength varies with the material and moment of inertia. **The rigidity (bending stiffness) of a plate is proportional to the thickness (*t*) to the third power (t^3).** Thus doubling plate thickness increases its bending stiffness eightfold. Plates are load-bearing devices and most effective when placed on a fracture's tension side. Types of plates include static compression (best in the upper extremity; can be stressed for compression), dynamic compression (e.g., tension band plate), neutralization (resists torsion), and buttress (protects bone graft). Stress concentration at open screw holes can lead to implant failure. **Screw holes that remain after removal of a plate and screws represent a stress riser and a site at risk for refracture.** Blade plates provide increased resistance to torsional deformation in subtrochanteric fractures.

c. **Intramedullary Nails**—Require a high polar moment of inertia to maximize torsional rigidity and strength. **In characterizing the mechanical characteristics of an IM nail, we describe the torsional rigidity and the bending rigidity. Torsional rigidity** is the amount of torque needed to produce torsional (rotational) deformation (a unit angle of torsional deformation). **Torsional rigidity of an IM nail** (cylinder) depends on both material properties (shear modulus) and structural properties (polar moment of inertia). **Bending rigidity** is the amount of force required to produce a unit amount of deflection. **Bending rigidity of an IM nail** also depends on both material properties (*E*) and structural properties (area moment of inertia, length). **Bending rigidity of an IM nail is related to the fourth power of the nail's radius**; increasing nail diameter by 10% increases bending rigidity by 50%. Reaming allows increased torsional resistance owing to the increased contact area and allows use of a larger nail with increased rigidity and strength. IM nails are better at resisting bending than rotational forces. Unslotted nails allow stronger fixation and a smaller diameter (at the expense of flexibility). **The greatest mechanical advantage of closed section IM nails over slotted nails is increased torsional stiffness.** During IM nail insertion for a femoral shaft fracture, the hoop stresses are lowest for a slotted nail with a thin wall made of titanium alloy. Posterior starting points for femoral nails decrease hoop stresses and iatrogenic comminution of fractures. Implant failure occurs more frequently with smaller-diameter, unreamed IM nails. **IM nails are load-sharing devices.**

d. External Fixators
   (1) **Conventional External Fixators—The most important factor for stability of fixation of a fracture treated with external fixation is allowing the fracture ends to come into contact. Other factors of the external fixator that may be used to enhance stability (rigidity) are**
      (a) **Larger diameter pins (the second most important factor)**—The bending rigidity of each pin is proportional to the fourth power of the pin diameter.
      (b) **Additional pins.**
      (c) **Decreased bone-rod distance**—The bending stiffness of each pin is proportional to the third power of the bone-rod distance.
      (d) **Pins in different planes** (pins separated by >45 degrees).
      (e) **Increased mass of the rods or stacked rods** (a second rod in the same plane provides increased resistance to bending moments in the sagittal plane).
      (f) **Rods in different planes.**
      (g) **Increased Spacing Between Pins**—Place central pins closer to the fracture site and peripheral pins further from the fracture site (near-near, far-far). For tibial shaft fractures, the use of additional lag screws with external fixation is associated with a higher refracture rate than external fixation alone.
   (2) **Circular (Ilizarov) External Fixators**—Thin wires (usually 1.8 mm in diameter) are fixed under tension (usually between 90 and 130 kg) to circular rings. Half-pins may also be used but offer better purchase in diaphyseal (not metaphyseal) bone. The optimal orientation of the implants on the ring is 90 degrees to each other to maximize stability (90 degrees is not always possible because of anatomic constraints [such as neurovascular structures]). The bending stiffness of the frame is independent of the loading direction because the frame is circular. Each ring should have at least two implants (wires or half-pins); the most stable construct when using two implants on a ring is an olive wire and a half-pin at 90 degrees to each other. When two wires are used on a ring, one wire should be positioned

superior to the ring and one should be positioned inferior to the ring (two tensioned wires on the same side of a ring can cause the ring to deform). Factors that enhance stability of circular external fixators include:

a. Larger diameter wires (and half-pins).
b. Decreased ring diameter.
c. The use of olive wires.
d. Additional wires and/or half-pins.
e. Wires (and/or half-pins) crossing at 90 degrees.
f. Increased wire tension (up to 130 kg).
g. Placement of the two central rings close to the fracture site.
h. Decreased spacing between adjacent rings.
i. Increased number of rings.

e. Total Hip Arthroplasty—Evolving design has reduced biomechanical constraints of THA. Femoral components are designed for use with and without cement. In cementless designs, the proximal porous coating should be circumferential to seal the diaphysis from wear debris. In cemented designs, a cement mantle <2 mm thick increases the incidence of crack formation. Stem length is directly related to rigidity. Metal femoral heads have greater neck-length options than do ceramics. A design with a broad medial surface, a broader lateral surface, and a large moment of inertia minimize compressive and tensile stresses in adjacent structures. Femoral component design must account for rotational forces. Rotational torque in retroversion is the force most responsible for the initiation of loosening in cemented femoral stems; these rotational torques are increased in femoral stems with a higher offset. **The femoral component should be in neutral or slight valgus position to decrease the moment arm, cement stress, and abductor length. Increasing femoral component offset moves the abductor attachment away from the joint center and increases the abductor moment arm; this reduces the abductor force required in normal gait and thus reduces the resultant hip joint reactive force. Unfortunately, increased offset also increases the bending moment on the implant (increased strain) and increases strain on the medial cement mantle. Femoral head size should be a compromise between small (22 mm) components, which decrease friction and torque and polyethylene volumetric wear but also decrease ROM and stability, and large (36 mm) components that increase friction and torque and polyethylene volumetric wear but also increase ROM and stability.** A 26- or 28-mm head seems to be the ideal size in most instances. The relatively poor survivorship of surface replacement hip arthroplasty is primarily due to volumetric wear of polyethylene, which is 4-10 times than that of a THA using a 28 mm head. Metal backing of acetabular components decreases the stress in cement and cancellous bone. Use of different metal alloys and titanium (with *E* closer to cortical bone) is being investigated. **Polyethylene on titanium makes a poor bearing surface because of excessive volumetric wear. The use of titanium on weight-bearing surfaces (poor resistance to wear, notch sensitivity) may lead to fretting, wear debris, and blackening of the soft tissues.** Histiocyte injection of submicron polyethylene debris has been associated with wear synovitis in TJA. UHMWPE serves as a "shock absorber" and should be at least 6 mm thick to prevent creep. **The lowest coefficient of friction is for a ceramic femoral head on a ceramic acetabulum. Wear rate of UHMWPE in the acetabulum is about 0.1 mm (100 micrometers) per year. By comparison, wear rate of metal-on-metal bearings for THA is approximately 0.002-0.005 mm (2-5 μm) per year. Ceramic bearing surfaces exhibit wear rates of only 0.0005-0.0025 mm (0.5-2.5 μm) per year.** Other new concepts include computer design of THA stems, modularity (increased corrosion at modular metallic junction sites [such as the junction of the head and stem]), custom designs, and more flexible stems. Forging of components appears to be superior to casting.

f. Total Knee Arthroplasty (TKA)—Design has evolved significantly after original design errors that did not take kinematics of the human knee into consideration (i.e., original hinge design). An appropriate compromise between total contact designs (high conformity) with excess stability (and less motion) but less wear and a low-contact design with less stability and increased wear is being approached. Metal alloys are typically used. **Cemented cruciate-substituting TKA designs are associated with low polyethylene wear rates and minimal osteolysis (due to the high degree of conformity of the tibiofemoral articulation).**

g. Compression Hip Screws—Demonstrate loading characteristics superior to blade plates. Higher-angled plates are subjected to lower bending loads but may be more difficult to insert. Sliding of the screw is proportional to the screw/side plate angle and the length of the screw in the barrel.

5. Implant Fixation—Three basic forms exist: interference fit, interlocking, and biologic.
   a. Interference Fit—Mechanical or press fit components rely on the formation of a fibrous tissue interface. Loosening can occur if stability is not maintained and high-E substances (leading to increased bone resorption/remodeling) are used.
   b. Interlocking Fit—PMMA (a grout with a low E) allows a gradual transfer of stresses to bone (microinterlocking of cement within cancellous bone). Microinterlock may not be achievable when doing a cemented revision of a previously cemented TKA. Aseptic loosening can occur over time. Careful technique with limiting of porosities and gaps and using a 3-5 mm cement thickness yields the best results. Other improvements include low-viscosity cement, better bone-bed preparation, plugging and pressurization, and better (vacuum) cement mixing.
   c. Biologic Fit—Tissue ingrowth makes use of fiber-metal composites, void metal composites, or microbeads to create **pore sizes of 100-400 μm (ideally 100-250 μm)**. Mechanical stability is required for ingrowth, which is most typically limited to 10-30% of the surface area. Problems include fiber/bead loosening, increased cost, proximal bone resorption (monocyte/macrophage-mediated), corrosion, and decreased implant fatigue strength. Bone ingrowth in the tibial component of an uncemented TKA occurs adjacent to fixation pegs and screws. Bone ingrowth of uncemented TJA components depends on the avoidance of micromotion (may be seen on follow-up radiographs as radiodense reactive lines about the prosthesis) at the bone-implant interface. Canal filling (maximal endosteal contact) of more fully coated femoral stems is an important factor for bone ingrowth.
6. Bone-Implant Unit—The integrated unit is a composite structure that has shared properties. The more accurately the bone cross-section is reconstructed with metallic support, the better the loading characteristics. Plates should act as tension bands. Materials with increased E may result in bone resorption, whereas materials with decreased E may result in implant failure. **Placement of the implant initiates a race between bone healing and implant failure.**

III. Biomechanics

A. Joint Biomechanics: General

1. Degrees of Freedom—Joint motion is described as rotations and translations occurring in the x, y, and z planes, thus requiring **six parameters, or degrees of freedom,** to describe motion. Fortunately, translations are usually relatively insignificant for most joints and can often be ignored in biomechanical analyses.
2. Joint Reaction Force (R)—Force generated within a joint in response to forces acting on the joint (both intrinsic and extrinsic). **Muscle contractions about a joint are the major contributory factor to the joint reaction force.** Values (of R) correlate with the predisposition to degenerative changes. Joint contact pressure (stress) can be minimized by decreasing R and increasing contact area.
3. Coupled Forces—In certain joints, rotation about one axis is accompanied by an obligatory rotation about another axis; such movements (and associated forces) are said to be coupled. For example, lateral bending of the spine is accompanied by axial rotation, and these movements/forces are coupled.
4. Joint Congruence—Relates to the fit of two articular surfaces and is a necessary condition for joint motion. It can be evaluated radiographically. High congruence increases joint contact area; low congruence decreases contact area. Movement out of a position of congruity causes increased stress in cartilage by allowing less contact area for distribution of the joint reaction force, predisposing the joint to degeneration.
5. **Instant Center of Rotation**—Point about which a joint rotates. **In joints such as the knee, the location of the instant center changes during the arc of motion (due to joint translation and morphology)**, following a curved path. The instant center normally lies on a line perpendicular to the tangent of the joint surface at all points of contact.
6. Rolling and Sliding (Fig. 1-98)—Almost all joints, during ROM, undergo simultaneous rolling and sliding in order to remain in congruence. Pure rolling occurs when the instant center of rotation is at the rolling surfaces and the contacting points have zero relative velocity (no "slipping" of one surface on the other). Pure sliding occurs with pure translation or rotation about a stationary axis; there is no angular change in position and no instant center of rotation ("slipping" of one surface on the other).
7. Friction and Lubrication—Friction is the resistance between two bodies as one slides over the other; it is not a function of the contact area. Lubrication decreases the coefficient of friction (0 = no friction) between surfaces.

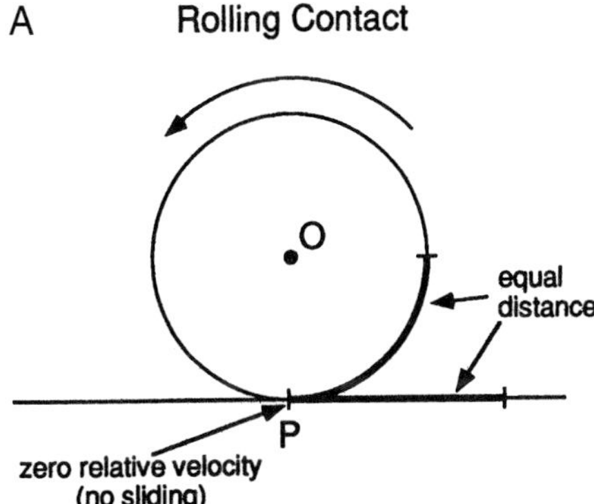

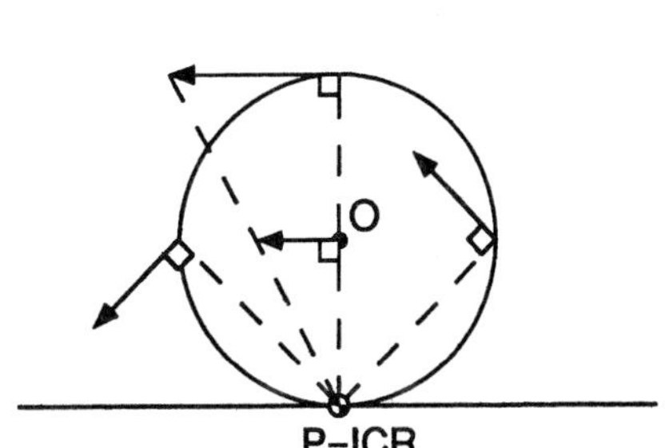

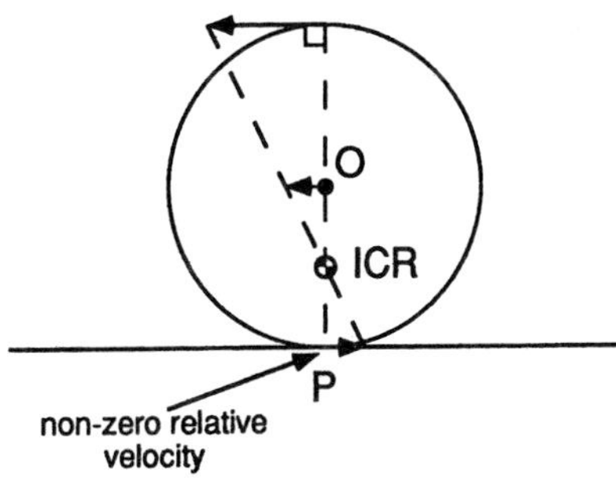

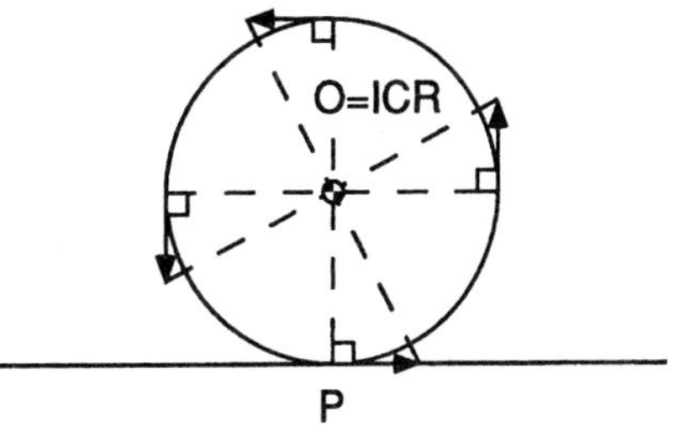

FIGURE 1-98 ■ *A*, Rolling contact occurs when the circumferential distance of the rolling object equals the distance traced along the plane. This can occur only when there is no sliding, that is, the relative velocity at the point of contact *(P)* is zero. *B*, For rolling contact, the point *P* of the wheel has zero velocity because it is in contact with the ground. Therefore *P* is the instant center of rotation (ICR) of the wheel. This diagram shows the actual velocity of points along the wheel as it rolls along the ground. *C*, Sliding contact occurs when the relative velocity at the contact point is not zero. *D*, Pure sliding occurs when the wheel rotates about a stationary axis, *O*. In this case, the wheel would have no forward motion. (From Buckwalter, J.A., Einhorn, T.A., and Simon, S.R.: Orthopaedic Basic Science: Biology and Biomechanics of the Musculoskeletal System, 2nd ed., Rosemont, IL, American Academy of Orthopaedic Surgeons, 2000, p. 146.)

Articular surfaces lubricated with synovial fluid have a coefficient of friction 10 times larger than the best synthetic systems. **The coefficient of friction of human joints is 0.002-0.04. The coefficient of friction for joint arthroplasty (metal on UHMWPE) is 0.05-0.15 (not as good as human joints). Elastohydrodynamic lubrication is the primary mechanism responsible for lubrication of articular cartilage during dynamic function.**

B. Hip Biomechanics
  1. Kinematics
     a. Range of Motion (Table 1-61)
     b. Instant Center—Simultaneous triplanar motion for this ball-and-socket joint makes analysis impossible.
  2. Kinetics—**The hip's *R* can reach three to six times body weight (*W*) and is primarily due to contraction of muscles crossing the hip.** This phenomenon can be demonstrated with the FBD in Figure 1-99. If $A = 5$ and $B = 12.5$, using standard FBD analysis

$\sum M = 0$ (the sum of the moments is 0)

$-5\ M_y + 12.5\ W = 0$

Table 1-61. HIP BIOMECHANICS: RANGE OF MOTION

MOTION	AVERAGE RANGE (DEGREES)	FUNCTIONAL RANGE (DEGREES)
Flexion	115	90 (120 squat)
Extension	30	
Abduction	50	20
Adduction	30	
Internal rotation	45	0
External rotation	45	20

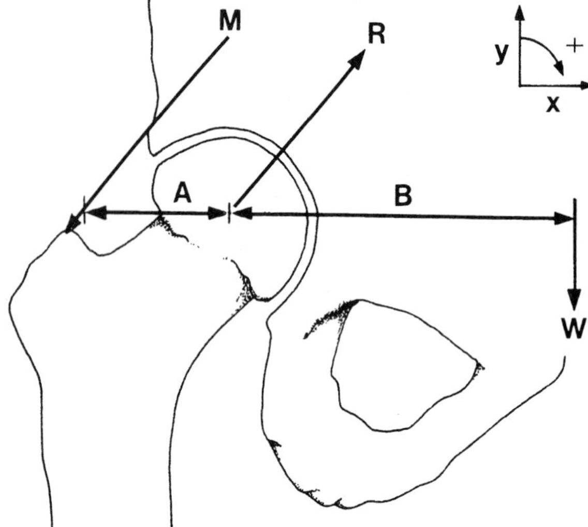

FIGURE 1-99 ■ Free body diagram (see text for explanation).

$M_y = 2.5\ W$

$\Sigma F_y = 0$ (the sum of the forces is 0)

$-M_y - W + R_y = 0$

$R_y = 3.5\ W$

$R = R_y/(\cos 30°)$

$R \cong 4\ W$

An increase in the ratio of A/B (e.g., with medialization of the acetabulum, with a long-neck prosthesis, or with lateralization of the greater trochanter) decreases R. If $A = 7.5$ and $B = 10, R \cong 2.3\ W$. ***R* and abductor moment are both reduced by shifting the body weight over the hip (Trendelenburg gait). A cane in the contralateral hand produces an additional moment and can reduce the joint reaction force up to 60% (carrying a load in the ipsilateral hand also decreases joint reaction force** at the hip). Energy expenditure is 264% of normal with a resection arthroplasty of the hip (such as after a THA infection). The hip and trunk generate approximately 50% (the largest component) of the force generated during a tennis serve.

3. Other Considerations
   a. Stability—Largely based on the intrinsic stability of the deep-seated "ball-and-socket" design.
   b. Sourcil—Condensation of subchondral bone under the superomedial acetabulum. At this point R is at maximum (Pauwels).
   c. Gothic Arch—Remodeled bone supporting the acetabular roof with the sourcil at its base (Bombelli).
   d. Neck-Shaft Angle—Varus angulation decreases R and increases shear across the neck. **Varus also leads to shortening of the lower extremity and alters the muscle tension resting length of the hip abductors, which may cause a persistent limp.** Valgus angulation increases R and decreases shear. Neutral or valgus is better for a THA because PMMA resists shear poorly.
   e. Arthrodesis—**The position for hip arthrodesis should be 25-30 degrees of flexion and 0 degrees of abduction and rotation (external rotation is better than internal rotation). If the hip is fused in an abducted position, the patient will lurch over the affected lower extremity with an excessive trunk shift, which will later result in lower back pain.** Hip arthrodesis increases oxygen consumption, decreases gait efficiency (to approximately 50% of normal), and increases transpelvic rotation of the contralateral hip.

C. Knee Biomechanics
   1. Kinematics
      a. Range of Motion—ROM of the knee is from 10 degrees of extension (recurvatum) to about 130 degrees of flexion. Functional ROM is from near full extension to about 90 degrees of flexion (117 degrees is required for squatting and lifting). Approximately 110 degrees of flexion is required to arise from a chair after TKA. Rotation varies with flexion: at full extension there is minimal rotation; at 90 degrees of flexion, 45 degrees of external rotation and 30 degrees of internal rotation are possible. Abduction/adduction is essentially 0 degrees (a few degrees of passive motion is possible at 30 degrees of flexion). Motion about the knee is a complex series of movements about a changing instant center of rotation (i.e., polycentric rotation). There is 0.5 cm of excursion of the medial meniscus and 1.1 cm of excursion of the lateral meniscus during a 0- to 120-degree arc of knee motion.
      b. Joint Motion—The instant center of rotation, when plotted, describes a J-shaped curve about the femoral condyle, moving posteriorly as the knee flexes. Flexion and extension of the knee involve both **rolling and sliding** motions. The femur internally rotates (external tibial rotation) during the last 15 degrees of extension (**"screw home" mechanism**, related to the size and convexity of the medial femoral condyle [MFC] and the musculature). **Posterior rollback of the femur on the tibia during knee flexion increases maximum knee flexion.** Normal femoral rollback is compromised when the PCL is sacrificed, as in some TKAs. The axis of rotation of the intact knee is in the MFC.

The patellofemoral joint is a sliding articulation (patella slides 7 cm caudally with full flexion), with an instant center near the posterior cortex above the condyles.

2. Kinetics—Extension via the quadriceps mechanism, through the patellar apparatus; flexion via the hamstring muscles.
   a. Knee Stabilizers—Although bony contours contribute to knee stability, it is the ligaments and muscles of the knee that play the major role (Table 1-62). The ACL is typically subjected to peak loads of 170 N during walking and up to 500 N with running. The ultimate strength of the ACL in young patients is about 1750 N. The ACL fails by serial tearing at 10-15% elongation. Cadaver studies have shown that sectioning the PCL increases contact pressures in the medial compartment and across the patellofemoral joint.
   b. Joint Forces
      (1) Tibiofemoral Joint—Knee joint surface loads are **three times body weight during level walking** and up to **four times body weight when climbing stairs.** Menisci help with load transmission (bear one third to one half of body weight), and removal of these structures increases contact stresses (up to four times load transfer to bone). The quadriceps muscle produces maximal anterior-directed force on the tibia at knee flexion of 0-60 degrees.
      (2) Patellofemoral Joint—The patella aids in knee extension by increasing the lever arm and in stress distribution. This joint has the thickest cartilage in the entire body because it must bear the greatest load—ranging from ½ *W* with normal walking to 7 times *W* with squatting and jogging. Loads are proportional to the quadriceps force/knee flexion ratio. **While descending stairs, the compressive force between the patella and the trochlea of the femur reaches 2-3 times body weight. After patellectomy, the length of the moment arm is decreased by the width of the patella (30% reduction) and the power of extension is decreased by 30%.** During TKA the following enhance patella tracking: external rotation of the femoral component, lateral placement of the femoral and tibial components, medial placement of the patellar component, and avoidance of malrotation of the tibial component (avoid internal rotation).
   c. Axes of the Lower Extremity (Fig. 1-100)
      (1) Mechanical Axis of the Lower Extremity—From the center of the femoral head to the center of the ankle. The mechanical axis of a normal lower extremity passes just medial to the medial tibial spine.
      (2) Vertical Axis—From the center of gravity to the ground.
      (3) Anatomic Axes—Along the shafts of the femur and tibia. There is a normal valgus angle where these two axes intersect at the knee.

Table 1-62. KNEE STABILIZERS

DIRECTION	STRUCTURES
Medial	Superficial MCL (1°), joint capsule, med. meniscus, ACL/PCL
Lateral	Joint capsule, IT band, LCL (mid), lat. meniscus, ACL/PCL (90°)
Anterior	ACL (1°), joint capsule
Posterior	PCL (1°), joint capsule; PCL tightens with IR
Rotatory	Combinations—MCL checks ER; ACL checks IR

IR, internal rotation; ER, external rotation; MCL, medial collateral ligament complex; LCL, lateral collateral ligament complex; IT, iliotibial; ACL, anterior cruciate ligament; PCL, posterior cruciate ligament.

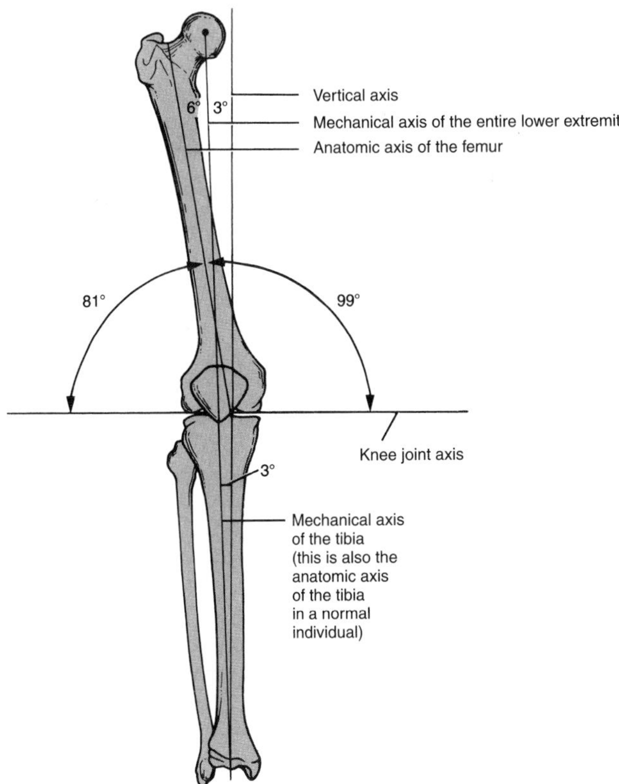

FIGURE 1-100 ■ Axes of the lower extremity. (Modified from Helfet, D.L.: Fractures of the distal femur. In Browner, B.D., Jupiter, J.B., Levine, A.M., et al., eds.: Skeletal Trauma. Philadelphia, WB Saunders, 1992, p. 1645.)

(4) Mechanical Axis of the Femur—From the center of the femoral head to the center of the knee.

(5) Mechanical Axis of the Tibia—From the center of the tibial plateau to the center of the ankle.

(6) Relationships—The mechanical axis of the lower extremity is in 3 degrees of valgus from the vertical axis. The anatomic axis of the femur is in 6 degrees of valgus from the mechanical axis (9 degrees versus the vertical axis). The anatomic axis of the tibia is in 2-3 degrees of varus from the mechanical axis.

d. Arthrodesis—**The position for knee arthrodesis should be 0-7 degrees of valgus and 10-15 degrees of flexion.**

D. Ankle and Foot Biomechanics

1. Ankle

a. Kinematics—Instant center of rotation is within the talus, and the lateral and posterior points are at the tips of the malleoli; they change slightly with movement. The talus is described as forming a cone with the body and trochlea wider anteriorly and laterally. Therefore the talus and fibula must externally rotate slightly with dorsiflexion. Ankle dorsiflexion and abduction are coupled movements in the ankle. Average ankle ROM is 25 degrees of dorsiflexion, 35 degrees of plantar flexion, and 5 degrees of rotation.

b. Kinetics—The tibial/talar articulation is the major weight-bearing surface of the ankle, supporting compressive forces up to 5 times body weight (*W*) on level surfaces and shear (backward-to-forward) forces up to *W*. A large weight-bearing surface area allows for decreased stress (force/area) at this joint. The fibula/talar joint transmits about one sixth of the force. The highest net muscle moment at the ankle occurs during the terminal stance phase of gait.

c. Other Considerations—Stability is based on the shape of the articulation (mortise that is maintained by the talar shape) and ligamentous support. The greatest stability is in dorsiflexion. During weight bearing (loaded), the tibial and talar articular surfaces contribute most to joint stability. A windlass action has been described in the ankle, where full dorsiflexion is limited by the plantar aponeurosis, and further tension on the aponeurosis (e.g., with toe dorsiflexion) causes the arch to rise. **A syndesmosis screw limits external rotation of the ankle. Arthrodesis of the ankle should be performed in neutral dorsiflexion, 5-10 degrees of external rotation, and 5 degrees of hindfoot valgus** (anticipate a loss of 70% of the sagittal plane motion of the foot).

2. Subtalar Joint (Talus-Calcaneus-Navicular)—The axis of rotation is 42 degrees in the sagittal plane and 16 degrees in the transverse plane. Described as functioning like an oblique hinge; its motions are also coupled with dorsiflexion, abduction, and eversion in one direction (pronation) and plantar flexion, adduction, and inversion (supination) in the other. Average ROM of pronation is 5 degrees; supination is 20 degrees. Functional ROM is approximately 6 degrees.

3. Transverse Tarsal Joint (Talus-Navicular, Calcaneal-Cuboid)—Motion is based on foot position with two axes of rotation (talonavicular and calcaneocuboid). With eversion of the foot (as during the early stance phase), the two joint axes are parallel and ROM is permitted. With foot inversion (late stance), external rotation of the lower extremity causes the joint axes to no longer be parallel, and motion is limited.

4. Foot—Transmits about 1.2 times *W* with walking and 3 times *W* with running. It is composed of three arches (Table 1-63). The second MT (Lisfranc) joint is "key-like" and stabilizes the second MT, allowing it to carry the most load with gait (the first MT bears the most load while standing). The expected life span of a Plastazote shoe insert in an active adult is <1 month (fatigues rapidly in both compression and shear). Therefore in a shoe

Table 1-63. ARCHES OF THE FOOT

ARCH	COMPONENTS	KEYSTONE	LIGAMENT SUPPORT	MUSCLE SUPPORT
Medial longitudinal	Calcaneus, talus, navicular, 3 cuneiforms, 1st–3rd metatarsals	Talus head	Spring (calcaneonavicular)	Tibialis post., flexor digitorum longus, flexor hallucis longus, adductor hallucis
Lateral longitudinal	Calcaneus, cuboid, 4th and 5th metatarsals		Plantar aponeurosis	Abductor digiti minimi, flexor digitorum brevis
Transverse	3 Cuneiforms, cuboid, metatarsal bases			Peroneus longus, tibialis post., adductor hallucis (oblique)

insert, Plastazote should be replaced frequently and/or supported with other materials such as Spenco or PPT.

E. Spine Biomechanics
   1. Kinematics—ROM varies with anatomic segment (Table 1-64). Analysis is based on the functional unit **(motion segment = two vertebrae and their intervening soft tissues). Six degrees of freedom exist about all three axes. Coupled motion** (simultaneous rotation, lateral bending, and flexion or extension) is also demonstrated, especially axial rotation with lateral bending. The instant center of rotation lies within the disc. The normal sagittal alignment of the lumbar spine (55-60 degrees of lordosis) exists because of the disc spaces (not the vertebrae); most of the lordosis is between L4 and S1. Loss of disc space height can cause a significant loss of the normal lumbar lordosis. Iatrogenic flat back syndrome of the lumbar spine is the result of a distraction force.
   2. Supporting Structures—Anterior supporting structures include the anterior longitudinal ligament, the posterior longitudinal ligament, and the vertebral disc. Posterior supporting structures include the intertransverse ligaments, capsular ligaments and facets, and ligamentum flavum (yellow ligament). The halo vest is the most effective device for controlling cervical motion (because of pin purchase in the skull).
      a. Apophyseal Joints—Resist torsion during axial loading, and the attached capsular ligaments resist flexion. They guide the motion of the motion segment. Direction of motion is determined by the orientation of the facets of the apophyseal joint, which varies with each level. **In the C-spine the facets are oriented 45 degrees to the transverse plane and parallel to the frontal plane. In the T-spine the facets are oriented 60 degrees to the transverse plane and 20 degrees to the frontal plane. In the L-spine the facets are oriented 90 degrees to the transverse plane and 45 degrees to the frontal plane** (i.e., they progressively tilt up [transverse plane] and in [frontal plane]). **Cervical facetectomy of greater than 50% causes a significant loss of stability in flexion and torsion. Torsional load resistance in the lumbar spine has a 40% contribution from the facets and a 40% contribution by the disc; the remaining 20% resistance to torsional load is contributed by the ligamentous structures.**
   3. Kinetics
      a. Disc—**Behaves viscoelastically and demonstrates creep (deforms with time) and hysteresis (absorbs energy with repeated axial loads and later decreases in function).** Compressive stresses are highest in the nucleus pulposus, and tensile stresses are highest in the annulus fibrosus. Stiffness of the disc increases with increasing compressive load. With higher loads, increased deformation and faster creep can be expected. Repeated torsional loading may separate the nucleus pulposus from the annulus and end-plate, forcing nuclear material out through an annular tear (produced by shear forces). Loads increase with bending and torsional stresses. **After subtotal discectomy, extension is the most stable loading mode. Disc pressures are lowest in the lying supine position on a flat surface. When carrying loads, disc pressures are lowest when the load is carried close to the body.**
      b. Vertebrae—Strength is related to the bone mineral content and vertebrae size (increased in the lumbar spine). Fatigue loading may lead to pars fractures. Compression fractures occur at the end-plate. Decreased vertebral body stiffness in osteoporosis is caused by loss of horizontal trabeculae. Increasing implant stiffness for an implant-augmented spinal arthrodesis results in an increased probability of a successful fusion but an increased likelihood of decreased bone mineral content of the bridged vertebrae.

Table 1-64. RANGE OF MOTION OF SPINAL SEGMENTS

LEVEL	FLEXION/EXTENSION (DEGREES)	LATERAL BENDING (DEGREES)	ROTATION (DEGREES)	INSTANT CENTER
Occiput-C1	13	8	0	Skull, 2-3 cm above dens
C1–C2	10	0	45	Waist of odontoid
C2–C7	10-15	8-10	10	Vertebral body below
T-spine	5	6	8	Vertebra below/disc centrum
L-spine	15-20	2-5	3-6	Disc annulus

F. Shoulder Biomechanics

1. Kinematics—The scapular plane is 30 degrees anterior to the coronal plane and is the preferred reference for ROM. Abduction requires external rotation of the humerus to prevent greater tuberosity impingement. With internal rotation contractures, patients cannot abduct >120 degrees. Abduction is a result of glenohumeral motion (120 degrees) and scapulothoracic motion (60 degrees) in a 2:1 ratio (although this ratio varies over first 30 degrees of motion). **Deceleration is the most violent phase of pitching; the rotator cuff is the principal decelerator and is susceptible to tensile failure from eccentric loading.** Movement at the AC joint is responsible for the early part of scapulothoracic motion, and sternoclavicular (SC) movement is responsible for the later portion, with clavicular rotation along the long axis. Surface joint motion in the glenohumeral joint is a combination of rotation, rolling, and translation.
2. Kinetics (Table 1-65)—The zero position (Saha)—165 degrees of abduction in the scapular plane—minimizes deforming forces about the shoulder. This position is ideal for reducing shoulder dislocations (or "fractures with traction"). Free-body analysis of the deltoid force (Fig. 1-101) reveals the following:

$$\Sigma M_0 = 0$$

$$3D - 0.05\ W(30) = 0$$

$$D = 0.5\ W$$

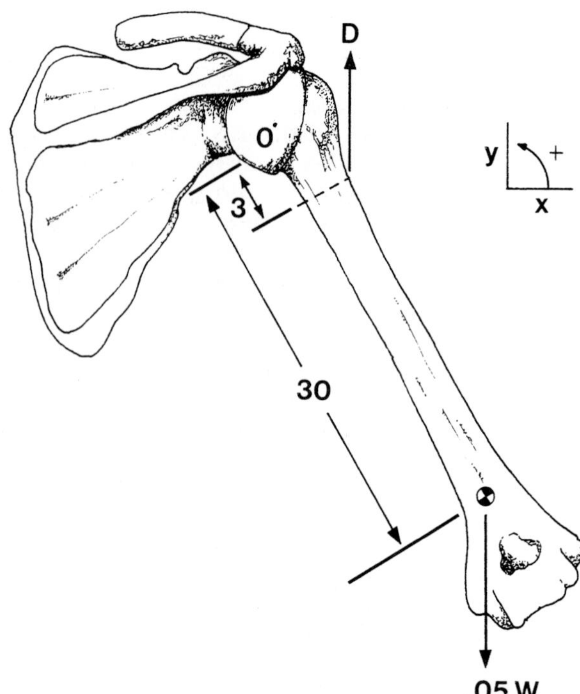

FIGURE 1-101 ■ Free body diagram (see text for explanation).

Table 1-65. SHOULDER BIOMECHANICS: MUSCLE FORCES

MOTION	MUSCLE FORCES	COMMENTS
Glenohumeral		
Abduction	Deltoid, supraspinatus	Cuff depresses head
Adduction	Latissimus dorsi, pectoralis major, teres major	
Forward flexion	Pectoralis major, deltoid (ant.), biceps	
Extension	Latissimus dorsi	
IR	Subscapularis, teres major	
ER	Infraspinatus, teres minor, deltoid (post.)	
Scapular		
Rotation	Upper trapezius, levator scapulae (ant.), serratus ant., lower trapezius	Works through a force couple
Adduction	Trapezius, rhomboid, latissimus dorsi	
Abduction	Serratus ant., pectoralis minor	

3. Stability—Limited about the glenohumeral joint. Humeral head surface area is larger than the glenoid (48 × 45 mm versus 35 × 25 mm). Bony stability is limited and relies only on inclination (125 degrees) and retroversion (25 degrees) of the humeral head and slight retrotilt of the glenoid. **The inferior glenohumeral ligament (superior band) is the most important static stabilizer about the shoulder.** The superior and middle glenohumeral ligaments are secondary stabilizers to anterior humeral translation. **Inferior subluxation of the humeral head is prevented by the shoulder's negative intra-articular pressure. The rotator cuff muscles provide a dynamic contribution to shoulder stability.** Stress on the posterior shoulder capsule is greatest during follow-through of throwing. **The position for arthrodesis of the shoulder is 15-20 degrees of abduction, 20-25 degrees of forward flexion, and 40-50 degrees of internal rotation (avoid excessive external rotation).**
4. Other Joints—The AC joint allows scapular rotation (through the conoid and trapezoid ligaments) and scapular motion (through the AC joint itself). The SC joint allows clavicular protraction/retraction in a transverse plane (through the coracoclavicular ligament), clavicular elevation and depression in the frontal plane (also through the coracoclavicular ligament), and clavicular rotation around the longitudinal axis.

G. Elbow Biomechanics

1. Introduction—The elbow serves three functions: (1) as a component joint of the lever arm when positioning the hand; (2) as a fulcrum for the forearm lever; and (3) as a weight-bearing joint in patients using crutches. During throwing, the elbow functions primarily as a positioner and a means of transferring energy from the shoulder and trunk. Most activities of daily living can be performed with an elbow range of motion of 30-130 degrees of flexion, 50 degrees of supination, and 50 degrees of pronation.
2. Kinematics—Motion about the elbow includes flexion and extension (0-150 degrees with **functional ROM 30-130 degrees**; the axis of rotation is the center of the trochlea) and pronation (P) and supination (S): P = 80 degrees and S = 85 degrees with a **functional P and S of 50 degrees each**; the axis is a line from the capitellum through the radial head and to the distal ulna (defines a cone). The normal carrying angle (valgus angle at the elbow) is 7 degrees for males and 13 degrees for females. This angle decreases with flexion.
3. Kinetics—The forces that act about the elbow have short lever arms and are relatively inefficient, resulting in large joint reaction forces that subject the elbow to degenerative changes. Flexion is primarily by the brachialis and biceps, extension by the triceps, pronation by the pronators (teres and quadratus), and supination by the biceps and supinator. Static loads approach, and dynamic loads exceed, body weight (W). The FBD in Figure 1-102 demonstrates the inefficiency of elbow flexion.

$$\Sigma M_0 = 0$$

$$-5B + 15W = 0$$

$$B = 3W$$

4. Stability—Provided partially by articular congruity. **The three necessary and sufficient constraints for elbow stability are the coronoid, lateral (ulnar) collateral ligament, and the anterior band of the medial collateral ligament (MCL)**. The **most important stabilizer is the MCL** (anterior oblique fibers). The MCL stabilizes the elbow to both valgus and distractional force with forearm flexion (90 degrees). **The most important secondary stabilizer to valgus stress at the elbow is the radial head.** The radial head provides about 30% of valgus stability and is more important in 0-30 degrees of flexion and pronation. Valgus extension overload of the elbow occurs during the late cocking and early acceleration phases of throwing. In extension, the capsule is the primary restraint to distractional forces. Laterally, stability is provided by the lateral collateral ligament (LCL), anconeus, and joint capsule. The position for unilateral arthrodesis is about 90 degrees of flexion; for bilateral arthrodesis one elbow is placed at 110 degrees of flexion (to reach the mouth) and the other at 65 degrees of flexion (for hygiene needs). Arthrodesis is difficult and, fortunately, rarely required.

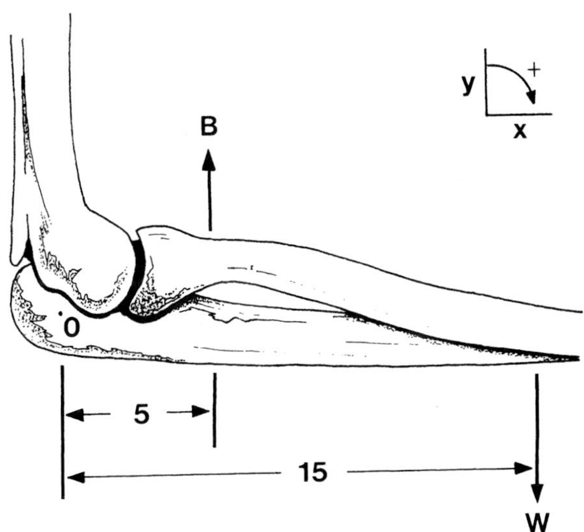

FIGURE 1-102 ■ Free body diagram (see text for explanation).

5. Forearm—About 17% of the axial load is transmitted by the ulna. The line of the center of rotation runs from the radial head to the distal ulna.

H. Wrist and Hand Biomechanics

1. Wrist—Part of an intercalated link system
   a. Kinematics—Motions about the wrist include flexion (65 degrees normal, 10 degrees functional), extension (55 degrees normal, 35 degrees functional), radial deviation (15 degrees normal, 10 degrees functional), and ulnar deviation (35 degrees normal, 15 degrees functional). Flexion and extension are primarily radiocarpal (two thirds), but intercarpal movement is also important (one third). Radial deviation is primarily due to intercarpal movement, whereas ulnar deviation relies on radiocarpal and intercarpal motion. The instant center for wrist motion is the head of the capitate but is variable.
   b. Columns—Three columns have been described for the wrist (Taleisnik) (Table 1-66).
   c. Link System—The carpus makes up a system of three links in a chain (Gilford): radius-lunate-capitate. This arrangement allows for less motion to be required at each link but adds to the instability of the "chain." Stability, however, is enhanced by

Table 1-66. COLUMNS OF THE WRIST

COLUMN	FUNCTION	COMMENTS
Central	Flexion-extension	Distal carpal row and lunate (link)
Medial	Rotation	Triquetrum
Lateral	Mobile	Scaphoid

strong volar ligaments and the scaphoid, which bridges both carpal rows.

d. Relationships—Carpal collapse can be evaluated based on the ratio of carpal height/third MC height (normally 0.54). Ulnar translation can be determined using the ulna-to-capitate length/third MC height ratio (normal is 0.30). The distal radius normally bears about 80% of the distal radioulnar joint load and the distal ulna 20%. Ulnar load-bearing can be increased with ulnar lengthening or decreased with ulnar shortening. Wrist arthrodesis is relatively common. A position of 10-20 degrees of dorsiflexion is good for a unilateral fusion; and if bilateral fusion is necessary (avoid if possible), the other wrist should be fused in 0-10 degrees of palmar flexion.

2. Hand
   a. Kinematics—ROM at the MCP joint (universal joint, 2 degrees of freedom) includes 100 degrees of flexion and 60 degrees of abduction-adduction. PIP joints usually have about 110 degrees of flexion and DIP joints 80 degrees.
   b. Arches—The hand has two transverse arches (proximal through the carpus and distal through the MC heads) and five longitudinal arches (through each of the rays).
   c. Stability—MCP joint stability is provided by the volar plate and the collateral ligaments. **The collateral ligaments of the MCP joints are taut in flexion and lax in extension.** The PIP joints and DIP joints rely more on joint congruity. Also there is a large ligament/articular surface ratio in these joints.
   d. Other Concepts—The pulleys in the hand prevent bowstringing and decrease tendon excursion. Bowstringing increases the moment arm to the joint instant center. The sagittal bands allow extension at the MCP joint. With hyperextension at the MCP joint, the intrinsics must function for PIP joint extension because the extensor tendon is lax. Normal grasp for males is 50 kg and for females is 25 kg (only 4 kg is required for daily function). Normal pinch for males is 8 kg and for females is 4 kg (1 kg is needed for daily activities).

Table 1-67. RECOMMENDED POSITIONS OF FLEXION FOR ARTHRODESIS OF THE JOINTS OF THE HAND

JOINT	DEGREES OF FLEXION	OTHER FACTORS
MCP	20-30	
PIP	40-50	Less radial than ulnar
DIP	15-20	
Thumb CMC		MC in opposition
Thumb MCP	25	
Thumb IP	20	

   e. Kinetics—Joint loading with pinch is mostly in the MCP joint, but because the MCP joints have a larger surface area, the contact pressures (joint load/contact area) at the MCP joints are less. The DIP joints have the most contact pressures and subsequently develop the most degenerative change with time (Heberden's nodes). Grasping contact pressures are less but focus on the MCP joint; therefore patients with MCP joint arthritis frequently have had occupations that required grasping activities. Compressive loads at the thumb with pinching include 3 kg at the interphalangeal (IP) joint, 5 kg at the MCP joint, and 12 kg at the thumb CMC joint (an unstable joint), which frequently leads to its degeneration.
   f. Arthrodesis—Recommended positions of flexion for arthrodesis of joints in the hand are shown in Table 1-67.

Selected Bibliography

HISTOLOGY OF BONE

RECENT ARTICLES

Athanasou, N.A.: Cellular biology of bone-resorbing cells. J. Bone Joint Surg. [Am.] 78:1096–1112, 1996.

Brinker, M.R., Lippton, H.L., Cook, S.D., et al.: Pharmacological regulation of the circulation of bone. J. Bone Joint Surg. [Am.] 72:964–975, 1990.

Doherty, W.J., DeRome, M.E., McCarthy, E., et al.: The effect of glucocorticoids on osteoblast function. J. Bone Joint Surg. [Am.] 77:396, 1994.

Dunlap, J.N., Brinker, M.R., and Cook, S.D.: A new in vivo method for the direct measurement of nutrient artery blood flow. Orthopedics 20:613–619, 1997.

Eyre, D.R.: Biochemical markers of bone turnover. In Primer on the Metabolic Bone Diseases and Disorders of Mineral Metabolism, 3rd ed., pp. 114–118. Philadelphia, Lippincott-Raven, 1996.

Hosoda K., Kanzaki S., Eguchi H., et al.: Secretion of osteocalcin and its propeptide from human osteoblastic cells: Dissociation of the secretory patterns of osteocalcin and its propeptide. J. Bone Min. Res. 8:553–565, 1993.

Hupel, T.M., Aksenov, S.A., and Schemitsch, E.H.: Cortical bone blood flow in loose and tight fitting locked unreamed intramedullary nailing: A canine segmental tibia fracture model. J. Orth. Trauma 12:127–135, 1998.

Iannotti, J.P.: Growth plate physiology and pathology. Orthop. Clin. North Am. 21:1–17, 1990.

Iannotti, J.P., Brighton, C.P., Iannotti, V., et al.: Mechanism of action of parathyroid hormone-induced proteoglycan synthesis in the growth plate chondrocyte. J. Orthop. Res. 8:136–145, 1990.

Jiranek, W.A., Machado M., et al.: Production of cytokines around loosened cemented acetablular components: Analysis with immunohistochemical techniques and in situ hybridization. J. Bone Joint Surg. [Am.] 75:863-879, 1993.

Kaysinger, K.K., Nicholson, N.C., Ramp, W.K., et al.: Toxic effects of wound irrigation solutions on cultured tibiae and osteoblasts. J. Orthop. Trauma 9:303-311, 1995.

Majeska, R., Ryaby, J., and Einhorn, T.: Direct modulation of osteoblastic activity with estrogen. J. Bone Joint Surg. [Am.] 76:713, 1994.

Mundy, G.R., and Yoneda T.: Facilitation and suppression of bone metastasis. Clin. Orthop. 312:34-44, 1995.

Schemitsch, E.H., Kowalski, M.J., Swiontkowski, M.F., et al.: Comparison of the effect of reamed and unreamed locked intramedullary nailing on blood flow in the callus and strength of union following fracture of the sheep tibia. J. Orth. Res. 13:382-389, 1995.

Smith, S.R., Bronk, J.R., and Kelly, P.J.: Effect of fracture fixation on cortical bone blood flow. J. Orthop. Res. 8:471-478, 1990.

Stuecker, R., Brinker, M.R., Bennett, J.T., et al.: Blood flow to the immature hip-ultrasonic measurements in pigs. Acta Orthop. Scand. 68:25-33, 1997.

Yoo, J.U., and Johnstone, B.: The role of osteochondral progenitor cells in fracture repair. Clin. Orthop. 355:S73-S81, 1998.

CLASSIC ARTICLES

Ash P., Loutit J.F., and Townsend, K.M.S.: Osteoclasts derived from haematopoietic stem cells. Nature 283:669-670, 1980.

Azuma, H.: Intraosseous pressure as a measure of hemodynamic changes in bone marrow. Angiology 15:396-406, 1964.

Branemark, P.: Experimental investigation of microcirculation in bone marrow. Angiology 12:293-306, 1961.

Bright, R.W., Burstein, A.H., and Elmore, S.M.: Epiphyseal-plate cartilage: A biomechanical and histological analysis of failure modes. J. Bone Joint Surg. [Am.] 56:688-703, 1974.

Brighton, C.T.: Clinical problems in epiphyseal plate growth and development. In American Academy of Orthopaedic Surgeons Instructional Course Lectures, XXIII, pp. 105-122. St. Louis, C.V. Mosby, 1974.

Brighton, C.T.: Structure and function of the growth plate. Clin. Orthop. 136:22-32, 1978.

Brookes, M.: The blood supply of bone: An approach to bone biology. London, Butterworth and Company, 1971.

Buck B.E., Malinin, T.I., Brown, M.D.: Bone transplantation and human immunodeficiency virus: An estimate of risk of acquired immunodeficiency syndrome (AIDS). Clin. Orthop. 240:129-136, 1989.

Buckwalter, J.A.: Proteoglycan structure in calcifying cartilage. Clin. Orthop. 172:207-232, 1983.

Houghton, G.R., and Rooker, G.D.: The role of the periosteum in the growth of long bones: An experimental study in the rabbit. J. Bone Joint Surg. [Br.] 61:218-220, 1979.

McPherson, A., Scales, J.T., and Gordon, L.H.: A method of estimating qualitative changes of blood-flow in bone. J. Bone Joint Surg. [Br.] 43:791-799, 1961.

Ogden, J.A.: Injury to the growth mechanisms of the immature skeleton. Skel. Radiol. 6:237-253, 1981.

Ponseti, I.V., and McClintock, R.: Pathology of slipping of the upper femoral epiphysis. J. Bone Joint Surg. [Am.] 38:71-83, 1956.

Rhinelander, F.W.: Effects of medullary nailing on the normal blood supply of diaphyseal cortex. In American Academy of Orthopaedic Surgeons Instructional Course Lectures, XXII, pp. 161-187. St. Louis, C.V. Mosby, 1973.

Rhinelander, F.W.: Tibial blood supply in relation to fracture healing. Clin. Orthop. 105:34, 1974.

Rhinelander, F.W., Phillips, R.S., Steel, W.M., et al.: Microangiography in bone healing. II: Displaced closed fractures. J. Bone Joint Surg. [Am.] 50:643-662, 1968.

Salter, R.B., and Harris, W.R.: Injuries involving the epiphyseal plate. J. Bone Joint Surg. [Am.] 45:587-622, 1968.

Shim, S.S.: Physiology of blood circulation. J. Bone Joint Surg. [Am.] 50:812-824, 1968.

REVIEW ARTICLES

Buckwalter, J.A., Glimcher, M.J., Cooper, R.R., et al.: Bone biology—Part II: Formation, form, modeling, remodeling, and regulation of cell function. J. Bone Joint Surg. [Am.] 77:1276-1283, 1995.

Buckwalter, J.A., Glimcher, M.J., Cooper, R.R., et al.: Bone biology—Part I: Structure, blood supply, cells, matrix and mineralization. J. Bone Joint Surg. [Am.] 77:1256-1272, 1995.

Frymoyer, J.W., ed.: Bone metabolism and metabolic bone disease. Orthopaedic Knowledge Update 4: Home Study Syllabus, p. 77. Rosemont, IL, American Academy of Orthopaedic Surgeons, 1993.

BOOK CHAPTERS

Bostrum, M.P.G., Boskey, A., Kaufman, J.J., et al.: Form and function of bone. In Buckwalter, J.A., Einhorn, T.A., and Simon, S.R., eds.: Orthopaedic Basic Science: Biology and Biomechanics of the Musculoskeletal System, 2nd ed., pp. 319-370. Rosemont, IL, American Academy of Orthopaedic Surgeons, 2000.

Day, S.M., Ostrum, R.F., Chao, E.Y.S., et al.: Bone injury, regeneration, and repair. In Buckwalter, J.A., Einhorn, T.A., and Simon, S.R., eds.: Orthopaedic Basic Science: Biology and Biomechanics of the Musculoskeletal System, 2nd ed., pp. 371-400. Rosemont, IL, American Academy of Orthopaedic Surgeons, 2000.

Frassica, F.J., Gitelis, S., and Sim, F.H.: Metastatic bone disease: General principles, pathophyisology, evaluation, and biopsy. In American Academy of Orthopaedic Surgeons, Instructional Course Lectures, XLI, pp. 293-300. St. Louis, C.V. Mosby, 1992.

Guyton, A.C.: Local control of blood flow by tissues, and nervous and humoral regulation. In Guyton, A.C., ed.: Textbook of Medical Physiology, 7th ed., pp. 230-243. Philadelphia, W.B. Saunders, 1986.

Iannotti, J.P., Goldstein, S., Kuhn, J., et al.: The formation and growth of skeletal tissues. In Buckwalter, J.A., Einhorn, T.A., and Simon, S.R., eds.: Orthopaedic Basic Science: Biology and Biomechanics of the Musculoskeletal System, 2nd ed., pp. 77-110. Rosemont, IL, American Academy of Orthopaedic Surgeons, 2000.

Simon, M.A., and Springfield, D.S., eds.: Surgery for Bone and Soft Tissue Tumors. Philadelphia, Lippincott-Raven, 1998.

Vaananen, K.: Osteoclast function: Biology and mechanisms. In Bilezikian, J.P., Raisz, L.G., and Rodan, G.A., eds.: Principles of Bone Biology, pp. 103-113. San Diego, Academic Press, 1996.

BONE INJURY AND REPAIR

RECENT ARTICLES

Brinker, M.R., Cook, S.D., Dunlap, J.N., et al.: Early changes in nutrient artery blood flow following tibial nailing with and without reaming: A preliminary study. J. Orthop. Trauma 13(2):129-133, 1999.

Bostrom, M.P.G., Lane, J.M., Berberian, W.S., et al.: Immunolocalization and expression of bone morphogenetic proteins 2 and 4 in fracture healing. J. Orthop. Res. 13:357-367, 1995.

Cook, S.D., Salkeld, S.L., Brinker, M.R., et al.: Use of an osteoinductive biomaterial (rhOP-1) in healing large segmental bone defects. J. Orthop. Trauma 12:407-417, 1998.

Cook, S.D., Wolfe, M.W., and Salkeld, S.L.: Effect of recombinant human osteogenic protein-1 on healing of segmental defects in non-human primates. J. Bone Joint Surg. [Am.] 77:734, 1995.

Einhorn, T.A.: Enhancement of fracture-healing. J. Bone Joint Surg. [Am.] 77:940-956, 1995.

Heckman, J.D., Ryaby, J.P., McCabe, J., et al.: Acceleration of tibial fracture-healing by non-invasive, low-intensity pulsed ultrasound. J. Bone Joint Surg. [Am.] 76:26, 1994.

Hietaniemi, K., Paavolainen, P., and Penttinen, R.: Connective tissue parameters in experimental nonunion. J. Orthop. Trauma 10:114-118, 1996.

Holbein, O., Neidlinger-Wilke, C., Suger, G., et al.: Ilizarov callus distraction produces systemic bone cell mitogens. J. Orthop. Res. 13:629-638, 1995.

Horowitz, M.C., and Friedlaender, G.E.: Induction of specific T-cell responsiveness to allogeneic bone. J. Bone Joint Surg. [Am.] 73:1157-1168, 1991.

Iwasaki, M., Nakahara, H., and Nakata, K.: Regulation of proliferation and osteochondrogenic differentiation of periosteum-derived cells by transforming growth factor-β and basic fibroblast growth factor. J. Bone Joint Surg. [Am.] 77:543, 1995.

Jazrawi, L.M., Majeska, R.J., Klein, M.L., et al.: Bone and cartilage formation in an experimental model of distraction osteogenesis. J. Orthop. Trauma 12:111-116, 1998.

Kurdy, N.M.G., Bowles, S., Marsh, D.R., et al.: Serology of collagen types I and III in normal healing of tibial shaft fractures. J. Orthop. Trauma 12:122-126, 1998.

Murray, J.H., and Fitch, R.D.: Distraction histiogenesis: Principles and indications. J. Am. Acad. Orthop. Surg. 4:317-327, 1996.

Porter, S.E., and Hanley, E.N.: The musculoskeletal effects of smoking. J. Am. Acad. Orthop. Surg. 9:9-17, 2001.

CLASSIC ARTICLES

Friedlaender, G.E.: Bone grafts: The basic science rationale for clinical applications. J. Bone Joint Surg. [Am.] 69:786-790, 1987.

Lane, J.M., Suda, M., von der Mark, K., et al.: Immunofluorescent localization of structural collagen types in endochondral fracture repair. J. Orthop. Res. 4:318-329, 1986.

Mankin, H.J., Doppelt, S.H., and Tomford, W.W.: Clinical experience with allograft implantation: The first ten years. Clin. Orthop. 174:69-86, 1983.

Mirels, H.: Metastatic disease in long bones: A proposed scoring system for diagnosing impending pathologic fractures. Clin. Orthop. 249:256-264, 1989.

McKibbin, B.: The biology of fracture healing in long bones. J. Bone Joint Surg. [Br.] 60:150-162, 1978.

Rhinelander, F.W.: Tibial blood supply in relation to fracture healing. Clin. Orthop. 105:34-81, 1974.

Springfield, D.S.: Massive autogenous bone grafts. Orthop. Clin. North Am. 18:249-256, 1987.

Stevenson, S., Dannucci, G.A., Sharkey, N.A., et al.: The fate of articular cartilage after transplantation of fresh and cryopreserved tissue-antigen-matched and mismatched osteochondral allografts in dogs. J. Bone Joint Surg. [Am.] 71:1297-1307, 1989.

Stevenson, S., Quing, L.X., and Martin, B.: The fate of cancellous and cortical bone after transplantation of fresh and frozen tissue-antigen-matched and mismatched osteochondral allografts in dogs. J. Bone Joint Surg. [Am.] 73:1143, 1991.

Sumner, D.R., Turner, T.M., Purchio, A.F., et al.: Enhancement of bone ingrowth by transforming growth factor-β. J. Bone Joint Surg. [Am.] 77:1135, 1995.

REVIEW ARTICLES

Brighton, C.T.: Principles of fracture healing. Part I: The biology of fracture repair. In Murray, J.A., ed.: American Academy of Orthopaedic Surgeons Instructional Course Lectures XXXIII, pp. 60-87. St. Louis, C.V. Mosby, 1984.

Burchardt, H.: The biology of bone graft repair. Clin. Orthop. 174:28-42, 1983.

Einhorn, T.A.: Current concepts review enhancement of fracture-healing. J. Bone Joint Surg. [Am.] 77:940-952, 1995.

Friedlaender, G.E.: Immune responses to osteochondral allografts: Current knowledge and future directions. Clin. Orthop. 174:58, 1983.

O'Sullivan, M.E., Chao, E.Y.S., and Kelly, P.J.: The effects of fixation on fracture-healing. J. Bone Joint Surg. [Am.] 71:306, 1989.

BOOK CHAPTERS

Bolander, M.E.: Inducers of osteogenesis. In Friedlaender, G.E., and Goldberg, V.M., eds.: Bone and Cartilage Allografts, pp. 75-83. Park Ridge, IL, American Academy of Orthopaedic Surgeons, 1991.

Bone grafts. In Frymoyer, J.W., ed.: Orthopaedic Knowledge Update 4: Home Study Syllabus, pp. 233-243. Rosemont, IL, American Academy of Orthopaedic Surgeons, 1993.

Day, S.M., Ostrum, R.F., Chao, E.Y.S., et al.: Bone injury, regeneration, and repair. In Buckwalter, J.A., Einhorn, T.A., and Simon, S.R., eds.: Orthopaedic Basic Science: Biology and Biomechanics of the Musculoskeletal System, 2nd ed., pp. 371-400. Rosemont, IL, American Academy of Orthopaedic Surgeons, 2000.

Friedlaender, G.E., Mankin, H.J., and Sell, K.W., eds.: Osteochondral Allografts: Biology, Banking, and Clinical Applications. Boston, Little, Brown, 1983.

CONDITIONS OF BONE MINERALIZATION, BONE MINERAL DENSITY, AND BONE VIABILITY

RECENT ARTICLES

Brinker, M.R., Rosenberg, A.G., Kull, L., et al.: Primary total hip arthroplasty using noncemented porous-coated femoral components in patients with osteonecrosis of the femoral head. J. Arthroplasty 9:457-468, 1994.

Byers, P.H., Wallis, G.A., and Willing, M.C.: Osteogenesis imperfecta: Translation of mutation to phenotype. J. Med. Genet. 28:433-442, 1991.

Delmas, P.D., and Mennier, P.J.: The management of Paget's disease of bone. N. Engl. J. Med. 336:558-566, 1997.

Emery, S.E., Brazinski, M.S., Koka, E., et al.: The biological and biomechanical effects of irradiation on anterior spinal bone grafts in a canine model. J. Bone Joint Surg. [Am.] 76:540-548, 1994.

Garland, D.E., Stewart, C.A., Adkins, R.H., et al.: Osteoporosis after spinal cord injury. J. Orthop. Res. 10:419-423, 1981.

Guerra, J.J., and Steinberg, M.E.: Distinguishing transient osteoporosis from avascular necrosis of the hip. J. Bone Joint Surg. [Am.] 77:616-624, 1995.

Healey, J.H.: Corticosteroid osteoporosis. Current Opinion in Orthopaedics 8:1-7, 1997.

Heckman, J.D., and Sassard, R.: Musculoskeletal considerations in pregnancy. J. Bone Joint Surg. [Am.] 76:1720-1730, 1994.

Kaplan, F.S., and Singer, F.R.: Paget's disease of bone: Pathophysiology, diagnosis, and management. J. Am. Acad. Orthop. Surg. 3:336-344, 1995.

Lane J.M., and Nydick, M.: Osteoporosis: current modes of prevention and treatment. J. Am. Acad. Orthop. Surg. 7:19-31, 1999.

Mankin, H.J.: Rickets, osteomalacia, and renal osteodystrophy: An update. Orthop. Clin. North. Am. 21:81-96, 1990.

Melton, L.J.: Epidemiology of spinal osteoporosis. Spine 22:2S-11S, 1997.

Mont, M.A., and Hungerford, D.S.: Non-traumatic avascular necrosis of the femoral head. J. Bone Joint Surg. [Am.] 77:459-474, 1995.

Pellegrini, V.D., and Gregoritch, S.J.: Preoperative irradiation for prevention of heterotopic ossification following total hip arthroplasty. J. Bone Joint Surg. [Am.] 78:870-881, 1996.

Schipani, E., Kruse, K., and Juppner, H.: A constitutively active mutant PTH-PTHrP receptor in Jansen-type metaphyseal chondrodysplasia. Science 268:98-100, 1995.

World Health Organization: Assessment of fracture risk and its application to screening of postmenopausal osteoporosis: Report of a WHO study group. World Health Organ. Tech. Rep. Ser. 843:1-129, 1994.

CLASSIC ARTICLES

Evans, G.A., Arulanantham, K., and Gage, J.R.: Primary hypophosphatemic rickets: Effect of oral phosphate and vitamin D on growth and surgical treatment. J. Bone Joint Surg. [Am.] 62:1130-1138, 1980.

Glimcher, M.J., and Kenzora, J.E.: The biology of osteonecrosis of the human femoral head and its clinical implications. I: Tissue biology. II: The pathological changes in the femoral head as an organ and in the hip joint. III: Discussion of the etiology and genesis of the pathological sequelae: Comments on treatment. Clin. Orthop. 138:284-309; 139:283-312; 140:273-312, 1979.

Kanis, J.A.: Vitamin D metabolism and its clinical application. J. Bone Joint Surg. [Br.] 64:542-560, 1982.

Kiel, D.P., Felson, D.T., Anderson, J.J., et al.: Hip fracture and the use of estrogens in postmenopausal women: The Framingham study. New Engl. J. Med. 317:1169-1174, 1987.

Lane, J.M., and Vigorita, V.J.: Osteoporosis. J. Bone Joint Surg. [Am.] 65:274-278, 1983.

Mankin, H.J.: Rickets, osteomalacia, and renal osteodystrophy: Part II. J. Bone Joint Surg. [Am.] 56:352-386, 1974.

Nordin, B.E.C., Horsman, A., Marshall, D.H., et al.: Calcium requirement and calcium therapy. Clin. Orthop. 140:216-239, 1979.

Sillence, D.: Osteogenesis imperfecta: An expanding panorama of variants. Clin. Orthop. 159:11-25, 1981.

Wallach, S.: Hormonal factors in osteoporosis. Clin. Orthop. 144:284-292, 1979.

REVIEW ARTICLES

Barth, R.W., and Lane, J.M.: Osteoporosis. Orthop. Clin. North Am. 19:845-858, 1988.

Boden, S.D., and Kaplan, F.S.: Calcium homeostasis. Orthop. Clin. North Am. 21:31-42, 1990.

Bullough, P.G., Bansal, M., and DiCarlo, E.F.: The tissue diagnosis of metabolic bone disease: Role of histomorphometry. Orthop. Clin. North Am. 21:65-79, 1990.

Kleerekoper, M.B., Tolia, K., and Parfitt, A.M.: Nutritional endocrine, and demographic aspects of osteoporosis. Orthop. Clin. North Am. 12:547–558, 1981.

Lotke, P., and Ecker, M.: Current concepts review: Osteonecrosis of the knee. J. Bone Joint Surg. [Am.] 70:470–473, 1988.

Mankin, H.J.: Rickets, osteomalacia, and renal osteodystrophy: An update. Orthop. Clin. North Am. 21:81–96, 1990.

Mankin, H.J.: Metabolic bone disease. J. Bone Joint Surg. [Am.] 76:760–788, 1994.

Mont, M.A., and Hungerford, D.S.: Current concepts review non-traumatic avascular necrosis of the femoral head. J. Bone Joint Surg. [Am.] 77:459–469, 1995.

BOOK CHAPTERS

Aglietti, P., and Bullough, P.G.: Osteonecrosis. In Insall, J.N., ed.: Surgery of the Knee, pp. 527–549. New York, Churchill-Livingstone, 1984.

Bilezikian, J.P.: Primary hyperparathyroidism. In Primer on the Metabolic Bone Diseases and Disorders of Mineral Metabolism, 3rd ed., p. 181. Philadelphia, Lippincott-Raven, 1996.

Bostrum, M.P.G., Boskey, A., Kaufman, J.J., et al.: Form and function of bone. In Buckwalter, J.A., Einhorn, T.A., and Simon, S.R., eds.: Orthopaedic Basic Science: Biology and Biomechanics of the Musculoskeletal System, 2nd ed., pp. 319–370. Rosemont, IL, American Academy of Orthopaedic Surgeons, 2000.

Broadus, A.E.: Mineral balance and homeostasis. In Primer on the Metabolic Bone Diseases and Disorders of Mineral Metabolism, 3rd ed., p. 57. Philadelphia, Lippincott-Raven, 1996.

Buckwalter, J.A., and Cruess, R.L.: Healing of the musculoskeletal tissues. In Rockwood, C.A., Jr., and Green, D.P., eds.: Fractures in Adults, pp. 181–264. Philadelphia, J.B. Lippincott, 1991.

Canale, S.T., and King, R.E.: Part II: Fractures of the hip. In Rockwood, C.A., Jr., Wilkins, K.E., and King, R.E., eds.: Fractures in Children, vol. 3, pp. 1046–1120. Philadelphia, J.B. Lippincott, 1991.

Day, S.M., Ostrum, R.F., Chao, E.Y.S., et al.: Bone injury, regeneration, and repair. In Buckwalter, J.A., Einhorn, T.A., and Simon, S.R., eds.: Orthopaedic Basic Science: Biology and Biomechanics of the Musculoskeletal System, 2nd ed., pp. 371–400. Rosemont, IL, American Academy of Orthopaedic Surgeons, 2000.

Frymoyer, J.W., ed.: Bone metabolism and metabolic bone disease. In Orthopaedic Knowledge Update 4: Home Study Syllabus, p. 77. Rosemont, IL, American Academy of Orthopaedic Surgeons, 1993.

Glorieux, F.H.: Hypophosphatemic vitamin D-resistant rickets. In Primer on the Metabolic Bone Diseases and Disorders of Mineral Metabolism, 3rd ed., p. 316. Philadelphia, Lippincott-Raven, 1996.

Greech, P., Martin, T.J., Barrington, N.A., et al.: Diagnosis of Metabolic Bone Disease. Philadelphia, W.B. Saunders, 1985.

Klein, G.L.: Nutritional rickets and osteomalacia. In Primer on the Metabolic Bone Diseases and Disorders of Mineral Metabolism, 3rd ed., p. 301. Philadelphia, Lippincott-Raven, 1996.

Liberman, U.A. and Marx, S.J.: Vitamin D-dependent rickets. In Primer on the Metabolic Bone Diseases and Disorders of Mineral Metabolism, 3rd ed., p. 311. Philadelphia, Lippincott-Raven, 1996.

Mankin H.J.: Metabolic bone disease. In Jackson, D.W., ed.: Instructional Course Lectures, pp. 3–29. Rosemont, IL, American Academy of Orthopaedic Surgeons, 1995.

Shane, E.: Hypercalcemia: Pathogenesis, clinical manifestations, differential diagnosis, and management. In Primer on the Metabolic Bone Diseases and Disorders of Mineral Metabolism, 3rd ed., p. 177. Philadelphia, Lippincott-Raven, 1996.

Whyte, M.P.: Hypophosphatasia. In Primer on the Metabolic Bone Diseases and Disorders of Mineral Metabolism, 3rd ed., p. 326. Philadelphia, Lippincott-Raven, 1996.

ARTICULAR TISSUES

RECENT ARTICLES

Arnoczky, S.P., Warren, R.F., and McDevitt, C.A.: Meniscal replacement using a cryopreserved allograft: An experimental study in the dog. Clin. Orthop. 252:121–128, 1990.

Cannon, W.D., and Morgan, C.D.: Meniscal repair. Part II: Arthroscopic repair techniques. J. Bone Joint Surg. [Am.] 76:294–311, 1994.

Chen, F.S., Frenkel, S.R., and DiCesare, P.E.: Repair of articular cartilage defects: Part I. Basic science of cartilage healing. Am. J. Orthop. 28:31–33, 1999.

Chen, F.S., Frenkel, S.R., and DiCesare, P.E.: Repair of articular cartilage defects: Part II. Treatment options. Am. J. Orthop. 28:88–96, 1999.

DeHaven, K.E., and Arnoczky, S.P.: Meniscal repair. Part I: Basic science, indications for repair and open repair. J. Bone Joint Surg. [Am.] 76:140–152, 1995.

Hardingham, T.E., and Fosang, A.J.: Proteoglycans: Many forms and many functions. FASEB J. 6:861–870, 1992.

Mente, P.L., and Lewis, J.L.: Elastic modulus of calcified cartilage is an order of magnitude less than that of subchondral bone. J. Orthop. Res. 12:637–647, 1994.

Müller, F.J., Setton, L.A., Manicourt, D.H., et al.: Centrifugal and biochemical comparison of proteoglycan aggregates from articular cartilage in experimental joint disuse and joint instability. J. Orthop. Res. 12:498–508, 1994.

O'Driscoll, S.W., Recklies, A.D., and Poole, A.R.: Chondrogenesis in periosteal explants. J. Bone Joint Surg. [Am.] 76:1042–1051, 1994.

Shapiro, F.R., Koide, S., and Glimcher, M.J.: Cell origin and differentiation in the repair of full-thickness defects of articular cartilage. J. Bone Joint Surg. [Am.] 75:532–553, 1993.

Swoboda, B., Pullig, O., and Kirsch, T.: Increased content of type VI collagen epitopes in human osteoarthritic cartilage: Quantitation by inhibition ELISA. J. Orthop. Res. 16:96–99, 1998.

Wakitani, S., Goto, T., Pineda, S.J., et al.: Mesenchymal cell-based repair of large, full-thickness defects of articular cartilage. J. Bone Joint Surg. [Am.] 76:579, 1994.

Walker, G.D., Fischer, M., Gannon, J., et al.: Expression of type-X collagen in osteoarthritis. J. Orthop. Res. 13:4–12, 1995.

Warman, M.L., Abbott, M., Apte, S.S., et al.: A type X collagen mutation causes Schmid metaphyseal chondrodysplasia. Nature Genet. 5:79–82, 1993.

CLASSIC ARTICLES

Arnoczky, S.P., and Warren, R.F.: Microvasculature of the human meniscus. Am. J. Sports Med. 10:90–95, 1982.

Buckwalter, J.A., Kuettner, K.E., and Thonar, E.J.: Age-related changes in articular cartilage proteoglycans: Electron microscopic studies. J. Orthop. Res. 3:251–257, 1985.

Fairbank, T.J.: Knee joint changes after meniscectomy. J. Bone Joint Surg. [Br.] 30:664–670, 1948.

Gannon, J.M., Walker, G., Fischer, M., et al.: Localization of type X collagen in canine growth plate and adult canine articular cartilage. J. Orthop. Res. 9:485–494, 1991.

Hardingham, T.E.: The role of link-protein in the structure of cartilage proteoglycan aggregates. Biochem. J. 177:237–247, 1979.

Heinegard, D., and Oldberg, A.: Structure and biology of cartilage and bone matrix noncollagenous macromolecules. FASEB J. 3:2042–2051, 1989.

Mankin, H.J., and Thrasher, A.Z.: Water content and binding in normal and osteoarthritic human cartilage. J. Bone Joint Surg. [Am.] 57:76–80, 1975.

Salter, R.B., Simmonds, D.F., Malcolm, B.W., et al.: The biological effect of continuous passive motion on the healing of full-thickness defects in articular cartilage: An experimental investigation in the rabbit. J. Bone Joint Surg. [Am.] 62:1232–1251, 1980.

Weiss, C., Rosenberg, L., and Helfet, A.J.: An ultrastructural study of normal young adult human articular cartilage. J. Bone Joint Surg. [Am.] 50:663–674, 1968.

REVIEW ARTICLES

Dehaven, K.E., and Arnoczky, S.P.: Meniscal repair. J. Bone Joint Surg. [Am.] 76:140–152, 1994.

Mankin, H.J.: Current concepts review: The response of articular cartilage to mechanical injury. J. Bone Joint Surg. [Am.] 64:460–466, 1982.

BOOK CHAPTERS

Arnoczky, S., Adams, M., DeHaven, K., et al.: Meniscus. In Woo, S.L.-Y., and Buckwalter, J.A., eds.: Repair of the Musculoskeletal Soft Tissues, pp. 487–537. Park Ridge, IL, American Academy of Orthopaedic Surgeons, 1988.

Arnoczky, S.P., and McDevitt, C.A.: The meniscus: Structure, function, repair, and replacement. In Buckwalter, J.A., Einhorn, T.A., and Simon, S.R., eds.: Orthopaedic Basic Science: Biology and Biomechanics of the Musculoskeletal System, 2nd ed., pp. 531-546. Rosemont, IL, American Academy of Orthopaedic Surgeons, 2000.

Buckwalter, J.A., and Hunziker, E.B.: Articular cartilage biology and morphology. In Mow, V.C., and Ratcliffe, A., eds.: Structure and Function of Articular Cartilage. Boca Raton, FL, CRC Press, 1993.

Buckwalter, J., Rosenberg, L. Coutts, R., et al.: Articular cartilage: Injury and repair. In Woo, S.L.-Y., and Buckwalter, J.A., eds.: Injury and Repair of the Musculoskeletal Soft Tissues, pp. 465-481. Park Ridge, IL, American Academy of Orthopaedic Surgeons, 1988.

Frymoyer, J.W., ed.: Arthritis. In Orthopaedic Knowledge Update 4: Home Study Syllabus, pp. 89-106. Park Ridge, IL, American Academy of Orthopaedic Surgeons, 1993.

Iannotti, J.P., Goldstein, S., Kuhn, J.L., et al.: The formation and growth of skeletal tissues. In Buckwalter, J.A., Einhorn, T.A., and Simon, S.R., eds.: Orthopaedic Basic Science: Biology and Biomechanics of the Musculoskeletal System, 2nd ed., pp. 77-110. Rosemont, IL, American Academy of Orthopaedic Surgeons, 2000.

Kasser, J.R., ed.: In Orthopaedic Knowledge Update 5, pp. 163-175. Rosemont, IL, American Academy of Orthopaedic Surgeons, 1996.

Mankin, H.J., and Brandt, K.D.: Biochemistry and metabolism of articular cartilage in osteoarthritis. In Moskowitz, R.W., Howell, D.S., Goldberg, V.M., et al., eds.: Osteoarthritis: Diagnosis and Medical/Surgical Management, 2nd ed., pp. 109-154. Philadelphia, W.B. Saunders, 1992.

Mankin, H.J., Mow, V.C., Buckwalter, J.A., et al.: Articular cartilage structure, composition, and function. In Buckwalter, J.A., Einhorn, T.A., and Simon, S.R., eds.: Orthopaedic Basic Science: Biology and Biomechanics of the Musculoskeletal System, 2nd ed., pp. 443-470. Rosemont, IL, American Academy of Orthopaedic Surgeons, 2000.

Mayne, R., and Irwin, M.H.: Collagen types in cartilage. In Kuettner, K.E., Schleyerbach, R., and Hascall, V.C., eds.: Articular Cartilage Biochemistry, pp. 23-38. New York, Raven Press, 1986.

Mow, V., and Rosenwasser, M.: Articular cartilage biomechanics. In Woo, S.L.-Y., and Buckwalter, J.A., eds.: Injury and Repair of the Musculoskeletal Soft Tissues, pp. 445-451. Park Ridge, IL, American Academy of Orthopaedic Surgeons, 1988.

Mow, V.C., and Soslowsky, L.J.: Friction, lubrication, and wear of diarthrodial joints. In Mow, V.C., and Hayes, W.C., eds.: Basic Orthopaedic Biomechanics, p. 263. New York, Churchill-Livingstone, 1988.

Mow, V.C., Zhu, W., and Ratcliffe, A.: Structure and function of articular cartilage and meniscus. In Mow, V.C., and Hayes, W.C., eds.: Basic Orthopaedic Biomechanics, pp. 143-198. New York, Raven Press, 1991.

Rosenberg, L.C., and Buckwalter, J.A.: Cartilage proteoglycans. In Kuettner, K.E., Schleyerbach, R., and Hascall, V.C., eds.: Articular Cartilage Biochemistry, pp. 39-58. New York, Raven Press, 1986.

Schenk, R.K., Eggli, P.S., and Hunziker, E.B.: Articular cartilage morphology. In Kuettner, K.E., Schleyerbach, R., and Hascall, V.C., eds.: Articular Cartilage Biochemistry, pp. 3-22. New York, Raven Press, 1986.

Woo, S.L., An, K., Frank, C.B., et al.: Anatomy, biology, and biomechanics of tendon and ligament. In Buckwalter, J.A., Einhorn, T.A., and Simon, S.R., eds.: Orthopaedic Basic Science: Biology and Biomechanics of the Musculoskeletal System, 2nd ed., pp. 581-616. Rosemont, IL, American Academy of Orthopaedic Surgeons, 2000.

Woo, S.L.-Y., and Buckwalter, J.A., eds.: Injury and Repair of the Musculoskeletal Soft Tissues. Park Ridge, IL, American Academy of Orthopaedic Surgeons, 1988.

ARTHROSES

RECENT ARTICLES

Brinker, M.R., Rosenberg, A.G., Kull, L., et al.: Primary noncemented total hip arthroplasty in patients with ankylosing spondylitis: Clinical and radiographic results at an average follow-up period of 6 years. J. Arthroplasty 11:808-812, 1996.

Rivard, G.E., Girard, M., Belanger, R., et al.: Synoviorthesis with colloidal 32P chromic phosphate for the treatment of hemophilic arthropathy. J. Bone Joint Surg. [Am.] 76:482, 1994.

Schaller, J.G.: Juvenile rheumatoid arthritis. Pediatr. Rev. 18:337-349, 1997.

CLASSIC ARTICLES

Ahlberg, A.K.M.: On the natural history of hemophilic pseudotumor. J. Bone Joint Surg. [Am.] 57:1133-1136, 1975.

Ansell, B.M., and Swann, M.: The management of chronic arthritis of children. J. Bone Joint Surg. [Br.] 65:536-543, 1983.

Byers, P.D., Cotton, R.E., Decon, O.W., et al.: The diagnosis and treatment of pigmented villonodular synovitis. J. Bone Joint Surg. [Br.] 50:290-305, 1968.

Chylack, L.T., Jr.: The ocular manifestations of juvenile rheumatoid arthritis. Arthritis Rheum. 20:217-223, 1977.

Cofield, R.H., Morrison, M.J., and Beabout, J.W.: Diabetic neuroarthropathy in the foot: Patient characteristics and patterns of radiographic change. Foot Ankle 4:15-22, 1983.

Culp, R.W., Eichenfield, A.H., Davidson, R.S., et al.: Lyme arthritis in children: An orthopaedic perspective. J. Bone Joint Surg. [Am.] 69:96-99, 1987.

Firooznia, H., Seliger, G., Genieser, N.B., et al.: Hypertrophic pulmonary osteoarthropathy in pulmonary metastases. Radiology 115:269-274, 1975.

Ishikawa, K., Masuda, I., Ohira, T., et al.: A histological study of calcium pyrophosphate dihydrate crystal-deposition disease. J. Bone Joint Surg. [Am.] 71:875-886, 1989.

Mankin, H.J., Dorfman, H., Lippiello, L., et al.: Biochemical and metabolic abnormalities in articular cartilage from osteo-arthritic human hips: II. Correlation of morphology with biochemical and metabolic data. J. Bone Joint Surg. [Am.] 53:523-537, 1971.

Mankin, H.J., Johnson, M.E., and Lippiello, L.: Biochemical and metabolic abnormalities in articular cartilage from osteoarthritic human hips: III. Distribution and metabolism of amino sugar-containing macromolecules. J. Bone Joint Surg. [Am.] 63:131-139, 1981.

Mankin, H.J., and Thrasher, A.Z.: Water content and binding in normal and osteoarthritic human cartilage. J. Bone Joint Surg. [Am.] 57:76-80, 1975.

McCarty, D.J., Halverson, P.B., Carrera, G.R., et al.: Milwaukee shoulder: Association of microspheroids containing hydroxyapatite, active collagenase and neutral protease with rotator cuff defects: I. Clinical aspects. 24:464-473, 1981.

Neer, C.S., Craig, E.V., and Fukuda, H.: Cuff-tear arthropathy. J. Bone Joint Surg. [Am.] 65:1232-1244, 1983.

Resnick, D.: Radiology of seronegative spondyloarthropathies. Clin. Orthop. 143:38-45, 1979.

Simmon, E.H.: The surgical correction of flexion deformity of the cervical spine in ankylosing spondylitis. Clin. Orthop. 86:132-143, 1972.

Williams, B.: Orthopaedic features in the presentation of syringomyelia. J. Bone Joint Surg. [Br.] 61:314-323, 1979.

REVIEW ARTICLES

Alpert, S.W., Koval, K.J., and Zuckerman, J.D.: Neuropathic arthropathy: Review of current knowledge. J. Am. Acad. Orthop. Surg. 4(2):100-108, 1996.

Barry, P.E., and Stillman, J.S.: Characteristics of juvenile rheumatoid arthritis: Its medical and orthopaedic management. Orthop. Clin. North Am. 6:641-651, 1975.

Ford, D.: The clinical spectrum of Reiter's syndrome and similar postenteric arthropathies. Clin. Orthop. 143:59-65, 1979.

BOOK CHAPTERS

Buchanan, W.W.: Clinical features of rheumatoid arthritis. In Scott, J.T., ed.: Copeman's Textbook of the Rheumatoid Diseases, 5th ed., pp. 318-364. Edinburgh, Churchill-Livingstone, 1978.

Calin, A.: Ankylosing spondylitis. In Kelley, W.N., Harris, E.D., Ruddy, S., et al., eds.: Textbook of Rheumatology, pp. 1021-1037. Philadelphia, W.B. Saunders, 1989.

Currey, H.L.F.: Aetiology and pathogenesis of rheumatoid arthritis. In Scott, J.T., ed.: Copeman's Textbook of the Rheumatoid Diseases, 5th ed., pp. 261-272. Edinburgh, Churchill-Livingstone, 1978.

Frymoyer, J.W., ed.: Arthritis. In Orthopaedic Knowledge Update 4: Home Study Syllabus, pp. 89-106. Rosemont, IL, American Academy of Orthopaedic Surgeons, 1993.

Gardner, D.L.: Pathology of rheumatoid arthritis. In Scott, J.T., ed.: Copeman's Textbook of the Rheumatoid Diseases, 5th ed., pp. 273-317. Edinburgh, Churchill-Livingstone, 1978.

Greene, W.B., and McMillan, C.W.: Nonsurgical management of hemophilic arthropathy. In Barr, J.S., ed.: Instructional Course Lectures XXXVIII, pp. 367-381. St. Louis, C.V. Mosby, 1989.

Guerra, J., Resnick, D.: Radiographic and scintigraphic abnormalities in seronegative spondylarthropathies and juvenile chronic arthritis. In Calin, A., ed.: Spondylarthropathies, pp. 339-382. Grune & Stratton, 1984.

Hockberg, M.C.: Epidemiology of rheumatoid disease. In Schumacher, H.R., Jr., ed.: Primer on the Rheumatic Diseases, 9th ed., pp. 48–51. Atlanta, Arthritis Foundation, 1988.

Jacobs, R.L.: Charcot foot. In Jahss, M.H., ed.: Disorders of the Foot and Ankle, 2nd ed., vol. 3, p. 2164. Philadelphia, W.B. Saunders, 1991.

Kasser J.R., ed.: Orthopaedic Knowledge Update 5, pp. 481–502. Rosemont, IL, American Academy of Orthopaedic Surgeons, 1996.

Kelley, W.N., and Fox, I.H.: Gout and related disorders of purine metabolism. In Kelley, W.N., Harris, E.D., Jr., Ruddy, S., et al., eds.: Textbook of Rheumatology, 2nd ed., p. 1382. Philadelphia, W.B. Saunders, 1985.

Mankin, H.J., and Brandt, K.D.: Biochemistry and metabolism of articular cartilage in osteoarthritis. In Moskowitz, R.W., Howell, V.C., Goldberg, V.M., et al., eds.: Osteoarthritis: Diagnosis and Medical/Surgical Management, 2nd ed., pp. 109–154. Philadelphia, W.B. Saunders, 1992.

Mankin, H.J., Mow, V.C., Buckwalter, J.A.: Articular cartilage repair and osteoarthritis. In Buckwalter, J.A., Einhorn, T.A., and Simon, S.R., eds.: Orthopaedic Basic Science: Biology and Biomechanics of the Musculoskeletal System, 2nd ed., pp. 471–488. Rosemont, IL, American Academy of Orthopaedic Surgeons, 2000.

Poss, R., ed.: Arthritis. In Orthopaedic Knowledge Update 3: Home Study Syllabus, p. 63. Park Ridge, IL, American Academy of Orthopaedic Surgeons, 1990.

Rana, N.: Rheumatoid arthritis, other collagen diseases, and psoriasis of the foot. In Jahss, M.H., ed.: Disorders of the Foot, pp. 1057–1058. Philadelphia, W.B. Saunders, 1982.

Rana, N.A.: Rheumatoid arthritis, other collagen diseases, and psoriasis of the foot. In Jahss, M.H., ed.: Disorders of the Foot and Ankle, 2nd ed., p. 1745. Philadelphia, W.B. Saunders, 1991.

Rodnan, G.P., and Schumacher, H.R., eds.: Primer on the Rheumatic Diseases, 8th ed., pp. 128–131. Atlanta, Arthritis Foundation, 1983.

Rogers, L.F.: Diseases of the Joints, 6th ed., pp. 125–127. Philadelphia, J.B. Lippincott, 1993.

Ryan, L.M., and McCarty, D.J.: Calcium pyrophosphate crystal deposition disease; pseudogout; articular chondrocalcinosis. In McCarty, D.J., and Koopmen, W.J., eds.: Arthritis and Allied Conditions, 12th ed., vol. 2, pp. 1835–1855. Philadelphia, Lea & Febiger, 1993.

Sammarco, G.J.: Diabetic arthropathy. In Sammarco, G.J., ed.: The Foot in Diabetes, pp. 153–172. Philadelphia, Lea & Febiger, 1991.

Schumacher, R.H., ed.: Primer of Rheumatic Disease, 9th ed., p. 149. Atlanta, Arthritis Foundation, 1988.

Smukler, N.: Arthritic disorders of the spine. In Rothman, R.H., and Simeone, F.A., eds.: The Spine, 2nd ed., pp. 906–941. Philadelphia, W.B. Saunders, 1982.

Recklies, A.D., Poole, A.R., Banerjee, S., et al.: Pathophysiologic aspects of inflammation in diarthrodial joints. In Buckwalter, J.A., Einhorn, T.A., and Simon, S.R., eds.: Orthopaedic Basic Science: Biology and Biomechanics of the Musculoskeletal System, 2nd ed., pp. 489–530. Rosemont, IL, American Academy of Orthopaedic Surgeons, 2000.

Rosier, R.N., Reynolds, P.R., and O'Keefe, R.J.: Molecular and cellular biology in orthopaedics. In Buckwalter, J.A., Einhorn, T.A., and Simon, S.R., eds.: Orthopaedic Basic Science: Biology and Biomechanics of the Musculoskeletal System, 2nd ed., pp. 19–76. Rosemont, IL, American Academy of Orthopaedic Surgeons, 2000.

Westring, D., Ries, M., and Dee, R.: Hematologic disorders. In Dee, R., Mango, E., and Hurst, L.C., eds.: Principles of Orthopaedic Practice, pp. 290–294. New York, McGraw-Hill, 1998.

SKELETAL MUSCLE AND ATHLETICS

RECENT ARTICLES

American Academy of Orthopaedic Surgeons Position Statement: Anabolic Steroids to Enhance Athletic Performance. Park Ridge, IL, American Academy of Orthopaedic Surgeons, 1991.

Beiner, J.M., Jokl, P., Cholewicki, J., Panjabi, M.M.: The effect of anabolic steroids and corticosteroids on healing of muscle contusion injury. Am. J. Sports Med. 27:2–9, 1999.

Hultman, E., Soderlund, K., Timmons, J.A., et al.: Muscle creatine loading in men. J. Appl. Physiol. 81:232–237, 1996.

Lutz, G.E., Palmitier, R.A., An, K.N., et al.: Comparison of tibiofemoral joint forces during open-kinetic-chain and closed-kinetic-chain exercises. J. Bone Joint Surg. [Am.] 75:732–739, 1993.

Nattiv, A., and Lynch, L.: Female athlete triad. Phys. Sports Med. 22:60–68, 1994.

Sapega, A.A.: Muscle performance evaluation in orthopaedic practice. J. Bone Joint Surg. [Am.] 72:1562–1574, 1990.

Sturmi, J.E., Diorio, D.J.: Anabolic agents. Clin. Sports Med. 17:261–282, 1998.

Voss, L.A., Fadale, P.D., and Hulstyn, M.J.: Exercise-induced loss of bone density in athletes. J. Am. Acad. Orthop. Surg. 6:349–357, 1998.

CLASSIC ARTICLES

Baldwin, K.M., Winder, W.W., and Holloszy, J.O.: Adaptation of actomyosin ATPase in different types of muscle to endurance exercise. Am. J. Physiol. 229:422–426, 1975.

Booth, F.W.: Physiologic and biochemical effects of immobilization on muscle. Clin. Orthop. 219:15–20, 1987.

Booth, F.W.: Physiologic and biochemical effects in immobilization of muscle. Clin. Orthop. 219:25–27, 1987.

Faulkner, J.A.: New perspectives in training for maximum performance. J.A.M.A. 205:741–746, 1968.

Gollnick, P.D., Armstrong, R.B., Saltin, B., et al.: Effect of training on enzyme activity and fiber composition of human skeletal muscle. J. Appl. Physiol. 34:107–111, 1973.

Holloszy, J.O.: Biochemical adaptations in muscle: Effects of exercise on mitochondrial oxygen uptake and respiratory enzyme activity in skeletal muscle. J. Biol. Chem. 242:2278–2282, 1967.

Huxley, H.E.: Electron microscope studies on the structure of natural and synthetic protein filaments from striated muscle. J. Mol. Biol. 7:281–308, 1963.

Huxley, H.E.: The mechanism of muscular contraction. Science 164:1356–1365, 1969.

Lowey, S., and Risby, D.: Light chains from fast and slow muscle myosins. Nature 234:81–85, 1971.

MacDougall, J.D., Elder, C.G., Sale, D.G., et al.: Effects of strength training and immobilization on human muscle fibres. Eur. J. Appl. Physiol. 43:25–34, 1980.

REVIEW ARTICLES

AMA Council on Scientific Affairs: Drug abuse in athletes: Anabolic steroids and human growth hormone. J.A.M.A. 259:1703–1705, 1988.

Haupt, H.A.: Current concepts: Anabolic steroids and growth hormone. Am. J. Sports Med. 21:468–474, 1993.

Kibler, W.B.: Physiology of exercising muscle. AAOS Instr. Course Lect. 43:3–4, 1994.

BOOK CHAPTERS

Asher, M.A., ed.: Health maintenance of the musculoskeletal system. In Orthopaedic Knowledge Update I: Home Study Syllabus, pp. 1–8. Park Ridge, IL, American Academy of Orthopaedic Surgeons, 1984.

Best, T.M., and Garret, W.E.: Basic science of soft tissue: Muscle and tendon. In DeLee, J., and Drez, D., eds.: Orthopaedic Sports Medicine: Principles and Practice, vol. 1, p. 17. Philadelphia, W.B. Saunders, 1994.

Bodine, S.C., and Lieber, R.L.: Peripheral nerve physiology, anatomy, and pathology. In Buckwalter, J.A., Einhorn, T.A., and Simon, S.R., eds.: Orthopaedic Basic Science: Biology and Biomechanics of the Musculoskeletal System, 2nd ed., pp. 617–682. Rosemont, IL, American Academy of Orthopaedic Surgeons, 2000.

Frymoyer, J.W., ed.: Bone metabolism and bone metabolic disease. In Orthopaedic Knowledge Update 4, p. 82. Rosemont, IL, American Academy of Orthopaedic Surgeons, 1993.

Garrett, W.E., and Best, T.M.: Anatomy, physiology, and mechanics of skeletal muscle. In Buckwalter, J.A., Einhorn, T.A., and Simon, S.R., eds.: Orthopaedic Basic Science: Biology and Biomechanics of the Musculoskeletal System, 2nd ed., pp. 683–716. Rosemont, IL, American Academy of Orthopaedic Surgeons, 2000.

Kibler, W.B., Chandler, T.J., and Reuter, B.H.: Advances in conditioning. In Griffin, L.Y., ed.: Orthopaedic Knowledge Update: Sports Medicine, pp. 65–73. Rosemont, IL, American Academy of Orthopaedic Surgeons, 1994.

Poss, R., ed.: Exercise and athletic conditioning. In Orthopaedic Knowledge Update 3: Home Study Syllabus, pp. 50–51. Park Ridge, IL, American Academy of Orthopaedic Surgeons, 1990.

Poss, R., ed.: Exercise and athletic conditioning: Drug use. In Orthopaedic Knowledge Update 3: Home Study Syllabus, p. 50. Park Ridge, IL, American Academy of Orthopaedic Surgeons, 1990.

Poss, R., ed.: General knowledge: Exercise and athletic conditioning; effect of warmup activities. In Orthopaedic Knowledge Update 3: Home Study Syllabus, p. 47. Park Ridge, IL, American Academy of Orthopaedic Surgeons, 1990.

Simon, S.R., ed.: Anatomy: Muscle. In Orthopaedic Science: A Resource and Self-Study Guide for the Practitioner, p. 28. Park Ridge, IL, American Academy of Orthopaedic Surgeons, 1986.

Simon, R.A., ed.: Biomechanics: Biomechanics of materials: musculoskeletal tissues. In Orthopaedic Science: A Resource and Self-Study Guide for the Practitioner, p. 163. Park Ridge, IL, American Academy of Orthopaedic Surgeons, 1986.

Waddler, G.I., and Hainline, B.: Drugs in the Athlete, p. 65. Philadelphia, F.A. Davis, 1989.

NERVOUS SYSTEM

RECENT ARTICLES

Bracken, M.B., Shepard, M.J., Holford, T.R., et al.: Administration of methylprednisolone for 24 or 48 hours or tirilazid mesylate for 48 hours in the treatment of acute spinal cord injury: Results of the Third National Acute Spinal Cord Injury Randomized Controlled Trial. National Acute Spinal Cord Injury Study. J.A.M.A. 277:1597-1604, 1997.

Bracken, M.B., Shepard, M.J., Collins, W.F., et al.: A randomized controlled trial of methylprednisolone or naloxone in the treatment of spinal cord injury: Results of the Second National Acute Spinal Cord Injury Study. N. Engl. J. Med. 322:1405-1411, 1990.

Koman, L.A., Mooney, J.F., Smith, B., et al.: Management of cerebral palsy with botulinum-A toxin: preliminary investigation. J. Pediatr. Orthop. 13:489-495, 1993.

Olmarker, K., and Rydevik, B.: Single versus double-level nerve root compression. Clin. Orthop. 279:35-39, 1992.

CLASSIC ARTICLE

Seddon, H.J.: Three types of nerve injuries. Brain 66:238-283, 1943.

REVIEW ARTICLES

Battista, A., and Lusskin, R.: The anatomy and physiology of the peripheral nerve. Foot Ankle 7:69, 1986.

Bracken, M.B.: Pharmacological treatment of acute spinal cord injury: Current status and future projects. J. Emerg. Med. 11:43-48, 1993.

Bruno, L.A., Gennarelli, T.A., and Torg., J.S.: Management guidelines for head injuries in athletics. Clin. Sports Med. 6:17-29, 1987.

BOOK CHAPTERS

Bodine, S.C., and Lieber, R.L.: Peripheral nerve physiology, anatomy, and pathology. In Buckwalter, J.A., Einhorn, T.A., and Simon, S.R., eds.: Orthopaedic Basic Science: Biology and Biomechanics of the Musculoskeletal System, 2nd ed., pp. 617-682. Rosemont, IL, American Academy of Orthopaedic Surgeons, 2000.

Brown, A.G., ed.: Organization in the Spinal Cord: The Anatomy and Physiology of Identified Neurones. Berlin, Springer-Verlag, 1981.

Lundborg, G., ed.: Nerve Injury and Repair, pp. 149-195. New York, Churchill-Livingstone, 1988.

Gelberman, R.H., Eaton R.G., and Urbaniak, J.R.: Peripheral nerve compression. In Schafer, M., ed.: Instructional Course Lectures, XXXIII, pp. 31-53. Rosemont, IL, American Academy of Orthopaedic Surgeons, 1994.

Gelberman, R.H., ed.: Operative Nerve Repair and Reconstruction. Philadelphia, J.B. Lippincott, 1991.

Guyton, A.C.: Basic Neuroscience: Anatomy and Physiology, 2nd ed. Philadelphia, W.B. Saunders, 1992.

McAfee, P.C.: Cervical spine trauma. In Frymoyer, J.W., ed.: The Adult Spine: Principles and Practice, vol. 2, p. 1079. New York, Raven Press, 1991.

Rall, W.: Core conductor theory and cable properties of neurons. In Kandel, E.R., ed.: Handbook of Physiology, Section 1: The Nervous System, pp. 39-97. Bethesda, MD, American Physiological Society, 1977.

CONNECTIVE TISSUES

RECENT ARTICLES

Terek, R.M., Jirnaek, W.A., Goldberg, M.J., et al.: The expression of platelet-derived growth factor gene in Dupuytren's contracture. J. Bone Joint Surg. [Am.] 77:1-9, 1995.

Wiggins, M.E., Fadale, P.D., Ehrlich, M.G., et al.: Effects of local injection of corticosteroids on the healing of ligaments. J. Bone Joint Surg. [Am.] 77:1682, 1995.

CLASSIC ARTICLES

Arnoczky, S.P.: Anatomy of the anterior cruciate ligament. Clin. Orthop. 172:19-25, 1983.

Butler, D.L., Grood, E.S., Noyes, F.R., et al.: Biomechanics of ligaments and tendons. Exerc. Sports Sci. Rev. 6:125-181, 1976.

Kurosaka, M., Yoshiya, S., and Andrish, J.T.: A biomechanical comparison of different surgical techniques of graft fixation in anterior cruciate ligament reconstruction. Am. J. Sports Med. 15:225-229, 1987.

Noyes, F.R., Butler, D.L., Grood, E.S., et al.: Biomechanical analysis of human ligament grafts used in knee ligament repairs and reconstructions. J. Bone Joint Surg. [Am.] 66:344-352, 1984.

Noyes, F.R., DeLucas, J.L., and Torvik, P.J.: Biomechanics of anterior cruciate ligament failure: An analysis of strain-rate sensitivity and mechanisms of failure in primates. J. Bone Joint Surg. [Am.] 56:236-253, 1974.

BOOK CHAPTERS

Frymoyer, J.W., ed.: Knee and leg: Soft-tissue trauma. In Orthopaedic Knowledge Update 4: Home Study Syllabus, pp. 593-602. Rosemont, IL, American Academy of Orthopaedic Surgeons, 1993.

Poss, R., ed.: Soft tissue implants. In Orthopaedic Knowledge Update 3: Home Study Syllabus, pp. 178-179. Park Ridge, IL, American Academy of Orthopaedic Surgeons, 1990.

Wood, S.L.: Ligament, tendon, and joint capsule insertions to bone. In Woo, S.L.-Y., and Buckwalter, J.A., eds.: Injury and Repair of the Musculoskeletal Soft Tissues. Park Ridge, IL, American Academy of Orthopaedic Surgeons, 1988.

Woo, S.L., An, K., Frank, C.B., et al.: Anatomy, biology, and biomechanics of tendon and ligament. In Buckwalter, J.A., Einhorn, T.A., and Simon, S.R., eds.: Orthopaedic Basic Science: Biology and Biomechanics of the Musculoskeletal System, 2nd ed., pp. 581-616. Rosemont, IL, American Academy of Orthopaedic Surgeons, 2000.

Woo, S.L.-Y., and Buckwalter, J.A., eds.: Injury and Repair of the Musculoskeletal Soft Tissues. Park Ridge, IL, American Academy of Orthopaedic Surgeons, 1988.

CELLULAR AND MOLECULAR BIOLOGY, IMMUNOLOGY AND GENETICS OF ORTHOPAEDICS

RECENT ARTICLES

D'Astous, J., Drouin, M.A., and Rhine, E.: Intraoperative anaphylaxis secondary to allergy to latex in children who have spina bifida: Report of two cases. J. Bone Joint Surg. [Am.] 74:1084-1086, 1992.

Jiranek, W., Jasty, M., and Wang, J.T.: Tissue response to particulate polymethylmethacrylate in mice with various immune deficiencies. J. Bone Joint Surg. [Am.] 77:1650, 1995.

Giunta, C., Superti-Furga, A., Spranger, S., et al.: Ehlers-Danlos syndrome type VII: Clinical features and molecular defects. J. Bone Joint Surg [Am.] 81:225, 1999.

Meehan, P.L., Galina, M.P., and Daftari, T.: Intraoperative anaphylaxis due to allergy to latex: Report of two cases. J. Bone Joint Surg. [Am.] 74:1087-1089, 1992.

Miyasaka, M.: Cancer metastasis and adhesion molecules. Clin. Orthop. 312:10-18, 1995.

Rousseau, F., Bonaventure, J., Legeai-Mallet, L., et al.: Mutations in the gene encoding fibroblast growth factor receptor-3 in achondroplasia. Nature 371:252-254, 1994.

Shiang, R., Thompson, L.M., Zhu, Y.Z, et al.: Mutations in the transmembrane domain of FGFR3 cause the most common genetic form of dwarfism, achondroplasia. Cell 78:335-342, 1994.

Tsipouras, P., Del Mastro, R., Sarfarazi, M., et al.: Genetic linkage of the Marfan syndrome, ectopia lentis, and congenital contractural arachnodactyly to the fibrillin genes on chromosomes 15 and 5:The International Marfan Syndrome Collaborative Study. N. Engl. J. Med. 326:905-909, 1992.

CLASSIC ARTICLES

Antonarakis, S.E.: Diagnosis of genetic disorders at the DNA level. N. Engl. J. Med. 320:151-163, 1989.

Harrod, M.J., Friedman, J.M., Currarino, G., et al.: Genetic heterogeneity in spondyloepiphyseal dysplasia congenita. Am. J. Med. Genet. 18:311-320, 1984.

McKusick, V.A.: Mapping and sequencing the human genome. N. Engl. J. Med. 320:910-915, 1989.

Turc-Carel, C., Aurias, A., Mugneret, F., et al.: Chromosomes in Ewing's sarcoma: An evaluation of 85 cases of remarkable consistency of t(11;22) (q24;q12). Cancer Genet. Cytogenet. 32:229-238, 1988.

White, R., and Lalouel, J.-M.: Chromosome mapping with DNA markers. Sci. Am. 258:40-48, 1988.

Veitch, J.M., and Omer, G.E.: Case report: Treatment of catbite injuries of the hand. J. Trauma 19:201-202, 1989.

Wahlig, H., Dingeldein, E., Bergmann, R., et al.: The release of gentamycin from polymethylmethacrylate beads: An experimental and pharmacokinetic study. J. Bone Joint Surg. [Br.] 60:270, 1978.

REVIEW ARTICLES

Beals, R.K., and Horton, W.: Skeletal dysplasias: An approach to diagnosis. J. Am. Acad. Orthop. Surg. 3:174-181, 1995.

Evans, C.H., and Robbins, P.D.: Current concepts review—possible orthopaedic applications of gene therapy. J. Bone Joint Surg. [Am.] 77:1103-1111, 1995.

Jaffurs, B.S., and Evans, C.: The Human Genome Project: Implications for the treatment of musculoskeletal disease. Am. Acad. Orthop. Surg. 6:1-14, 1998.

Tolo, V.T.: Spinal deformity in short stature syndromes. AAOS Instr. Course Lect. 39:399-405, 1990.

BOOK CHAPTERS

Alberts, B., Bray, D., Lewis, J., et al., eds.: Molecular Biology of the Cell, 2nd ed. New York, Garland Publishing, 1989.

DiDonato, S., DiMauro, S., Mamoli, A., et al.: Molecular Genetics of Neurological and Neuromuscular Disease, vol. 48. New York, Advances in Neurology, 1988.

Dietz, F.R., and Murray, J.C.: Update on the genetic basis of disorders with orthopaedic manifestations. In Buckwalter, J.A., Einhorn, T.A., and Simon, S.R., eds.: Orthopaedic Basic Science: Biology and Biomechanics of the Musculoskeletal System, 2nd ed., pp. 111-132. Rosemont, IL, American Academy of Orthopaedic Surgeons, 2000.

Rosier, R.N., Reynolds, P.R., and O'Keefe, R.J.: Molecular and cellular biology in orthopaedics. In Buckwalter, J.A., Einhorn, T.A., and Simon, S.R., eds.: Orthopaedic Basic Science: Biology and Biomechanics of the Musculoskeletal System, 2nd ed., pp. 19-76. Rosemont, IL, American Academy of Orthopaedic Surgeons, 2000.

Ross, D.W.: Introduction to Molecular Medicine, 2nd ed. New York, Springer-Verlag, 1996.

Watson, J.D., Tooze, J., and Kurtz, D.T.: Recombinant DNA: A Short Course. New York, Scientific American Books, 1983.

Wynbrandt, J., and Ludman, M.D.: The Encyclopedia of Genetic Disorders and Birth Defects. New York, 1991.

MUSCULOSKELETAL INFECTIONS

RECENT ARTICLES

Barrack, R., and Harris, W.: The value of aspiration of the hip joint before revision total hip arthroplasty. J. Bone Joint Surg. [Am.] 75:66-76, 1993.

Bass, J.W., Vincent, J.M., and Person, D.A.: The expanding spectrum of Bartonella infections: II. Cat-scratch disease. Pediatr. Infect. Dis. 16:163-179, 1997.

Brodsky, J.W., and Schneidler, C.: Diabetic foot infections. Orthop. Clin. North Am. 22:473-489, 1991.

Clarke, H.J., Jinnah, R.H., Byank R.P., et al.: Clostridium difficile infection in orthopaedic patients. J. Bone Joint Surg. [Am.] 72:1056-1059, 1990.

Feldman, D.S., Lonner, J.H., Desai, P., et al.: The role of intraoperative frozen sections in revision or total joint arthroplasty. J. Bone Joint Surg [Am.] 77:1807, 1995.

Gristina, A.G.: Implant failure and the immuno-incompetent fibro-inflammatory zone. Clin. Orthop. 298:106-118, 1994.

Hollmann, M.W., and Horowitz, M.: Femoral fractures secondary to low velocity missiles: Treatment with delayed intramedullary fixation. J. Orthop. Trauma 4:64-69, 1990.

Holton, P.D., Mader, J., Nelson, C.L., et al.: Antibiotics for the practicing orthopaedic surgeon. Price, C.T., ed.: American Academy of Orthopaedic Surgeons Instructional Course Lectures, XLIX, pp. 36-42. Park Ridge, IL, American Academy of Orthopaedic Surgeons, 2000.

Hospital Infection Control Practices Advisory Committee: Recommendations for preventing the spread of vancomycin resistance. Infect. Control Hosp. Epidemiol. 16:105-113, 1995.

Miclau, T., Edin, M.L., Lester, G.E., et al.: Bone toxicity of locally applied aminoglycosides. J. Orthop. Trauma 9:401-406, 1995.

Mills, W.J., and Swiontkowski, M.F.: Fatal group A streptococcal infection with toxic shock syndrome: Complicating minor orthopedic trauma. J. Orthop. Trauma 10:149-155, 1996.

Nelson, J.P., Fitzgerald, R.H., Jr., Jaspers, M.T., et al.: Prophylactic antimicrobial coverage in arthroplasty patients [editorial]. J. Bone Joint Surg. [Am.] 72:1, 1990.

Paiement, G.D., Hymes, R.A., LaDouceur, M.S., et al.: Postoperative infections in asymptomatic HIV seropositive orthopaedic trauma patients. J. Trauma 37:545-551, 1994.

Patzakis, M.J., Wilkins, J., Kumar, J., et al.: Comparison of the results of bacterial cultures from multiple sites in chronic osteomyelitis of long bones. J. Bone Joint Surg. [Am.] 76:664, 1994.

Sullivan, P.M., Johnston, R.C., and Kelky, S.S.: Late infection after total hip replacement, caused by an oral organism after dental manipulation. J. Bone Joint Surg. [Am.] 72:121-123, 1990.

Thelander, U., and Larsson, S.: Quantitation of C-reactive protein levels and erythrocyte sedimentation rate after spinal surgery. Spine 17:400-404, 1992.

Tomford, W.W.: Transmission of disease through transplantation of musculoskeletal allografts. J. Bone Joint Surg. [Am.] 77:1742-1754, 1995.

Travis, J.: Reviving the antibiotic miracle. Science 264:360-362, 1994.

Unkila-Kallio, L., Markku, K.J.T., and Peltola, H.: The usefulness of C-reactive protein levels in the identification of concurrent septic arthritis in children who have acute hematogenous osteomyelitis. J. Bone Joint Surg. [Am.] 76:848, 1994.

Wang, K.C., and Shih, C.H.: Necrotizing fascilitis of the extremities. J. Trauma 32:179-182, 1992.

Wilson, M.G., Kelley, K., and Thornhill, T.S.: Infection as a complication of total-knee replacement arthroplasty: Risk factors and treatment in sixty-seven cases. J. Bone Joint Surg. [Am.] 72:878-883, 1990.

Windsor, R.E., Insall, J.N., Urs, W.K., et al.: Two-stage reimplantation for the salvage of total knee arthroplasty complicated by infection: Further follow-up and refinement of indications. J. Bone Joint Surg. [Am.] 72:272-278, 1990.

CLASSIC ARTICLES

Aalto, K., Osterman, K., Peltola, H., et al.: Changes in erythrocyte sedimentation rate and C-reactive protein after total hip arthroplasty. Clin. Orthop. 184:118-120, 1984.

Bailey, J.P., Jr., Stevens, S.J., Bell, W.M., et al.: Mycobacterium marinum infection: A fishy story. J.A.M.A. 247:1314, 1982.

Bartlett, P., Reingold, A.L., Graham, D.R., et al.: Toxic shock syndrome associated with surgical wound infections. J.A.M.A. 247:1448-1451, 1982.

Brand, R.A., and Black, H.: Pseudomonas osteomyelitis following puncture wounds in children. J. Bone Joint Surg. [Am.] 56:1637-1642, 1974.

Buck B.E., Malinin, T.I., Brown, M.D.: Bone transplantation and human immunodeficiency virus: an estimate of risk of acquired immunodeficiency syndrome (AIDS). Clin. Orthop. 240:129-136, 1989.

Buchholz, H.W., Elson, R.A., Engelbrecht, E., et al.: Management of deep infection of total hip replacement. J. Bone Joint Surg. [Br.] 63:342-353, 1981.

Committee on Trauma, American College of Surgeons: Prophylaxis against tetanus in wound management. Am. Coll. Surg. Bull 69:22-23, 1984.

Dalinka, M.K., Dinnenberg, S., Greendyk, W.H., et al.: Roentgenographic features of osseous coccidioidomycosis and differential diagnosis. J. Bone Joint Surg. [Am.] 53:1157-1164, 1971.

Digby, J.M., and Kersley, J.B.: Pyogenic non-tuberculous spinal infection: An analysis of thirty cases. J. Bone Joint Surg. [Br.] 61:47-55, 1979.

Eismont, F.J., Bohlman, H.H., Soni, P.L., et al.: Pyogenic and fungal vertebral osteomyelitis with paralysis. J. Bone Joint Surg. [Am.] 65:19-29, 1983.

Fee, N.F., Dobranski, A., and Bisla, R.S.: Gas gangrene complicating open forearm fractures: Report of five cases. J. Bone Joint Surg. [Am.] 59:135-138, 1977.

Fielding, J.W., and Hawkins, R.J.: Atlanto-axial rotatory fixation. J. Bone Joint Surg. [Am.] 59:37-44, 1977.

Fitzgerald, R.H., and Cowan, J.D.E.: Puncture wounds of the foot. Orthop. Clin. North Am. 6:965-972, 1975.

Fitzgerald, R.H., Jr., Peterson, L.F., Washington, J.A., II, et al.: Bacterial colonization of wounds and sepsis in total hip arthroplasty. J. Bone Joint Surg. [Am.] 55:1242-1250, 1973.

Garcia, A., and Grantham, S.A.: Hematogenous pyogenic vertebral osteomyelitis. J. Bone Joint Surg. [Am.] 42:429-436, 1960.

Garvin, K.L., Salvati, E.A., and Brause, B.D.: Role of gentamicin-impregnated cement in total joint arthroplasty. Orthop. Clin. North Am. 19:605-610, 1988.

Goulet, J.A., Pellicci, P.M., Brause, B.D., et al.: Prolonged suppression of infection in total hip arthroplasty. J. Arthroplasty 3:109-116, 1988.

Grogan, T.J., Dorey, F., Rollins, J., et al.: Deep sepsis following total knee arthroplasty: Ten-year experience at the University of California at Los Angeles Medical Center. J. Bone Joint Surg. [Am.] 68:226-234, 1986.

Gustilo, R.B., Gruninger, R.P., and Davis, T.: Classification of type III (severe) open fractures relative to treatment and results. Orthopaedics 10:1781-1788, 1987.

Hawkins, L.G.: Pasteurella multocida infections. J. Bone Joint Surg. [Am.] 51:362-366, 1969.

Hill, C., Flamont, R., Mazas, F., et al.: Prophylactic cefazolin versus placebo in total hip replacement: Report of a multicentre double-blind randomized trial. Lancet 1:795-796, 1981.

Insall, J., Thompson, F., and Brause, B.: Two-stage reimplantation for the salvage of infected total knee arthroplasty. J. Bone Joint Surg. [Am.] 65:1087-1098, 1983.

Lange, R.H., Bach, A.W., Hansen, S.T., Jr., et al.: Open tibial fractures with associated vascular injuries: Prognosis for limb salvage. J. Trauma 25:203-208, 1985.

MacAusland, W.R., Jr.: The management of sepsis following intramedullary fixation for fractures of the femur. J. Bone Joint Surg. [Am.] 44:1643-1653, 1963.

McDonald, D.J., Fitzgerald, R.H., and Ilstrup, D.M.: Two-stage reconstruction of a total hip arthroplasty. J. Bone Joint Surg. [Am.] 71:828-834, 1989.

Mallouh, A., and Talab, Y.: Bone and joint infection in patients with sickle cell disease. J. Pediatr. Orthop. 5:158-162, 1985.

Nelson, J.D.: Antibiotic concentrations in septic joint effusions. N. Engl. J. Med. 284:349, 1971.

Nelson, J.D., and Koontz, W.C.: Septic arthritis in infants and children: A review of 117 cases. Pediatrics 92:131, 1978.

O'Connor, B.T., Steel, W.M., and Sanders, R.: Disseminated bone tuberculosis. J. Bone Joint Surg. [Am.] 52:537-542, 1970.

Pappas, A.M., Filler, R.M., Eraklis, A.J., et al.: Clostridial infections (gas gangrene): Diagnosis and early treatment. Clin. Orthop. 76:177-184, 1971.

Patzakis, M.J., Harvey, J.P., Jr., and Ivler, F.: The role of antibiotics in the management of open fractures. J. Bone Joint Surg. [Am.] 56:532-541, 1974.

Patzakis, M.J., Wilkins, J., and Bassett, R.L.: Surgical findings in clenched-fist injuries. Clin. Orthop. 220:237-240, 1987.

Patzakis, M.J., Wilkins, J., and Moor, T.M.: Considerations in reducing the infection rate in open tibial fractures. Clin. Orthop. 178:36-41, 1983.

Patzakis, M.J., Wilkins, J., and Wiss, D.A.: Infection following intramedullary nailing of long bones. Clin. Orthop. 212:182-191, 1986.

Riegler, H.F., and Rouston, G.W.: Complications of deep puncture wounds of the foot. J. Trauma 19:18-22, 1979.

Roberts, J.M., Drummond, D.S., Breed, A.L., et al.: Subacute hematogenous osteomyelitis in children: A retrospective study. J. Pediatr. Orthop. 2:249-254, 1982.

Rovner, R.A., Baird, R.A., and Malerick, M.M.: Fatal toxic shock syndrome as a complication of orthopaedic surgery: A case report. J. Bone Joint Surg. [Am.] 66:952-954, 1984.

Salvati, E.A., Callaghan, J.J., Brause, B.D., et al.: Reimplantation in infection: Elution of gentamicin from cement and beads. Clin. Orthop. 207:83-93, 1986.

Wahlig, H. Dingeldein, E., Bergmann, R., et al.: The release of gentamyscin from polymethylmethacrylate beads: An experimental and pharmacokinetic study. J. Bone Joint Surg. [Br.] 60:270, 1978.

Wopperer, J.M., White, J.J., Gillespie, R., et al.: Long term follow-up of infantile hip sepsis. J. Pediatr. Orthop. 8:322-325, 1988.

REVIEW ARTICLES

Chang, H.J., Luck, J.V., Jr., Bell, D.M., et al.: Transmission of human immunodeficiency virus infection in the surgical setting. J. Am. Acad. Orthop. Surg. 4:279-286, 1996.

Garvis, K.L., and Hanssen, A.D.: Current concepts review—infection after total hip arthroplasty. J. Bone Joint Surg. [Am.] 77:1576-1584, 1995.

Gustilo, R.B., Merkow, R.L., and Templeman, D.: The management of open fractures: Current concepts. J. Bone Joint Surg. [Am.] 72:299-304, 1990.

McLaughlin, T.P., Zemel, L., Fisher, R.L., et al.: Chronic arthritis of the knee in Lyme disease: Review of the literature and report of two cases treated by synovectomy. J. Bone Joint Surg. [Am.] 68:1057, 1986.

Tomford, W.W.: Current concepts review: Transmission of disease through transplantation of musculoskeletal allografts. J. Bone Joint Surg. [Am.] 77:1742-1750, 1995.

Waldvogel, F.A., and Papageorgiou, P.S.: Osteomyelitis: The past decade. N. Engl. J. Med. 303:360-370, 1980.

BOOK CHAPTERS

AAOS Task Force on AIDS and Orthopaedic Surgery: Recommendations for the Prevention of Human Immunodeficiency Virus (HIV) Transmission in the Practice of Orthopaedic Surgery. Park Ridge, IL, American Academy of Orthopaedic Surgeons, 1989.

Cierney, G., III: Chronic osteomyelitis: Results of treatment. Instr. Course Lect. 39:495-508, 1990.

Del Curling, O., Jr., Gower, J.D., and McWhorter, J.M.: Changing concepts in spinal epidural abscess: A report of 29 cases. Neurosurgery 27:185-192, 1990.

Fitzgerald, R.H., Jr., ed.: Infection. In Orthopaedic Knowledge Update 2: Home Study Syllabus, pp. 71-82. Park Ridge, IL, American Academy of Orthopaedic Surgeons, 1987.

Fitzgerald, R.H., Jr.: Orthopaedic sepsis in osteomyelitis: Antimicrobial therapy for the musculoskeletal system. Instr. Course Lect. 31:1-9, 1982.

Frymoryer, J.W., ed.: Orthopaedic Knowledge Update 4: Home Study Syllabus, p. 157. Rosemont, IL, American Academy of Orthopaedic Surgeons, 1993.

Frymoyer, J.W., ed.: Infection. In Orthopaedic Knowledge Update 4: Home Study Syllabus, p. 162. Rosemont, IL, American Academy of Orthopaedic Surgeons, 1993.

Gavin, K.L., Luck, J.V., Rupp, M.E., and Fey, P.D.: Infections in orthopaedics. In Buckwalter, J.A., Einhorn, T.A., and Simon, S.R., eds.: Orthopaedic Basic Science: Biology and Biomechanics of the Musculoskeletal System, 2nd ed., pp. 239-260. Rosemont, IL, American Academy of Orthopaedic Surgeons, 2000.

Gilbert, D.N., Moellering, R.C., and Sande, M.A.: The Sanford Guide to Antimicrobial Therapy, 32nd ed. Hyde Park, VT, Antimicrobial Therapy, Inc., 2002.

Gristina, A.J., Naylor, P.T., and Webb, L.X.: Molecular mechanisms in musculoskeletal sepsis: A race for the surface. In Greene, W.P., ed.: American Academy of Orthopaedic Surgeons Instructional Course Lectures, XXXIX, pp. 471-482. Park Ridge, IL, American Academy of Orthopaedic Surgeons, 1990.

Kind, A.C., and Williams, D.N.: Antibiotics in open fractures. In Gustillo, R.B., ed.: Management of Open Fractures and Their Complications, pp. 55-59. Philadelphia, W.B. Saunders, 1982.

Mader, J.T., and Calhoun, J.H.: Antimicrobial treatment of musculoskeletal infections. In Evarts, C.M., ed.: Surgery of the Musculoskeletal System, 2nd ed. New York, Churchill-Livingstone, 1990.

Morris, C.D., and Einhorn, T.A.: Principles of orthopaedic pharmacology. In Buckwalter, J.A., Einhorn, T.A., and Simon, S.R., eds.: Orthopaedic Basic Science: Biology and Biomechanics of the Musculoskeletal System, 2nd ed., pp. 217-238. Rosemont, IL, American Academy of Orthopaedic Surgeons, 2000.

Morrissy, R.T.: Bone and joint infections. In Morrissy, R.T., ed.: Lovell and Winter's Pediatric Orthopaedics, 3rd ed., vol. 1., pp. 539-561. Philadelphia, J.B. Lippincott, 1990.

Sande, M.A., Kapusnik-Ulner, J.E., and Mandell, G.L.: Antimicrobial agents. In Gilman, A.G., ed.: Goodman and Gilman's The Pharmacological Basis of Therapeutics, 8th ed., pp. 1103-1107. New York, McGraw, 1990.

Sande, M.A., and Mandell, G.L.: Antimicrobial agents: The aminoglycosides. In Gilman, Goodman, Gilman, eds.: The Pharmacological Basis of Therapeutics, 6th ed., pp. 1162-1180. New York, MacMillan, 1980.

Tachdjian, M.O.: Pediatric Orthopaedics, 2nd ed., vol. 2, pp. 1415-1441. Philadelphia, W.B. Saunders, 1990.

PERIOPERATIVE PROBLEMS

RECENT ARTICLES

Bierbaum, B.E., Callaghan, J.J., Galante, J.O., et al.: An analysis of blood management in patients having a total hip or knee arthroplasty. J. Bone Joint Surg. [Am.] 81:2-10, 1999.

Brinker, M.R., Reuben, J.D., Mull, J.R., et al.: Comparison of general and epidural anesthesia in patients undergoing primary unilateral total hip replacement. Orthopedics, 20:109-115, 1997.

Colwell, C.W., Spiro, T.E., Trowbridge, A.A., et al.: Use of enoxaparin, a low-molecular-weight heparin, and unfractionated heparin for the prevention of deep venous thrombosis after elective hip replacement: A clinical trial comparing efficacy and safety. J. Bone Joint Surg. [Am.] 76:3-14, 1995.

Fahmy, N., Chandler, H., and Danylchuk, K.: Blood gas and circulatory changes during total knee replacement: Role of the intramedullary alignment rod. J. Bone Joint Surg. [Am.] 72:19, 1990.

Faris, P.M., Ritter, M.A., Keating, E.M., et al.: Unwashed filtered shed blood collected after knee and hip arthroplasties: A source of autologous red blood cells. J. Bone Joint Surg. [Am.] 73:1169-1178, 1991.

Lieberman, J.R., and Geerts, W.H.: Prevention of venous thromboembolism after total hip and knee arthroplasty. J. Bone Joint Surg. [Am.] 76:1239-1250, 1994.

MacLennan, D.H., and Phillips, M.S.: Malignant hyperthermia. Science 256:789-794, 1992.

Pape, H.C., Regel, G., Dwenger, A., et al.: Influences of different methods of intramedullary femoral nailing on lung function in patients with multiple trauma. J. Trauma 35:709-716, 1993.

Webb, L.X., Rush, P.T., Fuller, S.B., et al.: Greenfield filter prophylaxis of pulmonary embolism in undergoing surgery for acetabular fractures. J. Orthop. Trauma 6:139-145, 1992.

CLASSIC ARTICLES

Aiach, M., Michaud, A., Balian, J.L., et al.: A new low molecular weight heparin derivative: In vitro and in vivo studies. Thromb. Res. 31:611-621, 1983.

Amato, J.J., Rheinlander, H.F., and Cleveland, R.J.: Post-traumatic adult respiratory distress syndrome. Orthop. Clin. North Am. 9:693-713, 1978.

Baker, J., Deitch, E., Berg, R., et al.: Hemorrhagic shock induces bacterial translocation from the gut. J. Trauma 28:896-905, 1988.

Barnes, R.W., Shanik, G.D., and Slaymaker, E.E.: An index of healing in below-knee amputation: Leg blood pressure by Doppler ultrasound. Surgery 79:13, 1976.

Culver, D., Crawford, J.S., Gardiner, J.H., et al.: Venous thrombosis after fractures of the upper end of the femur: A study of incidence and site. J. Bone Joint Surg. [Br.] 52:61-69, 1970.

DeLee, J.C., and Rockwood, C.A., Jr.: Current concepts review. The use of aspirin in thromboembolic disease. J. Bone Joint Surg. [Am.] 62:149-152, 1980.

Duis, J.H., Nijsten, M.W.N., Kalausen, H.J., et al.: Fat embolism in patients with an isolated fracture of the femoral shaft. J. Trauma 28:383-390, 1988.

Einhorn, T.A., Bonnarens, F., and Burstein, A.H.: The contributions of dietary protein and mineral to the healing of experimental fractures: A biomechanical study. J. Bone Joint Surg. [Am.] 68:1389-1395, 1986.

Jardon, O.M., Wingard, D.W., Barak, A.J., et al.: Malignant hyperthermia: A potentially fatal syndrome in orthopaedic patients. J. Bone Joint Surg. [Am.] 61:1064-1070, 1979.

Johnson, K.D., Cadambi, A., and Seibert, G.B.: Incidence of adult respiratory distress syndrome in patients with multiple musculoskeletal injuries: Effect of early operative stabilization of fractures. J. Trauma 24:375-384, 1985.

Kakkar, V.V., Hose, C.T., Flanc, C., et al.: Natural history of postoperative deep vein thrombosis. Lancet 2:230-232, 1969.

Knize, D.M., Weatherly-White, R.C.A., Paton, B.C., et al.: Prognostic factors in the management of frostbite. J. Trauma 9:749, 1969.

Matsen, F.A., and Clawson, D.K.: The deep posterior compartmental syndrome of the leg. J. Bone Joint Surg. [Am.] 57:34-39, 1975.

Matsen, F.A., III, Winquist, A., Krugmire, R.B., Jr.: Diagnosis and management of compartment syndromes. J. Bone Joint Surg. [Am.] 62:286-291, 1980.

REVIEW ARTICLES

Gellman, H., and Nichols, D.: Reflex sympathetic dystrophy in the upper extremity. J. Am. Acad. Orthop. Surg. 5:313-322, 1997.

Levy, D.: The fat embolism syndrome: A review. Clin. Orthop. 261:281-286, 1990.

Whitesides, T., Jr., and Heckman, M.M.: Acute compartment syndrome: Update on diagnosis and treatment. J. Am. Acad. Orthop. Surg. 4:209-218, 1996.

Zimlich, R.H., Fulbright, B.M., and Friedman, R.J.: Current status of anticoagulation therapy after total hip and total knee arthroplasty. J. Am. Acad. Orthop. Surg. 4:54-62, 1996.

BOOK CHAPTERS

Bone, L.B.: Emergency treatment of the injured patient. In Browner, B.D., Jupiter, J.B., Levine, A.M., et al., eds.: Skeletal Trauma: Fractures, Dislocations and Ligamentous Injuries, p. 138. Philadelphia, W.B. Saunders, 1992.

Frymoyer, J.W., ed.: Multiple trauma: Pathophysiology and management. In Orthopaedic Knowledge Update 4: Home Study Syllabus, pp. 141-153. Rosemont, IL, American Academy of Orthopaedic Surgeons, 1993.

Lotke, P.A., and Elia, E.A.: Thromboembolic disease after total knee surgery: A critical review. In Green, W.B., ed.: American Academy of Orthopaedic Surgeons Instructional Course Lectures XXXIX, pp. 409-412. Park Ridge, IL, American Academy of Orthopaedic Surgeons, 1990.

MacLean, L.D.: Shock: Causes and management of circulatory collapse. In Sabiston, D.C., Jr., ed.: Davis-Christopher Textbook of Surgery, 12th ed., pp. 58-90. Philadelphia, W.B. Saunders, 1981.

Morris, C.D., Creevy, W.S., and Einhorn, T.A.: Pulmonary distress and thromboembolitic conditions affecting orthopaedic practice. In Buckwalter, J.A., Einhorn, T.A., and Simon, S.R., eds.: Orthopaedic Basic Science: Biology and Biomechanics of the Musculoskeletal System, 2nd ed., pp. 307-318. Rosemont, IL, American Academy of Orthopaedic Surgeons, 2000.

Mubarak, S.J.: Compartment syndromes in operative technique. In Chapman, M.W., ed.: Operative Orthopaedics, vol. 1, pp. 179-202. Philadelphia, J.B. Lippincott, 1988.

Poss, R., ed.: Polytrauma. In Orthopaedic Knowledge Update 3: Home Study Syllabus, p. 88. Park Ridge, IL, American Academy of Orthopaedic Surgeons, 1990.

IMAGING AND SPECIAL STUDIES

RECENT ARTICLES

Clarke, H.D., Kitaoka, H.B., and Berquist, T.H.: Imaging of tendon injuries about the ankle. Orthopedics 20:639-643, 1997.

Moed, B.R., Kim, E.C., and van Holsbeeck, M.: Ultrasound for the early diagnosis of tibial fracture healing after static interlocked nailing without reaming: Histologic correlation using a canine model. J. Orthop. Trauma 12:200-205, 1998.

Moed, B.R., Subramanian, S., van Holsbeeck, M., et al.: Ultrasound for the early diagnosis of tibial fracture healing after static interlocked nailing without reaming: Clinical results. J. Orthop. Trauma 12:206-213, 1998.

Nerlich, A.G., Schleicher, E.D., and Boos, N.: Immunohistologic markers for age-related changes of human lumbar intervertebral discs. Spine 22:2781-2795, 1997.

Rizzo, P.F., Gould, E.S., Lyden, J.P., et al.: Diagnosis of occult fractures about the hip: Magnetic resonance imaging compared with bone scanning. J. Bone Joint Surg. [Am.] 75:395-401, 1993.

CLASSIC ARTICLES

Gilmer, P.W., Herzenberg, J., Frank, J.L., et al.: Computerized tomographic analysis of acute calcaneal fractures. Foot Ankle 6:184–193, 1986.

Guyer, B.H., Levinsohn, E.M., Fredericksohn, B.E., et al.: Computed tomography of calcaneal fractures: Anatomy, pathology, and clinical relevance. Am. J. Radiol. 145:911–919, 1985.

Hauzeur, J.P., Pasteels, J.L., Schoutens, A., et al.: The diagnostic value of magnetic resonance imaging in nontraumatic osteonecrosis of the femoral head. J. Bone Joint Surg. [Am.] 71:641–649, 1989.

Herzenberg, J.E., Goldner, J.L., Martinez, S., et al.: Computerized tomography of talocalcaneal coalition: A clinical and anatomic study. Foot Ankle 6:273–288, 1986.

Kneeland, J.B., Middleton, W.D., Carrera, G.F., et al.: MR imaging of the shoulder: Diagnosis of rotator cuff tears. A.J.R. 149:333–337, 1987.

Marchisello, P.J.: The use of computerized axial tomography for the evaluation of talocalcaneal coalition. J. Bone Joint Surg. [Am.] 69:609–611, 1987.

Pykett, I.L., Newhouse, J.H., Buonanno, F.S., et al.: Principles of nuclear magnetic resonance imaging. Radiology 143:157–168, 1982.

Robinson, H.J., Jr., Hartleben, P.D., Lund, G., et al.: Evaluation of magnetic resonance imaging in the diagnosis of osteonecrosis of the femoral head: Accuracy compared with radiographs, core biopsy, and intraosseous pressure measurements. J. Bone Joint Surg. [Am.] 71:650–653, 1989.

Watanabe, A.T., Carter, B.C., Tettelbaum, G.P., et al.: Common pitfalls in magnetic resonance imaging of the knee. J. Bone Joint Surg. [Am.] 71:857–862, 1989.

BOOK CHAPTERS

Aminoff, M.J., ed.: Electrodiagnosis in Clinical Neurology, 3rd ed. New York, Churchill-Livingstone, 1992.

Fitzgerald, R.H., Jr., ed.: Imaging of the musculoskeletal system: Orthopaedic Knowledge Update 2: Home Study Syllabus, p. 159. Park Ridge, IL, American Academy of Orthopaedic Surgeons, 1987.

Herzog, R.J.: Magnetic resonance imaging of the spine. In Frymoyer, J.W., ed.: The Adult Spine: Principles and Practice, pp. 457–510. New York, Raven Press, 1991.

Peterfy, C.G., Roberts, T.P.L., and Genant, H.K.: Magnetic resonance imaging of the musculoskeletal system: advances in musculoskeletal imaging. In Buckwalter, J.A., Einhorn, T.A., and Simon, S.R., eds.: Orthopaedic Basic Science: Biology and Biomechanics of the Musculoskeletal System, 2nd ed., pp. 261–278. Rosemont, IL, American Academy of Orthopaedic Surgeons, 2000.

Lane, J.M., and Healey, J.H.: Fractures of the hip. In Lane, J.M., ed.: Diagnosis and Mangement of Pathologic Fractures, pp. 122–127. New York, Raven Press, 1993.

Schneider, R., and Rapuano, B.: Radioisotopes in orthopaedics. In Buckwalter, J.A., Einhorn, T.A., and Simon, S.R., eds.: Orthopaedic Basic Science: Biology and Biomechanics of the Musculoskeletal System, 2nd ed., pp. 289–306. Rosemont, IL, American Academy of Orthopaedic Surgeons, 2000.

BIOMATERIALS AND BIOMECHANICS

RECENT ARTICLES

Collier, J.P., Sutula, L.C., Currier, B.H., et al.: Overview of polyethylene as a bearing material: comparison of sterilization methods. Clin. Orthop. 333:76–86, 1996.

Dye, S.F., Chew, M.H.: The use of scintigraphy to detect increased osseous metabolic activity about the knee. In Schafer, M., ed. American Academy of Orthopaedic Surgeons Instructional Course Lectures, XLIII, pp. 453–469. Park Ridge, IL, American Academy of Orthopaedic Surgeons, 1994.

Ebramzadeh, E., Sarmiento, A., McKellop, H.A., et al.: The cement mantle in total hip arthroplasty: analysis of long-term radiographic results. J. Bone Joint Surg. [Am.] 76:77–87, 1994.

Jasty, M., Goetz, D.D., Bragdon, C.R., et al.: Wear of polyethylene acetabular components in total hip arthroplasty: An analysis of one hundred and twenty-eight components retrieved at autopsy or revision operations. J. Bone Joint Surg. [Am.] 79:349–358, 1997.

King G.J., Morrey, B.F., and An, K.N.: Stabilizers of the elbow. J. Shoulder Elbow Surg. 2:165–174, 1993.

McKellop, H.A., Campbell, P., Park, S.H., et al.: The origin of submicron polyethylene wear debris in total hip arthroplasty. Clin. Orthop. 311:3–20, 1995.

McKellop, H., Shen, F.W., Lu, B., et al.: Development of an extremely wear-resistant ultrahigh molecular weight polyethylene for total hip replacements. J. Orthop. Res. 17:157–167, 1999.

O'Donnell, R.J., Springfield, D.S., Motwani, H.K., et al.: Recurrence of giant-cell tumors of the long bones after cutterage and packing with cement. J. Bone Joint Surg [Am.] 76:1827–1833, 1994.

Schmalzried, T.P., and Callaghan, J.J.: Wear in total hip and knee replacements. J. Bone Joint Surg. [Am.] 81:115–136, 1999.

Skyhar, M.J., Warren, R.F., Oriz, G.J., et al.: The effects of sectioning of the posterior cruciate liagment and the posterolateral complex on the articular contact pressures within the knee. J. Bone Joint Surg. [Am.] 75:694–669, 1993.

Tan, V., Klotz, M.J., Greenwald, A.S., and Steinberg, M.E.: Carry it on the bad side! Am J. Orthop. 27:673–677, 1998.

Urban, R.M., Jacobs, J.J., Sumner, D.R., et al.: The bone-implant interface of femoral stems with non-circumferential porous coating. J. Bone Joint Surg. [Am.] 78:1068–1081, 1996.

CLASSIC ARTICLES

Bobyn, J.D., Pilliar, R.M., Cameron, H.U., et al.: The optimum pore size for the fixation of porous-surfaced metal implants by bone ingrowth. Clin. Orthop. 150:263–270, 1980.

Burstein, A.J., Currey, J., Frankel, V.H., et al.: Bone strength: The effect of screw holes. J. Bone Joint Surg. [Am.] 54:1143–1156, 1972.

Carter, D.R., and Spengler, D.M.: Mechanical properties and composition of cortical bone. Clin. Orthop. 135:192–217, 1978.

Freedman, L., and Munro, R.H.: Abduction of the arm in the scapular plane: scapular and glenohumeral movements. J. Bone Joint Surg [Am.] 18:1503, 1966.

Hawkins, R.J., and Neer, C.S.: A functional analysis of shoulder fusions. Clin. Orthop. 223:65–76, 1987.

Krettek, C., Haas, N., and Tscherne, H.: The role of supplemental lag-screw fixation for open fractures of the tibial shaft treated with external fixation. J. Bone Joint Surg. [Am.] 73:893–897, 1991.

Morrey, B.F., Askew, L.J., and Chao, E.Y.: A biomechanical study of normal elbow motion. J. Bone Joint Surg. [Am.] 63:872–877, 1981.

Morrey, B.F., and Wiedeman, G.P.: Complications and long-term results of ankle arthrodeses following trauma. J. Bone Joint Surg. [Am.] 62:777–784, 1980.

Nachemson, A.L., and Morris, J.M.: Lumbar intradiscal pressure. Acta. Orthop. Scand. (Suppl.) 43, 1964.

Perry, J.: Anatomy and biomechanics of the hindfoot. Clin. Orthop. 177:9–15, 1983.

Rowe, C.R.: Re-evaluation of the position of the arm in arthrodesis of the shoulder in the adult. J. Bone Joint Surg. [Am.] 56:913–922, 1974.

REVIEW ARTICLES

Friedman, R.J., Black, J., Galante, J.O., et al.: Current concepts in orthopaedic biomaterials and implant fixation. J. Bone Joint Surg. [Am.] 75:1086–1109, 1993.

Li, S., and Burstein, A.H.: Current concepts review—ultra-high molecular weight polyethylene: The material and its use in total joint implants. J. Bone Joint Surg. [Am.] 76:1080–1089, 1994.

BOOK CHAPTERS

Black, J.: Orthopaedic Biomaterials in Research and Practice, pp. 57–81. New York, Churchill-Livingstone, 1988.

Burstein, A.H., and Wright, T.M.: Fundamentals of Orthopaedic Biomechanics, pp. 171–187. Baltimore, Williams & Wilkins, 1994.

Chao, E.Y.S., and Aro, H.T.: Biomechanics of fracture fixation. In Mow, V.C., and Hayes, W.C., eds.: Basic Orthopaedic Biomechanics. New York, Raven Press, 1991.

Charnley, J.: Acrylic Cement in Orthopaedic Surgery. Baltimore, Williams & Wilkins, 1970.

Frankel, V.H., and Burstein, A.H.: Orthopaedic Biomechanics. Philadelphia, Lea & Febiger, 1970.

Frankel, V.H., and Nordin, M.: Basic Biomechanics of the Skeletal System. Philadelphia, Lea & Febiger, 1980.

Fung, Y.C.: Biomechanics: Mechanical Properties of Living Tissues. New York, Springer-Verlag, 1981.

Fung, Y.C.: Biomechanics: Motion, Flow, Stress and Growth. New York, Springer-Verlag, 1990.

Hipp, J.A., Chapel, E.J., and Hayes, W.C.: Biomechanics of fractures. In Browner, B.J., Jupiter, J.B., Levine, A.M., et al., eds.: Skeletal Trauma. Philadelphia, W.B. Saunders, 1992.

Lemons, J.E.: Metals and alloys. In Petty, W., ed.: Total Joint Replacement, pp. 21-27. Philadelphia, W.B. Saunders, 1991.

Mow, V.C., Flatow, E.L., and Ateshian, G.A.: Biomechanics. In Buckwalter, J.A., Einhorn, T.A., and Simon, S.R., eds.: Orthopaedic Basic Science: Biology and Biomechanics of the Musculoskeletal System, 2nd ed., pp. 133-180. Rosemont, IL, American Academy of Orthopaedic Surgeons, 2000.

Mow, V.C., and Soslowsky, L.J.: Friction, lubrication and wear of diarthrodial joints. In Mow, V.C., and Hayes, W.C., eds.: Basic Orthopaedic Biomechanics, pp. 256-257, 285-286. New York, Raven Press, 1991.

Park, J.B.: Biomaterials Science and Engineering. New York, Plenum, 1984.

Pauwels, F.: Biomechanics in the Normal and Diseased Hip, p. 26. Berlin, Springer-Verlag, 1976.

Simon, S.R., Alaranta, H., An, K.N., et al.: Kinesiology. In Buckwalter, J.A., Einhorn, T.A., and Simon, S.R., eds.: Orthopaedic Basic Science: Biology and Biomechanics of the Musculoskeletal System, 2nd ed., pp. 730-827. Rosemont, IL, American Academy of Orthopaedic Surgeons, 2000.

Timoshenko, S., and Young, D.H.: Elements of Strength of Materials, 5th ed., pp. 70-74. New York, Van Nostrand Reinhold, 1968.

White, A.A., and Panjabi, M.M.: Clinical Biomechanics of the Spine. Philadelphia, J.B. Lippincott, 1978.

Wright, T.M., and Li, S.L.: Biomaterials. In Buckwalter, J.A., Einhorn, T.A., and Simon, S.R., eds.: Orthopaedic Basic Science: Biology and Biomechanics of the Musculoskeletal System, 2nd ed., pp. 181-216. Rosemont, IL, American Academy of Orthopaedic Surgeons, 2000.

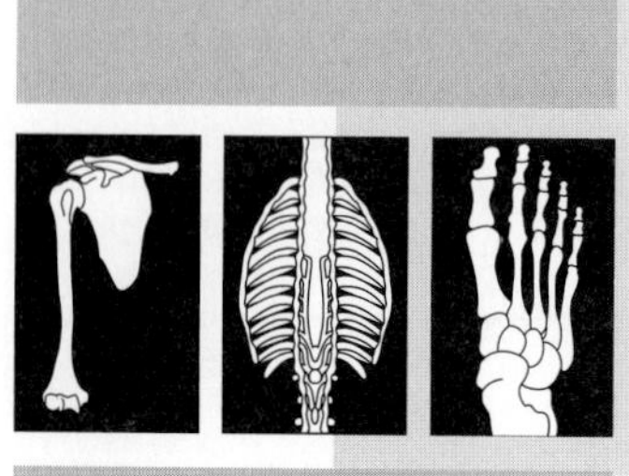

2 Pediatric Orthopaedics

TODD A. MILBRANDT
DANIEL J. SUCATO

I. Bone Dysplasias (Dwarfs)

A. Introduction—By definition, **dysplasia** means abnormal development. Bone dysplasias typically cause shortening of the involved bones affecting specific portions of the growing bone (Fig. 2-1), thereby leading to the term *dwarfism*. **Proportionate** dwarfism implies a symmetric decrease in both truncal and limb length (e.g., mucopolysaccharidoses). **Disproportionate** dwarfing conditions are subdivided into the short-trunk variety (e.g., Kniest's syndrome—spondyloepiphyseal dysplasia) or the short-limb variety (e.g., achondroplasia, diastrophic dysplasia). Short-limb dwarfism can be subdivided by the region of the limb that is short (e.g., rhizomelic-proximal, mesomelic-middle, acromelic-distal). The summation of all the dwarfisms are found in Table 2-1.

B. Achondroplasia

1. Introduction and Etiology—Achondroplasia is the most common form of disproportionate dwarfism. It is an *autosomal dominant (AD)* condition with an 80% prevalence of a spontaneous mutation in the fibroblast growth factor receptor 3 (**FGFR3**). This disproportionate, short-limbed form of dwarfism is caused by abnormal endochondral bone formation that is more affected than appositional growth. Anatomically, achondroplasia is categorized as a physeal dysplasia. The defect involves a failure in the cartilaginous **proliferative zone** of the physis. Achondroplasia is a quantitative, not a qualitative, cartilage defect. It may be associated with advanced paternal age.
2. Signs and Symptoms—Clinical features include a normal trunk and short limbs (rhizomelic). Typically, these patients have frontal bossing, button noses, small nasal bridges, **trident hands** (inability to approximate extended middle and ring fingers) (Fig. 2-2), thoracolumbar kyphosis (which usually resolves with ambulation) lumbar stenosis (**most likely to cause disability**) and excessive lordosis (short pedicles with decreased interpedicular distances), radial head subluxation, and hypotonia during the first year of life.

   Involved children have normal intelligence but delayed motor milestones. Although sitting height may be normal, standing height is below the third percentile. Radiographs show increasingly narrowed interpedicular distance in the distal spine (L1-S1); T12/L1 wedging; generalized posterior vertebral scalloping; delayed appearance of growth plates; and a pelvis that is wider than it is deep (**"champagne glass"** pelvic outlet). Achondroplasia may also be associated with radial or tibial bowing, coxa valga, genu varum (with disproportionately long fibula), and metaphyseal flaring with an inverted V-shaped distal femoral physis. Neurologic symptoms are usually related to nerve root or spinal cord compression, which can occur at any level, including the foramen magnum (which may cause periods of apnea).
3. Treatment—Nonoperative treatment includes weight loss, bracing, and exercises (unpredictable). Surgical options for symptomatic lumbar stenosis include decompression and fusion of the spine for a developing neurologic deficit (usually in children older than age 10). Symptomatic stenosis at the foramen magnum may require decompression. In rare cases, young children have progressive kyphosis without neurologic problems that fail bracing. In such cases, anterior fusion with strut grafting and posterior fusion are indicated for residual kyphosis >60 degrees by age 5 years. Fibular epiphysiodesis or tibial osteotomies, or both, are indicated for genu varum. Limb-lengthening procedures, including chondrodiatasis (lengthening through the growth plate) or callodiatasis

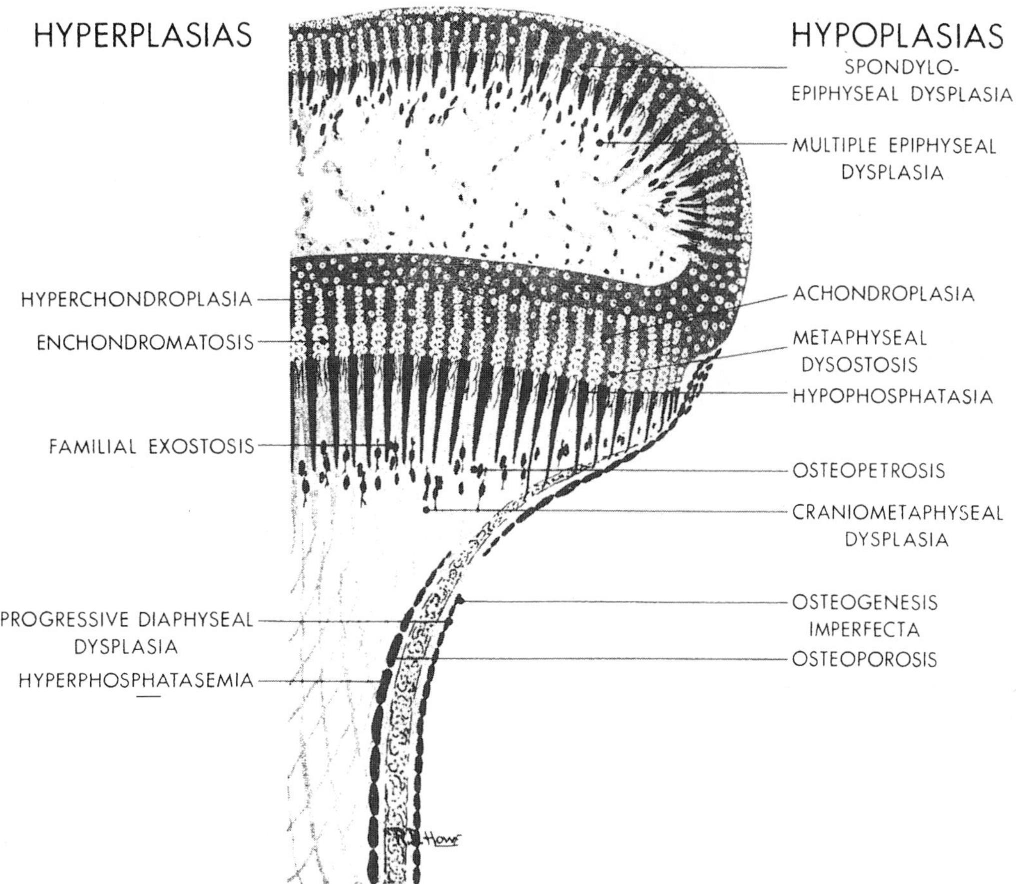

FIGURE 2-1 ■ Location of abnormalities leading to dysplasias. (From Rubin, P.: Dynamic Classification of Bone Dysplasias. Chicago, Year Book Medical Publishers, 1964.)

Table 2-1. SUMMATION OF MAJOR DWARFISMS

DWARFISM	GENETIC DEFECT	INHERITANCE	PATHONEUMONIC FEATURE
Achondroplasia	FGFR3	AD	Trident hands and lumbar kyphosis
Pseudoachondroplasia	COMP	AD	Normal facies and cervical instability
Spondyloepiphyseal Dysplasia	Type II collagen	Congenita-AD; tarda-X-linked recessive	Epiphyseal fragmentation with spine involvement
Kniest's Syndrome	Type II collagen	AD	Retinal detachment and dumbbell shaped bone
Jansen's	PTHRP	AD	Hypercalcemia with metaphyseal expansion
Schmid's	Type X collagen	AD	Coxa vara with proximal femur involvement
McKusick's Multiple Epiphyseal Dysplasia	Unknown COMP and Type II collagen	AR AD	Odontoid hypoplasia Bilateral hip involvement
Mucopolysaccharidosis (see Table 2-2)			
Diastrophic Dysplasia	Sulfate transport protein	AR	Cauliflower ears and kyphoscoliosis
Cleidocranial Dysplasia	CBFA1	AD	Aplasia of clavicles and coxa vara

FGFR3, fibroblast growth factor receptor 3; AD, autosomal dominant; COMP, cartilage oligometric matrix protein; PTHRP, parathyroid hormone related peptide; AR, autosomal recessive; CBFA1, transcription factor for osteocalcin.

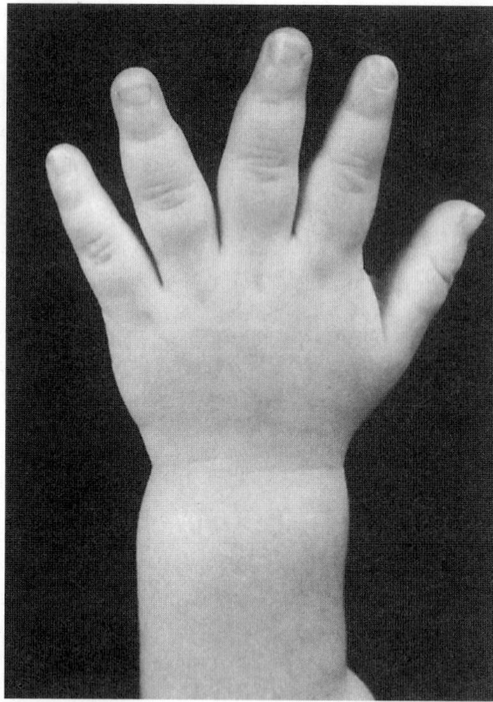

FIGURE 2-2 ■ Trident hand characteristic of achondroplasia. Note the space between the middle and the ring finger. (From Herring, T.: Tachdjian's Pediatric Orthopaedics, 3rd ed. Philadelphia, WB Saunders, 2002, p. 1511.)

(lengthening through a metaphyseal corticotomy), have been well described, with a low rate of complications. The patients still have the other underlying problems, however, and limb-lengthening procedures remain controversial in achondroplastic patients.

4. Pseudoachondroplasia—This disorder is clinically similar to achondroplasia. The inheritance pattern is AD with a defect on chromosome 19 within the cartilage oligometric matrix protein (**COMP**). In contrast to achondroplasia, the affected children have normal facies. Radiographs demonstrate metaphyseal flaring and delayed epiphyseal ossification. Orthopaedic manifestations of the disorder include **cervical instability**; scoliosis with increased lumbar lordosis; significant lower-extremity bowing; and hip, knee, and elbow flexion contractures with precocious osteoarthritis.

C. Spondyloepiphyseal Dysplasia—Two forms are generally recognized and must be differentiated from multiple epiphyseal dysplasia (MED). MED and spondyloepiphyseal dysplasia involve abnormal epiphyseal development in upper and lower extremities. The distinguishing feature of spondyloepiphyseal dysplasia is the added typical spine involvement and the genetic defect is within the gene encoding **type II collagen**.

1. Congenita Form—Short-trunked dwarfism associated with primary involvement of the vertebra (beaking) and epiphyseal centers (affects the proliferative zone), clinical heterogenicity, and **AD inheritance**. Clinically more severe than the tarda form. Delayed appearance of the epiphysis, flattened facies, platyspondyly (delayed ossification), kyphoscoliosis, odontoid hypoplasia, coxa vara, and genu valgum are common. Patients should also be screened for associated retinal detachment and myopia.
2. Tarda Form—These patients have an **X-linked recessive** inheritance and late (ages 8–10) manifestations of the disorder, which affects primarily the spine and large joints. Clinically less severe than the congenita form. Hips may be dislocated, and affected children are often susceptible to premature osteoarthritis (osteotomies may be helpful) and scoliosis (treated like idiopathic scoliosis). No lower-extremity angular deformities.

D. Chondrodysplasia Punctata—Characterized by multiple punctate calcifications seen on radiographs during infancy. The AD form (Conradi-Hunermann) has a wide variation of clinical expression. The severe autosomal recessive (AR) rhizomelic form is usually fatal during the first year of life. Cataracts, asymmetric limb shortening that may require surgical correction, and spinal deformities are common.

E. Kniest's Syndrome—AD, short-trunked, disproportionate dwarfism with joint stiffness/contractures, scoliosis, kyphosis, dumbbell-shaped femora, and hypoplastic pelvis and spine. The genetic abnormality is within the gene for **type II collagen**. Radiographs show osteopenia and dumbbell-shaped bones. Respiratory problems and cleft palate are common. Associated retinal detachment and myopia require an ophthalmology consult. Early therapy for joint contractures is required. Reconstructive procedures may be required for early hip degenerative arthritis. Otitis media and hearing loss are frequent.

F. Metaphyseal Chondrodysplasia—Heterogeneous group of disorders characterized by metaphyseal changes of tubular bones with *normal epiphyses*. The defect appears to be in the proliferative and hypertrophic zones of the physis. Several types are recognized, including the following:

1. Jansen's (Rare)—Most severe form. The genetic defect is in parathyroid hormone related peptide (**PTHRP**) AD, retarded, markedly short-limbed dwarf with wide eyes, monkey-like stance, and hypercalcemia. Striking bulbous metaphyseal expansion of long bones is a distinctive radiographic finding.
2. Schmid's—More common, less severe form. The genetic defect is in **type X collagen**. AD, short-limbed dwarf not diagnosed until patient is older, due to coxa vara and genu varum. Predominantly involves the proximal femur. Gait is often Trendelenburg, and patients suffer increased lumbar lordosis. Often confused with rickets, but laboratory test results are normal.

3. McKusick's—AR, *cartilage-hair dysplasia* (hypoplasia of cartilage and small diameter of hair) is seen most commonly among the Amish population and in Finland. Atlantoaxial instability is common (*odontoid hypoplasia*). Ankle deformity develops due to fibular overgrowth distally. These patients may have abnormal immunologic competence and have an increased risk for malignancies. In addition, they may suffer from intestinal malabsorption and megacolon.

G. MED—Short-limbed, disproportionate dwarfism that often does not manifest until between the ages 5–14. Must be differentiated from spondyloepiphyseal dysplasia. A mild form (Ribbing's) and a more severe form (Fairbank's) exist. MED is characterized by irregular, delayed ossification at multiple epiphyses (Fig. 2-3). Short, stunted metacarpals/metatarsals, irregular proximal femora, abnormal ossification (tibial **"slant sign"** and flattened femoral condyles, patella with **double layer**), valgus knees (consider early osteotomy), waddling gait, and early hip arthritis are common. The proximal femoral involvement can be confused with Perthes'; MED is bilateral and symmetric, has early acetabular changes, and does not have metaphyseal cysts.

H. Dysplasia Epiphysealis Hemimelica (Trevor's Disease)—Essentially an epiphyseal osteochondroma. Calcifications are seen within the joint. Most commonly seen at the knee. Usually affects only one joint. Partial excision of the prominent overgrowth (if symptomatic) and later osteotomies may be required. Recurrence is a common complication.

I. Progressive Diaphyseal Dysplasia (Camurati-Engelmann Disease)—AD; affected children are often "late walkers" (because of associated muscle weakness), with symmetric cortical thickening of long bones. Radiographs demonstrate widened, fusiform diaphyses with increased bone formation and sclerosis. The tibia, femur, and humerus are most often affected (in that order), affecting only the diaphyseal portion of bone. Symptomatic treatment includes salicylates, nonsteroidal anti-inflammatory drugs (NSAIDs), and steroids for refractory cases. Watch for leg-length inequality.

J. Mucopolysaccharidosis—In contrast to the aforementioned conditions, these forms of dwarfism are easily differentiated, based on the presence of complex sugars found in the urine. They produce a *proportionate* dwarfism caused by accumulation of mucopolysaccharides due to a hydrolase enzyme deficiency. Four main types include Morquio's, Hurler's, Hunter's, and Sanfilippo's syndromes (Table 2-2). **Morquio's syndrome (AR)** is the most common form and presents by age 18 months to 2 years with waddling gait, knock-knees, thoracic kyphosis, cloudy corneas, and *normal intelligence*. Morquio's syndrome is associated with urinary excretion of *keratan sulfate*. Bony changes include a thickening skull; wide ribs; anterior beaking of vertebrae; wide, flat pelvis;

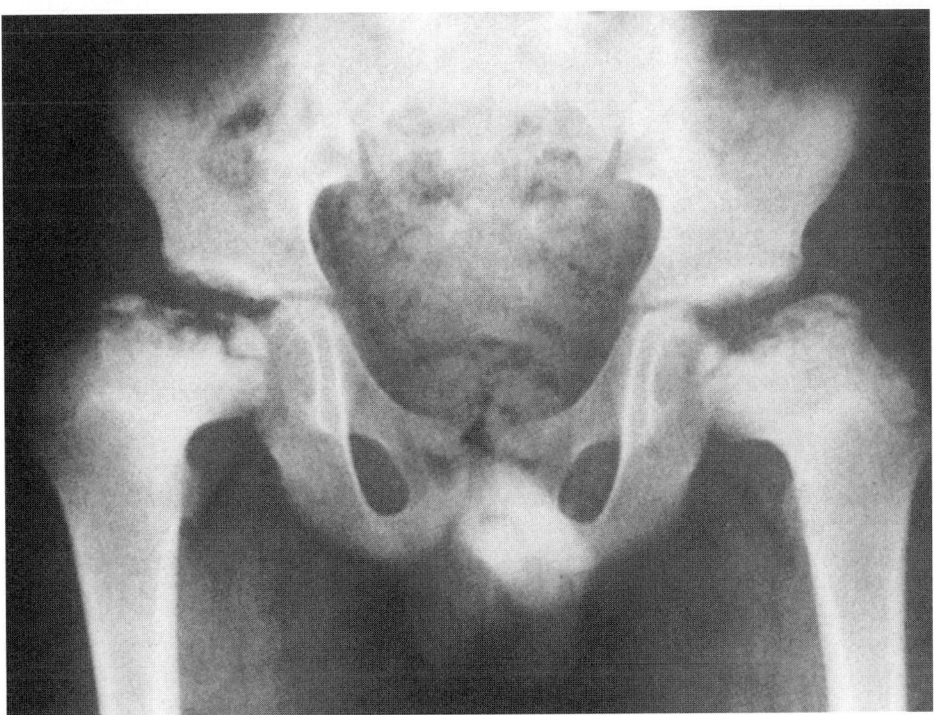

FIGURE 2-3 ■ Multiple epiphyseal dysplasia. Radiographs of the pelvis at 6 years old show abnormal bilateral femoral heads. (From Benson, M., Fixen, J., Macniol, M.: Children's Orthopaedics and Fractures, Churchill Livingstone, 1994, p. 52.)

Table 2-2. MAIN TYPES OF MUCOPOLYSACCHARIDOSIS

SYNDROME	INHERITANCE	INTELLIGENCE	CORNEA	URINARY EXCRETION	OTHER
Hurler's	AR	MR	Cloudy	Dermatan/heparin sulfate	Worst prognosis
Hunter's	XR	MR	Clear	Dermatan/heparin sulfate	
Sanfilippo's	AR	MR	Clear	Heparin sulfate	Normal until 2 years old
Morquio's	AR	Normal	Cloudy	Keratan sulfate	Most common

AR, autosomal recessive; MR, mentally retarded; XR, x-linked recessive.

coxa vara with unossified femoral heads; and bullet-shaped metacarpals. C1–C2 instability (due to odontoid hypoplasia) can be seen with Morquio's syndrome presenting with myelopathy and requiring decompression and cervical fusion. **Hurler's syndrome (AR)** is the most severe form and is associated with urinary excretion of *dermatan/heparan sulfate.* **Hunter's syndrome (sex-linked recessive)** is associated with urinary excretion of *dermatan/heparan sulfate.* **Sanfilippo's syndrome (AR)** is associated with urinary excretion of *heparan sulfate.* Hunter's, Hurler's, and Sanfilippo's syndromes are associated with *mental retardation.*

K. Diastrophic Dysplasia—AR; severe, short-limbed dwarfism associated with a deficiency in sulfate transport protein. This *"twisted"* dwarf classically has a cleft palate (59%), severe joint contractures (especially hip and knee), cauliflower ears (80%), hitchhiker thumb, rigid clubfeet, **cervical kyphosis** (often severe, requiring immediate treatment), thoracolumbar kyphoscoliosis (83%), spina bifida occulta, and atlantoaxial instability. Risk of quadriplegia is a major concern. Surgical release of clubfoot deformities, osteotomies for contractures, and spinal fusion are often required.

L. Cleidocranial Dysplasia (Dysostosis)—AD, proportionate dwarfism that affects bones formed by intramembranous ossification. Defect in **CBFA1** (a transcription factor for osteocalcin). Patients present with dwarfism and aplasia of a portion or the entire clavicle (Fig. 2-4). Usually unilateral, often the lateral part of the clavicle is missing (no intervention necessary), and there are delayed skull suture closure, frontal bossing, coxa vara (consider intertrochanteric valgus osteotomy if neck-shaft angle is <100 degrees), delayed ossification of the pubis, and wormian-type bone.

M. Dysplasias Associated with Benign Bone Growths—Include multiple hereditary exostosis (osteochondromatosis), fibrous dysplasia, Ollier's disease (enchondromatosis), and Maffucci's syndrome (enchondromatosis and hemangiomas). These entities are discussed in Chapter 8, Orthopaedic Pathology.

II. Chromosomal and Teratologic Disorders

A. Down's Syndrome (Trisomy 21)—*Most common chromosomal abnormality*; its incidence increases with maternal age. Usually associated with ligamentous laxity, hypotonia, mental retardation, *heart disease* (50%), endocrine disorders (hypothyroidism and diabetes), and premature aging. Orthopaedic problems include metatarsus primus varus, pes planus, spinal abnormalities (**atlantoaxial instability** [see Fig. 2-5], scoliosis [50%], spondylolisthesis [6%]), hip instability (*open reduction ± osteotomy* usually required), slipped capital femoral epiphysis (look for hypothyroidism), patellar dislocation, and symptomatic planovalgus feet. Atlantoaxial instability may be subtle in its presentation but commonly presents as a loss or change in motor milestones. Atlantoaxial instability is evaluated with flexion-extension radiographs of the C-spine. **Asymptomatic children with instability should avoid contact sports, diving, and gymnastics.**

B. Turner's Syndrome—45,XO females with short stature, sexual infantilism, web neck, and cubitus valgus. Idiopathic scoliosis is common. Growth hormone therapy can exacerbate scoliosis. Watch for osteoporosis. Genu valgum and shortening of the fourth and fifth metacarpals usually require no treatment. *Malignant hyperthermia* is common with anesthetic use. Must be differentiated from Noonan's syndrome (share appearance except for normal gonadal development, mental retardation, and more severe scoliosis).

C. Prader-Willi Syndrome—Partial chromosome 15 deletion (missing portion from father) causing a floppy, hypotonic infant who becomes an intellectually impaired, obese adult with an insatiable appetite. Growth retardation, hip dysplasia, hypoplastic genitalia, and juvenile-onset scoliosis are common.

D. Menkes' Syndrome—Sex-linked recessive disorder of copper transport that affects bone growth and causes characteristic "kinky" hair. May be differentiated from occipital horn syndrome (which also affects copper transport) by the characteristic bony projections from the occiput of the skull in that disorder.

E. Rett's Syndrome—*Progressive impairment* and stereotaxic abnormal hand movements (like autism) characterize this disorder. It is seen in *girls* at 6–18 months of age, who present with rapid developmental delay that stabilizes. This is different from cerebral palsy (CP) because the infants

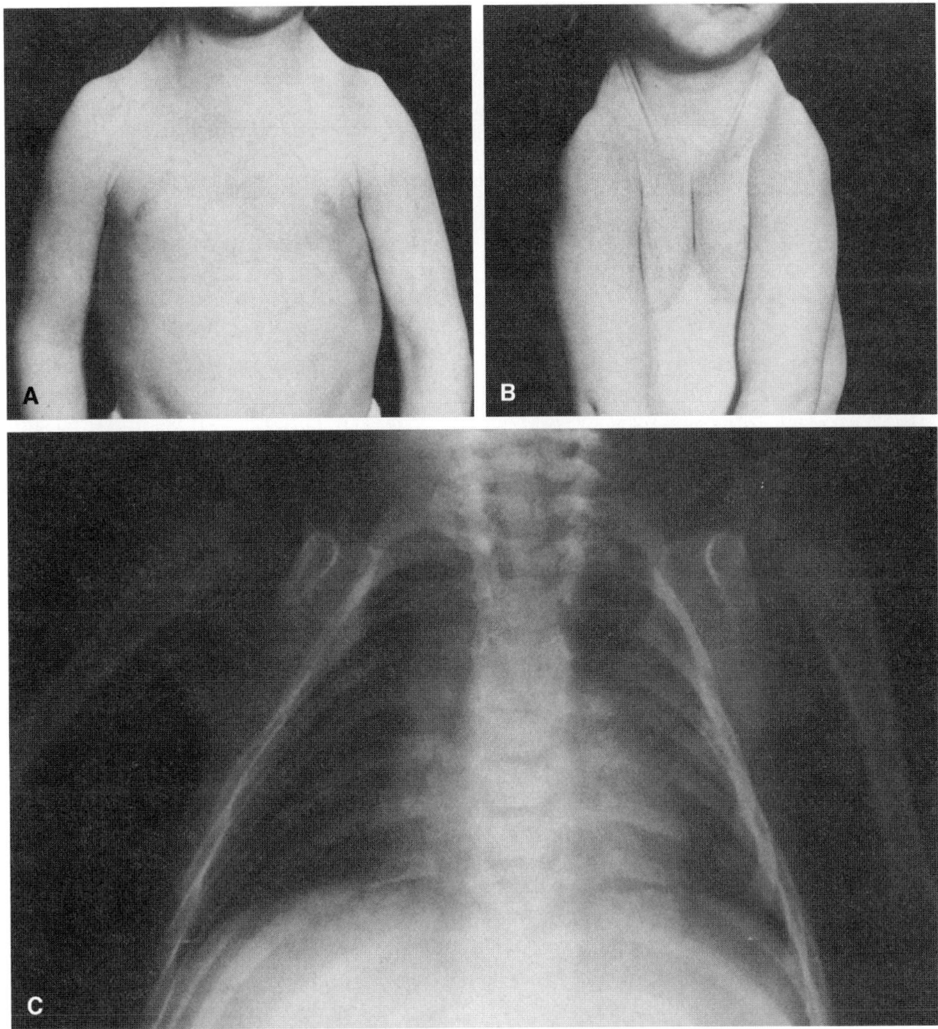

FIGURE 2-4 ■ *A*, Clinical photograph of cleidocranial dysostosis with the shoulders in normal position. *B*, Clinical photograph with the shoulders approximated. *C*, Radiograph of the chest and shoulders showing the aplasia of the clavicles bilaterally. (From Benson, M., Fixen, J., Macniol, M.: Children's Orthopaedics and Fractures, Churchill Livingstone, 1994, p. 364.)

have normal development for the first months of life and then decline. Affected children typically have *scoliosis* with a C-shaped curve unresponsive to bracing. Instrumentation must include all of the kyphosis and the scoliosis. Spasticity results in joint contractures, which are treated as in cerebral palsy patients.

F. Beckwith-Wiedemann Syndrome—The triad of organomegaly, omphalocele, and a large tongue defines this disorder. Orthopaedic manifestations include hemihypertrophy with spastic cerebral palsy. The spasticity is thought to be the result of infantile hypoglycemic episodes secondary to the pancreatic islet cell hypertrophy. There is a predisposition to *Wilms' tumor* (must be screened regularly).

G. Teratogens

1. Fetal Alcohol Syndrome—*Maternal alcoholism* can cause growth disturbances, central nervous system dysfunction, dysmorphic facies, hip dislocation, C-spine vertebral and upper-extremity congenital fusions, congenital scoliosis, and myelodysplasia. Contractures respond to physical therapy.
2. Maternal Diabetes—May lead to heart defects, **sacral agenesis**, and anencephaly. Careful management of pregnant diabetics is essential.
3. Other Teratogens—Include drugs (e.g., aminopterin, phenytoin, thalidomide), trace metals, maternal conditions, infections, and intrauterine factors; may also lead to orthopaedic manifestations in affected children.

III. Hematopoietic Disorders

A. Gaucher's Disease—Aberrant AR lysosomal storage disease characterized by accumulation of *cerebroside* in cells of the reticuloendothelial system. Cause is a deficiency of the enzyme ***beta-glucocerebrosidase***. There are three different types: type I most common, type II infantile,

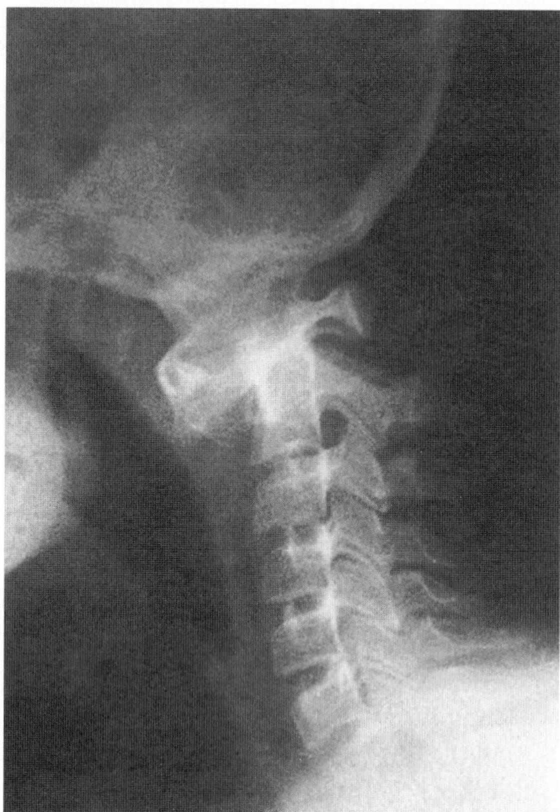

FIGURE 2-5 ■ Eleven-year-old with Down's syndrome with gross atlantoaxial instability. His gait was clumsy and he had poor coordination of his extremities and thus underwent posterior stabilization. (From Benson, M., Fixen, J., Macniol, M.: Children's Orthopaedics and Fractures, Churchill Livingstone, 1994, p. 590.)

and type II chronic neuronopathic. Type I is commonly seen in children of Ashkenazic Jewish descent; it is associated with osteopenia, metaphyseal enlargement (failure of remodeling), *femoral head necrosis* (may be confused with Perthes' or MED), "moth-eaten" trabeculae, patchy sclerosis, and **"Erlenmeyer's flask"** distal femora (70%). Affected patients may complain of bone pain (Gaucher crisis), and bleeding abnormalities are common. ***Hepatosplenomegaly*** is a characteristic finding. Histologic examination demonstrates characteristic lipid-laden histiocytes (Gaucher's cells). Treatment is basically supportive; new enzyme therapy is available but is extremely expensive.

B. Niemann-Pick Disease—AR disorder. It is caused by an accumulation of sphingomyelin in reticuloendothelial system cells. Seen commonly in eastern European Jews. Marrow expansion and cortical thinning are common in long bones; coxa valga is also seen.

C. Sickle Cell Anemia—Sickle cell disease (affects 1% of African Americans) is more severe but less common than sickle cell trait (8% prevalence). Crises usually begin at age 2–3, are caused by substance P, and may lead to characteristic *bone infarctions*. Growth retardation/skeletal immaturity, *osteonecrosis* of femoral and humeral heads, *osteomyelitis (often in diaphysis),* biconcave "fish" vertebrae, and septic arthritis are commonly seen in this disorder. *Salmonella* is more commonly seen in children with sickle cell disease. **Despite this tendency, *Staphylococcus aureus*** *is still the most common cause of osteomyelitis in sickle cell patients*. Dactylitis (acute hand/foot swelling) is also common. Aspiration and culture are necessary to differentiate infarction from osteomyelitis. Preoperative oxygenation and exchange transfusion are helpful for affected patients requiring surgery. Hydroxyurea has produced dramatic relief of pain when used for bone crises.

D. Thalassemia—It is similar to sickle cell anemia in presentation. Most commonly seen in people of Mediterranean descent. Common symptoms include bone pain and leg ulceration. Radiographs show long-bone thinning, metaphyseal expansion, osteopenia, and premature physeal closure.

E. Hemophilia—X-linked recessive disorder with decreased factor VIII (hemophilia A), abnormal factor VIII with platelet dysfunction (von Willebrand's disease), or factor IX (hemophilia B—Christmas disease); associated with bleeding episodes and skeletal/joint sequelae. Can be mild (5–25% of factor present), moderate (1–5% available), or severe (<1% of factor present).

Hemarthrosis presents with painful swelling and decreased range of motion (ROM) of affected joints. The knee is the most commonly affected joint. Deep intramuscular bleeding is also common and can lead to the formation of a *pseudotumor* (blood cyst), which can occur in soft tissue or bone. Intramuscular hematomas can lead to compression of adjacent nerves (e.g., an *iliacus hematoma may cause femoral nerve paralysis* and may mimic a bleed into the hip joint). Radiographic findings in hemophilia include *squaring* of the patellas and condyles, epiphyseal overgrowth with leg-length discrepancy, and generalized osteopenia with resulting fractures. Fractures heal in normal time with proper clotting. Cartilage atrophy due to enzymatic matrix degeneration and chondrocyte death is frequent.

Home transfusion therapy has reduced the severity of the arthropathy with the advantage of treatment when a bleed occurs. Treatment of the sequella includes contracture release, osteotomies, open synovectomy, arthroscopic synovectomy (better motion, shorter hospitalization), radiation synovectomy (useful in patients with antibody inhibitors and poor medical management), and total joint arthroplasty. Mild to moderate hemophilia A can be treated with desmopressin. Factor VIII levels should be increased for prophylaxis in the following situations: vigorous physical therapy (20%), treatment of hematoma (30%), acute hemarthrosis or soft-tissue surgery (>50%), and skeletal surgery (approach 100%

preoperatively and maintain >50% for 10 days postoperatively). Tourniquets, ligated vessels rather than cauterized vessels, and rigid fixation of fractures decrease postoperative bleeding. Immunoglobulin G **(IgG) antibody inhibitors** are present in 4–20% of hemophiliacs and **are a relative contraindication to surgery**. Large levels of factor VIII, or Autoplex (activated prothrombin), are required to offset these inhibitors. Because of the amount of blood component therapy required to treat this disorder, a large percentage of older hemophiliacs are *human immunodeficiency virus (HIV) positive*.

F. Leukemia—**The most common malignancy of childhood.** Acute lymphocytic leukemia (ALL) represents 80% of cases of leukemia. Peak incidence at 4 years. Causes demineralization of bones, periostitis, and occasionally lytic lesions. One fourth to one third of children have musculoskeletal complaints (back, pelvic, leg pains). Radiolucent "leukemia" lines may be seen in the metaphyses of affected bones in older children. Management of leukemia includes chemotherapy that may predispose to pathologic fractures.

G. AIDS—Caused by HIV. Children born with AIDS are becoming more common in neonatal units, and supportive care is indicated. Protection for surgeons with patients at risk (e.g., intravenous [IV] drug abusers, homosexuals, hemophiliacs) is essential (see Chapter 1, Basic Sciences).

IV. **Metabolic Disease/Arthritides** (see Chapter 1, Basic Sciences)

A. Rickets—Decrease in calcium (and sometimes phosphorus), affecting mineralization at the epiphyses of long bones. Classically, brittle bones with **physeal cupping/widening**, bowing of long bones, transverse radiolucent Looser's lines, ligamentous laxity, flattening of the skull, enlargement of costal cartilages (rachitic rosary), and dorsal kyphosis (cat back) characterize this disorder (Fig. 2-6). There are several varieties of rickets based on the underlying abnormality (e.g., gastrointestinal, kidney, diet, and organ), which are discussed in detail in Chapter 1. Histologically, **widened osteoid seams** and "Swiss cheese" trabeculae are characteristic in bone; at the growth plate there is gross distortion of the maturation zone (enlarged and distorted) and a poorly defined zone of provisional calcification.

B. Osteogenesis Imperfecta—Defect in **type I collagen** (COL1A2 gene) that causes abnormal cross-linking that leads to decreased collagen secretion, bone fragility (brittle "wormian" bone), short stature, scoliosis, tooth defects (dentinogenesis imperfecta), hearing defects, and ligamentous laxity. Four types have been identified (Sillence), although the disorder is probably best considered as a continuum with different inheritance patterns and severity (Table 2-3).

Radiographs demonstrate thin cortices and generalized osteopenia. Histologically, increased diameters of haversian canals and osteocyte lacunae, increased numbers of cells, and replicated cement lines are noted and result in the thin cortices seen on radiographs. Fractures are common; **the initial healing is normal**, but bone typically does not remodel. Fractures occur less frequently with advancing age (usually cease at puberty). Compression fractures (codfish vertebrae) are also common. The goal of treatment is fracture management and long-term rehabilitation. Bracing of extremities is indicated early to prevent deformity and minimize fractures. *Sofield's osteotomies* ("shish kebab" multiple long-bone osteotomies with either fixed-length Rush's rods or telescoping [Bailey-Dubow] intramedullary rods) are sometimes required for progressive bowing of long bones. Fractures in children younger than age 2 are treated similarly to those in children without osteogenesis imperfecta. After age 2 years, telescoping intramedullary rods can be considered. Although synthetic salmon calcitonin, calcium supplements, and pamitrondate have been suggested to decrease the number of fractures in some osteogenesis imperfecta patients, no medical therapy has been proved unequivocally effective. Scoliosis is common, and bracing is ineffective treatment. Surgery is necessary for scoliosis deformities exceeding 50 degrees.

C. Idiopathic Juvenile Osteoporosis—Rare, **self-limited** disorder that appears between the ages 8–14 with osteopenia, growth arrest, and bone and joint pain. Other manifestations can include multiple vertebral body microfractures that can be treated with bracing. Serum calcium and phosphorus levels are normal. Typically, there is spontaneous resolution 2–4 years after onset of puberty. This disorder must be differentiated from other causes of osteopenia (e.g., osteogenesis imperfecta, malignancy, Cushing's disease).

D. Osteopetrosis—Failure of *osteoclastic* resorption, probably secondary to a defect in the thymus, leading to dense bone *(marble bone),* "rugger jersey" spine (Fig. 2-7), *marble bone*, and an "Erlenmeyer flask" proximal humerus/distal femur. Loss of medullary canal can cause anemias, encroachment on the optic, and oculomotor nerves. Healing is normal but time to healing may be elongated. Mild form is AD; "malignant" form is AR. **Bone marrow transplant** may be helpful for treating the malignant form (see Chapter 1, Basic Sciences).

E. Infantile Cortical Hyperostosis (Caffey's Disease)—Soft-tissue swelling and bony cortical thickening (especially the jaw and ulna) that *follow a febrile illness* in infants 0–9 months old. Radiographs show characteristic periosteal reaction. This disorder may be differentiated from trauma

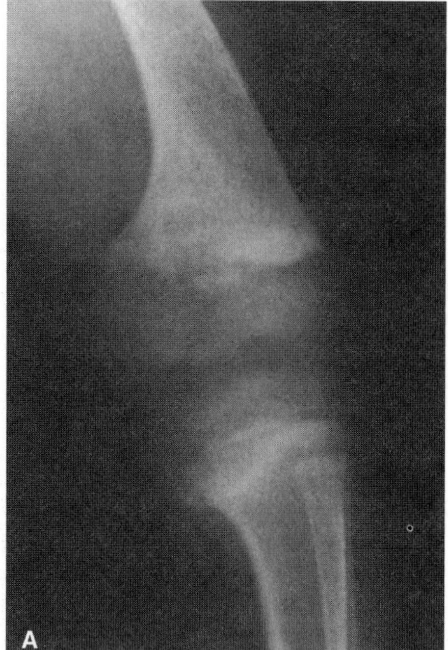

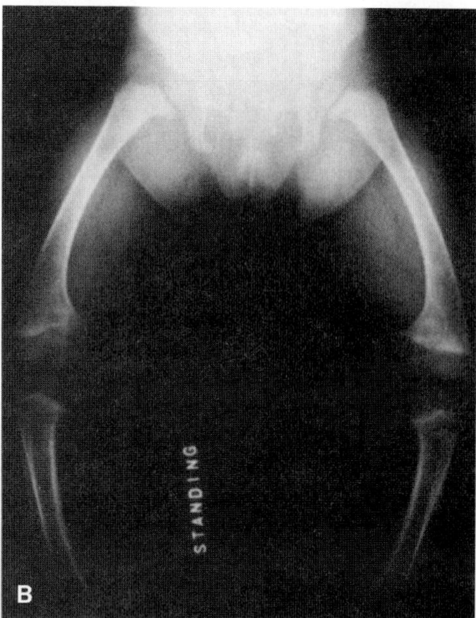

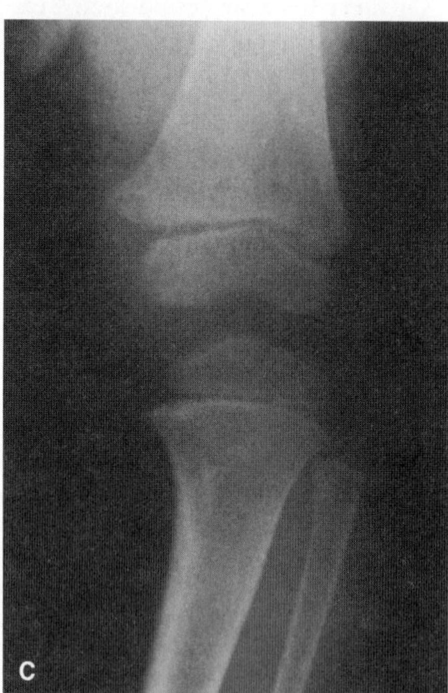

FIGURE 2-6 ■ *A,* Hazy metaphysis with cupping in a young boy with rickets. *B,* Accentuated genu barum is present. *C,* With vitamin D replacement therapy, the bony lesions healed in 6 months. (From Herring, T.: Tachdjian's Pediatric Orthopaedics, 3rd ed. Philadelphia, WB Saunders, 2002, p. 1688.)

(and child abuse) based on single-bone involvement. Infection, scurvy, and progressive diaphyseal dysplasia may also be in the differential diagnosis for children of all ages. Condition is benign and self limiting.

F. Connective Tissue Syndrome—A heterogeneous group of disorders with a broad spectrum of features.

1. Marfan's Syndrome—AD disorder of **fibrillin** associated with arachnodactyly (long, slender fingers), pectus deformities, scoliosis (50%), cardiac (valvular) abnormalities, and ocular findings ***(superior** lens dislocation in 60%).* Other abnormalities may include dural ectasia and meningocele. Joint laxity is treated conservatively. Scoliosis and spondylolisthesis

Table 2-3. OSTEOGENESIS IMPERFECTA TYPES

TYPE	INHERITANCE	SCLERAE	FEATURES
IA, IB	AD	Blue	Preschool age (tarda), hearing loss (IA = teeth involved; IB = teeth not affected)
II	AR	Blue	Lethal, concertina femur beaded ribs
III	AR	Normal	Fractures at birth, progressive short stature
IVA, IVB	AD	Normal	Milder form, normal hearing (IVA = teeth involved; IVB = teeth not affected)

are common. Bracing is ineffective. The presence of kyphosis with scoliosis requires anterior discectomy and fusion with posterior fusion and instrumentation.

2. Ehlers-Danlos Syndrome—AD disorder with *hyperextensibility* of "cigarette paper" skin, *joint hypermobility* and dislocation, soft-tissue/bone fragility, and soft-tissue calcification. Types II and III (of XI) are the most common and least disabling. Treatment consists of physical therapy, orthotics, and *arthrodesis*; soft-tissue procedures fail.
3. Homocystinuria—AR inborn error of *methionine metabolism* (decreased enzyme cystathionine beta-synthase). Accumulation of the intermediate metabolite homocysteine in the production of the amino acid cysteine can lead to osteoporosis, a marfanoid-like habitus (but with stiffening joints), and ***inferior*** *lens dislocation*. The diagnosis is made by demonstrating an increased homocysteine in urine (cyanide-nitroprusside test). This disorder is differentiated from Marfan's syndrome based on the direction of lens dislocation and the presence of osteoporosis in homocystinuria. Central nervous system effects, including mental retardation, are common in this disorder. Early treatment with vitamin B_6 and a decreased methionine diet is often successful.

G. Juvenile Idiopathic Arthritis (JID)—Includes both juvenile rheumatoid arthritis (JRA) and juvenile chronic arthritis. Persistent noninfectious arthritis lasting 6 weeks to 3 months and diagnosed after other possible causes have been ruled out. To confirm the diagnosis, one of the following is required: rash, presence of rheumatoid factor, iridocyclitis, C-spine involvement, pericarditis, tenosynovitis, intermittent fever, or morning stiffness.

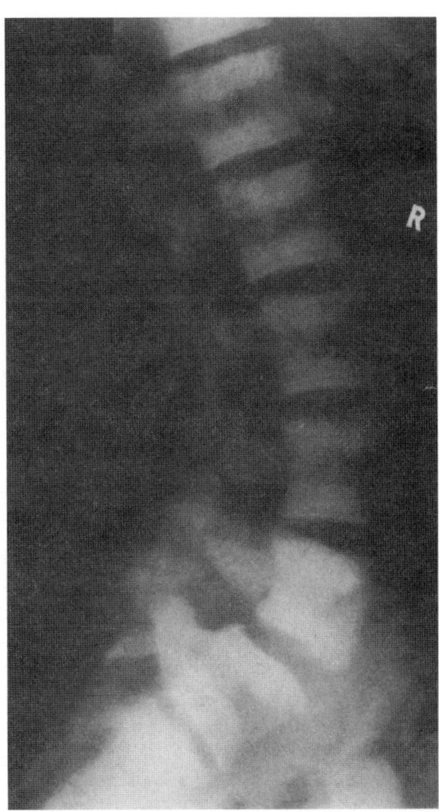

FIGURE 2-7 ■ Spine radiographs in osteopetrosis showing the "rugger jersey" pattern of ossification. (From Benson, M., Fixen, J., Macniol, M.: Children's Orthopaedics and Fractures, 1994, p. 86.)

JID affects girls more than boys and commonly involves the wrist (flexed and ulnar deviated) and hand (fingers extended, swollen, radially deviated). C-spine involvement can lead to kyphosis, facet ankylosis, and atlantoaxial subluxation. Lower-extremity problems include flexion contractures (hip and knee flexed, ankle dorsiflexed), subluxation, and other deformities (hip protrusio, valgus knees, equinovarus feet). Radiographs can show rarefaction of juxta-articular bone. In 50% of patients, symptoms resolve without sequelae; 25% are slightly disabled, and 20–25% have crippling arthritis/blindness. Therapy includes night splinting, salicylates and, rarely, synovectomy (for chronic swelling refractory to medical management). Arthrodesis and arthroplasty may be required for severe JID. Slit-lamp examination is required twice yearly, as progressive **iridocyclitis** can lead to rapid loss of vision if left untreated.

H. Ankylosing Spondylitis (AS)—Typically affects adolescent boys with asymmetric lower-extremity large-joint arthritis, heel pain, and sometimes, eye symptoms; hip and back pain (cardinal symptom) may develop later. **HLA-B27** test is positive in 90–95% of patients with AS or Reiter's syndrome but is also positive in 4–8% of all white Americans. Therefore HLA-B27 is not a good screening test for AS. **Limitation of chest-wall**

expansion is more specific than HLA-B27. Radiographs show bilateral, symmetric sacroiliac erosion, followed by joint space narrowing, later ankylosis, and late vertebral scalloping (bamboo spine). NSAIDs and physical therapy are the mainstays of treatment.

V. Birth Injuries

A. Brachial Plexus Palsy—Decreasing in severity as a result of better obstetric management, but still 2 per 1000 births have an injury associated with stretching or contusion of the brachial plexus. Occurs most commonly with *large babies, shoulder dystocia, forceps delivery, breech position, and prolonged labor*. Three types are commonly recognized (Table 2-4).

The key to therapy is maintaining passive ROM and awaiting return of motor function (up to 18 months). As many as 90% or more cases eventually resolve without intervention. However, **lack of biceps function 6 months after injury and Horner's syndrome** carry a poor prognosis. Late musculoskeletal surgery can improve functional motion. Options include releasing contractures (Fairbanks'), latissimus and teres major transfer to the shoulder external rotators (L'Episcopo's), tendon transfers for elbow flexion (Clarke's pectoral transfer and Steindler's flexorplasty), proximal humerus rotational osteotomy (Wickstrom's), and microsurgical nerve grafting. Reports have shown that release of the subscapularis tendon for internal rotation contracture, if performed by age 2 years, may result in improved active external rotation of the shoulder, with muscle transfer to assist in active external rotation.

B. Congenital Muscular Torticollis—A congenital deformity resulting from contracture of the sternocleidomastoid muscle. It is associated with other "molding disorders," such as *hip dysplasia and metatarsus adductus* (up to 20% association with hip dysplasia). The cause of congenital muscular torticollis remains uncertain, although most cases follow a difficult labor and delivery. Studies suggest that the muscle abnormality may be the result of an intrauterine compartment syndrome involving the sternocleidomastoid muscle compartment. Fibrosis of the muscle and a palpable mass are noted within the first 4 weeks of life. Most patients (90%) respond to passive stretching within the first year. Surgery (Z-plasty of the sternocleidomastoid) may be required if torticollis persists beyond the first year. Torticollis may also be associated with congenital atlanto-occipital abnormalities.

Table 2-4. BRACHIAL PLEXUS PALSY

TYPE	ROOTS	DEFICIT	PROGNOSIS
Erb Duchenne palsy	C5,6	Deltoid, cuff, elbow flexors, wrist and hand dorsiflexors; "waiter's tip" deformity	Best
Total plexus	C5,T1	Sensory and motor; flaccid arm	Worst
Klumpke	C8,T1	Wrist flexors, intrinsics; Horner's	Poor

C. Congenital Pseudarthrosis of the Clavicle—*Failure of union of the medial and lateral ossification centers of* ***the right clavicle*** (Fig. 2-8). Cause may be related to pulsations of the underlying subclavian artery. Presents as an enlarging, painless, nontender mass. Radiographs show rounded sclerotic bone at the pseudarthrosis site. *Surgery (open reduction/internal fixation with bone grafting) is indicated for unacceptable cosmetic deformities or with significant functional symptoms (mobility of the fragments and winging of the scapula) at ages 3–6.* Successful union is predictable (in contrast to congenital pseudarthrosis of the tibia).

VI. Cerebral Palsy

A. Introduction—**Nonprogressive** neuromuscular disorder with onset before age 2 years, resulting from injury to the immature brain. *The cause is most commonly not identifiable* but can include prenatal intrauterine factors, perinatal infections (toxoplasmosis, other infections, rubella, cytomegalovirus infection, and herpes simplex), *prematurity* (most common), anoxic injuries, and meningitis. This *upper motor neuron* disease results in a mixture of muscle weakness and spasticity. Initially, the abnormal muscle forces cause a dynamic deformity at joints. Persistent spasticity can lead to contractures, bony deformity, and ultimately joint subluxation/dislocation. MRI reveals periventricular leukomalacia.

B. Classification—CP can be classified based on physiology (according to the movement disorder) or anatomy (according to geographic distribution).

1. Physiologic Classification
   a. Spastic—Characterized by increased muscle tone and hyperreflexia with slow, restricted movements because of simultaneous contraction of agonist and antagonist. This form of CP is the *most common* and is most amenable to improvement of musculoskeletal function by operative intervention.
   b. Athetosis—Characterized by a constant succession of slow, writhing, involuntary movements, this form of CP is less common and more difficult to treat.
   c. Ataxia—Characterized by an inability to coordinate muscles for voluntary movement, resulting in an unbalanced, wide-based gait. Also less amenable to orthopaedic treatment.
   d. Mixed—Typically involves a combination of spasticity and athetosis with total body involvement.

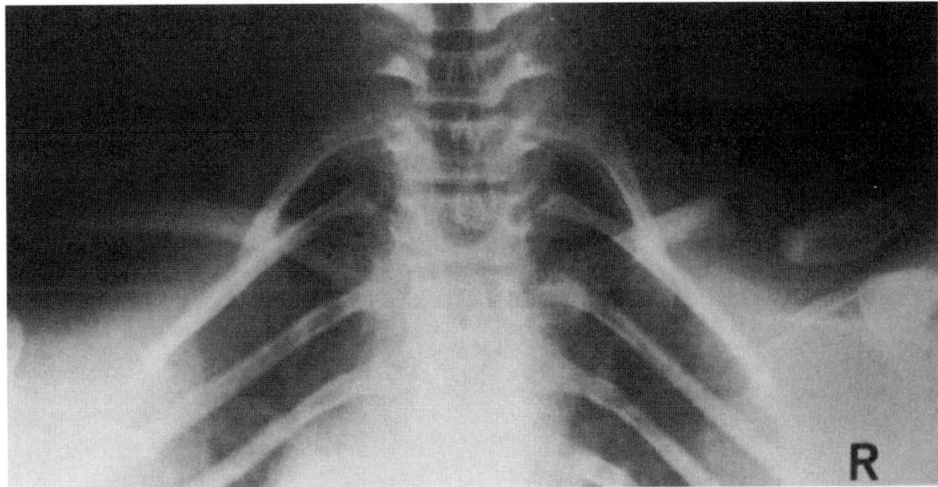

FIGURE 2-8 ■ Radiograph of bilateral clavicles in a case of congenital pseudarthrosis of clavicles. Note the pseudarthrosis is on the right side. (From Benson, M., Fixen, J., Macniol, M.: Children's Orthopaedics and Fractures, Churchill Livingstone, 1994, p. 362.)

2. Anatomic Classification
   a. Hemiplegia—Involves the upper and lower extremities on the same side, usually with spasticity. These children often develop early "handedness." All children with hemiplegia are eventually able to walk, regardless of treatment.
   b. Diplegia—Patients have more extensive involvement of the lower extremity than the upper extremity. Most diplegic patients eventually walk. IQ may be normal; strabismus is common.
   c. Total Involvement—These children have extensive involvement, low IQ, and high mortality rate; they usually are unable to walk.

C. Orthopaedic Assessment—Based on examination and thorough birth and developmental history. A patient's locomotor profile is based on the persistence of primitive reflexes; the presence of two or more usually means the child will be a nonambulator. Commonly tested reflexes include the Moro startle reflex (normally disappears by age 6 months) and the parachute reflex (normally appears by age 12 months). Surgery to improve function should be considered for a child more than 3 years old with spastic CP and voluntary motor control. Muscle imbalance yields later bony changes; therefore the general surgical plan is to perform *soft-tissue procedures early* and, if necessary, *bony procedures later*. Intramuscular botulinum A toxin can temporarily decrease dynamic spasticity. *The mechanism of action of botulinum toxin is a postsynaptic blockade at the neuromuscular junction.* Botulinum toxin effectiveness is limited to 6 months, and therefore it is not a permanent cure to spasticity. Instead, it is used to maintain joint motion during rapid growth when a child is too young for surgery. Selective dorsal root rhizotomy is a neurosurgical procedure designed to decrease lower-extremity spasticity. This treatment, indicated only for spastic CP, includes resection of dorsal rootlets not exhibiting a myographic or clinical response to stimulation. It may help reduce spasticity and complement orthopaedic management in spastic diplegic patients. It requires multilevel laminoplasty, which may lead to late instability and deformity. Discussion of hand disorders is included in Chapter 6, Hand and Microsurgery.

D. Gait Disorders—Probably the most common problem seen by orthopaedists. *Hemiplegics* usually present with *toe walking* only. The use of three-dimensional computerized gait analysis with dynamic electromyography and force-plate studies have allowed a more scientific approach to preoperative decision making and postoperative analysis of the results of CP surgery. Specific abnormal gait patterns have been identified, and surgical procedures have been devised to treat these patterns. The use of gait analysis has allowed a more individualized treatment plan for patients with CP. Lengthening of continuously active muscles and transfer of muscles out of phase is often helpful. Timing and indications for surgery require experience and skill because surgeries should often be done in tandem to best correct the problem (e.g., often, heel-cord lengthening alone exacerbates a crouched gait). In general, surgery is typically performed at 4–5 years old. A few generalized guidelines are given in Table 2-5.

Table 2-5. SURGICAL OPTIONS FOR GAIT DISORDERS

PROBLEM	DIAGNOSIS	SURGICAL OPTION
Hip flexion	Contraction (Thomas')	Psoas tenotomy or recession
Spastic hip	Decreased abduction/uncovered head	Adductor release, osteotomy (late)
Hip adduction	Scissoring gait	Adductor release
Femoral anteversion	Prone internal rotation increased	Osteotomy, VDRO, hamstring lengthening
Knee flexion	Contraction increased popliteal angle	Hamstring lengthening
Knee hypertension	Recurvatum	Rectus femoris lengthening
Stiff-leg gait	Electromyography—hamstring quadriceps continuous passive knee flexion decreased with hip extension	Distal rectus transfer to hamstrings
Talipes equines	Toe walking	Achilles lengthening
Talipes varus	Standing position	Split anterior or posterior tibialis transfer (based on EMG findings)
Talipes valgus	Standing position	Peroneal lengthening, Grice's subtalar fusion, calcaneal lengthening osteotomy
Hallux valgus	Examination/radiographs	Osteotomy, metatarsophalangeal fusion

VDRO, varus derotation osteotomy; EMG, electromyogram.

E. Spinal Disorders—Most commonly involve scoliosis, which can be severe, making proper wheelchair sitting difficult. **The risk for scoliosis is highest in children with total body involvement (spastic quadriplegic).** Surgical indications include curves >45–50 degrees or worsening pelvic obliquity. Two types of curves occur. Group I curves are double curves with thoracic and lumbar components and little pelvic obliquity. Group II curves are larger lumbar or thoracolumbar curves with marked pelvic obliquity (Fig. 2-9). Treatment is tailored to the needs of the patient. Custom-molded seat inserts allow better positioning but do not prevent curve progression. Small curves with no loss of function or large curves in severely involved patients may require observation alone. Group I curves in ambulants are treated as idiopathic scoliosis with posterior fusion and instrumentation. Group I curves in sitters and group II curves require *anterior and posterior fusion with segmental posterior instrumentation from the upper thoracic spine to the pelvis (Luque-Galveston technique).* The decision for one-stage versus two-stage anterior and posterior fusion is based on the surgeon's skill and speed, blood loss, and the presence of other factors. Kyphosis is also common and may require fusion and instrumentation. It is important to assess *nutritional status* (albumin <3.5 g/dL and white blood cell [WBC] count <1500 k/uL) preoperatively and consider gastrostomy tube placement before spinal surgery if indicated.

F. Hip Subluxation/Dislocation—Treated initially with a soft-tissue release (adductor/psoas) plus abduction bracing. Later, hip subluxation/dislocation may require femoral and/or acetabular osteotomies (Dega's) to maintain hip stability. The goal is to keep the hip reduced. Spastic dislocation often leads to painful arthritis, which is

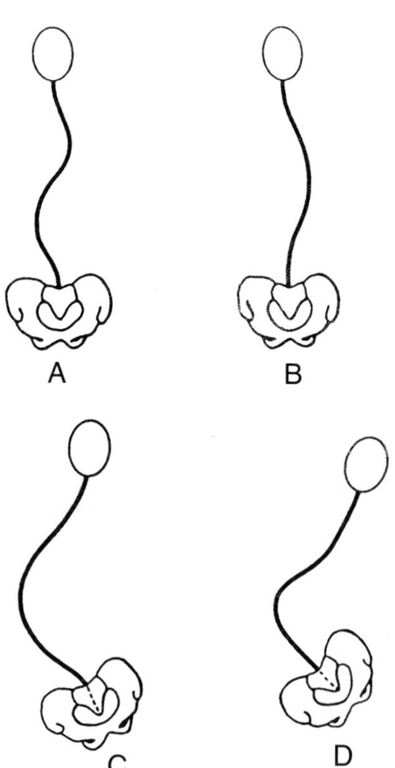

FIGURE 2-9 ■ Curve patterns of cerebral palsy scoliosis. Group I curves are double curves with thoracic and lumbar components. *A*, There is little pelvic obliquity; the curve may be well balanced; *B*, if the thoracic curve is more significant, there may be some imbalance. Group II curves are large lumbar or thoracolumbar curves with marked pelvic obliquity. *C*, There may be a short fractional curve between the end of the curve and the sacrum; *D*, the curve may continue into the sacrum, with the sacral vertebrae forming part of the curve. (From Weinstein, S.L.: The Pediatric Spine: Principles and Practice. New York, Raven Press, 1994.)

difficult to treat. This entity is characterized by four stages.

1. **Hip at Risk**—This situation is the only exception to the general rule of avoiding surgery in CP patients during the first 3 years of life. Characterized by abduction of <45 degrees, with partial uncovering of the femoral head on radiographs. May benefit from *adductor and psoas release*. Neurectomy of the anterior branch of the obturator nerve is now rarely performed because, by converting an upper motor neuron lesion to a lower motor neuron lesion, the muscle is made stiff and fibrotic.
2. **Hip Subluxation**—Best treated with adductor tenotomy in children with abduction of <20 degrees, sometimes with psoas release/recession. *Femoral or pelvic osteotomies* may be considered with femoral coxa valga and acetabular dysplasia, which is usually lateral and posterior.
3. **Spastic Dislocation**—May benefit from *open reduction, femoral shortening, varus derotation osteotomy, Dega's* (Fig. 2-10), *triple, or Chiari's osteotomy.* The type of pelvic osteotomy indicated is best determined by obtaining a three-dimensional computed tomographic (CT) scan, which will demonstrate the area of acetabular deficiency (anterior, lateral, or posterior) and the congruency of the joint surfaces. *Late dislocations* may best be left out or treated with a *Shanz abduction osteotomy* or a *Girdlestone resection arthroplasty* (resection below the lesser trochanter).
4. Windswept Hips—Characterized by abduction of one hip and adduction of the contralateral hip. Treatment is best directed at attempting to abduct the adducted hip with bracing or tenotomies and releasing the abduction contracture of the contralateral hip.

G. Knee Abnormalities—Usually includes hamstring contractures and decreased range of motion. Hamstring lengthening is often helpful (sometimes increases lumbar lordosis). Distal transfer of an out-of-phase rectus femoris muscle to semitendinosus or gracilis is indicated when there is loss of knee flexion during the swing phase of gait.

H. Foot and Ankle Abnormalities

1. Equinovalgus Foot—More commonly seen in spastic diplegia. *Caused by spastic peroneals, contracted heel cords, and ligamentous laxity.* Peroneus brevis lengthening is often helpful in correcting moderate valgus. Lateral column-lengthening calcaneal osteotomy is used to correct hindfoot valgus.

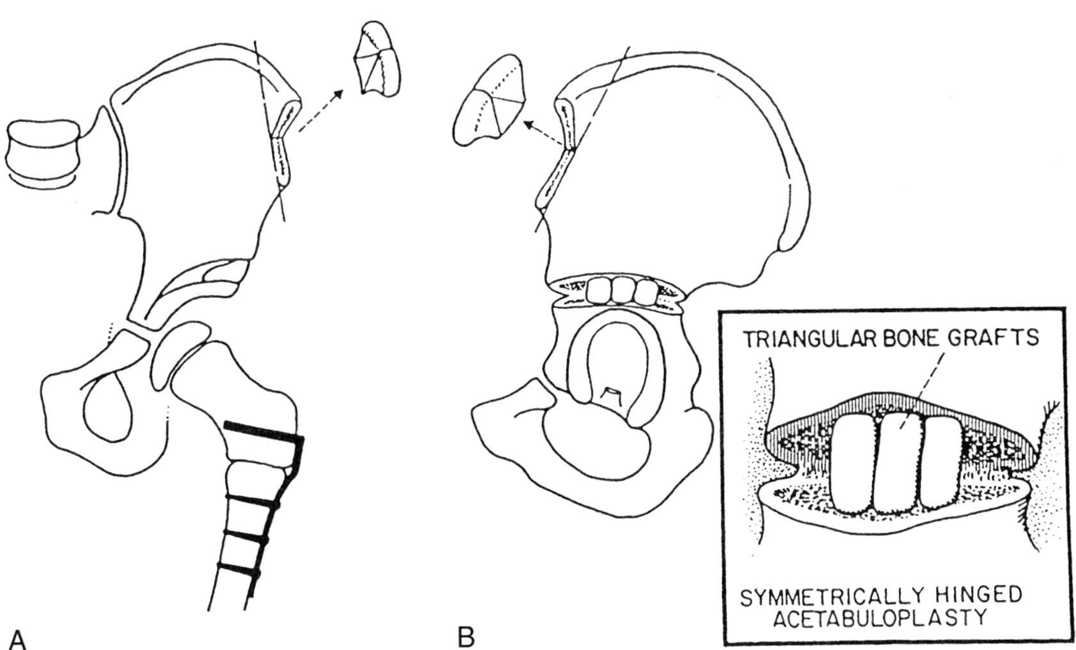

FIGURE 2-10 ■ Placement of graft for Dega's acetabuloplasty. *A*, A bone graft is obtained from the anterosuperior iliac crest and converted to three small triangles, with the base measuring 1 cm. *B*, The grafts are placed in the osteotomy site with the largest in the area where maximum improvement of coverage is desired. The triangular wedges are packed close to each other to prevent collapse, turning, or dislodgment; the result is a symmetric hinging on the **triradiate cartilage** (*inset*). With the medial wall of the pelvis maintained, the elasticity of the osteotomy keeps the wedges in place. No pins are necessary to maintain the osteotomy. (Adapted from Mubarak, S.J., Valencia, F.G., and Wenger, D.R.: One-stage reconstruction of the spastic hip. J. Bone Joint Surg. [Am.] 74:1352, 1992.)

2. Equinovarus Foot—More common in spastic hemiplegia, *caused by overpull of the posterior or anterior tibialis tendons (or both).* Lengthening of the posterior tibialis is rarely sufficient. Likewise, transfer of an entire muscle (posterior or anterior tibialis) is rarely recommended. **Split muscle transfers are helpful** in certain circumstances, especially **when the affected muscle is spastic during both stance and swing phases** of gait. The split posterior tibialis transfer (rerouting half of the tendon dorsally to the peroneus brevis) is used in cases with spasticity of the muscle, flexible varus foot, and weak peroneals. Complications include decreased foot dorsiflexion. Split anterior tibialis transfer (rerouting half of its tendon laterally to the cuboid) is used in patients with spasticity of the muscle and a flexible varus deformity. Most often it is coupled with an Achilles tendon lengthening and a posterior tibial tendon intramuscular lengthening (the Rancho procedure) to treat the fixed equinous contracture.

VII. Neuromuscular Disorders

A. Arthrogrypotic Syndromes

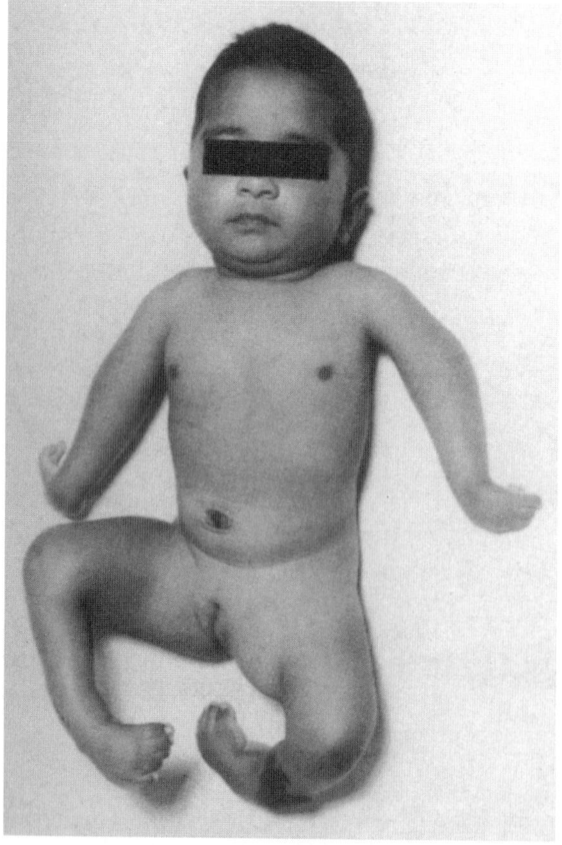

FIGURE 2-11 ■ Typical appearance of a child with arthrogryposis in all four limbs. Note the lack of creases at the elbows, the flexion contractures at the knees, and the severe clubfeet deformities. (From Benson, M., Fixen, J., Macniol, M.: Children's Orthopaedics and Fractures, Churchill Livingstone, 1994, p. 321.)

1. Arthrogryposis Multiplex Congenita (Amyoplasia)—*Nonprogressive* disorder with multiple congenitally rigid joints (Fig. 2-11). This disorder can be myopathic, neuropathic, or mixed and is associated with a decrease in *anterior horn cells* and other neural elements of the spinal cord. Intelligence is normal. Evaluation should include neurologic studies, enzyme tests, and muscle biopsy (at 3–4 months). *Affected patients typically have normal facies, normal intelligence, multiple joint contractures, and no visceral abnormalities.* Upper-extremity involvement usually includes adduction and internal rotation of the shoulder, extension of the elbow, and flexion and ulnar deviation of the wrist. The elbow has no creases. Treatment for the elbow deformities consists of passive manipulation and serial casting. Osteotomies are considered after 4 years of age to allow independent eating. One upper extremity should be left in extension at the elbow, for positioning and perineal care, and one elbow in flexion for feeding. *The lower-extremity deformities seen in arthrogryposis include teratologic hip dislocations, knee contractures, resistant clubfeet, and vertical talus.* Treatment includes early (6–9 months) soft-tissue releases (especially hamstrings) for knee contractures and medial open reduction with possible femoral shortening for hip dislocation. The foot deformities (clubfoot and vertical talus) are initially treated with a soft-tissue release, but later recurrences may need bone procedures (talectomy). The goal is a stiff, plantigrade foot that enables shoe wear and, possibly, ambulation. Knee contractures should be corrected before hip reduction in order to maintain the reduction. The spine may be involved with characteristic "C-shaped" (neuromuscular) scoliosis (33%). Fractures are also common (25%). These patients have an ability to adapt by using feet as functional appendages.
2. Distal Arthrogryposis Syndrome—AD disorder that predominantly affects hands and feet. Ulnarly deviated fingers (at metacarpal joints), metacarpal and proximal interphalangeal flexion contractures, and adducted thumbs with web-space thickening are common. *Clubfoot and vertical talus deformities* are common in the feet.
3. Larsen's Syndrome—Similar to arthrogryposis in clinical appearance, but joints are less rigid. The disorder is primarily associated with **multiple joint dislocations** (including bilateral congenital knee dislocations), flattened facies, scoliosis, clubfeet, and cervical kyphosis (watch for late myleopathy). These patients have normal intelligence.

4. Multiple Pterygium Syndrome—AR disorder that means "little wing" in Greek. It is characterized by cutaneous flexor surface webs (knee and elbow), congenital vertical talus, and scoliosis. Care must be taken when the webs are elongated because of the superficial nature of the neurovascular bundle.

B. Myelodysplasia (Spina Bifida)

1. Introduction—Disorder of incomplete spinal cord closure or secondary rupture of the developing cord secondary to hydrocephalus. Includes spina bifida occulta (defect in the vertebral arch with confined cord and meninges); meningocele (sac without neural elements protruding through the defect); myelomeningocele (spina bifida; protrusion of the sac with neural elements); and rachischisis (neural elements exposed with no covering). Can be diagnosed in utero (**increased alpha-fetoprotein**). Related to a folate deficiency in utero. Function is primarily related to the level of the defect and the associated congenital abnormalities. A type II Arlnold-Chirari malformation is the most common comorbidity. **Sudden changes in function (rapid increase of scoliotic curvature, spasticity, new neurologic deficit, or increase in urinary tract infections) can be associated with tethered cord, hydrocephalus (most common), or hydromyelia.** Head CT scans (70% of myelodysplastic patients have hydrocephalus) and myelography or spinal magnetic resonance imaging (MRI) are required. **Fractures are also common in myelodysplasia**, most often about the knee and hip in children 3 to 7 years old and frequently can be diagnosed only by noting **redness**, **warmth**, and **swelling**. Fractures are commonly misdiagnosed as infection in these patients. Treatment of fractures is conservative (avoid disuse). Fractures usually heal with abundant callus. The myelodysplasia level is based on the lowest functional level (Table 2-6). *L4 is a key level* because quadriceps can function and allow independent community ambulation (Fig. 2-12).

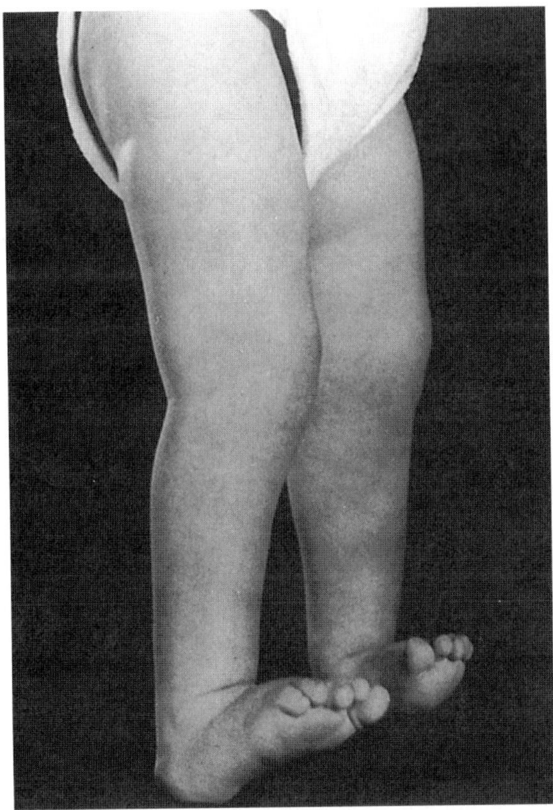

FIGURE 2-12 ■ Typical posture of the legs and feet in a child with myelodysplasia below L5. The feet assume a progressive calcaneus posture that demands surgical correction. (From Benson, M., Fixen, J., Macniol, M.: Children's Orthopaedics and Fractures, Churchill Livingstone, 1994, p. 281.)

2. Treatment Principles—Careful observation of patients with myelodysplasia is important. Several myelodysplasia "milestones" have been developed to assess progress (Table 2-7).

Treatment utilizes a team approach to allow maximum function consistent with the patient's level and other abnormalities. Proper use of orthotics is essential in myelodysplasia. Determination of ambulation potential is based on the level of the deficit. Surgery for myelodysplasia focuses on balancing of muscles and correction of deformities. Increased attention has been focused

Table 2-6. CHARACTERISTICS OF MYELODYSPLASIA LEVELS

LEVEL	HIP	KNEE	FEET	ORTHOSIS	AMBULATION
L1	External rotation/flexed		Equinovarus	HKAFO	Nonfunctional
L2	Adduction/flexed	Flexed	Equinovarus	HKAFO	Nonfunctional
L3	Adduction/flexed	Recurvatum	Equinovarus	KAFO	Household
L4	Adduction/flexed	Extended	Cavo varus	AFO	Household plus
L5	Flexed	Limited flexion	Calcaneal valgus	AFO	Community
S1			Foot deformities	Shoes	Near normal

HKAFO, hip-knee-ankle-foot orthosis; KAFO, knee-ankle-foot orthosis; AFO, ankle-foot orthosis.

Table 2-7. MILESTONES IN MYELODYSPLASIA

AGE (MONTHS)	FUNCTION	TREATMENT
4-6	Head control	Positioning
6-10	Sitting	Supports/orthotics
10-12	Prone mobility	Prone board
12-15	Upright stance	Standing orthosis
15-18	Upright mobility	Trunk/extremity orthosis

on **latex sensitivity** in myelodysplastic patients. Consideration should be given to providing a latex-free environment whenever surgical procedures are performed.

3. Hip Problems—Flexion contractures occur commonly in patients with thoracic/high lumbar myelomeningocele resulting from unopposed hip flexors or in patients who sit most of the time. Treatment for these patients consists of anterior hip release with tenotomy of the iliopsoas, sartorius, rectus femoris, and tensor fascia lata. For low-lumbar-level patients, the psoas should be preserved for independent ambulation. Hip abduction contracture can cause pelvic obliquity and scoliosis; it is treated with proximal division of the fascia lata and distal iliotibial band release (Ober-Yount procedure). Adduction contractures are treated with adductor myotomy. Hip dislocation occurs frequently in myelodysplastic patients because of paralysis of the hip abductors and extensors with unopposed hip flexors and adductors. **Hip dislocation is most common at the L3/L4 level.** Treatment of hip dislocation is controversial but, in general, containment is considered essential only in patients with a functioning quadriceps. Redislocation may occur no matter what treatment is used to maintain the reduction. Late dislocation at the low lumbar level may be due to a tethered cord, which must be released before reducing the hip.
4. Knee Problems—Usually includes quadriceps weakness (usually treated with knee-ankle-foot orthoses). Flexion deformities are not important in wheelchair-bound patients but can be treated with hamstring release and posterior capsular release. Recurvatum is rarely a problem and can be treated early with serial casting and knee-ankle-foot orthoses. Tenotomies (quadriceps lengthening) are sometimes required. Valgus deformities are usually not a problem. Sometimes iliotibial band release or late osteotomies are needed.
5. Ankle and Foot Deformities—Objectives are to obtain braceable, plantigrade feet and muscle balance. Affected patients may present with a valgus foot. Ankle-foot orthoses are often helpful, but clubfoot release, tendon release (anterior tibialis, Achilles), posterior tibialis lengthening, and other procedures may be required. Triple arthrodesis should be avoided in most myelodysplastic patients and is used only for severe deformities with sensate feet.

   Rigid clubfoot, secondary to retained activity or contracture of tibialis posterior and tibialis anterior, is common in L4-level patients. Treatment consists of complete subtalar release via a transverse (Cincinnati) incision, lengthening of tibialis posterior and Achilles tendons, and transfer of tibialis anterior tendon to the dorsal midfoot.
6. Spine Problems—Deformity can result from the spine disorder itself, resulting in an upper lumbar kyphosis or other congenital malformation of the spine due to a lack of segmentation or formation (i.e., hemivertebrae, diastomatomyelia, unsegmented bars). Scoliosis can also occur with severe lordosis as a result of muscular imbalance due to thoracic-level paraplegia. Spinal deformities are often severe and progressive. *Nearly all patients with thoracic-level paraplegia develop scoliosis.* Bracing is generally unsuccessful in treating these spinal deformities. **Rapid curve progression** can be associated with hydrocephalus or a **tethered cord**, which may manifest as lower-extremity spasticity or an increase in urinary tract infections. Severe, progressive curves require surgical treatment. Segmental Luque's sublaminar wiring with fixation to the pelvis (Galveston's technique) or fixation to the front of the sacrum (Dunn's technique) may be used. Kyphosis in myelodysplasia is a difficult problem. Resection of the kyphosis (kyphectomy) with local fusion (Figure 2-13 shows Lindseth's procedure) or fusion to the pelvis with instrumentation is required in severe cases. Infection rates are high because of frequent septicemia and poor skin quality over the lumbar spine.
7. Pelvic Obliquity—Can occur in myelodysplasia as a result of prolonged unilateral hip contractures or scoliosis. Custom seat cushions, thoracolumbosacral orthosis, spinal fusion, and ultimately pelvic osteotomies may be required for treatment.

C. Myopathies (Muscular Dystrophies)—Noninflammatory inherited disorders with progressive muscle weakness. Treatment focuses on physical therapy, orthotics, genetic counseling, and surgery for severe problems (tibialis posterior transfers, release of flexion contractures, and early fusion for neuromuscular scoliosis). Several types of muscular dystrophy are classified based on their inheritance pattern.

1. Duchenne's—*Sex-linked recessive* abnormality of young boys, manifested as clumsy walking, decreased motor skills, lumbar lordosis,

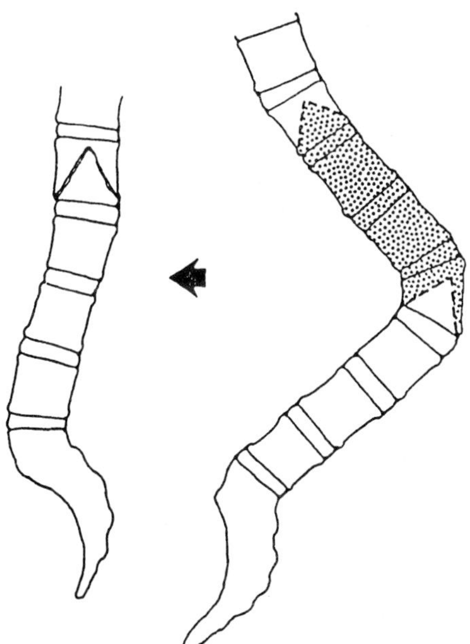

FIGURE 2-13 ■ Rigid S-shaped kyphosis is corrected by excising the vertebrae between the apex of the kyphosis and the lordosis and fusing the apical vertebrae. (From Lindseth, R.E.: Myelomeningocele. In Morrisey, R.T., ed.: Lovell and Winters' Pediatric Orthopaedics, 3rd ed. Philadelphia, JB Lippincott, 1990, p. 522.)

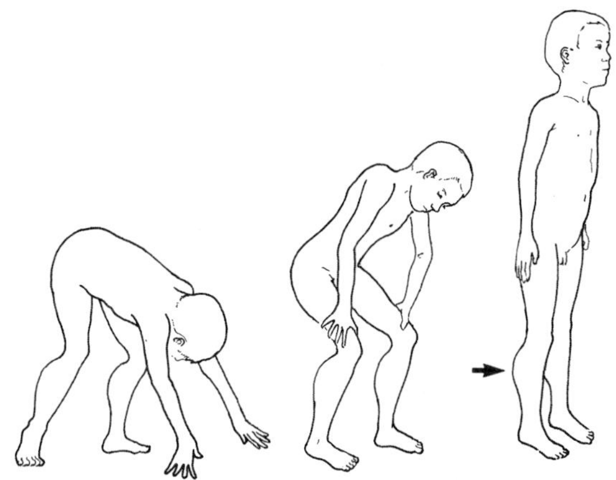

FIGURE 2-14 ■ Gowers' sign: the child arises from the floor by "walking up the thighs with his hands—a functional test for quadriceps muscle weakness. Note the bulky calf (*arrow*). (From Benson, M., Fixen, J., Macniol, M.: Children's Orthopaedics and Fractures, Churchill Livingstone, 1994, p. 305.)

calf pseudohypertrophy, positive Gowers' sign (rises by walking the hands up the legs to compensate for gluteus maximus and quadriceps weakness) (Fig. 2-14), **markedly elevated creatine phosphokinase (CPK)**, and **absent dystrophin protein** on muscle biopsy and DNA testing. *Hip extensors are typically the first muscle group affected.* Muscle biopsy sample shows foci of necrosis and connective tissue infiltration. Treatment is based on keeping patients ambulatory as long as possible. Patients lose independent ambulation by age 10; although controversial, the use of knee-ankle-foot orthoses and release of contractures can extend walking ability for 2–3 years. Patients are usually wheelchair bound by age 15 years. With no muscle support, scoliosis progresses rapidly between age 13–14 years. Patients can become bedridden by age 16 due to spinal deformity and are unable to sit for more than 8 hours. Scoliosis should be treated early (25–30 degrees of curvature) before pulmonary and cardiac function deteriorates. Surgical approach includes posterior spinal fusion with segmental instrumentation. These children usually die of cardiorespiratory complications before age 20. Differential diagnosis includes **Becker's** dystrophy (also sex-linked recessive with a decrease in dystrophin), which is often seen in red/green color-blind boys with a similar, but less severe, picture. Becker's dystrophy applies to all who live beyond age 22 years without respiratory support.

2. Fascioscapulohumeral—AD disorder typically seen in patients 6–20 years old with facial muscle abnormalities, normal CPK, and winging of the scapula (stabilized with scapulothoracic fusion).
3. Limb-Girdle—AR disorder; seen in patients 10–30 years old with pelvic or shoulder girdle involvement and increased CPK values.
4. Others—Gowers' (distal involvement, high incidence in Sweden); ocular, oculopharyngeal (high incidence in French Canadiens).

D. Polymyositis, Dermatomyositis—Characterized by a febrile illness that may be acute or insidious. Females predominate and typically exhibit photosensitivity and increased CPK and erythrocyte sedimentation rate values. Muscles are tender, brawny, and indurated. Biopsy demonstrates the *pathognomonic inflammatory response*.

E. Hereditary Neuropathies—Disorders associated with multiple central nervous system lesions, including the following:

1. Friedreich's Ataxia—AR disorder with problems with frataxin gene; spinocerebellar degenerative disease with mean onset between 7 and 15 years of age. Presents with staggering, wide-based gait; nystagmus; *cardiomyopathy; cavus foot* (treated with plantar release ± metatarsal and calcaneal osteotomies early, and triple arthrodesis later), *and scoliosis* (treated much like idiopathic scoliosis). **Involves motor and sensory defects with an increase in polyphasic potentials by EMG.** Ataxia forces use of a wheelchair by age 30, and death occurs between ages 40 and 50.

Table 2-8. MAJOR HEREDITARY MOTOR SENSORY NEUROPATHIES

TYPE	TERMINOLOGY	INHERITANCE	DESCRIPTION
I	Charcot-Marie-Tooth syndrome (hypertrophic form)	AD	Peroneal weakness, slow nerve conduction, absent reflexes
II	Charcot-Marie-Tooth syndrome (neuronal form)	Variable	Peroneal weakness, normal nerve conduction, and normal reflexes
III	Dejerine-Sottas disease	AR	Begins in infancy and more severe

2. Hereditary Sensory Motor Neuropathies (HSMNs)—A group of inherited neuropathic disorders with similar characteristics (Table 2-8).
3. Charcot-Marie-Tooth Disease (Peroneal Muscular Atrophy)—*AD* motor sensory demyelinating neuropathy. Two forms are described: a hypertrophic form with onset during the second decade of life, and a neuronal form with onset during the third or fourth decade but with more extensive foot involvement. Orthopaedic manifestations include pes cavus, hammer toes with frequent corns/calluses, peroneal weakness, and "stork legs." Low nerve conduction velocities with prolonged distal latencies are noted in peroneal, ulnar, and median nerves. Diagnosis is made most reliably by **DNA testing** for a duplication of a portion of chromosome 17. *Intrinsic wasting is noted in hands.* The most severely affected muscles are tibialis anterior, peroneous longus, and peroneous brevis. Treatment includes plantar release, posterior tibial tendon transfer (if hindfoot varus is flexible), triple arthrodesis (poor long-term results) versus calcaneal and metatarsal osteotomies (if bony deformity is fixed and foot not too short), Jones' procedure for hammer toes, and intrinsic procedures for hand deformity. **Involves motor defects much more than sensory defects.**
4. Dejerine-Sottas Disease—AR hypertrophic neuropathy of infancy. Delayed ambulation, pes cavus foot, footdrop, stocking-glove dysesthesia, and spinal deformities are common. Patient confined to wheelchair by third or fourth decade.
5. Riley-Day Syndrome (Dysautonomia)—One of five inherited (AR) sensory and autonomic neuropathies. This disease is found only in patients of *Ashkenazic Jewish ancestry*. Clinical presentation includes dysphagia, alacrima, pneumonia, excessive sweating, postural hypotension, and sensory loss.

F. Myasthenia Gravis—Chronic disease with insidious development of easy muscle fatigability after exercise. Caused by *competitive inhibition of acetylcholine receptors* at the motor endplate by antibodies produced in the thymus gland. Treatment consists of cyclosporin, antiacetylcholinesterase agents, or thymectomy.

G. Anterior Horn Cell Disorders
1. Poliomyelitis—Viral destruction of *anterior horn cells* in the spinal cord and brain stem motor nuclei; all but disappeared in the United States after vaccine was developed. Many surgical procedures still used were developed for treatment of polio. *The hallmark of polio is muscle weakness with normal sensation.*
2. Spinal Muscular Atrophy—AR; loss of horn cells from the spinal cord. There are three types (Table 2-9). Often associated with *progressive scoliosis* that is best treated surgically like Duchenne's muscular dystrophy curves, except that fusion may be required while patient is still ambulant (may result in loss of ambulatory ability). Patients have symmetric paresis with more involvement of the lower-extremity and proximal muscles.

H. Acute Idiopathic Postinfectious Polyneuropathy **(Guillain-Barré Syndrome)**—*Symmetric ascending motor paresis caused by demyelination following viral infection.* **Cerebrospinal fluid protein is typically elevated.** Usually self-limited; better prognosis with the acute form.

I. Overgrowth Syndromes
1. Proteus Syndrome—An overgrowth of the hands and feet with bizarre facial disfigurement, scoliosis, genu valgum, hemangiomas,

Table 2-9. TYPES OF SPINAL MUSCULAR ATROPHY

TYPE	DESCRIPTION	AGE OF PRESENTATION	PROGNOSIS
I	Acute Werdnig-Hoffman disease	less than 6 mo	Poor
II	Chronic Werdnig-Hoffman disease	6-24 mo	May live into 5th decade
III	Kugelberg-Welander disease	2-10 years	Good—may need respiratory support

lipomas, and nevi. Must be differentiated from neurofibromatosis and McCune-Albright.

2. Klippel-Trénaunay Syndrome—Overgrowth caused by underlying arteriovenous malformations. Associated with cutaneous hemangiomas and varicosities. Severely hypertrophied extremities often require amputation. Embolization is a treatment option in selected patients.
3. Hemihypertrophy—Can be caused by various syndromes, but most are idiopathic. Most commonly known cause is *neurofibromatosis.* This disorder is often associated with renal abnormalities (especially Wilms' tumor); **best evaluated with serial ultrasound until age 5 years**. Management of associated leg-length discrepancy is discussed below.

VIII. Pediatric Spine

B. Idiopathic Scoliosis

1. Introduction—A lateral deviation and rotational deformity of the spine without an identifiable cause. It may be related to a hormonal, brain stem, or proprioception disorder. Recent studies have suggested that hormonal factors *(melatonin)* may play a significant role in the cause. Most patients have a positive family history, but there is variable expressivity. The deformity is described as right or left based on the direction of the apical convexity. *Right-thoracic curves* are the most common, followed by double-major (right thoracic and left lumbar), left-lumbar, and right-lumbar curves. In adolescents *left-thoracic curves* are rare, and *evaluation of the spinal cord by MRI* is suggested to rule out cord abnormalities. Three distinct categories of idiopathic scoliosis have been identified: infantile, juvenile, and adolescent. The adolescent form is the most common. **Risk factors for curve progression include curve magnitudes (>20 degrees), younger age (<12 years), and skeletal immaturity [Risser stage (0–1)] at presentation** (Table 2-10). About 75% of immature patients with curves of 20–30 degrees will progress at least 5 degrees. Peak growth velocity is the best predictor of progression (predictions are based on age, menarchal status, and Risser's stage). Severe curves (>90 degrees) may be associated with cardiopulmonary dysfunction, early death, pain, and a decreased self-image.
2. Diagnosis—Patients are often referred from *school screening* where rotational deformities may be noted on forward flexion testing with a scoliometer. A threshold level of **7 degrees** is thought to be an acceptable compromise between over-referral and a high false-negative rate. Physical findings include shoulder elevation, waistline asymmetry, trunk shift, limb-length inequality, spinal deformity, and rib rotational deformity (rib hump). Careful neurologic examination for potential spinal cord disorder is important (especially with left thoracic curves). Abnormal neurologic examination (**especially aysmmetric abdominal reflexes** from syringomyelia) results warrant further work-up (MRI). Standing posteroanterior and lateral radiographs are obtained and curves are measured based on the Cobb method (Fig. 2-15). Typically, there is ***hypokyphosis*** of the apical vertebrae in the saggital plane because idiopathic scoliosis is a *lordoscoliotic deformity*. The potential coexistence of spondylolisthesis can also be noted on the lateral x-ray film.

Table 2-10. INCIDENCE OF PROGRESSION AS RELATED TO THE MAGNITUDE OF THE CURVE AND RISSER'S STAGE

	PERCENT OF CURVES THAT PROGRESSED	
Risser's Stage	*5–19 degrees (curves)*	*20–29 degrees (curves)*
0, 1	22%	68%
2, 3, 4	1.6%	23%

From Lonstein, J.E., and Carlson, J.M.: The prediction of curve progression in untreated idiopathic scoliosis during growth. J. Bone Joint Surg. [Am.] 66:1067, 1984.

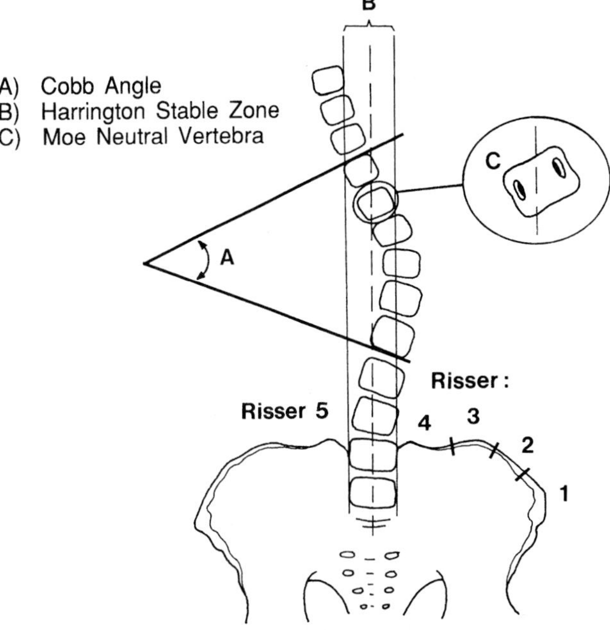

FIGURE 2-15 ■ Measurements for idiopathic scoliosis. Note *A*, Cobb's angle; *B*, Harrington's stable zone; *C*, Moe's neutral vertebra; and *1–5*, Risser's staging.

Inclusion of the iliac crest on radiographs allows determination of skeletal maturity based on the *Risser sign* (based on ossification of the iliac crest apophysis and graded 0–5). *An MRI scan is obtained for cases with noted structural abnormalities on plain films, excessive kyphosis, juvenile-onset scoliosis (age over 11 years), rapid curve progression, neurologic signs/symptoms, associated syndromes, and left thoracic/thoracolumbar curves.*

3. Treatment—*Based on the maturity of the patient (Risser stage and presence of menarche), magnitude of the deformity, and curve progression.* Treatment options include *observation, bracing, and surgery.* Exercise and electrical stimulation have not been shown to affect the natural history of curve progression. Bracing may help to halt or slow curve progression but does not reverse the magnitude of the deformity. The Milwaukee brace (cervicothoracolumbosacral orthosis) or Boston underarm brace with Milwaukee superstructure is used for curves with the apex at or above T7. The Boston-type underarm thoracolumbosacral orthosis brace is used for curves with the apex at T8 or below. Patients with thoracic lordosis or hypokyphosis are poor candidates for bracing. *The effectiveness of bracing patients with idiopathic scoliosis is dose related* (the more the brace is worn each day, the more effective it is). Although the efficacy of full-time wear has been well demonstrated, long-term prospective studies on part-time brace wear have not been done. *The basic options for the surgical treatment of idiopathic scoliosis are anterior spinal fusion (ASF) with instrumentation, posterior spinal fusion (PSF) with instrumentation, or both ASF and PSF.* **The indications for ASF and PSF in idiopathic scoliosis are severe deformities (>75 degrees) and crankshaft prevention (Risser's stage 0, girls <10 and boys <13 years old, before or during peak growth velocity).** The decision between ASF alone versus PSF is made on a case-by-case basis. *In general, ASF alone with instrumentation is used in thoracolumbar and lumbar cases since better coronal, axial, and saggital correction can be achieved while saving lumbar fusion levels.* Current research efforts are in progress to extend the use of ASF with instrumentation proximally into the thoracic spine. *The benefits of ASF with instrumentation are saving fusion levels and improved correction. The disadvantages are lumbar kyphosis, thoracic hyperkyphosis, and rod breakage (pseudarthrosis).* **PSF with instrumentation remains the gold standard for thoracic and double major curves.** With the newer instrumentation systems, it is generally not necessary to use postoperative bracing or casting.

4. Fusion Levels—Successful surgery is based on choosing appropriate fusion levels, among other considerations. Several methods have been developed to select the correct levels. The goal is to fuse the spinal levels necessary to establish a well-balanced spine in the coronal and sagittal planes. Harrington recommends fusion one level above and two levels below the end vertebrae if these levels fell within the **stable zone** (within parallel lines drawn vertically up from the lumbosacral facet joints). Moe recommends fusion to the **neutral vertebrae** (without rotation, pedicles symmetric). The **stable vertebra** is defined as the most proximal vertebrae that is most closely bisected by the center sacral line. It is almost never necessary to fuse to the pelvis in adolescent idiopathic scoliosis. Cochran identified a markedly *increased incidence of late, low back pain with fusion to L5 and some increase with fusion to L4.* Therefore every attempt should be made to **stop the fusion at L3** or above. **King, Moe, et al., identified five patterns** and treatment options (Fig. 2-16). These treatment options were developed in the Harrington instrumentation era. The newer segmental spinal instrumentation systems allow more powerful correction of these three-dimensional deformities. A new classification by **Lenke et al.**, defines six curve types, three lumbar modifiers, and thoracic sagittal plane analysis.

5. Complications—The most disastrous complication of spinal surgery is a *neurologic deficit.* Successful surgical intervention is based on careful technique (intraoperative monitoring [somatosensory-evoked potentials and motor-evoked potentials] is helpful ± Stagnara's wake-up test and clonus tests). It is especially useful in patients with congenital kyphoscoliosis. *Attempting excessive correction or placement of sublaminar wires is associated with an increased risk of neurologic damage.* Minimizing blood loss and maximizing the use of autologous blood is important to avoid transfusion-associated problems. *Surgical complications include pseudarthrosis (1–2%), early wound infection (1–2%), implant failure (early hook cutout and late rod breakage and pain from prominent hardware).* Late rod breakage frequently signifies failure of fusion. Only an asymptomatic pseudarthrosis (no pain or loss of curve correction) should be observed because the results of the late repair do not differ from those performed earlier. *Use of*

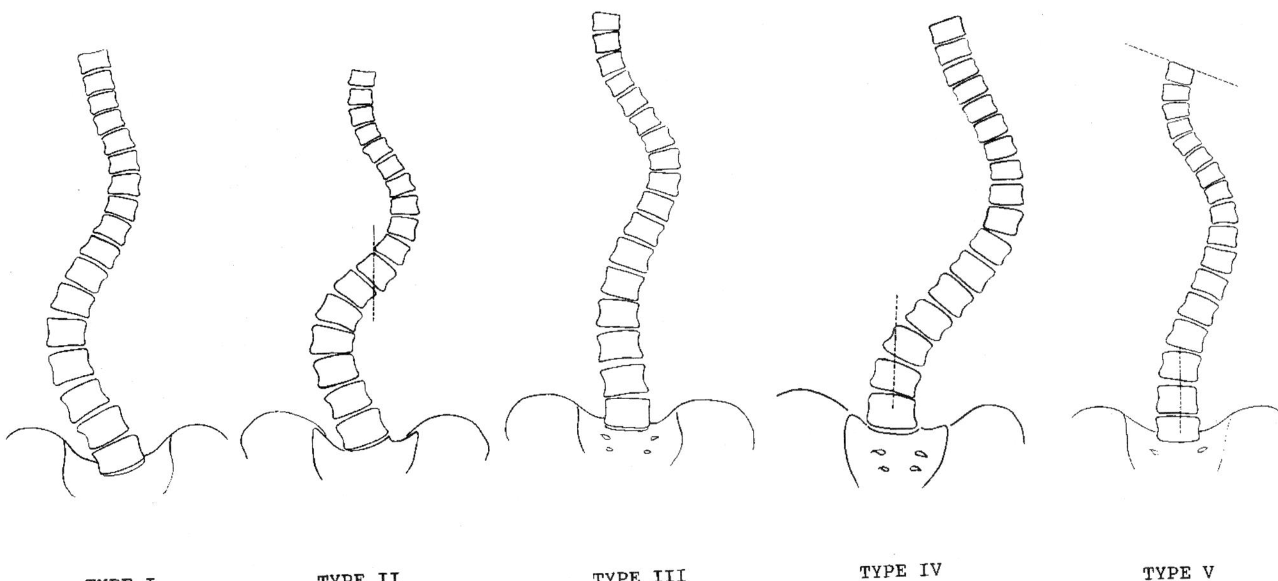

FIGURE 2-16 ■ Five types of scoliotic curves (I–V). See text for description. (From King, H.A., Moe, J.H., Bradford, D.S., et al.: The selection of fusion levels in thoracic idiopathic scoliosis. J. Bone Joint Surg. [Am.] 65:1302–1313, 1983.)

a compression implant facilitates pseudarthrosis repair. Creation of a **"flat back syndrome,"** or early fatigability and pain due to loss of lumbar lordosis, can be minimized with rod contouring in the saggital plane and effective use of compression and distraction devices. Treatment of this condition requires revision surgery with posterior closing wedge osteotomies. The results appear to be improved, with maintenance of correction, if anterior release and fusion precede the posterior osteotomies. **The crankshaft phenomenon** occurs in the setting of continued anterior spinal growth after posterior fusion in skeletally immature patients. It results in increased rotation and deformity of the spine as continued anterior growth causes a spin around the posterior tether (fusion mass). This situation is best avoided by anterior discectomy and fusion coupled with PSF as described previously.

6. Infantile Idiopathic Scoliosis—Presents at <3 years old with more commonly a **left-sided thoracic scoliosis, male predominance, plagiocephaly (skull flattening), and other congenital defects**. Most cases have been reported from Great Britain. The two factors most affecting progression are *curve magnitude and the apical rib-vertebral angle difference of Mehta*. Most curves <25 degrees with rib-vertebral angle of Mehta >20 degrees tend to resolve spontaneously, and observation is appropriate in these patients. Surgical options for severe curves include instrumentation ("growing rods") without fusion or ASF/PSF combination. Any child with infantile idiopathic scoliosis should have MRI preoperatively to rule out any possible spinal cord disease (20% incidence).
7. JID—Scoliosis in 3- to 10-year-olds is similar to adolescent scoliosis in terms of presentation and treatment. *A high risk of curve progression is seen*; 70% require treatment, with 50% needing bracing and 50% requiring surgery. Fusion should be delayed until the onset of the adolescent growth spurt if possible (unless curve magnitude is >50 degrees). The use of spinal instrumentation without fusion (as for infantile scoliosis) may facilitate this delay. In patients with severe deformities that require surgery, a careful assessment of their skeletal maturity should be done. In patients with multiple risk factors for skeletal immaturity, ASF and PSF with instrumentation should be performed to prevent the occurrence of crankshaft phenomenon.

B. Neuromuscular Scoliosis—Many children with neuromuscular disorders develop scoliosis or other spinal deformities. In contrast to idiopathic curves, neuromuscular curves are longer; involve more vertebrae; are less likely to have compensatory curves; *progress more rapidly and may progress after maturity; and are often associated with* ***pelvic obliquity****, bony deformities, and cervical involvement.* Pulmonary complications are also more frequent, including decreased pulmonary function, pneumonia, and atelectasis. For patients who are already wheelchair bound, curve progression may make them bedridden. Orthotic use is advised until age 10–12 years, at which time corrective fusion is usually performed to provide permanent stability in severe deformities. Underarm (Boston-type) braces are most often used. The surgical treatment of neuromuscular scoliosis often involves the fusion of more levels than for idiopathic curves. Fusion to the pelvis may be required for fixed pelvic obliquity. The ***Galveston technique*** of pelvic fixation has traditionally been used (bending the caudal end of the rods from the lamina of S1 to pass into the posterosuperior iliac spine and between the tables of the ilium just anterior to the sciatic notch). Other techniques include Dunn-McCarthy S rods and sacral and iliac screws. The goal of treatment is stability and truncal balance with a level pelvis. Patients with upper motor neuron disease (CP) are initially treated with wheelchair modifications or seat orthotics but require fusion for curve progression to >50 degrees. *Children with severe involvement require fusion to the sacrum and may require both anterior and posterior procedures.* Posterior fusion alone is associated with higher pseudarthrosis rates and development of the crankshaft phenomenon (delayed bone age is common in neuromuscular patients).

C. Congenital Spinal Disorders—Due to a developmental defect in the formation of the mesenchymal anlage during the 4th to 6th week of development. Three basic types of defect are noted: **failure of segmentation** (typically results in a vertebral bar), **failure of formation** (due to lack of material, may result in hemivertebrae), and **mixed**. Three-dimensional CT is helpful for defining the type (Fig. 2-17) of vertebral anomaly. Spinal MRI scans should be obtained before any surgery to assess for intraspinal anomalies. *Associated anomalies include genitourinary (25%), cardiac (10%), and dysraphism (25%, usually diastomatomyelia). Renal ultrasonography is used to rule out associated kidney abnormalities.*

1. Congenital Scoliosis—Most common congenital spinal disorder. Risk for progression is dependent on the morphology of the vertebrae. A fully segmented hemivertebra is free with normal disc spaces on both sides (higher risk of progression), whereas an unsegmented hemivertebra is fused above and below (lower risk) (see Fig. 2-17). An incarcerated hemivertebra (within the lateral margins of the vertebrae above and below) has a better prognosis than an unincarcerated (laterally positioned) hemivertebra. A unilateral unsegmented bar is a common disorder and is likely to progress. The best prognosis is with a block vertebra (bilateral failure of segmentation). **The worst prognosis (most likely to progress) is seen with *a unilateral unsegmented bar with a contralateral, fully segmented hemivertebra and is an indication for surgery at presentation.*** The treatment options include ASF and PSF in situ, or convex anterior and posterior hemiepiphysiodesis. *Other deformities should demonstrate progression before surgical options are considered.* Bracing may be effective for compensatory curves or for smaller, supple curves above a vertebral anomaly, but it is ineffective for controlling congenital curves. Anterior and posterior hemivertebral excision may be indicated for lumbosacral hemivertebrae associated with progressive curves and an oblique take-off (severe truncal imbalance). Isolated hemivertebral excision can destabilize the spine on the convex side and should be accompanied by anterior/posterior arthrodesis with instrumentation to stabilize the adjacent vertebrae. Anterior and posterior convex hemiepiphysiodesis/arthrodesis is safer, but correction of imbalance is less predictable.

Posterior fusion in situ is the gold standard of treatment for most progressive curves. In young patients (girls <10, boys <13 years old), the crankshaft phenomenon may occur because of continued anterior spinal growth; in these cases anterior/posterior fusion may be required. A summary of treatment recommendations for congenital scoliosis is found in Table 2-11.

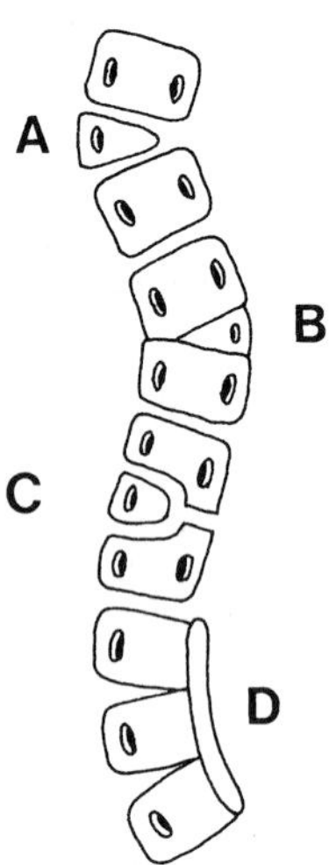

FIGURE 2-17 ■ Vertebral anomalies leading to congenital scoliosis. *A,* Fully segmented hemivertebra. *B,* Unsegmented hemivertebra. *C,* Incarcerated hemivertebra. *D,* Unilateral unsegmented bar.

Table 2-11. CONGENITAL SCOLIOIS PATTERNS AND THE RISK OF PROGRESSION

RISK OF PROGRESSION (HIGHEST TO LOWEST)	CHARACTER OF CURVE PROGRESSION	TREATMENT OPTIONS
Unilateral unsegmented bar with contralateral hemivertebra	Rapid and relentless	Posterior spinal fusion (add anterior fusion for girls age <10 years, boys <12)
Unilateral unsegmented bar	Rapid	Same
Fully segmented hemivertebra	Steady	Anterior spinal fusion Hemivertebra excision
Partially segmented hemivertebra	Less rapid; curve usually <40 degrees at maturity	Observation, hemivertebra excision
Incarcerated hemivertebra	May slowly progress	Observation
Nonsegmented hemivertebra	Little progression	Observation

2. Congenital Kyphosis—May be secondary to failure of formation (type I), failure of segmentation (type II), or mixed abnormalities (type III). **Failure of formation (type I, most common) has the worst prognosis** for progression (95% progress) and neurologic involvement of all spinal deformities. **Type I congenital kyphosis is also the most likely to result in paraplegia (neurofibromatosis is second)**. *The presence of significant congenital kyphosis secondary to failure of formation (type I) is an indication for surgery.* Posterior fusion is favored in young children (<5 years old) with curves <50 degrees. This is essentially a *posterior (convex) hemiepiphysiodesis*. Combined anterior/posterior fusion is reserved for older children or more severe curves. Anterior vertebrectomy, spinal cord decompression, and anterior fusion followed by posterior fusion are indicated for curves associated with neurologic deficits. A type II congenital kyphosis can be observed to document progression, but progressive curves should be fused posteriorly.

D. Neurofibromatosis—AD disorder of neural crest origin, often associated with neoplasia and skeletal abnormalities. It is characterized by neurofibromas and café-au-lait spots. *The spine is the most common site of skeletal involvement.* Careful screening of scoliosis radiographs for vertebral scalloping; **enlarged foramina**; penciling of transverse processes or ribs; severe apical rotation; **short, tight curves**; or a paraspinal mass may differentiate this condition from idiopathic scoliosis. Spinal deformity secondary to neurofibromatosis is characteristically kyphoscoliosis in the thoracic region with dystrophic changes, but nondystrophic scoliosis or cervical involvement may also be noted. Nondystrophic scoliosis is treated as appropriate for idiopathic scoliosis, but with **dystrophic deformities nonoperative treatment of curves >20 degrees is futile**. *Surgical treatment consists of anterior/posterior fusion with instrumentation for patients with progressive dystrophic deformities.* The reported pseudarthrosis rate is very high with PSF alone. If fusion is required in the juvenile age group, anterior and posterior fusion is routinely performed to avoid the crankshaft phenomenon. Neurologic involvement is common in neurofibromatosis and may be caused by the deformity itself: an intraspinal tumor, a soft-tissue mass, or dural ectasia. Therefore any patient with neurofibromatosis undergoing spinal surgery should have an **MRI** preoperatively. Because of a high pseudarthrosis rate, some authors recommend routine augmentation of the posterior fusion mass at 6 months postoperatively with repeat iliac crest bone graft. C-spine involvement includes kyphosis or atlantoaxial instability. Posterior fusion with autologous grafting and halo immobilization is recommended for severe C-spine deformity with instability. Isolated kyphosis of the T-spine is treated with anterior decompression of the kyphotic angular cord compression, followed by anterior and posterior fusion.

E. Other Spinal Abnormalities

1. Diastematomyelia—Fibrous, cartilaginous, or osseous bar creating a longitudinal cleft in the spinal cord (Fig. 2-18). More commonly occurs in the lumbar spine and can lead to tethering of the cord with associated neurologic deficits. Intrapedicular widening on plain radiographs is suggestive, and myelo-CT or MRI is necessary to fully define the disorder. A diastomatomyelia must be resected before correction of a spinal deformity, but if otherwise asymptomatic and without neurologic sequelae, it may be observed.
2. Sacral Agenesis—Partial or complete absence of the sacrum and lower lumbar spine. **Highly associated with maternal diabetes**, it is often accompanied by gastrointestinal, genitourinary, and cardiovascular abnormalities. Clinically, children have a prominent lower lumbar spine and atrophic

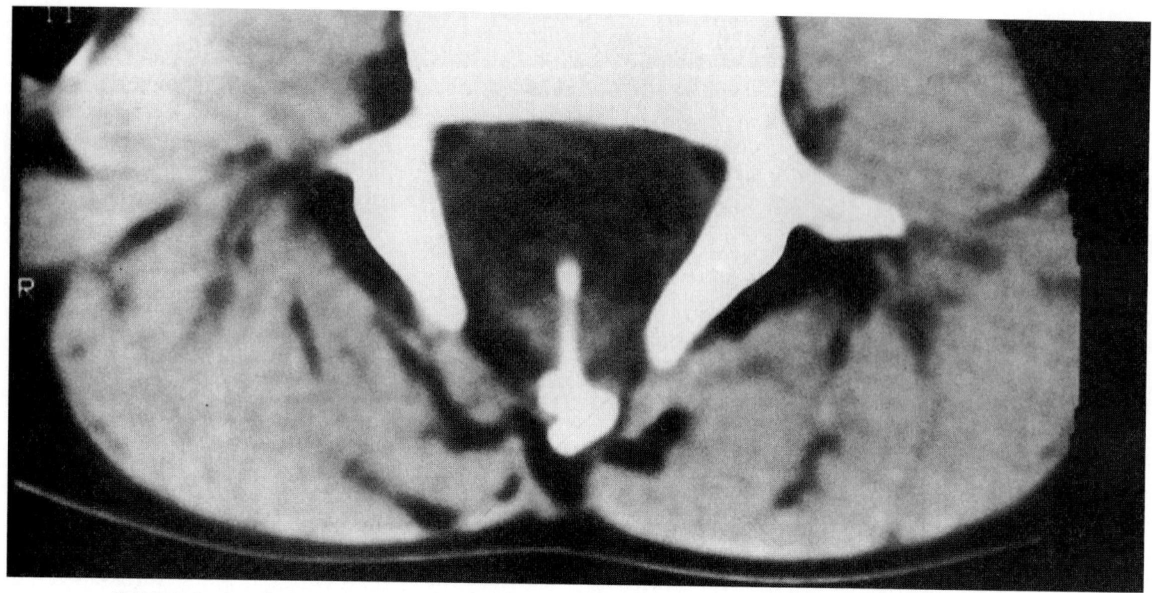

FIGURE 2-18 ■ Ten-year-old girl with diastematomyelia. Note the incomplete bony spur between the hemicords. (From Benson, M., Fixen, J., Macniol, M.: Children's Orthopaedics and Fractures, Churchill Livingstone, 1994, p. 299.)

lower extremities; they may sit in a "Buddha" position. Motor impairment is at the level of the agenesis, but sensory innervation is largely spared. Management may include amputation or spinal-pelvic fusion.

F. Low Back Pain (Table 2-12)—In children, complaints of low back pain and especially painful scoliosis should be taken seriously. Acute back pain can be associated with *discitis* (presents as refusal to sit or walk, increased ESR, and later disc-space narrowing with preservation of the endplates—takes 3 weeks to appear on plain films) or osteomyelitis (systemic illness, leukocytosis). Rang and Wenger discussed the difficulty of differentiating between discitis and osteomyelitis, and they recommended use of the term infectious spondylitis to describe disc-space infections in children. Occasionally, herniated nucleus pulposus, presenting as sciatica and back pain in older children, occurs and may require operative intervention but most resolve with time. *Spondylolysis* (stress fracture at the pars interartilularis) is common after athletic injuries, especially activities involving **repetitive hyperextension of the lumbosacral spine** (gymnastics, football lineman) and is best visualized with a CT scan or SPECT. Spondylolisthesis (forward slippage of the proximal vertebra on the distal vertebra) is most commonly seen at L5–S1. Can be lytic (from spondylosis) or dysplastic (congenital absence or dysplasia of the facets) and is defined by the degree of slip (**Meyerding classification**). Dysplastic spondylolisthesis is more at risk to progress especially in the skeletally immature patient. **The larger the slip the greater the chance of progression**. Asymptomatic slips should be observed. Conservative treatment, including avoiding the repetitive activity and bracing, is usually adequate. If conservative measures fail then fusion (if at L5) versus repair of pars defect (if at L4 or higher) is appropriate. Decompression (**Gill procedure**) must also be considered for neurologic compromise. Painful scoliosis often signifies a tumor (e.g., osteoid osteoma) or spinal cord anomaly and should be investigated aggressively. *A bone scan is an excellent screening method for a child or adolescent with back pain*.

Table 2-12. DIFFERENTIAL FOR LOW-BACK PAIN IN CHILDREN

CATEGORY	DISEASE
Mechanical	Muscle strain Herniated nucleus pulposis
Infectious & tumor	Discitis osteomyelitis Eosinophilic granuloma Osteoid osteoma Osteoblastoma Ewing's spinal cord tumor Metastatic disease
Developmental	Spondylosis Spondylosithesis Syringomyelia Tethered cord

G. Kyphosis
1. Congenital Kyphosis—See the previous discussion of congenital spinal disorders.
2. Scheuermann's Disease—Classic definition is increased thoracic kyphosis (>45 degrees)

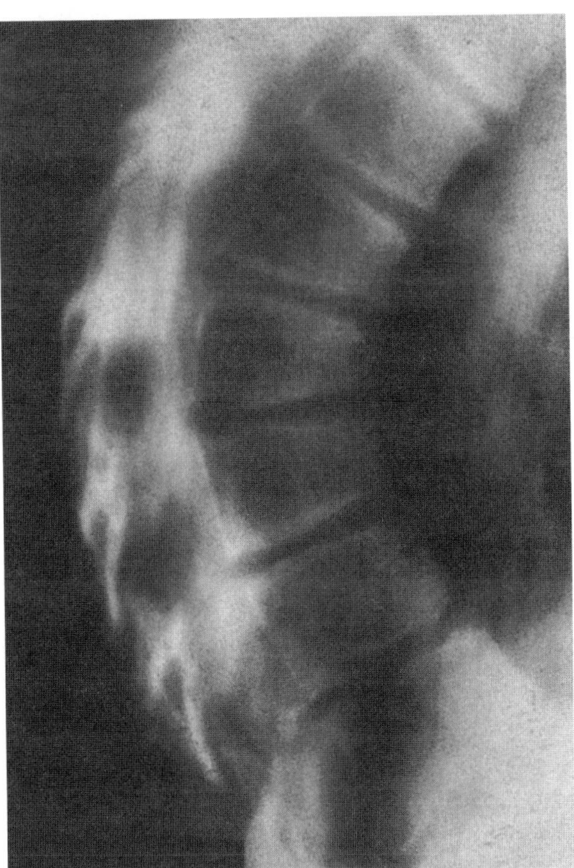

FIGURE 2-19 ■ Lateral radiograph of a patient with Scheuermann's thoracic hyperkyphosis. Note the anterior wedging at three sequential vertebra. (From Benson, M., Fixen, J., Macniol, M.: Children's Orthopaedics and Fractures, Churchill Livingstone, 1994, p. 19.)

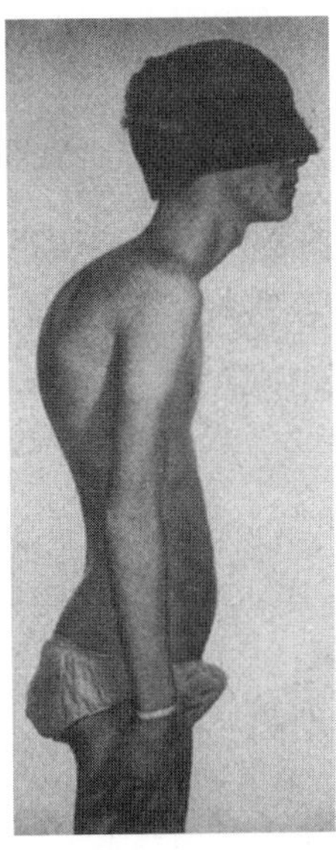

FIGURE 2-20 ■ Clinical photograph of Scheuermann's thoracic kyphosis. (From Benson, M., Fixen, J., Macniol, M.: Children's Orthopaedics and Fractures, Churchill Livingstone, 1994, p. 610.)

with 5 degrees or more anterior wedging at three sequential vertebrae. Other radiographic findings include disc narrowing, **endplate irregularities**, spondylolysis (30–50%), scoliosis (33%), and Schmorl's nodes (Sorenson) (Figs. 2-19 and 2-20). Scheuermann's disease is more common in males and typically presents in adolescents with poor posture and occasionally aching pain. Physical examination characteristically shows tight hamstrings and hyperkyphosis that does not reverse on attempts at hyperextension. Neurologic sequelae secondary to disc herniation or extradural spinal cysts are rare but have been reported. Treatment consists of **bracing** (a modified Milwaukee brace) for a progressive curve in a patient with 1 year or more of skeletal growth remaining (Risser's stage 3 or below). Bracing may effect 5–10 degrees of permanent curve correction but is less effective for kyphosis of >75 degrees. For the skeletally mature patient with severe kyphosis (>75 degrees), surgical correction may be indicated. *Posterior fusion with dual rods segmentally attached to compression instrumentation is the treatment of choice, preceded by anterior release and interbody fusion for curves of >75 degrees or those not correcting to <55 degrees on hyperextension.* Thorascopic anterior discectomy and interbody fusion have decreased the morbidity associated with thoracotomy for anterior release and fusion. Lumbar Scheuermann's disease is less common than the thoracic variety but more often causes back pain on a mechanical basis (more common in athletes and manual laborers). The pain is often self-limited. Lumbar Scheuermann's disease also demonstrates irregular vertebral end plates with Schmorl's nodes and decreased disc height, but it is not associated with vertebral wedging.

3. Postural Round Back—Also associated with kyphosis but does not demonstrate vertebral body changes. Forward bending demonstrates kyphosis, but there is no sharp angulation as in Scheuermann's disease. Correction with backward bending and prone hyperextension is typical. Treatment includes a hyperextension exercise program. Occasionally, bracing is required, but surgery is rarely indicated.
4. Other Causes of Kyphosis—Trauma, infections, spondylitis, bone dysplasias (mucopolysaccharidoses, Kniest's syndrome, diastrophic dysplasia), and neoplasms. Additionally, *postlaminectomy kyphosis (most often for spinal cord abnormalities) can be severe and requires anterior and posterior fusion early. Performance of total*

laminectomy in immature patients without stabilization is contraindicated.

H. Cervical Spine Disorders

1. Klippel-Feil Syndrome—Multiple abnormal cervical segments due to failure of normal segmentation or formation of cervical somites at 3–8 weeks' gestation. Often associated with congenital scoliosis, renal disease (aplasia 33%), synkinesis (mirror motions), Sprengel's deformity (30%), congenital heart disease, brainstem abnormalities, or congenital cervical stenosis. ***The classic triad of low posterior hairline, short "web" neck, and limited cervical ROM is seen in fewer than 50% of cases.*** Most therapy is conservative, but chronic pain with myelopathy associated with instability may require surgery. Disc degeneration occurs in almost 100% of cases. Affected children should avoid collision sports.
2. Atlantoaxial Instability
   a. Anteroposterior Instability—*Associated with Down's syndrome (trisomy 21), JRA, various osteochondrodystrophies, os odontoideum, and other abnormalities.* In patients with Down's syndrome and a normal neurologic examination, simple avoidance of contact sports is appropriate, but with any acute or progressive neurological symptoms posterior spinal fusion is indicated (high complication rate).
   b. Rotatory Atlantoaxial Subluxation—*May present with torticollis; can be caused by retropharyngeal inflammation (Grisel's disease).* It is probably caused by secondary ligamentous laxity and is best *treated with traction and bracing early.* Current diagnosis is by CT scans at the C1–C2 level with the head straight forward, in maximal rotation to the right, and then in maximum rotation to the left (Fig. 2-21). *Late diagnosis may require C1–C2 fusion.* Traumatic atlantoaxial subluxation may present as torticollis, which can be treated initially with a soft collar for up to 1 week. If symptoms persist past this point, cervical traction should be initiated. If discovered late (>1 month), fusion may be required for fixed rotary subluxation. *Rotary subluxation can also be seen in rheumatoid arthritis, AS, Down's syndrome, congenital anomalies, and cervical tumors.*
3. Os Odontoideum—Previously thought to be due to the failure of fusion of the base of the odontoid, it appears like a type II odontoid fracture. Evidence suggests that it may represent the residuals of an old traumatic process. Usually seen in place of the normal odontoid process (orthotopic type), but it may fuse to the clivus (dystopic type more often seen with neurologic compromise). *Treatment is conservative unless there is instability (>10 mm of Atlantol-Dens Interval [ADI] or <13 mm Space Available for the Cord [SAC]) or neurologic symptoms are present, which require a posterior C1–C2 fusion.*
4. Pseudosubluxation of the Cervical Spine—Subluxation of C2 on C3 (and occasionally of C3 on C4) of up to 40% or 4 mm can be normal in children <8 years old because of the orientation of the facets. Rapid resolution of pain, relatively minor trauma, lack of anterior swelling, continued alignment of the posterior interspinous distances and the posterior spinolaminar line (**Schwischuk's line**) on radiographs, and reduction of the subluxation with neck extension help differentiate this entity from more serious disorders.
5. Intervertebral Disc Calcification Syndrome—Pain, decreased range of motion, low-grade fevers, increased ESR, and radiographic disc calcification (within the annulus) without erosion characterize this disorder, which usually involves the C-spine. Conservative treatment is indicated for this self-limited condition.

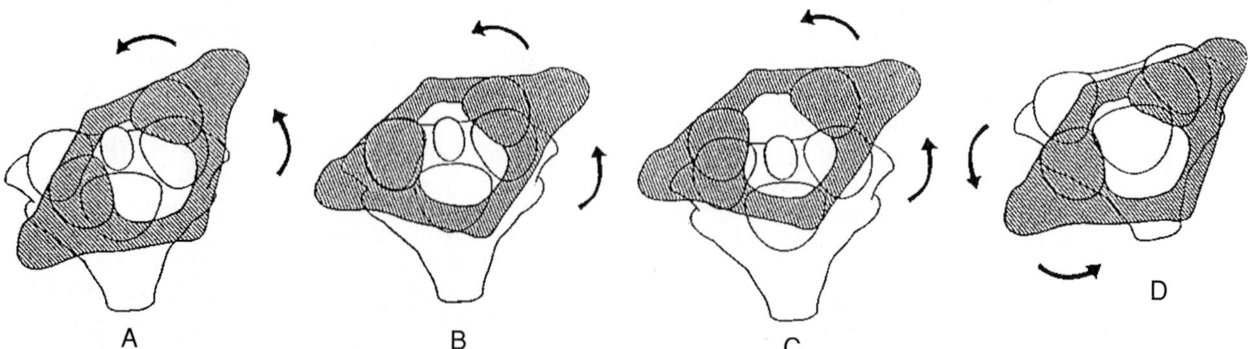

FIGURE 2-21 ■ Four types of rotary fixation. *A*, Type I: rotary fixation with no anterior displacement and the odontoid acting as the pivot. *B*, Type II: rotary fixation with anterior displacement of 3–5 mm, one lateral process acting as the pivot. *C*, Type III: rotary fixation with anterior displacement >5 mm. *D*, Type IV: rotary fixation with posterior displacement. (From Fielding, J.W., and Hawkins, R.J.: Atlantoaxial rotatory fixation. J. Bone Joint Surg. [Am.] 59:42, 1977.)

6. Basilar Impression/Invagination—Bony deformity at the base of the skull causes cephalad migration of the odontoid into the foramen magnum. Sagittal MRI scan best demonstrates impingement of the dens on the brain stem. Weakness, paresthesias, and hydrocephalus may result. Treatment is often operative and may include transoral resection of the dens, occipital laminectomy, and occipitocervical fusion and wiring.

IX. Upper-Extremity Problems (see Chapter 6, Hand and Microsurgery)

A. Sprengel's Deformity—*Undescended scapula often associated with winging, hypoplasia, and omovertebral connections (30%)* (Fig. 2-22). It is the most common congenital anomaly of the shoulder in children. Affected scapulae are usually small, relatively wide, and medially rotated. Increased association with Klippel-Feil syndrome, kidney disease, scoliosis, and diastematomyelia. Surgery for cosmetic or functional deformities (decreased abduction) includes distal advancement of the associated muscles and scapula (Woodward) or detachment and movement of the scapula (Schrock, Green). Clavicle osteotomy is needed to avoid brachial plexus injury due to stretch. Surgery is best done on 3- to 8-year-olds.

B. Deltoid Fibrotic Problems—Short, fibrous bands replace the deltoid muscle and cause abduction contractures at the shoulder, with elevation and winging of the scapula when the arms are adducted. Surgical resection of these bands is often required.

X. Lower-Extremity Problems

A. Introduction—Lower-extremity problems that are best considered as a whole are presented in this section to provide a basis for understanding and comparison.

B. Rotational Problems of the Lower Extremities—Include *femoral anteversion, tibial torsion, and metatarsus adductus*. All of these problems may be a result of intrauterine positioning and commonly present with an *intoeing gait*. These deformities are usually bilateral, and the clinician should be wary of asymmetric findings. Evaluation should include the measurements noted in Table 2-13 and illustrated in Figure 2-23.

1. Metatarsus Adductus—Forefoot is adducted at the tarsal-metatarsal joint. Usually seen during the first year of life. *May be associated with hip dysplasia (10–15%).* Approximately 85% of cases resolve spontaneously; feet that can be actively corrected to neutral require no treatment. Stretching exercises are used for

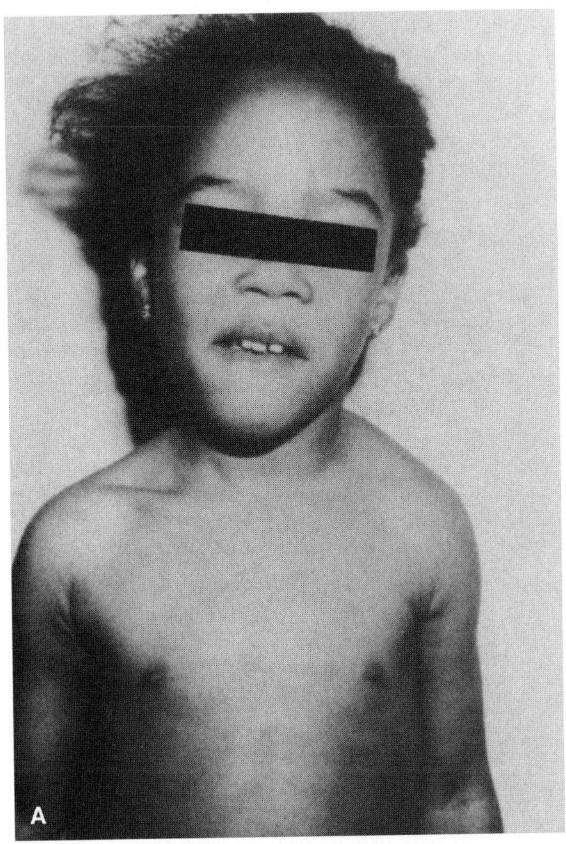

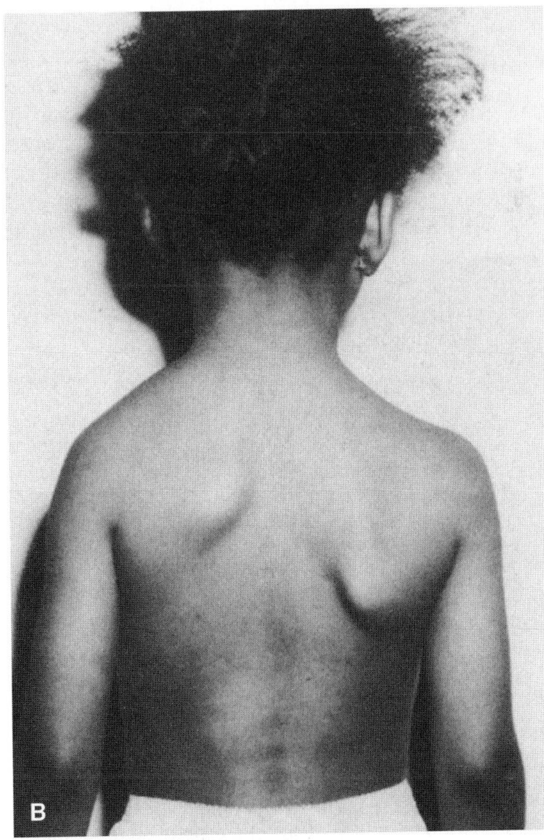

FIGURE 2-22 ■ Clinical photograph of a child with left Sprengel's shoulder: *A*, anterior view; *B*, posterior view. Note the elevation and rotation of the scapula. (From Benson, M., Fixen, J., Macniol, M.: Children's Orthopaedics and Fractures, Churchill Livingstone, 1994, p. 365.)

Table 2-13. EVALUATION OF ROTATIONAL PROBLEMS OF THE LOWER EXTREMITIES

MEASUREMENT	TECHNIQUE	NORMAL VALUES (DEGREES)	SIGNIFICANCE
Foot-progression angle	Foot vs. straight line	−5 to +20	Nonspecific rotation
Medial rotation	Prone hip ROM	20-60	>70 degrees; femoral anteversion
Lateral rotation	Prone hip ROM	30-60	<20 degrees; femoral anteversion
Thigh-foot angle	Knee bent; foot up	0-20	<−10 degrees; tibial torsion
Foot lateral border	Convex; medial crease	Straight; flexible	Metatarsus adductus

feet that can be passively corrected to neutral (heel bisector line lines up with the second metatarsal). Feet that cannot be passively corrected usually respond to serial casting. Cuneiform osteotomies and limited medial release are indicated in resistant cases. The best results with osteotomies are seen when the surgery is performed after 5 years of age. Rigidity and heel valgus should be identified and treated with early casting.

2. Tibial Torsion—*The most common cause of intoeing. Usually seen during the second year* of life and can be associated with metatarsus adductus. It is often bilateral and may be secondary to excessive medial ligamentous tightness. Internal rotation of the tibia causes the intoeing gait. This intrauterine "molding" deformity typically resolves spontaneously with growth. Operative correction is rarely necessary except in severe cases, which are addressed with a supramalleolar osteotomy.
3. Femoral Anteversion—Internal rotation of the femur, *seen in 3- to 6-year-olds.* Increased internal rotation and decreased external rotation are noted on examination of a child with an intoeing gait and whose patellas are internally rotated. Children with this problem classically *sit in a W position.* If associated with tibial torsion, femoral anteversion may lead to patellofemoral problems. This disorder usually corrects spontaneously by age 10, but in the older child with less than 10 degrees of external rotation, femoral derotational osteotomy (intertrochanteric is best) may be considered for cosmesis.

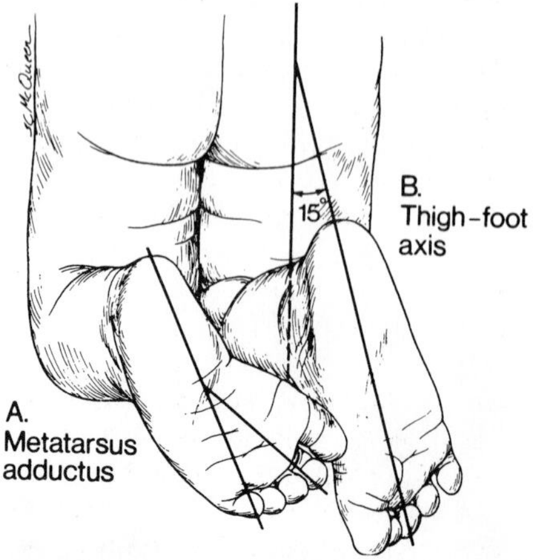

FIGURE 2-23 ■ *A,* Deviation of the forefoot in metatarsus adductus. *B,* Note also the normal thigh-foot angle (15 degrees); negative thigh-foot angles (<10 degrees) are seen in tibial torsion. (From Fitch, R.D.: Introduction to pediatric orthopedics. In Sabiston, D.C., Jr., ed.: Sabiston's Essentials of Surgery. Philadelphia, WB Saunders, 1987.)

XI. Hip and Femur

A. Developmental Dysplasia of the Hip (DDH)

1. Introduction—Previously called congenital dysplasia of the hip, this disorder represents abnormal development or dislocation of the hip secondary to capsular laxity and mechanical factors (e.g., intrauterine positioning). **Breech positioning, female sex, positive family history, and being a first born are risk factors.** Decreased intrauterine space explains the increased incidence of DDH in the first-born child. *Commonly associated with other "packaging problems," such as torticollis (20%) and metatarsus adductus (10%),* it is partially characterized by increased amounts of type III collagen. DDH is seen most commonly in the left hip (67%) in females (85%) with a positive family history (20% +), increased maternal estrogens, and breech births (30–50%). This disorder includes the spectrum of complete dislocation, subluxation, instability, and acetabular dysplasia.

   If left untreated, muscles about the hip become contracted, and the acetabulum becomes more dysplastic and filled with fibrofatty tissue (**pulvinar**). *Potential obstructions to obtaining a concentric reduction in DDH are iliopsoas tendon, pulvinar, contracted inferomedial hip capsule, and the transverse acetabular ligament.*

   The teratologic form is most severe and usually requires early surgery. The teratologic form of DDH is defined as those hips that present with a pseudoacetabulum at or near birth. Teratologic hip dislocations commonly present in association with syndromes such as arthrogryposis or Larsen's syndrome.
2. Diagnosis—Early diagnosis is possible with *Ortolani's test (elevation and abduction of*

femur relocates a dislocated hip) and Barlow's test (adduction and depression of femur dislocates a dislocatable hip). Three phases are commonly recognized: (1) **dislocated** (Ortolani-positive, early; Ortolani-negative, late, when femoral head cannot be reduced); (2) **dislocatable** (Barlow-positive); and (3) **subluxatable** (Barlow-suggestive). *Later diagnosis is made with limitation of hip abduction* in the affected hip as the laxity resolves and stiffness becomes more clinically evident. (*Caution:* Abduction may be decreased symmetrically with bilateral dislocations.) Another sign of dislocation includes a positive *Galeazzi sign,* demonstrated by the clinical appearance of foreshortening of the femur on the affected side. This clinical test is performed with the feet held together and knees flexed (a congenitally short femur can also cause a positive Galeazzi sign). Other clinical findings associated with DDH include asymmetric gluteal folds (less reliable) and a positive Trendelenburg stance (older child). Repeat examination, especially in an infant, is important because a child's irritability can prevent proper evaluation.

Radiographs may be helpful in the older child (>3 months), and measurement of the acetabular index (normal <25 degrees), measurement of Perkins' line (normally the ossific nucleus of femoral head is medial to this line), and evaluation of Shenton's line are useful (Fig. 2-24). Later, delayed ossification of the femoral head on the affected side may be seen. Dynamic ultrasonography is also useful for making the diagnosis, especially in young children before ossification of the femoral head (which occurs at age 4–6 months) (Fig. 2-25). It is also useful for assessing reduction in a Pavlik harness and diagnosing acetabular dysplasia or capsular laxity; however, it is operator dependent (normal alpha angle is >60 degrees and the femoral head is bisected by the line drawn down the ilium. Arthrography is helpful after closed reduction to determine concentric reduction.

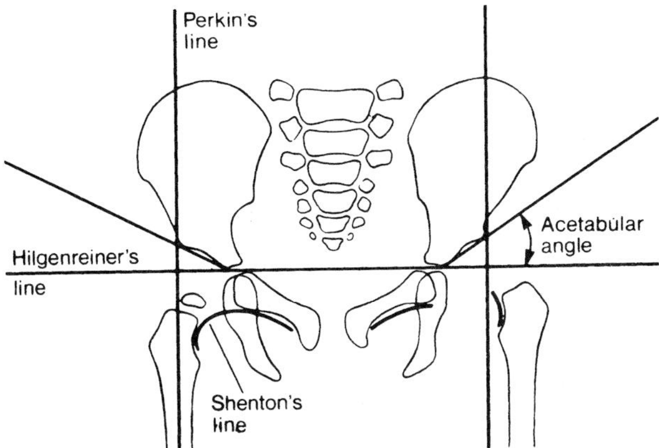

FIGURE 2-24 ■ Common measurements used to evaluate developmental dysplasia of the hip. Note the delayed ossification, disruption of Shenton's line, and increased acetabular index on the left dislocated hip. (From Fitch, R.D.: Introduction to pediatric orthopaedics. In Sabiston, D.C., Jr., ed.: Sabiston's Essentials of Surgery. Philadelphia, WB Saunders, 1987.)

3. Treatment (Fig. 2-26)—Based on achieving and maintaining early "concentric reduction" in order to prevent future degenerative joint disease. Specific therapy is based on the child's age and includes the *Pavlik harness,* which is designed to maintain infants (<6 months) reduced in about **100 degrees of flexion** and mild abduction (the "human position" [Salter]). The reduction should be confirmed by radiographs or ultrasound scans after placement in the harness and brace adjustment. The position of the hip should be within the *"safe zone"* of Ramsey (between maximum adduction before redislocation and excessive abduction causing a high risk of avascular necrosis). Impingement of the **posterosuperior retinacular branch of the medial femoral circumflex artery** has been implicated in osteonecrosis associated with DDH treated in an abduction orthosis. *Pavlik harness treatment is contraindicated in teratologic hip dislocations.* Patients with a narrow safe zone should be considered for an adductor tenotomy. *Excessive flexion may result in transient femoral nerve palsy.* Weaning from the harness is generally done over a period twice as long as the treatment duration. *Open reduction is reserved for children 12 to 18 months old who fail closed reduction, have an obstructive limbus, or have an unstable safe zone. Open reduction is also the initial treatment for children 18 months and older.* It is usually done through an anterior approach (less risk to the medial femoral circumflex artery) and includes capsulorrhaphy, adductor tenotomy, and perhaps femoral shortening. The major risk associated with both open and closed reductions is osteonecrosis (due to direct vascular injury or impingement versus disruption of the circulation from osteotomies). Failure of open reduction is difficult to treat surgically because of the high complication rate of revision surgery (50% osteonecrosis, 33% pain and stiffness in a recent study). *Diagnosis after age 8 years (younger in patients with bilateral DDH) may contraindicate reduction because the acetabulum has little chance to remodel,* although reduction may be indicated in conjunction with salvage procedures.
4. Osteotomies—May be required in toddlers and school-age children. *Osteotomies are indicated during open reduction in a child older than 2 years with residual hip dysplasia.* Osteotomies should be done only after congruent reduction, with satisfactory ROM, and after

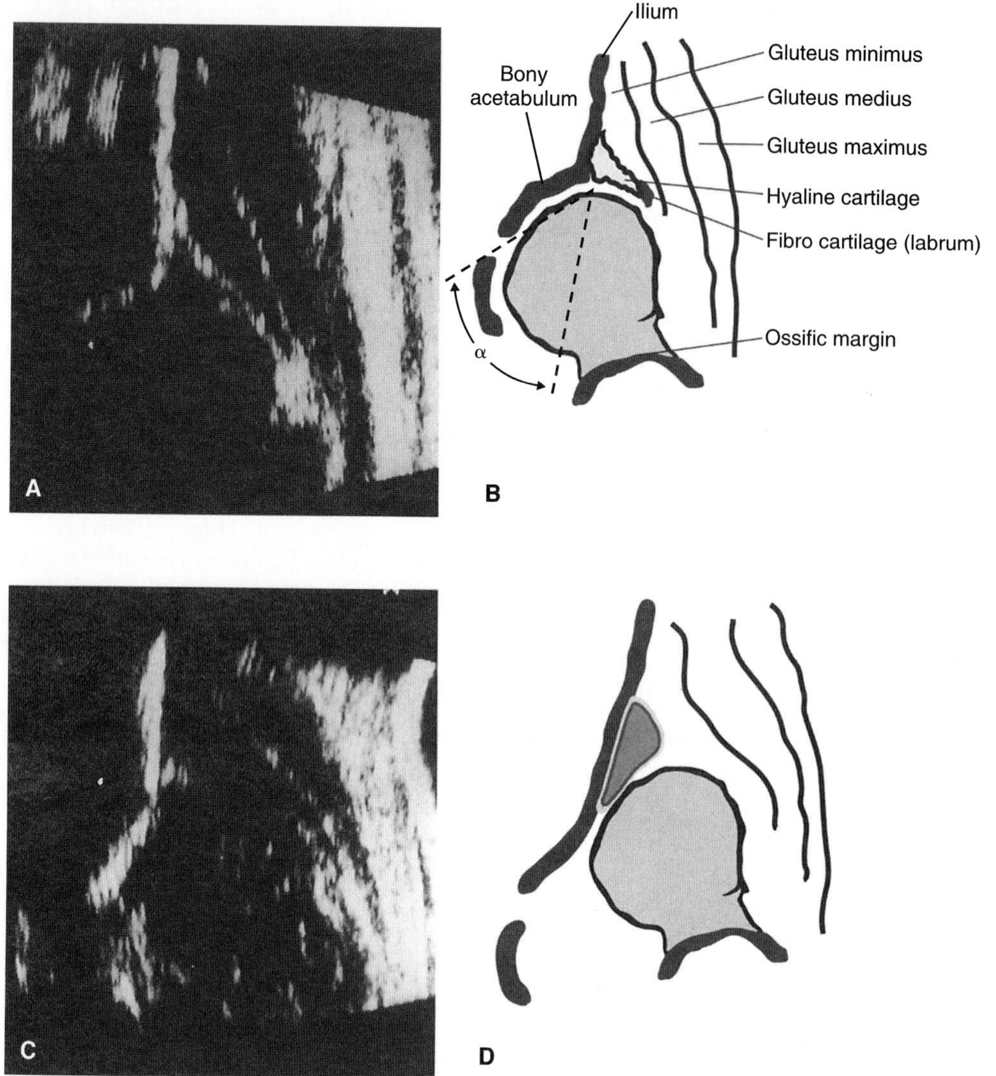

FIGURE 2-25 ■ Ultrasound evaluation of the neonate's hip. *A*, Ultrasound of normal hip. *B*, Graphic representation of the ultrasound. *C*, Ultrasound of a dislocated hip with poor bony roof. *D*, Graphic illustration of the dislocated hip. (Modified from Benson, M., Fixen, J., Macniol, M.: Children's Orthopaedics and Fractures, 2nd ed., WB Saunders, 2002, p. 364.)

reasonable femoral sphericity is achieved by closed or open methods. The choice of femoral versus pelvic osteotomy (Fig. 2-27) is sometimes a matter of the surgeon's choice. Some surgeons prefer to perform pelvic osteotomies after age 4 and femoral osteotomies before this age. *In general, pelvic osteotomies should be done when severe dysplasia is accompanied by significant radiographic changes on the acetabular side (i.e., increased acetabular index, failure of lateral acetabular ossification), whereas changes on the femoral side (e.g., marked anteversion, coxa valga) are best treated by femoral osteotomies.* Femoral osteotomies rarely correct hip dysplasia successfully after age 5 years. Table 2-14 lists common reconstructive osteotomies.

The Salter osteotomy may lengthen the affected leg up to 1 cm. *The Pemberton acetabuloplasty is a good choice for residual dysplasia because it reduces acetabular volume* (bends on triradiate cartilage). The Steel (triple) innominate osteotomy is favored for older children because their symphysis pubis does not rotate as well. *Dega's-type osteotomies are often favored for paralytic dislocations and patients with posterior acetabular deficiency.* This osteotomy is more versatile and is sometimes used for DDH. The Dial osteotomy is technically difficult and

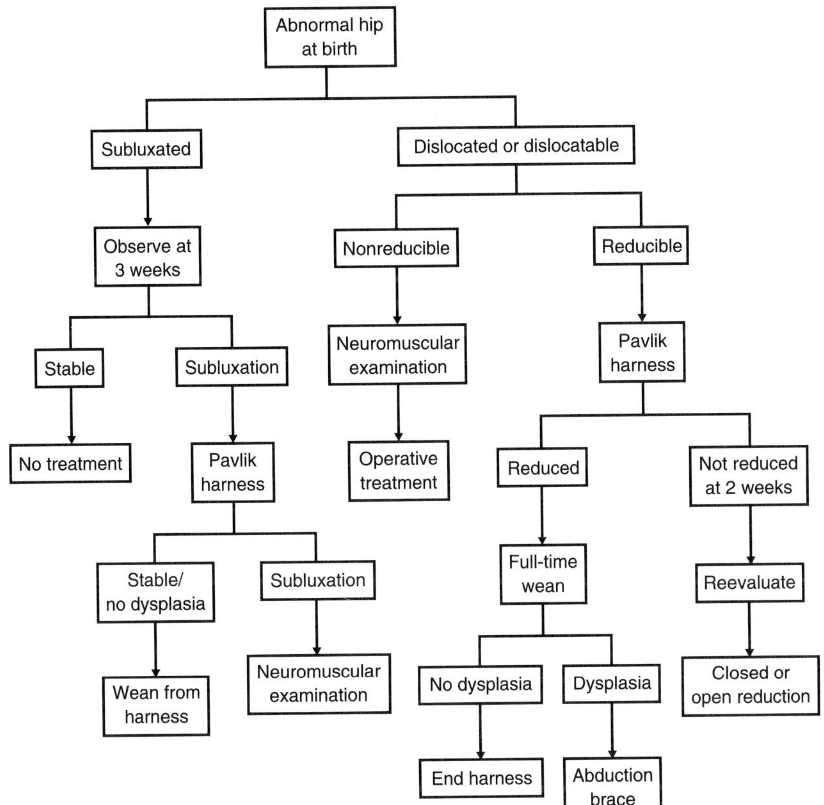

FIGURE 2-26 ■ Algorithm for the treatment of developmental dysplasia of the hip (From Guille, J.T., Pizzutillo, M.D., and MacEwen, G.D.: Developmental dysplasia of the hip from birth to six months. JAAOS 8:232–242, 2000.)

rarely used. *The Chiari osteotomy is recommended for patients with inadequate femoral head coverage and an incongruous joint but is considered a salvage procedure.* The Chiari osteotomy shortens the affected leg and requires periarticular soft-tissue metaplasia for success. Other procedures include the shelf lateral acetabular augmentation procedure for patients with inadequate lateral coverage or trochanteric advancement in a patient >8 years old with increased trochanteric overgrowth (improves hip abductor biomechanics). *The two pelvic osteotomies that depend on metaplastic*

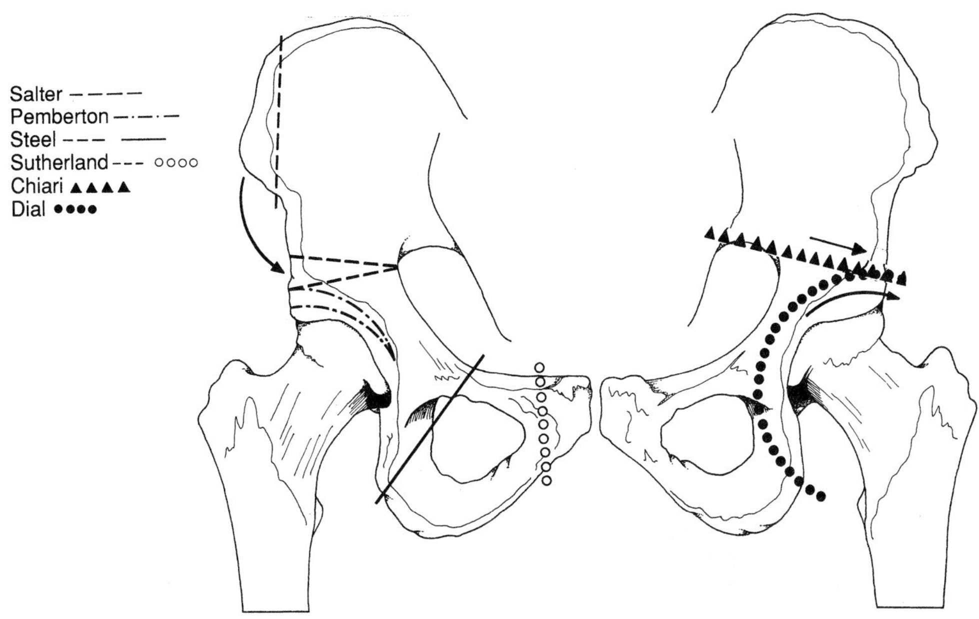

FIGURE 2-27 ■ Common pelvic osteotomies for treatment of developmental dysplasia of the hip.

Table 2-14. COMMON PELVIC OSTEOTOMIES

OSTEOTOMY	PROCEDURE	REQUIREMENT
Femoral	Intertrochanteric osteotomy (VDRO)	Concentric reduction <8 years of age
Salter's	Innominate osteotomy open wedge	Concentric reduction <8 years of age
Pemberton's	Through acetabular roof to triradiate cartilage	Concentric reduction <8 years of age
Sutherland's (double)	Salter's + pubic osteotomy	Concentric reduction Open triradiate
Steel's (triple)	Salter's + osteotomy of both rami	Concentric reduction Open triradiate
Ganz	Periacetabular osteotomy	Surgeon's experience Closed triradiate cartilage
Chiari's	Through ilium above acetabulum (makes new roof)	Salvage procedure for asymmetric incongruity
Shelf's	Slotted lateral acetabular augmentation	Salvage procedure for asymmetric incongruity

VDRO, varus derotation osteotomy.

tissue (fibrocartilage) for a successful result are the shelf and Chiari osteotomies. The Ganz provides improved three-dimensional correction since the cuts are close to the acetabulum, allows immediate weight bearing, spares stripping of the abductor muscles, allows for a capsulotomy to insect the joint and is performed through a single incision.

B. Congenital Coxa Vara—*Decreased neck-shaft angle due to a defect in ossification of the femoral neck.* It is bilateral in one third to one half of cases. Coxa vara can be congenital (noted at birth and differentiated from DDH by MRI), developmental (AD, progressive), or acquired (e.g., trauma, Legg-Calvé-Perthes, slipped capital femoral epiphysis). May present with a waddling gait (bilateral) or a painless limp (unilateral). *Radiographs classically demonstrate a triangular ossification defect in the inferomedial femoral neck in developmental coxa vara.* Evaluation of **Hilgenreiner's epiphyseal angle** (the angle between Hilgenreiner's line and a line through the proximal femoral physis) is the key to treatment. *An angle of <45 degrees spontaneously corrects, whereas an angle of 45–60 degrees requires close observation and >60 degrees (and a neck-shaft angle <110 degrees) usually requires surgery.* The surgical treatment is a corrective valgus osteotomy of the proximal femur. Proximal femoral (valgus) ± derotation osteotomy (Pauwel) is indicated for a neck-shaft angle <90 degrees, a vertically oriented physeal plate, progressive deformities, or significant gait abnormalities. Concomitant distal/lateral transfer of the greater trochanter may also be indicated to restore more normal hip abductor mechanics.

C. Legg-Calvé-Perthes Disease (Coxa Plana)—Noninflammatory deformity of the proximal femur secondary to a vascular insult, leading to *osteonecrosis of the proximal femoral epiphysis.* Usually seen in boys 4–8 years old with delayed skeletal maturation usually by 2 years of age. There is an increased incidence with a positive family history, low birth weight, and abnormal birth presentation. *Symptoms include pain (often knee pain), effusion (from synovitis), and limp. Decreased hip ROM (especially abduction and internal rotation) and a Trendelenburg gait are also common.* **Prognosis is dependent on bone age and radiographic appearance during fragmentation phase (lateral pillar classification).** *Patients who have a bone age >6 years and B or C lateral pillar have a significantly poorer prognosis.* Bilateral involvement may be seen in 12–15% of cases. However, in bilateral cases the involvement is asymmetric and virtually never simultaneous. *Bilateral involvement may mimic multiple epiphyseal dysplasia.* Differential diagnosis includes septic arthritis, blood dyscrasias, hypothyroidism, and epiphyseal dysplasia. Wallenstraam's classification determines the four stages that all cases follow; initial, fragmentation, reossification, healed or reossified. Pathologically, the osteonecrosis is followed by revascularization and resorption via creeping substitution that eventually allows remodeling and fragmentation. Radiographic findings vary with the stage of disease but include cessation of growth of the ossific nucleus, medial joint space widening, and development of a "crescent sign" representing subchondral fracture.

The classification that is most prognostic is Herring classification, which is based on the involvement of the lateral pillar of the capital femoral epiphysis (CFE) during the fragmentation stage (Fig. 2-28 and Table 2-15)

Maintaining the sphericity of the femoral head is the most important factor in achieving a good result. Use of circular templates (Mose) is helpful for evaluating this parameter. Early hip degenerative joint disease results from aspherical femoral heads. *Poor prognosis is associated with older children (bone age >6 years), female sex, and decreased hip ROM (decreased abduction).* Radiographic findings associated with poor prognosis (Catterall's "head at risk" signs) include *(1) lateral calcification, (2) Gage's sign (V-shaped defect at lateral physis), (3) lateral subluxation, (4) metaphyseal cyst formation, and (5) horizontal growth plate.*

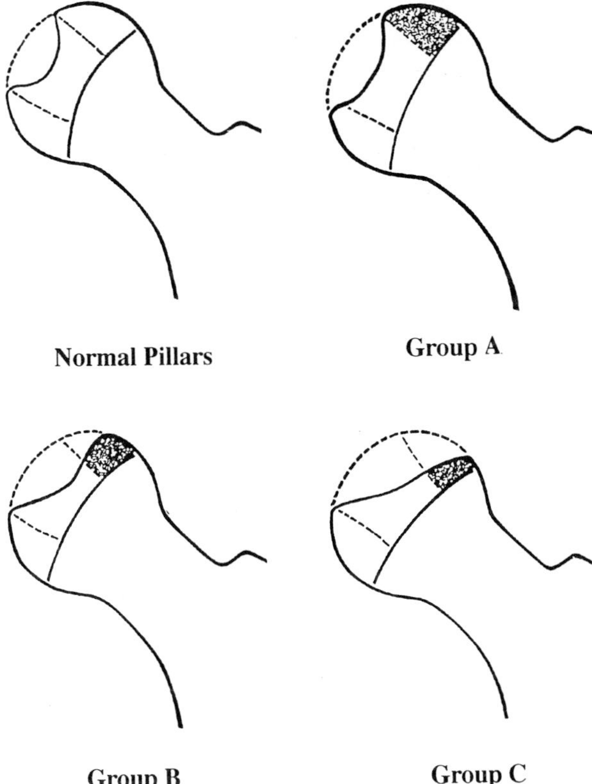

FIGURE 2-28 ■ Lateral pillar classification of Legg-Calvé-Perthes disease. *Normal pillars,* The pillars were derived by noting the lines of demarcation between the central sequestrum and the remainder of the epiphysis on the anteroposterior radiograph. *Group A,* Normal height of lateral pillar is maintained. *Group B,* More than 50% of height of lateral pillar is maintained. *Group C,* Less than 50% of height of lateral pillar is maintained. (Adapted from Herring, J.A., Neustadt, J.B., Williams, J.J., et al.: The lateral pillar classification of Legg-Calvé-Perthes disease. J. Pediatr. Orthop. 12:143–150, 1992.)

In general, the goals of treatment are relief of symptoms, restoration of ROM, and containment of the hip. Use of outpatient or inpatient traction, anti-inflammatory medications, and partial weight bearing with crutches for periods of 1-2 days to several weeks is helpful for relieving symptoms. ROM is maintained with traction, muscle releases, exercise, and/or use of a Petrie cast.

Table 2-15. LATERAL PILLAR CLASSIFICATION

GROUPS	PILLAR INVOLVEMENT	PROGNOSIS
Group A	Little or no involvement of the lateral pillar	Uniformly good outcome
Group B	>50% of lateral pillar height maintained	Good outcome in younger patients (bone age <6 years) but poorer outcome in older patients
Group C	<50% of lateral pillar height maintained	Poor prognosis in all age groups

Containment of the hip by use of traction, muscle releases, abduction bracing, or varus femoral versus pelvic osteotomy is helpful for maintaining hip sphericity. Herring has described a treatment plan based on age and the lateral pillar classification of disease involvement.

D. Slipped Capital Femoral Epiphysis (SCFE)—*Disorder of the proximal femoral epiphysis caused by weakness of the perichondral ring and slippage through the hypertrophic zone of the growth plate.* The femoral head remains in the acetabulum, and the neck displaces anteriorly and externally rotates. *SCFE is seen most commonly in African American, obese, adolescent boys (10-16 years old) with a positive family history. Up to 25% of cases are bilateral.* It is related to puberty. May be associated with hormonal disorders in young children, such as hypothyroidism or renal osteodystrophy. May present with coxalgic, externally rotated gait; decreased internal rotation; thigh atrophy; **and hip, thigh, or knee pain**. Symptoms vary with acuteness of the slip. On physical examination, all patients have obligate external rotation with flexion of the hip.

Loder described a classification of SCFE based on the patients' ability to bear weight at the time of presentation. **Stable slips** are those in which weight bearing with or without crutches is possible. **Unstable slips** are those in which weight bearing is not possible because of severe pain. No patients with stable slips developed osteonecrosis, whereas 50% of the patients with unstable slips developed it. Radiographs show the slip, which is classified based on the percentage of slip: grade I, 0-33%; grade II, 33-50%; and grade III, >50%. In mild cases, loss of the lateral overhang of the femoral ossific nucleus *(Klein's line)* and blurring of the proximal femoral metaphysis may be all that is seen on the anteroposterior film. **The recommended treatment is pinning in situ**. Forceful reduction before pinning is not indicated. Pin placement can be done percutaneously with **one pin** (Fig. 2-29). The pin should be started anteriorly on the femoral neck, ending in the central portion of the femoral head. The goal is to force the proximal femoral physis to close. *Patients presenting at less than 10 years of age should have an endocrine work-up. Prophylactic pinning of the opposite hip is controversial but is generally recommended in patients diagnosed with an endocrinopathy and young children (<10 years old).*

In severe SCFE, the residual proximal femoral deformity may remodel with the patient's remaining growth. Intertrochanteric (Kramer's) or subtrochanteric (Southwick's) osteotomies may be useful in treating the deformities caused by SCFE that fail to remodel. Cuneiform osteotomy at the femoral neck has the potential to correct a higher degree of deformity but remains controversial due

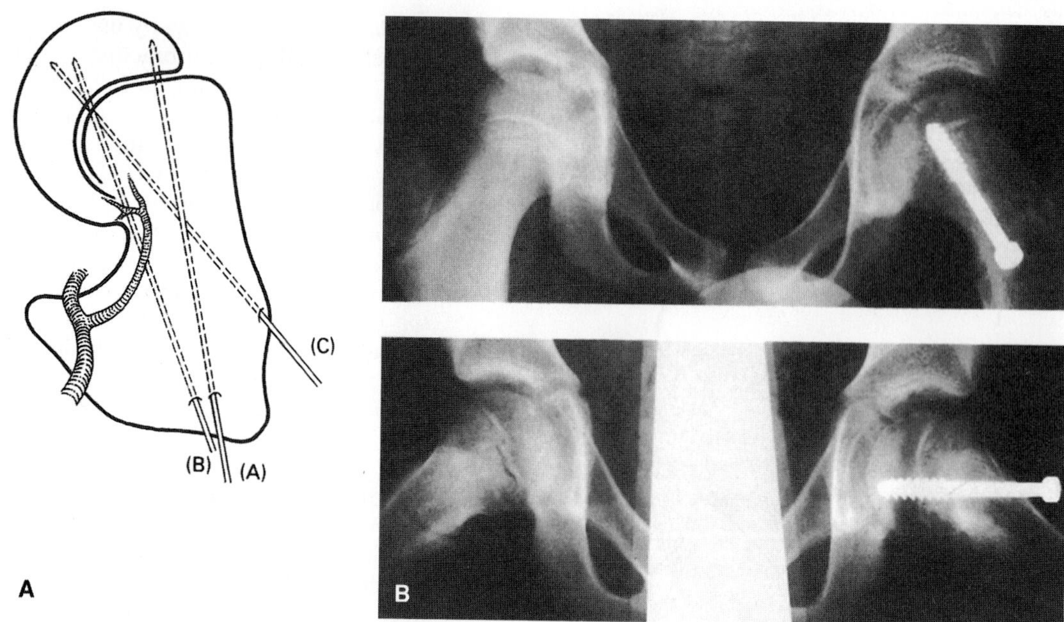

FIGURE 2-29 ■ *A*, Percutaneous pinning or screw fixation for slipped capital femoral epiphysis. Note the epiphysis slips posteriorly and inferiorly. The implant must be inserted into the anterior femoral neck and directed toward the center of the epiphysis. Pin C is optimally placed. *B*, Radiographs show satisfactory screw placement with the screw entering the anterior femoral neck. (From Benson, M., Fixen, J., Macniol, M.: Children's Orthopaedics and Fractures, Churchill Livingstone, 1994, p. 464.)

to the high reported rates of osteonecrosis (37%) and future osteoarthritis (37%). *Complications associated with SCFE include chondrolysis (narrowed joint space, pain, and decreased motion), osteonecrosis (higher incidence in unstable slips), and degenerative joint disease (pistol grip deformity of the proximal femur).*

E. Proximal Femoral Focal Deficiency (PFFD)—Developmental defect of the proximal femur recognizable at birth. Clinically, patients with PFFD have a short, bulky thigh that is flexed, abducted, and externally rotated. *PFFD is often associated with coxa vara or fibular hemimelia (50%).* Congenital knee ligamentous deficiency and contracture are also common. Treatment must be individualized based on leg-length discrepancy, adequacy of musculature, proximal joint stability, and the presence or absence of foot deformities. The percentage of shortening remains constant during growth. The Aiken classification divides PFFD into four groups (Fig. 2-30). Classes A and B both have a femoral head present, which potentially allows for reconstructive procedures including limb lengthening. Classes C and D do not have a femoral head and present a more difficult treatment dilemma. *Treatment options include amputation, femoral-pelvic fusion (Brown's procedure), Van Ness' rotationplasty, and limb lengthening.*

F. Leg-Length Discrepancy (LLD)—There are many causes of LLD, such as congenital disorders (e.g., hemihypertrophy, dysplasias, PFFD, DDH), paralytic disorders (e.g., spasticity, polio), infection (pyogenic disruption of the physis), tumors, and trauma. Long-term problems associated with LLD include inefficient gait, equinus contractures of the ankle, postural scoliosis, and low back pain. The discrepancy must be measured accurately (e.g., with blocks of set height under the affected side, scanogram) and can be tracked with the Green-Anderson or Mosely graph (with serial leg-length films or CT scanograms and bone age determinations). **In general, projected discrepancies at maturity of <2 cm are observed or treated with shoe lifts. Discrepancies of 2–5 cm can be treated with epiphysiodesis of the long side, shortening of the long side (ostectomy), or lengthening. Discrepancies of >5 cm are generally treated with lengthening.** Using standard techniques, lengthening of 1 mm/d is typical. The Illizarov principles are followed, including metaphyseal corticotomy (preserving the medullary canal and blood supply) followed by gradual distraction. Rarely, one can consider physeal distraction (chondrodiatasis). This procedure must be done near skeletal maturity because the physis almost always closes after this type of limb lengthening. **A gross estimation of LLD can be made using the following assumption of growth per year up to age 16 in boys and age 14 in girls: distal femur, 3/8 in/y (9 mm); proximal tibia, 1/4 in/y (6 mm); and proximal femur 1/8 in/y (3 mm).** *Use of the Mosely data gives more accurate data.*

G. Lower-Extremity Inflammation and Infection (see Chapter 1, Basic Sciences)

TYPE		FEMORAL HEAD	ACETABULUM	FEMORAL SEGMENT	RELATIONSHIP AMONG COMPONENTS OF FEMUR AND ACETABULUM AT SKELETAL MATURITY
A		Present	Normal	Short	Bony connection between components of femur Femoral head in acetabulum Subtrochanteric varus angulation, often with pseudarthrosis
B	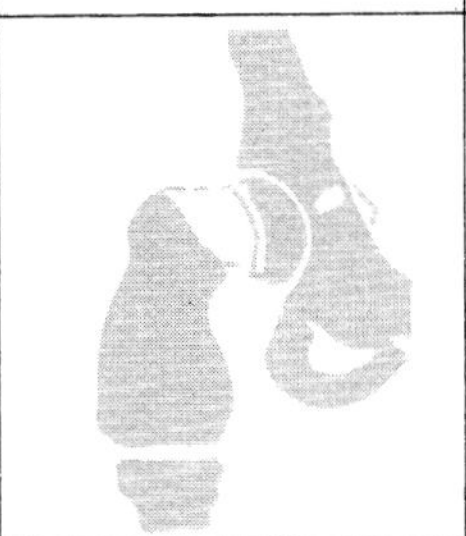	Present	Adequate or moderately dysplastic	Short, usually proximal bony tuft	No osseous connection between head and shaft Femoral head in acetabulum
C	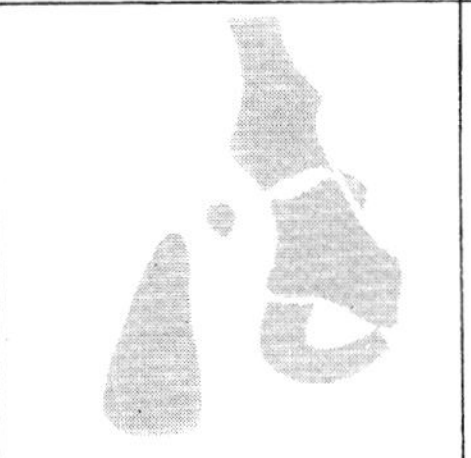	Absent or represented by ossicle	Severely dysplastic	Short, usually proximally tapered	May be osseous connection between shaft and proximal ossicle No articular relation between femur and acetabulum
D	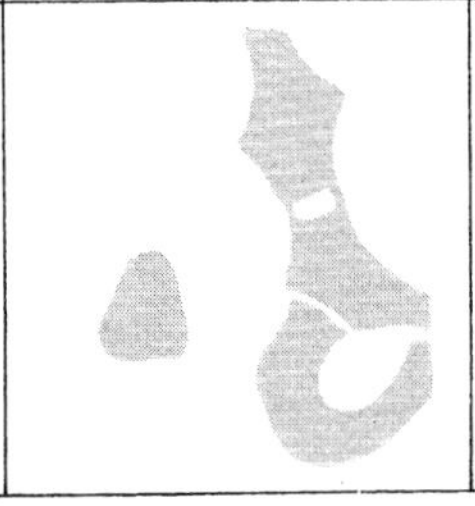	Absent	Absent Obturator foramen enlarged Pelvis squared in bilateral cases	Short, deformed	(none)

FIGURE 2-30 ■ Aiken's classification of proximal femoral focal deficiency. Note lack of femoral head in types C and D. (From Tachdjian, M.O.: Pediatric Orthopaedics, 2nd ed. Philadelphia, WB Saunders, 1990.)

1. Transient Synovitis—Most common cause of painful hips during childhood, but it is *a diagnosis of exclusion. Can be related to viral infection, allergic reaction, or trauma; however, cause is unknown*. Onset can be acute or insidious. Symptoms, which are self-limited, include voluntary limitation of motion and muscle spasm. With transient synovitis, the **ESR is usually <20 mm/h**. Rule out septic hip with aspiration (especially in children with fever, leukocytosis, or elevated ESR); then observe patient in Buck's traction for 24–48 hours.
2. Osteomyelitis—More common in children because of their rich metaphyseal blood supply and thick periosteum. Most common organism is ***Staphylococcus aureus*** *(except in neonates, in whom group B streptococcus is more common)*. With the advent of the ***Haemophilus influenzae*** **vaccination,** *H. influenzae* is now a much less common organism in musculoskeletal sepsis. A history of trauma is common in children with osteomyelitis. *Osteomyelitis in children usually begins through hematogenous seeding of a bony metaphysis in the small arterioles that bend just beyond the physis, where blood flow is sluggish and there is poor phagocytosis, creating a bone abscess* (Fig. 2-31). Pus lifts the thick periosteum and puts pressure on the cortex, causing coagulation. Chronic bone abscesses may become surrounded by thick, fibrous tissue and sclerotic bone (*Brodie's abscess*).

   Clinically, the child presents with a tender, warm, sometimes swollen area over a long-bone metaphysis. Fever may or may not be present. Laboratory tests may be helpful

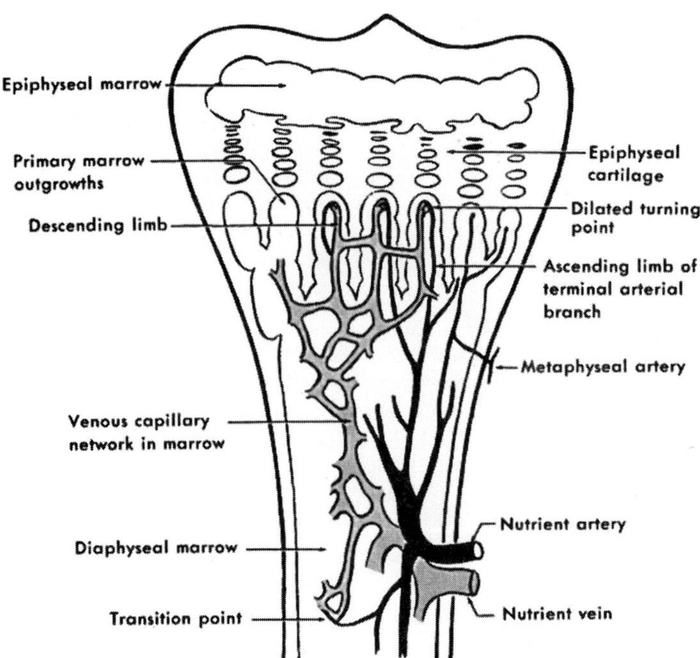

FIGURE 2-31 ■ Metaphyseal sinusoids where sluggish blood flow increases susceptibility to osteomyelitis. (From Tachdjian, M.O.: Pediatric Orthopaedics, 2nd ed. Philadelphia, WB Saunders, 1990.)

(blood cultures, WBC count, ESR, C-reactive protein), and radiologic studies are also useful (radiographs with only soft-tissue edema early, metaphyseal rarefaction late, and bone scans). Definitive diagnosis is made with *aspiration* (50% positive cultures). Intravenous antibiotics are the best initial treatment if osteomyelitis is diagnosed early, prior to radiographic changes or the development of a subperiosteal abscess. Initially, broad-spectrum antibiotics are chosen, followed by antibiotics specific for the organism cultured. *Failure to respond to antibiotics, frank pus on aspiration, or the presence of a sequestered abscess (not accessible to antibiotics) requires operative drainage and débridement.* Specimens should be sent for histology and culture. Antibiotics should be continued until the ESR (or C-reactive protein) returns to normal, usually at 4–6 weeks.

3. Septic Arthritis—Can develop from osteomyelitis (especially in neonates, in whom transphyseal vessels allow proximal spread into the joint) in joints with an intra-articular metaphysic (*hip, elbow, shoulder, and ankle*). Septic arthritis can also occur as a result of hematogenous spread of infection. Because pus is chondrolytic, septic arthritis in children is an acute surgical emergency. Organisms vary with age (Table 2-16).

   Septic arthritis presents as a much more acute process than osteomyelitis. Decreased ROM and severe pain with passive motion may be accompanied by systemic symptoms of infection. Radiographs may show widened joint space or even dislocation. *Joint fluid aspirate shows a high white blood cell count (>50,000), glucose level 50 mg/dL less than serum levels, and in patients with gram-positive cocci or gram-negative rod, a high lactic acid level.*

   Distinguishing a hip septic arthritis and transient synovitis is a common problem; however, when three of four of the following criteria are present the diagnosis of septic arthritis is >90%: WBC >12,000 cells/ml, ESR >40, inability to bear weight, and fever >101.5°F.

   Ultrasonography can be helpful for identifying the presence of an effusion. Aspiration should be followed by irrigation and débridement in major joints (especially in the hip, culture of synovium is also recommended). Lumbar puncture should be considered in a septic joint caused by *H. influenzae* because of increased incidence of meningitis. Prognosis is

Table 2-16. COMMON ORGANISMS BY AGE FOR SEPTIC ARTHRITIS

AGE	COMMON ORGANISMS	EMPIRIC ANTIBIOTICS
<12 mo	Staphylococcus, group B streptococcus	First generation cephalosporin
6 months-5 years	Staphylococcus, *H. influenzae*	Second- or third-generation cephalosporin
5-12 years	*S. aureus*	First-generation cephalosporin
12-18 years	*S. aureus*, *N. gonorrhoeae*	Oxacillin/cephalosporin

usually good except in patients with a delayed diagnosis. Patients with *Neisseria gonorrhoeae* septic arthritis usually have a preceding migratory polyarthralgia, small red papules, and multiple joint involvement. This organism typically elicits less WBC response (less than 50,000 cells/ml) and usually does not require surgical drainage. Large doses of penicillin are required to eliminate this organism.

XII. Knee and Leg

A. Leg—Normally, genu varum (bowed legs) evolves naturally to genu valgum (knock-knees) by age 2½ years, with a gradual transition to physiologic valgus by age 4 years.

1. Genu Varum (Bowed Legs)—Normal in children <2 years old. Radiographs in physiologic bowing typically show flaring of the tibia and femur in a symmetric fashion. *Pathologic conditions that can cause genu varum include osteogenesis imperfecta, osteochondromas, trauma, various dysplasias, and most commonly, Blount's disease.* **Blount's disease** (tibia varum) is best divided into two distinct entities: infantile (0–4 years of age) and adolescent (>10 years old).

   a. Infantile Blount's—More common, usually affects both extremities. It is more common in the overweight child who begins walking at less than one year of age and is associated with internal tibial torsion. Radiographs may show a *metaphyseal-diaphyseal angle abnormality and metaphyseal beaking*. Drennan's angle of >16 degrees is considered abnormal and is formed between the metaphyseal beaks (demonstrated in Fig. 2-32). The epiphyseal-metaphyseal angle is also useful (Fig. 2-33). Treatment is based on age and the stage of disease (Langinskiold's I–VI, with V and VI characterized by a metaphyseal-epiphyseal bony bridge). Early in the disease, bracing may be effective especially in the unilateral case. Proximal tibia/fibula valgus osteotomy to slightly overcorrect the deformity (since medial physeal growth abnormalities persist) is required for patients who don't respond to bracing or for a child older than age 4. Epiphysiolysis is also needed for stage V and VI disease.

   b. Adolescent Blount's—Less severe and more often unilateral. Initial treatment is lateral proximal tibial and fibular epiphyseodesis when growth remains. If residual deformity exists or the physes are closed proximally, tibia and fibular osteotomy is performed. When significant leg-length discrepancy is present, the Illizarov technique allows for deformity correction and lengthening.

2. Genu Valgum (Knock-Knees)—Up to 15 degrees at the knee is common in 2- to

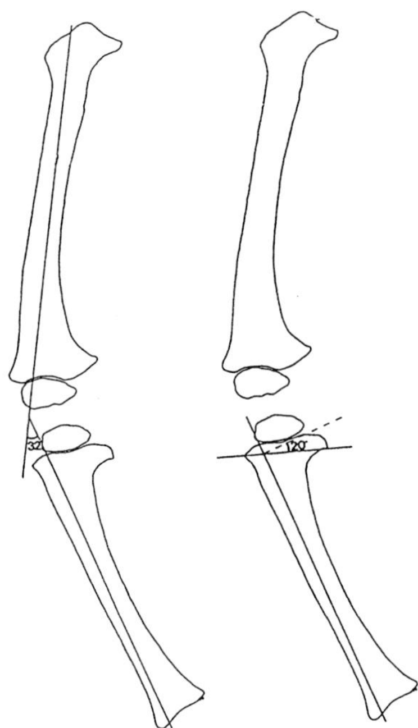

FIGURE 2-32 ■ Comparison of tibiofemoral angle with Levine and Drennan's metaphyseal-diaphyseal angle in tibia vara. The tibiofemoral angle method is used to determine the tibiofemoral angle. A line is drawn along the longitudinal axis of the tibia and the femur; the angle between the lines is the tibiofemoral angle (32 degrees). The metaphyseal-diaphyseal angle method is used to determine the metaphyseal-diaphyseal angle in the same extremity. A line is drawn perpendicular to the longitudinal axis of the tibia, and another is drawn through the two beaks of the metaphysis to determine the transverse axis of the tibial metaphysis. The metaphyseal-diaphyseal angle (12 degrees) is the angle bisected by the two lines. (Adapted from Levine, A.M., and Drennan, J.C.: Physiological bowing and tibia vara. J. Bone Joint Surg. [Am.] 64:1159, 1982.)

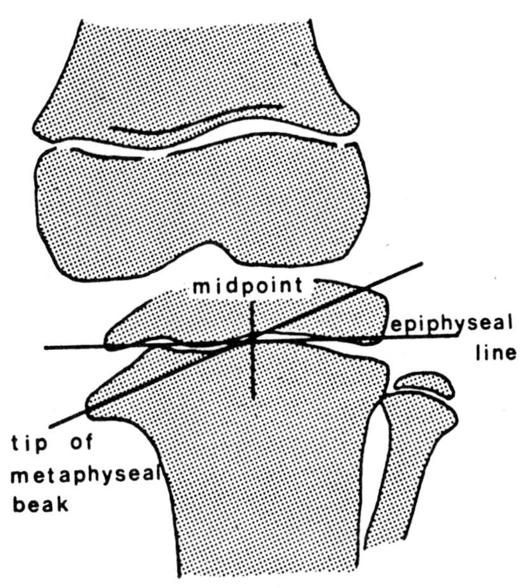

FIGURE 2-33 ■ Blount's disease and measurement of the epiphyseal-metaphyseal angle. (From Tachdjian, M.O.: Pediatric Orthopaedics, 2nd ed. Philadelphia, WB Saunders, 1990.)

6-year-old children. Patients within this physiologic range do not require treatment. *Pathologic genu valgum may be associated, for example, with renal osteodystrophy (most common cause if bilateral), tumors (e.g., osteochondromas), infections (may stimulate proximal asymmetric tibial growth), or trauma*. Conservative treatment is ineffective in pathologic genu valgum. Consider surgery at the site of the deformity in children >10 years old with >10 cm between the medial malleoli or >15–20 degrees of valgus. *Hemiepiphysiodesis or physeal stapling of the medial side is effective before the end of growth for severe deformities.*

B. Tibial Bowing—Three types (Table 2-17) based on the apex of the curve:
   1. Posteromedial—Physiologic bowing usually of the middle and distal thirds of the tibia may be the result of abnormal intrauterine positioning (Fig. 2-34). It is *commonly associated with calcaneovalgus feet and tight anterior structures*. Spontaneous correction is the rule, but follow the patient to evaluate LLD. The most common sequelae of posteromedial bowing is an **average LLD of 3-4 cm**, which may require an age-appropriate epiphysiodesis of the long limb. Tibial osteotomies are not indicated.
   2. Anteromedial Tibial Bowing—Typically caused by fibular hemimelia—a *congenital longitudinal deficiency of the fibula is the most common long-bone deficiency.* It is usually *associated with anteromedial bowing, ankle instability, equinovarus foot (± absent lateral rays), tarsal coalition, and femoral shortening.* Classically, skin dimpling is seen over the tibia. Significant LLD often results from this disorder. The fibular deficiency can be intercalary, which involves the whole bone (absent fibula), or terminal. Fibular hemimelia is frequently associated with femoral abnormalities such as coxa vara and PFFD. Radiographic findings include complete or partial absence of the fibula, ball-and-socket ankle (secondary to tarsal coalitions), and deficient lateral rays in the foot. Treatment varies from a simple shoe lift or bracing to Syme's amputation. *Treatment decisions are based on the degree of foot deformity and the degree of shortening of the limb.* Amputation is usually done to treat limbs with severe shortening and/or a stiff, nonfunctional foot at about 10 months of age. For less severe cases, reconstructive procedures, including lengthening, may be an

Table 2-17. TYPES OF TIBIAL BOWING

TIBIAL BOWING	CAUSE	TREATMENT
Posterior-medial	Physiologic	Observation
Anteromedial	Fibular hemimelia	Bracing vs. amputation for severe deformities
Anterolateral	Congenital pseudarthrosis	Total contact brace, IM fixation, vascularized bone graft, or amputation

IM, intramedullary.

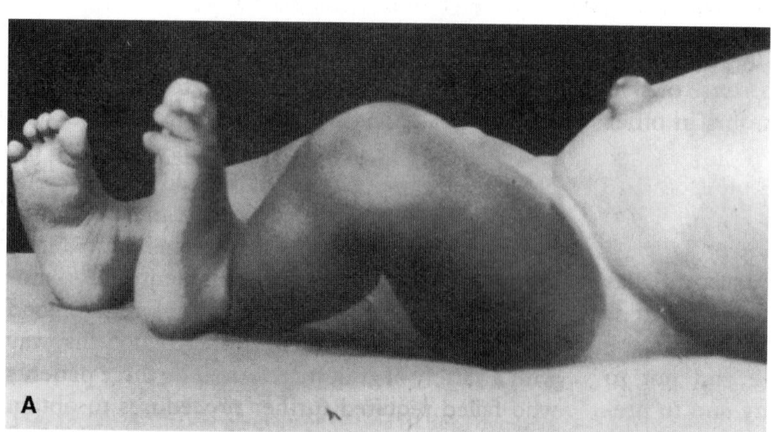

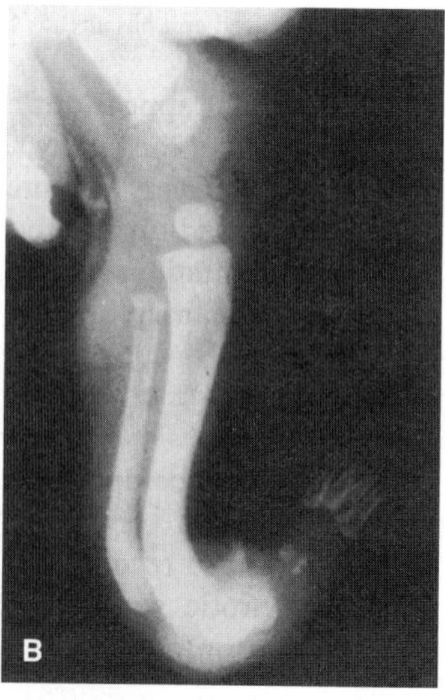

FIGURE 2-34 ■ *A*, Clinical radiograph of a child age 5 months with posterior medial angulation of the tibia. *B*, Lateral radiograph of the same patient. The appearance is dramatic, but these deformities are best treated with stretching and splinting into equinus. (From Benson, M., Fixen, J., Macniol, M.: Children's Orthopaedics and Fractures, Churchill Livingstone, 1994, p. 408.)

alternative. This procedure should include resection of the fibular anlage to avoid future foot problems.

3. Anterolateral Tibial Bowing—**Congenital pseudarthrosis of the tibia** is the most common cause of anterolateral bowing. It is often accompanied by *neurofibromatosis* (50%, but only 10% of patients with neurofibromatosis have this disorder). Classification (Boyd's) is based on bowing and the presence of cystic changes, sclerosis, or dysplasia; dysplasia and cystic changes are most common. **Initial treatment includes a total contact brace to protect from fractures.** Intramedullary fixation with excision of hamartomatous tissue and autogenous bone grafting are options for nonhealing fractures. Vascularized fibular graft or Illizarov's methods should also be considered if bracing fails. *Osteotomies to correct the anterolateral bowing are contraindicated*. Amputation (Syme's) and prosthetic fitting are indicated after two or three failed surgical attempts. Syme's amputation is preferred to below-knee amputation in these patients because the soft tissue available at the heel pad is superior to that in the calf as a weight-bearing stump. The soft tissue in the calf in these patients is often quite scarred and atrophic.
4. Other Lower-Limb Deficiencies—Include tibial hemimelia, an AD disorder that is a *congenital longitudinal deficiency of the tibia. Tibial hemimelia is the only long-bone deficiency with a known inheritance pattern (AD).* It is much less common than fibular hemimelia and is often associated with other bony abnormalities (especially lobster-claw hand). Clinically, the extremity is shortened and bowed anterolaterally with a prominent fibular head and equinovarus foot, with the sole of the foot facing the perineum. **The treatment for severe deformities with an entirely absent tibia is a knee disarticulation.** Fibular transposition (Brown's) has been unsuccessful, especially with absent quadriceps function and an absent proximal tibia. When the proximal tibia and quadriceps function are present, the fibula can be transposed to the residual tibia and create a functional below-knee amputation.

C. Osteochondritis Dissecans—An intra-articular condition common in 10- to 15-year-olds that can affect many joints, especially the *knee and elbow (capitellum)*. The lesion is thought to be secondary to trauma, ischemia, or abnormal epiphyseal ossification. ***The lateral intercondylar portion of the medial femoral condyle is most frequently involved.*** Classified into three categories based on age at appearance (Pappas).
Symptoms include activity-related pain, localized tenderness, stiffness, and swelling ± mechanical symptoms. Radiographs should include the tunnel (notch) view to evaluate the condyles. MRI can define if there is synovial fluid behind the lesion (worse prognosis for nonoperative healing). Differential diagnosis includes anomalous ossification centers. Treatment is bracing and restricted weight bearing if the patient has significant growth remaining. Surgical therapy is reserved for the adolescent with minimal growth left or a loose lesion. Operative treatment includes drilling with multiple holes, fixation of large fragments, and bone grafting of large lesions. Commonly treated arthroscopically. Poor prognosis is associated with lesions in the lateral femoral condyle and patella.

D. Osgood-Schlatter Disease—An osteochondrosis, or fatigue failure, of the tibia tubercle apophysis due to stress from the extensor mechanism in a growing child *(tibial tubercle apophysitis)*. Radiographs may show irregularity and fragmentation of the tibial tubercle. It is usually self-limiting and may require activity modification. Late excision of separate ossicles is occasionally required.

E. Discoid Meniscus—Abnormal development of the lateral meniscus leads to the formation of a disk-shaped (or hypertrophic), rather than the normal crescent-shaped, meniscus. Typically, radiographs demonstrate widening of the cartilage space on the affected side (up to 11 mm). If symptomatic and torn, discoid meniscus can be arthroscopically débrided. If not torn, they should be observed only.

XIII. Feet (Fig. 2-35)

A. Clubfoot (Congenital Talipes Equinovarus)—*Forefoot adductus and supination; hindfoot equinous and varus*. Talar neck deformity (medial and plantar deviation) with medial rotation of the calcaneus and medial displacement of the navicular and cuboid occurs. Clubfoot is more common in males, and half the cases are bilateral. It is associated with *shortened/contracted muscles (intrinsics, tendoachilles, tibialis posterior, flexor hallucis longus, flexor digitorum longus)*, joint capsules, ligaments, and fascia that lead to the associated deformities. *Can be associated with hand anomalies (Streeter's dysplasia), diastrophic dwarfism, arthrogryposis, prune belly, tibial hemimelia, and myelomeningocele*. Radiographs should include the **dorsiflexion lateral** view (Turco's), in which a talocalcaneal angle of >35 degrees is normal; a smaller angle with a flat talar head is seen with clubfoot. On the AP view a talocalcaneal (Kite's) angle of 20–40 degrees is normal (<20 degrees is seen with clubfoot). The talus-first metatarsal angle is normally 0–20 degrees, a negative talus-first metatarsal angle is seen with clubfoot (Fig. 2-36). ***"Parallelism"*** of the calcaneus and talus is seen

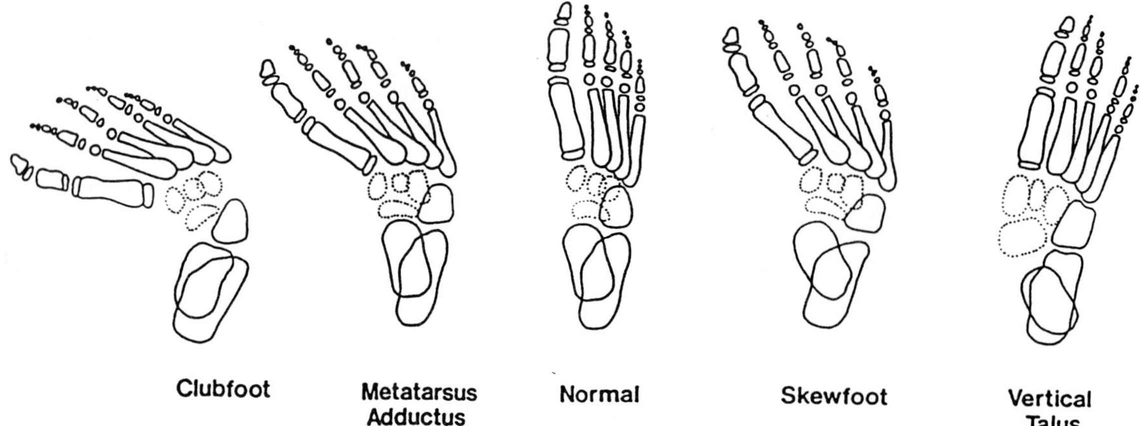

FIGURE 2-35 ■ Anteroposterior view of common childhood foot disorders. *A*, Varus position of hindfoot and adducted forefoot in clubfoot. *B*, Normal hindfoot and adducted forefoot in metatarsus adductus. *C*, Normal foot. *D*, Valgus hindfoot (with increased talocalcaneal angle) and adducted forefoot in skewfoot. *E*, Increased talocalcaneal angle and lateral deviation of the calcaneus in congenital vertical talus.

on both views. The **Ponsetti** method of serial casting has recently become more popular because of the more favorable long-term results.This method requires a series of long leg plaster casts and possible Achilles release, and it is followed by external rotation of the feet in boots and bars. Casting begins with correction of the cavus by aligning the first ray with the remaining metatarsals. Subsequent manipulation and casting utilizes lateral pressure on the distal talar head as a fulcrum to correct the forefoot adduction and heel varus. All deformities are corrected gradually. Residual equines requires tendoachilles release in >80%. Subsequent forefoot adduction/supination requires transfer of the anterior tibalis laterally in 25%. Some cases can be fully corrected with serial casts but many require corrective surgery. ***Surgical soft-tissue release with tendon lengthening is favored in resistant feet, usually at age 6–9 months*** (Table 2-18).

The posterior tibial artery must be carefully protected. Often, the dorsalis pedis artery is insufficient. Casting for several months is

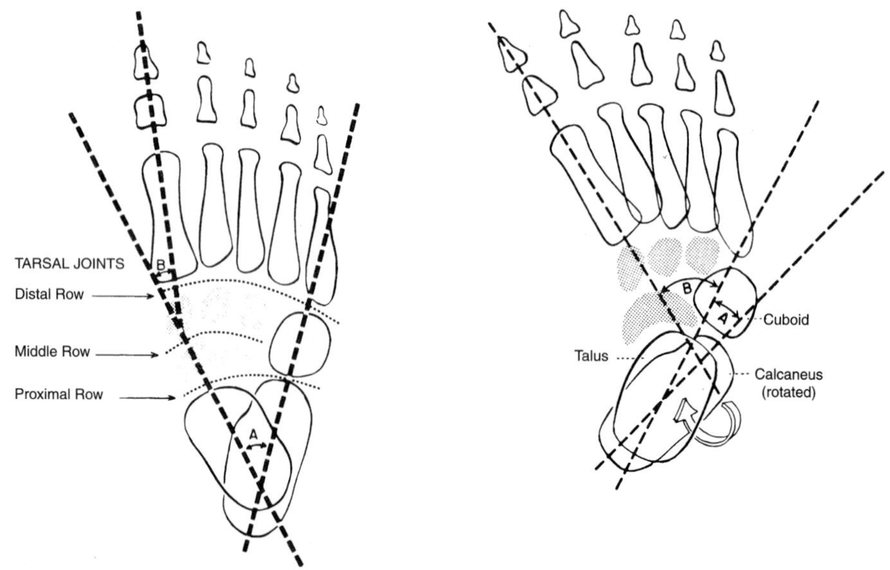

FIGURE 2-36 ■ Radiographic evaluation of clubfeet. Note the "parallelism" of the talus and calcaneus with a talocalcaneal angle *A* of <20 degrees and negative talus-first metatarsal angle *B* on the clubfoot side. (From Simons, G.W.: Analytical radiology of club feet. J. Bone Joint Surg. 59-B:485–489, 1977.)

Table 2-18. STRUCTURES TO BE ADDRESSED IN A SURGICAL CLUBFOOT CORRECTION

STRUCTURE	PROCEDURE
Achilles tendon	Z-lengthening
Calcaneal-fibular ligament	Release
Posterior talofibular ligament	Release
Posterior tibialis tendon	Z-lengthening
Flexor digitorum longus tendon	Z-lengthening
Superficial deltoid	Release
Flexor hallucis longus tendon	Z-lengthening
Tibiotalar, subtalar capsule	Complete release
Talonavicular tibionavicular (pseudo)	Release

Table 2-19. METATARSUS ADDUCTUS (MTA)

TYPE	FEATURES
Simple MTA	MTA
Complex MTA	MTA + lateral shift of midfoot
Skew foot	MTA + valgus hindfoot
Complex skew foot	MTA, lateral shift, valgus hindfoot

usually required postoperatively. In older patients (3–10 years old), medial opening or lateral column shortening osteotomy or cuboidal decancellization is recommended. For children who present with refractory clubfoot late (8–10 years old), triple arthrodesis is the only procedure possible for eliminating associated pain and deformity. Triple arthrodesis is contraindicated in patients with insensate feet because it causes a rigid foot that may lead to ulceration. Talectomy may be a better procedure in these patients.

B. Forefoot Adduction (Fig. 2-37)

1. Metatarsus Adductus—See the discussion on rotational problems of lower extremities in Lower Extremity Problems. *Adduction of the forefoot is commonly associated with DDH.* A simple clinical grading system has been described by Bleck, which is based on the heel bisector line (see Fig. 2-37). Normally, the heel bisector should line up with the second/third toe web space. Four subtypes have been identified (Berg) (Table 2-19).

   If peroneal muscle stimulation corrects metatarsus adductus, it usually responds to stretching. Otherwise, manipulation and special off-the-shelf orthotics or serial casting may be required. *Surgical options in refractory cases (usually those with a medial skin crease) include abductor hallucis longus recession (for an atavistic first toe), medial capsular release with Evans' calcaneal osteotomy (lateral column shortening), or medial opening cuneiform and lateral closing cuboid osteotomies, ± metatarsal osteotomies based on the severity of deformity.*

2. Medial Deviation of the Talar Neck—Benign disorder of the foot that generally corrects spontaneously.

3. Serpentine (Z) Foot (Complex Skew Foot)—Associated with residual *tarsometatarsal adductus, talonavicular lateral subluxation, and hindfoot valgus.* Nonoperative treatment is ineffective in correcting the deformity. Surgical treatment of this difficult problem is demanding and may include medial calcaneal sliding osteotomy (for hindfoot valgus), opening wedge cuboid osteotomy and

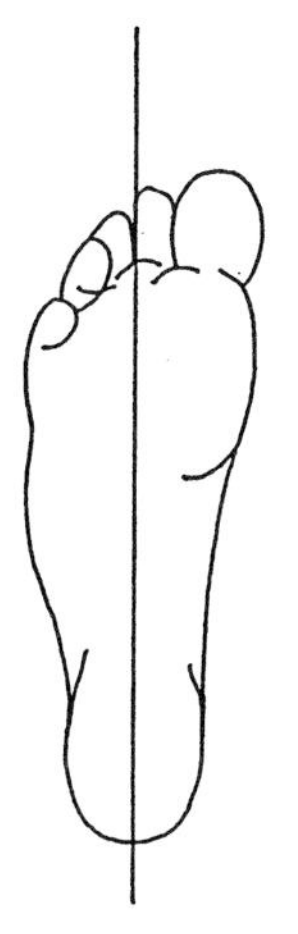

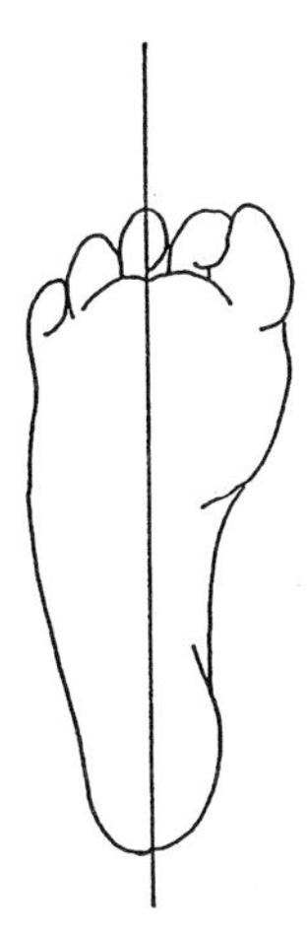

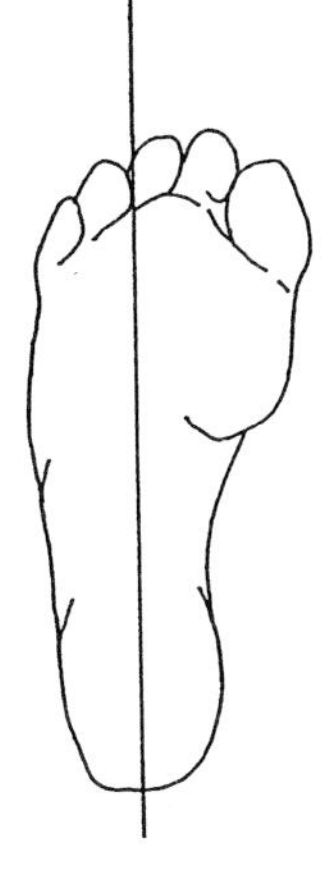

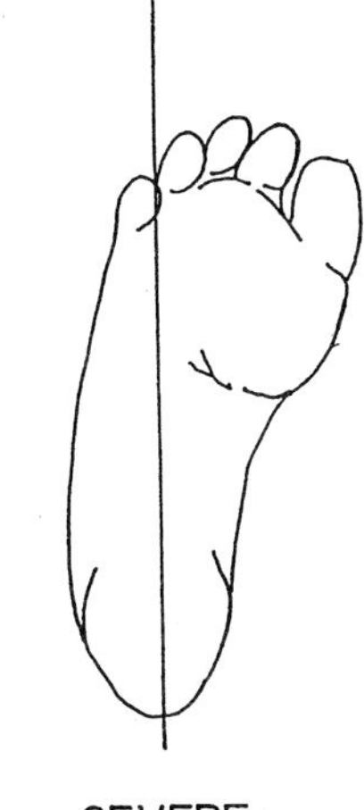

FIGURE 2-37 ■ Classification of metatarsus adductus. (From Bleck, E.E.: Metatarsus adductus: Classification and relationship to all kinds of treatment. J. Pediatr. Orthop. 3:2–9, 1983.)

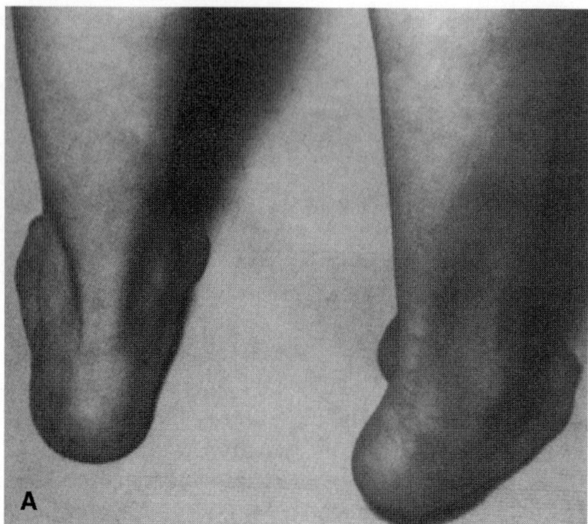

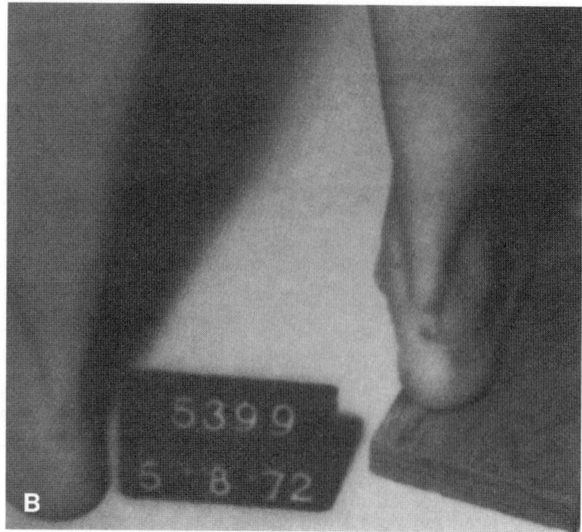

FIGURE 2-38 ■ Illustration of the Coleman block test to document hindfoot flexibility in a cavovarus foot. Posterior view of the foot of a 9-year-old boy with Charcot-Marie-Tooth disease. *A*, Note the heel varus. *B*, By placing the heel on a 3-cm block, the heel assumes a normal position and thus the calcaneus is spared from an osteotomy during surgical correction. (From Benson, M., Fixen, J., Macniol, M.: Children's Orthopaedics and Fractures, Churchill Livingstone, 1994, p. 563.)

closing wedge cuneiform osteotomy (to correct midfoot lateral subluxation), and metatarsal osteotomies (to correct forefoot adductus). Most cases can be treated symptomatically.

C. Pes Cavus—Cavus deformity of the foot (elevated longitudinal arch) due to fixed plantar flexion of the forefoot. **Pes cavus is commonly associated with neurologic disorders** including *polio, CP, Friedreich's ataxia, and Charcot-Marie-Tooth disease (an imbalance between tibialis anterior and peroneus longus*. Full neurologic work-up is mandatory. *Lateral block test (Coleman's)* assesses hindfoot flexibility of the cavovarus foot (a flexible hindfoot corrects to neutral with a lift placed under lateral aspect of foot) (Fig. 2-38). Nonoperative management is rarely successful. *Surgical options in supple deformities include plantar release, metatarsal osteotomies, and tendon transfers. If the lateral block test is abnormal (rigid deformity), a calcaneal osteotomy is done in addition.* In the past, triple arthrodesis has been used for rigid deformity in mature patients; the use of calcaneal sliding osteotomy, with multiple metatarsal extension osteotomies, may offer an alternative to subtalar fusion procedures.

D. Pes Calcaneovalgus

1. Congenital Vertical Talus (Convex Pes Valgus)—*Irreducible dorsal dislocation of the navicular on the talus with a fixed equinous hindfoot deformity.* Clinically, the talar head is prominent medially, the sole is convex, the forefoot is abducted and in dorsiflexion, and the hindfoot is in equinovalgus (Persian slipper foot) (Fig. 2-39). Patients may demonstrate a "peg-leg" gait (awkward gait with limited forefoot push-off). It is caused by a rigid flatfoot, *which can be isolated or can occur with chromosomal abnormalities, myeloarthropathies, or neurologic disorders.* **Plantar-flexion**

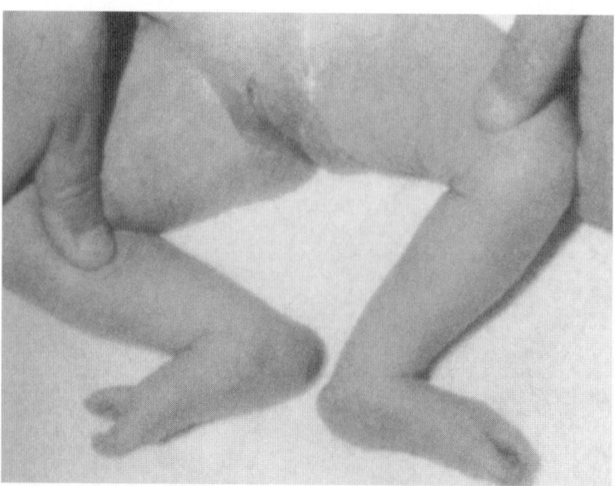

FIGURE 2-39 ■ Clinical photograph of typical calcaneovalgus feet in a newborn infant. (From Benson, M., Fixen, J., Macniol, M.: Children's Orthopaedics and Fractures, Churchill Livingstone, 1994, p. 519.)

lateral radiographs show that a line along the long axis of the talus passes below the first metatarsal-cuneiform axis (Meary's, tarsal-first metatarsal angle >20 degrees [normal 0–20 degrees dorsal tilt]). AP radiographs show a talocalcaneal angle of >40 degrees (normal 20–40 degrees). Differential diagnosis includes oblique talus (corrects with plantar flexion), tarsal coalition, and paralytic pes valgus. Three months of corrective casting (foot plantar flexed/ inverted) or manipulative stretching is tried initially. *Surgery when the patient is 6–12 months old includes soft-tissue release/ lengthening*. Talectomy may be required for resistant cases.

2. Oblique Talus—Talonavicular subluxation that reduces with plantar flexion of foot. Treatment is observation and sometimes a shoe insert University of California, Berkeley, Laboratory (UCBL). Some patients require pinning of the talonavicular joint in the reduced position and tendoachilles lengthening.

E. Tarsal Coalitions—A disorder of mesenchymal segmentation leading to *fusion of tarsal bones and rigid flatfoot. Most commonly occurs as a talocalcaneal or calcaneonavicular coalition and is the leading cause of peroneal spastic flatfoot.* Symptoms, which appear by age 10–12 years, include calf pain due to *peroneal spasticity, flatfoot, and limited subtalar motion.* Coalitions may be fibrous, cartilaginous, or osseous. ***Calcaneonavicular coalition is the most common in children ages 10–12 and subtalar is more common in 12–14 year olds.*** Lateral radiographs may demonstrate an elongated anterior process of the calcaneus (*"anteater" sign*). Talocalcaneal coalitions may demonstrate talar beaking on the lateral view (does not denote degenerative joint disease) or an irregular middle facet on Harris's axial view. The best study for identifying and measuring the cross-sectional area of a talocalcaneal coalition is a CT scan. Initial treatment for either type involves immobilization (casting) or orthotics. *Surgery is recommended in resistant cases. In calcaneonavicular coalitions, resection is commonly successful. For subtalar coalition a symptomatic bar involving <50% of the middle facet should be resected while if >50% of middle facet is involved then subtalar arthrodesis is preferred.* Before a patient undergoes resection of a calcaneonavicular coalition, a CT scan should be done to rule out the possibility of a coexisting subtalar coalition. Observation is reasonable for asymptomatic bars in young children. Advanced cases, and cases that fail attempts at resection, often require triple arthrodesis.

F. Calcaneovalgus Foot—Newborn condition associated with intrauterine positioning. It is common in first-born children. Presents with a dorsiflexed hindfoot with eversion and abduction of the hindfoot that is passively correctable to neutral. *Treatment is passive stretching and observation*. Also seen with myelomeningocele at the L5 level due to muscular imbalance between foot dorsiflexors/everters (L4 and L5 roots) and plantar flexors/inverters (S1 and S2 roots).

G. Juvenile Bunions—Often are bilateral and familial. This disorder is less common and usually less severe than the adult form. May be associated with ligamentous laxity and a hypermobile first ray. Usually found in adolescent girls. Wide shoes and arch supports help early. Surgery is indicated in symptomatic patients with an intermetatarsal angle of >10 degrees (metatarsus primus varus) and a hallux valgus angle of >20 degrees. Metatarsus primus varus may require proximal metatarsal osteotomy and distal capsular reefing. Complications include overcorrection and hallux varus. **Recurrence is frequent (>50%)**, especially when only soft-tissue procedures are performed. It is best to wait until maturity to reoperate.

H. Kohler's Disease—*Osteonecrosis of the tarsal navicular*; usually presents at about 5 years old. Pain is the typical presenting complaint. Radiographs show sclerosis of the navicular. Symptoms usually resolve spontaneously with decreased activity ± immobilization.

I. Flexible Pes Planus—Foot is flat only when standing and not with toe walking or foot hanging. This is frequently familial and almost always bilateral. Commonly associated with minor lower-extremity rotational problems and ligamentous laxity. Symptoms, including aching midfoot or pretibial pain, can occur. Lateral radiographic findings mimic those of vertical talus, but a plantar-flexed lateral view demonstrates that a line along the long axis of the talus passes above the metatarsal-cuneiform axis (Table 2-20). Treatment is observation only, with no special shoes. Sometimes, soft arch supports are helpful but not corrective. Thorough evaluation should be completed to

Table 2-20. RADIOLOGIC VIEWS FOR PES PLANUS

VIEW	ASSESSMENT
Standing AP	Talar head coverage, talocalcaneal angle
Standing lateral	Calcaneal/talar equinus, talocalcaneal angle
Oblique	To rule out coalition

rule out tight heel cords and decreased subtalar motion. UCBL heel cups are sometimes indicated for advanced cases with pain (symptomatic treatment only). Calcaneal osteotomy or select fusions may provide pain relief at the expense of inversion/eversion in adolescents with disabling pain refractory to every means of conservative treatment.

J. Habitual Toe Walker—Contracture of the Achilles tendon (often resolves with time). Usually responds to serial casting; sometimes requires tendoachilles lengthening.

K. Accessory Navicular—Normal variant seen in up to 12% of the population. Commonly associated with flat feet. Symptoms usually include medial arch pain with overuse. Symptoms usually resolve with activity restriction or immobilization. External oblique radiographic views are often helpful for the diagnosis. Most cases resolve spontaneously. Occasionally, excision of the accessory bone is done, which can correct symptoms (but not flatfoot) in most patients.

L. Ball and Socket Ankle—Abnormal formation with a spherical talus (ball) and a cup-shaped tibiofibular articulation (socket). *It usually requires no treatment but should be recognized because of its high association with tarsal coalition (50%), absent lateral rays (50%), fibular deficiency, and leg-length discrepancies.*

M. Congenital Toe Disorders
   1. Syndactyly—Fusion of the soft tissues (simple) and sometimes bone (complex) of the toes. Simple syndactyly usually does not require treatment; complex syndactyly is treated as it is in the hand.
   2. Polydactyly (Extra Digits) May be AD and usually involves the lateral ray in patients with a positive family history. Treatment includes ablation of the extra digit and any bony protrusion of the common metatarsal (typically, the border digit is excised, not the best formed digit). The procedure is usually done at age 9–12 months, but some rudimentary digits can be ligated in the newborn nursery.
   3. Oligodactyly—Congenital absence of the toes. May be associated with more proximal agenesis (i.e., fibular hemimelia) and tarsal coalition. The disorder usually requires no treatment.
   4. Atavistic Great Toe (Congenital Hallux Varus)—Great toe adduction deformity that is often associated with polydactyly. Must be differentiated from metatarsus adductus. Usually, the deformity occurs at the metatarsophalangeal joint and includes a short, thick first metatarsal and a firm band (abductor hallucis longus muscle) that may be responsible for the disorder. Surgery is sometimes required and includes release of the abductor hallucis longus muscle.
   5. Overlapping Toe—The fifth toe overlaps the fourth (usually bilaterally) and may cause problems with footwear. Initial treatment includes passive stretching and "buddy" taping. Surgical options include tenotomy, dorsal capsulotomy, and syndactylization to the fourth toe (McFarland).
   6. Underlapping Toe (Congenital Curly Toe)—Usually occurs at lateral three toes and is rarely symptomatic. **Surgery (flexor tenotomies) is occasionally indicated.**

Selected Bibliography

BONE DYSPLASIAS

Bassett, G.S.: Lower extremity abnormalities in dwarfing conditions. Instr. Course Lect. 39:389–397, 1991.

Bassett, G.S.: Orthopedic aspects of skeletal dysplasias. Instr. Course Lect. 39:381–387, 1991.

Beals, R.K., and Rolfe, B.: Current concepts review: Vater association: a unifying concept of multiple anomalies. J. Bone Joint Surg. [Am.] 71:948–950, 1989.

Bethem, D., Winter, R.B., Lutter, L., et al.: Spinal disorders of dwarfism. J. Bone Joint Surg. [Am] 63:1412–1425, 1981.

Brook, C.G., and de Vries, B.B: Skeletal dysplasias. Archives of Disease in Childhood. 79(3):285–289, 1998.

Dawe, C., Wynne-Davies, R., and Fulford, G.E.: Clinical variation in dyschondrosteosis: a report on 13 individuals in 8 families. J. Bone Joint Surg. [Br.] 64:377–381, 1982.

Dietz, F.R., and Mathews, K.D.: Update on the genetic bases of disorders with orthopaedic manifestations. J. Bone Joint Surg. [Am.] 78(10):1583–1598, 1996.

Goldberg, M.J.: The Dysmorphic Child: An Orthopedic Perspective. New York, Raven Press, 1987.

Hecht, J.T., Horton, W.A., Reid, C.S., et al.: Growth of the foramen magnum in achondroplasia. Am. J. Med. Genet. 32:528–535, 1989.

Jones, K.L., and Robinson, L.K.: An approach to the child with structural defects. J. Pediatr. Orthop. 3:238–244, 1983.

Kopits, S.E.: Orthopedic complications of dwarfism. Clin. Orthop. 114:153–179, 1976.

McKusick, V.A.: Heritable Disorders of Connective Tissue, 4th ed. St. Louis, C.V. Mosby, 1972.

Rubin, P.: Dynamic Classification of Bone Dysplasias. Chicago, Year Book Medical Publishers, 1964.

Stanscur, V., Stanscur, R., and Maroteaux, P.: Pathogenic mechanisms in osteochondrodysplasias. J. Bone Joint Surg. [Am.] 66:817–836, 1984.

Swanson, A.B.: A classification for congenital limb malformation. J. Hand Surg. 1:8–22, 1976.

Warman, M.L.: Human genetic insights into skeletal development, growth, and homeostasis. Clinical Orthopaedics and Related Research Suppl. (379):S40–54, 2000.

CHROMOSOMAL AND TERATOLOGIC DISORDERS

Doyle, J.S., Lauerman, W.C., Wood, K.B., and Krause, D.R.: Complications and long-term outcome of upper cervical spine arthrodesis in patients with Down syndrome. Spine 21(10):1223–1231, 1996.

Huang, T.J., Lubricky, J.P., and Hammerberg, K.W.: Scoliosis in Rhett syndrome. Orthop. Rev. 23:931–937, 1994.

Loder, R., Lee, C., and Richards, B.: Orthopedic aspects of Rhett syndrome: A multicenter review. J. Pediatr. Orthop. 9:557–562, 1989.

Rees, D., Jones, M.W., Owen, R., et al.: Scoliosis surgery in the Prader-Willi syndrome. J. Bone Joint Surg. [Br.] 71:685–688, 1989.

Segal, L.S., Drummond, D.S., Zanott, R.M., et al.: Complications of posterior arthrodesis of the cervical spine in patients who have Down syndrome. J. Bone Joint Surg. [Am.] 73:1547–1554, 1991.

Smith, D.W.: Recognizable Pattern of Human Malformation, 2nd ed. Philadelphia, WB Saunders, 1983.

Uno, K., Kataoka, O., and Shiba, R.: Occipitoatlantal and occipitoaxial hypermobility in Down syndrome. Spine 21(12):1430–1434, 1996.

HEMATOPOIETIC DISORDERS

Diggs, L.W.: Bone and joint lesions in sickle-cell disease. Clin. Orthop. 52:119–143, 1967.

Gill, J.C., Thometz, J.C., and Scott, J.P.: Musculoskeletal Problems in Hemophilia in the Child and Adult. New York, Raven Press, 1989.

Lofqvist, T., Nilsson, I.M., and Petersson, C.: Orthopaedic surgery in hemophilia. 20 years' experience in Sweden. Clinical Orthopaedics and Related Research (332):232–241, 1996.

Ribbans, W.J., Giangrande, P., and Beeton, K.: Conservative treatment of hemarthrosis for prevention of hemophilic synovitis. Clinical Orthopaedics and Related Research (343):12–18, 1997.

Triantafylluo, S., Hanks, G., Handal, J.A., et al.: Open and arthroscopic synovectomy in hemophilic arthropathy of the knee. Clin. Orthop. 283:196–204, 1992.

Thomas, H.B.: Some orthopaedic findings in ninety-eight cases of hemophilia. Clinical Orthopaedics and Related Research (343):3–5, 1997.

METABOLIC DISEASE/ARTHRITIDES

Albright, J.A., and Miller, E.A.: Osteogenesis imperfecta [editorial comment]. Clin. Orthop. 159:2, 1981.

Birch, J.G., and Herring, J.A.: Spinal deformity in Marfan syndrome. J. Pediatr. Orthop. 7:546–552, 1987.

Certner, J.M., and Root, L.: Osteogenesis imperfecta. Orthop. Clin. North Am. 21:151–162, 1990.

Cole, W.G.: Advances in osteogenesis imperfecta. Clinical Orthopaedics and Related Research (401):6–16, 2002.

Gamble, J.G., Strudwick, W.J., Rinsky, L.A., et al.: Complications of intramedullary rods in osteogenesis imperfecta: Bailey-Dubow rods versus nonelongating rods. J. Pediatr. Orthop. 8:645–649, 1989.

Hensinger, R.N., DeVito, P.D., and Ragsdale, C.G.: Changes in the cervical spine in juvenile rheumatoid arthritis. J. Bone Joint Surg. [Am.] 68:189–199, 1986.

Kulas, D.T., and Schanberg, L.: **Juvenile** idiopathic arthritis. Current Opinion in Rheumatology. 13(5):392–398, 2001.

Mankin, H.J.: Rickets, osteomalacia and renal osteodystrophy: an update. Orthop. Clin. North Am. 21:81–96, 1990.

Robelo, I., Peredra, D.A., Silva, L., et al.: Effects of synthetic salmon calcitonin therapy in children with osteogenesis imperfecta. J. Int. Med. Res. 17:401–405, 1989.

Schaller, J.G.: Chronic arthritis in children: juvenile rheumatoid arthritis. Clin. Orthop. 182:79–89, 1984.

Shapiro, F.: Consequences of an osteogenesis imperfecta diagnosis for survival and ambulation. J. Pediatr. Orthop. 5:456–462, 1985.

Sherry, D.D.: What's new in the diagnosis and treatment of juvenile rheumatoid arthritis. J. Pediatr. Orthop. 20(4):419–420, 2000.

Sillence, D.O.: Osteogenesis imperfecta: An expanding panorama of variance. Clin. Orthop. 159:11, 1981.

Sofield, H.A., and Miller, E.A.: Fragmentation realignment and intramedullary rod fixation of deformities of the long bones in children. J. Bone Joint Surg. [Am.] 41:1371, 1959.

Tortolani, P.J., McCarthy, E.F., and Sponseller, P.D.: Bone mineral density deficiency in children. Journal of the American Academy of Orthopaedic Surgeons 10(1):57–66, 2002.

BIRTH INJURIES

Bellew, M., Kay, S.P., Webb, F., and Ward, A.: Developmental and behavioural outcome in obstetric brachial plexus palsy Journal of Hand Surgery [Br.] 25(1):49–51, 2000.

Canale, S.T., Griffin, T.W., and Hubbard, C.N.: Congenital muscular torticollis: a long-term follow-up. J. Bone Joint Surg. [Am.] 64:810–816, 1982.

Davids, J.R., Wenger, D.R., and Mubarak, S.J.: Congenital muscular torticollis: Sequelae of intrauterine or perinatal compartment syndrome. J. Pediatr. Orthop. 13:141–147, 1993.

Gilbert, A., Brockman, R., and Carlioz, H.: Surgical treatment of brachial plexus birth palsy. Clin. Orthop. 264:39–47, 1991.

Hentze, V.R., and Meyer, R.D.: Brachial plexus microsurgery in children. Microsurgery 12:175–185, 1991.

Jahnke, A.H., Bovill, D.F., McCarroll, H.R., et al.: Persistent brachial plexus birth palsies. J. Pediatr. Orthop. 11:533–537, 1991.

Quinlan, W.R., Brady, P.G., and Regan, B.F.: Congenital pseudarthrosis of the clavicle. Acta Orthop. Scand. 51:489–492, 1980.

Waters, P.M.: Comparison of the natural history, the outcome of microsurgical repair, and the outcome of operative reconstruction in brachial plexus birth palsy. J. Bone Joint Surg. [Am.] 81(5):649–659, 1999.

CEREBRAL PALSY

Albright, A.L., Barron, W.B., Fasick, M.P., et al.: Continuous intrathecal baclofen infusion for spasticity of cerebral origin. J.A.M.A. 270:2475–2477, 1993.

Barnes, M.J., and Herring, J.A.: Combined split anterior tibial-tendon transfer and intramuscular lengthening of the posterior tibial tendon. J. Bone Joint Surg. [Am.] 73:734–738, 1991.

Bell, K.J., Ounpuu, S., DeLuca, P.A., and Romness, M.J.: Natural progression of gait in children with cerebral palsy. J. Pediatr. Orthop. 22(5):677–682, 2002.

Bleck, E.E.: Current concepts review: management of the lower extremities in children who have cerebral palsy. J. Bone Joint Surg. [Am.] 72:140, 1990.

Bleck, E.E.: Orthopedic Management of Cerebral Palsy. Philadelphia, JB Lippincott, 1987.

Coleman, S.S., and Chestnut, W.J.: A simple test for hindfoot flexibility in the cavovarus foot. Clin. Orthop. 123:60–62, 1977.

Dobson, F., Boyd, R.N., Parrott, J., Nattrass, G.R., et al.: Hip surveillance in children with cerebral palsy. Impact on the surgical management of spastic hip disease. J. Bone Joint Surg. [Br.] 84(5):720–726, 2002.

Elmer, E.B., Wenger, D.R., Mubarak, S.J., et al.: Proximal hamstring lengthening in the sitting cerebral palsy patient. J. Pediatr. Orthop. 12:329–336, 1992.

Ferguson, R.L., and Allen, B.L.: Considerations in the treatment of cerebral palsy patients with spinal deformities. Orthop. Clin. North Am. 19:419–425, 1988.

Gage, J.R.: Gait analysis: an essential tool in the treatment of cerebral palsy. Clin. Orthop. 288:126–134, 1993.

Gage, J.R.: The clinical use of kinetics for evaluation of pathologic gait in cerebral palsy. J. Bone Joint Surg. [Am.] 76:622–631, 1994.

Koman, L.A., Mooney, J.F., Goodman, A.: Management of valgus hindfoot deformity in pediatric cerebral palsy patients by medial displacement osteotomy. J. Pediatr. Orthop. 13:180–183, 1993.

Koman, L.A., Mooney, J.F., Smith, B.P., et al.: Management of spasticity in cerebral palsy with botulinum-A toxin: report of preliminary, randomized, double-blind trial. J. Pediatr. Orthop. 14:299–303, 1994.

Mubarak, S.J., Valencia, F.G., and Wenger, D.R.: One stage correction of the spastic dislocated hip. J. Bone Joint Surg. [Am.] 74:1347–1357, 1994.

Ounpuu, S., Muik, E., Davis, R.B., et al.: Rectus femoris surgery in children with cerebral palsy. Part II. A comparison between the effect of transfer and release of the distal rectus femoris on knee motion. J. Pediatr. Orthop. 13:331–335, 1993.

Rang, M., Silver, R., de la Garza, Jr., et al.: Cerebral palsy. In Lovell, R., and Winter, R., eds.: Pediatric Orthopedics, 2nd ed. Philadelphia, JB Lippincott, 1986.

Rang, M., and Wright, J.: What have 30 years of medical progress done for cerebral palsy? Clin. Orthop. 247:55–60, 1989.

Renshaw, T.S., Green, N.E., Griffin, P.P., and Root, L.: Cerebral palsy: orthopaedic management. Instr. Course Lect. 45:475–490, 1996.

Sutherland, D.H., and Davids, J.R.: Common gait abnormalities of the knee in cerebral palsy. Clin. Orthop. 288:139–147, 1993.

Thomas, S.S., Aiona, M.D., Buckon, C.E., Piatt, J.H., Jr.: Does gait continue to improve 2 years after selective dorsal rhizotomy? J. Pediatr. Orthop. 17(3):387–391, 1997.

NEUROMUSCULAR DISORDERS

Allen, B.L., Jr., and Ferguson, R.L.: The Galveston technique of pelvic fixation with Luque-rod instrumentation of the spine. Spine 9:388–394, 1984.

Babat, L.B., and Ehrlich, M.G.: A paradigm for the age-related treatment of knee dislocations in Larsen's syndrome. J. Pediatr. Orthop. 20(3):396–401, 2000.

Banta, J.V., Drummond, D.S., and Ferguson, R.L.: The treatment of neuromuscular scoliosis. Instr. Course Lect. 48:551–562, 1999.

Drennan, J.C.: Foot deformities in myelomeningocele. Instr. Course Lect. 40:287–291, 1991.

Drennan, J.C.: Current concepts in myelomeningocele. Instr. Course Lect. 48:543–550, 1999.

Drummond, D.S., Moreau, M., and Cruess, R.L.: The results and complications of surgery for the paralytic hip and spine in myelomeningocele. J. Bone Joint Surg. [Br.] 62:49–53, 1980.
Emans, J.B.: Current concepts review: allergy to latex in patients who have myelodysplasia. J. Bone Joint Surg. [Am.] 74:1103–1109, 1992.
Evans, G.A., Drennan, J.C., and Russman, B.S.: Functional classification and orthopedic management of spinal muscular atrophy. J. Bone Joint Surg. [Br.] 63:516–522, 1981.
Greene, W.B.: Treatment of hip and knee problems in myelomeningocele. Instr. Course Lect. 48:563–574, 1999.
Hall, J.G.: Arthrogryposis multiplex congenita: etiology, genetics, classification, diagnostic approach, and general aspects. Journal of Pediatric Orthopaedics, Part B. 6(3):159–166, 1997.
Hoffer, M.M., Feiwell, E., Perry, R., et al.: Functional ambulation in patients with myelomeningocele. J. Bone Joint Surg. [Am.] 55:137–148, 1973.
Lindseth, R.E.: Spine deformity in myelomeningocele. Instr. Course Lect. 40:273–279, 1991.
Mazur, J.M., Shurtleff, D., Menelaus, M., et al.: Orthopedic management of high-level spina bifida: early walking compared with early use of a wheelchair. J. Bone Joint Surg. [Am.] 71:56, 1989.
Mendell, J.R., and Sahenk, Z.: Recent advances in diagnosis and classification of Charcot-Marie-Tooth disease. Curr. Opin. Orthop. 4:39–45, 1993.
Shapiro, F., and Bresnan, M.J.: Orthopedic management of childhood neuromuscular disease. Part II. Peripheral neuropathies, Friedreich's ataxia, and arthrogryposis multiplex congenita. J. Bone Joint Surg. [Am.] 64:949–953, 1982.
Shapiro, F., and Specht, L.: Current concepts review: the diagnosis and orthopedic management of inherited muscular disorders of childhood. J. Bone Joint Surg. [Am.] 75:439–454, 1993.
Sodergard, J., and Ryoppy, S.: Foot deformities in arthrogryposis multiplex congenita. J. Pediatr. Orthop. 14:768–772, 1994.
Sussman M.: Duchenne muscular dystrophy. Journal of the American Academy of Orthopaedic Surgeons 10(2):138–151, 2002.

PEDIATRIC SPINE

Bellah, R.D., Summerville, D.A., Treves, S.T., et al.: Low-back pain in adolescent athletes: detection of stress injury to the pars interarticularis with SPECT. Radiology 180:509–512, 1991.
Betz, R.R., and Shufflebarger, H.: Anterior versus posterior instrumentation for the correction of thoracic idiopathic scoliosis. Spine 26(9):1095–1100, 2001.
Bollini, G., Bergion, M., Labriet, C., et al.: Hemivertebrae excision and fusion in children aged less than 5 years. J. Pediatr. Orthop. 1 (part B):95–101, 1993.
Bradford, D.S., Ahmed, K.B., Moe, J.H., et al.: The surgical management of patients with Scheuerman's disease: a review of twenty-four cases managed by combined anterior and posterior spine fusion. J. Bone Joint Surg. [Am.] 62:705–712, 1980.
Bradford, D.S., and Hensinger, R.M., eds.: The Pediatric Spine. New York, Thieme-Stratton, 1985.
Bradford, D.S., Lonstein, J.E., Ogilvie, J.B., et al., eds.: Moe's Textbook of Scoliosis and Other Spinal Deformities, 2nd ed. Philadelphia, WB Saunders, 1987.
Bridwell, K.H., McAllister, J.W., Betz, R.R., et al.: Coronal decompensation produced by Cotrel-Dubousset "derotation" maneuver for idiopathic right thoracic scoliosis. Spine 16:769–777, 1991.
Carr, W.A., Moe, J.H., Winter, R.B., et al.: Treatment of idiopathic scoliosis in the Milwaukee brace. J. Bone Joint Surg. [Am.] 62:599–612, 1980.
Crawford, A.H., and Schorry, E.K.: Neurofibromatosis in children: the role of the orthopaedist. Journal of the American Academy of Orthopaedic Surgeons 7(4):217–230, 1999.
Denis, F.: Cotrel-Dubousset instrumentation in the treatment of idiopathic scoliosis. Orthop. Clin. North Am. 19:291–311, 1988.
Dobbs, M.B., and Weinstein, S.L.: Infantile and juvenile scoliosis. Orthopedic Clinics of North America 30(3):331–341, vii, 1999.
Dimeglio, A.: Growth of the spine before age 5 years. J. Pediatr. Orthop. 1 (part B):102–107, 1993.
Engler, G.L.: Preoperative and intraoperative considerations in adolescent idiopathic scoliosis. Instr. Course Lect. 38:137–141, 1989.
Fielding, J.W., and Hawkins, R.J.: Atlantoaxial rotatory fixation. J. Bone Joint Surg. [Am.] 59:37–44, 1977.
Fielding, J.W., Hensinger, R.N., and Hawkins, R.J.: Os odontoideum. J. Bone Joint Surg. [Am.] 62:376–383, 1980.
Fitch, R.D., Turi, M., Bowman, B.E., et al.: Comparison of Cotrel-Dubousset and Harrington rod instrumentation in idiopathic scoliosis. J. Pediatr. Orthop. 10:44–47, 1990.
Karachalios, T., Roidis, N., Papagelopoulos, P.J., and Karachalios, G.G.: The efficacy of school screening for scoliosis. Orthopedics 23(4):386–391, 2000.
King, H.A., Moe, J.H., Bradford, D.S., et al.: The selection of fusion levels in thoracic idiopathic scoliosis. J. Bone Joint Surg. [Am.] 65:1302–1313, 1983.
Koop, S.E., Winter, R.B., and Lonstein, J.E.: The surgical treatment of instability of the upper part of the cervical spine in children and adolescents. J. Bone Joint Surg. [Am.] 66:403–411, 1984.
Lenke, L.G., Bridwell, K.H., Baldus, C., et al.: Cotrel-Dubousset instrumentation for idiopathic scoliosis. J. Bone Joint Surg. [Am.] 74:1056–1068, 1992.
Lenke, L.G., Betz, R.R., Clements, D., et al.: Curve prevalence of a new classification of operative adolescent idiopathic scoliosis: does classification correlate with treatment. Spine 27(6):604–611, 2002.
Lonstein, J.E., and Carlson, J.M.: The prediction of curve progression in untreated idiopathic scoliosis during growth. J. Bone Joint Surg. [Am.] 66:1061–1071, 1984.
Lonstein, J.E.: Congenital spine deformities: scoliosis, kyphosis, and lordosis. Orthopedic Clinics of North America 30(3):387–405, viii, 1999.
Lowe, T.G.: Current concepts review: Scheuermann's disease. J. Bone Joint Surg. [Am.] 72:940–945, 1990.
Lowe, T.G., Edgar, M., Margulies, J.Y., Miller, N.H., et al.: Etiology of idiopathic scoliosis: current trends in research. J. Bone Joint Surg. [Am.] 82 A(8):1157–1168, 2000.
Luque, E.R.: Segmental spinal instrumentation for correction of scoliosis. Clin. Orthop. 163:192–198, 1982.
McMaster, M.J., and Ohtsuka, K.: The natural history of congenital scoliosis: A study of two hundred and fifty-one patients. J. Bone Joint Surg. [Am.] 64:1128–1137, 1982.
Mehta, M.H.: The rib-vertebra angle in the early diagnosis between resolving and progressive infantile scoliosis. J. Bone Joint Surg. [Br.] 54:230–243, 1972.
Miller, N.H.: Cause and natural history of adolescent idiopathic scoliosis. Orthopedic Clinics of North America 30(3):343–352, vii, 1999.
Montgomery, S., and Hall, J.: Congenital kyphosis: surgical treatment at Boston Children's Hospital. Orthop. Trans. 5:25, 1981.
Pang, D., and Wilberger, J.E., Jr.: Spinal cord injury without radiographic abnormalities in children. J. Neurosurg. 57:114–129, 1982.
Picetti, G.D., III, Ertl, J.P., Bueff, H.U.: Anterior endoscopic correction of scoliosis. Orthopedic Clinics of North America 33(2):421–429, 2002.
Ring, D., and Wenger, D.R.: Magnetic resonance imaging scans in discitis: sequential studies in a child who needed operative drainage; a case report. J. Bone Joint Surg. [Am.] 76:596–601, 1994.
Schrock, R.D.: Congenital abnormalities at the cervicothoracic level. Inst. Course Lect. 6:1949.
Scoles, P.V., and Quinn, T.P.: Intervertebral discitis in children and adolescents. Clin. Orthop. 162:31–36, 1982.
Sorenson, K.H.: Scheuermann's Juvenile Kyphosis. Copenhagen, Munksgaard, 1964.
Tolo, V.T.: Surgical treatment of adolescent idiopathic scoliosis. Instr. Course Lect. 38:143–156, 1989.
Tredwell, S.J., Newman, D.E., and Lockitch, G.: Instability of the upper cervical spine in Down syndrome. J. Pediatr. Orthop. 10:602–606, 1990.
Tucker, S.K., Noordeen, M.H., and Pitt, M.C.: Spinal cord monitoring in neuromuscular scoliosis. Journal of Pediatric Orthopaedics, Part B 10(1):1–5, 2001.
Weinstein, S.L., and Ponseti, I.V.: Curve progression in idiopathic scoliosis. J. Bone Joint Surg. [Am.] 65:447–455, 1983.
Weinstein, S.L.: Natural history. Spine 24(24):2592–2600, 1999.
Winter, R.B., Lonstein, J.E., Drogt, J., et al.: The effectiveness of bracing in the nonoperative treatment of idiopathic scoliosis. Spine 11:790–791, 1986.
Winter, R.B., Moe, J.H., and Lonstein, J.E.: The incidence of Klippel-Feil syndrome in patients with congenital scoliosis and kyphosis. Spine 9:363–366, 1984.
Winter, R.B., Moe, J.H., and Lonstein, J.E.: The surgical treatment of congenital kyphosis: a review of 94 patients age 5 years or older, with 2 years or more follow-up in 77 patients. Spine 10:224–231, 1985.

UPPER EXTREMITY PROBLEMS

Carson, W.G., Lovell, W.W., and Whitesides, T.E., Jr.: Congenital elevation of the scapula: surgical correction by the Woodward procedure. J. Bone Joint Surg. [Am.] 62:1199–1207, 1981.

Green, W.T.: The surgical correction of congenital elevation of the scapula (Sprengel's deformity). J. Bone Joint Surg. [Am.] 149, 1957.

Liebovic, S.J., Erlich, M.G., and Zaleske, D.J.: Sprengel deformity. J. Bone Joint Surg. [Am.] 72:192–197, 1990.

Woodward, J.W.: Congenital elevation of the scapula: Correction by release and transplantation of muscle origins. J. Bone Joint Surg. [Am.] 43:219–228, 1961.

LOWER EXTREMITY PROBLEMS

Berg, E.F.: A reappraisal of metatarsus adductus and skewfoot. J. Bone Joint Surg. [Am.] 68:1185–1196, 1986.

Bleck, E.E.: Metatarsus adductus: Classification and relationship to outcomes of treatment. J. Pediatr. Orthop. 3:2–9, 1983.

Crawford, A.H., and Gabriel, K.R.: Foot and ankle problems. Orthop. Clin. North Am. 18:649–666, 1987.

Green, W.B.: Metatarsus adductus and skewfoot. Instr. Course Lect. 43:161–178, 1994.

Kling, T.F., and Hensinger, R.N.: Angular and torsional deformities of the lower limbs in children. Clin. Orthop. 176:136–147, 1983.

Staheli, L.T., Clawson, D.K., and Hubbard, D.D.: Medial femoral torsion: experience with operative treatment. Clin. Orthop. 146:222–225, 1980.

Staheli, L.T., Corbett, M., Wyss, C., et al.: Lower extremity rotational problems in children: normal values to guide management. J. Bone Joint Surg. [Am.] 67:39–47, 1985.

HIP AND FEMUR

Blanco, J.S., Taylor, B., and Johnston, C.E., II: Comparison of single pin vs. multiple pin fixation in treatment of slipped capital femoral epiphysis. J. Pediatr. Orthop. 12:384–389, 1992.

Canale, S.T., Harkness, R.M., Thomas, P.A., et al.: Does aspiration of bones and joints affect results of later bone scanning? J. Pediatr. Orthop. 5:23–26, 1985.

Chiari, K.: Medial displacement osteotomy of the pelvis. Clin. Orthop. 98:55–71, 1974.

Christensen, F., Soballe, K., Ejsted, R., et al.: The Catterall classification of Perthes disease: an assessment of reliability. J. Bone Joint Surg. [Br.] 68:614–615, 1986.

Daoud, A., and Saighi-Bouaouina, A.: Treatment of sequestra, pseudarthroses, and defects in the long bones of children who have chronic hematogenous osteomyelitis. J. Bone Joint Surg. [Am.] 71:1448–1468, 1989.

Epps, C.H., Jr.: Current concepts review: proximal femoral focal deficiency. J. Bone Joint Surg. [Am.] 65:867–870, 1983.

Fabry, F., and Meire, E.: Septic arthritis of the hip in children: Poor results after late and inadequate treatment. J. Pediatr. Orthop. 3:461–466, 1983.

Faciszewski, T., Coleman, S.S., and Biddolpf, G.: Triple innominate osteotomy for acetabular dysplasia. J. Pediatr. Orthop. 13:426–430, 1993.

Faciszewski, T., Keifer, G., and Coleman, S.S.: Pemberton osteotomy for residual acetabular dysplasia in children who have congenital dislocation of the hip. J. Bone Joint Surg. [Am.] 5:643–649, 1993.

Gage, J.R., and Winter, R.B.: Avascular necrosis of the capital femoral epiphysis as a complication of closed reduction of congenital dislocation of the hip: a critical review of twenty years' experience at Gillette Children's Hospital. J. Bone Joint Surg. [Am.] 54:373–388, 1972.

Galpin, R.D., Roach, J.W., Wenger, D.R., et al.: One-stage treatment of congenital dislocation of the hip in older children, including femoral shortening. J. Bone Joint Surg. [Am.] 71:734–741, 1989.

Gillingham, B.L., Sanchez, A.A., and Wenger, D.R.: Pelvic osteotomies for the treatment of hip dysplasia in children and young adults. Journal of the American Academy of Orthopaedic Surgeons 7(5):325–337, 1999.

Green, N.E., and Edwards, K.: Bone and joint infections in children. Orthop. Clin. North Am. 18:555–576, 1987.

Green, S.A.: Patient management during limb lengthening. Instr. Course Lect. 46:547–554, 1997.

Guille, J.T., Pizzutillo, P.D., and MacEwen, G.D.: Development dysplasia of the hip from birth to six months. Journal of the American Academy of Orthopaedic Surgeons 8(4):232–242, 2000.

Harke, H.T., and Grissom, L.E.: Performing dynamic ultrasonography of the infant hip. A. J.R. Am. J. Roentgenol. 155:837–844, 1990.

Haynes RJ. Developmental dysplasia of the hip: etiology, pathogenesis, and examination and physical findings in the newborn. Instr. Course Lect. 50:535–540, 2001.

Herndon, W.A., Knaur, S., Sullivan, J.A., et al.: Management of septic arthritis in children. J. Pediatr. Orthop. 6:576–578, 1986.

Herring, J.A., Neustadt, J.B., Williams, J.J., et al.: The lateral pillar classification of Legg-Calvé-Perthes disease. J. Pediatr. Orthop. 12:143–150, 1992.

Kocher, M.S., Zurakowski, D., and Kasser J.R.: Differentiating between septic arthritis and transient synovitis of the hip in children: an evidence-based clinical prediction algorithm. J. Bone Joint Surg. [Am.] 81(12):1662–1670, 1999.

Jackson, M.A., and Nelson, J.D.: Etiology and medical management of acute suppurative bone and joint infections in pediatric patients. J. Pediatr. Orthop. 2:313–323, 1982.

Loder, R.T., Aronsson, D.D., Dobbs, M.B., and Weinstein, S.L.: Slipped capital femoral epiphysis. Instr. Course Lect. 50:555–570, 2001.

Matan, A.J., and Smith, J.T.: Pediatric septic arthritis. Orthopedics 20(7):630–635, 1997.

Mausen, J.P.G.M., Rozing, P.M., and Obermann, W.R.: Intertrochanteric corrective osteotomy in slipped capital femoral epiphysis: a long-term follow-up study of 26 patients. Clin. Orthop. 259:100–109, 1990.

Morrissey, R.T., ed.: Lovell and Winter's Pediatric Orthopedics, 3rd ed. Philadelphia, JB Lippincott, 2000.

Moseley, C.F.: Assessment and prediction in leg length discrepancy. Instr. Course Lect. 38:325–330, 1989.

Moseley, C.F.: Developmental hip dysplasia and dislocation: management of the older child. Instr. Course Lect. 50:547–553, 2001.

Mubarak, S.J., Beck, L.R., and Sutherland, D.H.: Home traction in the management of congenital dislocation of the hips. J. Pediatr. Orthop. 6:721–723, 1986.

Mubarak, S.J., Garfin, S., Vance, R., et al.: Pitfalls in the use of the Pavlik harness for treatment of congenital dysplasia, subluxation, and dislocation of the hip. J. Bone Joint Surg. [Am.] 63:1239–1248, 1981.

Norlin, R., Hammerby, S., and Tkaczuk, H.: The natural history of Perthes disease. Int. Orthop. 15:13–16, 1991.

Paley, D.: Current techniques of limb lengthening. J. Pediatr. Orthop. 8:73–92, 1988.

Price, C.T.: Metaphyseal and physeal lengthening. Instr. Course Lect. 38:331–336, 1989.

Richardson, E.G., and Rambach, B.E.: Proximal femoral focal deficiency: A clinical appraisal. South. Med. J. 72:166–173, 1979.

Ritterbusch, J.F., Shantharam, S.S., and Gelinas, C.: Comparison of lateral pillar classification and Catterall classification of Legg-Calvé-Perthes disease. J. Pediatr. Orthop. 13:200–202, 1993.

Salter, R.B., Hansson, G., and Thompson, G.H.: Innominate osteotomy in the management of residual congenital subluxation of the hip in young adults. Clin. Orthop. 182:53–68, 1984.

Southwick, W.O.: Compression fixation after biplane intertrochanteric osteotomy for slipped capital femoral epiphysis. J. Bone Joint Surg. [Am.] 55:1218–1224, 1973.

Song, J., Letts, M., and Monson, R.: Differentiation of psoas muscle abscess from septic arthritis of the hip in children. Clinical Orthopaedics and Related Research (391):258–265, 2001.

Staheli, L.T., and Chew, D.E.: Slotted acetabular augmentation in childhood and adolescence. J. Pediatr. Orthop. 12:569–580, 1992.

Steele, H.H.: Triple osteotomy of the innominate bone. J. Bone Joint Surg. [Am.] 55:343–350, 1973.

Sutherland, D.H., and Greenfield, R.: Double innominate osteotomy. J. Bone Joint Surg. [Am.] 59:1082–1091, 1977.

Suzuki, S., and Yamamuro, T.: Avascular necrosis in patients treated with Pavlik harness for congenital dislocation of the hip. J. Bone Joint Surg. [Am.] 72:1048–1055, 1990.

Tachdjian, M.O.: Pediatric Orthopedics, 3rd ed. Philadelphia, WB Saunders, 2001.

Thompson, G.H., Price, C.T., Roy, D., Meehan, P.L., et al.: Legg-Calve-Perthes disease: current concepts. Instr. Course Lect. 51:367–384, 2002.

Vitale, M.G., and Skaggs, D.L.: Developmental dysplasia of the hip from six months to four years of age. Journal of the American Academy of Orthopaedic Surgeons 9(6):401–411, 2001.

Willis, R.B.: Developmental dysplasia of the hip: assessment and treatment before walking age Instr. Course Lect. 50:541–545, 2001.

KNEE AND LEG

Brown, F.W., and Pohnert, W.H.: Construction of a knee joint in meromelia tibia (congenital absence of the tibia): a 15-year follow-up study. J. Bone Joint Surg. [Am.] 54:1333, 1972.

Cain, E.L., and Clancy, W.G.: Treatment algorithm for osteochondral injuries of the knee. Clinics in Sports Medicine 20(2):321–342, 2001.

Dickhaut, S.C., and DeLee, J.C.: The discoid lateral meniscus syndrome. J. Bone Joint Surg. [Am.] 64:1068–1073, 1982.

Jacobsen, S.T., Crawford, A.H., Miller, E.A., et al.: The Syme amputation in patients with congenital pseudarthrosis of the tibia. J. Bone Joint Surg. [Am.] 65:533–537, 1983.

Johnston, C.E, 2nd: Congenital pseudarthrosis of the tibia: results of technical variations in the charnley-williams procedure. J. Bone Joint Surg. [Am.] 84 A(10):1799–1810, 2002.

Laville, J.M., Chau, E., Willemen, L., Kohler, R., et al.: **Blount's disease**: classification and treatment. Journal of Pediatric Orthopaedics, Part B 8(1):19–25, 1999.

Langenskiold, A.: Tibia vara: Osteochondrosis deformans tibiae: Blount's disease. Clin. Orthop. 158:77–82, 1981.

Letts, M., and Vincent, N.: Congenital longitudinal deficiency of the fibula (fibular hemimelia): Parental refusal of amputation. Clin. Orthop. 287:160–166, 1993.

Roach, J.W., Shindell, R., and Green, N.E.: Late onset pseudarthrosis of the dysplastic tibia. J. Bone Joint Surg. [Am.] 75:1593–1601, 1993.

FEET

Coleman, S.S.: Complex Foot Deformities in Children. Philadelphia, Lea & Febiger, 1983.

Crawford, A.H., Marxen, J.L., and Osterfeld, D.L.: The Cincinnati incision: a comprehensive approach for surgical procedures of the foot and ankle in childhood. J. Bone Joint Surg. [Am.] 64:1355–1358, 1982.

Cummings, R.J., Davidson, R.S., Armstrong, P.F., Lehman, W.B.: Congenital clubfoot. Instr. Course Lect. 51:385–400, 2002.

Cummings, R.J., Davidson, R.S., Armstrong, P.F., Lehman, W.B.: Congenital clubfoot. J. Bone Joint Surg. [Am.] 84 A(2):290–308, 2002.

Drennan, J.C.: Congenital vertical talus. Instr. Course Lect. 45:315–322, 1996.

Drennan, J.C.: Tarsal coalitions. Instr. Course Lect. 45:323–329, 1996.

Jacobs, R.F., Adelman, L., Sack, C.M., et al.: Management of Pseudomonas osteochondritis complicating puncture wounds of the foot. Pediatrics 69:432–435, 1982.

McHale, K.A., and Lenhart, M.K.: Treatment of residual clubfoot deformity, the "bean-shaped" foot, by opening wedge medial cuneiform osteotomy and closing wedge cuboid osteotomy: clinical review and cadaver correlations. J. Pediatr. Orthop. 11:374–381, 1991.

Mosca VS. The cavus foot. J. Pediatr. Orthop. 21(4):423–424, 2001.

Onley, B.W., and Asher, M.A.: Excision of symptomatic coalition of the middle facet of the talocalcaneal joint. J. Bone Joint Surg. [Am.] 69:539–544, 1987.

Pentz, A.S., and Weiner, D.S.: Management of metatarsus adductovarus. Foot Ankle 14:241–246, 1993.

Peterson, H.A.: Skewfoot (forefoot adduction with heel valgus). J. Pediatr. Orthop. 6:24–30, 1986.

Piqueres, X., de Zabala, S., Torrens, C., Marin, M.: Cubonavicular coalition: a case report and literature review. Clinical Orthopaedics and Related Research (396):112–114, 2002.

Simons, G.W.: Analytical radiography of club feet. J. Bone Joint Surg. [Br.] 59:485–489, 1974.

Sullivan, J.A.: Pediatric flatfoot: evaluation and management. Journal of the American Academy of Orthopaedic Surgeons 7(1):44–53, 1999.

Turco, V.J.: Resistant congenital clubfoot: one-stage posteromedial release with internal fixation: a follow-up report of a 15 year experience. J. Bone Joint Surg. [Am.] 61:805–814, 1979.

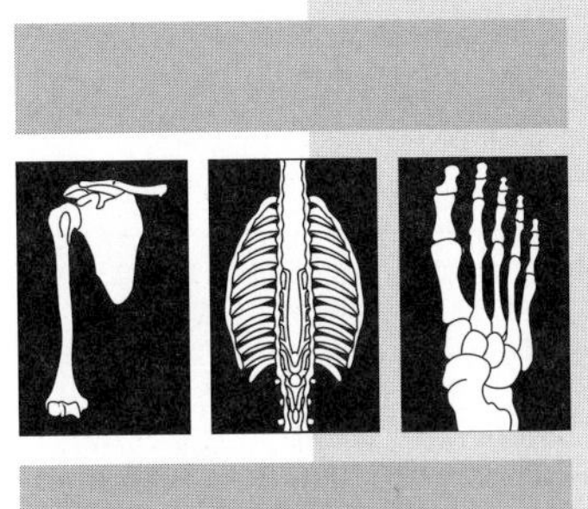

3

Sports Medicine

ANIKAR CHHABRA
LEONID I. KATOLIK
RAYMOND PAVLOVICH, JR.
BRIAN J. COLE
MARK D. MILLER

SECTION 1

Knee

I. Basic Sciences

A. Anatomy—The knee is much more than a simple hinge joint, because both gliding and rolling are essential to its kinematics. An understanding of the interactions of ligaments, menisci, capsular structures, and musculature is imperative. Although a thorough discussion of anatomy is included in Chapter 11, Anatomy, a brief review of knee anatomy is relevant.

1. Ligaments—Four major ligaments and several other supporting ligaments and structures provide stability to the knee joint.

a. Despite being the subject of intensive research, the function and anatomy of the ***anterior cruciate ligament (ACL)*** is still debated. The tibial insertion is a broad, irregular, oval-shaped area just anterior to and between the intercondylar eminences of the tibia. The femoral attachment is a semicircular area on the posteromedial aspect of the lateral femoral condyle (Fig. 3-1). The ACL is approximately 33 mm long and 11 mm in diameter. The ACL is often said to be composed of two "bundles"—***an anteromedial bundle that is tight in flexion and a posterolateral bundle that is tight in extension***. The ACL is composed of 90% type I collagen and 10% type III collagen. The blood supply to both cruciate ligaments is via branches of the middle geniculate artery and the fat pad. Mechanoreceptor nerve fibers within the ACL have been found and may have a proprioceptive role.

b. The **posterior cruciate ligament (PCL)** originates from a broad, crescent-shaped area anterolaterally on the medial femoral condyle and ***inserts on the tibia in a sulcus that is below the articular surface*** (see Fig. 3-1). It is also composed of two bundles—an ***anterolateral portion that is tight in flexion and a posteromedial portion that is tight in extension***. The PCL is approximately 38 mm in length and 13 mm in diameter. Variable meniscofemoral ligaments (Humphry's—anterior; Wrisberg's—posterior) originate from the posterior horn of the lateral meniscus and insert into the substance of the PCL. The neurovascular supply of the PCL is similar to the ACL.

c. The **medial collateral ligament (MCL)** is composed of superficial and deep fibers. The superficial MCL (tibial collateral ligament) lies deep to the gracilis and semitendinosus tendons, originates from the medial femoral epicondyle, and inserts onto the periosteum of the proximal tibia, deep to the pes anserinus. The anterior fibers of the superficial MCL tighten during the first 90 degrees of motion, while the posterior fibers tighten in extension. The deep portion of the ligament (medial capsular ligament) is a capsular thickening that blends with the superficial fibers and is intimately associated with the medial meniscus (coronary ligaments).

d. The **lateral collateral ligament (LCL)**, or fibular collateral ligament, is a cord-like

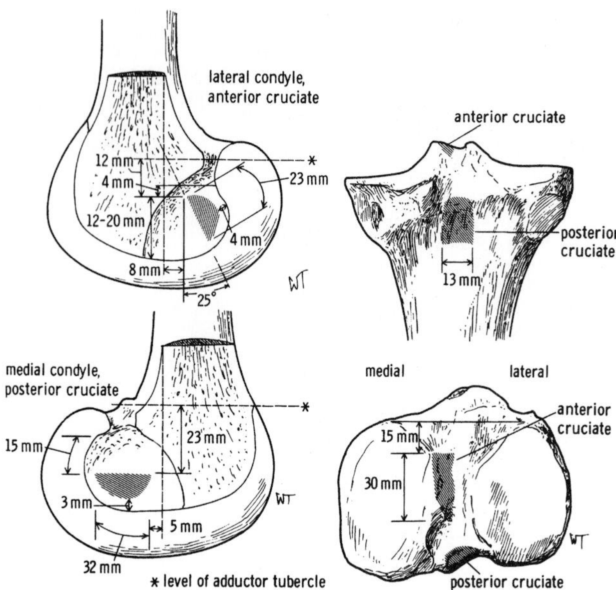

FIGURE 3-1 ■ Origins and insertions of the anterior cruciate ligament and posterior cruciate ligament. (From Girgis, F.G., Marshall, J.L., and Al Monajem, A.R.S.: The cruciate ligaments of the knee joint: Anatomical, functional, and experimental analysis. Clin. Orthop. 106:216–231, 1975.)

structure that originates on the lateral femoral epicondyle ***posterior and superior to the insertion of the popliteus tendon*** and inserts on the lateral aspect of the fibular head. Since it is located behind the axis of knee rotation, the LCL is tight in extension and lax in flexion.

e. The posteromedial corner, a structure deep to the MCL, is important to rotary stability. The capsular thickening of the ***multiple insertions of the semimembranosus***; ***the posterior oblique ligament (POL)***, which originates on the adductor tubercle; and ***the oblique popliteal ligament***, or thickening of the posterior capsule, make up the posteromedial corner.

f. The posterolateral corner is becoming increasingly important in treating the multiple ligament-injured knee. It consists of the ***popliteus*** (which originates on the back of the tibia, and inserts medial, anterior, and distal to the LCL); the ***popliteofibular ligament***; the ***lateral capsule***; the ***arcuate ligament***, which is contiguous with the oblique popliteal ligament medially; and the ***fabellofibular ligament***.

2. Medial Structures of the Knee—The medial structures of the knee are composed of three layers (Table 3-1) (Fig. 3-2).
3. Lateral Structures of the Knee—The lateral structures of the knee are also composed of three layers (Table 3-2) (see Fig. 3-2).

Table 3-1. MEDIAL STRUCTURES OF KNEE

LAYER	COMPONENTS
I	Sartorius and fascia
II	Superficial MCL, posterior oblique ligament, semimembranosus
III	Deep MCL, capsule

Note: The gracilis, semitendinosis, and saphenous nerves run between layers I and II.

MCL, medial collateral ligament.

4. The menisci are crescent-shaped fibrocartilaginous structures that are triangular in cross-section. Only the ***peripheral 20-30% of the medial menisci and 10-25% of the lateral meniscus are vascularized*** (medial and lateral genicular arteries). The medial meniscus is more C-shaped, and the lateral meniscus is more circular in shape (see Fig. 3-1). These structures, which deepen the articular surfaces of the tibial plateau and have a role in stability, lubrication, and nutrition, are connected anteriorly by the transverse (intermeniscal) ligament and are attached peripherally via the coronary ligaments.
5. Joint Relationships—The height of the lateral femoral condyle is greater than that of the medial condyle. The alignment of the condyles is also different; the lateral condyle is relatively straight, but the medial condyle is curved (allowing the medial tibial plateau to rotate externally in full extension—***the "screw home mechanism"***). The lateral condyle can also be identified by its terminal sulcus and groove of the popliteus insertion (Fig. 3-3). The patellofemoral joint is composed of the patella (with variably sized medial and lateral facets) and the femoral trochlea. The patella is restrained in the trochlea by the valgus axis of the quadriceps mechanism ***(Q angle)***, the

Table 3-2. LATERAL STRUCTURES OF KNEE

LAYER	COMPONENTS
I	Iliotibial tract, biceps, fascia
II	Patellar retinaculum, patellofemoral ligament
III	Arcuate ligament, fabellofibular ligament, capsule, LCL

Note: The inferior lateral geniculate artery is deep to the LCL, and is at risk with aggressive meniscal resection.

LCL, lateral collateral ligament.

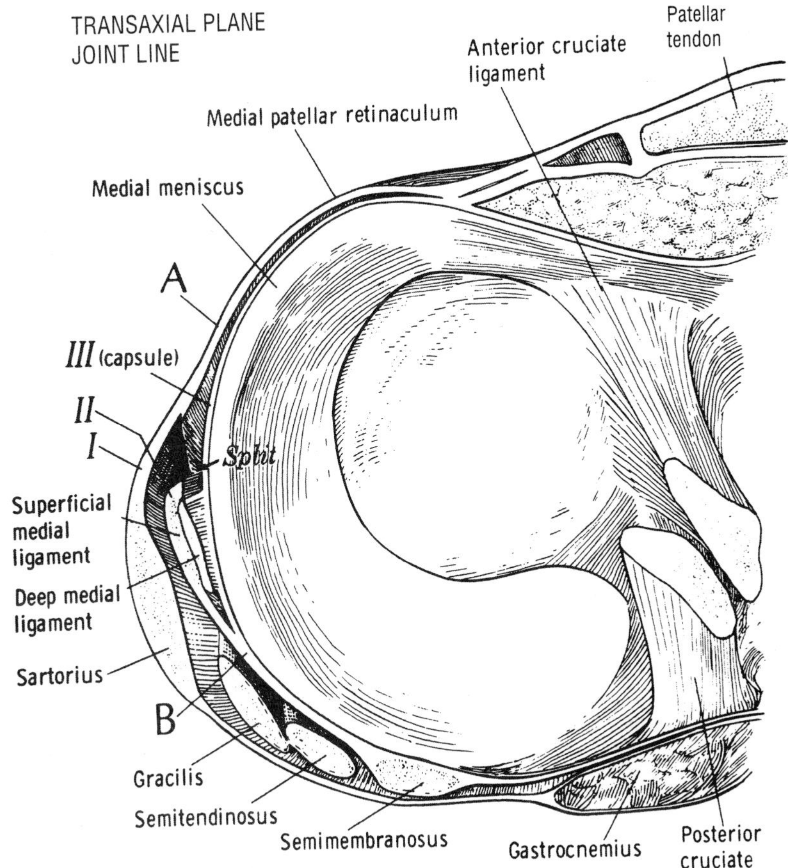

A

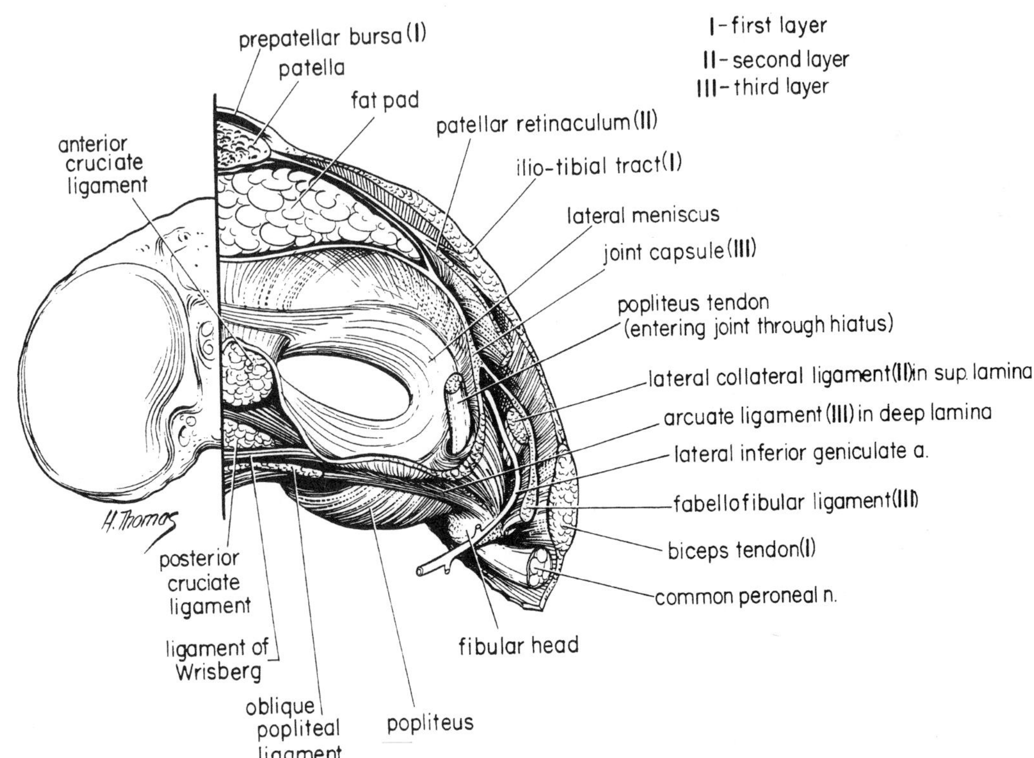

B

FIGURE 3-2 ■ Medial and lateral supporting structures of the knee. *A,* Medial structures of the knee include the sartorius and its fascia and the patellar retinaculum (layer I), the hamstring tendons and superficial medial collateral ligament (MCL) (layer II), and the deep MCL (layer III). (From Warren, L.F., and Marshal, J.L.: The supporting structures and layers of the medial side of the knee. J. Bone Joint Surg. [Am.] 61:56–62, 1979.) *B,* Lateral structures of the knee include the iliotibial tract and biceps (layer I), patellar retinaculum (layer II), and capsule and lateral collateral ligament (layer III). (From Seebacher, J.R., Ingilis, A.E., Marshall, J.L., et al.: The structure of the posterolateral aspect of the knee. J. Bone Joint Surg. [Am.] 64:536–541, 1982.)

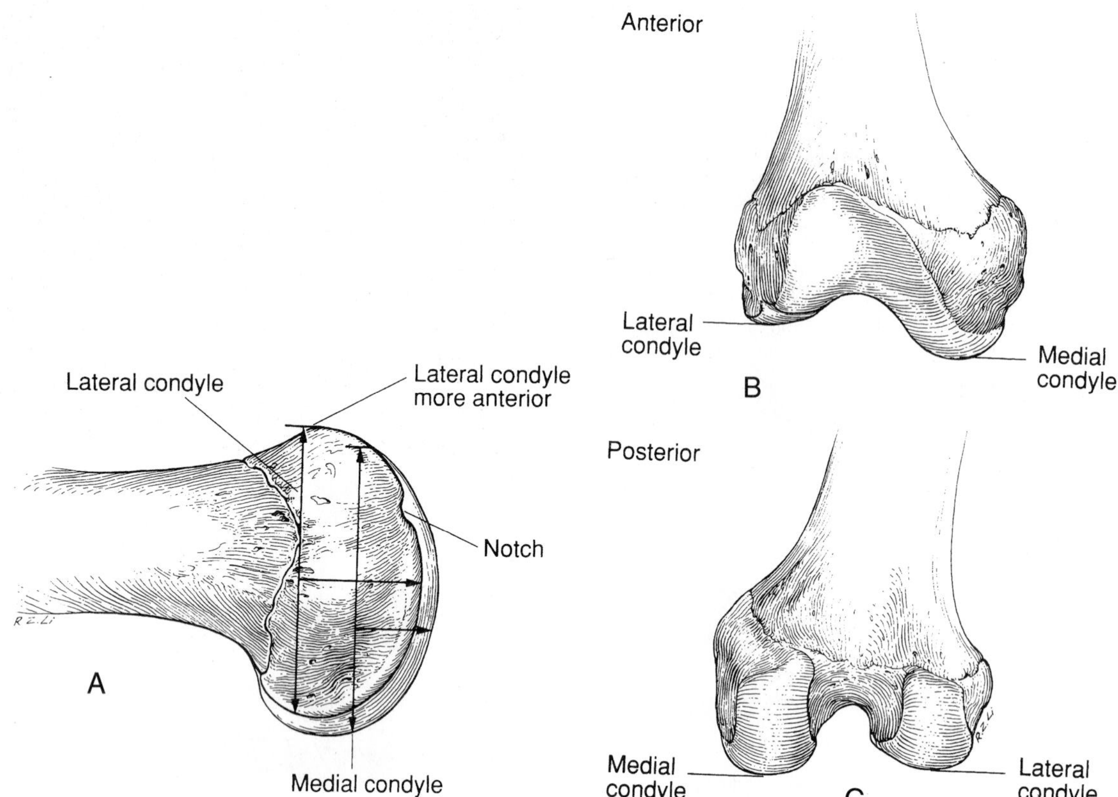

FIGURE 3-3 ■ Relationships of the femoral condyles. *A,* On the lateral projection, the lateral condyle projects more anteriorly and is notched. Anteroposterior *(B)* and posteroanterior *(C)* view demonstrate the difference in size and curvature of the medial femoral condyle. (From Tria, A.J., and Klein, K.S.: An Illustrated Guide to the Knee. New York, Churchill Livingstone, 1992, p. 5.)

oblique fibers of the vastus medialis and lateralis muscles (and their extensions—the patella retinacula), and the patellofemoral ligaments. The articular surface of the patella is thickest in the body, and the patella can withstand forces several times the body weight. The ***medial patellofemoral ligament (MPFL)***, which originates from the adductor tubercle and inserts into the medial border of the patella, has a major role in preventing lateral displacement of the patella (Fig. 3-4).

B. Biomechanics
   1. Ligamentous Biomechanics—The role of the ligaments of the knee is to provide passive restraints to abnormal motion (Table 3-3).
   2. Structural Properties of Ligaments—The tensile strength of a ligament, or maximal stress that a ligament can sustain before failure, has been characterized for all knee ligaments. However, it is important to consider age, orientation, preparation of specimen, and other factors prior to graft use. The ACL's tensile strength is approximately 2200 N and up to 2500 N in young individuals. The tensile strength of a 10-mm patellar tendon graft (young specimen) is more than 2900 N and is about 30% stronger

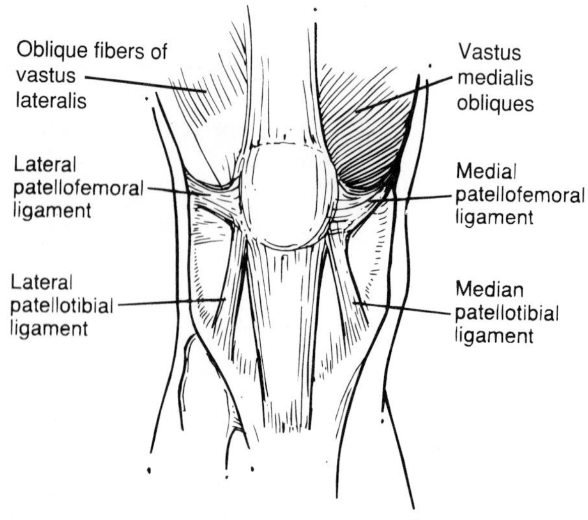

FIGURE 3-4 ■ Patellar restraints include the patellofemoral and patellotibial ligaments as well as the oblique fibers of the vastus medialis and lateralis. (From Walsh, W.M.: Patellofemoral joint. In DeLee, J.C., and Drez, D., Jr., eds.: Orthopaedic Sports Medicine: Principles and Practice. Philadelphia, WB Saunders, 1994, p. 1168.)

Table 3-3. LIGAMENTOUS BIOMECHANICS

LIGAMENT	RESTRAINT
ACL	Anterior translation of the tibia relative to the femur (85%)
PCL	Posterior tibial displacement (95%)
MCL	Valgus angulation
LCL	Varus angulation
MCL and LCL	Act in concert with posterior structures to control axial rotation of the tibia on the femur
PCL and posterolateral corner	Act synergistically to resist posterior translation and posterolateral rotary instability

ACL, anterior cruciate ligament; PCL, posterior cruciate ligament; MCL, medial collateral ligament; LCL, lateral collateral ligament.

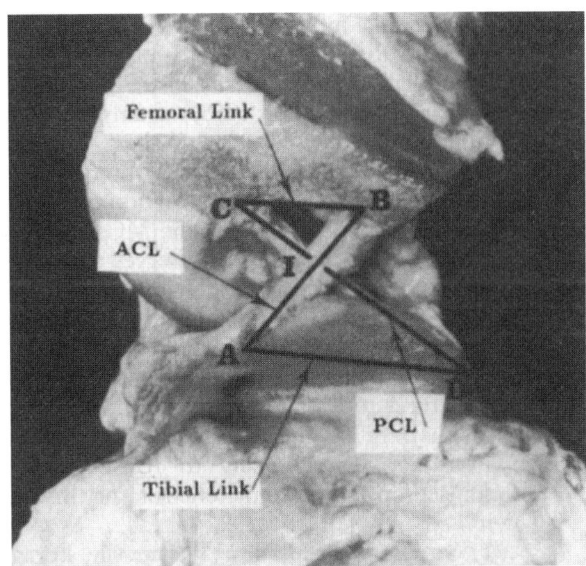

FIGURE 3-5 ■ The four-bar linkage system consists of the anterior cruciate ligament *(AB)*, the posterior cruciate ligament *(CD)*, the femoral link *(CB)*, and the tibial link *(AD)*. (From O'Connor, J., Shercliff, T., Fitzpatrick, D., et al.: Geometry of the Knee. In Daniels, D.M., Akeson, W.H., O'Connor, J.J., eds.: Knee Ligaments, Structure, Function, Injury, and Repair. New York, Raven Press, 1990, pp. 163–199. Reprinted with permission from the Institution of Mechanical Engineers, London.)

when rotated 90 degrees. However, this strength quickly diminishes in vivo. Studies suggest that the quadrupled hamstring graft is even greater but is very dependent on graft fixation. The PCL is thought to have a higher tensile strength than the ACL, but its value is disputed. The MCL has approximately twice the stiffness and tensile strength as the ACL, whereas the strength of the LCL is approximately 750 N.

3. Kinematics—The motion of the knee joint and interplay of ligaments has been described as a four-bar cruciate linkage system (Fig. 3-5). As the knee flexes, the center of joint rotation (intersection of the cruciate ligaments) moves posteriorly, causing rolling and gliding to occur at the articulating surfaces. The concept of ligament "isometry" remains controversial. Reconstructed ligaments should reapproximate normal anatomy and lie within the flexion axis in all positions of knee motion. Ligaments anterior to the flexion axis stretch as the joint flexes and ligaments posterior to the axis shorten. Although many instruments have been designed to achieve isometry, other considerations such as graft impingement and avoiding flexion contractures may be more important during light reconstructions.
4. Meniscal Biomechanics—The collagen fibers of the menisci are arranged radially and longitudinally (Fig. 3-6). The longitudinal fibers help dissipate the hoop stresses in the menisci, and the combination of fibers allows the meniscus to expand under compressive forces and increase the contact area of the joint. The lateral meniscus has twice the excursion of the medial

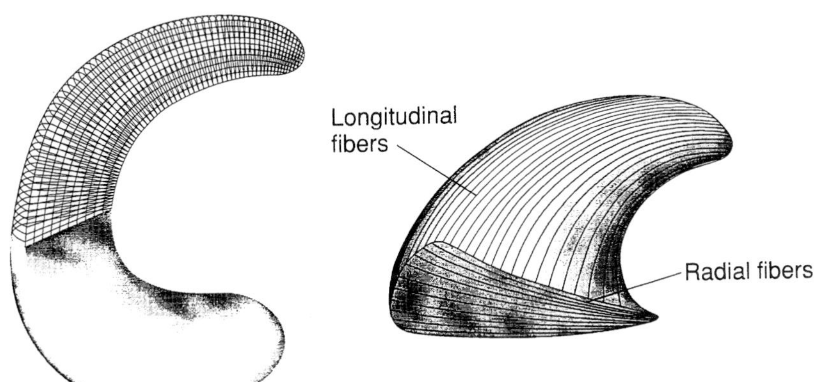

FIGURE 3-6 ■ Longitudinal and radial fibers of the menisci. (From Tria, A.J., and Klein, K.S.: An Illustrated Guide to the Knee. New York, Churchill Livingstone, 1992, p. 37.)

meniscus during knee range of motion (ROM) and rotation. Studies have shown that an ACL deficiency may result in abnormal meniscal strain, particularly in the posterior horn of the medial meniscus.

5. ***The patellofemoral joint*** must withstand forces that are more than three times that of body weight. ***The main restraint to lateral displacement of the patella is the medial patellofemoral ligament***, contributing 53–60% of the restraining force.

II. Diagnostic Techniques

A. History—A complete history and clarification of mechanism is essential. The age of the patient is important, since younger patients with traumatic injuries often have meniscal or ligamentous injuries, whereas older patients are more likely to have degenerative conditions. Several key historical points should be sought (Table 3-4).

B. Physical Examination—The following are key examination points, and some may be best elicited with an examination under anesthesia (Table 3-5).

C. Instrumented Knee Laxity Measurement—KT-1000 and KT-2000 (MED-metric, San Diego) is the most commonly accepted device for standardized laxity measurement. ACL laxity is measured with the knee in slight flexion and the foot externally rotated 10–30 degrees. The manual maximum anterior displacements are the most commonly reported values and are based on side-to-side comparison (>3 mm significant). PCL laxity can also be measured with this device, although it is less accurate.

D. Imaging the Knee

1. Standard Radiographs—Standard plain films include an anteroposterior (AP) view, 45 degree posteroanterior (PA) view, lateral view, and a Merchant's or Laurin's view of the patella. Additional views include long-cassette lower-extremity views, obliques, and stress radiographs. Several findings and their significance are listed in Table 3-6. Normal bony anatomy is demonstrated in Figure 3-7*A*. Many of these findings are illustrated in Figure 3-7*B*. Evaluation of patella height is accomplished by one of three commonly used methods (Fig. 3-7*C*).
2. Nuclear Imaging—Technetium 99m bone scans are useful in diagnosing stress fractures, early degenerative joint disease (DJD), and reflex sympathetic dystrophy (RSD).
3. Magnetic Resonance Imaging (MRI)—This has become the imaging modality of choice for diagnosis of ligament injuries, meniscal pathology, avascular necrosis (AVN), and articular cartilage defects and has replaced the use of arthrograms.
4. Computed Tomography—CT has largely been replaced by MRI, but it is still useful in evaluation of bony tumors, patellar tilt, and fractures.
5. Arthrography—This technique historically was useful for the diagnosis of MCL tears, and has been supplanted by MRI. However, it is useful when MRI is not available or tolerable.
6. Tomography—Tomograms are preferred to CT in evaluation of tibial plateau fractures at some medical centers.
7. Ultrasonography—This technique is useful for soft tissue lesions about the knee, including patellar tendonitis, hematomas, and extensor mechanism ruptures in some centers.

E. **Knee Arthroscopy—*The gold standard for diagnosis of knee pathology.*** The benefits of arthroscopic versus open techniques include smaller incisions, less morbidity, improved visualizations, and decreased recovery time.

1. Portals—Standard portals include a superomedial or superolateral inflow portal (made with the knee in extension) and inferomedial and inferolateral portals (made with the knee in flexion) for instruments and the arthroscope, respectively (Fig. 3-8). Accessory portals, sometimes helpful for visualizing the posterior horns of the menisci and PCL, include the posteromedial portal (1 cm above the joint line behind the MCL [avoid saphenous nerve branches]) and the posterolateral portal (1 cm above the joint line between the LCL and biceps tendon [avoiding the common peroneal nerve]). The transpatellar portal (1 cm distal to the patella, splitting the patellar tendon fibers) can be used for central viewing or grabbing but should be avoided in patients requiring subsequent autogenous patellar tendon harvesting. Other less commonly used portals include the medial and lateral midpatellar portals; the proximal superomedial portal (4 cm proximal to the patella), which is used for anterior compartment visualization; and

Table 3-4. KEY HISTORICAL POINTS THAT INDICATE MECHANISM

HISTORY	SIGNIFICANCE
Pain after sitting/stair climbing	Patellofemoral etiology
Locking/pain with squatting	Meniscal tear
Noncontact injury with "pop"	ACL tear, patellar dislocation
Contact injury with "pop"	Collateral ligament, meniscus, fracture
Acute swelling	ACL, peripheral meniscus tear, osteochondral fx, ± capsule tear
Knee "gives way"	Ligamentous laxity, patellar instability
Anterior force—**dorsiflexed foot**	Patellar injury
Anterior force—**plantar-flexed foot**	PCL injury
Dashboard injury	PCL or patellar injury
Hyperextension, varus, and tibial external rotation	Posterolateral corner injury

ACL, anterior cruciate ligament; PCL, posterior cruciate ligament; fx, fracture.

Table 3-5. KEY EXAMINATION POINTS

EXAMINATION	METHOD	SIGNIFICANCE
Standing/gait	Observe gait	Based on pathology
Deformity	Observe patient standing	Based on pathology
Effusion	Patella: ballot/milk	Ligament/meniscus injury (acute), arthritis (chronic)
Point of maximum tenderness	Palpate for tenderness	Based on location **(joint line tenderness = meniscus tear)**
Range of motion (ROM)	Active and passive	Block = meniscus injury (bucket handle), loose body, ACL tear impinging
Patella crepitus	With passive ROM	Patellofemoral pathology
Patella grind	Push patella with quadriceps contraction	Patellofemoral pathology
Patella apprehension	Push patella lat. at 20–30 degree flexion	**Patella subluxation/dislocation**
Q angle	ASIS-patella-tibial tubercle	Increased with patella malalignment (normal <15 degrees)
Flexion Q Angle	ASIS-patella-tibial tubercle	Increased with patella malalignment
J sign	Lateral deviation of the patella in extension	Patellar instability
Patella tilt	Tilt up laterally	>15 degrees = lax, <0 degrees = tight lateral constraint
Patella glide	Like apprehension	>50 degrees = increased medial constraint laxity
Active glide	Lat. excursion with quad. contraction	Lat. > prox. excursion = increased functional Q angle quadriceps
Quadriceps circumference	10 cm (VMO), 15 cm (quad.)	Atrophy from inactivity
Symmetric extension	Back of knee from ground or prone heel height difference	Contracture, displaced meniscal tear, or other mechanical block
Varus/valgus stress	30 degrees	MCL/LCL laxity (grade I: opening 1-5 mm; grade II: opening 6-10 mm; grade III [complete]: opening >10 mm)
Varus/valgus stress	0 degrees	MCL/LCL and PCL
Apley's	Prone-flexion compression	DJD, meniscal pathology
Lachman	Tibia forward at 30 degrees flexion	ACL injury (most sensitive)
Finacetto	Lachman with tibia subluxing beyond post. horns of menisci	ACL injury (severe)
Ant. drawer	Tibia forward at 90 degrees flexion	ACL injury
Internal rotation drawer	Foot int. rotated with drawer	Tighter = (normal), looser = ACL injury
External rotation drawer	Foot ext. rotated with drawer	Loose (normal), looser = ACL/MCL injury
McMurray	Varus/valgus stress and tibial rotation while extending knee	Meniscal pathology
Pivot shift	Flexion with int. rotation and valgus	ACL injury (EUA)
Pivot jerk	Extension with int. rotation and valgus	ACL injury (EUA)
Posterior drawer	Tibia backward at 90 degrees flexion	PCL injury
Tibia sag	Flex 90 degrees, observe	PCL
90 degrees quad. active test	Extend flexed knee	PCL
Asymmetric external rotation	"Dial" feet externally at 30 degree and 90 degree flexion	Asymmetric increased external rotation >10 degrees –15 degrees = posterolateral corner (PLC) injury if asymmetric at 30 degrees only; if asymmetric at both 30 degrees and 90 degrees = PCL + PCL
Ext. rotation recurvatum	Pick up great toes	PCL injury
Reversed pivot	Extension with ext. rotation and valgus	PCL injury
Posterolateral drawer	Post. drawer, lat. > med.	PCL injury

ACL, anterior cruciate ligament; ASIS, anterior superior iliac spine; lat., lateral; quad., quadriceps; prox., proximate; VMO, vastus medialis obliqus; MCL, medial collateral ligament; LCL, lateral collateral ligament; PCL, posterior cruciate ligament; DJD, degenerative joint disease; post., posterior; int., internally; ext., externally; ant., anterior; EUA, exam under anasthesia; med., medial.

Table 3-6. RADIOGRAPH FINDINGS

VIEW/SIGN	FINDING	SIGNIFICANCE
Lateral-high patellar	Patella alta	Patellofemoral pathology
Congruence angle	$\mu = -6$ degrees $SD = 11$ degrees	Patellofemoral pathology
Tooth sign	Irregular ant. patella	Patellofemoral chondrosis
Varus/valgus stress view	Opening	Collateral ligament injury; Salter-Harris fracture
Lateral capsule (Segund) sign	Small tibial avulsion off lateral tibia	ACL tear
Pellegrini-Stieda lesion	Med. femoral condyle avulsion	Chronic MCL injury
Lateral stress view—Stress to anterior tibia with knee 70 degrees flexed	Asymmetric posterior tibial displacement	PCL injury
PA flexion weight-bearing		Early DJD, OCD, notch evaluation
Fairbank's changes	Square condyle, peak eminences, ridging, narrowing	Early DJD (postmeniscectomy)
Square lateral condyle	Thickened joint space	Discoid meniscus

SD, standard deviation; ACL, anterior cruciate ligament; MCL, medial collateral ligament; PA, posteroanterior; OCD, osteochondral defect.

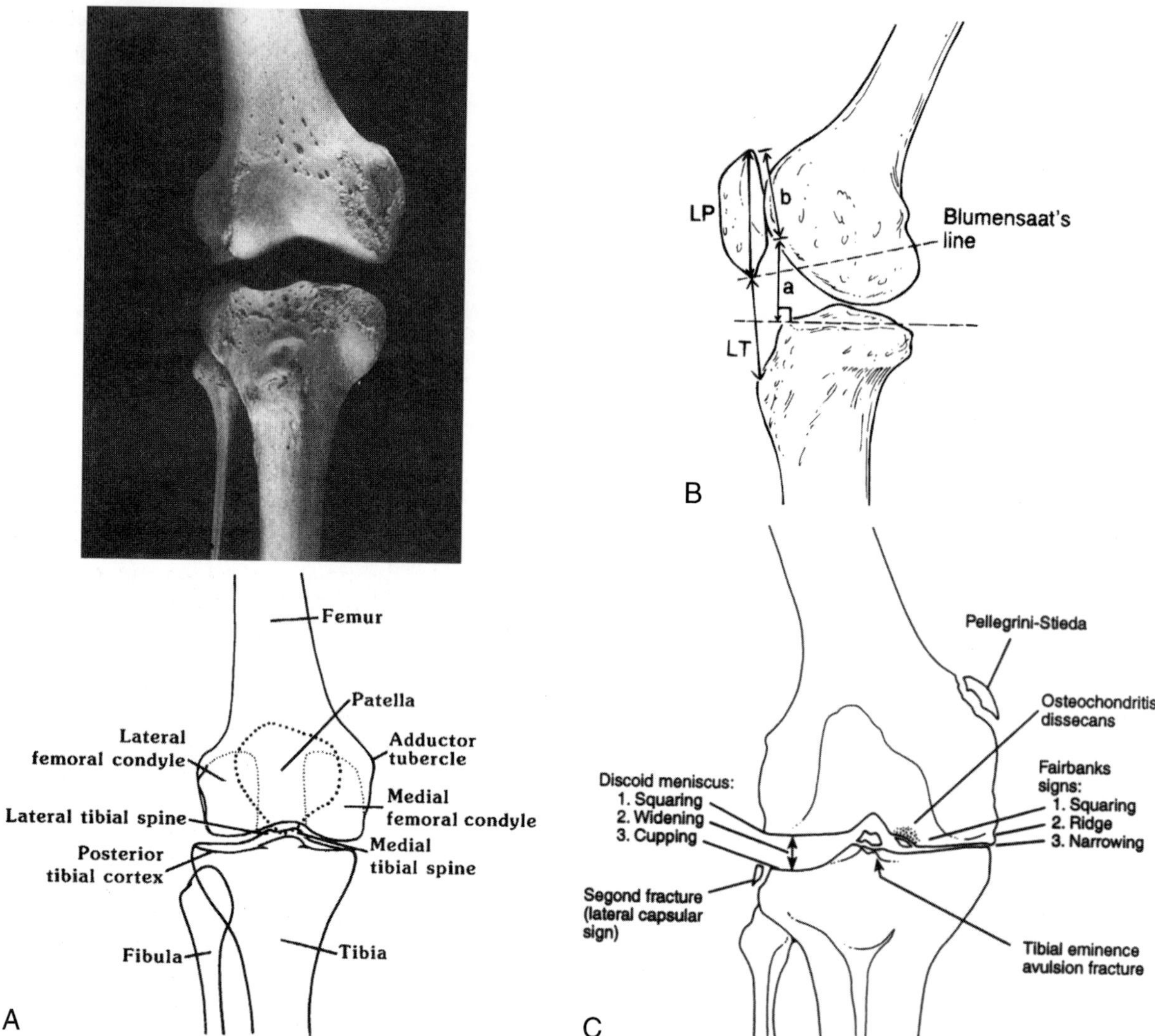

FIGURE 3-7 ■ *A,* Anterior view and drawing demonstrating the bones of the knee. (From Weissman, B.N.W., and Sledge, C.B.: Orthopedic Radiology. Philadelphia, WB Saunders, 1986, p. 498.) *B,* Three popular methods for evaluating patella alta and baja. (1) ***Blumensaat's line***: With the knee flexed 30 degrees, the lower border of the patella should lie on a line extended from the intercondylar notch. (2) ***Insall-Salvati index***: Patella tendon length *(LT)* to patella length *(LP)* ratio, or index, should be 1.0. An index of >1.2 is alta and <0.8 is baja. (3) ***Blackburne-Peel index***: Ratio of the distance from the tibial plateau to the inferior articular surface of the patella *(a)* to the length of the patella articular surface *(b)* should be 0.8. An index of >1.0 is alta. (From Harner, C.D., Miller, M.D., and Irrgang, J.J.: Management of the stiff knee after trauma and ligament reconstruction. In Siliski, J.M., ed.: Traumatic Disorders of the Knee. New York, Springer-Verlag, 1994, p. 364.) *C,* Common radiographic abnormalities.

the far medial and far lateral portals, which are used for accessory instrument placement (loose-body removal).

2. Technique—A systematic examination of the knee should include evaluation of the patellofemoral joint, medial and lateral gutters, medial and lateral compartments, and the notch. The posteromedial corner can best be visualized with a 70 degree arthroscope placed through the notch (modified Gillquist's view). Each knee arthroscopy should include an evaluation of the suprapatellar pouch, patellofemoral joint and tracking, medial and lateral gutters, medial compartment including the medial meniscus and the articular surface, the lateral compartment including the lateral menisci and the articular surface, and the intercondylar notch to visualize the ACL and PCL.
3. **Arthroscopic Complications—The most common arthroscopic complication is iatrogenic articular cartilage damage.** Additional complications include instrument breakage, hemarthrosis, infection, and neurovascular injury.

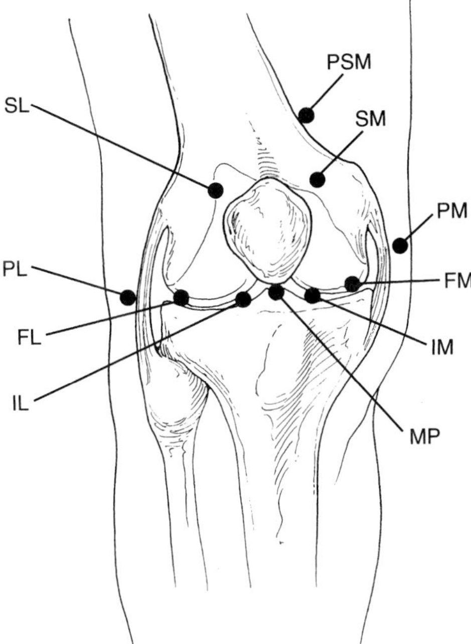

FIGURE 3-8 ■ Arthroscopic portals. PSM, proximal superomedial; FM, far medial; IM, inferomedial; MP, midpatellar; IL, inferolateral; FL, far lateral; PL, posterolateral; SL, superolateral. (From Miller, M.D., Osborne J.R., Warner J.J.P., et al.: MRI-Arthroscopy Correlative Atlas. Philadelphia, WB Saunders, 1997, p. 50.)

III. Menisci

A. Meniscal Tears

1. Meniscal tear is the most common injury to the knee that requires surgery. ***The medial meniscus is torn approximately three times as often as the lateral meniscus.*** Traumatic meniscal tears are common in young patients with sports-related injuries. Degenerative tears usually occur in older patients and can have an insidious onset. Meniscal tears can be classified based on their location in relation to the vascular supply (and healing potential), their position (anterior, middle, or posterior third), and their appearance and orientation (Fig. 3-9).

a. Treatment

(1) Partial Meniscectomy—Tears that are not amenable to repair (e.g., peripheral, longitudinal tears), excluding tears that do not require any treatment (e.g., partial-thickness tears, tears <5 mm in length, and tears that cannot be displaced >1–2 mm), are best treated by partial menisectomy. In general, complex, degenerative, and central/radial tears are resected with minimal normal meniscus being resected. A motorized shaver is helpful for creating a smooth transition zone (Fig. 3-10). The role of lasers or other devices for this purpose is still under investigation. There is some concern about possible iatrogenic chondral injury caused by lasers.

(2) Meniscal Repair—Should be done for all peripheral longitudinal tears, especially in young patients and in conjunction with an ACL reconstruction. Augmentation techniques (fibrin clot, vascular access channels, synovial rasping) may extend the indications for repair. Four techniques are commonly used: open, "outside-in," "inside-out," and "all-inside" (Fig. 3-11). Newer techniques for all-inside repairs (arrows, darts, staples, screws, etc.) are popular because of their ease of use; however, they are probably not as reliable as vertical mattress sutures. ***The gold standard for meniscal repair remains the inside-out technique with vertical mattress sutures.*** Regardless of the technique used, it is essential to ***protect the saphenous nerve branches during medial repairs and the peroneal nerve during lateral repairs*** (Fig. 3-12).

(3) Meniscal Repair Results—Several studies report 80–90% success rates with meniscal repairs. However, this depends on location, type of tear, and chronicity. It is accepted that the results of meniscal repair are best with acute, peripheral tears in young patients undergoing concurrent ACL reconstruction.

B. Meniscal Cysts—Most commonly occur in conjunction ***with horizontal cleavage tears of the lateral meniscus*** (Fig. 3-13). Operative treatment consisting of arthroscopic partial meniscectomy and decompression through the tear (sometimes including "needling" of the cyst) has been shown to be effective. En bloc excision is no longer favored for most meniscal cysts. Popliteal (Baker's) cysts are also related to meniscal disorder and will usually resolve with treatment. They are usually ***located between the semimembranosus and medial head of the gastrocnemius***.

C. Discoid Menisci ("Popping Knee Syndrome")—Can be classified as (1) incomplete, (2) complete, or (3) Wrisberg's variant (Fig. 3-14). Patients may develop mechanical symptoms, or "popping," with the knee in extension. Plain radiographs may demonstrate a widened joint space, squaring of the lateral condyle, cupping of the lateral tibial plateau, and a hypoplastic lateral intercondylar spine. MRI can be helpful and can also show associated tears. Treatment includes partial meniscectomy (saucerization) for tears, meniscal repair for peripheral detachments (Wrisberg's variant), and ***observation for discoid menisci without tears***.

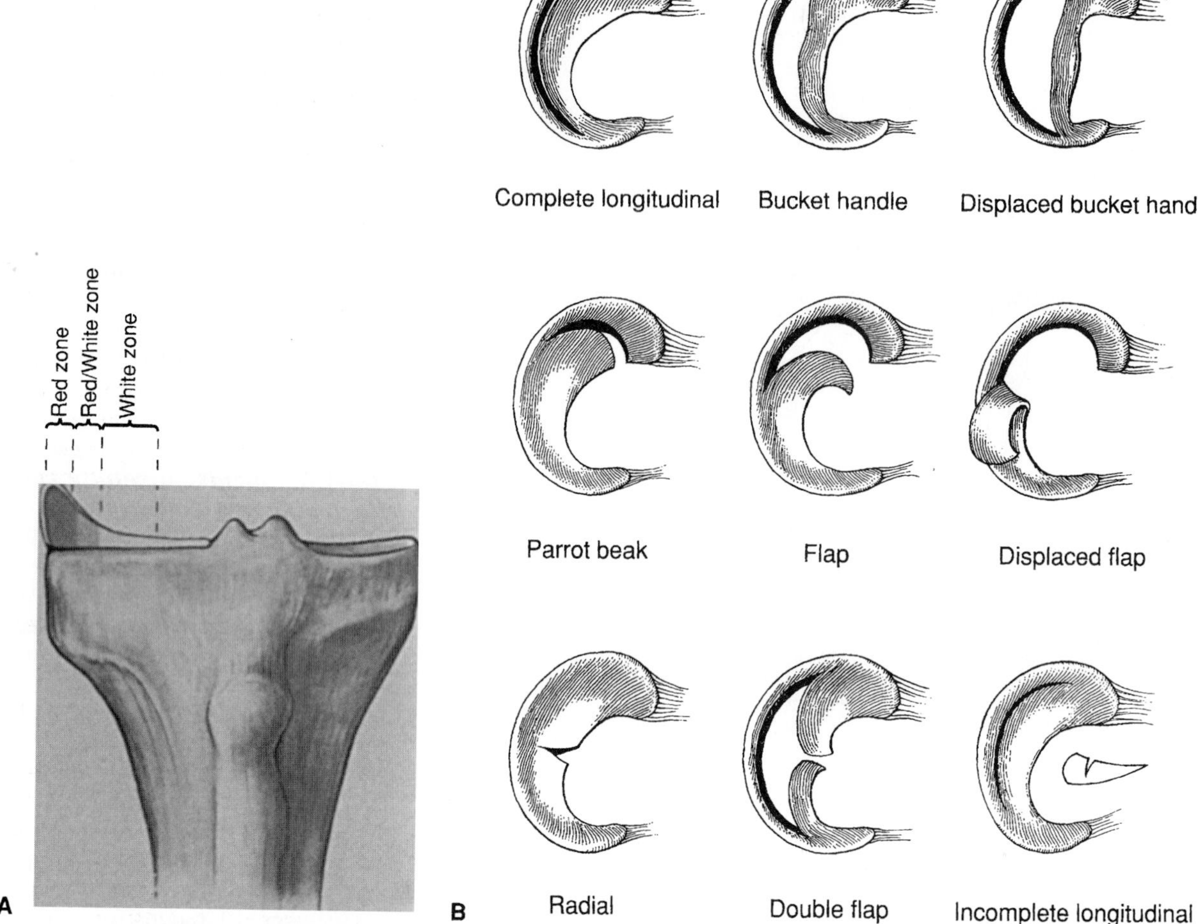

FIGURE 3-9 ■ Classification of meniscal tears. *A,* Vascular zones. The red-red zone has the highest potential for meniscal healing, and the white-white zone has essentially no potential for healing without enhancement. (Modified from Miller, M.D., Warner, J.J.P., and Harner, C.D.: Meniscal repair. In Fu, F.H., Harner, C.D., and Vince, K.G., eds.: Knee Surgery. Baltimore, Williams & Wilkins, 1994, p. 616.) *B,* Common meniscal tear appearance and orientation. (From Tria, A.J., and Klein, K.S.: An Illustrated Guide to the Knee. New York, Churchill Livingstone, 1992.)

D. Meniscal Transplantation—Remains controversial but may be indicated for young patients who have had near-total meniscectomy (especially lateral meniscectomy) and who have early chondrosis. Results are excellent in animal models, but are still preliminary in humans. Indications and graft choices are evolving. The preferred technique is arthroscopically with the meniscus being introduced through the contralateral portal.

IV. Ligamentous Injuries

A. ACL Injury

1. Introduction—Controversy continues regarding the development of late arthritis in ACL-deficient versus reconstructed knees. Nevertheless, chronic ACL deficiency is associated with a higher incidence of complex meniscal tears not amenable to repair. Although the arthritis issue remains controversial, ACL-deficient knees have an increased incidence of chondral injury and meniscal tears over time. Bone bruises (trabecular microfractures) occur in more than half of acute ACL injuries and are typically located near the sulcus terminalis on the lateral femoral condyle and the posterolateral aspect of the tibia. Although the long-term significance of these injuries is unknown, they may be related to late cartilage injury. Treatment decisions should be individualized based on age, activity level, instability, associated injuries, and other factors (Fig. 3-15). The ACL injury rate is higher in female than in male individuals and is thought to be due to smaller notches, smaller ligaments, and different landing biomechanics.
2. History and Physical Exam—ACL injuries are often the result of noncontact pivoting

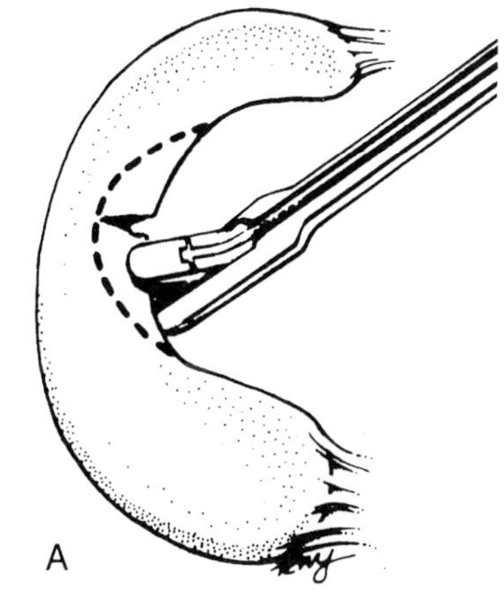

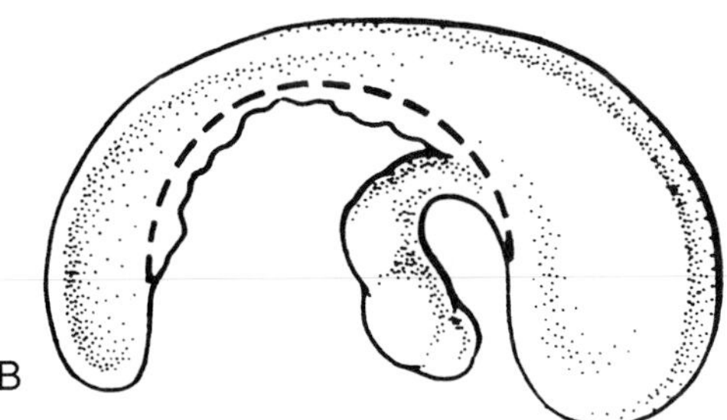

FIGURE 3-10 ■ Outlines of partial menisectomies necessary for a radial tear *(A)*, and a degenerative flap tear *(B)*. (From Ciccotti, M.G., Shields, C.L., El Attrache, N.: Menisectomy. In Fu, F.H., Harner, C.D., and Vince, K.G., eds.: Knee Surgery. Baltimore, Williams & Wilkins, 1994.)

injuries and are commonly associated with an audible "pop" with immediate hemarthrosis. Associated injuries, including meniscal tears (75%) are common. The ***Lachman test is the most sensitive examination for acute ACL injuries***. The pivot shift or jerk is helpful in evaluating an ACL-deficient knee, especially in an exam under anesthesia. The KT-1000 or KT-2000 is useful in quantifying laxity. Plain radiographs are essential in evaluating ACL injuries, and MRI has become a useful adjunct to diagnosis.

3. Treatment—Intra-articular reconstruction is currently favored for patients who meet the criteria indicated in Figure 3-14. Graft selection is dependent on patient factors and surgeon preference and most commonly includes (1) bone-patella, tendon-bone autograft, (2) four-strand hamstring autograft, (3) quadriceps tendon, or (4) allograft. Primary repair of ACL tears is not currently recommended. Primary and extra-articular repair are used mostly in revision situations and in children.
4. Partial ACL Tears—The existence and treatment of "partial" ACL tears is also controversial, although clinical examination and functional stability remain the most important factors for need of reconstruction.
5. Postoperative Rehabilitation—Rehabilitation has evolved, and early motion and weight bearing are encouraged in most protocols. Closed-chain rehabilitation has been emphasized because it allows physiologic cocontraction of the musculature around the knee.
6. Complications—Complications in ACL surgery most commonly are a result of aberrant tunnel placement (often the femoral tunnel is anteriorly placed too far, limiting flexion) and early surgery (resulting in knee stiffness). ***Arthrofibrosis, which can occur more commonly with acute ACL reconstruction***, and aberrant hardware placement (interference screw divergence of >30 degrees [for endoscopic femoral tunnels] and >15 degrees [for tibial tunnels]) can also result in complications.

B. PCL Injury
1. Treatment is controversial, although reports suggest that nonoperative management may result in late patellar and medial femoral condyle chondrosis. Injuries occur most commonly as a result of a direct blow to the anterior tibia with the knee flexed (the "dashboard injury") or ***hyperflexion with a plantar-flexed foot*** without a blow; hyperextension injuries can also result in PCL rupture. The ***key examination is the posterior drawer test*** with an absent or posteriorly directed tibial "step-off." Nonoperative treatment is favored for most isolated PCL injuries. ***Bony avulsion fractures can be repaired primarily with good results***, although primary repair of midsubstance PCL (and ACL) injuries has not been successful. ***Chronic PCL deficiency can result in late chondrosis of the patellofemoral compartment and/or medial femoral condyle.*** PCL reconstruction is recommended for functionally unstable or combined injuries (Fig. 3-16).

C. Collateral Ligament Injury
1. MCL Injury—Occurs as a result of valgus stress to the knee. Pain and ***instability with valgus stress testing at 30 degrees of flexion*** (and not in full extension) is diagnostic. Injuries most commonly occur at the femoral insertion of the ligament. ***Nonoperative treatment (hinged knee brace)*** is highly successful for isolated MCL injuries. Prophylactic bracing may be helpful for football players. Rarely, advancement and reinforcement of the ligament are necessary for chronic injuries that do not respond to conservative treatment (Fig. 3-17). Chronic injuries may have calcification at the medial femoral condyle insertion (Pellegrini-Stieda *sign*). Pellegrini-Stieda *syndrome*, which can occur with chronic MCL injury, usually responds to a brief period of immobilization followed by motion.

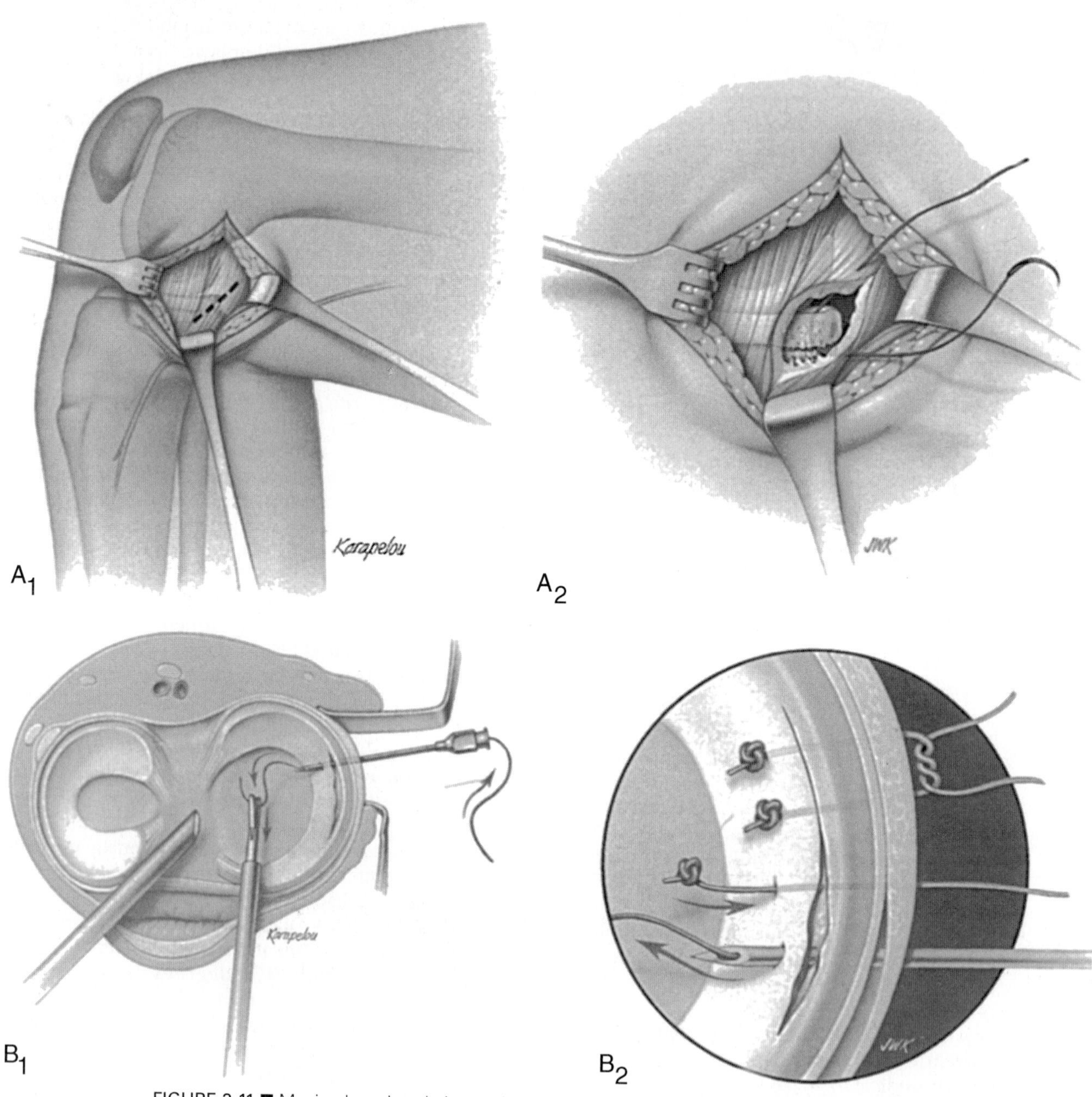

FIGURE 3-11 ■ Meniscal repair techniques. *A,* Open repair of the medial meniscus (right knee). *B,* "Outside-in" medial meniscal repair (right knee).

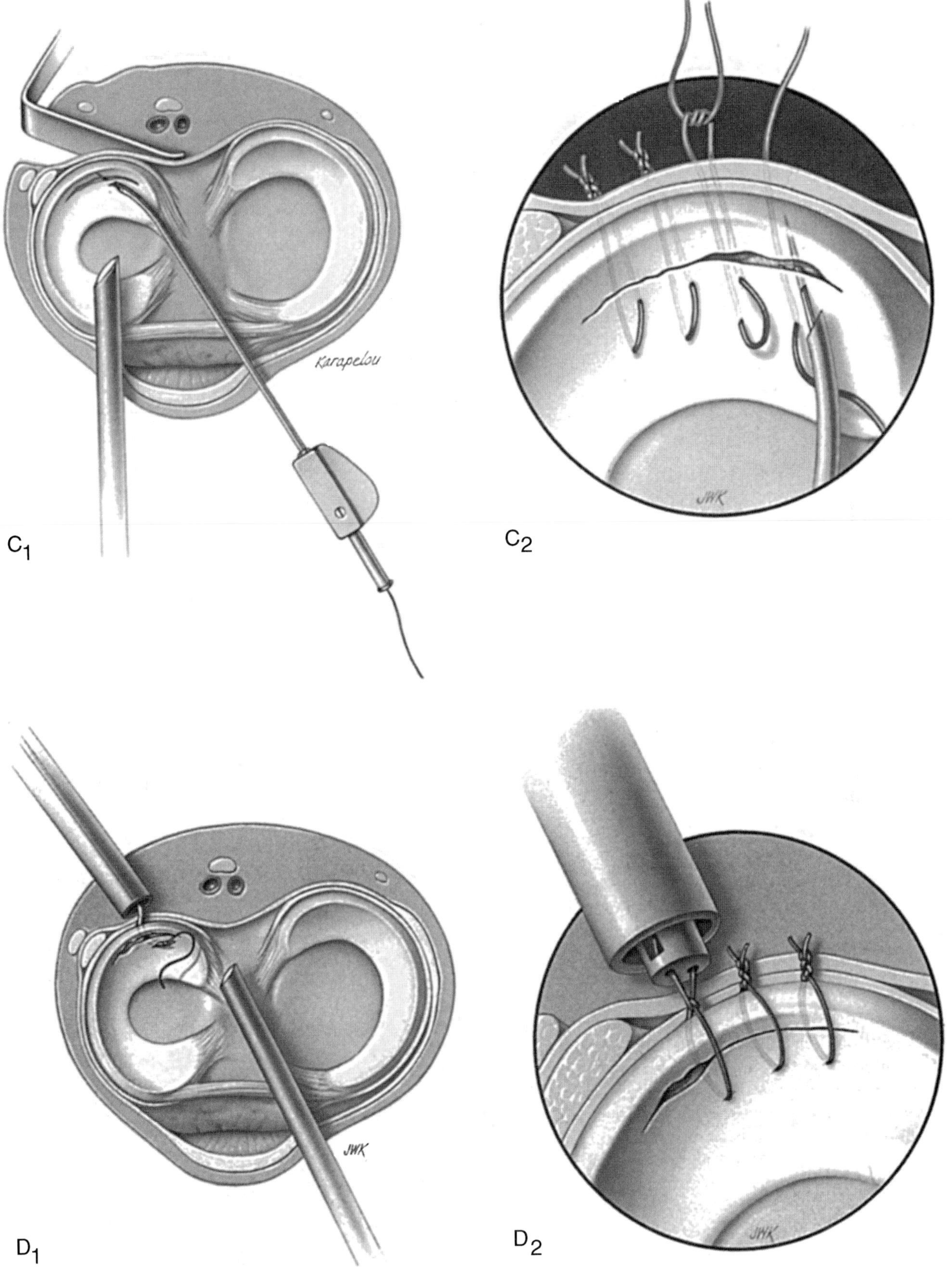

FIGURE 3-11 Cont'd ■ *C,* "Inside-out" lateral meniscal repair (right knee). *D,* "All inside" lateral meniscal repair (right knee). (From Miller, M.D.: Atlas of meniscal repair. Op. Tech. Orthop. 5(1):70–71, 1995.)

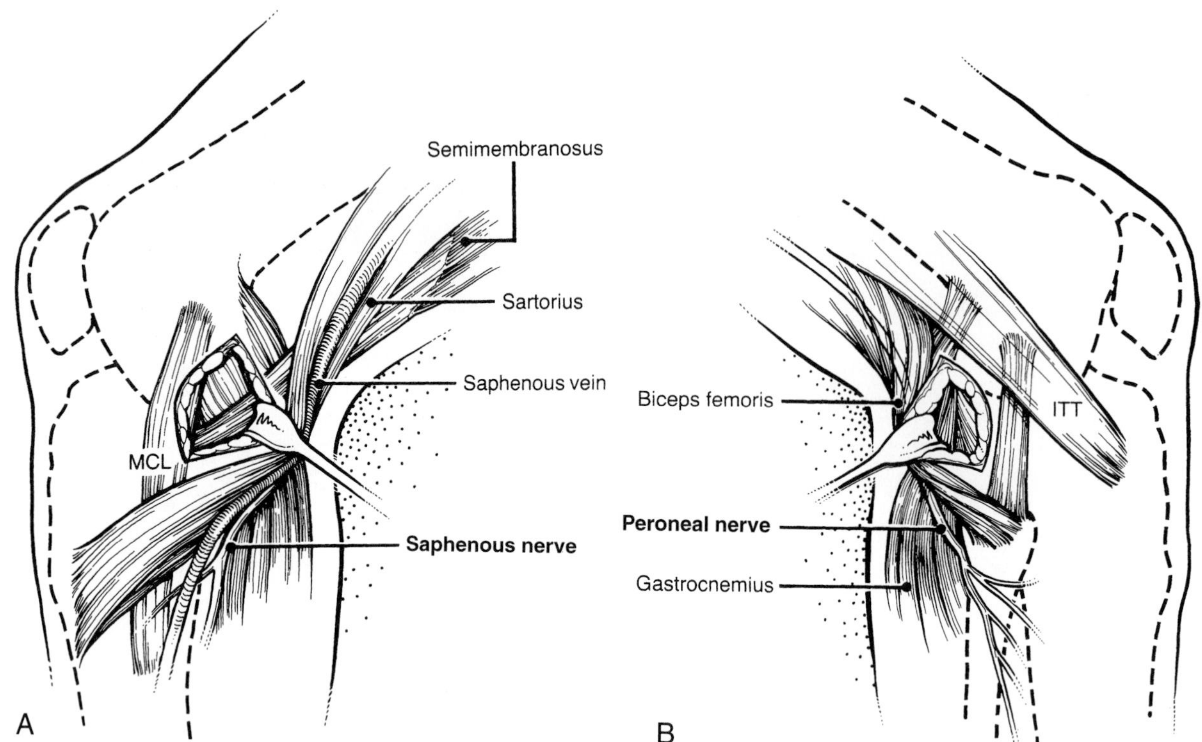

FIGURE 3-12 ■ Incisions for meniscal repair must be planned to allow for retraction and protection of the saphenous nerve branches during medial meniscal repairs *(A)* and the peroneal nerve during lateral meniscal repairs *(B)*. MCL, medial cruciate ligament; ITT, iliotibial tract. (From Scott, W.N., ed.: Arthroscopy of the Knee: Diagnosis and Treatment. Philadelphia, WB Saunders, 1990.)

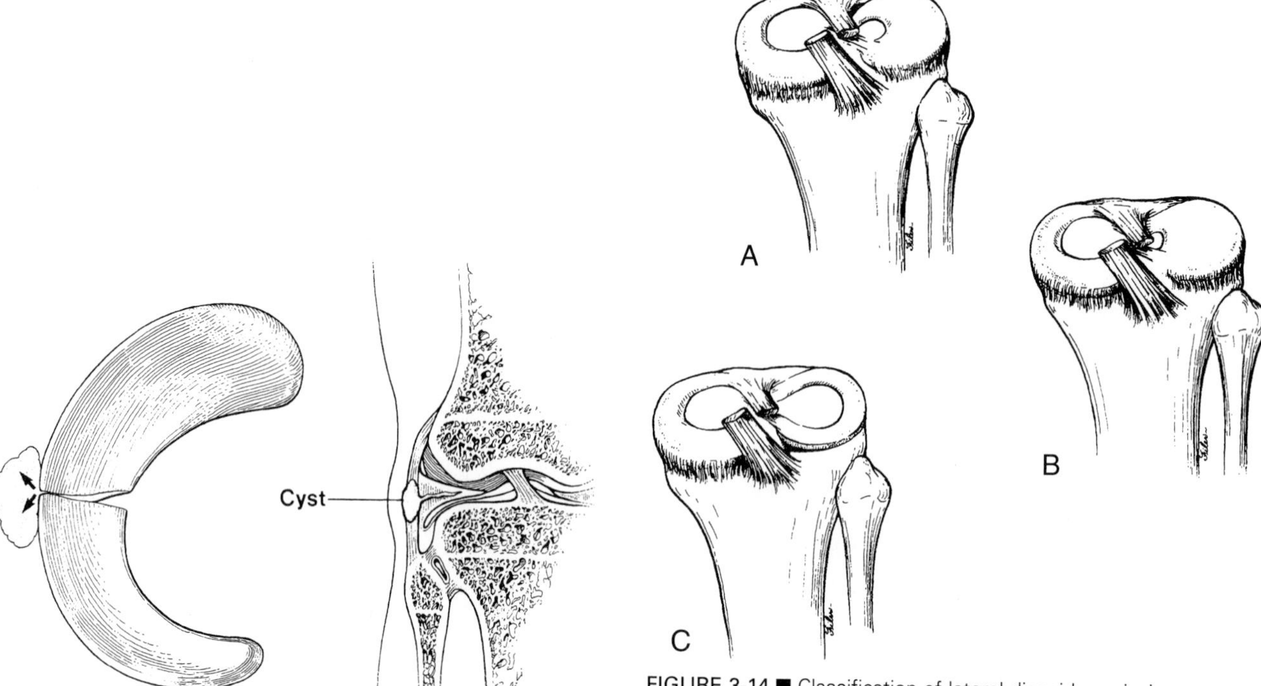

FIGURE 3-13 ■ Meniscal cysts most commonly involve the lateral meniscus. (From Tria, A.J., and Klein, K.S.: An Illustrated Guide to the Knee. New York, Churchill Livingstone, 1992, p. 101.)

FIGURE 3-14 ■ Classification of lateral discoid menisci. *A,* Incomplete. *B,* Complete. *C,* Wrisberg's ligament variant. (From Neuschwander, D.C.: Discoid lateral meniscus. In Fu, F.H., Harner, C.D., and Vince, K.G., eds.: Knee Surgery. Baltimore, Williams & Wilkins, 1994, p. 394.)

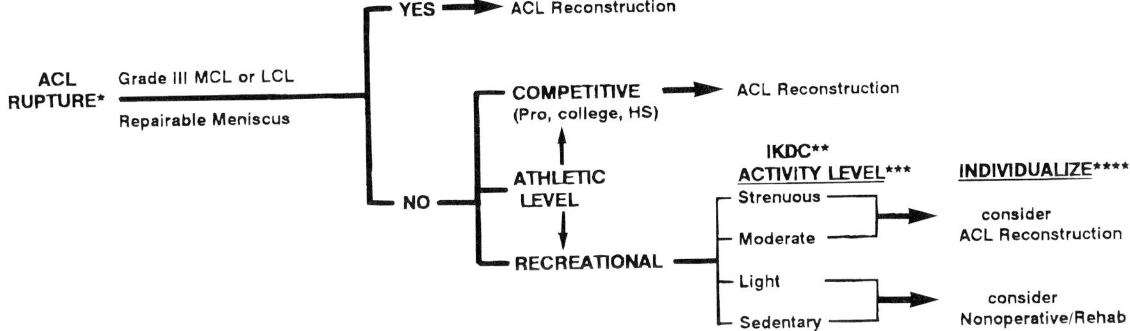

FIGURE 3-15 ■ Algorithm for the treatment of anterior cruciate ligament ruptures. *midsubstance tears; **IKDC (International Knee Documentation Committee); *** strenuous (jumping/pivoting sports), moderate (heavy manual work, skiing), light (manual work, running), sedentary (activities of daily living); ****individualize based on age, arthritis, occupation, activity modification, other medical conditions. MCL, medial cruciate ligament; LCL, lateral collateral ligament. (From Spindler, K.P., and Walker, R.N.: General approach to ligament surgery. In Fu, F.H., Harner, C.D., and Vince, K.G., eds.: Knee Surgery. Baltimore, Williams & Wilkins, 1994, p. 652.)

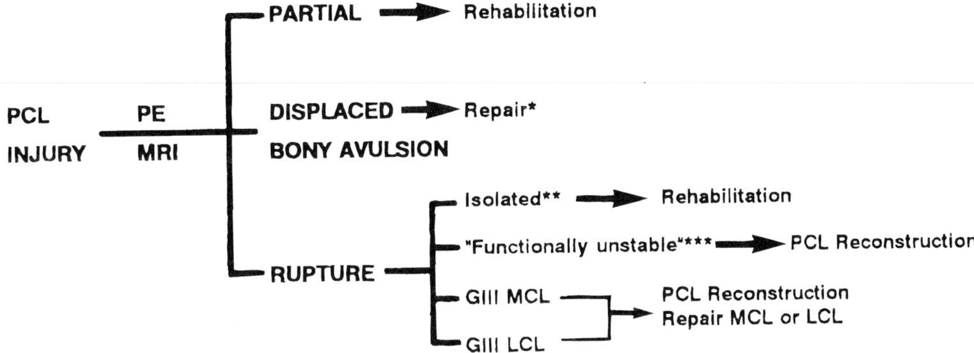

FIGURE 3-16 ■ Algorithm for treatment of posterior cruciate ligament injuries. *with an intact ligament; **without posterolateral injury or combined ligamentous injury; ***failed rehabilitation or unstable/symptomatic with activities of daily living. MCL, medial cruciate ligament; LCL, lateral collateral ligament. (From Spindler, K.P., and Walker, R.N.: General approach to ligament surgery. In Fu, F.H., Harner, C.D., and Vince, K.G., eds.: Knee Surgery. Baltimore, Williams & Wilkins, 1994, p. 655.)

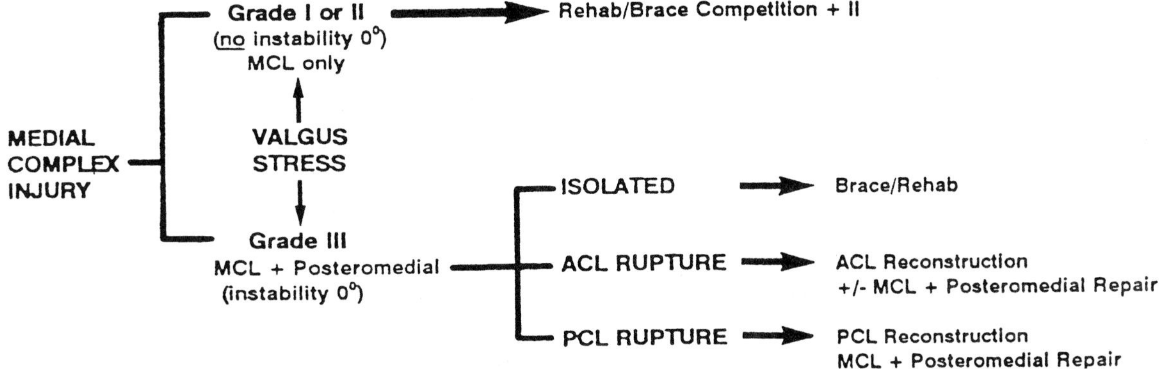

FIGURE 3-17 ■ Algorithm for treatment of medial collateral ligament injuries. ACL, anterior cruciate ligament; PCL, posterior cruciate ligament. (From Spindler, K.P., and Walker, R.N.: General approach to ligament surgery. In Fu, F.H., Harner, C.D., and Vince, K.G., eds.: Knee Surgery. Baltimore, Williams & Wilkins, 1994.)

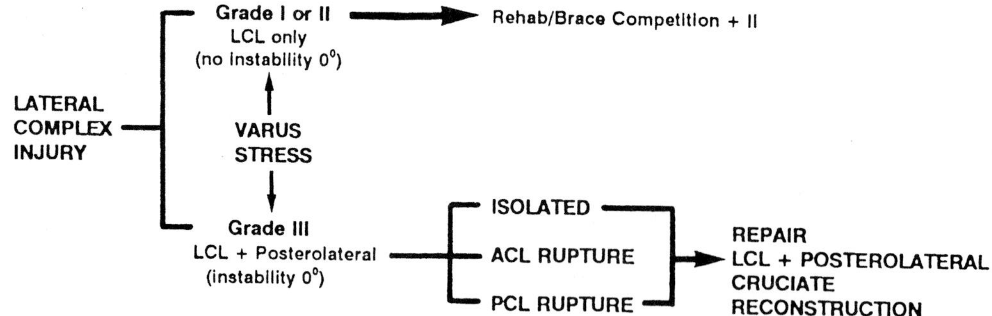

FIGURE 3-18 ■ Algorithm for treatment of lateral collateral ligament injuries. ACL, anterior cruciate ligament; PCL, posterior cruciate ligament. (From Spindler, K.P., and Walker, R.N.: General approach to ligament surgery. In Fu, F.H., Harner, C.D., and Vince, K.G., eds.: Knee Surgery. Baltimore, Williams & Wilkins, 1994.)

2. LCL Injuries—***Varus instability in 30 degrees of flexion is diagnostic only for an isolated LCL ligament injury.*** Isolated injuries to the LCL ligament are uncommon, and should be managed nonoperatively if laxity is mild (Fig. 3-18).

D. Posterolateral Corner Injuries

1. These injuries occur rarely as isolated injuries but more commonly are associated with other ligamentous injuries (especially the PCL). Because of poor results with chronic reconstructions, ***acute repair is advocated. Examination for increased external rotation***, external rotation recurvatum test, posterolateral drawer test, and reverse pivot shift test are important. Early anatomic repair is often successful, but these injuries are frequently missed. Procedures recommended for chronic injuries include posterolateral corner advancement, popliteus bypass, two- and three-tailed reconstruction, biceps tenodesis, and more recently, "split" grafts, which are used to reconstruct both the LCL and the popliteus/posterolateral corner (Figs. 3-19 and 3-20).

E. Multiple-Ligament Injuries

1. Combined ligamentous injuries (especially ACL-PCL injuries) can be a result of a knee dislocation, and neurovascular injury must be suspected. ***The incidence of vascular injury following anterior knee dislocation is 30% to 50%.*** Liberal use of vascular studies is recommended early (Fig. 3-21).

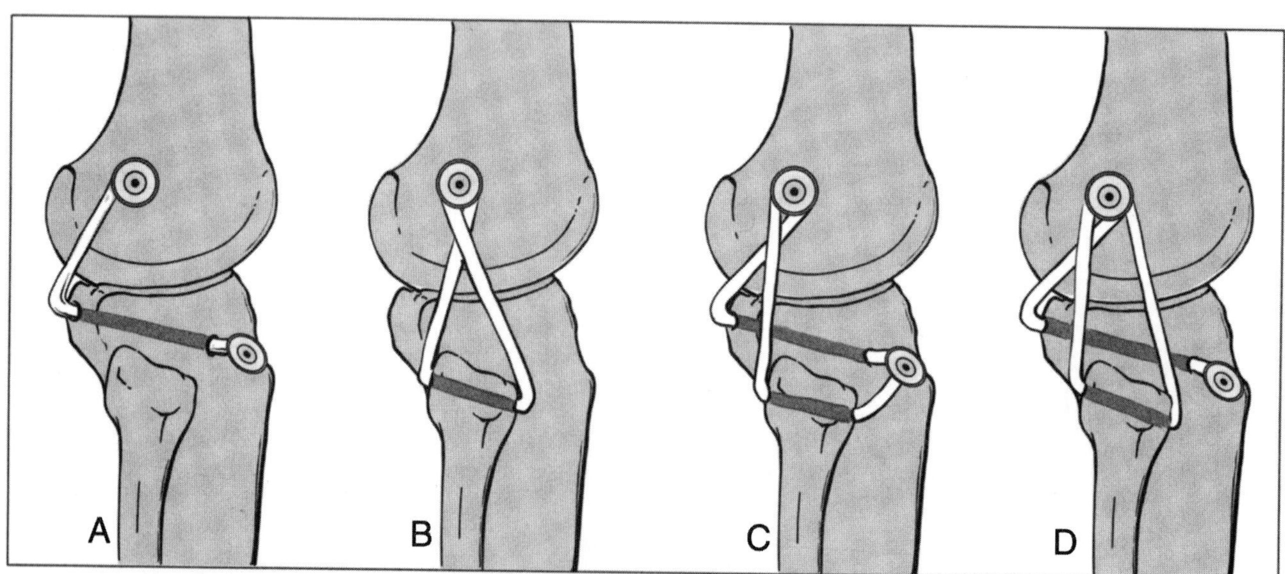

FIGURE 3-19 ■ Techniques for posterolateral corner reconstruction. *(A)*, Popliteal bypass (Muller). *(B)*, figure eight (Larsen). *(C)*, Two-tailed (Warren). *(D)*, Three-tailed (Warren/Miller). (From Miller, M.D., Cooper, D.E., and Warner, J.J.P.: Review of Sports Medicine and Arthroscopy, 2nd ed. Philadelphia, WB Saunders, 2002.)

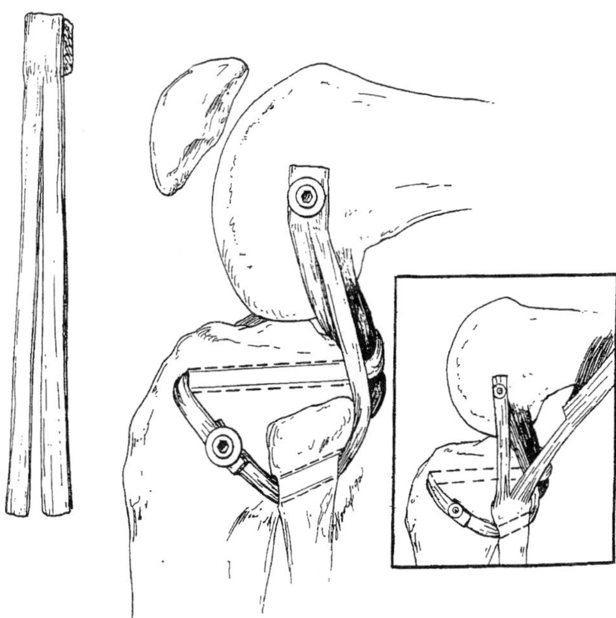

FIGURE 3-20 ■ Split posterolateral corner graft. (From McKernan, D.J., and Paulos, L.E.: Graft selection. In Fu, F.H., Harner, C.D., and Vince, K.G., eds.: Knee Surgery. Baltimore, Williams & Wilkins, 1994, p. 669.)

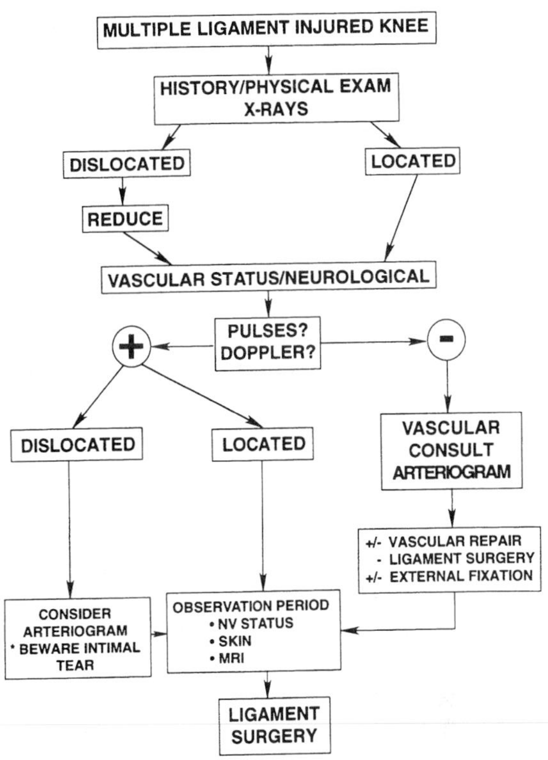

FIGURE 3-21 ■ Algorithm for treatment of multiple knee-ligament injuries. (From Marks, P.H., and Harner, C.D.: The anterior cruciate ligament in the multiple ligament–injured knee. Clin. Sports Med. 12:825–838, 1993.)

Dislocations are classified based on the direction of tibial displacement (Fig. 3-22). Treatment is usually operative. Emergent surgical indications include popliteal artery injury, open dislocations, and irreducible dislocations. Most surgeons recommend delaying surgery 5–12 days to ensure that there is no vascular injury. The use of the arthroscope, especially with a pump, must be limited during these procedures because of the risk of fluid extravasation. Avulsion injuries can be repaired primarily; however, interstitial injuries must be reconstructed. Early motion is critical to avoid a high incidence of a stiff knee after these combined procedures.

V. Osteochondral Lesions

A. Osteochondritis Dissecans

1. Introduction—Involves subchondral bone and overlying cartilage separation, most likely as a result of occult trauma. The lesion most often involves the ***lateral aspect of the medial femoral condyle***.
2. Diagnosis—Patients usually have poorly localized, vague complaints. Radiographs, nuclear imaging, and MRI can be helpful in determining the size and location of the lesion.

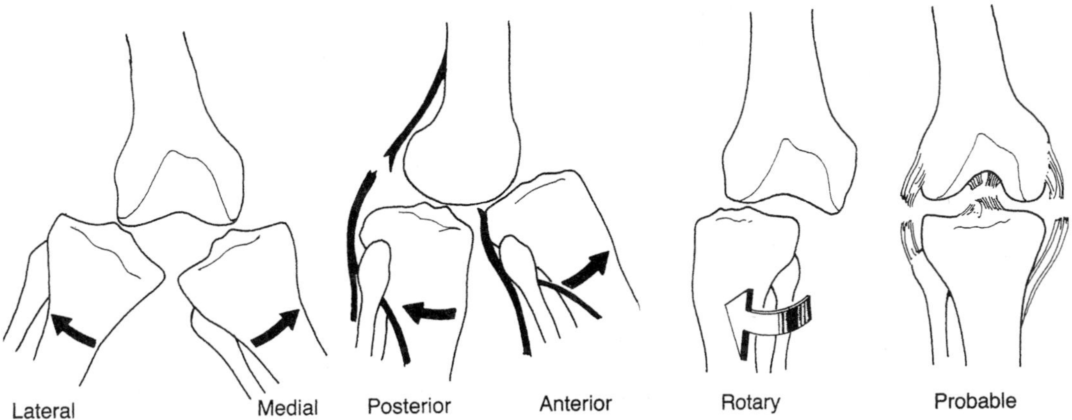

FIGURE 3-22 ■ Classification of knee dislocations. (From Miller, M.D., Cooper, D.E., and Warner, J.J.P.: Review of Sports Medicine and Arthroscopy. Philadelphia, WB Saunders, 1995, p. 51.)

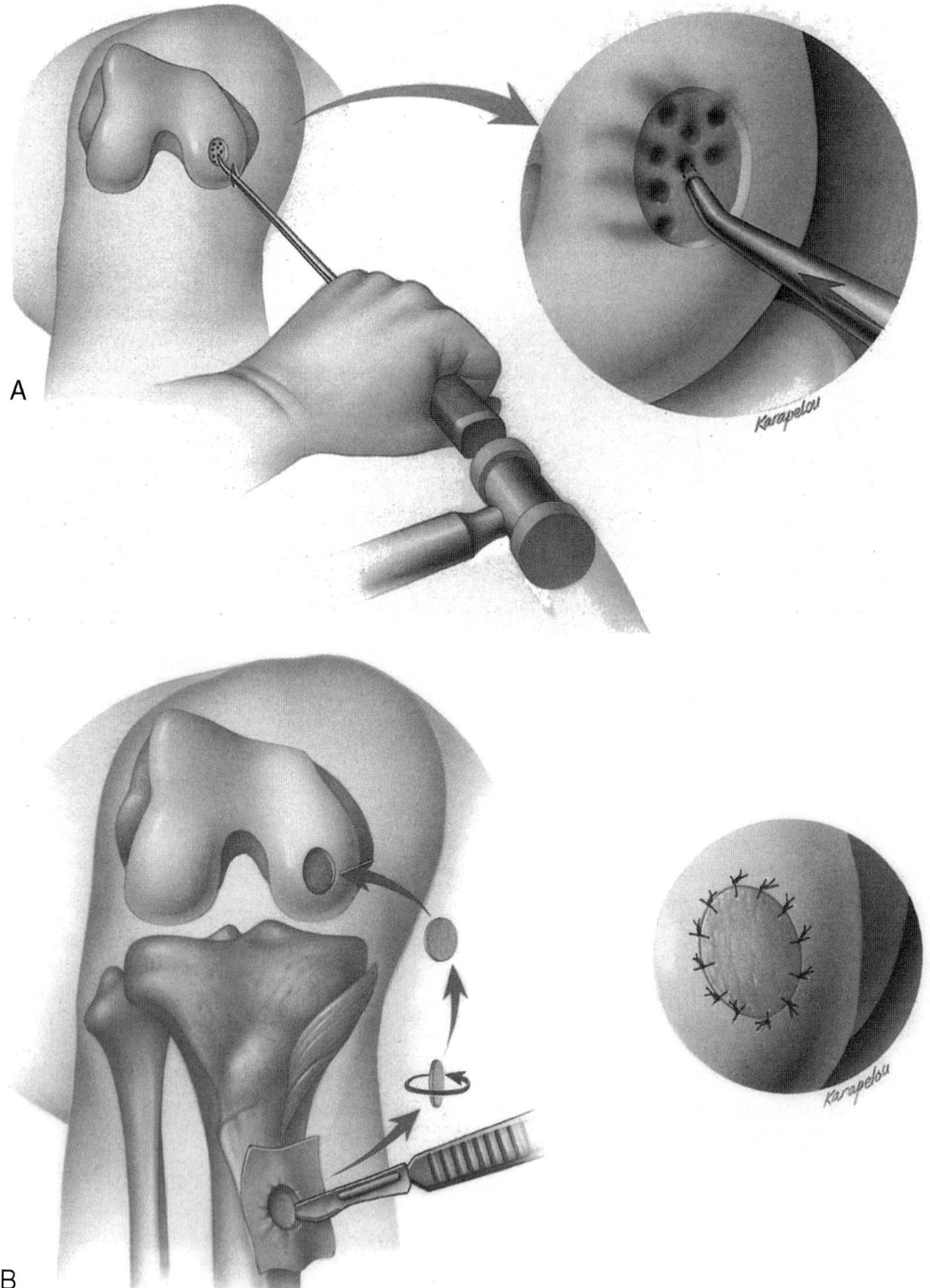

FIGURE 3-23 ■ Treatment of chondral injuries. *A,* Microfracture. Awls, with various degrees of angulation, are introduced throughout the ipsilateral arthroscopic portal and are used to penetrate the subchondral bone and encourage stem cell production of "cartilage-like" tissue. *B,* Periosteal graft. Periosteum is used as a "patch" The inner cambium layer is rotated so that it is facing outward. The patch is carefully sewn in place, and "cartilage" may grow out from the undifferentiated cambium layer of the graft.

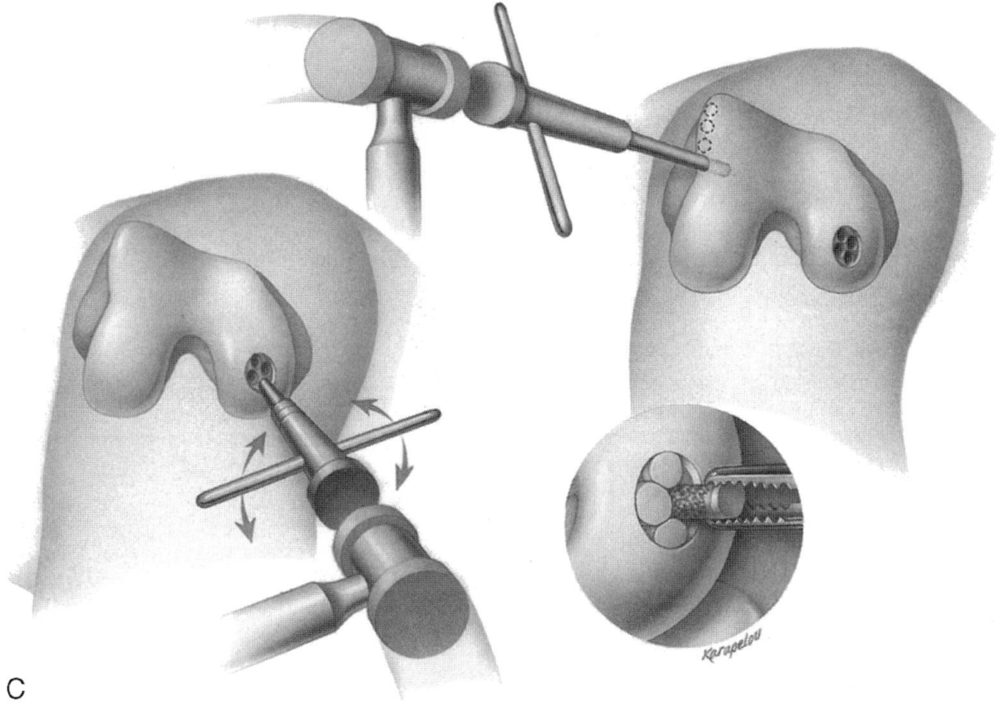

FIGURE 3-23 cont'd ■ *C,* Osteochondral plugs. Cylindrical "plugs" of exposed bone are removed from the defect. Plugs of normal non–weight-bearing cartilage and bone are harvested and placed into the defect. (From Miller, M.D.: Atlas of chondral injury treatment. Op. Tech. Orthop. 7[4]:289–294, 1997.)

3. Treatment and Prognosis—Children with open growth plates have the best prognosis, and often these lesions can be observed simply. In situ lesions can be treated with retrograde drilling. Detached lesions may require abrasion chondroplasty or newer, more aggressive, techniques.Osteochondritis dissecans (OCD) in adults usually is symptomatic and leads to DJD if left untreated.

B. Articular Cartilage Injury

1. The distinction between articular cartilage injury and OCD is not often clear, but articular cartilage injury occurs as a result of rotational forces in direct trauma. It usually occurs on ***the medial femoral condyle***. The lesions are classified according to their arthroscopic appearance. Débridement and chondroplasty are currently recommended for symptomatic lesions. Displaced osteochondral fragments can sometimes be replaced and secured with small recessed screws or absorbable pins. Several treatment options for discrete, isolated, full-thickness cartilage injuries are in clinical use. These include microfracture, periosteal patches (±chondrocyte implantation), and osteochondral transfer (plugs) (Fig. 3-23). Donor-site problems and the creation of true articular cartilage at the recipient site are still challenges.

C. Degenerative Joint Disease

1. Diffuse chondral damage is usually not considered "sports medicine," but treatment modalities include medications, nutritional supplements, hyaluronic acid injections, arthroscopic débridements, osteotomies, and arthroplasty. These treatment modalities are addressed in detail in Chapter 4, Adult Reconstruction.

D. Osteonecrosis

1. Atraumatic osteonecrosis is similar to AVN of the hip. Risk factors are similar to that of the hip and are common in elderly females.
2. Spontaneous Osteonecrosis of the Knee (SONK) is thought to represent a subchondral insufficiency fracture and is a self-limiting condition.

VI. Synovial Lesions

A. Pigmented Villonodular Synovitis—Patients may present with pain and swelling and may have a palpable mass. Synovectomy is effective, but there is a high recurrence rate. Arthroscopic techniques are just as effective as traditional open procedures.

B. Synovial Chondromatosis—This proliferative disease of the synovium is associated with cartilaginous metaplasia, resulting in multiple intra-articular loose bodies.

C. Other synovial lesions that respond to synovectomy include (osteo) chondromatosis, pauciarticular juvenile rheumatoid arthritis, and hemophilia. Additional arthroscopic portals are required for complete synovectomy.

D. Plicae—Synovial folds that are embryologic remnants. Occasionally, they are pathologic,

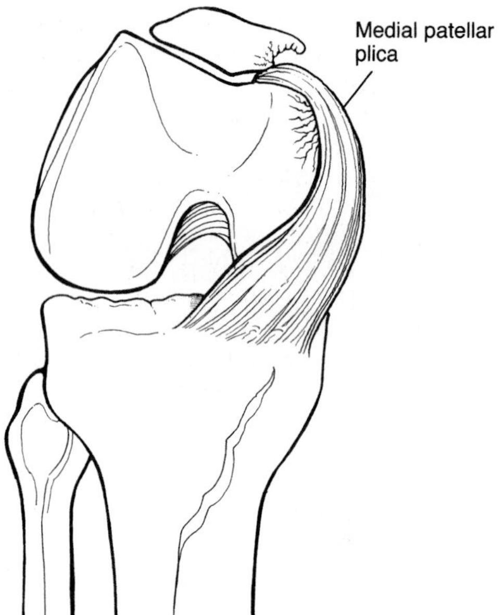

FIGURE 3-24 ■ Medial patellar plica with associated chondromalacia of the medial femoral condyle and patella. (From Miller, M.D., Cooper, D.E., and Warner, J.J.P.: Review of Sports Medicine and Arthroscopy, 2nd ed. Philadelphia, WB Saunders, 2002.)

particularly the medial patellar plica. This plica can cause abrasion of the medial femoral condyle and sometimes responds to arthroscopic excision (Fig. 3-24).

VII. Patellofemoral Disorders

A. Introduction—Anterior knee pain is classified based on etiologic factors (Table 3-7). The term *chondromalacia* should be replaced with a specific diagnosis based on this classification.

B. Trauma—Includes fractures of the patella (discussed in Chapter 10 Adult Trauma,) and tendon injuries.

1. Tendon Ruptures—Quadriceps tendon ruptures are more common than patellar tendon ruptures and occur most commonly in patients more than 40 years old with indirect trauma. Patellar tendon ruptures occur in young patients with direct or indirect trauma. Both types of tendon rupture are more common in patients with underlying disorders of the tendon. A palpable defect and inability to extend the knee are diagnostic. Primary repair with temporary stabilization is indicated.

2. Repetitive Trauma: Overuse Injuries

a. Patellar Tendinitis (Jumper's Knee)—This condition, most common in athletes who participate in sports such as basketball and volleyball, is associated with pain and tenderness near the inferior border of the patella (worse in extension than flexion).

Table 3-7. CLASSIFICATION OF PATELLOFEMORAL DISORDERS

I. Trauma (conditions caused by trauma in the otherwise normal knee)
  A. Acute trauma
    1. Contusion (924.11)
    2. Fracture
      a. Patella (822)
      b. Femoral trochlea (821.2)
      c. Proximal tibial epiphysis (tubercle) (823.0)
    3. Dislocation (rare in the normal knee) (836.3)
    4. Rupture
      a. Quadriceps tendon (843.8)
      b. Patellar tendon (844.8)
  B. Repetitive trauma (overuse syndromes)
    1. Patellar tendinitis ("jumper's knee") (726.64)
    2. Quadriceps tendinitis (726.69)
    3. Peripatellar tendinitis (e.g., anterior knee pain of the adolescent due to hamstring contracture) (726.699)
    4. Prepatellar bursitis ("housemaid's knee") (726.65)
    5. Apophysitis
      a. Osgood-Schlatter disease (732.43)
      b. Sinding-Larsen-Johansson disease (732.42)
  C. Late effects of trauma (905)
    1. Post-traumatic chondromalacia patellae
    2. Post-traumatic patellofemoral arthritis
    3. Anterior fat pad syndrome (post-traumatic fibrosis)
    4. Reflex sympathetic dystrophy of the patella
    5. Patellar osseous dystrophy
    6. Acquired patella infera (719.366)
    7. Acquired quadriceps fibrosis
II. Patellofemoral dysplasia
  A. Lateral patellar compression syndrome (LPCS) (718.365)
    1. Secondary chondromalacia patellae (717.7)
    2. Secondary patellofemoral arthritis (715.289)
  B. Chronic subluxation of the patella (CSP) (718.364)
    1. Secondary chondromalacia patellae (717.7)
    2. Secondary patellofemoral arthritis (715.289)
  C. Recurrent dislocation of the patella (RDP) (718.361)
    1. Associated fractures (822)
      a. Osteochondral (intra-articular)
      b. Avulsion (extra-articular)
    2. Secondary chondromalacia patellae (717.7)
    3. Secondary patellofemoral arthritis (715.289)
  D. Chronic dislocation of the patella (718.362)
    1. Congenital
    2. Acquired
III. Idiopathic chondromalacia patellae (717.7)
IV. Osteochondritis dissecans
  A. Patella (732.704)
  B. Femoral trochlea (732.703)
V. Synovial plicae (727.8916) (anatomic variant made symptomatic by acute or repetitive trauma)
  A. Medial patellar ("shelf") (727.89161)
  B. Suprapatellar (727.89163)
  C. Lateral patellar (727.89165)

From Merchant, A.C.: Classification of patellofemoral disorders. Arthroscopy 4:235, 1988.

Note: Orthopaedic ICD-9-CM Expanded Diagnostic Codes in parentheses.

Treatment includes nonsteroidal anti-inflammatory drugs (NSAIDs), physical therapy (strengthening and ultrasound), and orthotics (rarely surgery—excision of necrotic tendon fibers).

b. Quadriceps Tendinitis—Less common but just as painful. Patients may note painful clicking and localized pain. Operative treatment is occasionally necessary.

c. Prepatellar Bursitis (Housemaid's Knee)—It is the most common form of bursitis of the knee and is associated with a history of prolonged kneeling. Supportive treatment (knee pads, occasional steroid injections) and (although rarely) bursal excision are recommended.

d. Iliotibial Band Friction Syndrome—Can occur in runners (especially running hills) and cyclists and is a result of abrasion between the iliotibial band and the lateral femoral condyle. Localized tenderness, worse with the knee flexed 30 degrees, is common. The Ober test (patient lies in a lateral decubitus position and abduction and hyperextension of the hip demonstrate tightness of the iliotibial band) is helpful in making the diagnosis. Rehabilitation is usually successful. Surgical excision of an ellipse of the iliotibial band is occasionally necessary.

e. Semimembranosus Tendinitis—Most common in male athletes in their early thirties, this condition can be diagnosed with nuclear imaging and responds to stretching and strengthening.

C. Late Effects of Trauma

1. Patellofemoral Arthritis—Injury and malalignment can contribute to patellar DJD. Lateral release may be beneficial early; however, other procedures may be required for advanced patellar arthritis. Options include anterior or anteromedial transfer of the tibial tubercle, or patellectomy for severe cases.

2. Anterior Fat Pad Syndrome (Hoffa's Disease)—Trauma to the anterior fat pad can lead to fibrous changes and pinching of the fat pad, especially in patients with genu recurvatum. Activity modification, ice, and knee padding can be helpful. Occasionally, arthroscopic excision is beneficial.

3. Reflex Sympathetic Dystrophy—Characterized by ***pain out of proportion to physical findings***, RSD is an exaggerated response to injury. Three stages, progressing from swelling, warmth, and hyperhidrosis to brawny edema and trophic changes, and finally to glossy, cool, dry skin and stiffness, are typical. Patellar osteopenia and a "***flamingo gait***" are also common. Treatment includes nerve stimulation, NSAIDs, and sympathetic or epidural blocks, which can be both diagnostic and therapeutic.

D. Patellofemoral Dysplasia

1. Lateral Patellar Facet Compression Syndrome—This problem is associated with a tight lateral retinaculum and excessive lateral tilt without excessive patellar mobility. Treatment includes activity modification, NSAIDs, and vastus medialis obiquus strengthening. Arthroscopy and ***lateral release*** are occasionally required. The ***best candidates have a neutral or negative tilt and medial patellar glide less than one quadrant with a lateral patellar glide less than three quadrants***. Arthroscopic visualization through a superior portal demonstrates that the patella does not articulate medially by 40 degrees of knee flexion. Lateral release requires care to ensure that ***adequate hemostasis*** is achieved postoperatively and that the patella can be passively tilted 80 degrees.

2. Patellar Instability

a. Recurrent subluxation/dislocation of the patella can be characterized by lateral displacement of the patella, a shallow intercondylar sulcus, or patellar incongruence. When associated with femoral anteversion, genu valgum, and pronated feet, the symptoms can be exacerbated, especially in adolescents ("miserable malalignment syndrome"). Extensive rehabilitation is often curative. Surgical procedures include proximal and/or distal realignment procedures. Acute, first-time patella dislocations may be best treated with arthroscopic evaluation/débridement and acute repair of the medial patellofemoral ligament (usually at the medial epicondyle).

b. Abnormalities of Patellar Height—Patella alta (high-riding patella) and baja (low-riding patella) are determined based on various measurements made on lateral radiographs of the knee (see Fig. 3-7). Patella alta can be associated with patellar instability because the patella may not articulate with the sulcus, which normally constrains the patella. Patella baja is often the result of fat pad and tendon fibrosis and may require proximal transfer of the tubercle for refractory cases.

E. Idiopathic Chondromalacia Patellae—Although this term has fallen into disfavor, articular damage and changes to the patella are common. Treatment is usually symptomatic and has a heavy emphasis on physical therapy. Débridement procedures are of questionable benefit. The Outerbridge classification system is still in common use today (Fig. 3-25).

VIII. Pediatric Knee Disorders

A. Physeal Injuries—Most commonly involve Salter-Harris II fractures of the distal femoral physis. Pain, swelling, and an inability to ambulate are common. ***Stress radiographs may be necessary to make the diagnosis***. Open reduction and internal fixation are indicated for Salter-Harris III and IV fractures and Salter-Harris I and II fractures that cannot be

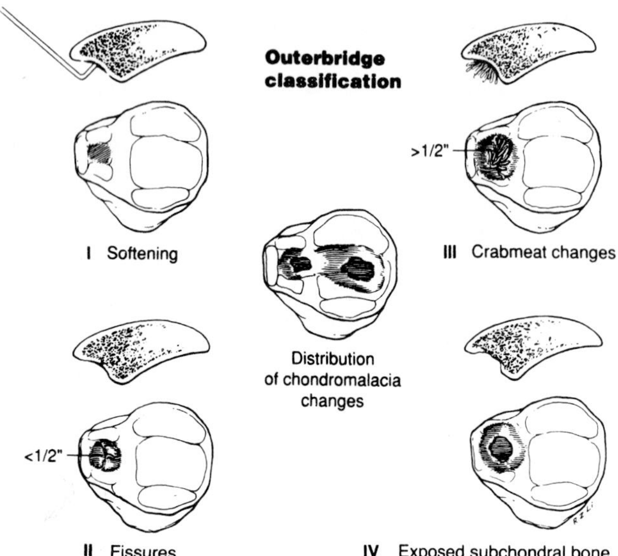

FIGURE 3-25 ■ Outerbridge classification of chondromalacia. (From Tria, A.J., and Klein, K.S.: An Illustrated Guide to the Knee. New York, Churchill Livingstone, 1992.)

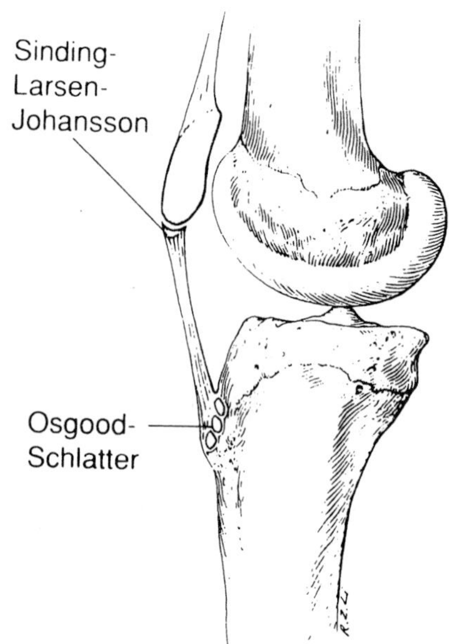

FIGURE 3-26 ■ Two types of traction apophysitis affecting adolescent knees. (From Miller, M.D., Cooper, D.E., and Warner, J.J.P.: Review of Sports Medicine and Arthroscopy, 2nd ed. Philadelphia, WB Saunders, 2002.)

adequately reduced. It is important to counsel the parents that, unlike other type II fractures, knee physeal injuries may have a worse prognosis.

B. Ligament Injuries—Most ligament injuries are treated like those in adults. Midsubstance ACL injuries in skeletally immature individuals remain a subject of considerable debate. Procedures that do not violate the growth plate are usually recommended for patients who fail nonoperative management. Avulsion fractures of the intercondylar eminence of the tibia are treated with closed treatment; if this treatment fails, arthroscopic reduction and fixation of the fragment are undertaken. Midsubstance injuries may be best addressed with procedures that avoid the physis, especially on the femoral side.

C. Traction Apophysitis—Includes Osgood-Schlatter disease and Sinding-Larsen-Johansson disease; it is usually treated symptomatically. Occasionally, procedures such as ossicle excision are indicated for refractory cases (Fig. 3-26).

SECTION 2

Thigh, Hip, and Pelvis

I. Contusions

A. Iliac Crest Contusions—Direct trauma to this area can occur in contact sports; known commonly as a ***hip pointer***. An avulsion of the iliac apophysis should be ruled out in adolescent athletes. Treatment consists of ice, compression, pain control, and placing the affected leg on maximum stretch. Occasionally, corticosteroid injections have been advocated. Additional padding is indicated after the acute phase.

B. Groin Contusions—An avulsion fracture of the lesser trochanter, traumatic phlebitis, thrombosis, or femoral neuropathy must be ruled out before supportive treatment.

C. Quadriceps Contusions—Can result in hemorrhage and late myositis ossificans. Acute management includes cold compression and ***immobilization in flexion***. Close monitoring for compartment syndrome is indicated in the acute phase.

II. Muscle Injuries

A. Hamstring Strain—This common injury is often the result of sudden stretch on the musculotendinous junction during sprinting. These injuries can occur anywhere in the posterior thigh. Treatment is supportive, followed by stretching and strengthening. To prevent recurrence, return to play (RTP) should be delayed until strength is approximately 90% of the opposite side.

B. Adductor Strain—Common in sports such as soccer, these injuries must be differentiated from subtle hernias. The adductor longus is most frequently injured. Pain and inflammation due to repetitive microtrauma or acute trauma to the tendinous origin of the adductor musculature has been termed ***"athletic pubalgia."***

C. Rectus Femoris Strain—Acute injuries are usually located more distally on the thigh, but chronic injuries are more commonly near the muscle origin. Pain is elicited with resisted hip flexion or extension. Treatment includes ice and stretching/strengthening.

III. Bursitis

A. Trochanteric Bursitis—Occurs frequently in female runners and associated with training on banked surfaces. Treatment includes oral anti-inflammatory drugs, stretching, and rest. Occasionally, corticosteroid injections are advocated.

B. Iliopsoas Bursitis—A cause of anterior hip pain in athletes, and often associated with mechanical irritation of the iliopsoas tendon.

C. Ischial Bursitis—Caused by direct trauma or prolonged sitting, and hard to distinguish from hamstring injuries.

IV. Nerve Entrapment Syndromes

A. Ilioinguinal Nerve Entrapment—This nerve can be constricted by hypertrophied abdominal muscles as a result of intensive training. Hyperextension of the hip may exacerbate the pain that patients experience, and hyperesthesia symptoms are common. Surgical release is occasionally necessary.

B. Obturator Nerve Entrapment—Can lead to chronic medial thigh pain, especially in athletes with well-developed hip adductor muscles (e.g., skaters). Nerve conduction studies are helpful for establishing the diagnosis. Treatment is usually supportive.

C. Lateral Femoral Cutaneous Nerve Entrapment—Can lead to a painful condition termed ***meralgia paresthetica***. Tight belts and prolonged hip flexion may exacerbate symptoms. Release of compressive devices, postural exercises, and NSAIDs are usually curative.

D. Sciatic Nerve Entrapment—Can occur anywhere along the course of the nerve, but the two most common locations are at the level of the ischial tuberosity or by the piriformis muscle, termed ***"piriformis syndrome."***

V. Bone Disorders

A. Stress Fractures—A history of overuse with an insidious onset of pain and localized tenderness and swelling are typical. Bone scan can be diagnostic, even with normal plain radiographs. ***MRI is the most specific test for detecting stress fractures.*** Treatment includes protected weight bearing, rest, cross-training, analgesics, and therapeutic modalities.

1. Femoral Neck Stress Fractures—Tension, or transverse, fractures are more serious than compression fractures (on medial side of the neck) and may require operative stabilization.
2. Femoral Shaft Stress Fractures—Usually respond to protected weight bearing but can progress to complete fractures if unrecognized.
3. Pelvic Stress Fractures—Stress fractures to the sacrum and pubis can occur, but are rare.

B. Fractures

1. Proximal Femoral Fractures—Can occur in athletes, especially cross-country skiers (***skier's hip***). Release bindings may reduce the incidence of these injuries.

C. Avascular Necrosis—Traumatic hip subluxation can disrupt the arterial blood supply to the hip and result in avascular necrosis. Early recognition of these injuries, seen in football players, is essential. A search for other causative factors (alcohol, catabolic steroids, and decompression sickness) should be made.

D. Osteitis Pubis—Repetitive trauma can cause an inflammation of the symphysis. It occurs frequently in soccer, hockey, and running. Conservative management is usually curative.

E. Tumors—Because more than 10% of all musculoskeletal tumors occur in the hip and pelvis, they must be suspected for cases of unexplained pain.

VI. Intra-articular Disorders

A. Loose Bodies—Often result from trauma or diseases, such as synovial chondromatosis. They must be removed, either open or arthroscopically, to prevent third-body wear.

B. Labral Tears—Often a cause of mechanical hip pain presenting with vague symptoms. MRI is often used for diagnosis, but arthroscopy is the gold standard (Fig. 3-27). ***The highest incidence of labral tears is present is patients with acetabular dysplasia.***

C. Chondral Injuries—Articular surface injury is often a cause of mechanical hip pain. Microfracture is effective in treatment of focal lesions.

D. Ruptured Ligamentum Teres—Associated with mechanical hip pain as the ruptured ligamentum catches within the joint following a hip dislocation. Débridement is often necessary. ***The viability of the femoral head is not in jeopardy with a ruptured ligamentum teres.***

VII. Hip Arthroscopy

A. Indications—As techniques improve, so do the indications. Currently, hip arthroscopy is effective for treatment of loose bodies, labral tears, chondral injuries, AVN, synovial disease, ruptured ligamentum teres, impinging osteophytes, or unexplained mechanical symptoms.

B. Setup—Typically is performed in the supine or lateral position with approximately 50 lb of traction with a well padded perineal post.

C. Portals—Three portals are commonly used for instrumentation—one on each side of the greater trochanter and an additional anterior portal (Fig. 3-28).

D. Complications—Complications are rare but are associated with traction injuries, iatrogenic chondral injuries, and neurovascular injury due to aberrant portal placement.

VIII. Other Hip Disorders

A. Snapping Hip—Condition in which the iliotibial band abruptly catches on the greater trochanter, or by iliopsoas impingement on the hip capsule. The iliotibial condition, more common in females with wide pelvis and prominent trochanters, can be exacerbated by running on banked surfaces. The snapping may be reproduced with passive hip flexion from an adducted position. Stretching/strengthening modalities, such as ultrasonography and, occasionally, surgical release, may relieve the snapping. This condition must be differentiated from the less common snapping iliopsoas tendon, which can be diagnosed with extension and internal rotation of the hip from a flexed and externally rotated position. Arthrography and/or bursography may also be helpful in making the diagnosis.

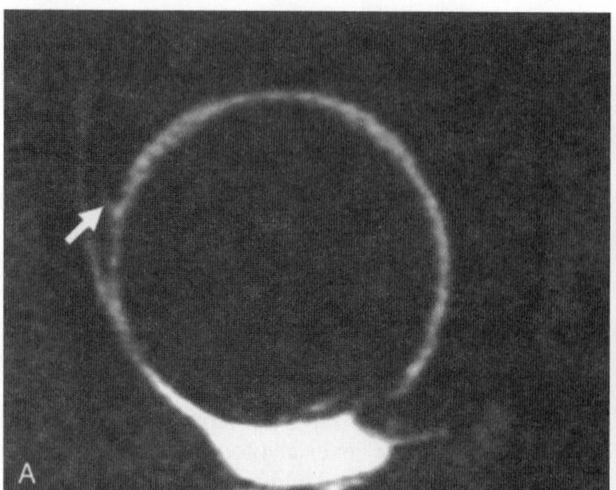

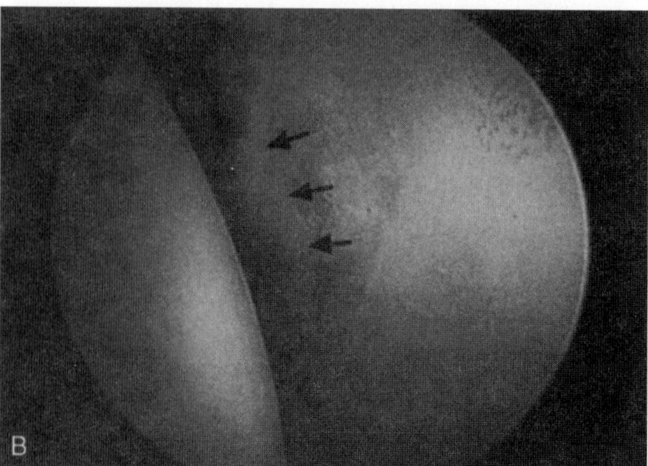

FIGURE 3-27 ■ A 27-year-old with mechanical symptoms in the left hip. *(A)* Sagittal MRI with gadolinium arthrography reveals a tear of the anterior labrum *(arrow)*. *(B)* Arthroscopic picture showing the anterior labral tear. (From Miller, M.D., Cooper, D.E., and Warner, J.J.P.: Review of Sports Medicine and Arthroscopy, 2nd ed. Philadelphia, WB Saunders, 2002.)

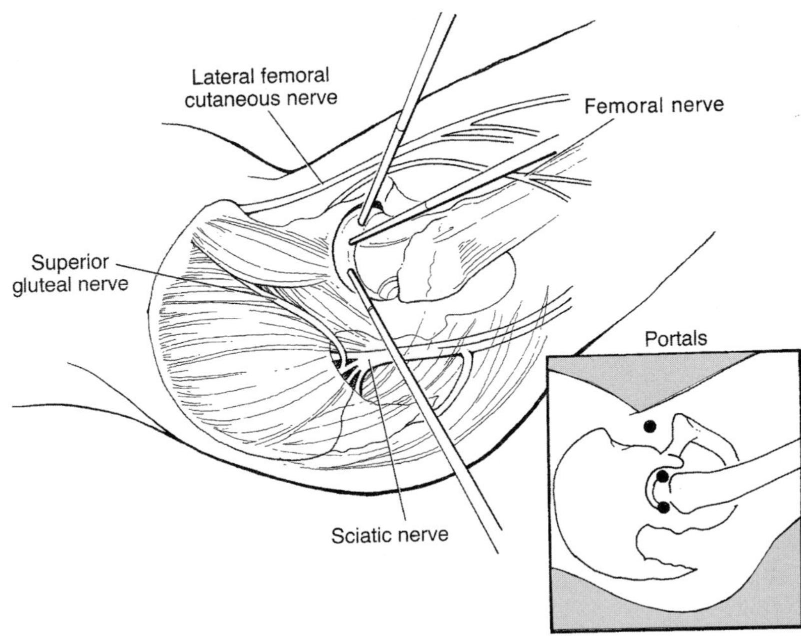

FIGURE 3-28 ■ Portals for hip arthroscopy include the anterior portal and two portals adjacent to the greater trochanter. (From Miller, M.D., Cooper, D.E., and Warner, J.J.P.: Review of Sports Medicine and Arthroscopy. Philadelphia, WB Saunders, 1995, p. 107.)

SECTION 3

Leg, Foot, and Ankle

I. Nerve Entrapment Syndromes

A. Saphenous Nerve Entrapment—When compressed at Hunter's canal or in the proximal leg, this nerve can cause painful symptoms inferior and medial to the knee.

B. Peroneal Nerve Entrapment—The common peroneal nerve can be compressed behind the fibula or injured by a direct blow to this area. The superficial peroneal nerve can be entrapped about 12 cm proximal to the tip of the lateral malleolus, where it exits the fascia of the anterolateral leg, as a result of inversion injuries. ***Fascial defects*** can be present as well, contributing to the problem. Compartment release is sometimes indicated. The deep peroneal nerve can be compressed by the inferior extensor retinaculum, leading to ***anterior tarsal tunnel syndrome***, sometimes necessitating release of this structure.

C. Tibial Nerve Entrapment—When the tibial nerve is compressed under the flexor retinaculum behind the medial malleolus, it may result in ***tarsal tunnel syndrome***. Electromyography/nerve-conduction evaluation is helpful, and surgical release is sometimes indicated. Distal entrapment of the ***first branch of the lateral plantar nerve (to the adductor digiti quinti)***, between the fascia of the abductor hallucis longus and the medial side of the quadratus plantae, has also been described.

D. Medial Plantar Nerve Entrapment—Occurs at the point where the flexor digitorum longus and flexor hallucis longus cross (knot of Henry) and is most commonly caused by external compression by orthotics. Commonly called ***jogger's foot***, this condition usually responds to conservative measures.

E. Sural Nerve Entrapment—Can occur anywhere along its course but is most vulnerable 12–15 mm distal to the tip of the fibula as the foot rests in equinus. Surgical release is usually effective.

F. Interdigital Nerve—Commonly called ***Morton's neuroma***, entrapment can occur during the push-off phase while running in athletes. It usually occurs between the third and fourth metatarsals plantar to the transverse metatarsal ligament and responds to surgical resection if conservative measures fail.

II. Muscle Injuries

A. Gastrocnemius-Soleus Strain—Nicknamed ***tennis leg*** because of its common association with that sport, this injury is probably much more common than rupture of the plantaris tendon. Supportive treatment is indicated.

III. Tendon Injuries

A. Peroneal Tendon Injuries

1. Subluxation/Dislocation—Violent dorsiflexion of the inverted foot can result in injury of the fibro-osseous peroneal tendon sheath. Diagnosis is confirmed by observing the subluxation or dislocation by means of eversion and dorsiflexion of the foot. Plain radiographs may demonstrate a rim fracture of the lateral aspect of the distal fibula. Treatment of acute injuries includes restoration of the normal anatomy (Fig. 3-29). Chronic reconstruction involves groove-deepening procedures, tissue transfers, or bone block techniques.
2. Tenosynovitis—These injuries are being recognized more frequently with MRI and often lead to tears of the peroneal tendons.
3. Longitudinal Tears of the Peroneal Tendons (Especially Brevis Tendon)—Recognized with increasing frequency. Repair and decompression are generally recommended.

B. Posterior Tibialis Tendon Injury—This injury can occur in older athletes. Patients complain of midarch foot pain, with difficulty pushing off. Débridement of partial ruptures and flexor digitorum longus transfer for chronic injuries are recommended.

C. Anterior Tibialis Tendon Injury—Rupture is uncommon, but has been reported in elderly athletes. Repair is recommended.

D. Achilles Tendon Injuries

1. Tendinitis—Overuse injury to the Achilles tendon usually responds to rest and physical therapy modalities. Progression to partial rupture may necessitate surgical excision of scar and granulation tissue.
2. Rupture—Complete rupture of the tendon is caused by maximal plantar flexion with the foot planted. Patients may relate that they felt as if they were "shot." The Thompson test (squeezing the calf results in plantar flexion of the foot normally) is helpful for confirming the diagnosis. **Treatment remains controversial; however, recurrence rates are reduced with primary repair.**

IV. Chronic Exertional Compartment Syndrome

A. Although more commonly encountered with trauma, sports-related compartment syndrome is becoming more frequently diagnosed. Athletes (especially runners and cyclists) may note pain that has a gradual onset during exercise, ultimately restricting their performance. Compartment pressures taken before, during, and after exercise

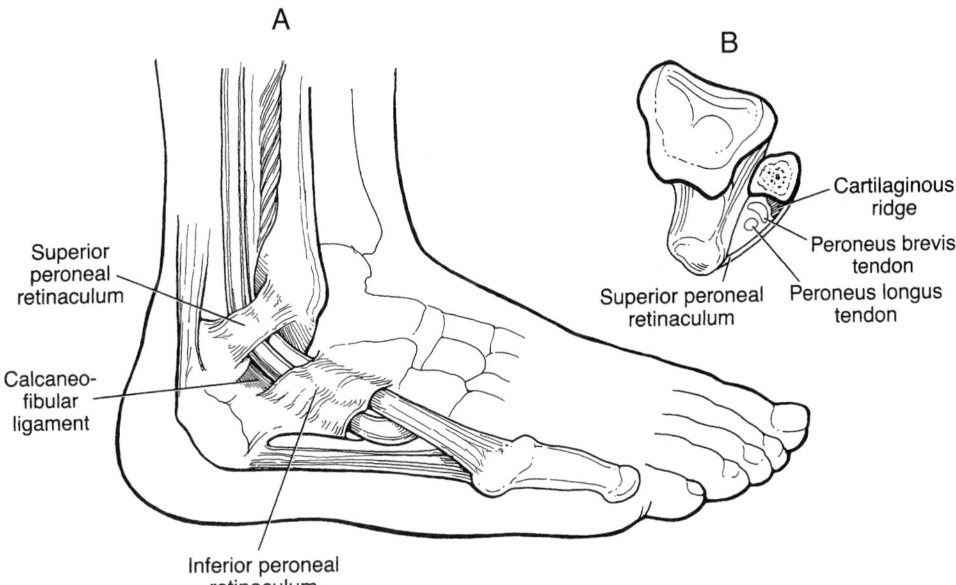

FIGURE 3-29 ■ Normal relationship of the peroneal tendons. Note the superior and inferior retinacula and the cartilaginous ridge on the posterolateral fibula. *A*, Lateral view. *B*, Superior view. (From Miller, M.D., Cooper, D.E., and Warner, J.J.P.: Review of Sports Medicine and Arthroscopy. Philadelphia, WB Saunders, 1995, p. 82.)

(pressures >15 mm Hg 15 minutes after exercise, or absolute values above 15 mm Hg while resting or above 30 mm Hg after exercise) can help establish the diagnosis. The anterior and deep posterior compartments of the leg are most often involved. Fasciotomy is sometimes indicated for refractory cases (Fig. 3-30).

V. Fractures

A. Stress Fractures—Common in athletes who have undergone a change in their training routine and in female endurance athletes (must ask about a menstrual history). Usually responds to rest and activity modification. Recalcitrant fractures may need operative fixation.

1. Tibial Shaft Fractures—Can be difficult. Persistence of the ***"dreaded black line"*** (Fig. 3-31) for more than 6 months, especially with a positive bone scan, can be an indication for bone grafting.
2. Tarsal Navicular Fractures—Often found in basketball players. Immobilization and ***no weight bearing*** are important during the early management of these stress fractures.
3. ***Freiberg Infarction***—Flattening of the second metatarsal head, usually due to stress overloading in a child's foot. Conservative management is indicated unless patient is having mechanical symptoms.

B. Jones Fractures—Fractures at the metaphyseal-diaphyseal junction of the fifth metatarsal in an athlete can be ***treated more aggressively with early open reduction and internal fixation to allow an earlier return to conditioning activities.***

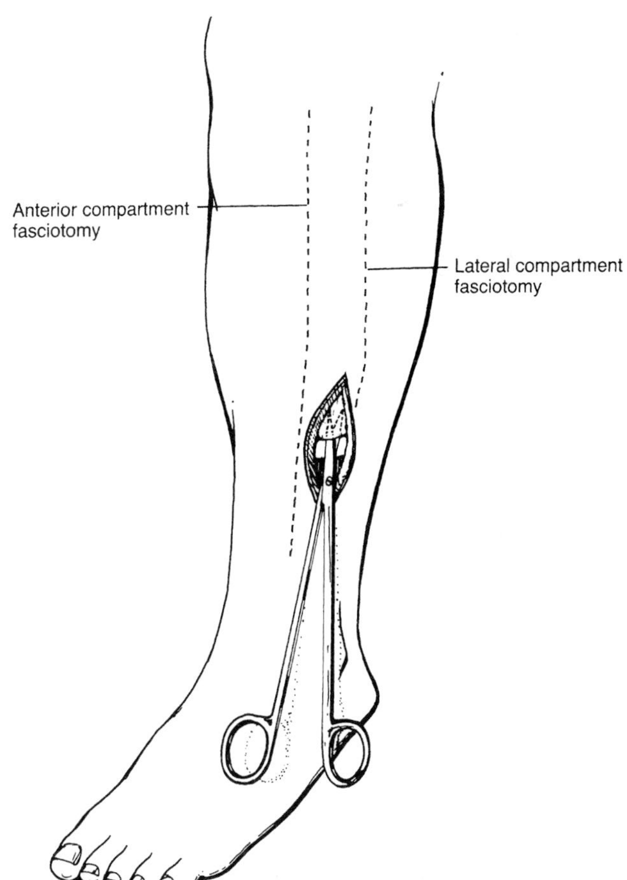

FIGURE 3-30 ■ Anterior and lateral compartment release. (From DeLee, J.C., and Drez, D., Jr.: Orthopaedic Sports Medicine: Principles and Practice. Philadelphia, WB Saunders, 1994, p. 1618.)

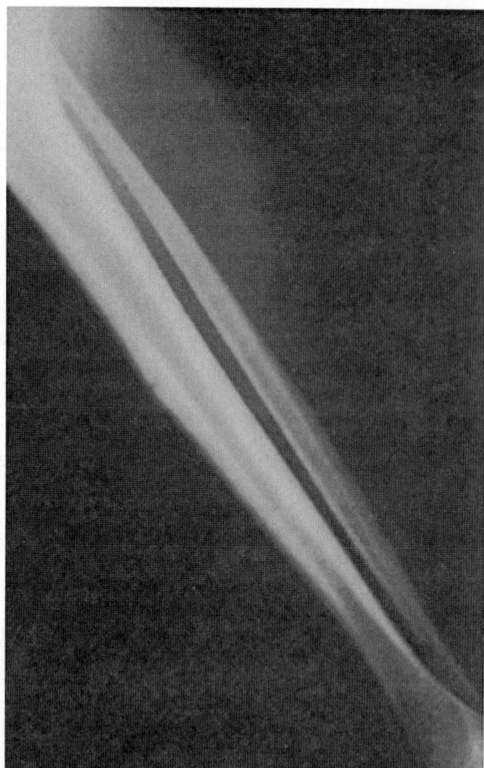

FIGURE 3-31 ■ Radiograph demonstrating the "dreaded black line" associated with an impending complete fracture of the tibial shaft. (From Miller, M.D., Cooper, D.E., and Warner, J.J.P.: Review of Sports Medicine and Arthroscopy. Philadelphia, WB Saunders, 1995, p. 81.)

VI. Ankle Arthroscopy

A. Indications include treatment of osteochondral injuries of the talus, débridement of post-traumatic synovitis, anterolateral impingement, removal of anterior tibiotalar spurring, and cartilage débridement in conjunction with ankle fusions. Supine positioning with the leg over a well-padded bolster and an external traction device are currently popular. Five portals have been suggested (Fig. 3-32), but most surgeons avoid the posteromedial portal, because of risk to the posterior tibial artery and tibial nerve, and the anterocentral portal, because of risk to the dorsalis pedis and deep peroneal nerve. The "nick and spread" method is advocated for the ***anterolateral portal (superficial peroneal nerve) and the anteromedial portal (saphenous vein)***. Treatment of osteochondral injuries of the talus, including drilling of the base of these lesions and fixation of replaceable lesions, has been advocated. ***Lateral lesions are usually traumatic, shallow, and anterior; medial lesions are atraumatic, deeper, and posterior.*** The Loomer and co-workers modification to the Berndt and Harty classification scheme (Fig. 3-33) is helpful in the management of these osteochondral lesions of the talus.

VII. Other Foot and Ankle Disorders

A. Plantar Fasciitis—Inflammation of the plantar fascia, usually in the central to medial subcalcaneal region, is common in runners. Rest, orthotics, stretching, and NSAIDs are helpful. Occasionally, plantar fasciotomy is necessary, but recovery can be protracted.

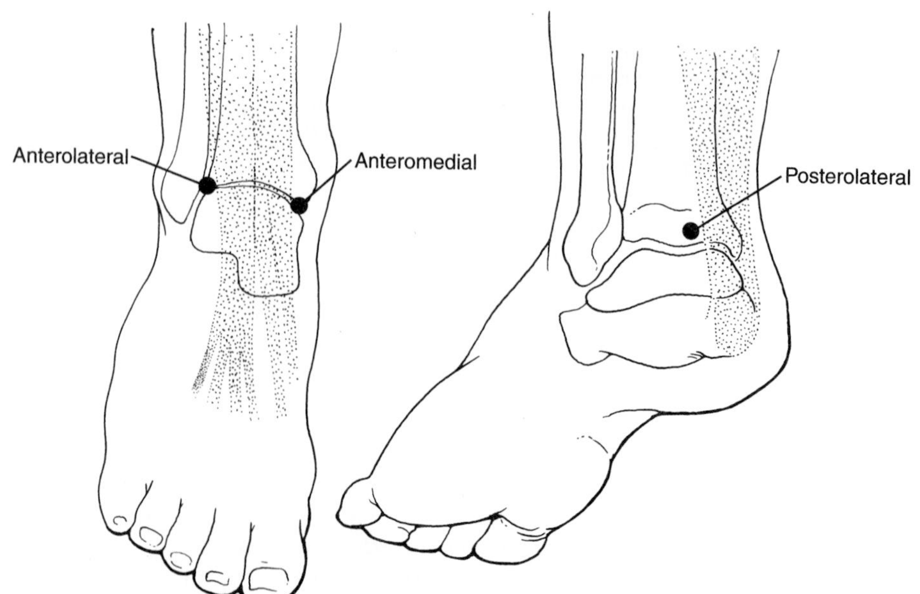

FIGURE 3-32 ■ Portals for ankle arthroscopy are the anteromedial, anterolateral, and posterolateral. (From Miller, M.D., Osborne J.R., Warner J.J.P., et al.: MRI-Arthroscopy Correlative Atlas, Philadelphia, WB Saunders, 1997, p. 134.)

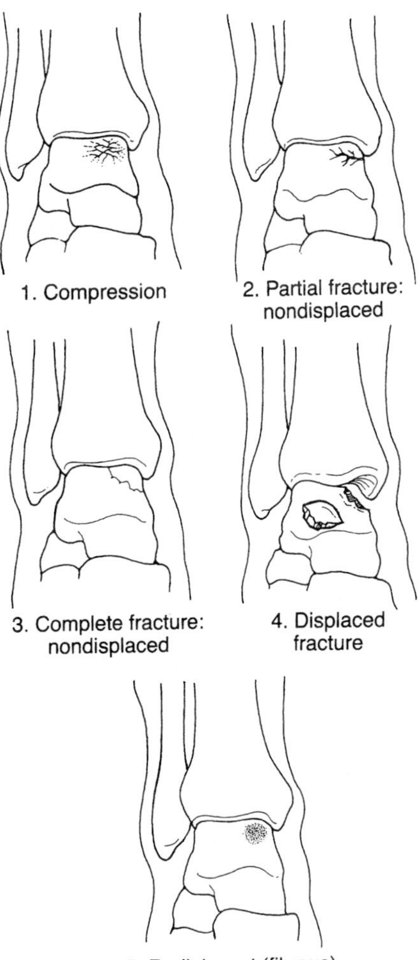

FIGURE 3-33 ■ Loomer and co-workers' modification to the Berndt and Harty classification of osteochondral lesions of the talus. (From Miller, M.D., Cooper, D.E., and Warner, J.J.P.: Review of Sports Medicine and Arthroscopy. Philadelphia, WB Saunders, 1995, p. 95.)

B. Os Trigonum—An unfused fractured os trigonum can cause impingement with plantar flexion of the foot, especially in ballet dancers. Treatment may include local anesthetic injection and other supportive measures. Surgical excision of the offending bone is occasionally necessary.

C. Ankle Sprains and Instability—These injuries are common in athletes and most often ***involve the anterior talofibular ligament (ATFL)***. Other lateral ligaments, the calcaneofibular ligament (CFL) and the posterior talofibular ligament (PTFL), can also be involved. The Ottawa ankle rules indicate that radiographs are required only in patients with distal (especially posterior) tibia or fibula tenderness, tenderness at the base of the fifth metatarsal or navicular, and an inability to bear weight. Surgical treatment is reserved for recurrent, symptomatic ankle instability with excessive tilt and drawer on examination/stress radiographs that has not responded to orthotics and peroneal strengthening over an extended period. Anatomic procedures (Brostrom's) are usually successful. Involvement of the subtalar joint requires tendon rerouting procedures that include this joint. Patients with "high" ankle sprains involving the syndesmosis require recovery periods almost twice those for common ankle sprains.

D. Turf Toe—Severe dorsiflexion of the metatarsophalangeal (MTP) joint of the great toe can result in a tender, stiff, swollen toe. Treatment includes motion, ice, and taping. If symptoms persist, a stress fracture of the proximal phalanx should be ruled out with a bone scan.

SECTION 4

Shoulder

I. Anatomy and Biomechanics—Refer to Chapter 11, Anatomy, for a more detailed description of shoulder anatomy. The shoulder consists of three bones and four joints.

A. Osteology

1. Clavicle—An S-shaped bone, it is the last to ossify (the medial growth plate fuses in the early twenties).
2. Scapula—Serves as the insertion site for 17 muscles. It has two important prominences: the coracoid process and the acromion. Os acromiale, an unfused secondary ossification, occurs with a 3% incidence and 60% bilaterality. Most common location is at the ***junction of the meso- and meta-acromion***.
3. Humeral Head—It is approximately spheroidal in shape in 90% of individuals and has an average diameter of 43 mm. It is normally retroverted an average of ***30 degrees*** to the transepicondylar axis of the distal humerus with its articular surface inclined an average of ***130 degrees*** superiorly relative to the shaft.
4. Glenoid—The shoulder "socket," or glenoid cavity, is a lateral thickening of the scapula. Its rim is surrounded by a fibrocartilaginous thickening known as the labrum, which serves to both deepen the socket (acting as a chock block) and anchor the inferior glenohumeral ligament complex. Its surface is pear-shaped with an average upward tilt of 5 degrees and an average range in version of 7 degrees of retroversion to 10 degrees of anteversion.

B. Articulations—The shoulder consists of four joints: glenohumeral (GH), sternoclavicular (SC), acromioclavicular (AC), and scapulothoracic (ST) joints.

1. GH Joint—A spheroidal (ball and socket) joint, it is the principle articulation of the shoulder and is stabilized by both static and dynamic restraints (see the following discussion on biomechanics). Part of the static restraints, the GH ligaments are discrete capsular thickenings that act as checkreins to limit excessive humeral head rotation or translation. The capsuloligamentous structures include ***the superior GH ligament*** (SGHL), ***coracohumeral ligament*** (CHL), ***middle GH ligament*** (MGHL), and ***inferior GH ligament complex*** (IGHLC) (Fig. 3-34). Additional capsular elements include the posterior capsule, which is the thinnest portion of the shoulder (<1 mm)

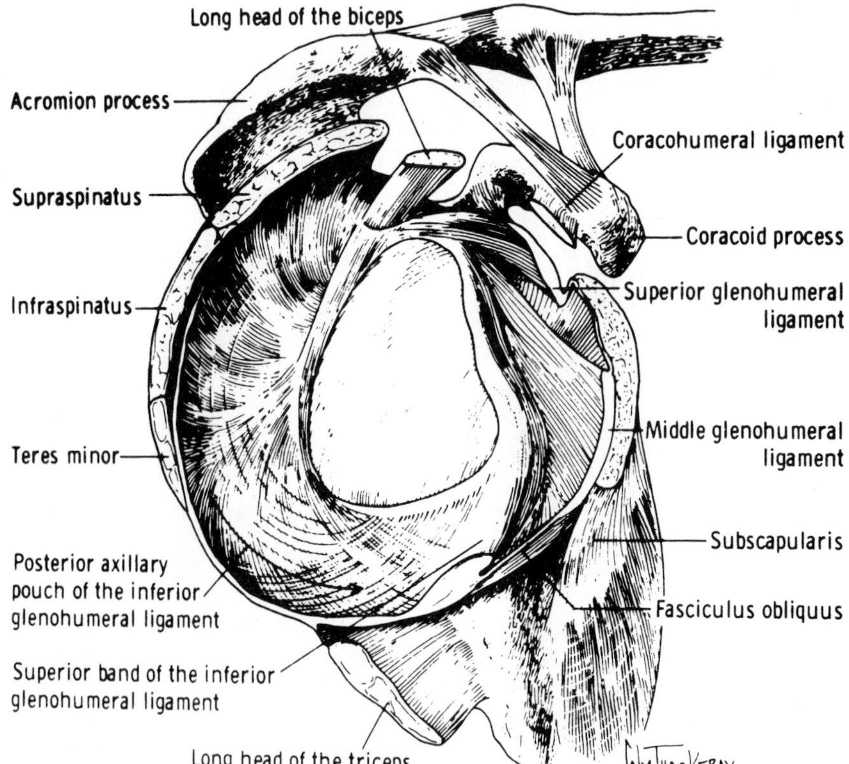

FIGURE 3-34 ■ Important ligaments of the shoulder. (From Turkel, S.J., Panio, M.W., Marshall, J.L., et al.: Stabilizing mechanisms preventing anterior dislocation of the glenohumeral joint. J. Bone Joint Surg. [Am.] 63:1209, 1981.)

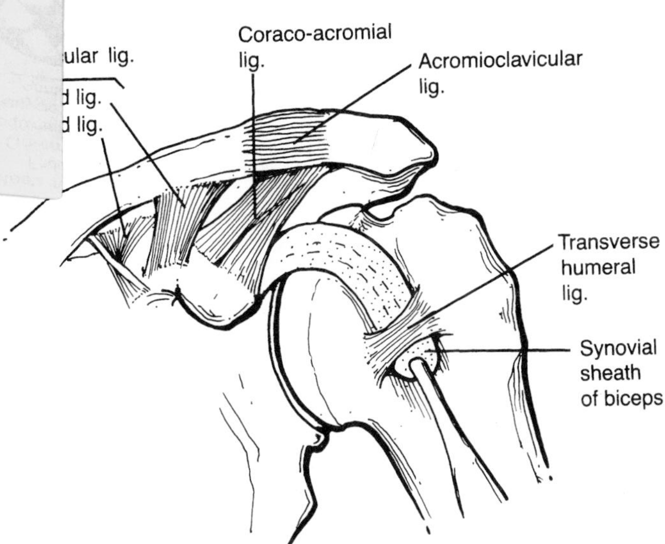

FIGURE 3-35 ■ Acromioclavicular joint anatomy. (From Tibone, J., Patek, R., Jobe, F.W., et al.: Functional anatomy, biomechanics, and kinesiology: The shoulder. In DeLee, J.C., and Drez, D., Jr., eds.: Orthopaedic Sports Medicine: Principles and Practice. Philadelphia, WB Saunders, 1994, p. 465.)

capsule and the ***rotator interval***. This interval includes the capsule and CHL that bridge the gap between the supraspinatus and the subscapularis. It is bounded medially by the lateral coracoid base, superiorly by the anterior edge of the supraspinatus, and inferiorly by the superior border of the subscapularis. The transverse humeral ligament forms its apex laterally.

2. SC Joint—A gliding joint with a disc. Serves to anchor the shoulder girdle to the chest wall. Elevation of the arm from 0 degrees to 90 degrees produces clavicular rotation about its longitudinal axis and elevation at the SC joint of 0 degrees to 40 degrees.
3. AC Joint—The articulation of the scapula with the clavicle occurs through a diarthrodial joint containing an incomplete intra-articular disc. It is stabilized by ***the AC ligaments, which primarily resist anteroposterior translation***, and the ***coracoclavicular (CC) ligaments, which prevent inferior translation of the coracoid and acromion from the clavicle*** (Fig. 3-35).
4. ST Joint—The medial border of the scapula articulates with the posterior aspect of the second to seventh ribs. It is angled 30 degrees toward the anterior and has a 3 degree upward tilt. There are two major ST bursae. The ***ratio of GH to ST motion during shoulder abduction is approximately 2:1***.

C. Supporting Structures—It is helpful to consider the shoulder in layers (Fig. 3-36).

D. Biomechanics—The shoulder is stabilized by both static and dynamic restraints.

1. Static Restraints—These include the glenoid labrum, articular version, articular conformity, negative intra-articular pressure, capsule (posterior capsule and rotator interval), and capsuloligamentous structures. Imbrication of the rotator interval decreases inferior and posterior translation while its release produces increased forward flexion and external rotation. The SGHL and CHL are reinforcing structures of the rotator interval, ***limiting inferior translation and external rotation when the arm is adducted and posterior translation when the arm is forward flexed, adducted, and internally rotated***. The MGHL acts to ***limit external rotation of the adducted humerus, inferior translation of the adducted and externally rotated humerus, and anterior and posterior translation of the partly abducted (45 degrees) and externally rotated arm***. The IGHLC serves as ***the primary restraint to anterior, posterior, and inferior GH translation for 45–90 degrees of GH elevation***.
2. Dynamic Restraints—These include joint concavity compression produced by synchronized contraction of the rotator cuff (RTC) acting to stabilize the humeral head within the glenoid, increased capsular tension produced by direct attachments of the RTC to the capsule, the scapular stabilizers that act to maintain a stable glenoid platform ("ball on a seal's nose"), and proprioception.

E. Throwing—Significant forces are generated when throwing and can result in injury. The five phases of throwing are shown in Figure 3-37. Maximum torque is generated during two points, at maximal external rotation (late cocking) and just after ball release (deceleration).

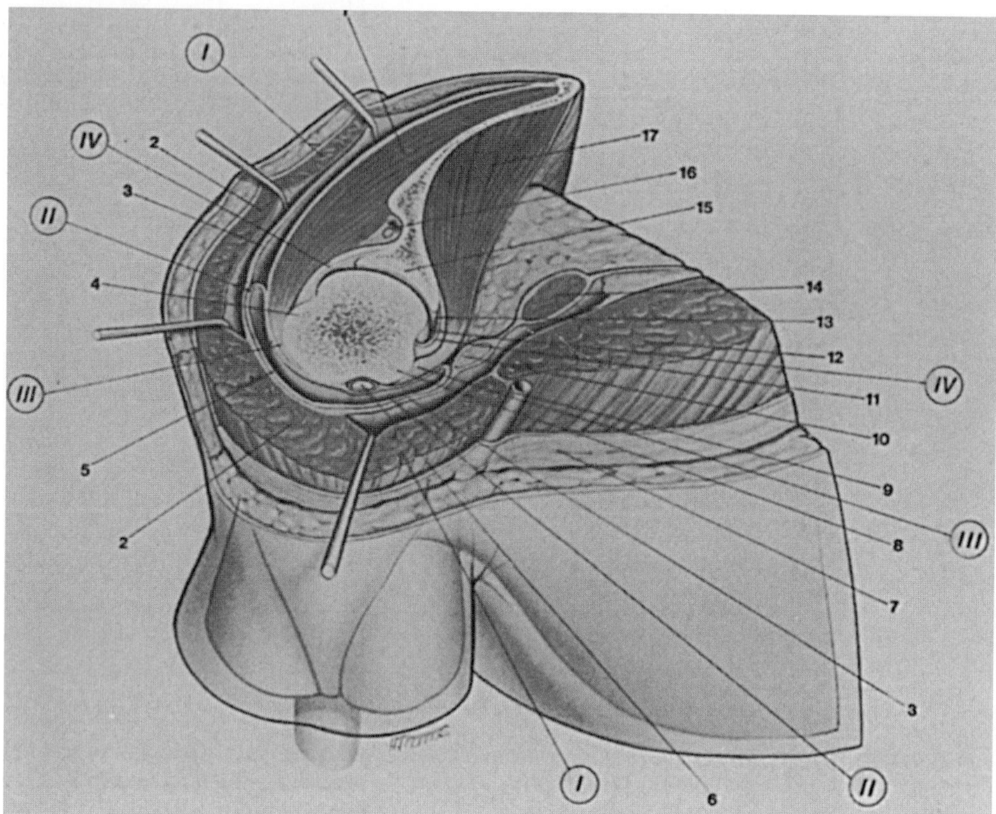

FIGURE 3-36 ■ Cross-sectional view of the right shoulder at the level of the lesser tuberosity. Note the four layers of the shoulder and their components: *I*—deltoid *(2)*, pectoralis major *(12)*, cephalic vein *(9)*; *II*—conjoined tendon *(10)*, pectoralis minor *(14)*, claviopectoral fascia *(7)*; *III*—subdeltoid bursa *(5)*, rotator cuff muscles *(1, 17)*, glenohumeral capsule *(11)*, greater tuberosity *(4)*, long head of biceps *(6)*, lesser tuberosity *(8)*, fascia *(3)*, synovium *(13)*, glenoid *(15)*. (From Cooper, D.E., O'Brien, S.J., and Warren, R.F.: Supporting layers of the glenohumeral joint: An anatomic study. Clin. Orthop. 289:151, 1993.)

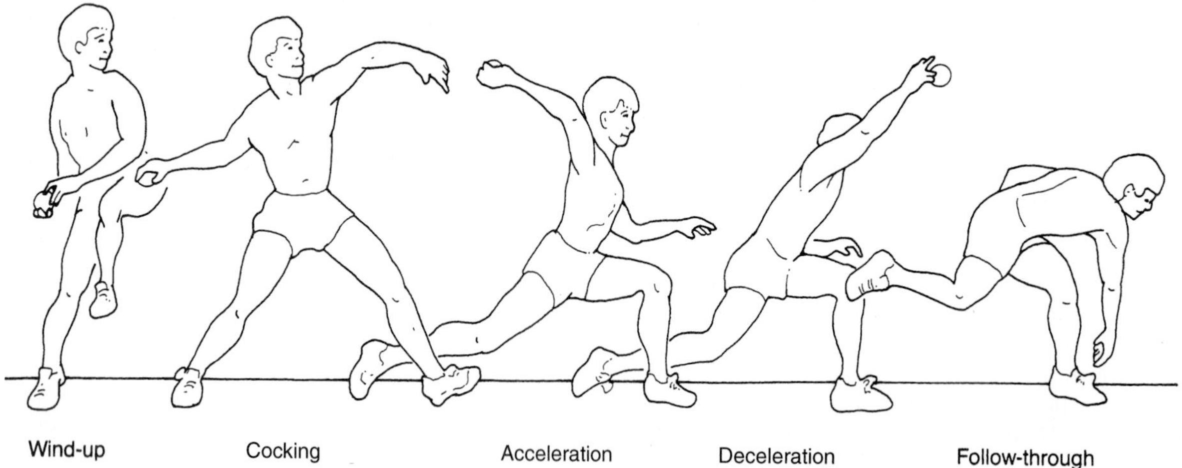

FIGURE 3-37 ■ The five phases of throwing. (From Miller, M.D., Cooper, D.E., and Warner, J.J.P.: Review of Sports Medicine and Arthroscopy. Philadelphia, WB Saunders, 1995, p. 123.)

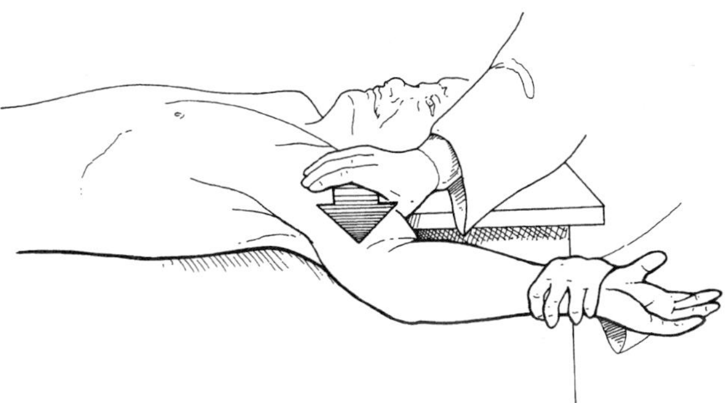

FIGURE 3-38 ■ Relocation test. Anterior pressure on the proximal arm relocates the humerus and causes relief of apprehension. (From Miller, M.D., Cooper, D.E., and Warner, J.J.P.: Review of Sports Medicine and Arthroscopy. Philadelphia, WB Saunders, 1995, p. 128.)

II. History and Physical Examination

A. History—Age and chief complaint are two important considerations. Instability, AC injuries, and distal clavicle osteolysis are more common in young patients. RTC tears, arthritis, and proxim fractures are more common in olde Direct blows are usually responsible for tions. Instability is related to injury to the externally rotated arm. Chronic overh and night pain are associated with RTC

B. Physical Examination—Observation, p and strength testing can lead to important diagnostic clues. This includes range and quality of motion (forward flexion of 150-180 degrees, external rotation with the arm adducted 30-60 degrees, and internal rotation reaching T4-T8 are considered normal) as well as specific muscle testing (Table 3-8).

III. Imaging the Shoulder

Imaging the Shoulder—The trauma series of radiographs includes a "true" anteroposterior view (plate is placed parallel to the scapula, about 45 degrees from the plane of the thorax) and an axillary lateral view. Other views that are sometimes helpful include a scapular Y or transscapular view and anteroposterior radiographs in internal and external rotation. Special radiographic views have

Table 3-8. MUSCLE TESTING FOR SHOULDER INJURIES

EXAMINATION	TECHNIQUE	SIGNIFICANCE
Impingement/RTC		
Impingement sign	Passive FF >90 degrees	Pain = impingement syndrome
Impingement test	Same after subacromial injection	Relief of pain = impingement syndrome
Hawkins test	Passive FF 90 degrees and IR	Pain = impingement syndrome
Jobe test	Resisted pronation/FF 90 degrees	Pain = supraspinatus lesion
Drop arm test	Maintain FF in plane of scapula	Inability = supraspinatus lesion
Hornblower sign	Resisted max ER/abd 90 degrees	Pain = infraspinatus/(post) supraspinatus lesion
Rubber band sign	Resisted max ER/slight abd	Pain = infraspinatus lesion
Lift-off test	Arm IR behind back	Inability to elevate from back = subscapularis lesion
Modified lift-off test	Resisted arm held off back	Inability to keep elevated off back = subscapularis lesion
Belly-push test	Elbow held ant with abd pressure	Inability to hold elbow forward = subscapularis lesion
Instability		
Apprehension test	Supine abd 90 degrees and ER	Apprehension = ant instability
Relocation test (Fig. 3-38)	Apprehension with posterior force	Relief of apprehension = ant instability
Load-and-shift test	Ant/post force on humeral head	degree of translation = laxity vs. instability (see grading)
Modified load-and-shift test	Supine load/shift with elbow bending	degree of translation = laxity vs. instability (see grading)
Jerk test	Post force w/ arm addr and FF	"clunk" = posterior subluxation
Sulcus sign	Inferior force w/arm at side	increased acromiohumeral interval = inf laxity vs. instability (see sulcus grading)
Labrum/Biceps		
Active compression test	10 degrees add, 90 degrees FF, max pronation	pain with resistance = SLAP lesion
Anterior slide test	Hand on hip, joint loading	pain with resistance = SLAP lesion
Crank test	Full abd, humeral loading, rotation	pain = SLAP lesion
Speed test	Resisted FF in scapular plane	pain = bicipital tendonitis
Yerguson test	Resisted supination	pain = bicipital tendonitis
Miscellaneous		
Spurling maneuver (Fig. 3-39)	Lat. flexion, rotation, cervical loading	Cervical spine pathology
Wright's test	Ext-abd-ER of arm w/neck rotated away	Loss of pulse and reproduction of sx = thoracic outlet syndrome

RTC, rotator cuff; FF, forward flexion; IR, internal rotation; ER, external rotation; abd, abductor; ant, anterior; post, posterior; add, adduction; ext, extension; inf, inferior; max, maximum; SLAP, superior labrum from anterior to posterior; lat, lateral; sx, symptom.

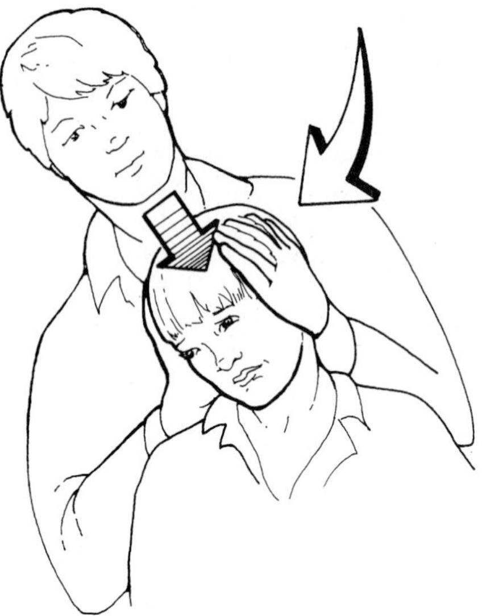

FIGURE 3-39 ■ Spurling's test. Lateral flexion and rotation with some compression may cause nerve root encroachment and pain on the ipsilateral side in patients with cervical nerve root impingement. (From Miller, M.D., Cooper, D.E., and Warner, J.J.P.: Review of Sports Medicine and Arthroscopy. Philadelphia, WB Saunders, 1995, p. 129.)

also been developed for certain other abnormalities. For example, the supraspinatus outlet view is helpful in the evaluation of impingement (Fig. 3-40) (Table 3-9).

IV. Shoulder Arthroscopy

A. Portals—standard portals include the posterior portal (2 cm distal and medial to the posterolateral border of the acromion, primarily used for viewing), anterior portal (lateral and inferior to the coracoid process), and the lateral portal (1–2 cm distal to the lateral acromial edge). Additional portals include the supraspinatus (Neviaser) portal for anterior glenoid visualization, anterolateral (port of Wilmington) and posterolateral portals, which are useful for labral or superior labrum from anterior to posterior (SLAP) and RTC repair, anteroinferior (5 o'clock position) portal for Bankart repair and stabilization procedures, and the posteroinferior (7 o'clock position) portal again for stabilization procedures (Fig. 3-41).

B. Technique—Orderly evaluation of intra-articular structures should be performed. As the number and variety of arthroscopic procedures grows, so does the opportunity for iatrogenic injury. Maintaining adequate visualization through hemostasis, avoiding chondral abrasion, maintaining adequate flow when using thermal devices, and preventing fluid extravasation by preserving muscle fascial layers will help minimize risk.

V. Shoulder Instability

A. Diagnosis—Due to the shoulder's extensive ROM, it is prone to instability and is the most commonly dislocated joint in the body. Instability is a pathologic condition manifesting as pain due to

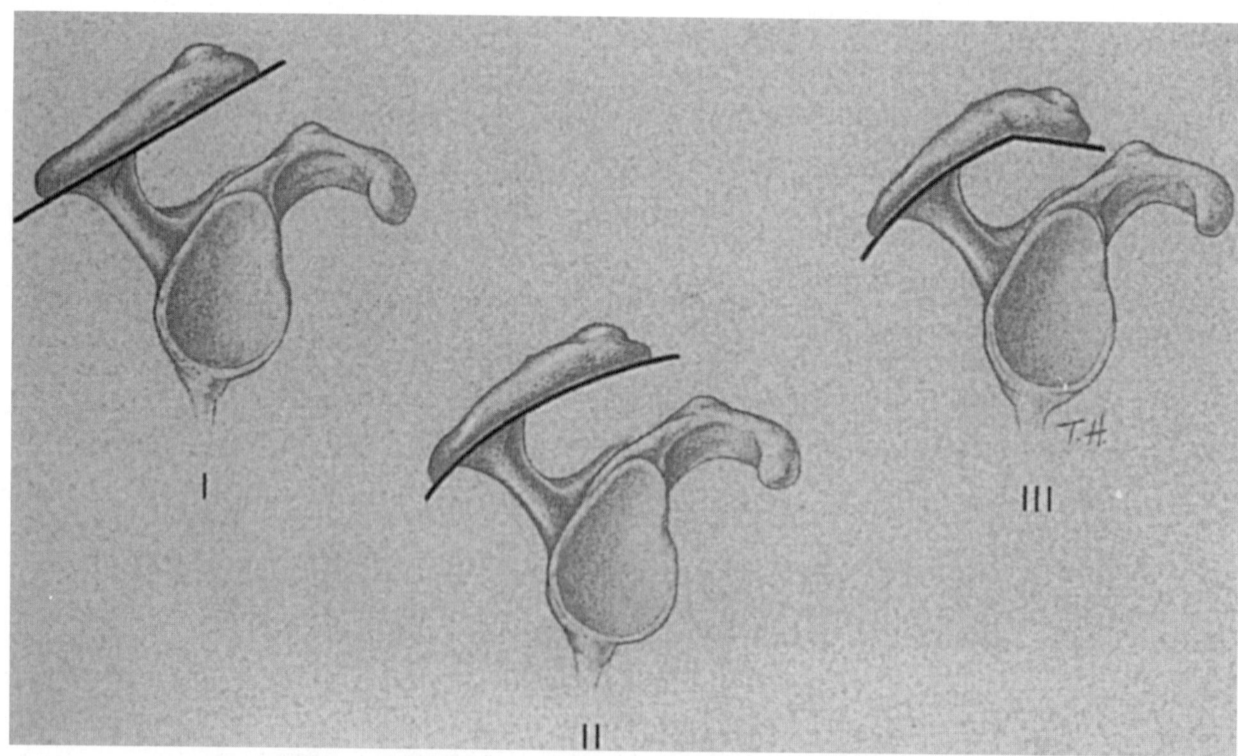

FIGURE 3-40 ■ Acromion morphology is classified on the basis of the supraspinatus outlet view as originally described by Bigliani. (From Esch, J.C.: Shoulder arthroscopy in the older age group. Op. Tech. Orthop. 1:200, 1991.)

Table 3-9. RADIOGRAPHIC VIEWS

VIEW/SIGN	FINDINGS	SIGNIFICANCE
Supraspinatus outlet view (Fig. 3-40)	Acromial morphology (type I-III)	Type III acromion associated with impingement
30 degree caudal tilt view	Subacromial spurring	Area below level of clavicle = impingement area
Zanca 10 degree cephalic tilt	AC joint pathology	AC DJD, distal clavicle osteolysis
West Point	Anteroinferior glenoid evaluation	Bony Bankart lesion seen with instability
Garth view	Anteroinferior glenoid evaluation	Bony Bankart
Stryker notch	Humeral head evaluation	Hill-Sachs impression fracture
AP IR	Humeral head evaluation	**Hill-Sachs defect**
Hobbs view	Sternoclavicular injury	AP dislocations
Serendipity view	Sternoclavicular injury	Ant-post dislocation
45 degree Abduction true AP	Glenohumeral space	Subtle DJD
Arthrography	Rotator cuff injuries	Dye above cuff = tear
CT	Fractures	Classification easier
MRI ± arthro-MRI	Soft-tissue evaluation	Labral, cuff, muscle tears

AC, acromioclavicular; DJD, degenerative joint disease; IR, internal rotation; ant, anterior; post, posterior; AP, anteroposterior; CT, computed tomography; MRI, magnetic resonance imaging.

excessive translation of the humeral head on the glenoid during active shoulder motion representing a spectrum of injury to the shoulder stabilizers. Diagnosis is based on history, physical exam, and imaging. *T*raumatic *U*nilateral dislocations with a *B*ankart lesion often require *S*urgery (*TUBS*) because they typically occur in young patients and have recurrence rates of up to 80-90% with nonoperative management. *A*traumatic *M*ultidirectional *B*ilateral shoulder dislocation/subluxation often responds to *R*ehabilitation, and sometimes an *I*nferior capsular shift is required (*AMBRI*). Clinical evidence of instability includes positive ***load-and-shift, modified load-and-shift, and apprehension-relocation testing as well as a sulcus sign (see Table 3-8)***. Grading of instability is shown in Table 3-10.

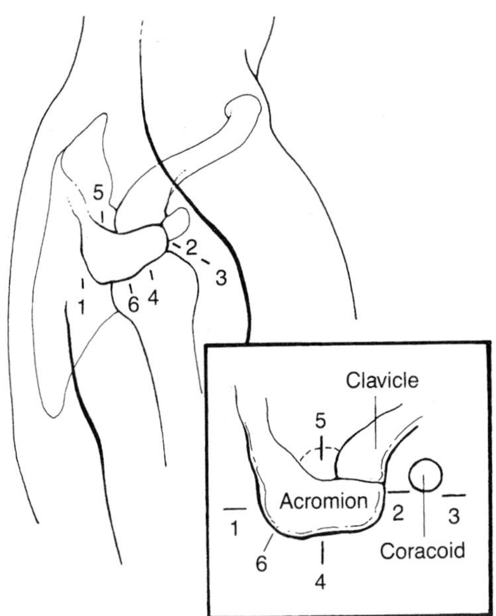

FIGURE 3-41 ■ Arthroscopic portals of the shoulder. *1*, posterior; *2*, anterosuperior; *3*, anteroinferior; *4*, lateral; *5*, supraspinatus (Neviaser's); *6*, port of Wilmington. (From Miller, M.D., Cooper, D.E., and Warner, J.J.P.: Review of Sports Medicine and Arthroscopy. Philadelphia, WB Saunders, 1995, p. 135.)

B. Treatment—Several open and arthroscopic techniques have been developed to address instability. These procedures have been broadened to address both capsuloligamentous laxity (e.g., capsular plication, rotator interval closure), in addition to labral pathology via a variety of instruments, suture passage and knot tying techniques, and fixation devices (both absorbable and nonabsorbable). ***Complications of open procedures include subscapularis overtightening (Z-lengthening required) or rupture (repair ± pectoralis transfer required) and hardware problems.*** Although the role for arthroscopic treatment of instability is being broadened, clinical studies have not yet established a clear role for the treatment of instability in the contact athlete. Additionally, the role of thermal capsular shrinkage has yet to be clearly elucidated (Table 3-11).

C. Posterior Instability—Patients may exhibit positive load-and-shift and ***jerk*** testing. Although less common and less amenable to surgery than anterior dislocations, posterior dislocations respond well, when recognized, to acute reduction and immobilization. Patients may present with their arm internally rotated with observable coracoid and posterior prominence. An ***axillary lateral radiograph*** is extremely helpful in making the diagnosis and must be obtained. Rehabilitation focuses on external rotator and deltoid strengthening with surgical management (posterior capsular shift) reserved for refractory cases.

VI. Impingement Syndrome/RTC Disease—

Subacromial impingement is a continuum of pathology and clinical symptoms that in its final stages may

Table 3-10. GRADES OF INSTABILITY

GRADE	ANTEROPOSTERIOR GRADING SCHEME*
Grade 0:	Normal small amount of humeral head translation
Grade 1+:	Humeral head translation to, but not over, the glenoid rim
Grade 2+:	Humeral head translation over the glenoid rim with spontaneous reduction when the applied force is withdrawn
Grade 3+:	Humeral head translation with locking over the glenoid rim
GRADE	**SULCUS GRADING SCHEME†**
Grade 1+:	Acromiohumeral interval <1 cm
Grade 2+:	Acromiohumeral interval 1-2 cm
Grade 3+:	Acromiohumeral interval >2 cm

* Abnormal (vs. contralateral shoulder): Anterior instability—1+ or greater; posterior instability—3+ or greater.
† Abnormal (vs. contralateral shoulder): Grade 2+ or greater.

Table 3-11. INSTABILITY CORRECTION PROCEDURES

PROCEDURE	ESSENTIAL FEATURES	COMPLICATIONS
Bankart	Reattachment of labrum (and IGHLC) to glenoid	Gold standard
Staple capsulorraphy	Capsular reattachment and tightening	Staple migration/articular injury
Putti-Platt	Subscapularis advancement capsular coverage	Decreased external rotation, DJD
Magnuson-Stack	Subscapularis transfer to greater tuberosity	Decreased external rotation
Boyd-Sisk	Transfer of biceps laterally and posteriorly	Nonanatomic, recurrence
Bristow	Coracoid transfer to inferior glenoid	Nonunion, migration, labral tears
Bone block osteotomy	Anterior bone block	Nonunion, migration, articular injury
Capsular shift	Inferior capsule shifted superiorly—"pants over vest"	Overtightening, gold standard for MDI

IGHLC, inferior glenohumeral ligament complex; DJD, degenerative joint disease; MDI, multidirectional instability.

be associated with full-thickness RTC tears. Tears associated with chronic impingement syndrome typically begin on the bursal surface or within the tendon substance, in contrast to those that occur on the articular surface because of tension failure in younger overhead athletes (Table 3-12).

A. Diagnosis—Patients typically present with the insidious onset of pain exacerbated by overhead activities. Complaints of night discomfort, pain in the deltoid insertion, selected muscular weakness, and differences in active versus passive ROM are common, with more significant weakness and loss of motion indicating a higher degree of cuff involvement. Acute pain and weakness may be seen following traumatic RTC rupture. In young athletes it is critical to exclude GH instability causing a secondary impingement (nonoutlet impingement) from primary impingement syndrome (pathology within the subacromial space). **For specific testing refer to Table 3-8.**
   1. Radiographs—May demonstrate classic changes within the acromion or coracoacromial ligament (spurring and calcification), in addition to cystic changes within the greater tuberosity. With chronic RTC pathology, superior migration of the humeral head with extensive degenerative change may be present.

B. Treatment
   1. Nonoperative treatment—Initially indicated for impingement syndrome, chronic atraumatic cuff tears, noncompliant patients, medical

Table 3-12. ROTATOR CUFF TEARS

STAGE	AGE (YEARS)	PATHOLOGY	CLINICAL COURSE	TREATMENT
I	<25	Edema and hemorrhage	Reversible	Conservative
II	25-40	Fibrosis and tendinitis	Activity-related pain	Therapy/operative
III	>40	AC spur and cuff tear	Progressive disability	Acromioplasty/repair

contraindications to surgery, RTC arthropathy, and athletes with a combined picture of instability or cuff tearing resulting from articular-sided partial thickness failure. Activity modification, avoiding repeated forward flexion beyond 90 degrees, and an aggressive rotator-cuff and scapular-stabilizer-strengthening program are initiated. Additionally, oral anti-inflammatory medications, therapeutic modalities, and judicious use of subacromial steroid injections may be implemented.

2. Chronic Impingement Syndrome—Without an RTC tear that is refractory to a minimum of 4 and, preferably, 6 months of nonoperative treatment, may respond favorably to subacromial decompression. Similarly, patients indicated for RTC repair will often require concomitant subacromial decompression at the time of repair. Exceptions include massive irreparable RTC tears, which may benefit from débridement with preservation of the coracoacromial arch to prevent anterosuperior humeral migration. Additional exceptions include the acute traumatic RTC tear or the overhead-movement athlete, who may benefit from limited acromial smoothing and bursectomy required only for visualization and to minimize postoperative irritation of the repair site.
3. RTC Surgery—Reliably decreases pain and improves motion and function as well as general health status. The operative approach has evolved from a classic open approach to a "mini-open," or deltoid sparing, to an all-arthroscopic technique. Independent of the technique, the rate-limiting step for recovery is the biologic healing of the RTC tendon to the humerus, estimated to require a minimum of 8–12 weeks. Treatment of partial-thickness articular-side tears with débridement versus repair remains controversial and considers the depth of the tear, the pattern of the tear (avulsion versus degenerative), and the activity level of the patient. Patients with a preponderance of impingement findings and a less than 50% thickness tear may benefit from débridement and subacromial decompression.

C. Subscapularis Tears—May occur after anterior dislocations and anterior shoulder surgery (e.g., shoulder arthroplasty). Symptoms are increased external rotation and presence of a ***lift-off***, modified lift-off, or belly-push sign. Surgical treatment, either open or arthroscopic, is generally indicated, with chronic cases occasionally requiring a pectoralis transfer.

D. RTC Arthropathy—Massive RTC tears combined with a fixed superior migration of the humeral head and severe GH arthrosis presumably due to chronic loss of the concavity-compression effect. Hemiarthroplasty may be helpful if the anterior deltoid is preserved. Use of reverse shoulder prostheses remains controversial.

E. Subcoracoid Impingement—Patients with long or excessively laterally placed coracoid processes may have impingement of this process on the proximal humerus with forward flexion (120–130 degrees) and internal rotation of the arm. This condition may occur following surgery that causes posterior capsular tightness and loss of internal rotation. Local anesthetic injection should relieve these symptoms. CT scan performed with the arms crossed on the chest is helpful to evaluate this problem. Treatment of chronic symptoms involves resection of the lateral aspect of the coracoid process and reattachment of the conjoined tendon to the remaining coracoid.

F. Internal Impingement—Impingement of the posterior labrum and cuff can occur in throwing-motion athletes with external rotation and anterior translation (secondary impingement). Treatment may include arthroscopic labral débridement/repair.

VII. Superior Labral and Biceps Tendon Injuries

A. Superior Labrum Lesions—SLAP lesions have been classified into many varieties (Fig. 3-42) with specific types associated with instability and RTC disease. Patients may exhibit a ***positive active compression*** (O'Brien's test), ***anterior slide***, or ***crank test***, as well as biceps tendon tenderness (Table 3-13).

B. Biceps Tendonitis—Often associated with impingement, RTC tears (subscapularis and leading-edge supraspinatus tears), and stenosis of the bicipital groove. Diagnosis is made by direct palpation with the arm internally rotated 10 degrees and confirmed with ***Speed*** and ***Yerguson tests***. Initial management includes strengthening and local injection (around, not into, the tendon) with surgical release (with or without tenodesis) being reserved for refractory cases.

C. Biceps Tendon Subluxation—Most commonly associated with a ***subscapularis tear***, a tear of the CHL or transverse humeral ligament may produce tendon subluxation as well. Arm abduction and external rotation may produce a palpable click with palpation as the tendon subluxates or dislocates outside of the groove. Nonoperative treatment is similar to that for tendonitis, whereas operative treatment includes tendon repair, groove deepening, or release/tenodesis.

VIII. AC and SC Injuries

A. AC Separation—Typically caused by a direct blow to the shoulder, it is a common athletic injury and can be classified into six types (Fig. 3-43). Management of type III injuries is controversial with some advocating surgical reduction and repair or reconstruction. Types IV–VI should be treated surgically.

B. AC DJD—Due to the transmission of large loads through a small surface area, the AC joint may begin to degenerate as early as the second

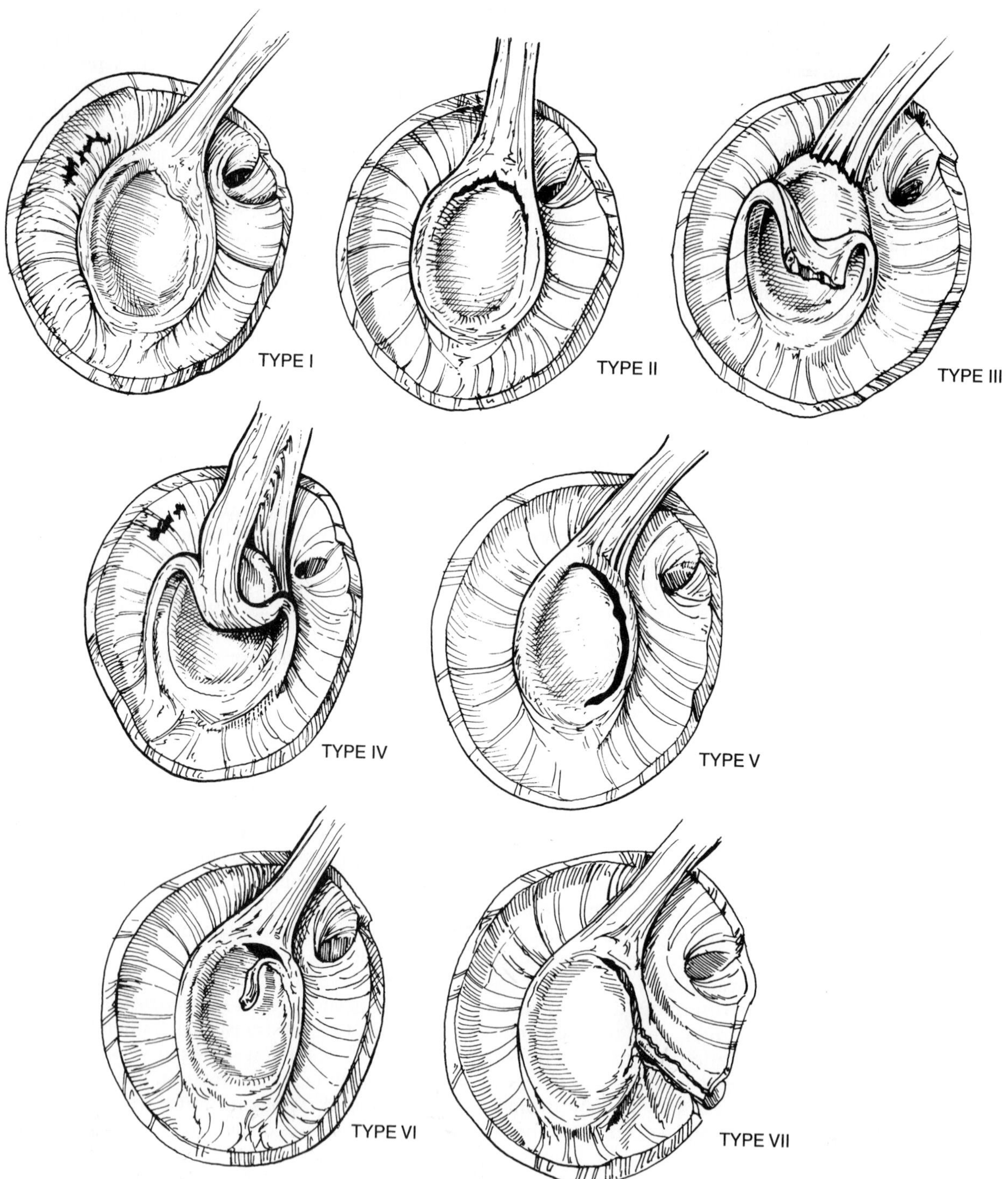

FIGURE 3-42 ■ Superior labraanterior and posterior lesions types I–IV and types V–VII. (From Miller, M.D., Osborne J.R., Warner J.J.P., et al.: MRI-Arthroscopy Correlative Atlas. Philadelphia, WB Saunders, 1997, p. 157.)

Table 3-13. SUPERIOR LABRAL AND BICEPS TENDON INJURIES

TYPE	DESCRIPTION	TREATMENT
I	Biceps fraying, intact anchor on superior labrum	Arthroscopic débridement
II	Detachment of biceps anchor	Reattachment/stabilization
III	Bucket-handle superior labral tear; biceps intact	Arthroscopic débridement
IV	Bucket-handle tear of superior labrum into biceps	Repair or tenodesis of tendon based on symptoms and condition of remaining tendon
V	Labral tear + SLAP	Stabilize both
VI	Superior flap tear	Débride
VII	Capsular injury + SLAP	Repair and stabilize

SLAP, superior labrum from anterior to posterior.

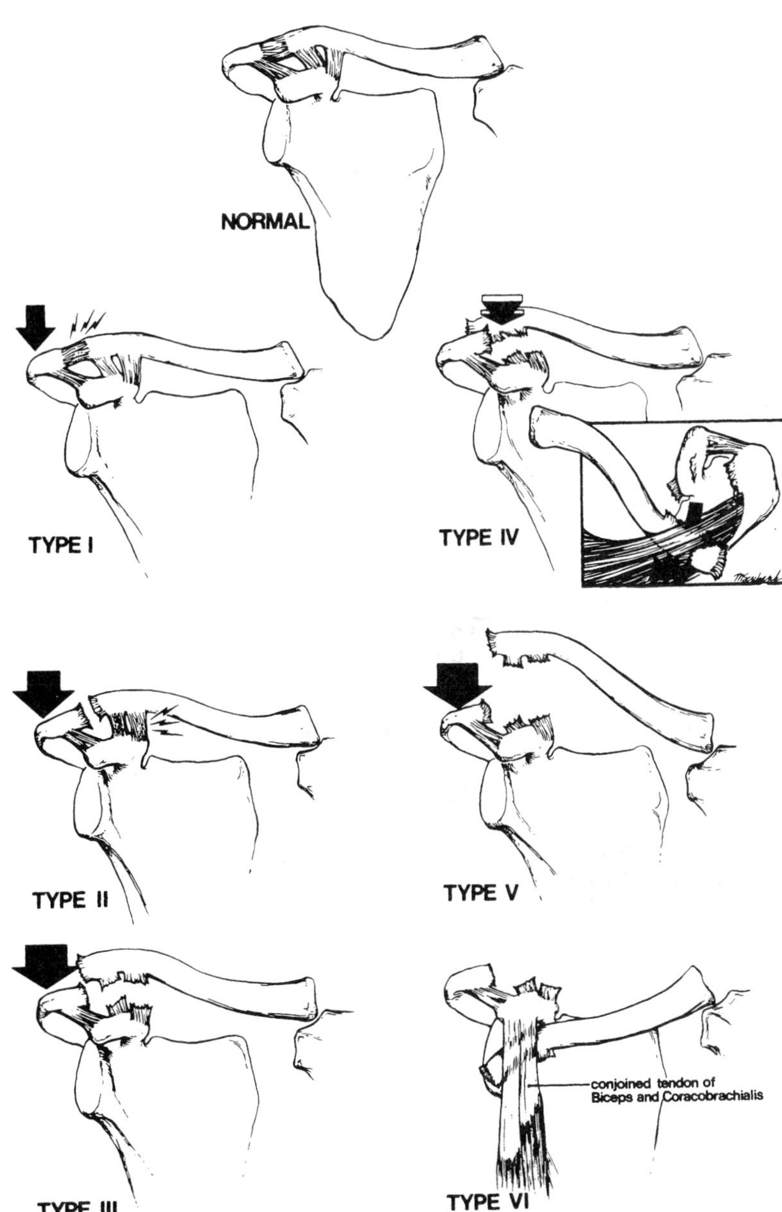

FIGURE 3-43 ■ Classification of acromioclavicular (AC) separations. Type I injuries involve only an AC sprain. Type II injuries are characterized by complete AC tear but intact coracoclavicular (CC) ligaments. Type III injuries involve both the AC and CC ligaments with a CC distance of 125-200% of the opposite shoulder. Type IV injuries are associated with posterior displacement of the clavicle through the trapezius muscle. Type V injuries involve superior displacement with a CC distance of more than twice the opposite side. This injury is usually associated with rupture of the deltotrapezial fascia, leaving the distal end of the clavicle subcutaneous. Type VI injuries are rare and are defined based on inferior displacement of the clavicle below the coracoid. (From Rockwood, C.A., Jr., and Young, D.C.: Disorders of the acromioclavicular joint. In Rockwood, C.A., Jr., and Matsen, F.A., III, eds.: The Shoulder, 2nd ed. Philadelphia, WB Saunders, 1998, p. 495.)

decade. Additionally, direct blows or AC separation may cause post-traumatic arthritis. Diagnosis is made with direct palpation, pain with crossed-chest adduction, radiographic evidence of osteophytes and joint-space narrowing, and relief with selective AC joint injection. Treatment includes both open and arthroscopic distal clavicle resection (Mumford procedure).

C. Distal Clavicle Osteolysis—Common in weight lifters and those with a history of traumatic injury. Radiographs of the distal clavicle reveal osteopenia, osteolysis, tapering, and cystic changes. After failure of selective corticosteroid injection, NSAIDs, and activity modification, this condition responds favorably to AC joint excision.

D. SC Subluxation/Dislocation: Often caused by motor vehicle accidents or direct trauma, this injury can be best diagnosed by CT. Plain imaging includes the Hobbs and ***Serendipity*** views. Closed reduction is often successful. Hardware should be avoided.

IX. Muscle Ruptures

A. Pectoralis Major—Injury to this muscle is caused by excessive tension on a maximally eccentrically contracted muscle, often in weight lifters. Localized swelling and ecchymosis, a palpable defect, and weakness with adduction and internal rotation are characteristic. Surgical repair to bone is usually necessary. Iatrogenic injury may occur during open RTC repair with some cases requiring deltoidplasty consisting of mobilization and anterior transfer of the middle third of the deltoid.

B. Deltoid—Complete rupture of this muscle is unusual, and injuries are most often strains or partial tears. Repair to bone is required for complete ruptures. Occasionally, iatrogenic injury may occur during open RTC repair with some cases requiring deltoidplasty consisting of mobilization and anterior transfer of the middle third of the deltoid.

C. Triceps—Most often associated with systemic illness (e.g., renal osteodystrophy) or steroid use. Primary repair of avulsions is indicated.

D. Latissimus Dorsi Rupture—Very rare condition exhibiting local tenderness and pain with shoulder adduction and internal rotation. Although nonoperative treatment may allow for resumption of activities, operative repair has been described for the high-demand athlete.

X. Calcifying Tendonitis and Shoulder Stiffness

A. Calcifying Tendinitis—A self-limiting condition of unknown etiology predominantly affecting the supraspinatus tendon in women. Radiographs demonstrate characteristic calcification within the tendon. Three stages have been elucidated: precalcific, calcific, and postcalcific. Nonoperative treatment is the rule, consisting of physical therapy, modalities, and injections. Occasionally, open removal of the deposit is necessary.

B. Shoulder Stiffness

1. Adhesive Capsulitis—This disorder (also known as "frozen shoulder") is characterized by pain and restricted GH joint motion. Factors associated with the development of adhesive capsulitis include trauma following chest or breast surgery, ***diabetes***, prolonged immobilization, thyroid disease and other medical conditions. Arthrography may demonstrate a loss of the normal axillary recess revealing contracture of the joint capsule.Three clinical and four arthroscopic stages have been defined (Table 3-14).
2. Post-Traumatic Shoulder Stiffness—Asymmetrical loss of GH motion secondary to a post-traumatic or post surgical complication due to excessive scar formation. Motion loss is related to the area of surgery or trauma and may involve the humeroscapular motion interface between the proximal humerus and overlying deltoid and conjoined tendon, as well as contracture of the RTC and capsule.
3. Treatment—For idiopathic adhesive capsulitis, a supervised physical therapy program combined with anti-inflammatory medications and/or steroid injections will successfully treat the majority of patients within 12 weeks. Post-traumatic shoulder stiffness lasting more than 24 months is unlikely to respond to nonsurgical treatment. If no improvement is seen after 12–16 weeks of nonsurgical treatment, operative intervention is recommended. Operative treatment consists of manipulation under anesthesia and/or arthroscopic and open release.

XI. Nerve Disorders

A. Brachial Plexus Injury—Minor traction and compression injuries, commonly known by football players as "burners" or "stingers," can be serious if they are recurrent or persist for more than a

Table 3-14. STAGES OF SHOULDER STIFFNESS

STAGE	CHARACTERISTICS
Clinical	
Painful	Gradual onset of diffuse pain
Stiff	Decreased ROM; affects activities of daily living
Thawing	Gradual return of motion
Arthroscopic	
1	Patchy fibrinous synovitis
2	Capsular contraction, fibrinous adhesions, synovitis
3	Increased contraction, resolving synovitis
4	Severe contracton

ROM, range of motion.

short time. Injury results from compression of the plexus between the shoulder pad and the superior medial scapula when the pad is compressed into Erb's point superior to the clavicle. Complete resolution of symptoms is required before RTP. ***If burners occur more than one time, the player should be removed from competition until cervical spine radiographs can be obtained.*** Three grades of nerve injury are commonly recognized. (Table 3-15).

B. Thoracic Outlet Syndrome—Compression of the nerves and vessels that pass through the scalene muscles and first rib can result in this disorder. This condition can be associated with cervical rib, scapular ptosis, or scalene muscle abnormalities. Patients may note pain and ulnar paresthesias. ***The Wright test*** (Table 3-8) and neurologic evaluation can be diagnostic. First-rib resection is occasionally required.

C. Long Thoracic Nerve Palsy—Injury to this nerve can result in scapular winging secondary to serratus anterior dysfunction. Simple observation is usually called for because many of these injuries spontaneously resolve within 18 months. Treatment with a modified thoracolumbar brace may be beneficial and, rarely, pectoralis major transfer may be required for chronic palsies that do not recover.

D. Suprascapular Nerve Compression—Compressed by various structures including a ganglion in the spinoglenoid notch, suprascapular notch or fracture callus in the area of the transverse scapular ligament. Weakness and atrophy of the supraspinatus (proximal lesions) and infraspinatus are present along with pain over the dorsal aspect of the shoulder. Electrodiagnostic studies and MRI may confirm and elucidate the nature of the nerve compression. Compression due to a cyst associated with a SLAP lesion may respond to arthroscopic decompression. In the absence of a structural lesion, ligament release may provide relief.

E. Other Nerve Injuries—Other injuries, including those of the axillary nerve, the spinal accessory nerve, and the musculocutaneous nerve, are usually the result of surgical injury to these structures. Several months of observation is appropriate before considering exploration and repair of the affected nerve.

Table 3-15. GRADES OF NERVE INJURY

GRADE	DESCRIPTION	PATHOPHYSIOLOGY
1	Neuropraxia	Selective demyelination of the axon sheath
2	Axonotmesis	Axon and myelin sheath disruption
3	Neurotmesis	Epineurium and endoneurium disruption

XII. Other Shoulder Disorders

A. GH DJD—Although more common in older patients, athletes who engage in throwing may develop arthritis at a younger age than usual. Arthritis may also be associated with other shoulder disorders, including instability and RTC disease. Certain iatrogenic factors may also contribute to the development of osteoarthritis of the shoulder, including the use of hardware in and around the shoulder and overtightening of the shoulder capsule during shoulder reconstruction. Radiographs, including a true AP view taken in abduction can be helpful in characterizing the amount of arthritis. In some cases, arthroscopic débridement may be a temporizing measure before considering joint arthroplasty. Progressive pain, decreased ROM, and inability to perform activities of daily living are reasonable indications for considering prosthetic replacement.

B. Scapulothracic crepitus—Also known as ***"snapping scapula syndrome."*** The presentation is that of painful scapulothoracic crepitance associated with elevation of the arm. Scapulothoracic diskinesis may be present, and the pain is generally relieved with manual stabilization of the scapula. Many possible causes of symptomatic crepitus exist. Patients may respond to scapular strengthening exercises, local injections, or anti-inflammatory medications. For more refractory cases, open or arthroscopic bursectomy and sometimes resection of the medial scapular border is necessary.

C. Scapular Winging—This can occur as a result of a nerve injury, bony abnormality, muscle contracture, intra-articular pathology, or voluntarily. Nerve injuries include the spinal accessory (trapezius palsy; ***lateral winging***), long thoracic (serratus anterior palsy, ***medial winging***), and dorsal scapular (rhomboideus palsy). Osseous origins include osteochondromas and fracture malunions. Selective muscle strengthening may improve winging. Surgical treatment includes lateral transfer of the levator scapulae and rhomboids (Edan-Lange procedure) for lateral winging and pectoralis major transfer for medial winging.

D. Complex Regional Pain Syndrome—(also known as "reflex sympathetic dystrophy") As in the knee, this condition is fraught with a poor response to both conservative and surgical treatments and, in a litigious medico-legal environment, is often associated with malingering and issues of secondary gain.

E. Little Leaguer's Shoulder—This disorder, actually a Salter-Harris type I fracture of the proximal humerus, responds ***to rest and activity modification***. Radiographs may demonstrate widening of the proximal humeral physis.

SECTION 5

Elbow Injuries

I. Tendon Injuries

A. Lateral Epicondylitis (Tennis Elbow)—Occurs commonly with activities that involve repetitive pronation and supination of the forearm with the elbow in near extension (backhand in tennis). Initiated as a microtear at the origin of the ***extensor carpi radialis brevis*** (ECRB) but may also involve the origin of the extensor carpi radialis longus (ECRL) and extensor carpi ulnaris (ECU). Microscopic evaluation of this tissue evidences angiofibroblastic hyperplasia. Diagnosis is clinical with reproducible localized tenderness at the extensor origin, with reproduction of symptoms with resisted wrist extension. Treatment is predominantly nonoperative with activity modification (slower playing surfaces, more flexible racquet, lower string tension, larger grip), physical therapy (stretching, ultrasound), anti-inflammatory medications, counterforce bracing, and up to three corticosteroid injections to the site of maximal tenderness, all achieving up to 95% success. Recalcitrant cases require open or arthroscopic débridement of the ECRB origin (Fig. 3-44).

B. Medial Epicondylitis (Golfer's Elbow)—Overuse syndrome of the flexor/pronator mass. Much less common and more difficult to treat than tennis elbow. Pain is worsened by resisted forearm pronation and wrist flexion. Treatment is similar to that for lateral epicondylitis. Multiple corticosteroid injections and medial epicondylectomy should be avoided.

C. Distal Biceps Tendon Rupture—Occurs almost exclusively in men following forceful eccentric overload of the partially flexed elbow. Up to 50% loss of supination power has been documented following rupture. Intraosseous tendon reattachment using the two-incision (Boyd-Anderson) technique has been traditionally favored. Care must be taken not to disrupt the syndesmosis. Complications include neurovascular injury, loss of motion, and heterotopic ossification. The latter may be reduced using a single-incision repair with an endobutton.

D. Distal Triceps Tendon Avulsion—This extremely uncommon injury results from a deceleration force to the outstretched elbow and is associated with multiple corticosteroid injections or chronic olecranon bursitis. Repair with transosseous tunnels is mandatory for the restoration of extension power.

II. Ligament Injuries

A. Ulnar Collateral Ligament (UCL) Injury: Repetitive, high velocity, valgus stress to the medial aspect of the elbow results in attenuation or rupture of the ***anterior band of the UCL***. The late cocking and acceleration phases of throwing are periods of highest stress generation. Patients present with acute or chronic medial elbow tenderness, and frequently, associated ulnar nerve symptoms. The pain is localized to the course of the ligament from the medial epicondyle to the sublime tubercle. Valgus instability is demonstrable in only 50% of patients because this is usually a dynamic phenomenon (Fig. 3-45). MRI is useful for confirmation of the diagnosis. Initial treatment is with rest, physical therapy, and the maintenance of joint motion. Surgery is only required in high-level athletes who desire a return to sport. Ligament reconstruction is favored over direct repair and treatment of chronic injuries enjoys better results than of acute injuries. The ligament is reconstructed using palmaris tendon graft woven in a figure-eight fashion ("docking procedure") (Fig. 3-46). Nearly 80% of patients return to sport at the same or better level at one year after reconstruction. Complications include loss of motion, graft site morbidity, and neurologic injury.

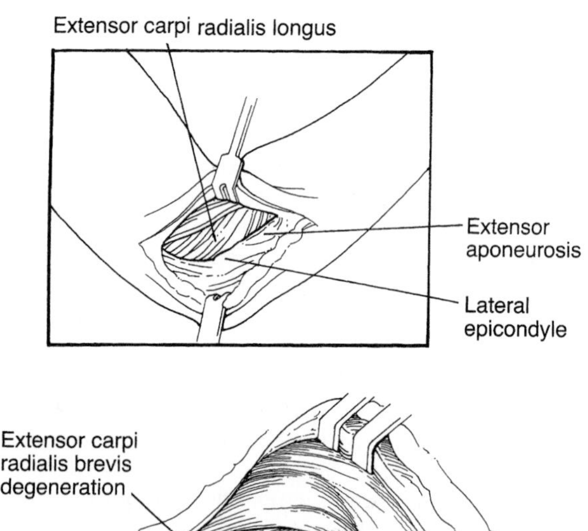

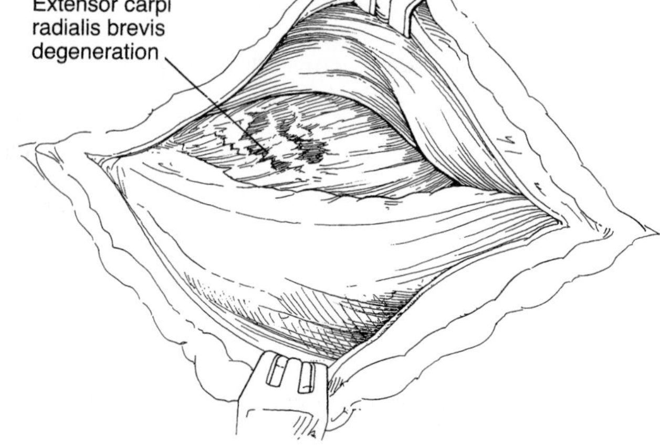

FIGURE 3-44 ■ Operative exposure for lateral epicondylitis. (From Miller, M.D., Cooper, D.E., and Warner, J.J.P.: Review of Sports Medicine and Arthroscopy. Philadelphia, WB Saunders, 1995, p. 178.)

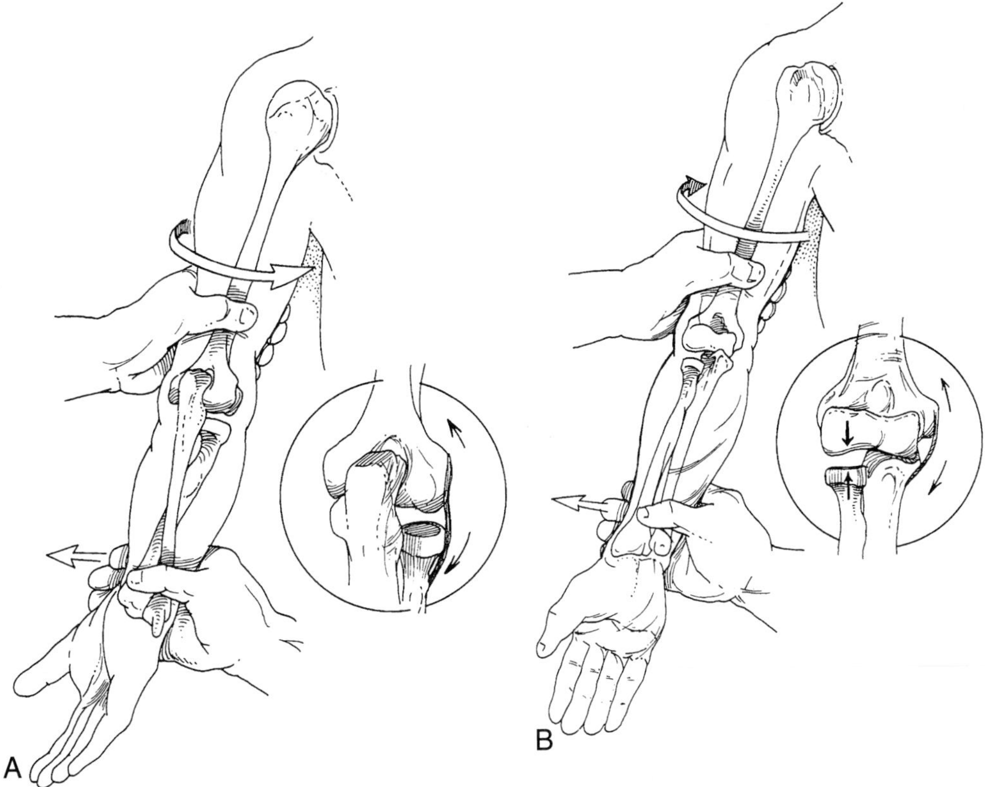

FIGURE 3-45 ■ Varus *(A)* and valgus *(B)* instability testing of the elbow. Note the position and rotation of the arm. (From Morrey, B.F.: The Elbow and Its Disorders, 2nd ed. Philadelphia, WB Saunders, 1994, p. 83.)

B. LCL Injury: This is typically the first ligament disrupted in elbow dislocation. Patients with LCL insufficiency may complain of clicking or locking with elbow extension, and often demonstrate posterolateral rotatory instability (Fig. 3-47). Surgical reconstruction with palmaris longus autograft and capsular plication is indicated for patients with recurrent instability, pain, or mechanical symptoms (Fig. 3-48).

III. Articular Injuries

A. Osteochondritis Dissecans: Occurs typically in the capitellum of the adolescent athlete engaged in repetitive overhead or upper extremity weight-bearing activities. The cause is thought to be related to vascular insufficiency and repetitive microtrauma. Plain radiographs and activity modification confirm the diagnosis. If the fragment is stable, this condition can be treated with activity modification and supportive methods. Separated fragments may be arthroscopically reduced and stabilized or excised and the defects drilled. Osteochondrosis of the capitellum is seen in young patients (Panner's disease) and is associated with a more benign course.

B. Little Leaguer's Elbow—Stress fracture of the medial epicondyle in adolescents due to repetitive valgus loading with throwing. Rest and limitation of number of innings pitched per week help to reduce the incidence of complete fracture.

C. Osteoarthritis—Primary elbow osteoarthritis disproportionately affects football linemen, participants in racquet sports, and throwers. These patients present with a decreased arc of motion and pain at the extremes of motion. Plain radiographs demonstrating joint-space narrowing and osteophytic spurring confirm the diagnosis. Surgical treatment consists of arthroscopic débridement, soft-tissue release, and loose body removal. Persistent symptoms are treated with distraction/interposition arthroplasty, ulnohumeral arthroplasty, or total elbow arthroplasty.

IV. Elbow Stiffness

A. Generally presents with loss of motion and function resulting from capsular contracture, olecranon, coronoid, and radial fossa overgrowth or heterotopic ossification about the elbow following a single acute injury or because of degenerative disease. Treatment is open surgical débridement using a collateral ligament–sparing approach (Hastings-Cohen), olecranon fossa fenestration and débridement (Outerbridge-Kashiwagi procedure) (Fig. 3-49), or arthroscopic débridement. Success is largely dependent on a motivated patient.

V. Elbow Arthroscopy

A. Arthroscopy—Typically indicated for diagnostic confirmation of suspected elbow pathology; removal of loose bodies; the treatment of osteochondritis

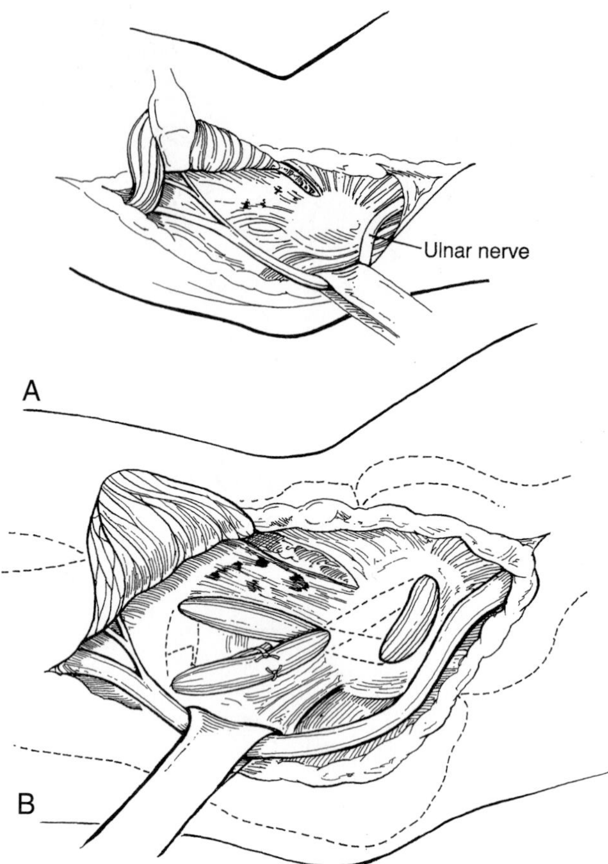

FIGURE 3-46 ■ Reconstruction of the (medial) ulnar collateral ligament. (From Miller, M.D., Cooper, D.E., and Warner, J.J.P.: Review of Sports Medicine and Arthroscopy. Philadelphia, WB Saunders, 1995, p. 179.)

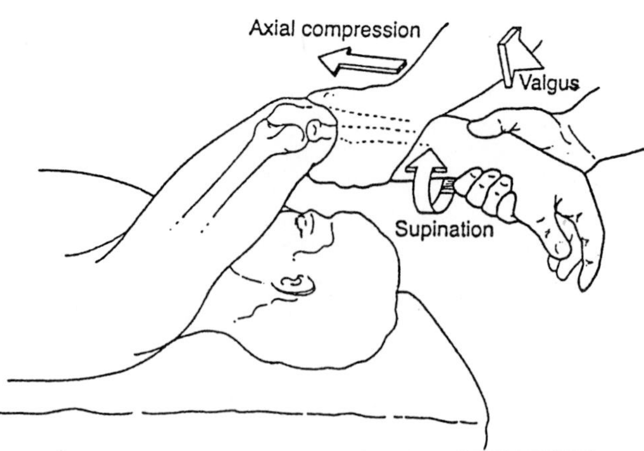

FIGURE 3-47 ■ Lateral pivot shift test of the elbow for posterolateral rotatory instability. (Redrawn from O'Driscoll, S.W., Bell, D.F., and Morrey, B.F.: Posterolateral instability of the elbow. J. Bone Joint Surg. [Am.] 73:440–446, 1991.)

dissecans of the capitellum; osteophyte débridement (as seen with chronic valgus overload in pitchers); capsular release and olecranon, radial, and coronoid fossa débridement in the stiff elbow; and synovectomy. Successful arthroscopic intervention depends on technical expertise in elbow arthroscopy and thorough anatomic familiarity because vital neurovascular structures are proximal to the intra-articular space and are thus prone to injury, particularly with overexuberant débridement.

B. Portals—The "nick and spread" method of portal placement is used to minimize inadvertent neurovascular injury. The utilization of far proximal portals may decrease these risks.

C. Common Portals (Fig. 3-50)
   1. **Anterolateral Portal**—Placed after joint distention 1 cm distal and 1 cm anterior to the lateral epicondyle. **The lateral antebrachial cutaneous and radial nerves are at risk.**
   2. **Anteromedial Portal**—Placed under direct visualization 2 cm distal and 2 cm anterior to the medial epicondyle. **The medial antebrachial cutaneous and median nerves are at risk.**
   3. **Posterolateral Portal**—Placed 2 cm proximal to the olecranon and just lateral to the triceps tendon.

FIGURE 3-48 ■ *(A)* Imbrication and advancement of the ulnar band of the radial collateral ligament and radial part of the radial collateral ligament. *(B)* Palmaris longus tendon through the ulnar and humeral tunnels and tied to itself. (From Canale, S.T., ed.: Campbell's Operative Orthopaedics, 9th ed. St. Louis, C.V. Mosby, 1998, p. 1397.)

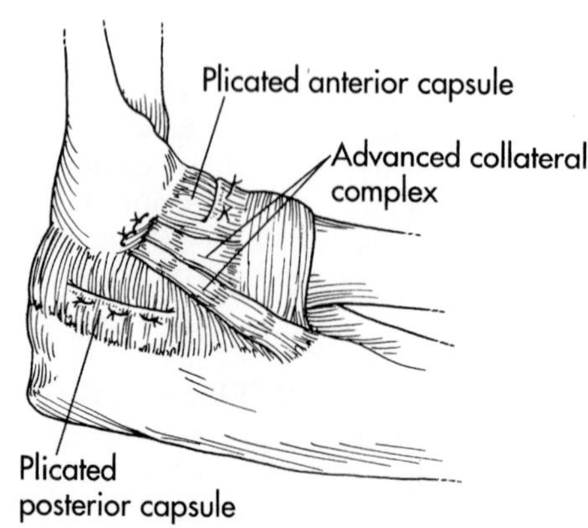

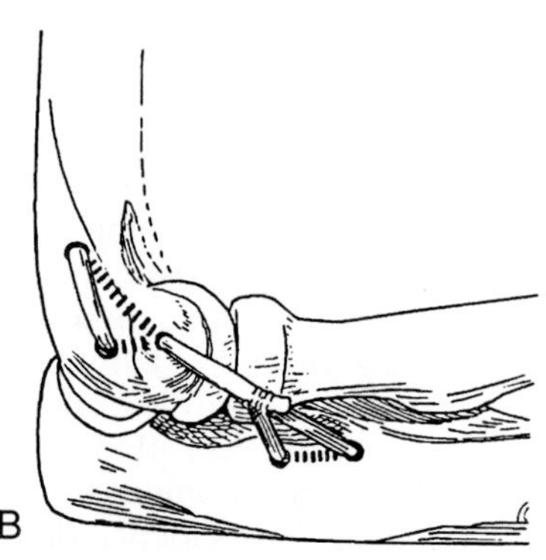

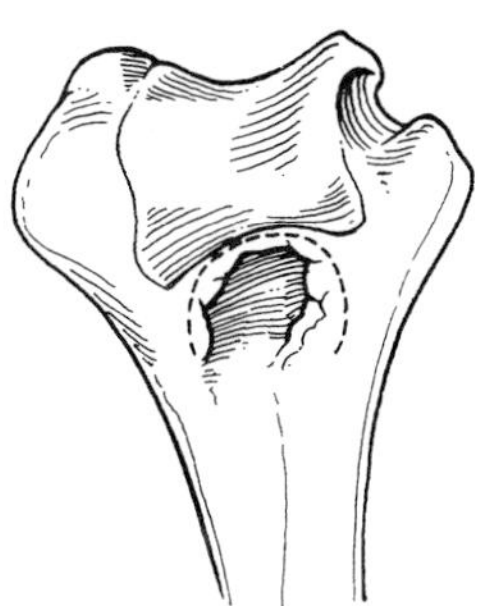
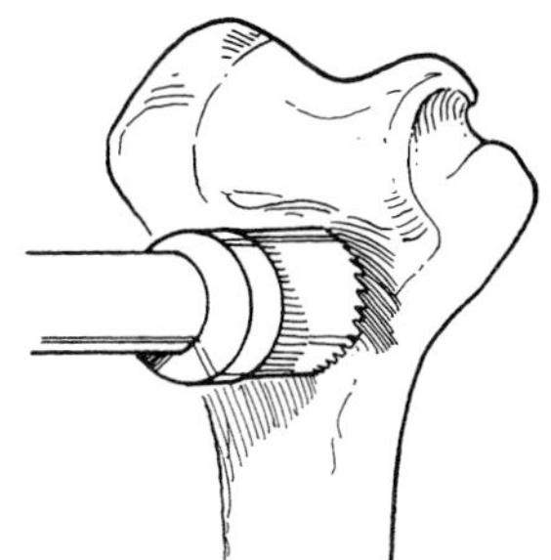
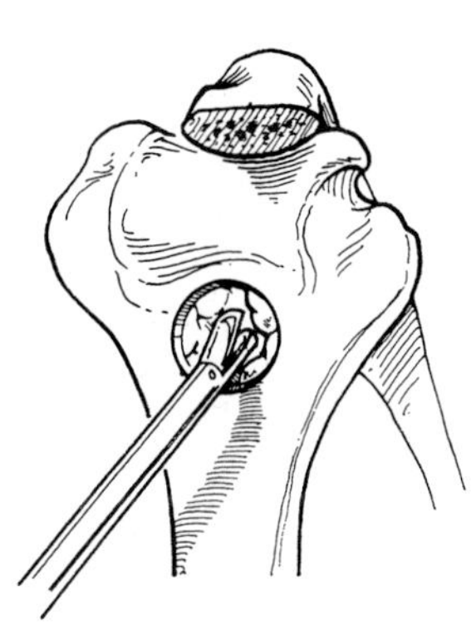

FIGURE 3-49 ■ Outerbridge-Kashiwagi arthroplasty, performed through a triceps-splitting approach. The coronoid is approached through a Cloward drill hole in the olecranon fossa. The olecranon can also be débrided with this approach. (From Miller, M.D., Cooper, D.E., and Warner, J.J.P.: Review of Sports Medicine and Arthroscopy. Philadelphia, WB Saunders, 1995, p. 180.)

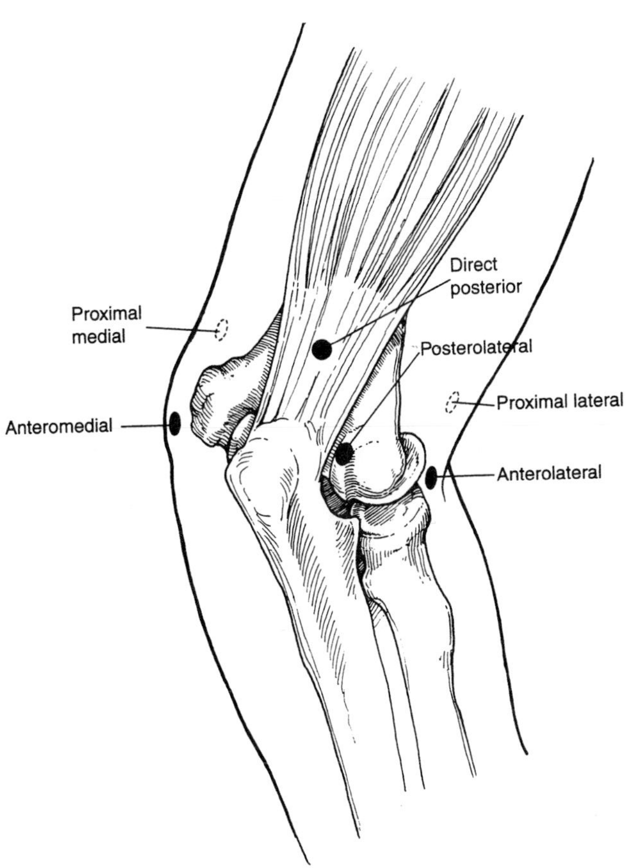

FIGURE 3-50 ■ Arthroscopic portals for elbow arthroscopy. (From Miller, M.D., Osborne J.R., Warner, J.J.P., et al.: MRI-Arthroscopy Correlative Atlas, Philadelphia, WB Saunders, 1997, p. 197.)

SECTION 6

Hand and Wrist Injuries

I. Tendon Injuries (Fig. 3-51)

A. De Quervain's Disease—Refers to stenosing tenosynovitis of the first dorsal wrist compartment (abductor pollicis longus [APL] and extensor pollicis brevis [EPB]). Occurs typically in racquet sports or in golfers. Ulnar deviation of the wrist with the thumb in the palm (Finkelstein's test) generally reproduces patient symptoms. Treatment includes activity modification, splinting, local corticosteroid injection, and occasionally surgical release (Fig. 3-52). The APL and EPB may lie in separate subsheaths in the first dorsal compartment, and care must be taken to release both.

B. Flexor Carpi Radialis/Flexor Carpi Ulnaris Tendonitis—Wrist flexor tendonitis is common and is associated with overuse. Activity modification, splinting, and NSAIDs are generally effective. Surgical tenolysis is rarely necessary.

C. Extensor Carpi Ulnaris Tendonitis—Tendonitis or subluxation of the sixth dorsal compartment is most common in tennis players. Patients experience painful snapping with forearm supination (tendon subluxates) and pronation (tendon reduces). This condition must be distinguished from other ulnar wrist disorders. Long arm cast immobilization in pronation may allow healing. Occasionally, surgical débridement of the sixth dorsal compartment and reconstruction of the fibro-osseous tunnel with a slip of extensor retinaculum is necessary (Fig. 3-53).

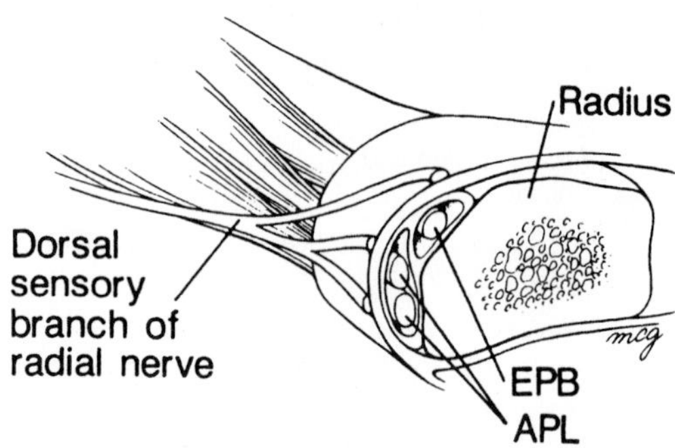

FIGURE 3-52 ■ Surgical release of the first compartment for refractory de Quervain's syndrome should include preservation of the dorsal sensory branch of the radial nerve. EPB, extensor pollicis brevis; APL, abductor pollicis longus. (From Kiefhaber, T.R., Stern, P.J.: Upper extremity tendinitis and overuse syndromes in the athlete. Clin. Sports Med. 11:44, 1992.)

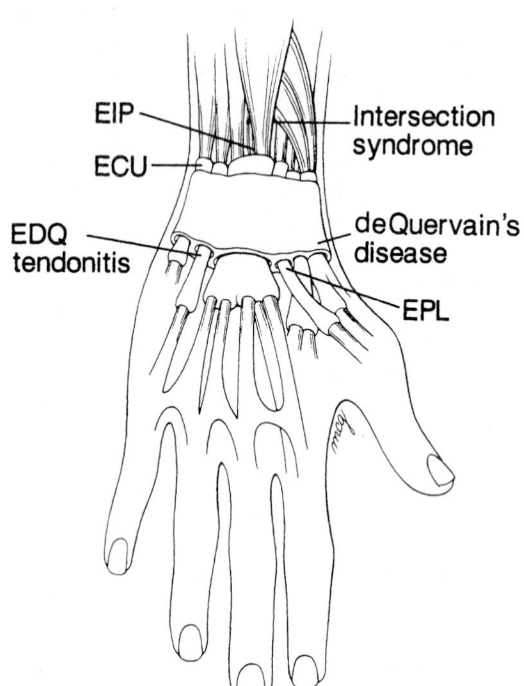

FIGURE 3-51 ■ Location of common sites of tendinitis about the wrist. EIP, extensor indicis proprius; ECU, extensor carpi ulnaris; EDQ, extensor digiti quinti; EPL, extensor pollicis longus. (From Kiefhaber, T.R., and Stern, P.J.: Upper extremity tendinitis and overuse syndromes in the athlete. Clin. Sports Med. 11:43, 1992.)

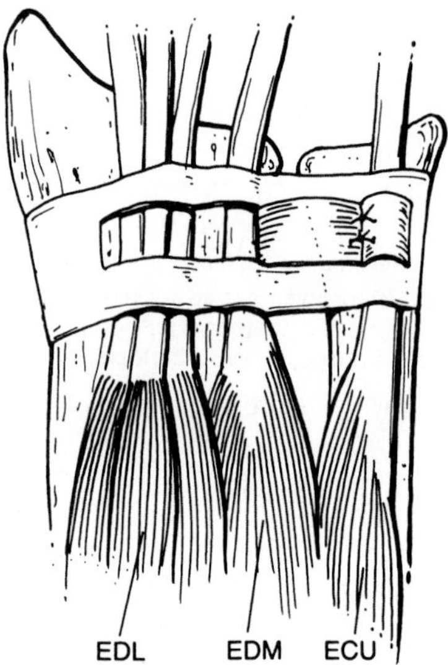

FIGURE 3-53 ■ Stabilization of the extensor carpi ulnaris (ECU) with a flap of the extensor retinaculum. extensor digitorum longus (EDL), extensor digiti minimi (EDM). (From Spinner, M., Kaplan, E.B.: Extensor carpi ulnaris. Clin. Orthop. 68:124–129, 1970.)

D. Intersection Syndrome—Painful crepitus at the dorsal forearm due to irritation and inflammation of the crossing point of the first dorsal compartment (APL and EPB) with the second dorsal compartment (ECRL and ECRB). Typically seen in rowers and weight lifters. Splinting and local injections are typically effective for this self-limited condition. Rarely, surgical decompression of the crossing point is necessary.

E. Other Extensor Tendon Tendinitis—May affect the extensor pollicis longus (EPL), extensor indicis proprius (EIP), or extensor digiti quinti (EDQ). Usually responsive to local measures and to surgical release if indicated.

F. "Jersey Finger"—Refers to an avulsion injury of the flexor digitorum profundus tendon from its insertion at the base of the proximal interphalangeal joint (PIP). These injuries require retrieval of the retracted tendon and reattachment to the base of the PIP. Arthrodesis is generally favored over late (>3 months) repair due to finger stiffness following tendon grafting.

G. "Mallet Finger"—Refers to avulsion of the terminal extensor tendon. These injuries are typically treated with prolonged (>6 weeks) extension splinting. Results are almost uniformly good. Chronic injuries may result in significant swan-neck deformities due to chronic overpull of the extensor tendon at the PIP with flexion of the distal interphalangeal joint (DIP). Chronic deformities in young patients with preserved passive finger motion may be corrected by restoring the balance between extensors and flexors.

H. Sagittal Band Rupture—("Boxer's knuckle") Typically occurs in pugilists due to forceful subluxation of the extensor tendon. Acute injuries are treated with extension splinting for 4 weeks. Chronic injury will lead to persistent extensor tendon subluxation and should be repaired or reconstructed with a slip of extensor tendon looped around the collateral ligament.

II. Ligament Injuries

A. Scapholunate (SL) Ligament Injury—Most common wrist ligament injury. Patients experience snuffbox tenderness following hyperextension of a pronated wrist, such as after a fall. Radial deviation of the hand with volar stabilization of the lunate (Watson test) may reproduce pain. Radiographic hallmarks include an increased SL interval (>2 mm), a cortical ring sign (proximal and distal poles of scaphoid overlap on PA projection), and an increased SL angle (>70 degrees) on lateral projection. Persistent SL dissociation with attenuation of extrinsic structures leads to an extended posture of the lunate [dorsal intercalated instability (DISI)] (Fig. 3-54) that unloads its articulation with the radius and increases contact forces at the radioscaphoid articulation leading to progressive arthrosis. Treatment is by either closed reduction and percutaneous pinning of the SL joint for 8–10 weeks or open reduction and internal fixation of the articulation combined with a capsulodesis.

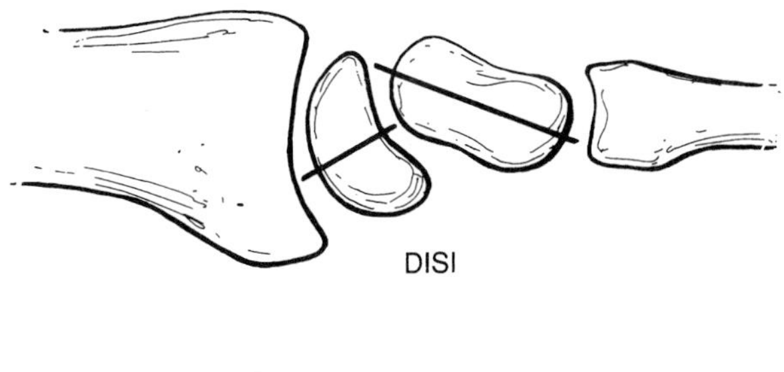

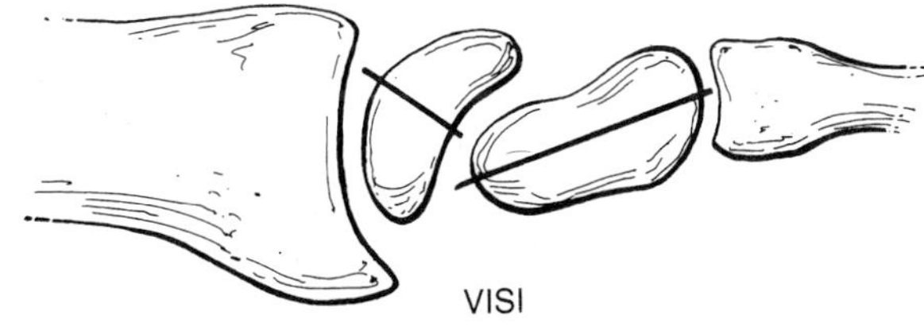

FIGURE 3-54 ■ Scapholunate instability is associated with a dorsal intercalated instability (DISI) pattern. Triquetrolunate instability may have a volar intercalated instability pattern. Note the increased scapholunate angle (>60 degrees) with the DISI pattern (normal 30 degrees).volar intercalated segmental instability (VISI). (From McCue, F.C., and Bruce, J.F.: The wrist. In DeLee, J.C., and Drez, D., Jr., eds.: Orthopaedic Sports Medicine: Principles and Practice. Philadelphia, WB Saunders, 1994, p. 918.)

B. Lunotriquetral (LT) Ligament Injury—Less common than SL ligament injury. Patients describe ulnar-sided wrist pain following a fall that is worse with pronation and ulnar deviation (power grip). Examination seeks to distinguish LT injuries from the spectrum of injuries that usually accompany them (chondral lesions, triangular fibrocartilage complex [TFCC] tears). Pain is reproduced with ballotment or schuck of the LT articulation. Radiographic hallmarks include widening of the LT interval, volar flexion of the lunate, increase in the capitolunate angle, and decrease in the scapholunate angle. MRI enjoys limited utility. Treatment following failure of conservative care is through débridement of the LT ligament. Arthrodesis is useful for refractory cases.

C. Hand Ligament Injury
   1. Digital Collateral Ligament Injury—Often the result of a "jammed finger." Simple tears are managed with buddy taping for 3 weeks whereas complete tears should be buddy taped for 6 weeks. Radial collateral ligament injury of the index finger PIP should be surgically repaired due to the need for pinch stability of this joint.
   2. PIP Dislocation—Typically occurs in a dorsal direction and results in a volar plate injury. Reduction is typically accomplished by the athlete. Incomplete reduction is due to volar plate interposition. Following reduction the finger is buddy taped to the adjacent digit for

3-6 weeks. A flexion contracture of the PIP joint (pseudoboutonnière) may develop late, but generally is resolved with therapy and appropriate splinting. Volar PIP dislocation is unusual. It generally results in a tear of the central slip insertion. Treatment includes 6-8 weeks of immobilization with the PIP joint in extension.

3. Collateral Ligament Injury of the Thumb—Includes radial and ulnar collateral ligament injuries; "gamekeeper's thumb." Incomplete ulnar injuries may be immobilized. Injuries with >15 degrees of side-to-side difference or greater than 45 degrees of opening require operative intervention since the aponeurosis of the adductor becomes interposed between the ends of the torn ligament (Stener's lesion) (Fig. 3-55). Aponeurotic interposition does not occur on the radial side. These rare injuries are often treated closed.

III. Fractures

A. Scaphoid Fracture—Occurs frequently in contact sports. Since the vascular supply enters distally, proximal fractures have a high rate of nonunion and avascular necrosis. Acute and subacute nondisplaced fractures less than 8 weeks old may be treated in a long arm-thumb-spica cast. Displaced fractures should be managed operatively either with percutaneous or limited open fixation. Nonunion may be managed with local vascularized bone graft with internal fixation.

B. Hamate Fracture—Hook-of-hamate fractures typically occur in a golfer or baseball batter following repeated direct contact. Diagnosis is confirmed by a carpal tunnel view. Treatment is either through cast immobilization or through excision of the hook. The latter allows more rapid RTP.

C. Metacarpal and Phalanx Fractures—Many of these fractures heal with closed reduction and immobilization. Displaced fractures, fractures involving the joints, and fractures resulting in rotational malalignment should be treated surgically. Early motion is the key to successful rehabilitation. Fractures involving the base of the thumb carpal-metacarpal (CMC) joint (Bennett's fracture, Rolando's fracture) often require operative reduction and stabilization.

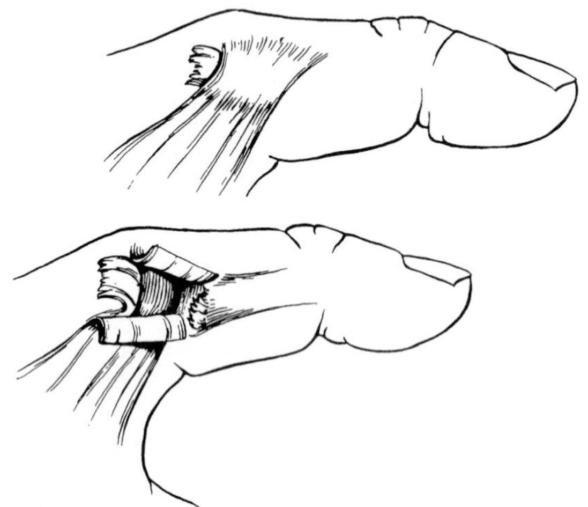

FIGURE 3-55 ■ Stener's lesion. The adductor aponeurosis separates the two ends of the ulnar collateral ligament, and the aponeurosis must be incised to repair the ligament. (From Green, D.P., and Strickland, J.W.: The hand. In DeLee, J.C., and Drez, D., Jr., eds.: Orthopaedic Sports Medicine: Principles and Practice. Philadelphia, WB Saunders, 1994, p. 976.)

IV. Ulnar Wrist Pain

Ulnar Wrist Pain—The differential diagnosis of ulnar-sided wrist pain in athletes includes TFCC tear, pisotriquetral arthritis, fracture (ulnar styloid, hook of hamate), lunotriquetral ligament injury, extensor carpi ulnaris subluxation or tendonitis, ulnar nerve entrapment at Guyon's canal, ulnar artery thrombosis (hypothenar Hammer syndrome), chondral lesions, and wrist ganglia.

A. TFCC/DRUJ (Distal radioulnar joint): Patients seek treatment following a fall onto a pronated, extended wrist, or following a traction injury to the ulnar aspect of the wrist. Point tenderness is present at the base of the ***"ulnar snuffbox,"*** between the triquetrum and ulnar styloid. Symptoms are reproduced with ulnar deviation (compresses TFCC) or radial deviation (applies tension to peripheral tear). Arthography and MRI may help diagnosis tear, but both are highly user dependent and have a high rate of false-positive results (Table 3-16). Arthroscopy is the diagnostic gold standard. Treatment is based on tear type, presence of DRUJ instability/arthritis, and ulnar variance. See Figure 3-56 for treatment algorithm.

B. Ulnocarpal Abutment Syndrome: Typically occurs in patients with ulnar positive variance. Pain is exacerbated with rotation or ulnar loading of wrist. Sclerotic and cystic changes may be seen in the lunate and ulnar head. If supportive measures fail, ulnar shortening (wafer procedure, ulnar shortening osteotomy) provide predictable pain relief. Ulnar head resection (Darrach), hemiresection with interpositional arthroplasty, and prosthetic ulnar head replacement are useful if significant arthritis is present.

V. Post-Traumatic Dysfunction of the Wrist and Hand

A. Scaphoid Avascular Necrosis —Common due to its tenuous blood supply. Bone grafting and internal fixation is usually curative. Unrecognized injuries may lead to the development of scapholunate advanced collapse, which in turn requires radial styloid excision, scaphoid excision and partial wrist arthrodesis (four-corner fusion), proximal row carpectomy, or total wrist fusion.

Table 3-16. CLASSIFICATION OF INJURIES OF THE TFCC

CLASS	DESCRIPTION	TREATMENT
1A	Horizontal tear adjacent to sigmoid notch	Débridement
1B	Avulsion from ulna ± ulnar styloid fracture	Suture repair
1C	Avulsion from carpus; exposes pisiform	Débridement
1D	Avulsion from sigmoid notch	Débridement
2A	Thinning of TFCC without perforation	
2B	Thinning of disc with chondromalacia	
2C	Perforation of disc with chondromalacia	
2D	Perforation of disc, chondromalacia, partial tear of lunotriquetral ligament	
2E	Perforation of disc, chondromalacia, complete tear of lunotriquetral ligament, ulnocarpal degenerative joint disease	

Note: Type 1: traumatic lesions; type 2: degenerative lesions. Treatment for degenerative lesions includes débridement of loose degenerated discs, intra-articular resection of the ulnar head, and débridement of lunotriquetral ligament tears with percutaneous pinning of the lunotriquetral joint based on the pathology present. From Miller M.D., Cooper D.E., Warner J.J.P., et al.: Review of Sports Medicine and Arthroscopy, p. 188. Philadelphia, WB Saunders, 1995.

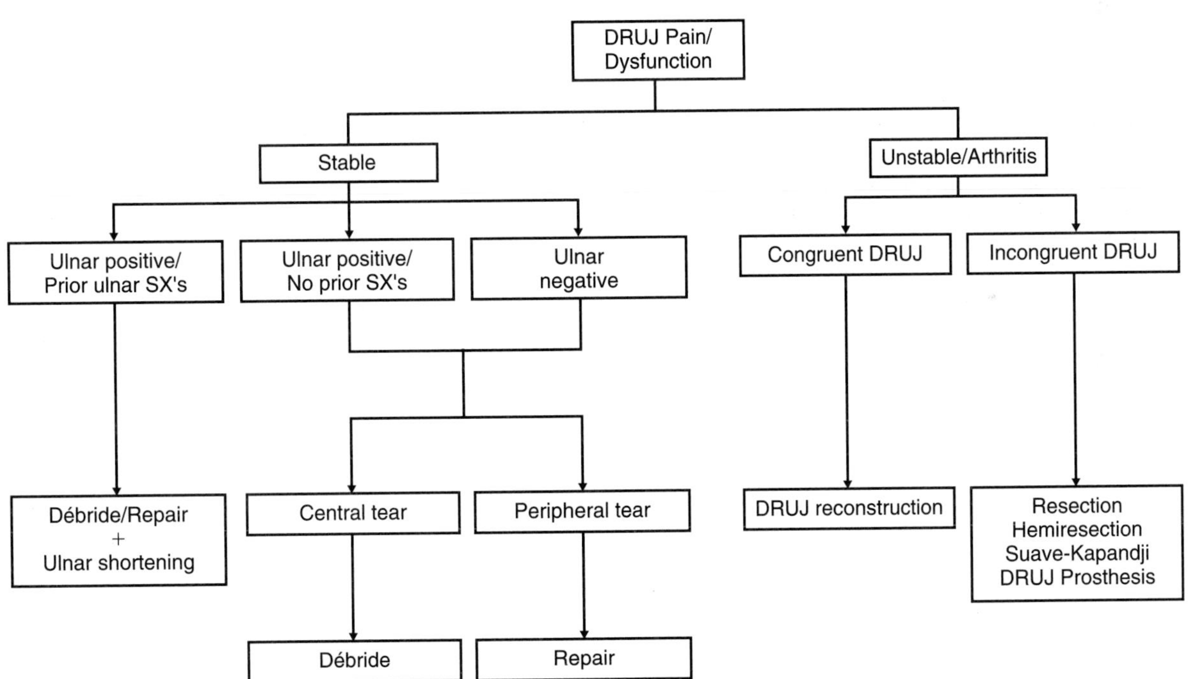

FIGURE 3-56 ■ Algorithmic approach to treatment of TFCC injuries.

B. Osteochondrosis of the Capitate—Commonly found in gymnasts and may respond to débridement or to limited wrist fusions.

C. Keinbock's Disease—Avascular necrosis and collapse of the lunate is likely related to overuse and to ulnar negative wrist variance. Early in the disease process, ulnar lengthening or radial shortening may be helpful in arresting progression to collapse. Limited wrist fusions may be necessary for cases of advanced collapse.

VI. Wrist Arthroscopy

A. Introduction—Serves as a useful diagnostic and staging adjunct and as an alternative to arthrotomy for the manipulation of intra-articular structures. It is indicated for the establishment of a diagnosis for unexplained wrist pain, treatment of mechanical symptoms secondary to interosseous ligament injuries or TFCC tears, assistance in the anatomic reduction and fixation of intra-articular fractures, débridement of chondral lesions, removal of loose bodies, or synovectomy.

B. Technique—The wrist is placed in a traction apparatus and a 2.5- or 3.0-mm scope is used. Portals are named in relation to the dorsal wrist compartments (Fig. 3-57). The 3-4 portal is established first and the 4-5 portal is used for instrumentation. The 6R portal serves as a useful adjunct for visualization and instrumentation. The midcarpal portals are necessary for complete carpal visualization and, often, confirmation of pathology visualized through the radiocarpal portals. The scaphotrapeziotrapezoid (STT) portal is typically used by advanced arthroscopists to evaluate localized pathology.

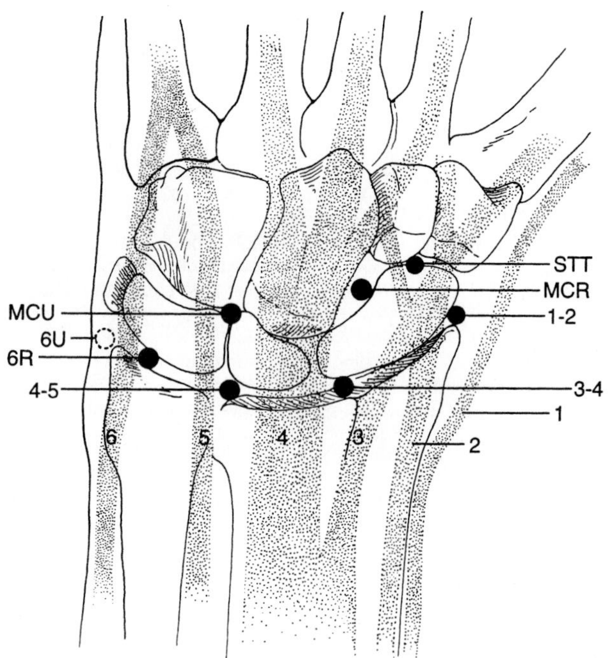

FIGURE 3-57 ■ Arthroscopic wrist portals. Numbers indicate wrist extensor compartments and associated portals. R, radial; U, ulnar; MCU, midcarpal ulnar; MCR, midcarpal radial; STT, scaphotrapeziotrapezoid. (From Miller, M.D., Osborne J.R., Warner J.J.P., et al.: MRI-Arthroscopy Correlative Atlas, Philadelphia, WB Saunders, 1997, p. 220.)

SECTION 7

Head and Spine Injuries

I. Head Injuries

A. Diffuse Brain Injuries—Include mild and "classic" cerebral concussion and diffuse axonal injury. Mild concussions occur without loss of consciousness and can be subdivided into three grades, shown in Table 3-17.

1. Postconcussion Syndrome—Characterized by persistent headaches, irritability, confusion, and difficulty concentrating, can occur with grade 2 and 3 mild concussions. "Classic" concussion includes a period of loss of consciousness. If it lasts >5 minutes, head CT should be obtained. Delay in RTP should be 1 week to 1 month after the first episode and for the entire season for a second episode. Diffuse axonal injury occurs with loss of consciousness lasting >6 hours, and athletes who suffer this injury should consider total avoidance of future contact sports. This condition is often fatal in young athletes.

B. Focal Brain Syndromes—Include contusions, intracranial hematomas, epidural hematomas, and subdural hematomas. CT scanning is helpful for distinguishing these entities (Fig. 3-58). Although epidural hematomas classically are said to be characterized by a period of lucidity followed by loss of consciousness, this sequence may not occur. Neurosurgical consultation and intensive care unit monitoring are necessary. Surgical treatment of intracranial hematomas may be indicated, followed by seizure prophylaxis.

C. Prevention—Head protection, especially with contact sports, equestrian events, hockey, boxing, skating, and skiing, should be encouraged.

Table 3-17. GRADES OF MILD CONCUSSIONS

GRADE	SYMPTOMS	DURATION	RECOMMENDED RTP
1	Confusion, no amnesia	Minutes	When symptoms resolve
2	Retrograde amnesia	Hours to days	1 wk
3	Amnesia after impact	Days	1 mo

RTP, return to play.

II. Cervical Spine Injuries

A. Introduction—Catastrophic injury to the cervical spine is unfortunately an all too common event in contact sports (especially football and rugby). Soft-tissue injuries of the C-spine, as well as fractures and dislocations in athletes, are treated as any traumatic injuries to the spine (See Chapter 7, Spine). Underlying cervical stenosis, or narrowing of the AP diameter of the spine, can make these injuries worse (Fig. 3-59). Recommendations for RTP for athletes with cervical stenosis with transient symptoms are controversial. Football players who repeatedly use poor tackling techniques can develop a condition known as ***spear tackler's spine***, which includes developmental cervical stenosis, loss of lordosis, and other radiographic abnormalities. Return to contact sports should be avoided.

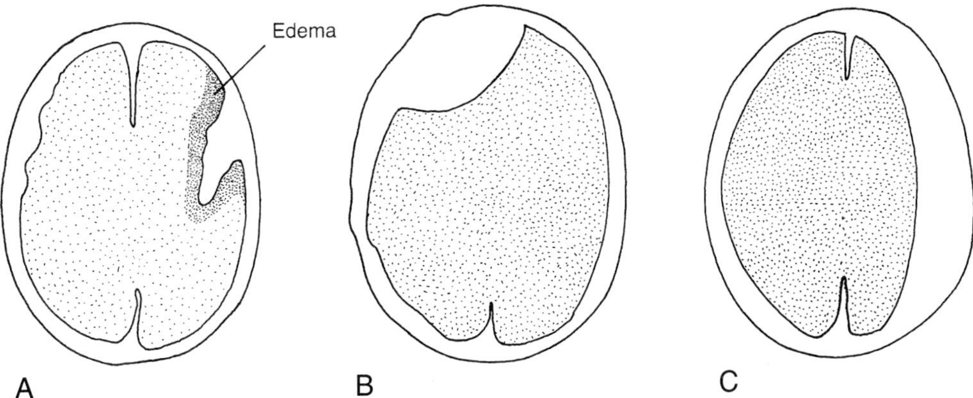

FIGURE 3-58 ■ CT findings. *A*, Contusion includes a hemorrhagic area and surrounding edema. *B*, Epidural hematomas typically have a biconvex appearance. *C*, Subdural hematomas have a concave or crescentic appearance. (From Miller, M.D., Cooper, D.E., and Warner, J.J.P.: Review of Sports Medicine and Arthroscopy. Philadelphia, WB Saunders, 1995, p. 204.)

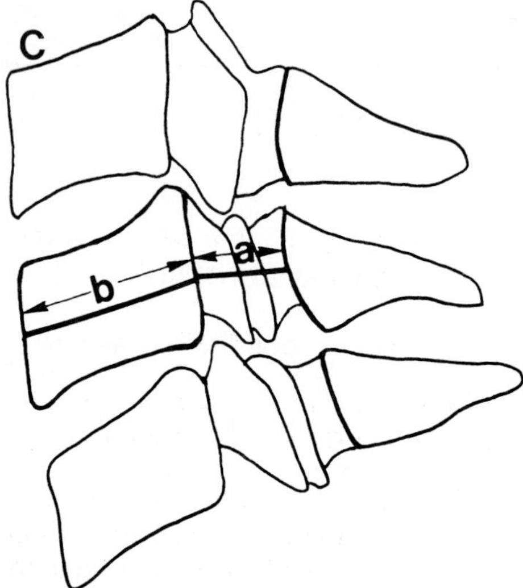

FIGURE 3-59 ■ Pavlov's ratio (*a/b*) of <0.8 is consistent with cervical stenosis. (Note that this ratio may not apply to larger individuals.) (From Pavlov, H., and Porter, I.S.: Criteria for cervical instability and stenosis. Op. Tech. Sports Med. 1:170, 1993.)

B. On-Field Management—As in any trauma victim, careful handling of the patient and immobilization is critical. In football, the helmet and shoulder pads should not be removed. If an emergent airway is needed, the face mask should be removed, with the helmet kept in place.

III. Thoracic and Lumbar Spine Injuries

A. See Chapter 7, Spine, for a more complete description of these injuries. Injuries commonly associated with sports include muscle injury, fractures, disc disease, and spondylolysis/spondylolisthesis. The latter condition is common in football interior line positions and gymnasts. Oblique radiographs, bone scan, and CT are all helpful for establishing the diagnosis. Treatment includes activity modification, bracing, and fusion for high-grade slips.

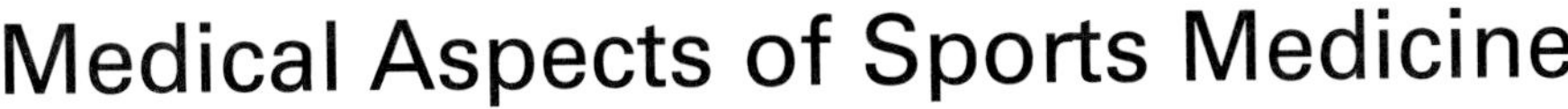

SECTION 8

Medical Aspects of Sports Medicine

I. Muscle Physiology

A. There are three types of muscle, types I, IIA, and IIB. Type I muscle is slow-twitch/aerobic and is helpful in endurance sports. Training can increase the number of mitochondria and increase capillary density. Types IIA and IIB muscle are fast-twitch/anaerobic and are helpful for sprinters. They have high contraction speeds, quick relaxation, and low triglycerine stores. Mode of energy utilization differentiates type IIA muscle from type IIB: IIA has both aerobic and anaerobic capabilities, whereas IIB is primarily anaerobic. Immobilization of muscle results in a shorter position with a decreased ability to generate tension.

II. Exercise

Exercise—Done on a regular basis, exercise can decrease heart rate and blood pressure (hypertension), decrease insulin requirements in diabetics, decrease cardiovascular risk, and increase lean body mass. It has also been shown to reduce cancer risk, osteoporosis, and hypercholesterolemia. The aerobic threshold can be determined by measuring oxygen consumption and is useful for evaluating endurance athletes. Sports-specific conditioning involves aerobic and anaerobic conditioning if different proportions are based on the season and the sport. In the off-season, long-distance runs can be helpful to sprinters to increase aerobic recovery capability following sprints. Several exercise categories have been described. Stretching has also been shown to have a beneficial effect (Table 3-18).

III. Cardiac Abnormalities in Athletes

A. Sudden Cardiac Death—Usually related to an underlying heart condition, especially ***hypertrophic cardiomyopathy in young athletes and coronary artery disease in older athletes***. Screening including electrocardiography can identify this problem early.

B. Commotio cordis—Cardiac contusion from a direct blow to the chest (e.g., in Little League baseball) has a poor prognosis, even when immediately recognized and treated.

IV. Metabolic Issues in Athletes

A. Dehydration—Fluid and electrolyte loss can lead to decreased cardiovascular function and work capacity. Absorption is increased with solutions with low osmolarity (<10%).

B. Nutritional Supplements—These continue to be a source of controversy. Creatine, one of the more popular supplements, increases the water retention in cells. In-season use can increase the incidence of dehydration and cramps.

V. Ergogenic Drugs

A. Anabolic Steroids—Derivatives of testosterone are abused by athletes attempting to increase muscle mass and strength and increase erythropoiesis. Adverse effects include liver dysfunction, hypercholesterolemia, cardiomyopathy, testicular atrophy, gynecomastia, and ***irreversible alopecia***. Urine sampling has been the standard for evaluation by the International Olympic Committee.

B. Human Growth Hormone (HGH)—Made from recombinant DNA; illegal use of this drug is common. Athletes attempting to increase muscle size and weight abuse this drug, which has side effects similar to those of steroids as well as hypertension and gigantism. Insulin-like growth factor-1 (IGF-1) has effects similar to HGH.

C. Prohormones—Derivatives of testosterone, dehydroepiandrosterone (DHEA) and androstenedione have been used as anabolic agents. However, their effects are controversial.

D. Other Commonly Abused Drugs—Include amphetamines, blood doping, diuretics, and laxatives.

VI. Female-Athlete-Related Issues

A. Physiologic Differences—Women are typically smaller, lighter, and have greater body fat. Lower

Table 3-18. EXERCISE TYPES

EXERCISE	DESCRIPTION	BENEFIT
Isometric	Muscle tension without change in unit length	Muscle hypertrophy; not endurance
Isotonic	Weight training with a constant resistance through arc of motion	Improved motor
Isokinetic	Weight training with a constant velocity, variable resistance	Increase strength; less time-consuming but more expensive
Plyometric	Rapid shortening	Power generation
Functional	Aerobic fitness	Easily performed

maximum oxygen consumption (MV_{O2}), cardiac output, hemoglobin, and muscular mass/strength are also important considerations. Other differences contribute to the increased incidence of patellofemoral disorders, stress fractures, and knee ACL injuries in females (especially with basketball, soccer, and rugby).

B. Amenorrhea—This problem may be related to a low body fat percentage and/or stress. The incidence approaches 50% in elite runners and is related to stress fractures ***(osteopenia) and eating disorders (female athlete triad)***. Dietary management and birth control pills are helpful for treating this problem.

VII. Other Sports-Related Injuries

A. Blunt Trauma—Can injure solid organs. These injuries may be subtle and require a high index of suspicion. ***The kidney is the most commonly injured organ (especially in boxing), followed by the spleen (injured in football).***

B. Chest Injuries—Can be serious and require immediate on-field action. Decreased breath sounds and hypotension may signify a tension pneumothorax. Treatment entails placing a 14-gauge intravenous needle in the second intercostal space at the midclavicular line and also placing a chest tube. Airway obstructions must also be anticipated and treated. Rib fractures may also occur in contact sports. More commonly, the player may have "had the air knocked out." This is usually related to a problem with the diaphragm.

C. Eye injuries—These injuries are best avoided with proper protection. A hyphema (blood in the eye) is associated with a vitreous or retinal injury in more than 50% of cases.

D. Heat Illness—Heat stroke, common in the football preseason, is characterized by collapse with neurological deficits, tachycardia, tachypnea, hypotension, and anhidrosis. Treatment involves rapidly cooling the body's core temperature. ***Heat stroke is the second leading cause of fatality in football players.***

E. Exercise-Induced Bronchospasm—Transient airway obstruction caused after exertion. ***Inhaled B2 agonists*** are the first-line treatment.

Selected Bibliography

GENERAL

Buckwalter, J.A., Einhorn, T.A., and Simon, S.R., eds.: Orthopaedic Basic Science: Biology and Biomechanics of the Musculoskeletal System, 2nd ed. Rosemont, IL, American Academy of Orthopaedic Surgeons, 2000.

Koval, K.J., ed.: Orthopaedic Knowledge Update 7. American Academy of Orthopaedic Surgeons, 2002.

KNEE

ANATOMY AND BIOMECHANICS

Arnoczky, S.P.: Anatomy of the anterior cruciate ligament. Clin. Orthop. 172:19–25, 1983.

Arnoczky, S.P., and Warren, R.F.: Microvasculature of the human meniscus. Am. J. Sports Med. 10:90–95, 1982.

Chhabra, A., Elliot, C., Miller, M.D.: Normal anatomy and biomechanics of the knee. Sports Medicine and Arthroscopy Review 9:166–177, 2002.

Cooper, D.E., Deng, X.H., Burnstein, A.L., et al.: The strength of the central third patellar tendon graft: A biomechanical study. Am. J. Sports Med. 21:818–824, 1993.

Daniel, D.M., Akeson, W.H., and O'Connor, J.J., eds.: Knee Ligaments: Structure, Function, Injury, and Repair. New York, Raven Press, 1990.

Fu, F.H., Harner, C.D., Johnson, D.L., et al.: Biomechanics of knee ligaments: Basic concepts and clinical application. J. Bone Joint Surg. 75:1716–1725, 1993.

Girgis, F.G., Marshall, J.L., and Al Monajem, A.R.S.: The cruciate ligaments of the knee joint: Anatomical, functional and experimental analysis. Clin. Orthop. 106:216–231, 1975.

Noyes, F.R., Butler, D.L., Grood, E.S., et al.: Biomechanical analysis of human ligament grafts used in knee-ligament repairs and reconstructions. J. Bone Joint Surg. [Am.] 66:344–352, 1984.

Seebacher, J.R., Inglis, A.E., Marshall, J.L., et al.: The structure of the posterolateral aspect of the knee. J. Bone Joint Surg. [Am.] 64:536–541, 1982.

Thompson, W.O., Theate, F.L., Fu, F.H., et al.: Tibial meniscal dynamics using three-dimensional reconstruction of magnetic resonance images. Am. J. Sports Med. 19:210–216, 1991.

Warren, L.F., and Marshall, J.L.: The supporting structures and layers of the medial side of the knee. J. Bone Joint Surg. [Am.] 61:56–62, 1979.

Warren, R., Arnoczky, S.P., and Wickiewicz, T.L.: Anatomy of the knee. In Nicholas, J.A., and Hershman, E.B., eds.: The Lower Extremity and Spine in Sports Medicine, St. Louis, C.V. Mosby, 1986, pp. 657–694.

HISTORY AND PHYSICAL EXAMINATION

Fetto, J.F., and Marshall, J.L.: Injury to the anterior cruciate ligament producing the pivot shift sign. J. Bone Joint Surg. [Am.] 61:710–714, 1979.

Fulkerson, J.P., Kalenak, A., Rosenberg, T.D., et al.: Patellofemoral pain. Instr. Course Lect. 41:57–71, 1992.

Galway, R.D., Beaupre, A., and MacIntosh, D.L.: Pivot shift. J. Bone Joint Surg. [Br.] 54:763, 1972.

Hosea, T.M., and Tria, A.J.: Physical examination of the knee: Clinical. In Scott, W.N., ed.: Ligament and Extensor Mechanism Injuries of the Knee: Diagnosis and Treatment. St. Louis, C.V. Mosby, 1991.

Ritchie, J.R., Miller, M.D., and Harner, C.D.: History and physical examination of the knee. In Fu, F.H., Harner, C.D., and Vince, K.G., eds.: Knee Surgery. Baltimore, Williams & Wilkins, 1994.

Slocum, D.B., and Larson, R.L.: Rotatory instability of the knee. J. Bone Joint Surg. [Am.] 50:211, 1968.

IMAGING

Blackburne, J.S., and Peel, T.E.: A new method of measuring patellar height. J. Bone Joint Surg. [Br.] 59:241–242, 1977.

Blumensaat, C.: Die lageabweichunger and verrenkungen der kniescheibe. Ergeb. Chir. Orthop. 31:149–223, 1938.

Insall, J., and Salvati, E.: Patella position in the normal knee joint. Radiology 101:101–104, 1971.

Jackson, D.W., Jennings, L.D., Maywood, R.M., et al.: Magnetic resonance imaging of the knee. Am. J. Sports Med. 16:29–38, 1988.

Jackson, R.W.: The painful knee: Arthroscopy or MR imaging. J. Am. Acad. Orthop. Surg. 4:93–99, 1996.

Merchant, A.C., Mercer, R.L., Jacobsen, R.H., et al.: Roentgenographic analysis of patellofemoral congruence. J. Bone Joint Surg. [Am.] 56:1391–1396, 1974.

Newhouse, K.E., and Rosenberg, T.D.: Basic radiographic examination of the knee. In Fu, F.H., Harner, C.D., and Vince, K.G., eds.: Knee Surgery. Baltimore, Williams & Wilkins, 1994, pp. 313–324.

Rosenberg, T.D., Paulos, L.E., Parker, R.D., et al.: The forty-five degree posteroanterior flexion weight-bearing radiograph of the knee. J. Bone Joint Surg. [Am.] 70:1479–1483, 1988.

Thaete, F.L., and Britton, C.A.: Magnetic resonance imaging. In Fu, F.H., Harner, C.D., and Vince, K.G., eds.: Knee Surgery. Baltimore, Williams & Wilkins, 1994.

KNEE ARTHROSCOPY

DeLee, J.C.: Complications of arthroscopy and arthroscopic surgery: Results of a national survey. Arthroscopy 4:214–220, 1988.

DiGiovine, N.M., and Bradley, J.P.: Arthroscopic equipment and set-up. In Fu, F.H., Harner, C.D., and Vince, K.G., eds.: Knee Surgery. Baltimore, Williams & Wilkins, 1994.

Gillquist, J.: Arthroscopy of the posterior compartments of the knee. Contemp. Orthop. 10:39-45, 1985.

Johnson, L.L.: Arthroscopic Surgery: Principles and Practice, 3rd ed. St. Louis, C.V. Mosby, 1986.

O'Connor, R.L.: Arthroscopy in the diagnosis and treatment of acute ligament injuries of the knee. J. Bone Joint Surg. [Am.] 56:333-337, 1974.

Rosenberg, T.D., Paulos, L.E., Parker, R.D., et al.: Arthroscopic surgery of the knee. In Chapman, M.W., ed.: Operative Orthopaedics. Philadelphia, JB Lippincott, 1988, pp. 1585-1604.

Small, N.C.: Complications in arthroscopy: The knee and other joints. Arthroscopy 2:253-258, 1986.

Wantanabe, M., and Takeda, S.: The number 21 arthroscope. J. Jpn. Orthop. Assoc. 34:1041, 1960.

MENISCUS

Arnoczky, S.P., Warren, R.F., and Spivak, J.M.: Meniscal repair using an exogenous fibrin clot—An experimental study in dogs. J. Bone Joint Surg. [Am.] 70:1209-1220, 1988.

Baratz, M.E., Fu, F.H., and Mengato, R.: Meniscal tears: The effect of meniscectomy and of repair on intra-articular contact areas and stresses in the human knee. Am. J. Sports Med. 14:270-275, 1986.

Belzer J.P., and Cannon W.D.: Meniscus tears: Treatment in the stable and unstable knee. J. Am. Acad. Orthop. Surg. 1:41-47, 1993.

Boenisch, U.W., Faber, K.J., et. al.: Pull out strength and stiffness of meniscal repair using absorbable arrows or Ti-cron verticle and horizontal loop sutures. Am. J. Sports Med. 27:626-631, 1999.

Carter, T.R.: Meniscal allograft transplantation. Sports Med. Arthrosc. Rev. 7:51-62, 1999.

Cannon, W.D., and Vittori, J.M.: The incidence of healing in arthroscopic meniscal repairs in anterior cruciate ligament reconstructed knees versus stable knees. Am. J. Sports Med. 20:176-181, 1992.

DeHaven, K.E., Black, K.P., and Griffiths, H.J.: Open meniscus repair: Technique and two to nine year results. Am. J. Sports Med. 17:788-795, 1989.

DeHaven, K.E.: Meniscus Repair. Am. J. Sports Med. 27:242-250, 1999.

Dickhaut, S.C., and DeLee, J.C.: The discoid lateral meniscus syndrome. J. Bone Joint Surg. [Am.] 64:1068-1073, 1982.

Fairbank, T.J.: Knee joint changes after meniscectomy. J. Bone Joint Surg. [Br.] 30:664-670, 1948.

Henning, C.E., Lynch, M.A., Yearout, K.M., et al.: Arthroscopic meniscal repair using an exogenous fibrin clot. Clin. Orthop. 252:64, 1990.

Jordan M.R.: Lateral meniscal variants: Evaluation and treatment. J. Am. Acad. Orthop. Surg. 4:191-200, 1996.

Miller, M.D., Ritchie, J.R., Royster, R.M., et al.: Meniscal repair: An experimental study in the goat. Am. J. Sports Med. 23(1):124-128, 1995.

Miller, M.D., Warner, J.J.P., and Harner, C.D.: Mensical repair. In Fu, F.H., Harner, C.D., and Vince, K.G., eds.: Knee Surgery. Baltimore, Williams & Wilkins, 1994.

Neuschwander, D.C., Drez, D., and Finney, T.P.: Lateral meniscal variant with absence of the posterior coronary ligament. J. Bone Joint Surg. [Am.] 74:1186-1190, 1992.

Parisien, J.S.: Arthroscopic treatment of cysts of the menisci: A preliminary report. Clin. Orthop. 257:154-158, 1990.

Warren, R.F.: Meniscectomy and repair in the anterior cruciate ligament-deficient patient. Clin. Orthop. 252:55-63, 1990.

OSTEOCHONDRAL LESIONS

Bauer, M., and Jackson, R.W.: Chondral lesions of the femoral condyles: A system of arthroscopic classification. Arthroscopy 4:97-102, 1988.

Buckwalter, J.A., Restoration of injured or degenerated articular cartilage. J. Am. Acad. Orthop. Surg. 2:192-201, 1994.

Buckwalter, J.A., and Mankin, H.J., Articular cartilage (parts I&II). Instructional Course Lectures. J. Bone Joint Surg. 79A:600-632, 1997.

Bugbee, W.D., Convery, F.R.: Osteochondral allograft transplantation. Clin. Sports Med. 18:67-75, 1999.

Cahill, B.R.: Osteochondritis dissecans of the knee: Treatment of juvenile and adult forms. J. Am. Acad. Orthop. Surg. 3:237-247, 1995.

Ecker, M.L., and Lotke, P.A.: Spontaneous osteonecrosis of the knee. J. Am. Acad. Orthop. Surg. 2:173-178, 1994.

Guhl, J.: Arthroscopic treatment of osteochondritis dissecans. Clin. Orthop. 167:65-74, 1982.

Mandelbaum, B.R., Browne, J.E., Fu, F.H., et al.: Articular cartilage lesions of the knee: Current concepts. Am. J. Sports Med. 26:853-861, 1998.

Menche, D.S., Vangsness, C.T., Pitman, M, et al.: The treatment of isolated articular cartilage lesions in the young individual. AAOS Instr. Course Lect. 47:505-515, 1998.

Murray, P.B., and Rand, J.A.: Symptomatic valgus knee: The surgical options. J. Am. Acad. Orthop. Surg. 1:1-9, 1993.

Newman, A.P.: Articular cartilage repair: Current concepts. Am. J. Sports Med. 26:309-324, 1998.

O'Driscoll, S.W.: Current concepts review: The healing and regeneration of articular cartilage. J. Bone Joint Surg. 80A:1795-1812, 1998.

Schenck, R.C., and Goodnight, J.M.: Current concepts review: Osteochondritis dissecans. J. Bone Joint Surg. 78A:439-456, 1996.

SYNOVIAL LESIONS

Curl, W.W.: Popliteal cysts: Historical background and current knowledge. J. Am. Acad. Orthop. Surg. 4:129-133, 1996.

Ewing, J.W.: Plica: Pathologic or not? J. Am. Acad. Orthop. Surg. 1:117-121, 1993.

Flandry, F., and Hughston, J.C.: Current concepts review: Pigmented villonodular synovitis. J. Bone Joint Surg. [Am.] 69:942, 1987.

KNEE LIGAMENT INJURIES

Almekinders, L.C., and Dedmond, B.T.: Outcomes of operatively treated knee dislocations. Clin. Sports Med. 19:503-518, 2000.

Albright, J.P., and Brown, A.W.: Management of chronic posterolateral rotatory instability of the knee: Surgical technique for the posterolateral corner sling procedure. AAOS Instr. Course Lect. 47:369-378, 1998.

Carson, E.W., Simonian, P.T., Wickiewicz, T.L., et al: Revision anterior cruciate ligament reconstruction. AAOS Instr. Course Lect. 47:361-368, 1998.

Chen, F.S., Rokito, A.S., and Piutman, M.I.: Acute and chronic posterolateral rotary instability of the knee. J Am Acad Orthop Surg 8:97-110, 2000.

Clancy, W.G., Ray, J.M., and Zoltan, D.J.: Acute tears of the anterior cruciate ligament: Surgical versus conservative treatment. J. Bone Joint Surg. [Am.] 70:1483-1488, 1988.

Cooper, D.E., Warren, R.F., and Warner, J.J.P.: The posterior cruciate ligament and posterolateral structures of the knee: Anatomy, function, and patterns of injury. Instr. Course Lect. 40:249-270, 1991.

Dye, S.F., Wojtys, E.M., Fu, F.H., et al.: Factors contributing to function of the knee joint after injury or reconstruction of the anterior cruciate ligament. J. Bone Joint Surg. 80A:1380-1393, 1998.

Fowler, P.J., and Messieh, S.S.: Isolated posterior cruciate ligament injuries in athletes. Am. J. Sports Med. 15:553-557, 1987.

France, E.P., and Paulos, L.E.: Knee bracing. J. Am. Acad. Orthop. Surg. 2:281-287, 1994.

Frank, C.B.: Ligament healing: Current knowledge and clinical applications. J. Am. Acad. Orthop. Surg. 4:74-83, 1996.

Frank, C.B., and Jackson, D.W.: Current concepts review: The science of reconstruction of the anterior cruciate ligament. J. Bone Joint Surg. 79A:1556-1576, 1997.

Frassica, F.J., Sim, F.H., Staeheli, J.W., et al.: Dislocation of the knee. Clin. Orthop. 263:200-205, 1991.

Fu, F.H., Bennett, C.H., et. al.: Current trends in anterior cruciate ligament reconstruction, Part I. Am. J. Sports Med. 27:821-830, 1999.

Fu, F.H., Bennett, C.H., et. al.: Current trends in anterior cruciate ligament reconstruction, Part II. Am. J. Sports Med. 28:124-130, 2000.

Good, L., and Johnson, R.J.: The dislocated knee. J. Am. Acad. Orthop. Surg. 3:284-292, 1995.

Harner, C.D., and Hoher, J.: Evaluation and treatment of posterior cruciate ligament injuries: Current concepts. Am. J. Sports Med. 26:471-482, 1998.

Harner, C.D., Irrgang, J.J., Paul, J., et al.: Loss of motion following anterior cruciate ligament reconstruction. Am. J. Sports Med. 20:507-515, 1992.

Howell, S.M., and Taylor, M.A.: Failure of reconstruction of the anterior cruciate ligament due to impingement by the intercondylar roof. J. Bone Joint Surg. [Am.] 75:1044-1055, 1993.

Indelicato, P.A., Isolated medial collateral ligament injuries in the knee. J. Am. Acad. Orthop. Surg. 3:9-14, 1995.

Indelicato, P.A., Hermansdorfer, J., and Huegel, M.: Nonoperative management of complete tears of the medial collateral ligament of the knee in intercollegiate football players. Clin. Orthop. 256:174–177, 1990.
Larson, R.L., and Taillon, M.: Anterior cruciate ligament insufficiency: Principles of treatment. J. Am. Acad. Orthop. Surg. 2:26–35, 1994.
Miller, M.D., Bergfeld, J.A., et al.: The posterior cruciate ligament injured knee: Principles of evaluation and treatment, AAOS Instr Course Lecture. 48:199–207, 1999.
Miller, M.D., Osbourne, J.R., et. al.: The natural histories of bone bruises. Am. J. Sports Med. 26:15–19, 1998.
Myers, M.H., and Harvey, J.P.: Traumatic dislocation of the knee joint: A study of eighteen cases. J. Bone Joint Surg. [Am.] 53:16–29, 1971.
Noyes, F.R., Barber-Westin, S.D., Butler, D.L., et al.: The role of allografts in repair and reconstruction of knee joint ligaments and menisci. AAOS Instr. Course Lect. 47:379–396, 1998.
O'Brien, S.J., Warren, R.F., Pavlov, H., et al.: Reconstruction of the chronically insufficient anterior cruciate ligament with the central third of the patellar ligament. J. Bone Joint Surg. [Am.] 73:278–286, 1991.
Paulos, L.E., Rosenberg, T.D., Drawbert, J., et al.: Infrapatellar contracture syndrome: An unrecognized cause of knee stiffness with patellar entrapment and patella infera. Am. J. Sports Med. 15:331–341, 1987.
Shelbourne, K.D., and Nitz, P.: Accelerated rehabilitation after anterior cruciate ligament reconstruction. Am. J. Sports Med. 18:292–299, 1990.
Shelton, W.R., Treacy, S.H., Dukes, A.D., et al.: Use of allografts in knee reconstruction. J. Am. Acad. Orthop. Surg. 6:165–175, 1998.
Sisto, D.J., and Warren, R.F.: Complete knee dislocation: A follow-up study of operative treatment. Clin. Orthop. 198:94–101, 1985.
Sitler, M., Ryan, J., Hopkinson, W., et al.: The efficacy of a prophylactic knee brace to reduce knee injuries in football: A prospective, randomized study at West Point. Am. J. Sports Med. 18:310–315, 1990.
Veltri, D.M., and Warren, R.F.: Isolated and combined posterior cruciate ligament injuries. J. Am. Acad. Orthop. Surg. 1:67–75, 1993.

ANTERIOR KNEE PAIN

Boden, B.P., Pearsall, A.W., Garrett, W.E., et al.: Patellofemoral instability: Evaluation and management. J. Am. Acad. Orthop. Surg. 5:47–57, 1997.
Cooper, D.E., and DeLee, J.C.: Reflex sympathetic dystrophy of the knee. J. Am. Acad. Orthop. Surg. 2:79–86, 1994.
Cramer, K.E., and Moed, B.R.: Patellar fractures: Contemporary approach to treatment. J. Am. Acad. Orthop. Surg. 5:323–331, 1997.
Fulkerson, J.P.: Anteromedialization of the tibial tuberosity for patellofemoral malalignment. Clin. Orthop. 177:176–181, 1983.
Fulkerson, J.P.: Patellofemoral pain disorders: Evaluation and management. J. Am. Acad. Orthop. Surg. 2:124–132, 1994.
Fulkerson, J.P., and Shea, K.P.: Disorders of patellofemoral alignment: Current concepts review. J. Bone Joint Surg. [Am.] 72:1424–1429, 1990.
Gambardella, R.A.: Technical pitfalls of patellofemoral surgery. Clin. Sports Med. 18:897–903, 1999.
James, S.L.: Running injuries to the knee. J. Am. Acad. Orthop. Surg. 3:309–318, 1995.
Kelly, M.A.: Algorithm for anterior knee pain. AAOS Instr. Course Lect. 47:339–343, 1998.
Kilowich, P., Paulos, L., Rosenberg, T., et al.: Lateral release of the patella: Indications and contraindications. Am. J. Sports Med. 18:361, 1990.
Larson, R.L., Cabaud, H.E., Slocum, D.B., et al.: The patellar compression syndrome: Surgical treatment by lateral retinacular release. Clin. Orthop. 134:158–167, 1978.
Matava, M.J.: Patellar tendon ruptures. J. Am. Acad. Orthop. Surg. 4:287–296, 1996.
Merchant, A.: Classification of patellofemoral disorders. Arthroscopy 4:235–240, 1988.
Merchant, A.C., Mercer, R.L., Jacobsen, R.J., et al.: Roentgenographic analysis of patellofemoral congruence. J. Bone Joint Surg. [Am.] 56:1391–1396, 1974.
Post, W.R.: Clinical evaluation of patients with patellofemoral disorders. Arthroscopy 15:841–851, 1999.

CHILDHOOD AND ADOLESCENT KNEE DISORDERS

Andrish, J.T.: Meniscal injuries in children and adolescents: Diagnosis and management. J. Am. Acad. Orthop. Surg. 5:231–237, 1996.
Aronowitz, E.R., Ganley, T.J. et al.: Anterior cruciate ligament reconstruction in adolecscents with open physes. Am. J. Sports Med. 28:168–875, 2000.
Baxter, M.P., and Wiley, J.J.: Fractures of the tibial spine in children: An evaluation of knee stability. J. Bone Joint Surg. [Br.] 70:228–230, 1988.
Edwards, P.H., and Grana, W.A.: Physical fractures about the knee. J. Am. Acad. Orthop. Surg. 3:63–69, 1995.
Lo, I.K.Y., Bell, D.M., and Fowler, P.J.: Anterior cruciate ligament injuries in the skeletally immature patient. AAOS Instr. Course Lect. 47:351–359, 1998.
McCarroll, J.R., Rettig, A.C., and Shelbourne, K.D.: Anterior cruciate ligament injuries in the young athlete with open physes. Am. J. Sports Med. 16:44–47, 1988.
Meyers, M.H., and McKeever, F.M.: Fractures of the intercondylar eminence of the tibia. J. Bone Joint Surg. [Am.] 41:209–222, 1959.
Micheli, L.J., and Foster, T.E.: Acute knee injuries in the immature athlete. Instr. Course Lect. 42:473–481, 1993.
Ogden, J.A., Tross, R.B., and Murphy, M.J.: Fractures of the tibial tuberosity in adolescents. J. Bone Joint Surg. [Am.] 62:205–215, 1980.
Parker, A.W., Drez, D., and Cooper, J.L.: Anterior cruciate ligament injuries in patients with open physes. Am. J. Sports Med. 22:44–47, 1994.
Riseborough, E.J., Barrett, I.R., and Shapiro, F.: Growth disturbances following distal femoral physeal fracture-separations. J. Bone Joint Surg. [Am.] 65:885–893, 1983.
Stanitski, C.L.: Anterior cruciate ligament injury in the skeletally immature patient: Diagnosis and treatment. J. Am. Acad. Orthop. Surg. 3:146–158, 1995.
Stanitski, C.L.: Patellar instability in the school age athlete. AAOS Instr. Course Lect. 47:345–350, 1998.

OTHER LOWER EXTREMITY SPORTS MEDICINE PROBLEMS

NERVE ENTRAPMENT SYNDROMES

Baxter, D.E.: Functional nerve disorders in the athlete's foot, ankle, and leg. Instr. Course Lect. 42:185–194, 1993.
Beskin, J.L.: Nerve entrapments of the foot and ankle. J. Am. Acad. Orthop. Surg. 5:261–269, 1997.
Styf, J.: Entrapment of the superficial peroneal nerve: Diagnosis and results of decompression. J. Bone Joint Surg. [Br.] 71:131–135, 1989.

CONTUSIONS

Jackson, D.W., and Feagin, J.A.: Quadriceps contusions in young athletes. J. Bone Joint Surg. [Am.] 55:95–105, 1973.
Renstrom, P.A.H.F.: Tendon and muscle injuries in the groin area. Clin. Sports Med. 11:815–831, 1992.
Ryan, J.B., Wheeler, J.H., Hopkinson, W.J., et al.: Quadriceps contusions: West Point update. Am. J. Sports Med. 19:299–304, 1991.

MUSCLE INJURY

Garrett, W.E.: Muscle strain injuries. Am. J. Sports Med. 24:S2–S8, 1996.
Zarins, B., and Ciullo, J.V.: Acute muscle and tendon injuries in athletes. Clin. Sports Med. 2:167, 1983.

TENDON INJURIES

Almekinders, L.C.: Tendinitis and other chronic tendinopathies. J. Am. Acad. Orthop. Surg. 6:157–164, 1998.
Bassett, F.H., and Speer, K.P.: Longitudinal rupture of the peroneal tendons. Am. J. Sports Med. 21:354–357, 1993.
Biedert, R.: Dislocation of the tibialis posterior tendon. Am. J. Sports Med. 20:775–776, 1992.
Brage, M.E., and Hansen, S.T.: Traumatic subluxation/dislocation of the peroneal tendons. Foot Ankle 13:423–430, 1992.
Jones, D.C.: Tendon disorders of the foot and ankle. J. Am. Acad. Orthop. Surg. 1:87–94, 1993.
Millar, A.P.: Strains of the posterior calf musculature ("tennis leg"). Am. J. Sports Med. 7:172–174, 1979.
Myerson, M.S., and McGarvey, W.: Disorders of the insertion of the achilles tendon and achilles tendinitis. J. Bone Joint Surg. 80A:1814–1824, 1998.
Ouzounian, T.J., and Myerson, M.S.: Dislocation of the posterior tibial tendon. Foot Ankle 13:215–219, 1992.
Saltzman, C.L., and Tearse, D.S.: Achilles tendon injuries. J. Am. Acad. Orthop. Surg. 6:316–325, 1998.

Sobel, M., Geppert, M.J., Olson, E.J., et al.: The dynamics of peroneus brevis tendon splits: A proposed mechanism, technique of diagnosis, and classification of injury. Foot Ankle 13:413–421, 1992.

Teitz C.C., Garrett W.E. Jr., Miniaci A., et al: Tendon problems in athletic individuals. Instr Course Lect 46:569-82, 1997.

Williams, J.G.P.: Achilles tendon lesions in sport. Sports Med. 3:114–135, 1986.

COMPARTMENT SYNDROME

Beckham, S.G., Grana, W.A., Buckley, P., et al.: A comparison of anterior compartment pressures in competitive runners and cyclists. Am. J. Sports Med. 21:36–40, 1993.

Eisele, S.A., and Sammarco, G.J.: Chronic exertional compartment syndrome. Instr. Course Lect. 42:213–217, 1993.

Pedowitz, R.A., Horgens, A.R., Mubarak, S.J., et al.: Modified criteria for the objective diagnosis of compartment syndrome of the leg. Am. J. Sports Med. 18:35–40, 1990.

Rorabeck, C.H., Bourne, R.B., and Fowler, P.J.: The surgical treatment of exertional compartment syndromes in athletes. J. Bone Joint Surg. [Am.] 65:1245, 1983.

Rorabeck, C.H., Fowler, P.J., and Nitt, L.: The results of fasciotomy in the management of chronic exertional compartment syndrome. Am. J. Sports Med. 16:224–227, 1986.

STRESS FRACTURES

Anderson, E.G.: Fatigue fractures of the foot. Injury 21:274–279, 1990.

Blickenstaff, L.D., and Morris, J.M.: Fatigue fracture of the femoral neck. J. Bone Joint Surg. [Am.] 48:1031, 1966.

Green, N.E., Rogers, R.A., and Lipscomb, A.B.: Nonunions of stress fractures of the tibia. Am. J. Sports Med. 13:171–176, 1985.

Khan, K.M., Fuller, P.J., Brukner, P.D., et al.: Outcome of conservative and surgical management of navicular stress fracture in athletes: Eighty-six cases proven with computerized tomography. Am. J. Sports Med. 20:657–661, 1992.

McBryde, A.M.: Stress fractures in athletes. J. Sports Med. 3:212, 1973.

Rettig, A.C., Shelbourne, K.D., McCarroll, J.R., et al.: The natural history and treatment of delayed union stress fractures of the anterior cortex of the tibia. Am. J. Sports Med. 16:250–255, 1988.

Shin, A.Y., and Gillingham, B.L.: Fatigue fractures of the femoral neck in athletes. J. Am. Acad. Orthop. Surg. 5:293–302, 1997.

OTHER HIP DISORDERS

Allen, W.C., and Cope, R.: Coxa saltans: The snapping hip revisited. J. Am. Acad. Orthop. Surg. 3:303–308, 1995.

Buckwalter, J.A., and Lane, N.E.: Athletics and osteoarthritis. Am. J. Sports Med. 25:873–881, 1997.

Clanton, T.O., and Coupe, K.J.: Hamstring strains in athletes: Diagnosis and treatment. J. Am. Acad. Orthop. Surg. 6:237–248, 1998.

Cooper, D.E., Warren, R.F., and Barnes, R.: Traumatic subluxation of the hip resulting in aseptic necrosis and chondrolysis in a professional football player. Am. J. Sports Med. 19:322–324, 1991.

Holmes, J.C., Pruitt, A.L., and Whalen, N.J.: Iliotibial band syndrome in cyclists. Am. J. Sports Med. 21:419–424, 1993.

Martens, M., Libbrecht, P., and Burssens, A.: Surgical treatment of the iliotibial band friction syndrome. Am. J. Sports Med. 17:651–654, 1989.

OTHER FOOT AND ANKLE DISORDERS

Baxter, D.E., and Zingas, C.: The foot in running. J. Am. Acad. Orthop. Surg. 3:136–145, 1995.

Churchill, J.A., and Mazur, J.M.: Ankle pain in children: Diagnostic evaluation and clinical decision-making. J. Am. Acad. Orthop. Surg. 3:183–193, 1995.

Colville, M.R.: Surgical treatment of the unstable ankle. J. Am. Acad. Orthop. Surg. 6:368–377, 1998.

Donahue S.W., and Sharkey N.A.: Strains in the metatarsals during the stance phase of gait: Implications for stress fractures. J. Bone Joint Surg. [Am.] 81:1236–1244, 1999.

Garrick, J.G., and Requa, R.K.: The epidemiology of foot and ankle injuries in sports. Clin. Sports Med. 7:29–36, 1988.

Gill, L.H.: Plantar fasciitis: Diagnosis and conservative management. J. Am. Acad. Orthop. Surg. 5:109–117, 1997.

Hamilton, W.G., Thompson, F.M., and Snow, S.W.: The modified Brostrom procedure for lateral ankle instability. Foot Ankle 14:1–7, 1993.

Hopkinson, W.J., St. Pierre, P., Ryan, J.B., et al.: Syndesmosis sprains of the ankle. Foot Ankle 10:325–330, 1990.

Lynch, S., Renstrom, P.: Treatment of acute lateral ankle ligament rupture in the athlete: Conservative vs. surgical treatment. Sports Med. 27:61–71, 1999.

Marotta, J.J., and Micheli, L.J.: Os trigonum impingement in dancers. Am. J. Sports Med. 20:533–536, 1992.

Miller, C.M., Winter, W.G., Bucknell, A.L., et al.: Injuries to the midtarsal joint and lesser tarsal bones. J. Am. Acad. Orthop. Surg. 6:249–258, 1998.

Mizel, M.S., and Yodlowski, M.L.: Disorders of the lesser metatarsophalangeal joints. J. Am. Acad. Orthop. Surg. 3:166–173, 1995.

Renstrom, P.A.F.H.: Persistently painful sprained ankle. J. Am. Acad. Orthop. Surg. 2:270–280, 1994.

Rodeo, S.A., O'Brien, S., Warren, R.F., et al.: Turf toe: An analysis of metatarsal phalangeal joint pain in professional football players. Am. J. Sports Med. 18:280–285, 1990.

Thacker, S., Stroup, D., et al.: The prevention of ankle sprains in sports: A systematic review of the literature. Am. J. Sports Med. 27:753–760, 1999.

Wuest, T.K.: Injuries to the distal lower extremity syndesmosis. J. Am. Acad. Orthop. Surg. 5:172–181, 1997.

HIP AND ANKLE ARTHROSCOPY

Angermann, P., and Jensen, P.: Osteochondritis dissecans of the talus: Long-term results of surgical treatment. Foot Ankle 10:161–163, 1989.

Basset, F.H., Billy, J.B., and Gates, H.S.: A simple surgical approach to the posteromedial ankle. Am. J. Sports Med. 21:144–146, 1993.

Ferkel, R.D., and Scranton, P.E.: Current concepts review: Arthroscopy of the ankle and foot. J. Bone Joint Surg. [Am.] 75:1233–1243, 1993.

Glick, J.M., Sampson, T.G., Gordon, R.B., et al.: Hip arthroscopy by the lateral approach. Arthroscopy 3:4–12, 1987.

Loomer, R., Fisher, C., Lloyd-Smith, R., et al.: Osteochondral lesions of the talus. Am. J. Sports Med. 21:13–19, 1993.

McCarroll, J.R., Schrader, J.W., Shelbourne, K.D., et al.: Meniscoid lesions of the ankle in soccer players. Am. J. Sports Med. 15:257, 1987.

McCarthy, J.C., Day, B., and Busconi, B.: Hip arthroscopy: Applications and technique. J. Am. Acad. Orthop. Surg. 3:115–122, 1995.

Meislin, R.J., Rose, D.J., Parisien, S., et al.: Arthroscopic treatment of synovial impingement of the ankle. Am. J. Sports Med. 21:186–189, 1993.

Ogilvie-Harris, D.J., Lieverman, I., and Fitsalos, D.: Arthroscopically assisted arthrodesis for osteoarthritic ankles. J. Bone Joint Surg. [Am.] 75:1167–1174, 1993.

Stetson, W.B., and Ferkel, R.D.: Ankle arthroscopy. J. Am. Acad. Orthop. Surg. 4:17–34, 1996.

Stone, J.W.: Osteochondral lestions of the talar dome. J. Am. Acad. Orthop. Surg. 4:63–73, 1996.

Thein, R., and Eichenblat, M.: Arthroscopic treatment of sports-related synovitis of the ankle. Am. J. Sports Med. 20:496–499, 1992.

SHOULDER

ANATOMY AND BIOMECHANICS

Cooper, D.E., Arnoczsky, S.P., O'Brien, S.J., et al.: Anatomy, histology, and vascularity of the glenoid labrum. J. Bone Joint Surg. [Am.] 74:46–52, 1992.

Cooper, D.E., O'Brien, S.J., and Warren, R.F.: Supporting layers of the glenohumeral joint: An anatomic study. Clin. Orthop. 289:144–155, 1993.

Ferrari, D.A.: Capsular ligaments of the shoulder: Anatomical and functional study of the anterior superior capsule. Am. J. Sports Med. 18:20–24, 1990.

Flatow, E.L.: The biomechanics of the acromioclavicular, sternoclavicular, and scapulothoracic joints. Instr. Course Lect. 42:237–245, 1993.

Harryman, D.T., Sidles, J.A., Harris, S.L., Matsen, F.A.: The role of the rotator interval capsule in passive motion and stability of the shoulder. J. Bone Joint Surg. [Am.] 74:53–66, 1992.

Harryman, D.T., II: Common surgical approaches to the shoulder. Instr. Course Lect. 41:3–11, 1992.

Iannotti, J.P., Gabriel, J.P., Schneck, S.L., et al.: The normal glenohumeral relationships: An anatomical study of one hundred and forty shoulders. J. Bone Joint Surg. [Am.] 74:491-500, 1992.

Kibler, W.B.: The role of the scapula in athletic shoulder function: Current concepts. Am. J. Sports Med. 26:325-337, 1998.

O'Brien, S.J., Neves, M.C., Rozbruck, S.R., et al.: The anatomy and histology of the inferior glenohumeral ligament complex of the shoulder. Am. J. Sports Med. 18:449, 1990.

O'Connell, P.W., Nuber, G.W., Mileski, R.A., et al.: The contribution of the glenohumeral ligaments to anterior stability of the shoulder joint. Am. J. Sports Med. 18:579-584, 1990.

Sher, J.S.: Anatomy, biomechanics, and pathophysiology of rotator cuff disease. In Iannotti, J.P., and Williams, G.R., eds.: Disorders of the Shoulder: Lippincott Williams and Wilkins, 1999.

Speer, K.P.: Anatomy and pathomechanics of shoulder instability. Clin. Sports Med. 14:751-7650, 1995.

Warner, J.J.P., Deng, X.H., Warren, R.F., et al.: Static capsuloligamentous restraints to superior-inferior translation of the glenohumeral joint. Am. J. Sports Med. 20:675-685, 1992.

Warner, J.J.P., Deng, X.H., Warren, R.F., et al.: Superior-inferior translation in the intact and vented glenohumeral joint. J. Shoulder Elbow Surg. 2:99-105, 1993.

HISTORY AND PHYSICAL EXAMINATION

Altchek, D.W., and Dines, D.M.: Shoulder injuries in the throwing athlete. J. Am. Acad. Orthop. Surg. 3:159-165, 1995.

Gerber, C., and Ganz, R.: Clinical assessment of instability of the shoulder with special reference to anterior and posterior drawer tests. J. Bone Joint Surg. [Br.] 66:551-556, 1984.

Hawkins, R.J., Hobeika, P.: Physical exam of the shoulder. Orthopaedics 6:1270-1278, 1983.

Neer, C.S., and Welsh, R.P.: The shoulder in sports. Orthop. Clin. North Am. 8:583-591, 1977.

IMAGING OF THE SHOULDER

Beltran, J.: The use of magnetic resonance imaging about the shoulder. J. Shoulder Elbow Surg. 1:287-295, 1992.

Bigliani, L.U., Morrison, D., and April, E.W.: The morphology of the acromion and its relationship to rotator cuff tears. Orthop. Trans. 10:228, 1986.

Garth, W.P., Jr., Slappey, C.E., and Ochs, C.W.: Roentgenographic demonstration of instability of the shoulder: The apical oblique projection—a technical note. J. Bone Joint Surg. [Am.] 66:1450-1453, 1984.

Herzog, R.J.: Magnetic resonance imaging of the shoulder. J. Bone Joint Surg. 79A:934-953, 1997.

Hill, H.A., and Sachs, M.D.: The grooved defect of the humeral head: A frequently unrecognized complication of dislocations of the shoulder joint. Radiology 35:690-700, 1940.

Hobbs, D.W.: Sternoclavicular joint: A new axial radiographic view. Radiology 90:801-802, 1968.

Kozo, O., Yamamuro, T., and Rockwood, C.A.: Use of a thirty-degree caudal tilt radiograph in the shoulder impingement syndrome. J. Shoulder Elbow Surg. 1:246-252, 1992.

Zanca, P.: Shoulder pain: Involvement of the acromioclavicular joint: Analysis of 1000 cases. AJR Am. J. Roentgenol. 112:493-506, 1971.

ARTHROSCOPY OF THE SHOULDER

Altchek, D.W., and Carson, E.W.: Arthroscopic acromioplasty: Indications and technique. AAOS Instr. Course Lect. 47:21-28, 1998.

Bell, R.H.: Arthroscopic distal clavicle resection. AAOS Instr. Course Lect. 47:35-41, 1998.

Caborn, D.M., and Fu, F.H.: Arthroscopic approach and anatomy of the shoulder. Op. Tech. Orthop. 1:126-133, 1991.

Lintner, S.A., and Speer, K.P.: Traumatic anterior glenohumeral instability: The role of arthroscopy. J. Am. Acad. Orthop. Surg. 5:233-239, 1997.

Nisbet, J.K., and Paulos, L.E.: Subacromial bursoscopy. Op. Tech. Orthop. 1:221-228, 1991.

Skyhar, M.J., Altchek, D.W., Warren, R.F., et al.: Shoulder arthroscopy with the patient in the beach chair position. Arthroscopy 4:256-259, 1988.

Wolf, E.M.: Anterior portals in shoulder arthroscopy. Arthroscopy 5:201-208, 1989.

SHOULDER INSTABILITY

Altchek, D.W., Warren, R.F., Skyhar, M.J., et al.: T-plasty modification of the Bankart procedure for multidirectional instability of the anterior an inferior types. J. Bone Joint Surg. [Am.] 73:105-112, 1991.

Arciero, R.A., Wheeler, J.H., III, Ryan, J.B., et al.: Arthroscopic Bankart repair for acute, initial anterior shoulder dislocations. Am. J. Sports Med. 22:589-594, 1994.

Black K.P. et al.: Biomechanics of a Bankart Repair: Relationship between glenohumeral translation and labral fixation site. Am. J. Sports Med. 27:339-344, 1999.

Cole B.J., Warner, J.J.P.: Arthroscopic vs. open Bankart repair for traumatic anterior shoulder instability: Decision making and results. Clin. Sports Med. 19:19-47, 2000.

Cole, B.J., Romeo, A.A., and Warner, J.J.P.: The use of bioabsorbable implants to treat shoulder instability. Tech. Sports Med. 8:197-205, 2000.

Cooper, R.A., and Brems, J.J.: The inferior capsular shift procedure for multidirectional instability of the shoulder. J. Bone Joint Surg. [Am.] 74:1516-1521, 1992.

Grana, W.A., Buckley, P.D., and Yates, C.K.: Arthroscopic Bankart suture repair. Am. J. Sports Med. 21:348-353, 1993.

Harryman, D.T., II, Sidles, J.A., Harris, S.L., et al.: Laxity of the normal glenohumeral joint: A quantitative in vivo assessment. J. Shoulder Elbow Surg. 1:66-76, 1992.

Lippit, S., and Matsen, F.A., III: Mechanisms of glenohumeral joint stability. Clin. Orthop. 291:20-28, 1993.

Morgan, C.D., and Bodenstab, A.B.: Arthroscopic Bankart suture repair: Techniques and early results. Arthroscopy 3:111-112, 1982.

Neer, C.S., II, and Foster, C.R.: Inferior capsular shift for involuntary inferior and multidirectional instability of the shoulder: A preliminary report. J. Bone Joint Surg. [Am.] 62:897-908, 1980.

Pollock, R.G., and Bigliani, L.U.: Glenohumeral instability: Evaluation and treatment. J. Am. Acad. Orthop. Surg. 1:24-32, 1993.

Rowe, C.R., Patel, D., and Southmayd, W.W.: The Bankart procedure: A long-term end-result study. J. Bone Joint Surg. [Am.] 55:445-460, 1973.

Schenk, T.J., and Brems, J.J.: Multidirectional instability of the shoulder: Pathophysiology, diagnosis, and management. J. Am. Acad. Orthop. Surg. 6:65-72, 1998.

Turkel, S.J., Panio, M.W., Marshall, J.L., et al.: Stabilizing mechanisms preventing anterior dislocation of the glenohumeral joint. J. Bone Joint Surg. [Am.] 63:1208-1217, 1981.

Zuckerman, J.D., and Matsen, F.A., III: Complications about the glenohumeral joint related to the use of screws and staples. J. Bone Joint Surg. [Am.] 66:175-180, 1984.

IMPINGEMENT SYNDROME/ROTATOR CUFF

Bigliani, L.U., Cordasco, F.A., McIlveen, S.J., et al.: Operative treatment of failed repairs of the rotator cuff. J. Bone Joint Surg. [Am.] 74:1505-1515, 1992.

Bigliani, L.U., and Levine, W.N.: Current concepts review: Subacromial impingement syndrome. J. Bone Joint Surg. 79A:1854-1868, 1997.

Budoff, J.E., Nirschl, R.P., and Guidi, E.J.: Current concepts review: Débridement of partial-thickness tears of the rotator cuff without acromioplasty. J. Bone Joint Surg. 80A:733-748, 1998.

Caspari, R.B., and Thal, R.: A technique for arthroscopic subacromial decompression. Arthroscopy 8:23-20, 1992.

Cordasco, F.A., and Bigliani, L.U.: The treatment of failed rotator cuff repairs. AAOS Instr. Course Lect. 47:77-86, 1998.

Ellman, H., Kay, S.P., and Worth, M.: Arthroscopic treatment of full-thickness rotator cuff tears: Two to seven year follow-up study. Arthroscopy 9:301-314, 1993.

Flatow, E.L., and Warner, J.J.P.: Instability of the shoulder: Complex problems and failed repairs (part I). J. Bone Joint Surg. 80A:122-140, 1998.

Flatow, E.L., Miniaci, A., Evans, P.J., et al.: Instability of the shoulder: Complex problems and failed repairs (part II). J. Bone Joint Surg. 80A:284-298, 1998.

Gartsman, G.M.: Arthroscopic management of rotator cuff disease. J. Am. Acad. Orthop. Surg. 6:259-266, 1998.

Gerber, C., Terrier, F., and Ganz, R.: The role of the coracoid process in the chronic impingement syndrome. J. Bone Joint Surg. [Br.] 67:703-708, 1985.

Holsbeeck, E.: Subacromial impingement: Open versus arthroscopic decompression. Arthroscopy 8:173-178, 1992.

Ianotti, J.P.: Full-thickness rotator cuff tears: Factors affecting surgical outcome. J. Am. Acad. Orthop. Surg. 2:87-95, 1994.

McConville, O.R., and Iannotti, J.P.: Partial-thickness tears of the rotator cuff: Evaluation and management. J. Am. Acad. Orthop. Surg. 7:32-43, 1999.

Neer, C.S. II: Anterior acromioplasty for the chronic impingement syndrome in the shoulder. J. Bone Joint Surg. [Am.] 54:41-50, 1972.

Norberg, F.B., Field, L.D., and Savoie, F.H., III: Repair of the rotator cuff: Mini open and arthroscopic repairs. Clin. Sports Med. 19:77-99, 2000.

Rockwood, C.A., Jr., and Lyons, F.R.: Shoulder impingement syndrome: Diagnosis, radiographic evaluation, and treatment with a modified Neer acromioplasty. J. Bone Joint Surg. [Am.] 75:409-424, 1993.

Speer, K.P., Lohnes, J., and Garrett, W.C.: Arthroscopic subacromial decompression: Results in advanced impingement syndrome. Arthroscopy 7:291-296, 1991.

Williams, G.R.: Painful shoulder after surgery for rotator cuff disease. J. Am. Acad. Orthop. Surg. 5:97-108, 1997.

Zeman, C.A., Arcand, M.A., Cantrell, J.S., et al.: The rotator cuff-deficient arthritic shoulder: Diagnosis and surgical management. J. Am. Acad. Orthop. Surg. 6:337-348, 1998.

BICEPS INJURIES

Andrews, J., Carson, W., and McLeod, W.: Glenoid labrum tears related to the long head of the biceps. Am. J. Sports Med. 13:337-341, 1985.

Froimson, A.I., and Oh, I.: Keyhole tenodesis of biceps origin at the shoulder. Clin. Orthop. 112:245-249, 1974.

Gartsman, G.M., Hammerman, S.M.: Superior labrum, anterior and posterior lesions. Clin. Sports Med. 19:115-124, 2000.

Mileski, R.A., and Snyder, S.J.: Superior labral lesions in the shoulder: Pathoanatomy and surgical management. J. Am. Acad. Orthop. Surg. 6:121-131, 1998.

Resch, H., Golser, K., Thoeni, H., et al.: Arthroscopic repair of superior glenoid labral detachment (the SLAP lesion). J. Shoulder Elbow Surg. 2:147-155, 1993.

Snyder, S.J., and Wuh, H.C.K.: Arthroscopic evaluation and treatment of the rotator cuff and superior labrum anterior posterior lesion. Op. Tech. Orthop. 1:207-220, 1991.

Tennent, T.D., Beach, W.R., Meyers, J.F.: Clinical sports medicine update. A review of the special tests associated with shoulder examination: Part II: Laxity, instability, and superior labral anterior and posterior (SLAP) lesions. Am. J. Sports Med. 31:301-307, 2003.

ACROMIOCLAVICULAR AND STERNOCLAVICULAR INJURIES

Cahill, B.R.: Osteolysis of the distal part of the clavicle in male athletes. J. Bone Joint Surg. [Am.] 64:1053-1058, 1982.

Gartsman, G.M.: Arthroscopic resection of the acromioclavicular joint. Am. J. Sports Med. 21:71-77, 1993.

Lemos, M.J.: The evaluation and treatment of the injured acromioclavicular joint in athletes: Current concepts. Am. J. Sports Med. 26:137-144, 1998.

Nuber, G.W., and Bowen, M.K.: Acromioclavicular joint injuries and distal clavicle fractures. J. Am. Acad. Orthop. Surg. 5:11-18, 1997.

Richards, R.R.: Acromioclavicular joint injuries. Instr. Course Lect. 42:259-269, 1993.

Rockwood, C.A., Jr., and Young, D.C.: Disorders of the acromioclavicular joint. In Rockwood, C.A., Jr., and Matsen, F.A., III, eds.: The Shoulder, pp. 413-476. Philadelphia, WB Saunders, 1990.

Scavenius, M., and Iverson, B.F.: Nontraumatic clavicular osteolysis in weight lifters. Am. J. Sports Med. 20:463-467, 1992.

Wirth, M.A., and Rockwood, C.A., Jr.: Acute and chronic traumatic injuries of the sternoclavicular joint. J. Am. Acad. Orthop. Surg. 4:268-278, 1996.

MUSCLE RUPTURES

Caughey, M.A., and Welsh, P.: Muscle ruptures affecting the shoulder girdle. In Rockwood, C.A., Jr., and Matsen, F.A., III, eds.: The Shoulder, pp. 863-873. Philadelphia, WB Saunders, 1991.

Gerber, C., and Krushell, R.J.: Isolated rupture of the tendon of the subscapularis muscle. J. Bone Joint Surg. [Br.] 73:389-394, 1991.

Kretzler, H.H., Jr., and Richardson, A.B.: Rupture of the pectoralis major muscle. Am. J. Sports Med. 17:453-458, 1989.

Miller, M.D., Johnson, D.L., Fu, F.H., et al.: Rupture of the pectoralis major muscle in a collegiate football player. Am. J. Sports Med. 21:475-477, 1993.

Wolfe, S.W., Wickiewics, T.L., and Cananaugh, J.T.: Ruptures of the pectoralis major muscle: An anatomic and clinical analysis. Am. J. Sports Med. 20:587-593, 1992.

CALCIFIC TENDINITIS AND ADHESIVE CAPSULITIS

Ark, J.W., Flock, T.J., Flatow, E.L., et al.: Arthroscopic treatment of calcific tendinitis of the shoulder. Arthroscopy 8:183-188, 1992.

Coventry, M.B.: Problem of the painful shoulder. J.A.M.A. 151:177-185, 1953.

Faure, G., and Daculsi, G.: Calcified tendinitis: A review. Ann. Rheum. Dis. (Suppl) 42:49-53, 1983.

Grey, R.G.: The natural history of "idiopathic" frozen shoulder. J. Bone Joint Surg. [Am.] 60:564, 1978.

Harmon, H.P.: Methods and results in the treatment of 2580 painful shoulders: With special reference to calcific tendinitis and the frozen shoulder. Am. J. Surg. 95:527-544, 1958.

Harryman, D.T., II: Shoulders: Frozen and stiff. Instr. Course Lect. 42:247-257, 1993.

Leffert, R.E.: The frozen shoulder. Instr. Course Lect. 34:199-203, 1985.

Miller, M.D., Wirth, M.A., and Rockwood, C.A., Jr.: Thawing the frozen shoulder: The "patient" patient. Orthopedics (in press).

Murnaghan, J.P.: Adhesive capsulitis of the shoulder: Current concepts and treatment. Orthopaedics 2:153-158, 1988.

Murnaghan, J.P.: Frozen shoulder. In Rockwood, C.A., Jr., and Matsen, F.A., III, eds.: The Shoulder. Philadelphia, WB Saunders, 1990.

Neviaser, J.S.: Adhesive capsulitis and the stiff and painful shoulder. Orthop. Clin. North Am. 2:327-331, 1980.

Neviaser, T.J.: Adhesive capsulitis. In McGinty, J.B., ed.: Operative Arthroscopy, pp. 561-566. New York, Raven Press, 1991.

Neviaser, R.J., and Neviaser, T.J.: The frozen shoulder: Diagnosis and management. Clin. Orthop. 223:59-64, 1987.

Shaffer, B., Tibone, J.E., and Kerlan, R.K.: Frozen shoulder: A long-term follow-up. J. Bone Joint Surg. [Am.] 74:738-746, 1992.

Uthoff, H.K., and Loehr, J.W.: Calcific tendinopathy of the rotator cuff: Pathogenesis, diagnosis, and management. J. Am. Acad. Orthop. Surg. 5:183-191, 1997.

Warner, J.J.P.: Frozen shoulder: Diagnosis and management. J. Am. Acad. Orthop. Surg. 5:130-140, 1997.

Warner, J.J.P., and Greis, P.E.: The treatment of stiffness of the shoulder after repair of the rotator cuff. J. Bone Joint Surg. 79A:1260-1269, 1997.

NERVE DISORDERS

Black, K.P., and Lombardo, J.A.: Suprascapular nerve injuries with isolated paralysis of the infraspinatus. Am. J. Sports Med. 18:225, 1990.

Burkhead, W.Z., Scheinberg, R.R., and Box, G.: Surgical anatomy of the axillary nerve. J. Shoulder Elbow Surg. 1:31-36, 1992.

Drez, D.: Suprascapular neuropathy in the differential diagnosis of rotator cuff injuries. Am. J. Sports Med. 4:443, 1976.

Fechter, J.D., and Kuschner, S.H.: The thoracic outlet syndrome. Orthopedics 16:1243-1254, 1993.

Kauppila, L.I.: The long thoracic nerve: Possible mechanisms of injury based on autopsy study. J. Shoulder Elbow Surg. 2:244-248, 1993.

Leffert, R.D.: Neurological problems. In Rockwood, C.A., Jr., and Matsen, F.A., III, eds.: The Shoulder, pp. 750-773. Philadelphia, WB Saunders, 1990.

Leffert, R.D.: Thoracic outlet syndrome. J. Am. Acad. Orthop. Surg. 2:317-325, 1994.

Markey, K.L., DiBeneditto, M., and Curl, W.W.: Upper trunk brachial plexopathy: The stinger syndrome. Am. J. Sports Med. 23:650-655, 1993.

Marmor, L., and Bechtal, C.O.: Paralysis of the serratus anterior due to electric shock relieved by transplantation of the pectoralis major muscle. J. Bone Joint Surg. [Am.] 45:156-160, 1983.

Post, M., and Grinblat, E.: Suprascapular nerve entrapment: Diagnosis and results of treatment. J. Shoulder Elbow Surg. 2:190-197, 1993.

Vastamaki, M., and Kauppila, L.I.: Etiologic factors in isolated paralysis of the serratus anterior muscle: A report of 197 cases. J. Shoulder Elbow Surg. 2:244-248, 1993.

Warner, J.J.P., Krushell, R.J., Masquelet, A., et al.: Anatomy and relationships of the suprascapular nerve: Anatomical constraints to mobilization of the supraspinatus and infraspinatus muscles in the management of massive rotator cuff tears. J. Bone Joint Surg. [Am.] 74A:36-45, 1992.

OTHER SHOULDER DISORDERS

Carson, W.G., Gasser, S.I.: Little leaguer's elbow: A report of 23 cases. Am. J. Sports Med. 26:575-580, 1998.

Fees, M., Decker, T., Snyder-Mackler, L, et al.: Upper extremity weight-training modifications for the injured athlete: Current concepts. Am. J. Sports Med. 26:732-742, 1998.

Goss, T.P.: Scapular fractures and dislocations: Diagnosis and treatment. J. Am. Acad. Orthop. Surg. 3:22-33, 1995.

Green, A.: Current concepts of shoulder arthroplasty. AAOS Instr. Course Lect. 47:127-133, 1998.

Kuhn, J.E., Plancher, K.D., and Hawkins, R.J.: Scapular winging. J. Am. Acad. Orthop. Surg. 3:319-325, 1995.

Kuhn, J.E., Plancher, K.D., and Hawkins, R.J.: Symptomatic scapulothoracic crepitus and bursitis. J. Am. Acad. Orthop. Surg. 6:267-273, 1998.

Matthews, L.S., Wolock, B.S., and Martin, D.F.: Arthroscopic management of degenerative arthritis of the shoulder. In McGinty, J.B., ed.: Operative Arthroscopy, pp. 567-572. New York, Raven Press, 1991.

Miller, M.D., and Warner, J.J.P.: The abduction (weight bearing) radiograph of the shoulder. Poster. American Academy of Orthopaedic Surgeons 61st Annual Meeting, New Orleans, 1994.

Schlegel, T.F., and Hawkins, R.J.: Displaced proximal humeral fractures: Evaluation and treatment. J. Am. Acad. Orthop. Surg. 2:54-66, 1994.

Simpson, N.S., and Jupiter, J.B.: Clavicular nonunion and malunion: Evaluation and surgical management. J. Am. Acad. Orthop. Surg. 4:1-8, 1996.

ELBOW AND WRIST

GENERAL ELBOW

Ball, C.M., Galatz, L.M.; and Yamaguchi, K.: Elbow instability: treatment strategies and emerging concepts. Instr. Course Lect. 51:53-61, 2002.

Bradley, J.P., and Petrie, R.S.: Osteochondritis dissecans of the humeral capitellum. Diagnosis and treatment. Clin. Sports Med. 20(3):565-590, 2001.

Burra, G., and Andrews, J.R.: Acute shoulder and elbow dislocations in the athlete. Orthop. Clin. North Am. 33(3):479-495, 2002.

Ciccotti, M.G.: Epicondylitis in the athlete. Instr. Course Lect. 48:375-381, 1999.

Ciccotti, M.G., and Jobe, F.W.: Medial collateral ligament instability and ulnar neuritis in the athlete's elbow. Instr. Course Lect. 48:383-391, 1999.

Field, L.D., and Savoie, F.H.: Common elbow injuries in sport. Sports Med. 26(3):193-205, 1998.

Grana, W.: Medial epicondylitis and cubital tunnel syndrome in the throwing athlete. Clin. Sports Med. 20(3):541-548, 2001.

Izzi, J., Dennison, D., Noerdlinger, M., Dasilva, M., et al.: Nerve injuries of the elbow, wrist, and hand in athletes. Clin. Sports Med. 20(1):203-217, 2001.

Kelly, E.W., Morrey, B.F., and O'Driscoll, S.W.: Complications of elbow arthroscopy. J. Bone Joint Surg [Am.] 83-A(1):25-34, 2001.

Lee, D.H.: Posttraumatic elbow arthritis and arthroplasty. Orthop. Clin. North Am. 30(1):141-162, 1999.

Maloney, M.D., Mohr, K.J., and el Attrache, N.S.: Elbow injuries in the throwing athlete. Difficult diagnoses and surgical complications. Clin. Sports Med. 18(4):795-809, 1999.

Moskal, M.J.: Arthroscopic treatment of posterior impingement of the elbow in athletes. Clin. Sports Med. 20(1):11-24, 2001.

Norberg, F.B., Savoie, F.H., 3rd, and Field, L.D.: Arthroscopic treatment of arthritis of the elbow. Instr. Course Lect. 49:247-253, 2000.

Oka, Y.: Débridement arthroplasty for osteoarthrosis of the elbow: 50 patients followed mean 5 years. Acta Orthop. Scand. 71(2):185-190, 2000.

Ramsey, M.L.: Elbow arthroscopy: basic setup and treatment of arthritis. Instr. Course Lect. 51:69-72, 2002.

Reddy, A.S., Kvitne, R.S., Yocum, L.A., Elattrache, N.S., et al.: Arthroscopy of the elbow: A long-term clinical review. Arthroscopy 16(6):588-594, 2000.

Rettig, A.C.: Traumatic elbow injuries in the athlete. Orthop. Clin. North Am. 33(3):509-522, v, 2002.

Rettig, A.C., Sherrill, C., Snead, D.S., Mendler, J.C., et al.: Nonoperative treatment of ulnar collateral ligament injuries in throwing athletes. Am. J. Sports Med. 29(1):15-7, 2001.

Rizio, L., and Uribe, J.W.: Overuse injuries of the upper extremity in baseball. Clin. Sports Med. 20(3):453-468, 2001.

Savoie, F.H., 3rd, Nunley, P.D., and Field, L.D.: Arthroscopic management of the arthritic elbow: Indications, technique, and results. J. Shoulder Elbow Surg. 8(3):214-219, 1999.

Schickendantz, M.S.: Diagnosis and treatment of elbow disorders in the overhead athlete. Hand Clin. 18(1):65-75, 2002.

Sevier, T.L., and Wilson, J.K.: Treating lateral epicondylitis. Sports Med. 28(5):375-380, 1999.

Sofka, C.M., and Potter, H.G.: Imaging of elbow injuries in the child and adult athlete. Radiol. Clin. North Am. 40(2):251-265, 2002.

Stubbs, M.J., Field, L.D., and Savoie, F.H., 3rd: Osteochondritis dissecans of the elbow. Clin. Sports Med. 20(1):1-9, 2001.

GENERAL WRIST

Berger, R.A.: Arthroscopic anatomy of the wrist and distal radioulnar joint. Hand Clin. 15(3):393-413, vii, 1999.

Chou, C.H., and Lee, T.S.: Peripheral tears of triangular fibrocartilage complex: results of primary repair. Int. Orthop. 25(6):392-395, 2001.

Cober, S.R., and Trumble, T.E.: Arthroscopic repair of triangular fibrocartilage complex injuries. Orthop. Clin. North Am. 32(2):279-294, viii, 2001.

Dailey, S.W., and Palmer, A.K.: The role of arthroscopy in the evaluation and treatment of triangular fibrocartilage complex injuries in athletes. Hand Clin. 16(3):461-476, 2000.

De Smet, L.: Ulnar variance and its relationship to ligament injuries of the wrist. Acta Orthop. Belg. 65(4):416-417, 1999.

Geissler, W.B.: Carpal fractures in athletes. Clin. Sports Med. 20(1):167-188, 2001.

Grechenig, W., Peicha, G., Fellinger, M., Seibert, F.J., and Weiglein, A.H.: Anatomical and safety considerations in establishing portals used for wrist arthroscopy. Clin. Anat. 12(3):179-185, 1999.

Haims, A.H., Schweitzer, M.E., Morrison, W.B., Deely, D., et al.: Limitations of MR imaging in the diagnosis of peripheral tears of the triangular fibrocartilage of the wrist. AJR Am. J. Roentgenol, 178(2):419-422, 2002.

Hanker, G.J.: Radius fractures in the athlete. Clin. Sports Med. 20(1):189-201, 2001.

Hester, P.W., and Blazar, P.E.: Complications of hand and wrist surgery in the athlete. Clin. Sports Med. 18(4):811-829, 1999.

Izzi, J., Dennison, D., Noerdlinger, M., Dasilva, M., and Akelman, E.: Nerve injuries of the elbow, wrist, and hand in athletes. Clin. Sports Med. 20(1):203-217, 2001.

Kocher, M.S., Waters, P.M., and Micheli, L.J.: Upper extremity injuries in the paediatric athlete. Sports Med. 30(2):117-135, 2000.

Le, T.B., and Hentz, V.R.: Hand and wrist injuries in young athletes. Hand Clin. 16(4):597-607, 2000.

Mastey, R.D., Weiss, A.P., and Akelman, E.: Primary care of hand and wrist athletic injuries. Clin. Sports Med. 16(4):705-724, 1997.

Morgan, W.J., and Slowman, L.S.: Acute hand and wrist injuries in athletes: evaluation and management. J. Am. Acad. Orthop. Surg. 9(6):389-400, 2001.

Morley, J., Bidwell, J., and Bransby-Zachary, M.: A comparison of the findings of wrist arthroscopy and magnetic resonance imaging in the investigation of wrist pain. J. Hand Surg. [Br.], 26(6):544-546, 2001.

Nakamura, T., Takayama, S., Horiuchi, Y., and Yabe, Y.: Origins and insertions of the triangular fibrocartilage complex: a histological study. J. Hand Surg. [Br.] 26(5):446-454, 2001.

Potter, H.G., and Weiland, A.J.: Magnetic resonance imaging of triangular fibrocartilage complex lesions. J. Hand Surg. [Am.]. 27(2):363-364, author reply 364, 2002.

Shih, J.T., Lee, H.M., and Tan, C.M.: Early isolated triangular fibrocartilage complex tears: Management by arthroscopic repair. J. Trauma. 53(5):922-927, 2002.

Stamos, B.D., and Leddy, J.P.: Closed flexor tendon disruption in athletes. Hand Clin. 16(3):359-365, 2000.

Strickland, J.W.: Considerations for the treatment of the injured athlete. Clin. Sports Med. 17(3):397-400, 1998.

Tomaino, M.M., and Weiser, R.W.: Combined arthroscopic TFCC débridement and wafer resection of the distal ulna in wrists with triangular fibrocartilage complex tears and positive ulnar variance. J. Hand Surg. [Am.]. 26(6):1047-1052, 2001.

Treihaft, M.M.: Neurologic injuries in baseball players. Semin. Neurol. 20(2):187-193, 2000.

Westkaemper, J.G., Mitsionis, G., Giannakopoulos, P.N., and Sotereanos, D.G.: Wrist arthroscopy for the treatment of ligament and triangular fibrocartilage complex injuries. Arthroscopy. 14(5):479-483, 1998.

TENDON INJURIES OF THE ELBOW AND WRIST

Boyd, H.B., and Anderson, L.D.: A method for reinsertion of the distal biceps brachii tendon. J. Bone Joint Surg. [Am.] 43:1041-1043, 1961.

Boyd, H.B., and McLeod, A.C.: Tennis elbow. J. Bone Joint Surg. [Am.] 55:1183, 1973.

Burhkhart, S.S., Wood, M.B., and Linscheid, R.L.: Posttraumatic recurrent subluxation of the extensor carpi ulnaris tendon. J. Hand Surg. 7:1, 1982.

Conrad, R.W.: Tennis elbow. Instr. Course Lect. 35:94-101, 1986.

D'Alessandro, D.F., Shields, C.L., Tibone, J.E., et al.: Repair of distal biceps tendon ruptures in athletes. Am. J. Sports Med. 21:114, 1993.

Froimson, A.I.: Treatment of tennis elbow with forearm support band. J. Bone Joint Surg. [Am.] 53:183, 1971.

Gabel, G.T., and Morrey, B.F.: Tennis elbow. AAOS Instr. Course Lect. 47:165-172, 1998.

Green, D.P., and Strickland, J.W.: The hand. In DeLee, J.C., and Drez, D., Jr., eds.: Orthopaedic Sports Medicine, pp. 945-1017. Philadelphia, WB Saunders, 1993.

Ilfeld, F.W.: Can stroke modification relieve tennis elbow? Clin. Orthop. 276:182-185, 1992.

Jobe, F.W., and Ciccotti, M.G.: Lateral and medial epicondylitis of the elbow. J. Am. Acad. Orthop. Surg. 2:1-8, 1994.

Kiefhaber, T.R., and Stern, P.J.: Upper extremity tendinitis and overuse syndromes in the athlete. Clin. Sports Med. 11:39-55, 1992.

Leddy, J.P.: Soft tissue injuries of the hand in the athlete. AAOS Instr. Course Lect. 47:181-186, 1998.

Leddy, J.P., and Packer, J.W.: Avulsion of the profundus tendon insertion in athletes. J. Hand Surg. 2:66-69, 1977.

Morrey, B.F.: Reoperation of failed surgical treatment of refractory lateral epicondylitis. J. Shoulder Elbow Surg. 1:47-55, 1992.

Moss, J.G., and Steingold, R.F.: The long-term results of mallet finger injury: A retrospective study of one hundred cases. Hand 15:151-154, 1983.

Nirschl, R.P.: Sports and overuse injuries to the elbow. In Morrey, B.F., ed.: The Elbow and Its Disorders, 2nd ed., pp. 537-552. Philadelphia, WB Saunders, 1993.

Nirschl, R.P., and Pettrone, F.: Tennis elbow: The surgical treatment of lateral epicondylitis. J. Bone Joint Surg. [Am.] 61:832, 1979.

Regan, W., Wold, L.E., Conrad, R., and Morrey, B.F.: Microscopic histopathology of chronic refractory lateral epicondylitis. Am. J. Sports Med. 20:746-749, 1992.

Rettig, A.C.: Closed tendon injuries of the hand and wrist in the athlete. Clin. Sports Med. 11:77-99, 1992.

Strickland, J.W.: Management of acute flexor tendon injuries. Orthop. Clin. North Am. 14:827-849, 1983.

Tarsney, F.F.: Rupture and avulsion of the triceps. Clin. Orthop. 83:177-183, 1972.

Wood, M.B., and Dobyns, J.H.: Sports-related extraarticular wrist syndromes. Clin. Orthop. 202:93-102, 1986.

LIGAMENTOUS INJURIES OF THE ELBOW AND WRIST

Alexander, C.E., and Lichtman, D.M.: Ulnar carpal instabilities. Orthop. Clin. North Am. 15:307-320, 1984.

Bednar, J.M., and Osterman, A.L.: Carpal instability: Evaluation and treatment. J. Am. Acad. Orthop. Surg. 1:10-17, 1993.

Bennett, J.B., Green, M.S., and Tullos, H.S.: Surgical management of chronic medial elbow instability. Clin. Orthop. 278:62-68, 1992.

Berger, R.A.: Radial-sided carpal instability. AAOS Instr. Course Lect. 47:219-228, 1998.

Betz, R.R., Browne, E.Z., Perry, G.B., et al.: The complex volar metacarpophalangeal-joint dislocation. J. Bone Joint Surg. [Am.] 64:1374-1375, 1982.

Campbell, C.S.: Gamekeepers thumb. J. Bone Joint Surg. [Br.] 37:148-149, 1955.

Conway, J.E., Jobe, F.W., Glousman, R.E., et al.: Medial instability of the elbow in throwing athletes: Surgical treatment by ulnar collateral ligament repair or reconstruction. J. Bone Joint Surg. [Am.] 74:67, 1992.

Cooney, W.P., III, Linscheid, R.L., and Dobyns, J.H.: Carpal instability: Treatment of ligament injuries of the wrist. Instr. Course Lect. 41:33-44, 1992.

Eaton, R.G., and Malerich, M.M.: Volar plate arthroplasty of the proximal interphalangeal joint: A review of ten years' experience. J. Hand Surg. 5:260-268, 1980.

Green, D.P., and Strickland, J.W.: The hand. In DeLee, J.C., and Drez, D., Jr., eds.: Orthopaedic Sports Medicine, pp. 945-1017. Philadelphia, WB Saunders, 1993.

Habernek, H., and Ortner, F.: The influence of anatomic factors in elbow joint dislocation. Clin. Orthop. 274:226-230, 1992.

Heyman, P.: Injuries to the ulnar collateral ligament of the thumb metacarpophalangeal joint. J. Am. Acad. Orthop. Surg. 5:224-229, 1997.

Hinterman, B., Holzach, P.J., Schultz, M., et al.: Skier's thumb: The significance of bony injuries. Am. J. Sports Med. 21:800-804, 1993.

Isani, A., and Melone, C.P., Jr.: Ligamentous injuries of the hand in athletes. Clin. Sports Med. 5:757-772, 1986.

Jobe, F.W., and Kvitne, R.S.: Elbow instability in the athlete. Instr. Course Lect. 40:17, 1991.

Kaplan, E.B.: Dorsal dislocation of the metacarpophalangeal joint of the index finger. J. Bone Joint Surg. [Am.] 39:1081-1086, 1957.

Kozin, S.H.: Perilunate injuries: Diagnosis and treatment. J. Am. Acad. Orthop. Surg. 6:114-120, 1998.

Light, T.R.: Buttress pinning techniques. Orthop. Rev. 10:49-55, 1981.

Lubahn, J.D., and Cermak, M.B.: Uncommon nerve compression syndromes of the upper extremity. J. Am. Acad. Orthop. Surg. 6:378-386, 1998.

McCue, F.C., and Bruce, J.F.: The wrist. In DeLee, J.C., and Drez, D., Jr., eds.: Orthopaedic Sports Medicine, pp. 913-944. Philadelphia, WB Saunders, 1993.

McElfresh, E.C., Dobyns, J.H., and O'Brien, E.T.: Management of fracture-dislocation of the proximal interphalangeal joints by extension-block splinting. J. Bone Joint Surg. [Am.] 54:1705-1711, 1972.

McLaughlin, H.L.: Complex "locked" dislocation of the metacarpalphalangeal joints. J. Trauma 5:683-688, 1965.

Miller, C.D., and Savoie, F.H., III: Valgus extension injuries of the elbow in the throwing athlete. J. Am. Acad. Orthop. Surg. 2:261-269, 1994.

Morrey, B.F.: Acute and chronic instability of the elbow. J. Am. Acad. Orthop. Surg. 4:117-128, 1996.

Morrey, B.F.: Complex instability of the elbow. J. Bone Joint Surg. 79A:460-469, 1997.

O'Driscoll, S.W., and Morrey, B.F.: Arthroscopy of the elbow: Diagnostic and therapeutic benefits and hazards. J. Bone Joint Surg. [Am.] 74:84-94, 1992.

O'Driscoll, S.W., Morrey, B.F., Korinek, S., et al.: Elbow subluxation and dislocation: A spectrum of instability. Clin. Orthop. 280:17-28, 1992.

Palmer, A.K., and Louis, D.S.: Assessing ulnar instability of the metacarpophalangeal joint of the thumb. J. Hand Surg. 3:542-546, 1978.

Redler, I., and Williams, J.T.: Rupture of a collateral ligament of the proximal interphalangeal joint of the fingers: Analysis of eighteen cases. J. Bone Joint Surg. [Am.] 49:322-326, 1967.

Short, W.H.: Wrist instability. AAOS Instr. Course Lect. 47:203-208, 1998.

Stener, B.: Displacement of the ruptured collateral ligament of the metacarpophalangeal joint of the thumb: A clinical and anatomical study. J. Bone Joint Surg. [Br.] 44:869-879, 1962.

Viegas, S.F.: Ulnar-sided wrist pain and instability. AAOS Instr. Course Lect. 47:215-218, 1998.

Watson, H.K., and Ballet, F.L.: The SLAC wrist: Scapholunate advanced collapse pattern of degenerative arthritis. J. Hand Surg. 9A:358-365, 1984.

Wilson, F.D., Andrews, J.R., Blackburn, T.A., et al.: Valgus extension overload in the pitching elbow. Am. J. Sports Med. 11:83, 1983.

ARTICULAR INJURIES OF THE ELBOW AND WRIST

Armstead, R.B., Linscheid, R.L., Dobyns, J.H., et al.: Ulnar lengthening in the treatment of Kienbock's disease. J. Bone Joint Surg. [Am.] 64:170-178, 1982.

Aulicino, P.L., and Siegel, L.: Acute injuries of the distal radioulnar joint. Hand Clin. 7:283-293, 1991.

Bauer, M., Jonsson, K., Josefsson, P.O., and Linden, B.: Osteochondritis dissecans of the elbow: A long-term follow-up study. Clin. Orthop. 284:156-160, 1992.

Bennett, J.B.: Articular injuries in the athlete. In Morrey, B.F., ed.: The Elbow and Its Disorders, 2nd ed., pp. 581–595. Philadelphia, WB Saunders, 1993.

DeHaven, K.E., and Evarts, C.M.: Throwing injuries of the elbow in athletes. Orthop. Clin. North Am. 1:801, 1973.

Dell, P.C.: Traumatic disorders of the distal radioulnar joint. Clin. Sports Med. 11:141–159, 1991.

Gelberman, R.H., Salamon, P.B., Jurist, J.M., et al.: Ulnar variance in Kienbock's disease. J. Bone Joint Surg. [Am.] 57:674–676, 1975.

Morrey, B.F.: Primary arthritis of the elbow treated by ulno-humeral arthroplasty. J. Bone Joint Surg. [Br.] 74:409, 1992.

Murakami, S., and Nakajima, H.: Aseptic necrosis of the capitate bone. Am. J. Sports Med. 12:170–173, 1984.

Nalebuff, E.A., Poehling, G.G., Siegel, D.B., et al.: Wrist and hand: Reconstruction. In Frymoyer, J.W., ed.: Orthopaedic Knowledge Update 4 Home Study Syllabus, pp. 389–402. Rosemont, IL, American Academy of Orthopaedic Surgeons, 1993.

Osterman, A.L.: Arthroscopic débridement of triangular fibrocartilage complex tears. Arthroscopy 6:120–124, 1990.

Palmer, A.K.: Triangular fibrocartilage disorders: Injury patterns and treatment. Arthroscopy 6:125–132, 1990.

Singer, K.M., and Roy, S.P.: Osteochondrosis of the humeral capitellum. Am. J. Sports Med. 12:351–360, 1984.

Watson, H.K., Ryu, J., and DiBella, W.S.: An approach to Kienbock's disease: Triscaphe arthrodesis. J. Hand Surg. 10A:179–187, 1985.

Woodward, A.H., and Bianco, A.J.: Osteochondritis dissecans of the elbow. Clin. Orthop. 110:35, 1975.

ARTHROSCOPY OF THE ELBOW AND WRIST

Adams, B.D.: Endoscopic carpal tunnel release. J. Am. Acad. Orthop. Surg. 2:179–184, 1994.

Andrews, J.R., and Carson, W.G.: Arthroscopy of the elbow. Arthroscopy 1:97, 1985.

Boe, S.: Arthroscopy of the elbow: Diagnosis and extraction of loose bodies. Acta Orthop. Scand. 57:52, 1986.

Carson, W.: Arthroscopy of the elbow. Instr. Course Lect. 37:195, 1988.

Chidgey, L.K.: The distal radioulnar joint: Problems and solutions. J. Am. Acad. Orthop. Surg. 3:95–108, 1995.

Cooney, W.P., Dobyns, J.H., and Linscheid, R.L.: Arthroscopy of the wrist: Anatomy and classification of carpal instability. Arthroscopy 6:133–140, 1990.

Guhl, J.: Arthroscopy and arthroscopic surgery of the elbow. Orthopedics 8:1290, 1985.

Lindenfeld, T.N.: Medial approach in elbow arthroscopy. Am. J. Sports Med. 18:413–417, 1990.

Lynch, G., Meyers, J., Whipple, T., et al.: Neurovascular anatomy and elbow arthroscopy: Inherent risks. Arthroscopy 2:191, 1986.

Osterman, A.L.: Arthroscopic débridement of triangular fibrocartilage complex tears. Arthroscopy 6:120–124, 1990.

Poehling, G.G., Siegel, D.B., Koman, L.A., et al.: Arthroscopy of the wrist and elbow. In DeLee, J.C., and Drez, D., Jr., eds.: Orthopaedic Sports Medicine, pp. 189–214. Philadelphia, WB Saunders, 1993.

Roth, J.H., Poehling, G.G., and Whipple, T.L.: Arthroscopic surgery of the wrist. Instr. Course Lect. 37:183–194, 1988.

Whipple, T.L.: Diagnostic and surgical arthroscopy of the wrist. In Nichols, J.A., and Hershman, E.B., eds.: The Upper Extremity in Sports Medicine, pp. 399–418. St. Louis, C.V. Mosby, 1990.

OTHER UPPER EXTREMITY PROBLEMS

O'Driscoll, S.W.: Elbow arthritis: Treatment options. J. Am. Acad. Orthop. Surg. 2:106–116, 1993.

Rettig, A.C.: Fractures in the hand in athletes. AAOS Instr. Course Lect. 47:187–190, 1998.

Simonian, P.T., and Trumble, T.E.: Scaphoid nonunion. J. Am. Acad. Orthop. Surg. 2:185–191, 1994.

Szabo, R.M., and Steinberg, D.R.: Nerve entrapment syndromes in the wrist. J. Am. Acad. Orthop. Surg. 2:115–123, 1994.

HEAD AND SPINE INJURIES

HEAD INJURIES

Bruno, L.A.: Focal intracranial hematoma. In Torg, J.S., ed.: Athletic Injuries to the Head, Neck and Face, 2nd ed. St. Louis, Mosby–Year Book, 1991.

Cantu, R.C.: Criteria for return to competition after a closed head injury. In Torg, J.S., ed.: Athletic Injuries to the Head, Neck and Face, 2nd ed., St. Louis, Mosby–Year Book, 1991.

Cantu, R.C.: Guidelines to return to sports after cerebral concussion. Phys. Sports Med. 14:76, 1986.

Gennarelli, T.A.: Head injury mechanisms, and cerebral concussion and diffuse brain injuries. In Torg, J.S., ed.: Athletic Injuries to the Head, Neck and Face, 2nd ed. St. Louis: Mosby–Year Book, 1991.

Jordan, B.D., Tsairis, P., and Warren, R.F.: Sports Neurology. Rockville, MD, Aspen Press, 1989.

Lindsay, K.W., McLatchie, G., Jennett, B.: Serious head injuries in sports. B.M.J. 281:789–791, 1980.

Wojtys, E., Hovda, D., et al.: Current concepts: Concussion in sports. Am. J. Sports Med. 27:676–687, 1999.

CERVICAL SPINE INJURIES

Albright, J.P., Moses, J.M., Feldich, H.G., et al.: Non-fatal cervical spine injuries in interscholastic football. J.A.M.A. 236:1243–1245, 1976.

Bracken, M.D., Shepard, M.J., Collins, W.F., et al.: A randomized, controlled trial of methylprednisolone or naloxone in the treatment of acute spinal cord injury. N. Engl. J. Med. 322:1405, 1990.

Pavlov, H., Torg, J.S., Robie, B., et al.: Cervical spinal stenosis: Determination with vertebral body radio method. Radiology 164:771–775, 1987.

Thompson, R.C.: Current concepts in management of cervical spine fractures and dislocations. Am. J. Sports Med. 3:159, 1975.

Torg, J.S., and Gennarelli, T.A.: Head and cervical spine injuries. In DeLee, J.C., and Drez, D., Jr., eds.: Orthopaedic Sports Medicine: Principles and Practice, pp. 417–462. Philadelphia, WB Saunders, 1994.

Torg, J.S., Pavlov, H., Genuario, S.E., et al.: Neuropraxia of the cervical spinal cord with transient quadriplegia. J. Bone Joint Surg. [Am.] 68:1354–1370, 1986.

Torg, J.S., Sennett, B., Pavlov, H., et al.: Spear tackler's spine: An entity precluding participation in tackle football and collision activities that expose the cervical spine to axial energy inputs. Am. J. Sports Med. 21:640–649, 1993.

Torg, J.S., Sennett, B., Vegso, J.J., et al.: Axial loading injuries to the middle cervical spine segment: An analysis and classification of twenty-five cases. Am. J. Sports Med. 19:6–20, 1991.

Torg, J.S., Vegso, J.J., O'Neill, J., et al.: The epidemiologic, pathologic, biomechanical and cinematographic analysis of football-induced cervical spine trauma. Am. J. Sports Med. 18:50–57, 1990.

Waninger, K.: On field management of potential cervical spine injury in helmeted football players: Leave the helmet on! Clin. J. Sports Med. 8:124–129, 1998.

White, A.A., Johnson, R.M., and Panjabi, M.M.: Biomechanical analysis of clinical stability in the cervical spine. Clin. Orthop. 109:85–93, 1975.

THORACIC AND LUMBAR SPINE INJURIES

Bradford, D.S., and Boachie-Adjei, O.: Treatment of severe spondylolisthesis by anterior and posterior reduction and stabilization: A long-term follow-up study. J. Bone Joint Surg. [Am.] 72:1060, 1990.

Eismont, F.J., and Currier, B.: Surgical management of lumbar intervertebral disc disease. J. Bone Joint Surg. [Am.] 71:1266, 1989.

Eismont, F.J., and Kitchel, S.H.: Thoracolumbar spine. In DeLee, J.C., and Drez, D., Jr., eds.: Orthopaedic Sports Medicine, pp. 1018–1062. Philadelphia, WB Saunders, 1994.

Jackson, D., Wiltse, L., Dingeman, R., et al.: Stress reactions involving the pars interarticularis in young athletes. Am. J. Sports Med. 9:305, 1981.

Keene, J.S., Albert, M.J., Springer, S.L., et al.: Back injuries in college athletes. J. Spinal Disord. 2:190–195, 1989.

Mundt, D.J., Kelsey, J.L., Golden, A.L., et al.: An epidemiological study of sports and weightlifting as possible risk factors for herniated lumbar and cervical discs. Am. J. Sports Med. 21:854–860, 1993.

MEDICAL ASPECTS

DRUGS

Beiner, J.M., Jokl P., Cholewicki, J., et al.: The effect of anabolic steroids and corticosteroids on healing of muscle contusion injury. Am. J. Sports Med. 27:2–9, 1999.

Berger, R.G.: Nonsteroidal anti-inflammatory drugs: Making the right choices. J. Am. Acad. Orthop. Surg. 2:255–260, 1994.

Fadale, P.D., and Wiggins, M.E.: Corticosteroid injections: Their use and abuse. J. Am. Acad. Orthop. Surg. 2:133–140, 1994.

ERGOGENIC DRUGS

Aronson, V.: Protein and miscellaneous ergogenic aids. Physician Sports Med. 14:209–212, 1986.

Brien, A.J., and Simon, T.L.: The effects of red blood cell infusion on 10-km race time. J.A.M.A. 257:2761, 1987.

Cowart, V.S.: Human growth hormone: The latest ergogenic aid? Physician Sports Med. 16:175, 1988.

Haupt, H.A.: Anabolic steroids and growth hormone: Current concepts. Am. J. Sports Med. 21:468–474, 1993.

Perlmutter, G., and Lowenthal, D.T.: Use of anabolic steroids by athletes. Am. Fam. Physician 32:208, 1985.

Pope, H.G., Katz, D.L., and Champoux, R.: Anabolic-androgenic steroid use among 1,010 college men. Physician Sports Med. 16:75, 1988.

Robinson, J.B.: Ergogenic drugs in sports. In DeLee, J.C., and Drez, D., Jr., eds.: Orthopaedic Sports Medicine, pp. 294–306. Philadelphia, WB Saunders, 1994.

CARDIOVASCULAR

Abraham, P., Chevalier, J-M, Leftheriotis, G., et al.: Lower extremity arterial disease in sports. Am. J. Sports Med. 25:581–584, 1997.

Alpert, S.A., et al.: Athletic heart syndrome. Physician Sports Med. 12:103–107, 1989.

Basilico, F.C.: Cardiovascular disease in athletes: Current concepts. Am. J. Sports Med. 27:108–121, 1999.

Braden, D.S., and Strong, W.B.: Preparticipation screening for sudden cardiac death in high school and college athletes. Physician Sports Med. 16:128–140, 1988.

Finney, T.P., and D'Ambrosia, R.D.: Sudden cardiac death in an athlete. In DeLee, J.C., and Drez, D., Jr., eds.: Orthopaedic Sports Medicine, pp. 404–416. Philadelphia, WB Saunders, 1994.

James, T.N., Froggatt, P., and Marshall, T.K.: Sudden death in young athletes. Ann. Intern. Med. 67:1013–1021, 1967.

Maron, B.J., Epstein, S.E., and Roberts, W.C.: Causes of sudden death in competitive athletes. J. Am. Coll. Cardiol. 7:204–214, 1986.

Maron, B.J., Roberts, W.C., McAllister, H.A., et al.: Sudden death in young athletes. Circulation 62:218–229, 1980.

Van Camp, S.P.: Exercise-related sudden deaths: Risks and causes. Physician Sports Med. 16:97–112, 1988.

EXERCISE PHYSIOLOGY

Almekinders, L.C., and Oman, J.: Isokinetic muscle testing: It is clinically useful? J. Am. Acad. Orthop. Surg. 2:221–225, 1994.

Cahill, B.R., Misner, J.E., and Boileau, R.A.: The clinical importance of the anaerobic energy system and its assessment in human performance: Current concepts. Am. J. Sports Med. 25:863–872, 1997.

Fleck, S.J., and Schutt, R.C.: Types of strength training. Clin. Sports Med. 4:159–168, 1985.

Galloway M., and Jikl, P.: Aging successfully: The importance of physical activity in maintaining health and function. J. Am. Acad. Orthop. Surg. 8:37–44, 2000.

Katch, F.I., and Drumm, S.S.: Effects of different modes of strength training on body composition and arthropometry. Clin. Sports Med. 5:413–459, 1986.

Kirkendall, D.T., and Garrett, W.E., Jr.: The effects of aging and training on skeletal muscle: Current concepts. Am. J. Sports Med. 26:598–602, 1998.

Latzka W., and Montain S.: Water and electrolyte requirements for exercise. Clin. Sports Med. 18:513–524, 1999.

Lephart, S.M., Pincivero, D.M., Giraldo, J.L., et al.: The role of proprioception in the management and rehabilitation of athletic injuries. Am. J. Sports Med. 25:130–137, 1997.

Paulos, L.E., and Grauer, J.D.: Exercise. In DeLee, J.C., and Drez, D., Jr., eds.: Orthopaedic Sports Medicine: Principles and Practice, pp. 228–243. Philadelphia, WB Saunders, 1994.

Pipes, T.V.: Isokinetic vs isotonic strength training an adult men. Med. Sci. Sports 7:262–274, 1975.

Taylor, D.C., Dalton, J.D., Seaber, A.V., et al.: Viscoelastic properties of muscle-tendon units: The biomechanical effects of stretching. Am. J. Sports Med. 18:300–309, 1990.

Yamamoto, S.K., Hartman, C.W., Feagin, J.A., et al.: Functional rehabilitation of the knee: A preliminary study. J. Sports Med. 3:228–291, 1976.

FEMALE ATHLETES

Barrow, G., and Saha, S.: Menstrual irregularity and stress fractures in collegiate female distance runners. Am. J. Sports Med. 16:209–215, 1988.

Eisenberg, T., and Allen, W.: Injuries in a women's varsity athletic program. Physician Sports Med. 6:112–116, 1978.

Hunter, L., Andrews, J., Clancy, W., et al.: Common orthopaedic problems of the female athlete. Instr. Course Lect. 31:126–152, 1982.

Otis, C., Drinkwater, B., et al.: American College of Sportsmedicine position stand: The female athlete triad. Med. Sci. Sports Exerc. 29:1–9, 1997

Powers, J.: Characteristic features of injuries in the knee in women. Clin. Orthop. 143:120–124, 1979.

Protzman, R.: Physiologic performance of women compared to men: Observations of cadets at the United States Military Academy. Am. J. Sports Med. 7:191–194, 1979.

Tietz, C.C., Hu, S.S., and Arendt, E.A.: The female athlete: Evaluation and treatment of sports-related problems. J. Am. Acad. Orthop. Surg. 5:87–96, 1997.

Voss, L.A., Fadale, P.D., and Hulstyn, M.J.: Exercise-induced loss of bone density in athletes. J. Am. Acad. Orthop. Surg. 6:349–357, 1998.

Whiteside, P.: Men's and women's injuries in comparable sports. Physician Sports Med. 8:130–140, 1980.

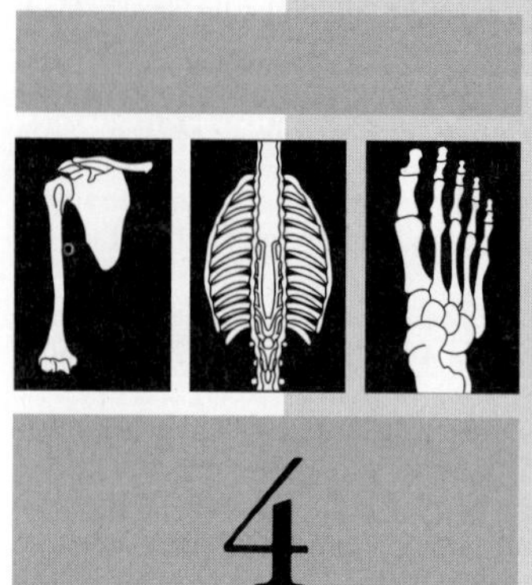

4 Adult Reconstruction

EDWARD J. MCPHERSON

I. Hip Replacement Surgery

A. Fixation—Total Hip Replacement. The method of long-term fixation of component parts for prosthetic joint replacement is either with cement or biologic interdigitation of bone to the prosthetic interface. The stated reasoning for the trend toward noncemented fixation in total hip replacement (THR) is the reported higher rates of loosening in young active patients. It is thought that the increased cycles and higher stresses applied to the hip joint in young, more active patients lead to a more rapid failure of cemented components.

1. Cement Fixation—With cement fixation, there is mechanical interlock of methylmethacrylate to the interstices of bone, which is static. If microfractures occur with continued cyclic loading, the cement cannot remodel and will ultimately loosen. In contrast, with noncemented components, there is a biologic fixation to the prosthesis that is dynamic. If microfractures occur with cyclic loading in this system, there is the potential for bone remodeling. This produces a potentially life-lasting bond. Furthermore, removing cement from the system provides one less interface that can fail.
2. Biologic Fixation—The methods of biologic fixation are either by a porous-coated metallic surface that provides bone *ingrowth* fixation or by a grit-blasted metallic surface that provides bone *ongrowth* fixation.
   a. With a porous-coated surface, pores are created on the metallic surface that allow bone to grow in and secure the prosthesis to host bone. Successful bone ingrowth requires an optimum *pore size* from 50 to 350 μm (preferably 50–150 μm). *Porosity* of the porous-coated surface is important to allow bone to fill into a significant area of the prosthesis, and it should be 40–50%. Increased porosity above this is detrimental, because the porous-coated surface would be at risk of shearing off. In addition, *pore depth* is a factor in the strength of the bone-prosthetic interlock. A deeper pore depth into the prosthesis provides greater interface shear strength with loading. Finally, *gaps* between the prosthesis and bone must be kept less than 50 μm.
   b. Grit Blasting. With a grit-blasted surface, a metallic surface is roughened with an abrasive spray of particles that pits the metallic surface. The resultant peaks and valleys in the metal surface provide areas for bone to interdigitate and provide a stable construct. With this method, the success of the bone ongrowth fixation is related to *surface roughness*. Surface roughness is defined as the average distance from peak to valley on the roughened surface. An increasing surface roughness is directly related to an increase in interface shear strength. The drawback of a grit-blasted surface is that bone fixation occurs only on the surface and therefore requires a more extensive area of coating to secure the prosthesis. Typically, the entire prosthesis needs to be grit-blasted to ensure adequate fixation.
3. Techniques of Fixation
   a. Rigid Fixation. Successful bone ingrowth or ongrowth requires initial rigid fixation. Micromotion of the prosthesis must be kept below 150 μm (preferably 50–100 μm) or the prosthesis will be secured only by fibrous tissue (fibrous ingrowth). This will allow continued prosthetic micromotion and pain. If gross motion is allowed, the prosthesis will be encapsulated with fibrous tissue rather than fibrous ingrowth, and this will cause the prosthesis to settle and remain mechanically unstable. The technique for

insertion of noncemented components, therefore, is very important. *Initial rigid fixation* of porous-coated implants is usually accomplished by the *press-fit technique*, in which the bone prepared for the acetabular cup or the femoral stem is sized slightly smaller in diameter (usually 1–2 mm undersized). When the component is inserted, the bone expands around the prosthesis, generating *hoop stresses* that keep the prosthesis in position and minimize micromotion. The other technique is a *line-to-line* fit in which the bone is prepared to the same size as the implant and is secured with additional measures. In the cup, a line-to-line technique requires screws for additional fixation. For the femoral stem, an extensive porous coating along the entire stem is required to obtain an interference fit. This provides a rough surface over a large area and prevents excessive motion.

b. Cortical Bone Seating. Another important factor for stable bone ingrowth is to have the implant seated against cortical bone rather than cancellous bone. Although cancellous bone will provide bone ingrowth, it is now known that the mechanical strength of an implant seated onto cortical bone is much stronger. Therefore in the acetabulum it is important to achieve a good cortical rim fit of the acetabular cup. On the femoral side, it is important that the implant design and surgical preparation allow for cortical contact with the porous-coated or grit-blasted surface.

c. Surface Coating. Hydroxyapatite (HA) has been used as an adjuvant surface coating on porous-coated and grit-blasted surfaces. HA is an *osteoconductive* agent that allows for more rapid closure of gaps. The HA surface readily receives osteoblasts, and thus it provides a bidirectional closure of gaps (i.e., bone to prosthesis and prosthesis to bone). HA has been reported to delaminate off the prosthetic interface, and its use may be better suited to porous-coated surfaces where the bone-HA bond is not the sole means of fixation. Successful use of HA as an adjuvant surface coating requires high *crystallinity* and optimal thickness (approximately 50 μm).

d. Extent of Porous Coating. The recommended amount of porous coating on a femoral stem is controversial. With proximal porous coating, the porous surface is kept in the metaphyseal and upper metadiaphyseal regions of the femur. With this design concept, proximal bone ingrowth allows proximal bone loading and less stress shielding (Fig. 4-1). Conversely, an extensively coated stem has a porous coating over its entire surface. Most bone ingrowth occurs in the diaphysis, and the weight-bearing forces bypass the proximal femur. The classic radiographic finding of a well-fixed extensively porous-coated stem is the *spot weld.* Radiographically, increased bone density is seen surrounding the distal extent of the porous coating (but *not* below the tip). As a result, the proximal femur is stress-shielded,

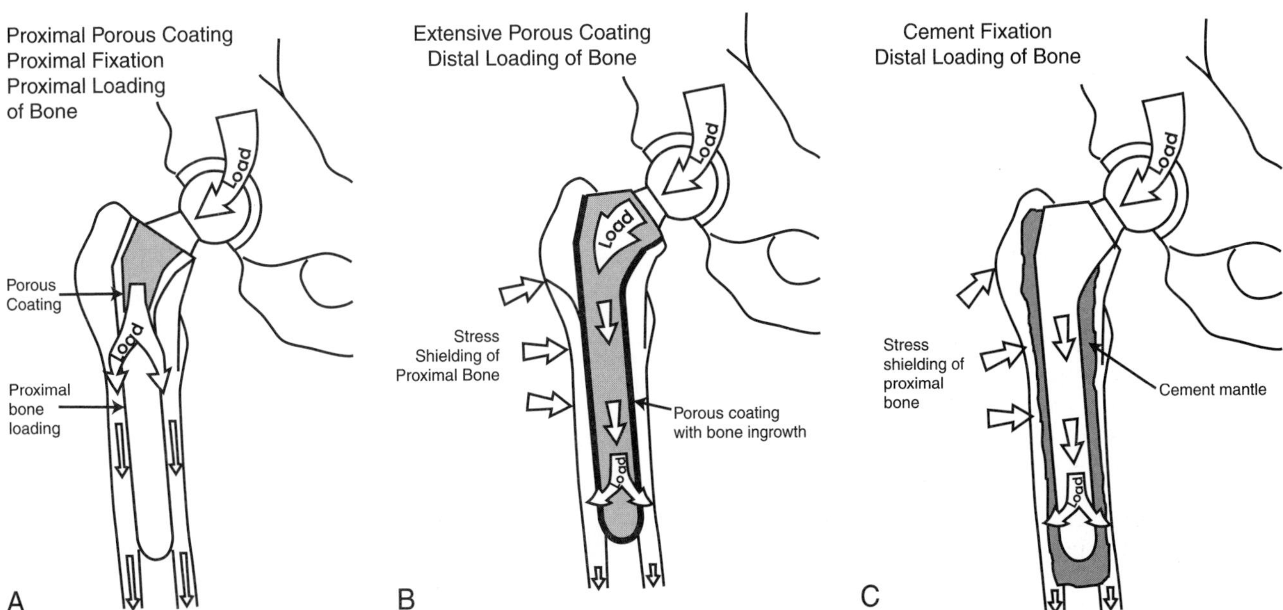

FIGURE 4-1 ■ Diagram of bone loading in relation to femoral stem fixation. *A*, Proximal porous coating, no cement. *B*, Extensive porous coating, no cement. *C*, Cement.

leading to loss of bone density. Although stress shielding has been noted in the clinical setting, this observation has not detracted from the long-term success of extensively coated implants. A similar distal loading scenario is seen with cemented femoral stems whereby most load bypasses the proximal femur and exits distally. Dual-energy x-ray absorption studies have confirmed proximal bone density loss with extensively coated uncemented femoral stems and with cemented femoral stems.

Stress shielding of porous-coated stems is related to several factors: (1) stem stiffness (most important), (2) extent of porous coating, and (3) metal alloy (Young's modulus). Stress shielding is seen more with extensively porous-coated stems, but it is thought that *stem stiffness* is a more important factor evoking the stress-shielding phenomenon. Stem stiffness is related to *modulus* (Co-Cr alloy will be stiffer than Ti alloy) and to the fourth power of stem *radius* (r^4). Stem stiffness is also related to stem geometry. Solid round stems are more stiff than stems with metallic relief (i.e., flutes, slots, tapers, splines). Therefore an extensively porous-coated solid stem made of Co-Cr alloy of large diameter (>15 mm) is much more likely to cause stress shielding.

e. Cement Fixation. Cement fixation for hip replacement surgery requires good technique to provide optimal interdigitation of cement to bone. The technique for cement preparation has undergone several generations of development and is summarized in Table 4-1. With cemented THR, it is usually the acetabular socket that fails first from loosening. Ranawat states that if the subgroups of patients with rheumatoid arthritis (or other similar inflammatory conditions), protrusio deformity, hip dysplasia, and excessive bleeding are excluded, the long-term results of cemented sockets are comparable to those of uncemented sockets.

For femoral stem implantation, an alternative cement technique is that of using a highly polished tapered stem with square edges and no centralizer (Ling's technique). With this technique, careful studies have documented that the stem settles within the cement mantle and, over time, finds a stable mechanical state. It is thought that this technique reduces mechanical stresses on the cement-bone mantle, which may reduce stem loosening rates in the long term.

f. Size of Cement Mantle. The size of the cement mantle surrounding the femoral stem is controversial. It is suggested that a minimum of 2 mm of cement thickness be allowed between prosthesis and bone. This would be impractical in narrow canals where a very small stem diameter would be required. A more practical approach is the two-thirds rule. With this technique, two thirds of the canal is displaced by the femoral stem and the other third by cement. Cement *mantle defects* should be avoided. A mantle defect where the prosthesis touches bone creates an area of concentrated stress and is associated with a higher loosening rate (Fig. 4-2).

4. Choice of Fixation

a. Cemented or Noncemented. The recommended fixation for primary hip arthroplasty remains controversial. The National Institutes of Health (NIH) consensus statement for total hip arthroplasty, in summary, recommends that a cemented femoral component using modern cementing technique, paired with a porous-coated hemispherical acetabular component, can give excellent long-term results. This is based on the data showing a higher loosening rate with cemented acetabular sockets compared with those of porous-coated noncemented sockets. On the other hand, there are so many different uncemented femoral stem designs and variations of coatings that there is no identified superiority of uncemented femoral stem fixation over cemented femoral stems. The general tendency, however, is to use uncemented femoral stems in younger active patients where cemented

Table 4-1. CEMENT TECHNIQUE—TOTAL HIP REPLACEMENT

1ST GENERATION	2ND GENERATION (BEGAN 1975)	3RD GENERATION (BEGAN 1982)
• Finger packing • No canal preparation • No cement plug • No cement gun • No pressurization • Cast stem • Narrow medial border on stem • Sharp edges on stem	• Cement gun (began 1971) • Pulsatile lavage • Canal preparation (brush and dry) • Cement restrictor • Super alloy stem (forged) • Broad and round medial border • Collar on stem	• Porosity reduction (vacuum) • Pressurization cement • Precoat stem • Rough surface finish on stem • Stem centralizer

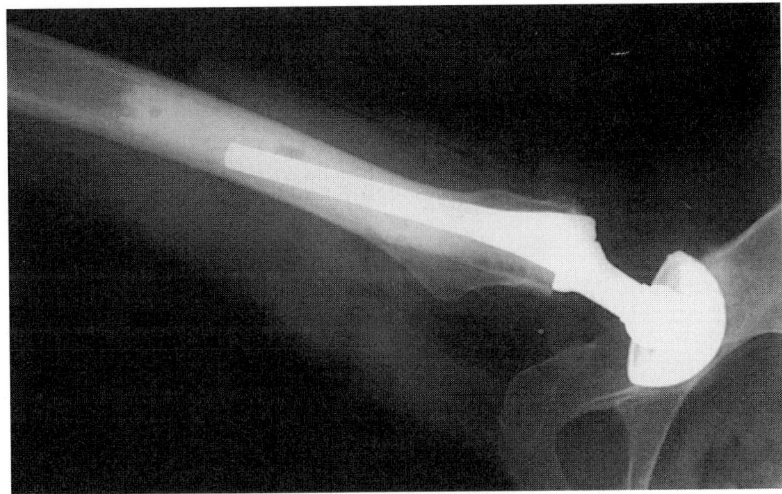

FIGURE 4-2 ■ Lateral radiograph of cemented femoral stem with mantle defect. Note distal stem tip that touches bone.

stems in this situation have a reported higher loosening rate in long-term follow-up.

B. Hip Stability—Primary and Revision Surgery
   1. Dislocation of THR—Evaluation of a dislocated THR is complex and often multifactorial. An understanding of the factors involved in an unstable total hip can provide value to the surgeon in both primary and revision arthroplasty. The dislocation incidence after primary THR averages 1-2%, but it has been reported to be as high as 9.5%. Dislocation after revision is higher and is reported as high as 26% in cases of multiple revisions. The highest incidence of dislocation in primary hip arthroplasty is in the subgroup of elderly patients (>80 years old) converted to total hip after failed osteosynthesis for femoral neck fracture. In this subgroup, dislocation incidence in one European study was 82%.
   2. Assessment of Hip Stability—The assessment of hip stability involves four major areas: (1) component design, (2) component alignment, (3) soft-tissue tensioning, and (4) soft-tissue function.
      a. Component Design. In the area of component design, the ball cup articulation is most important. The *primary arc range* defines the amount of arc the ball and cup articulation moves before impinging and levering out (Fig. 4-3). The major determinant of primary arc range is the *head-neck ratio*. The head-neck ratio is defined as the ratio of the femoral head diameter to the femoral neck diameter. A larger head-neck ratio allows further arc of motion before primary impingement (Fig. 4-4). Another factor affecting component stability is *excursion distance*. At the point of primary impingement, the head will begin to lever out of the cup. The distance a head must travel to dislocate is defined as excursion. The greater the

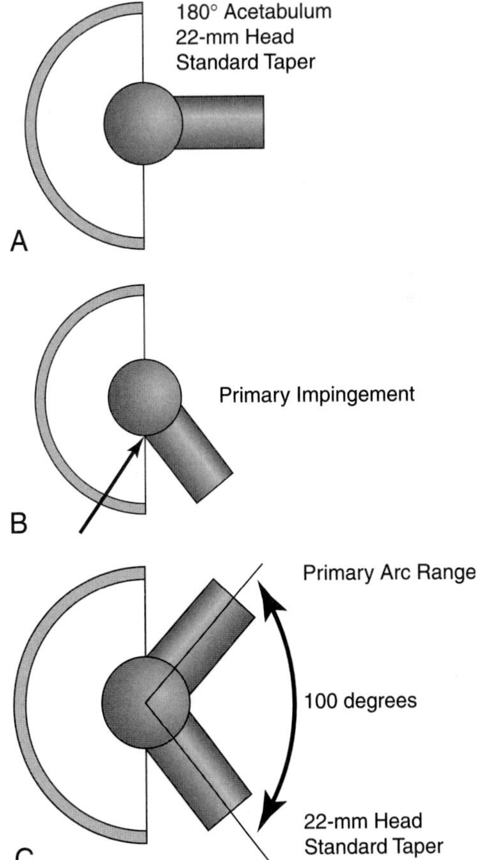

FIGURE 4-3 ■ Diagram of THR articulation demonstrating primary arc range. *A*, 22-mm head articulating with 180 degrees polyethylene. *B*, At the end of range, primary impingement occurs. *C*, Primary arc range is the arc of motion allowed between the two ends of primary impingement.

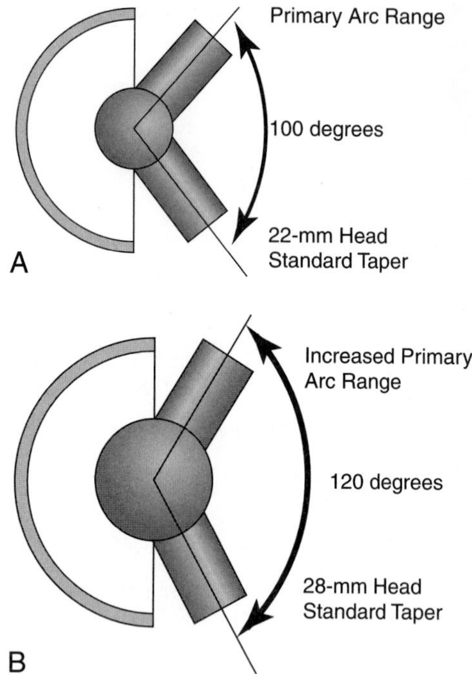

FIGURE 4-4 ■ Comparison of primary arc range between 22-mm head and 28-mm head. *A*, Primary arc range with 22-mm head. *B*, Primary arc range with 28-mm head. The only change in this illustration is head size. This increases the head-to-neck ratio, which in turn allows for an increased arc range.

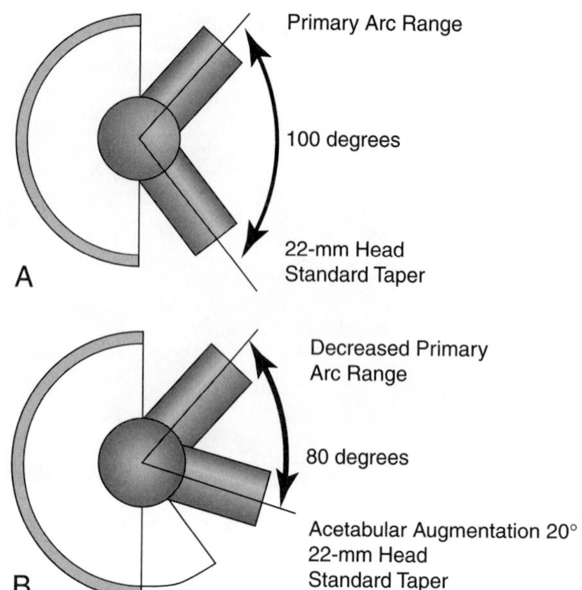

FIGURE 4-5 ■ Comparison of primary arc range between non-hooded and hooded acetabular liner. *A*, Primary arc range with 22-mm head. *B*, Primary arc range with augmented acetabular liner (i.e., hood). Primary arc range is reduced as a result of the augmented liner.

excursion a ball must travel to dislocate when levered out, the more stable the hip. Excursion distance is usually half the diameter of the femoral head. Comparing a 32-mm head with a 22-mm head shows that excursion distance is 16 mm compared with 11 mm. In addition, a 32-mm head is more stable because of a more favorable head-neck ratio. Taken to the extreme, a hemiarthroplasty head is the most inherently stable head because of a very favorable head-neck ratio.

It is important to know the details of total hip design as it relates to hip stability. The size of the morse taper affects stability by affecting the head-neck ratio. Narrow neck tapers provide more stability via a more favorable head-neck ratio. Conversely, the addition of a collar on a modular femoral head (seen in long neck lengths) increases neck diameter and adversely affects head-neck ratio. Augmented acetabular liners (i.e., hoods) decrease the primary arc range because the primary arc range is less than the typical 180 degree arc (Fig. 4-5). The larger the hood, the more likely there will be impingement and excursion. Large hoods should be avoided. A constrained liner that covers almost the entire femoral head provides inherent stability but at a cost. The primary arc range is dramatically reduced (Fig. 4-6).

If the patient consistently exceeds this primary arc range, the acetabulum can fail from early mechanical failure. The repetitive impingement imparts a levering force on the acetabular component, leading to early loosening.

b. Component Alignment. This is another important area in hip stability. Because the patient's native femoral head is much larger than a prosthetic THR head, it is more stable and has a larger primary arc range than a prosthetic replacement. Therefore when inserting acetabular and femoral components, the goal is to center the prosthetic primary arc range in the middle of the patient's functional range (Fig. 4-7). By doing so, if the primary arc range is exceeded, there is still

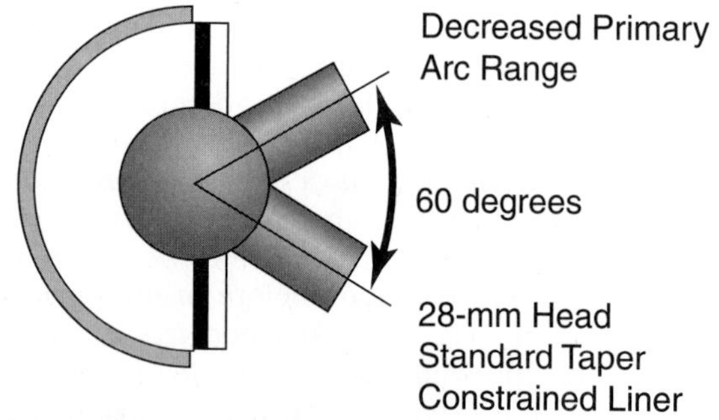

FIGURE 4-6 ■ Diagram of constrained acetabular liner. A constrained liner covers the femoral head past its equator. This keeps the ball from coming out of socket. This has the adverse effect of severely restricting primary arc range.

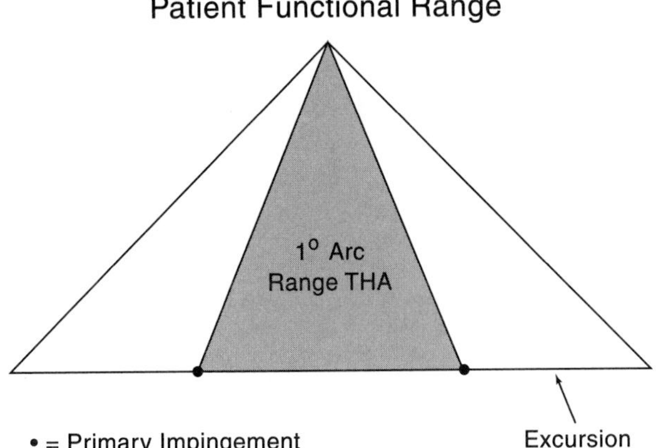

FIGURE 4-7 ■ Diagram illustrating difference in patient's functional hip range of motion compared with prosthetic range. Because of the smaller heads used in prosthetic replacement, the prosthetic arc range is smaller than native hip range. The prosthetic arc range should be centered within the patient's functional range to minimize dislocation. THA, total hip arthroscopy.

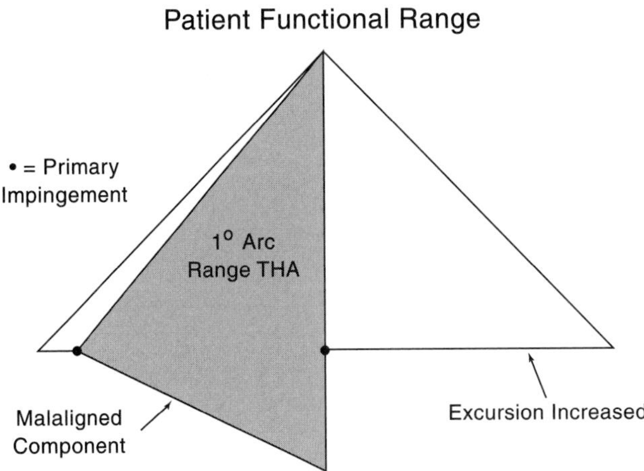

FIGURE 4-8 ■ Diagram illustrating prosthetic malalignment. In this instance, the prosthetic arc range is positioned to one side of the patient's functional range. On one side of the range, the hip will be very stable. However, on the other side, the patient's arc range will exceed the prosthetic arc range. Primary impingement will occur, followed by head levering, head excursion, and dislocation. If the patient is unwilling to accept limitation of functional range, then recurrent dislocation will result. THA, total hip arthroscopy.

some stability with prosthetic excursion distance. Malaligned components do not decrease primary arc range; it is just not centered in the patient's functional range. As a result, on one side of the arc range, the head will suffer excessive excursion and hip dislocation (Fig. 4-8). Because surgeon preference and training vary, there is no one correct answer for the proper component position. On the acetabulum, anteversion should be 15–30 degrees, and the theta angle (i.e., coronal tilt) should be 35–45 degrees (Fig. 4-9). Intraoperative trialing is important to ensure that component placement is optimum. The hip must be taken through all extremes of end range to assure stability.

c. Soft-Tissue Tensioning. This factor also plays a critical role in hip stability. Components properly placed may still dislocate if there is inadequate soft-tissue tension to hold the components in place. The major key to hip stability is the *abductor complex*. This consists primarily of the gluteus medius and minimus. Maintaining the correct tension of this complex will provide optimal stability. *Preoperative templating* should assess *head offset* and *neck length* so that when the prosthetic stem is inserted, appropriate neck length and offset are restored (Fig. 4-10). Restored hip mechanics confers hip stability via optimized abductor tension. Conversely, reduced hip length and offset can lead to instability. A THR left short in neck length results in a lax abductor complex and may not generate the force required to keep the hip in place. Additionally, a short neck length can cause trochanteric impingement, with abduction and rotation causing the hip to lever out of the socket. Hip stability can also be affected by a decreased offset. With a *narrow offset*, the greater trochanter can again impinge, allowing the hip to lever out of socket. The worst-case scenario would be a THR with a shortened neck length and a narrow offset. It is very important to template x-rays preoperatively to see if neck length and offset can be adequately restored. If not, a different prosthetic system may be required. In a related issue, greater trochanter deficiency or trochanteric escape (seen after trochanteric osteotomy) often leads to hip instability. With loss of the greater trochanter attachment to the femur, there is loss of abductor power and loss of hip compressive forces. Also, with loss of the greater trochanter, the hip is allowed a greater range of motion, leading to prosthetic neck impingement, head excursion, and dislocation.

d. Soft-Tissue Function. This is the last area of concern. What controls the abductor complex and surrounding soft tissues of the hip is the synchronized neurologic firing from the brain delivered through the peripheral nervous system. Any disruption in this system can adversely affect function and hip stability. Soft-tissue function can be broken into two main issues: central and peripheral. *Central issues* involve the brain, brain stem, and spinal cord. Problems in this area can be numerous and include such problems as stroke, cerebellar dysfunction, Parkinson's disease, multiple sclerosis, dementia, cervical stenosis/myelopathy, and psychiatric disorder. The issue common to all of these is the coordinated firing of muscles to keep the

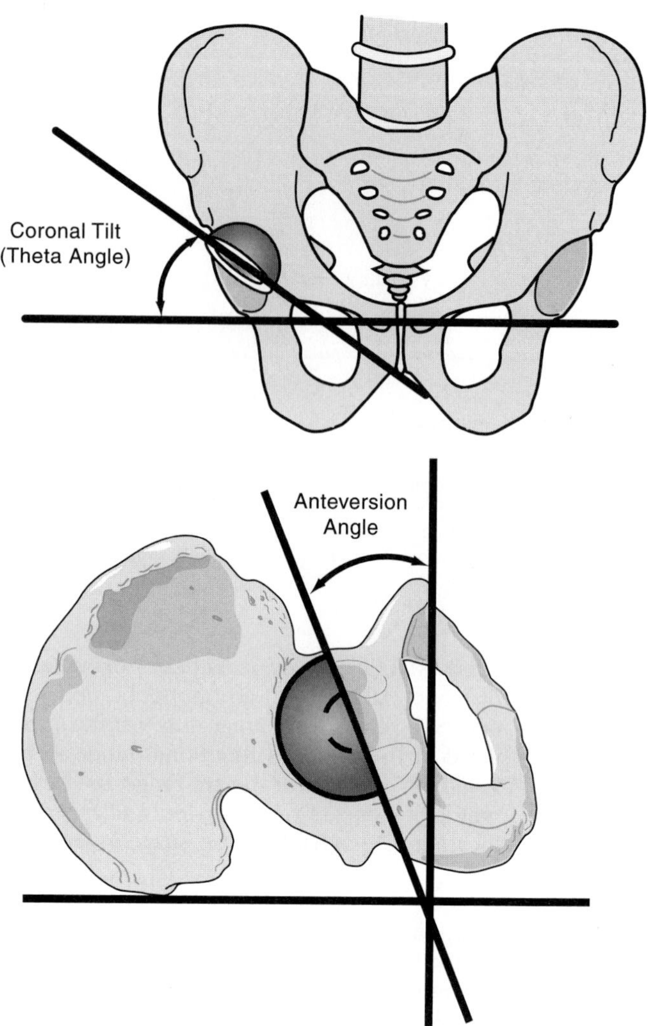

FIGURE 4-9 ■ Diagram showing acetabular cup position in coronal and sagittal plane. Coronal tilt (also known as theta angle) should be 35–45 degrees. In the sagittal plane, cup anteversion should be 15–30 degrees.

hip stable. The problem could be from paralysis, spasticity, or loss of coordinated movements of the surrounding hip musculature. *Peripheral issues* involve the area of the peripheral nerves and muscles that support the hip. Peripheral issues that can affect hip stability include lumbar stenosis, peripheral neuropathy, myopathy, localized soft-tissue trauma, and radiation therapy. The cause of poor soft-tissue function may be multifactorial in an elderly patient. Sometimes, it is difficult preoperatively to ascertain the extent of soft-tissue dysfunction, and it is only after multiple dislocations that one appreciates the significance of these deficits.

3. Management of the Dislocated THR—Treatment of the dislocated THR depends on the reason for dislocation. Approximately two thirds of patients with a dislocated THR can be treated successfully with a closed reduction and a period of hip immobilization. Immobilization can be by means of either a spica cast or brace. A knee immobilizer is effective as well; it keeps the patient from putting the hip in a compromised position. However, immobilization in a brace or cast allows a better chance for soft tissues to heal in a more contracted position. During closed reduction, it is important to take the hip through a full range and assess the positions that make the hip dislocate. If the dislocating positions noted are near the extremes of end range, the prognosis for long-term stability is good. On the other hand, if the hip dislocates easily within the patient's functional range, then revision surgery is more likely necessary. As a general rule, if the hip dislocates more than two times, recurrent dislocation is likely, and the hip should be revised to enhance stability.

The surgical options to repair recurrent dislocation depend on the cause of the dislocation. Although, in many circumstances, the cause of recurrent dislocation is multifactorial, there is usually one main area that stands out. If the THR components are malaligned, they should be revised, even if they are well fixed. The choice of implants for revision surgery should take

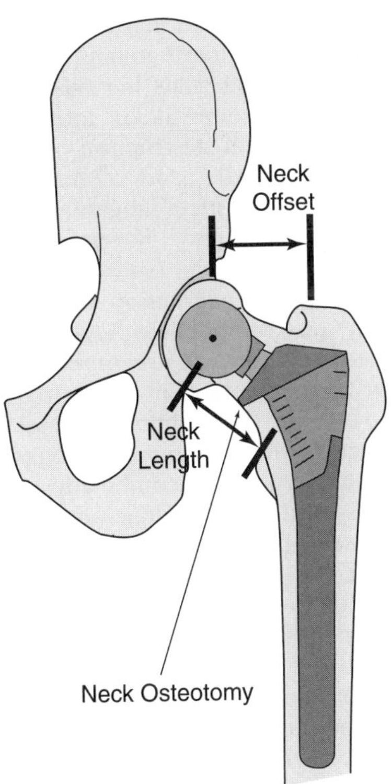

FIGURE 4-10 ■ Diagram illustrating preoperative templating for proper femoral stem positioning. Prosthetic stem should be positioned such that femoral stem offset (center of head to greater trochanter) matches the native hip. Also, femoral neck length must be restored. Restoring head offset and neck length optimizes abductor tension, providing stability.

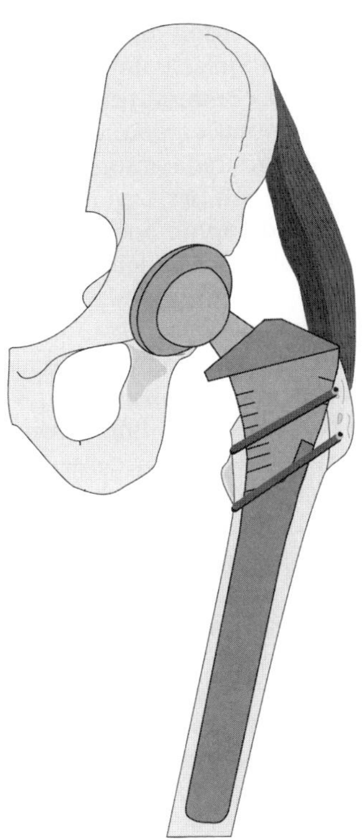

FIGURE 4-11 ■ Diagram depicting trochanteric advancement. Distal advancement tightens hip abductor complex, restoring compressive force to hip joint.

into account factors that restore normal hip offset and neck length, and provide an optimal arc range. Optimizing head-neck ratio with a larger head should take priority over polyethylene (PE) thickness, if this provides the stability needed for a successful outcome. In some situations, where hip component parts are reasonably aligned, trochanteric osteotomy with distal advancement is a good option (Fig. 4-11). Distal advancement places the abductor complex under tension, providing more hip compressive force. Trochanteric advancement, if performed, is usually accompanied by postoperative immobilization in a spica brace or cast. In the scenario where a prior trochanteric osteotomy has detached and migrated proximally, reattaching the greater trochanter is not often successful. In the abductor-deficient patient, hip stability may be achieved only by using a larger femoral head and/or a constrained PE liner.

Conversion of a THR to a hemiarthroplasty with a large femoral head is another solution for hip instability and is more often used when there is soft-tissue deficiency or dysfunction. Conversion to a monopolar or bipolar head cannot be used where the acetabular bone is compromised (i.e., segmental deficiencies). If acetabular wall deficiences are present, there is a high likelihood of pelvic migration. If the hemiarthroplasty can be seated firmly on the bony acetabular rim and there is acceptable remaining bone stock, then conversion to a hemiarthroplasty is an option. A constrained PE liner is used in a similar fashion where soft-tissue deficiency and dysfunction are the main problem. The advantage of a constrained liner is that it can be used in the reconstructed acetabulum where there is acetabular deficiency. The main problem with a constrained liner is the very limited range of motion it provides. If a patient is not compliant with the limited range, then the acetabular cup may rapidly become mechanically loose from levering forces. Conversion to a constrained liner should not be the first surgical option if other surgical options will take care of the problem. The last surgical option is resection arthroplasty. This option is used when other options have been exhausted. Resection arthroplasty is usually used in the multiply revised patient with significant soft-tissue deficiency along with significant bone loss. Resection arthroplasty is also used for the psychiatric patient who purposely dislocates the hip for secondary gratification (e.g., narcotics, hospitalization).

C. Hip Loosening—Aseptic femoral and acetabular loosening are the most common indications for revision surgery. In cemented hip replacement, the most common reason for revision is failure of the cemented acetabular component. In uncemented THR, the most common reason for revision is failure of the femoral component (usually from osteolysis). Standard radiographs taken in the same rotational position are required to assess interval changes. Radiographic analysis is based on dividing the acetabular and femoral components into radiographic zones. The acetabulum is divided into three zones as described by DeLee and Charnley. The femoral component is divided into seven zones as described by Gruen (Fig. 4-12). The development of radiolucent lines around these zones (either with cemented or cementless implants) in a progressive fashion suggests loosening. It is important to distinguish progressive radiolucent lines in the femur from the typical age-related expansion of the femoral canal and cortical thinning, which may give the appearance of a progressively widening radiolucency. Age-related radiolucent zones generally do not have the associated sclerotic line seen about loose femoral stems. In addition, radiolucent lines associated with osteolysis tend to be more irregular, with variable areas of cortical thinning and ectasia. With cemented femoral implants, Gruen describes four modes of failure, which are defined and diagrammed in Table 4-2. The acetabular cup is considered loose if there is a radiolucency >2 mm in all three zones, progressive radiolucent lines in zones 1 and 2, or a change in component position.

D. Revision THR—Revision hip surgery is often difficult and complex. The results are less satisfactory than in primary hip replacement. Postoperative complications of infection, dislocation, nerve palsy, cortical perforation, fracture, and deep vein thrombosis are higher than in primary hip replacement. The surgical goals in revision hip replacement are (1) removal of loose components without significant destruction of host bone and tissue, (2) reconstruction of bone defects with bone graft and/or metal augmentation, (3) stable revision implants, and (4) restoration of normal hip center of rotation.

Acetabular reconstruction first requires defining the extent of bone loss. Acetabular defects are classified as follows: (1) *segmental* (type I)—loss of part of the acetabular rim or medial wall; (2) *cavitary* (type II)—volumetric loss in the bony substance of the acetabular cavity; (3) *combined deficiency* (type III)—combination of segmental bone loss and cavitary deficiency; (4) *pelvic discontinuity* (type IV)—complete separation between the superior and inferior acetabulum, usually due to combined deficiencies and fracture; and (5) *arthrodesis* (type V)—obliteration of the acetabulum due to fusion.

1. Revision of Acetabulum—In revision of the acetabulum, a porous-coated hemisphere cup secured with superior screws is the preferred choice, provided that the rim is intact. The acetabular rim in the revision situation provides the stability for the acetabular cup when inserted with a press fit technique. Because acetabular bone stock is weakened in revision surgery, superior screws should be placed to augment stability. The correct placement of acetabular screws is important. Figure 4-13 diagrams the safe zones for correct screw placement. Incorrect screw placement can lead

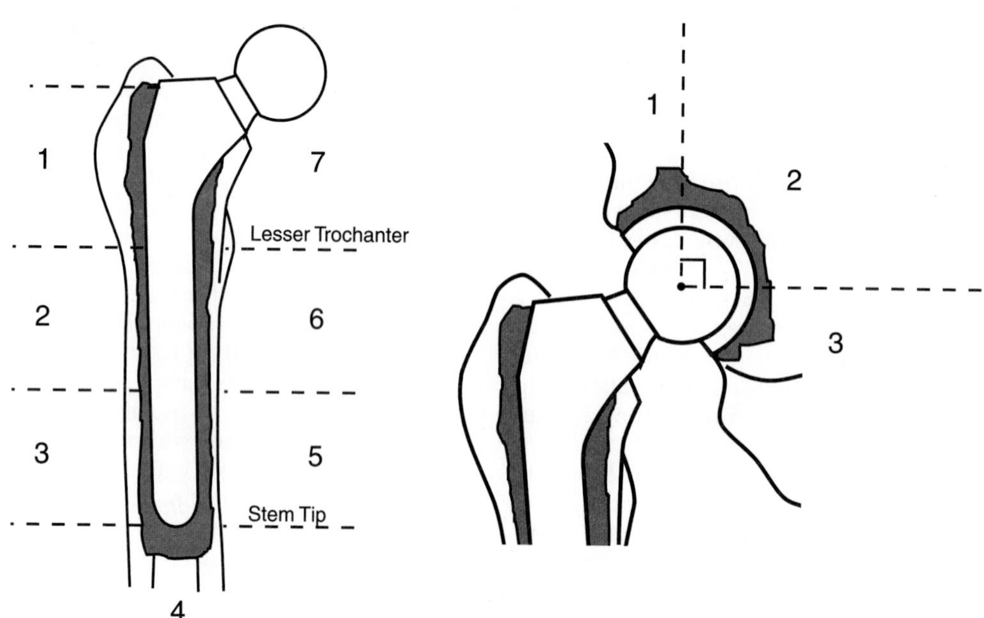

FIGURE 4-12 ■ Diagram of seven Gruen zones for femoral stem and three DeLee-Charnley zones for acetabular cup.

Table 4-2. MODES OF CEMENTED FEMORAL STEM LOOSENING

MODE	MECHANISM	CAUSE	FINDINGS
IA	Pistoning behavior	• Subsidence of stem within cement	• RLL between stem and cement in zones 1 and 2 • Distal cement fracture • Stem displaced distally in cement
IB	Pistoning behavior	• Subsidence of cement mantle and stem within bone	• RLL all 7 zones
II	Medial stem pivot	• Lack of superomedial and inferolateral cement support	• Medial migration proximal stem • Lateral migration distal tip • Cement fracture zones 2 and 6
III	Calcar pivot	• Medial and lateral toggle of distal stem • "Hang up" of stem collar on medial cortex • "Windshield wiper" reaction at distal stem	• Sclerosis and thickening of bone at stem tip • RLL zones 4 and 5
IV	Cantilever bending	• Loss of proximal cement support leaving distal stem still fixed; allows for proximal cantilever bending	• Stem crack or fracture • RLL zones 1 and 2, 6 and 7

RLL, radiolucent lines.

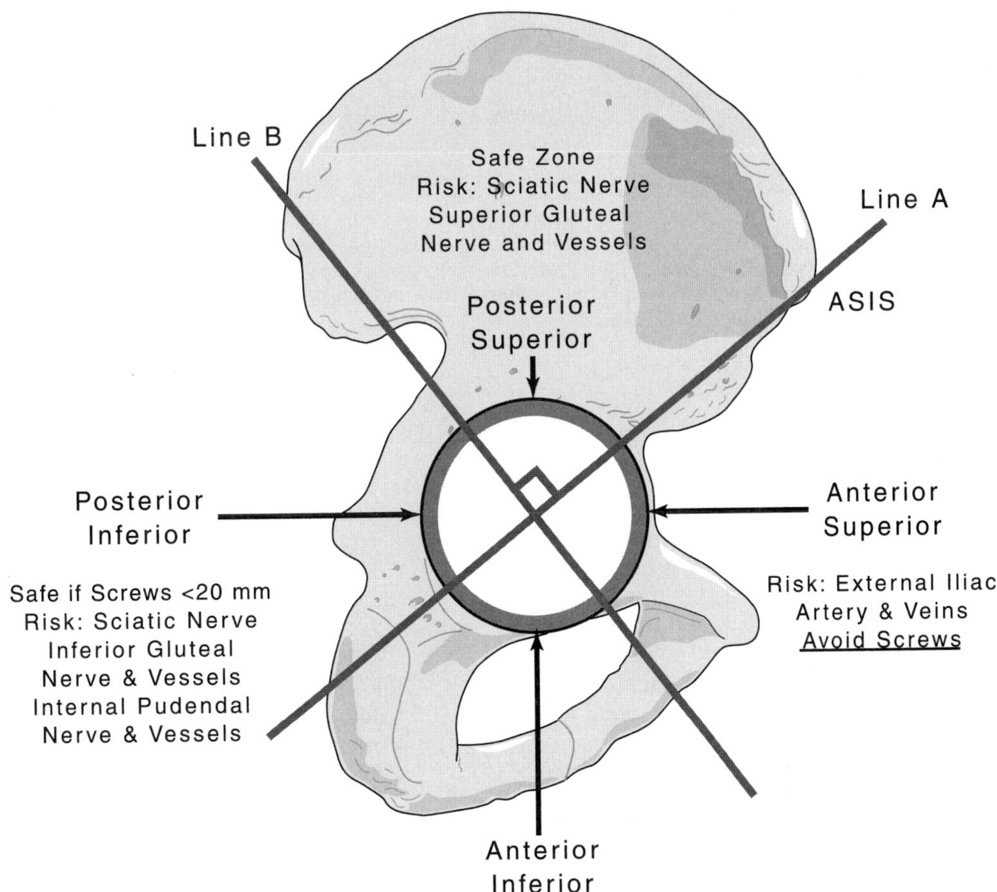

FIGURE 4-13 ■ Acetabular zones for screw insertion. Line *A* is formed by drawing line from the anterior superior iliac spine (ASIS) to center of acetabular socket. Line *B* is then drawn perpendicular to *A*, also passing through center of socket. The posterior-superior quadrant is the preferred zone for screw insertion.

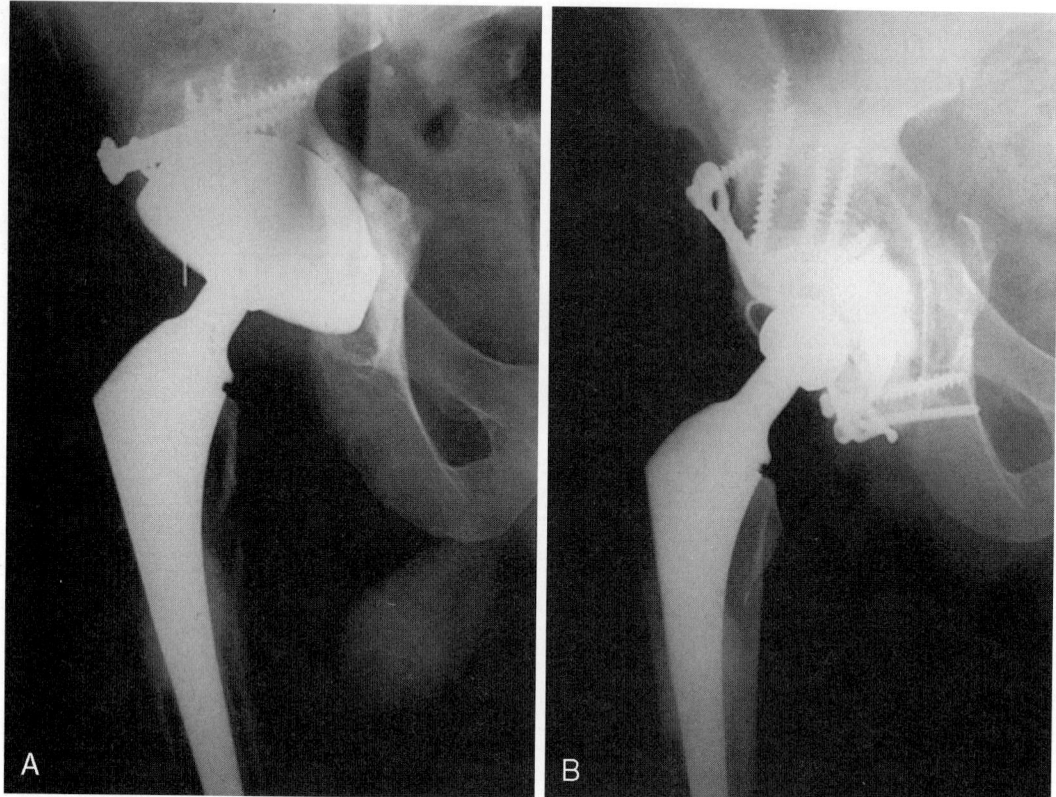

FIGURE 4-14 ■ X-ray films demonstrating acetabular reconstruction with reconstruction cage and bulk support allograft. *A*, Preoperative radiograph of loose jumbo cup with collapse of superior bone graft. *B*, Postoperative 1 year x-ray film of Birch-Schneider acetabular reconstruction cage for the large segmental acetabular deficiency. A structural allograft is placed superiorly. The cage is secured with screws to the ilium and ischium. A polyethylene acetabular component is then cemented into the cage. This construct enables weight-bearing forces to be partly distributed from the cage to the ilium, allowing allograft to remodel and incorporate to host bone.

to catastrophic vascular injury or neurologic damage.

A porous-coated hemisphere cup can still be used with segmental deficiency of the acetabular rim. As a general rule, a hemisphere cup can be utilized if at least *two thirds* of the rim is remaining and there is still a good "rim fit." The cup must be secured with screws. Cavitary deficiencies with an intact rim are filled with particulate graft, and the acetabular cup will hold the graft in place.

Acetabular deficiencies that are rim deficient and/or have large cavitary deficiencies will require structural and/or particulate allograft. A structural allograft (as opposed to particulate graft) is a large solid piece of bone that supports weight-bearing stress. If a cup is placed into a large structural allograft, the failure rate is high. Failure is usually due to graft resorption and subsequent component migration. Failure of cementless components with a large structural allograft is 40–60%. Failure rate with a cemented socket is 40%. A much higher success rate is achieved when the structural deficiencies are reinforced by a reconstruction cage (Fig. 4-14). A structural allograft supported by a reconstruction cage is the preferred revision construct if a large structural allograft is to be used. If a reconstruction cage is used, generally an all-PE acetabular component is cemented into the cage. More recently, all metal cups (metal-metal bearing) can be cemented into the reconstruction cage.

2. Femoral Bone Defects—Femoral bone defects, like acetabular defects, are primarily either segmental or cavitary. The complete classification of femoral bone deficiencies is as follows (1) *segmental* (type I)—any loss of bone of the supporting shell of the femur; (2) *cavitary* (type II)—loss of endosteal bone but an intact cortical shell; (3) *combined deficiency* (type III)—combined segmental and cavitary defects; (4) *malalignment* (type IV)—loss of normal femoral geometry due to prior surgery, trauma, or disease; (5) *stenosis* (type V)—occlusion of canal from trauma, fixation devices, or bony hypertrophy; and (6) *femoral discontinuity* (type VI)—loss of femoral integrity from fracture or nonunion.

With femoral stem revision, the most commonly utilized technique is an uncemented extensively porous-coated (or porous coating/grit blast combination) long-stem prosthesis. The revision stem should pass 2–3 cm below the original stem. This is to bypass stress risers that may occur from stem extraction or osteolysis. If there is a femoral cortical violation, the revision stem should pass at least *two shaft diameters* below the defect. Ectatic, cavitary lesions can be grafted with particulate graft. Segmental deficiencies are usually reconstructed with cortical onlay struts secured with cerclage wires or multifilament cables (Fig. 4-15).

Impaction bone grafting (Ling's technique) can be used in some revision cases where there is a large ectatic canal and narrow, thin cortices (destroyed by osteolysis). This technique uses morselized fresh-frozen allograft packed tightly into the ectatic proximal femur. A smooth tapered stem is cemented into the allograft. This technique requires an intact cortical tube, although small segmental defects can be patched with a wire mesh. The most common complication of this technique is stem settling.

E. Periprosthetic Fracture: Hip—The management of periprosthetic femur fractures depends on the location of the fracture and whether the stem is well-fixed or loose. Femurs with bone ingrowth prosthesis tend to fracture within the first 6 months after implantation. The reason is probable stress risers created by reaming and broaching of the femoral canal. Cemented implants tend to fracture late (5 years on average). Fractures in cemented implants occur most commonly about the stem tip or distal to the prosthesis. In revision cases, fractures tend to occur at the site of a cortical defect from previous operations. Fractures also occur when the new stem does not bypass a cortical defect by greater than two cortical diameters.

Fractures that occur where there is a loose prosthesis (cemented or cementless) should be revised using a noncemented ingrowth long-stem prosthesis that bypasses the last cortical defect by two diameters of the femoral shaft.

Treatment of fractures with an intact prosthetic interface depends on the site of fracture and the extent of fracture involvement. A fracture classification (Beals and Tower) with recommended treatments is reviewed in Table 4-3.

F. Heterotopic Ossification—Heterotopic ossification (HO) after hip replacement surgery most commonly affects males. Predisposing risk factors include hypertrophic osteoarthritis, ankylosing spondylitis, diffuse idiopathic skeletal hyperostosis (DISH), post-traumatic arthritis, prior hip fusion, and history of previous development of heterotopic ossification. HO is seen more often with the direct lateral approach to the hip (Harding Approach). If HO is seen in the contralateral hip, the incidence of HO with the ipsilateral hip is high.

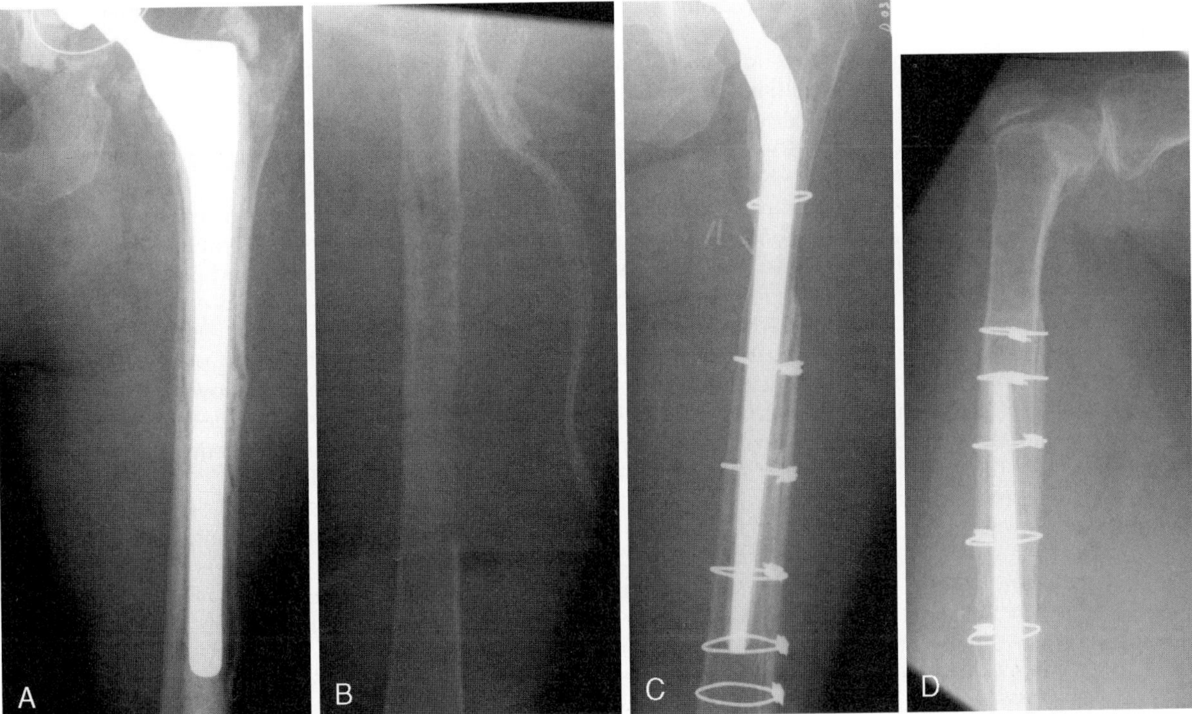

FIGURE 4-15 ■ X-ray film of long-stem revision femoral stem *(A-D)*. Cortical allograft onlay struts are secured with multifilament cables to enforce segmental and cavitary deficiencies.

Table 4-3. PERIPROSTHETIC FEMUR FRACTURE CLASSIFICATION AND TREATMENT

STABLE PROSTHETIC INTERFACE		
Fracture Type	*Fracture Location*	*Recommended Treatment*
I	Trochanteric region	Nonoperative
II	Proximal metaphysis/diaphysis not involving stem tip	Nonoperative or cerclage fixation
IIIA	Diaphyseal fracture at stem tip Disruption of prosthetic interface (<25%)	Long-stem ingrowth revision or ORIF: Plate with screws ± cerclage ORIF: Cortical struts with cerclage cables
IIIB	Diaphyseal fracture at stem tip Disruption of prosthetic interface (>25%)	Cemented stem: long-stem ingrowth revision Ingrowth stem: long-stem ingrowth revision or ORIF: Plate with screws ± cerclage ORIF: Cortical struts with cerclage cables
IIIC	Supracondylar fracture at tip of a long-stem prosthesis	Nonoperative if stable or ORIF: Plate with screws ± cerclage ORIF: Custom IM rod extension to prosthesis
IV	Supracondylar fracture distant to stem tip	Nonoperative if stable or ORIF: Plate with screws (must extend proximal to stem tip) ORIF: Supracondylar intramedullary nail
Loose prosthetic interface		Long-stem ingrowth revision

ORIF, open reduction internal fixation.

Heterotopic ossification limits hip motion when pronounced, but it generally does not cause pain or muscle weakness. Reoperation to remove HO is not recommended unless there is severe restriction of hip range or severe pain from impingement. Recurrence is likely unless prophylactic measures are taken. Once HO is seen radiographically, there is no treatment to prevent further progression. Instead, treatment for HO is directed toward identifying those patients at high risk for developing HO and treating this subgroup prophylactically.

Prophylactic treatment with low-dose radiation or with certain nonsteroidal anti-inflammatory drugs (NSAIDs) are the two effective treatments for HO. A single dose of 600–750 cGy (Rad) is considered the lowest effective dose for HO. Treatment must be delivered within 72 hours of surgery (preferably within the first 48 hours) to be effective. If noncemented prosthetic components are used, these areas should be shielded from the radiation beam so as not to reduce bone ingrowth potential. Indomethacin is the most commonly used NSAID for heterotopic ossification. Other NSAIDs have also shown effectiveness. The recommended indomethacin dose is 75 mg per day for 6 weeks. The efficacy of indomethacin in preventing recurrent HO after excision is not well documented.

II. Osteolysis and Wear in Prosthetic Joint Replacement—Osteolysis at this time remains the most vexing problem in total joint arthroplasty. In its most basic form, it represents a histiocytic response to wear debris. The process begins with *wear sources* that generate particulate debris, which initiates the osteolytic reaction. The potential wear sources are listed in Figure 4-16. Although any particle can serve as a source of wear debris and cause osteolysis, debris that is known to elicit an enhanced histiocytic response includes ultrahigh molecular-weight polyethylene (UHMWPE), polymethylmethacrylate (PMMA), cobalt chrome (Co-Cr), and titanium (Ti). Because PE is relatively softer than other materials used in joint replacement surgery, it is considered the major source of the osteolytic process by virtue of the volume of PE generated, as compared with other sources. As a result of particle ingestion by the macrophages, the activated macrophage liberates osteolytic factors, including osteoclast-activating factor, oxide radicals, hydrogen peroxide, acid phosphatase, interleukins, and prostaglandins. These factors together assist in the dissolution of bone from around the prosthesis, allowing for prosthetic micromotion that leads to further generation of wear debris. Additional lysis of bone allows for prosthetic macromotion, loosening, and pain.

Once particulate debris is generated and the osteolytic process begins, the inflammatory response generated within the joint produces an increased hydrostatic pressure that allows for dissemination of particulate debris within the *effective joint space*. The effective joint space comprises the potential space where joint fluid can be pumped and thereby allow particle debris to travel (Fig. 4-17). The effective joint space comprises the joint itself along with the surfaces where the prosthesis (or cement) contacts host bone. The size of the particles implicated in osteolysis is very small. The particles are micron or submicron size (0.2 μm to 7 μm). McKellop suggests that the main culprit in osteolysis is submicron particles of PE.

Wear particles can be generated by *abrasive* wear, in which particles are generated by rough articular

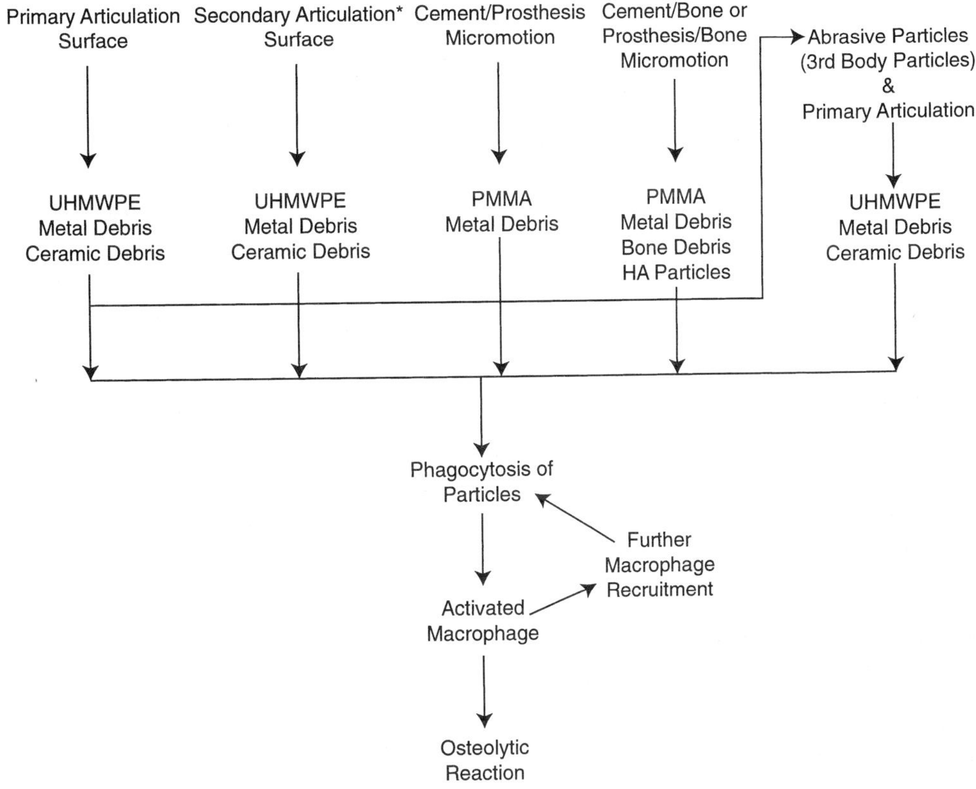

FIGURE 4-16 ■ Wear in total replacement.

surfaces (e.g., scratches, carbide asperites), either at the primary articulation or other secondary surfaces (backside of PE insert with metal backed shell). *Third-body particles* can generate debris through an abrasive process at articulating surfaces. McKellop also describes the loss of PE at the primary articulation via a process of *adhesive wear*. PE is produced by the heating of small PE beads into a congealed mass. On its surface, the small submicron beads can be pulled off by the passing of the adjacent articulation surface.The generation of these small particles is significant (Fig. 4-18). The combination of abrasive wear and adhesive wear can generate many billions of particles that are then disseminated throughout the effective joint space. Efforts to minimize osteolysis in total joint replacement are primarily focused on minimizing adhesive wear at the primary articulation and also at minimizing abrasive wear within the total joint construct.

The sterilization process of PE has been implicated as a factor causing high wear rates and rapid PE failure. PE components sterilized via radiation and stored in an oxygen environment generate oxidized PE that, under repetitive cyclic loading, can excessively wear, delaminate, and crack, leading to PE failure. The pathways of irradiated PE are outlined in Figure 4-19. Irradiated PE undergoes an intermediate step of free radical formation. At this point, there are four pathways that can be taken: *recombination, unsaturation, chain scission,* or *cross-linking***.** The two important pathways concerning PE wear are chain scission and cross-linking. In the presence of an oxygen environment, oxidized PE is favored. In an environment without oxygen, *cross-linking* is favored. Cross-linked PE has *improved* resistance to adhesive and abrasive wear and improves wear rates in wear simulator data.The disadvantage of cross-linking PE is that it does diminish the mechanical properties.

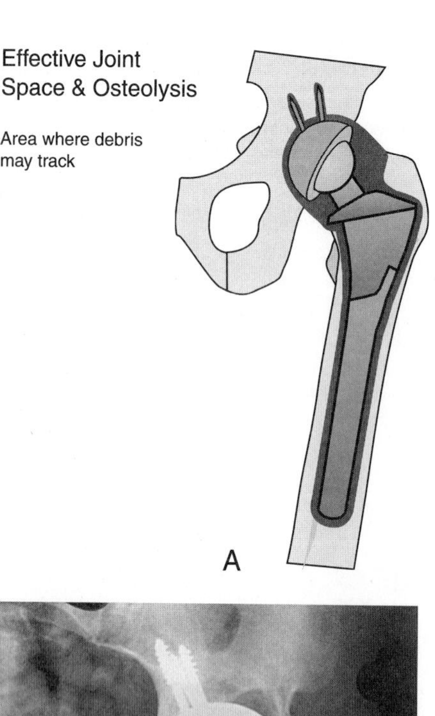

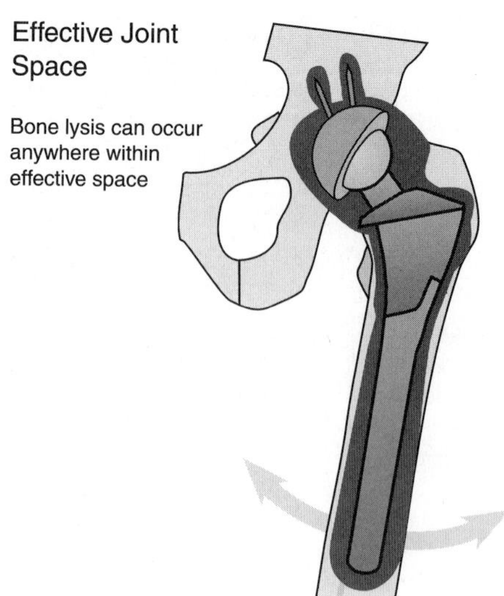

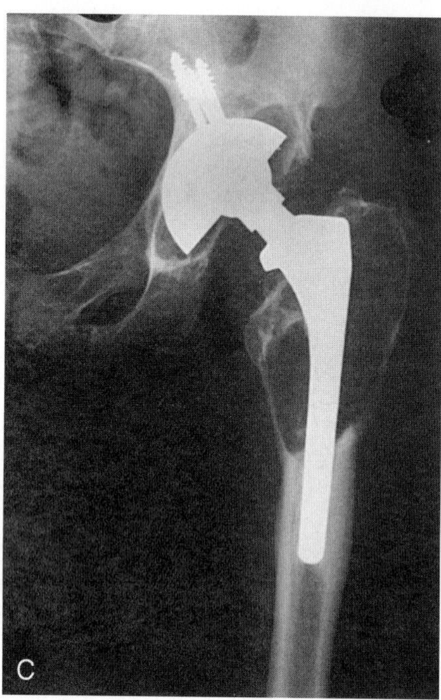

FIGURE 4-17 ■ Diagram showing effective joint space. *A*, Area of effective joint space, which includes any area around prosthetic construct, including screws. *B*, Osteolysis can occur in any region of the effective joint space. Particles are pumped via the path of least resistance. *C*, X-ray film example of massive osteolysis. Note eccentric position of femoral head indicating polyethylene wear.

Therefore cross-linked PE may fail catastrophically if excessive stresses are applied. Conversely, oxidized PE causes *subsurface delamination* and cracking, leading to accelerated PE failure. Oxidized PE should be avoided. If PE is irradiated, modern packaging techniques employ packing in an environment free of oxygen. This is achieved via argon, nitrogen, or vacuum packaging. The other methods of sterilization are ethylene oxide gas sterilization or peroxide gas plasma sterilization. The disadvantage of ethylene oxide gas sterilization is that residues left by the gas sterilization process may have deleterious effects on the surrounding human tissues.

III. Prosthetic Articular Bearing

A. Hip and Shoulder Bearings. In hip and shoulder replacement surgery, the traditional bearing has been a "hard-on-soft couple." "Hard-on-soft" bearing couples include metallic heads (Co-Cr alloy or Ti alloy) mated to a polyethylene (PE) cup. The other hard-on-soft couple is a ceramic head (alumina ceramic or zirconia ceramic) mated to a PE cup. Of the metallic head options, the Co-Cr-PE couple is considered the best couple. For hip and shoulder replacement, Ti alloy heads should be avoided. This metallic bearing is susceptible to scratching from third-body debris. A rough scratched surface will cause rapid wear of the PE surface.

For both Co-Cr-PE and ceramic-PE couples, optimum wear is related to the *roughness* of the head surface and its *sphericity*. In Co-Cr heads, residual roughness is a result of carbide asperites that stick up from the surface after polishing.

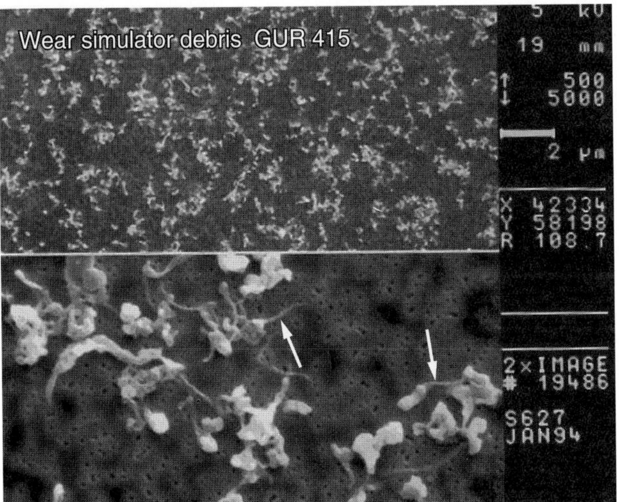

FIGURE 4-18 ■ Scanning electron microscope of polyethylene (PE) heads at bottom of wear simulator. The top photograph shows a 2-µm guide to right. Note that most of the PE particles are submicron size. In bottom photograph, arrows point to "tails" on PE heads indicating these PE are being pulled off surface via adhesive wear. (Courtesy Harry McKellop, PhD.)

For ceramic heads, residual pits within the surface cause the surface to be rough.

The lubrication regime for a hard-on-soft bearing in the hip is always *boundary lubrication*. In this regime, the lubricant (i.e., synovial fluid) is not thick enough to prevent contact between the asperites (i.e., high points on the bearing surface) of the two opposing surfaces. However, the boundary lubricant (i.e., synovial fluid with its long-chain protein molecules) can separate the two surfaces enough to prevent severe wear.

B. Knee Replacement Bearings. For knee replacement surgery the vast majority of prosthetic components manufactured employ a Co-Cr alloy femoral surface mated to a PE tibial surface. Similar to the hip and shoulder, Ti alloy is not used, because this metal alloy is susceptible to scratching from third-body debris. The rare exception for using a Ti alloy femoral component would be a patient with a documented nickel allergy. The Co-Cr alloys used for prosthetic implants contain a small percentage of nickel. Ceramic femoral components for total knee replacement (TKR) are much less commonly

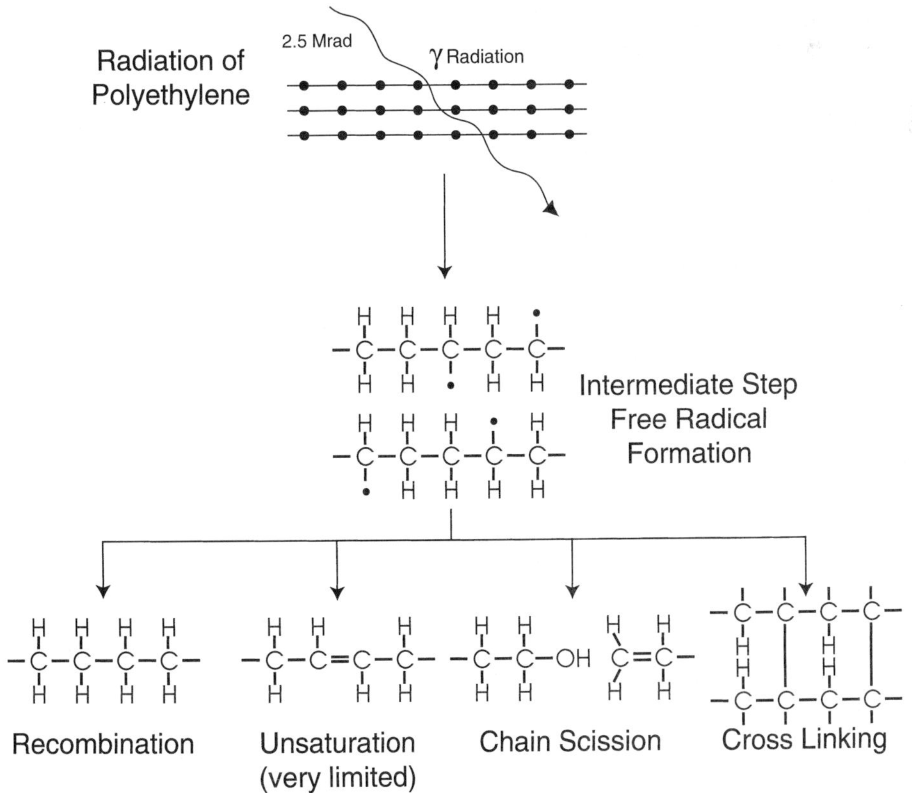

FIGURE 4-19 ■ Effect of gamma radiation on polyethylene.

used. Ceramic femoral components have the advantage of greater scratch resistance than Co-Cr alloy, but have the disadvantage of being more brittle, which may lead to prosthetic breakage.

C. Polyethylene. On the PE side of the hard-on-soft bearing couple, the PE used is ultrahigh molecular weight polyethylene (UHMWPE). Wear of PE is the major factor in causing osteolysis and prosthetic failure in all hard-on-soft bearing couples. PE wear is related to several factors: (1) PE manufacturing, (2) postprocessing sterilization, and (3) shelf storage time (i.e., how long the PE product has sat on the shelf unused).

UHMWPE for prosthetic devices in general is made by four different manufacturing techniques. These are (1) ram bar extrusion with secondary machining into the desired product (Fig. 4-20), (2) hot isostatic pressing into large sheets with secondary machining into the desired product, (3) compression molding into bars with secondary machining into the desired product, and (4) direct-compression molding from PE powder to the desired product. Better wear of UHMWPE has been consistently achieved with the *direct-compression molding* process.

In addition, the additive *calcium stearate* should not be used in the production of PE. Calcium stearate prevents PE caking on processing equipment and acts as a corrosion inhibitor to protect processing equipment. Studies have shown that calcium stearate added to PE adversely affects PE consolidation by creating areas with unfused PE particles (fusion defects). These *fusion defect* areas significantly diminish the mechanical properties of finished PE implants.

The postprocess sterilization of PE significantly affects PE performance and wear characteristics. PE sterilization techniques involve either nonenergetic (i.e., no irradiation) processes, or energetic (i.e., radiation) processes. The nonirradiation techniques are gas plasma sterilization or ethylene oxide sterilization. Irradiation of UHMWPE for sterilization is performed at two different levels: (1) the traditional low-dose (2.5–4.5 Mrad) irradiation and (2) the newer high-dose (5–15 Mrad) irradiation.

UHMWPE treated with low-dose irradiation in an inert environment *without* oxygen favors cross-linking of PE. Cross-linking of UHMWPE is good because it improves resistance to adhesive and abrasive wear. In addition, cross-linked PE improves bearing wear rates. The reason for employing the newer techniques of high-dose irradiation is to further increase cross-linking of PE to further improve PE wear rates. UHMWPE treated with high-dose irradiation is named highly cross-linked PE. Remember that irradiation of UHMWPE in an oxygen environment promotes oxidation of PE, and this is detrimental. Oxidation of PE causes molecular chain scission, which causes accelerated PE wear and failure. The techniques of gas plasma and ethylene oxide sterilization have no effect upon the cross-linking of UHMWPE. When these techniques are used alone, the wear rates of UHMWPE are generally higher than cross-linked PE.

There are at least four different methods to produce highly cross-linked PE (HCLPE) with high-dose irradiation. The key factor in all of these techniques is maintaining optimum *crystallinity* of the PE. PE in a manufactured implant exists in two different phases: crystalline phase and amorphous phase (Fig. 4-21). With postprocessing irradiation, only the amorphous areas cross-link. Crystallinity of PE >70% is associated with higher PE failure rates. When using high-dose irradiation

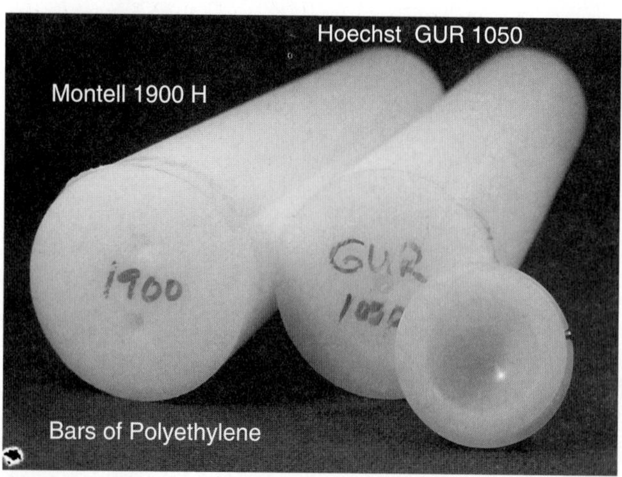

FIGURE 4-20 ■ Diagram of ram bar extruded polyethylene. Samples are from Hoechst GUR 1050 and Montell 1900 H. From these bars hip and knee polyethylene products are cut and machined.

TWO PHASES OF POLYETHYLENE

• Polyethylene has 2 different phases: Crystalline and Amorphous

• Only amorphous areas crosslink

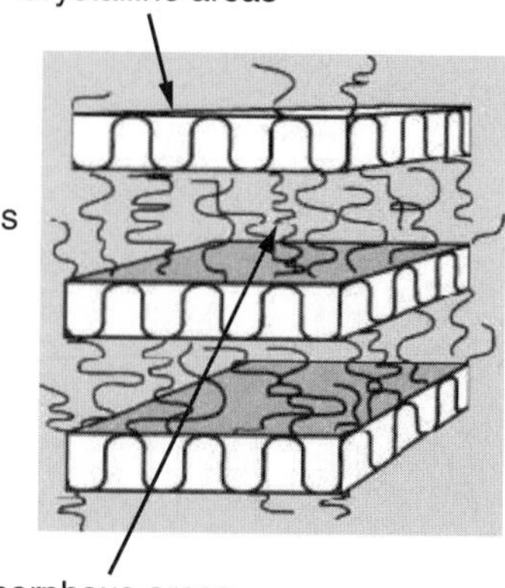

FIGURE 4-21 ■ Diagram of the molecular structure of UHMWPE. There are two distinct phases. One phase is the crystalline phase, which coexists with the adjacent amorphous regions. It is the amorphous regions that are cross-linked with irradiation treatment.

techniques, the manufacturing techniques must keep the crystalline phase to 50–56%.

The secondary processes involved in high-dose irradiation of PE generally involve the heating of PE to remove remaining free radicals. *Heat annealing* is the process of heating PE to close to the melting point to remove free radicals. If the heating is kept below the melting point, there is little reordering of the PE structure. If heating is taken above the melting point, there is structural reordering of the PE chains, which can increase crystallinity of PE with certain techniques.

It is important to remember that cross-linking of PE has disadvantages. Increasing cross-linking results in *diminished* mechanical properties of PE. Highly cross-linked PE has shown a significant reduction in Young's modulus, yield strength, and fracture toughness. HCLPE also has a diminished fatigue-crack resistance. HCLPE may not be desirable in the knee because the diminished mechanical properties may lead to macroscopic failure of the PE if high stresses are applied. An example of this situation in the knee would be edge loading of the femoral component onto the PE. Finally, HCLPE has not yet been shown to reduce osteolysis and improve implant survival because there are no long-term outcome studies with these devices.

PE performance can be adversely affected by its *shelf storage time* (the time the PE product sits on the shelf before implantation). The extent of PE degradation while sitting on the shelf depends on two major factors: (1) extent of radiation treatment and (2) type of packaging.

Irradiation of PE produces *free radicals*. If PE products are packaged and irradiated in an oxygen-free environment, oxidation of PE is minimized. However, if PE products are allowed to sit on the shelf and age, oxygen diffusion into the PE can occur, resulting in oxidation. The extent of oxygen diffusion into PE depends on the type of packaging. In experimental studies, free radicals are known to survive within PE for as long as 2–3 years. The higher the radiation dose, the more free radicals that are produced. Therefore a long shelf life can adversely affect PE performance via *on-the-shelf* oxidation. A PE product that has been on the shelf a long time may have already developed significant oxidative structural changes before implantation. The worst-case scenario is irradiated PE packaged in air (i.e., oxygen) and allowed to sit for years on the shelf. This occurs with odd lot sizes (i.e., very small or very large product sizes that are infrequently used). PE wear rates in these odd lot parts once implanted may be severe. It is recommended that irradiated PE products sit on the shelf no longer than several years. Nonirradiated PE products are not affected significantly by shelf storage time.

D. Hard on Hard Bearings. The "hard-on-hard" bearing couple has been reintroduced as an alternative bearing for THR. The main impetus for employing the hard-on-hard bearing surface is the associated structural bone damage and prosthetic failure incurred from PE-particulate-induced osteolysis. The particle size of 0.2 μm to 7 μm has been demonstrated to trigger the immune response, which leads to the osteolytic reaction. For hard-on-hard bearings, the particulate debris generated is much smaller in size (0.015–0.12 μm). It is believed that these smaller-sized particles induce a much less intense osteolytic reaction. Ironically, even though hard-on-hard bearings show very low *linear wear rates* and low wear volumes, the number of particles generated is still greater than hard-on-soft bearing couples. The reason is that the particles are so much smaller compared with PE particles that the calculated total particle aggregate is greater.

The very small particle sizes generated with hard-on-hard bearing couples changes the physiologic clearance of debris. These very small particles are absorbed regionally and are disseminated throughout the body via lymphatic channels. This is a concern with metal-metal (i.e., Co-Cr alloy) bearings. With metal-metal bearings, increased cobalt and chromium levels in blood and urine have been documented. At present, the primary concern of long-term induction of neoplasia is unfounded. Several long-term studies have shown no increase in cancer levels associated with metal on metal hip bearings. Ceramic particles within the body are essentially inert and the cancer risk with ceramic-ceramic bearings is not an issue.

The lubrication regime for a hard-on-hard bearing is *mixed lubrication*. This means that part of the time the lubrication regimen is *boundary lubrication*, and part of the time the lubrication regimen is *hydrodynamic* (also known as fluid-film lubrication). With hydrodynamic lubrication, the two opposing bearing surfaces are completely separated by the lubricant. Hydrodynamic lubrication occurs only during parts of the walking cycle, because hydrodynamic lubrication requires continuous motion of the bearing. Hydrodynamic lubrication is preferred, as bearing wear with this regime is low.

The success of hard-on-hard bearing couples depends on several important factors. These are *surface roughness, sphericity,* and *radial clearance* (i.e., clearance difference). Radial clearance is defined as the difference in radius of the head and cup. If the radius of the head is larger than the cup, bearing contact is *equatorial*. An equatorial bearing has high frictional torques, because there is no space for lubricant ingress and egress. If the diameter of the head is smaller than the cup, bearing contact is *polar*. Polar contact with low conformity (i.e., high radial

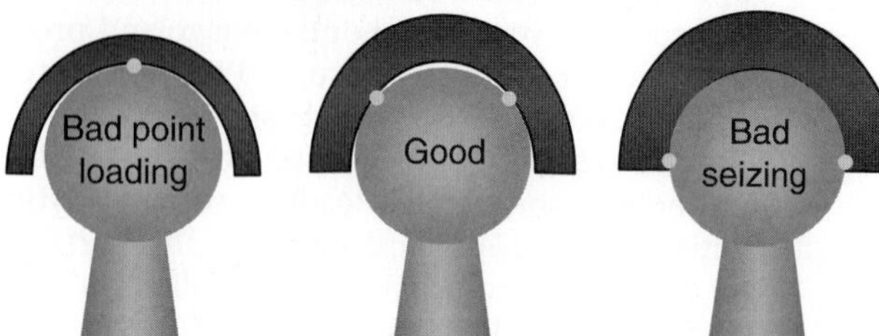

FIGURE 4-22 ■ Diagram of the three different areas of bearing contact that can be employed for a hard-on-hard bearing couple for hip replacement. Polar contact allows fluid lubrication but contact stress at the pole is high, causing high friction and wear. Mid-polar contact is the best as contact loads are optimized and there is good bearing lubrication. Equatorial contact prevents fluid lubrication and is bad.

clearance) also causes high friction and wear. The small bearing contact area causes high stress resulting in poor lubrication. The optimum design is polar contact with high-bearing conformity (Fig. 4-22). In this situation, the radial clearance is small (typically <150 μm). The low radial clearance is still enough to allow ingress and egress of lubricant into the bearing.

For optimum lubrication, a hard-on-hard bearing surface must be very smooth. The rougher the surface, the more difficult it is to separate with lubricant. Metal (i.e., Co-Cr alloy) surfaces have a surface roughness (Ra) of 0.05 μm. Ceramic surfaces have an Ra of 0.02 μm. In comparison, machined UHMWPE has an Ra of several hundred μms. Sphericity also affects bearing lubrication. Sphericity should be kept below 10 μm. Sphericity variation creates small high points on the surface. This causes localized stress points that can adversely affect lubrication and increase wear.

Hard-on-hard bearings have a phenomenon of *"run-in" wear*. Typically, within the first million cycles of wear, there is a higher wear rate that, after the run-in period, diminishes to a lower steady-state wear rate. It is thought that during the run-in period, high stress points (i.e., sphericity discrepancies) and the larger surface asperites are polished out of the bearing couple.

IV. Knee Replacement Surgery

A. Surgical Technique—The technical goals of knee replacement surgery are (1) restoration of *mechanical* alignment, (2) preservation (or restoration) of the joint line, (3) balanced ligaments, and (4) maintaining or restoring a normal Q angle.

Table 4-4. RECOMMENDED PREOPERATIVE RADIOGRAPHS IN KNEE REPLACEMENT SURGERY

- Standing full-length anteroposterior radiograph from hip to ankle
- Standing extension lateral on large cassette (14" × 17")
- Flexion lateral on large cassette
- Merchant's view

Consistent clinical results are predicated on good preoperative planning, which includes a good clinical examination of the knee along with preoperative radiographs. Preoperative radiographs are used to identify corrections needed in alignment and defects in bone that will require bone grafting or augmentation. Table 4-4 lists the recommended series of preoperative radiographs.

1. Mechanical Alignment—Restoring a neutral mechanical alignment ensures that the forces through the leg pass through the center of the hip, knee, and ankle. Restoring a neutral mechanical alignment in knee replacement surgery allows optimum load share through medial and lateral sides of the prosthetic components. In a knee replacement where mechanical alignment is not restored, a net varus or valgus moment is created. This places excessive stress on one side of the knee, leading to excessive wear and early failure. Identifying the mechanical axis on preoperative radiographs and with intraoperative instrumentation is essential. Figure 4-23 defines the anatomic and mechanical axes of the femur and tibia. In the femur, the anatomic axis is defined by the medullary canal and most often exits in the intercondylar notch region. The exit of the anatomic axis at the distal end of the femur defines the medullary entry point for the intramedullary rod of the femoral jigs used to prepare the femur. In some cases, the anatomic axis may be located just medial or lateral to the intercondylar notch due to distal femoral bowing deformities. A preoperative standing, full-length radiograph can be used to identify the anatomic axis and femoral entry point. The femoral *mechanical axis* starts from the center of the femoral head and ends at the point of intersection, with the femoral anatomic axis at the intercondylar notch. The angle measured between the femoral anatomic axis and mechanical axis is called the *valgus cut angle*. This can be measured in each case using a standing, anteroposterior full-length radiograph of the leg; in most cases it measures 5–7 degrees. The goal is to cut the distal femur at an angle perpendicular to the *mechanical axis*. By cutting the distal femur by the valgus cut angle, the femoral prosthesis

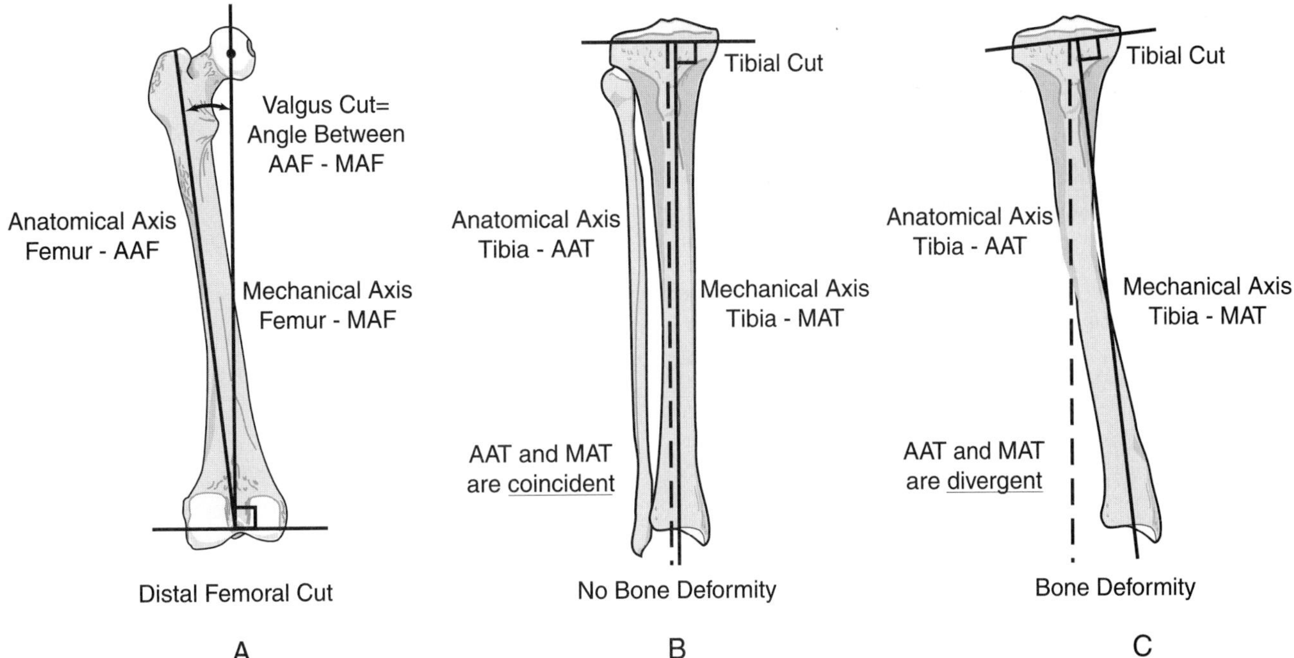

FIGURE 4-23 ■ Diagram showing mechanical axis and anatomic axis of leg. *A*, In the femur, the anatomic axis follows the femoral shaft, whereas the mechanical axis lies along the line from hip center to knee center (mechanical axis and anatomic axis intersect at knee). *B*, In the tibia, the anatomic axis follows the tibial shaft. Mechanical axis runs from knee center to ankle-joint center. When deformities are absent, the tibial anatomic axis and mechanical axis are usually coincident. *C*, When deformities are present, these axes are divergent.

will point toward the center of the femoral head and will be in a mechanically neutral position. Cases in which the valgus cut angle should be measured with a full-length radiograph are patients who are very tall or short, patients who have post-trauma deformities of the femur, and patients who have congenital femoral bow deformities. Patients who are very tall will often have a valgus cut angle less than 5 degrees, whereas patients who are very short may have a valgus cut angle more than 7 degrees.

The anatomic axis of the tibia is the line defining the medullary canal, and in the majority of cases it is coincident with the mechanical axis. The cases in which the tibial anatomic and mechanical axes are disparate are in post-traumatic and congenital bow deformities. The goal in either case is to cut the tibial surface perpendicular to the *mechanical axis* such that leg stresses are passed evenly through the medial and lateral sides of the prosthetic tibial surface. When the tibial anatomic and mechanical axes are coincident, an intramedullary rod will readily assist in determining the correct cut. However, in a post-traumatic tibia deformity the medullary rod may not pass. In this instance, an extra medullary guide device placed over the center of the ankle up to the center of the tibia or center of the tibial tubercle will be necessary.

2. Bone Cuts and Alignment—The next technical aspect in knee replacement surgery is to remove sufficient amount of bone so that the prosthesis, when placed, will re-create the original thickness of cartilage and bone. This ensures that the *joint line is re-created*, because knee ligaments play a vital role in prosthetic knee kinematics. Knee function is optimized when the joint line is preserved. Current total knee instrumentation is capable of providing precise bone cuts, but the surgeon should never be lulled into a sense of complacency; cutting jigs can be pinned improperly or may shift as sawing occurs, causing inaccurate cuts. The surgeon should always double-check cuts and alignment during the trialing process. Furthermore, during the bone-cut and trialing process, bone defects should be identified and restored. If not, malalignment may occur. If bone defects are small (<1 cm deep), they can be filled with cement. Larger defects may require bone grafts or, more commonly, metallic augmentation, which is provided with many modular knee replacement systems.
3. Maintenance of Q Angle—The next important factor in knee replacement surgery is avoiding techniques that result in an increased Q angle. The most common complication in TKR involves the patellofemoral articulation. An increased Q angle leads to increased lateral

subluxation forces, which can adversely affect patellofemoral tracking. A following section addresses the technical factors in avoiding abnormal patellofemoral maltracking.

4. Ligament Balancing—Knee ligament balancing is the final important aspect for successful knee replacement. In the degenerative process, ligaments may become scarred and contracted, or they may become stretched from excessive bow deformities. Ligaments must be balanced to provide optimum function and wear for the prosthesis. Balancing must be accomplished in the coronal plane and in the sagittal plane.
   a. Coronal Plane. In the coronal plane, the two deformities are varus and valgus. The basic principle in coronal plane balancing is to *release* on the *concave* side of the deformity and to fill up the convex side until the ligament is taut. Figure 4-24 illustrates the principle for varus and valgus deformities. Table 4-5 lists the structures to be released for varus and valgus deformities. Typically for varus deformities, release of osteophytes and the deep medial collateral ligament (MCL) is all that is required to make the medial and lateral compartments symmetric in size. More significant deformities require the release of the posterior-medial corner along with the attachment of the semimembranosus. For more significant deformities, sequential subperiosteal elevation of the superficial MCL (at the pes anserine region) is required. The ligament cannot be fully released, or it will become incompetent. If over-release occurs, a constrained knee device is required. The posterior cruciate ligament (PCL) in rare instances may be a deforming factor in significant varus deformities, and one should consider release of the PCL if other releases fail to achieve proper balance. For valgus deformities, release of osteophytes

Table 4-5. KNEE LIGAMENT BALANCING CORONAL PLANE

VARUS DEFORMITY MEDIAL RELEASE	VALGUS DEFORMITY LATERAL RELEASE
Osteophytes	Osteophytes
Deep meniscotibial ligament	Lateral capsule
Posteromedial corner with semimembranosus	Iliotibial band if tight in extension
Superficial meniscotibial ligament (pes anserine complex)	Popliteus if tight in flexion
Posterior cruciate ligament (rare occasions)	Lateral collateral ligament

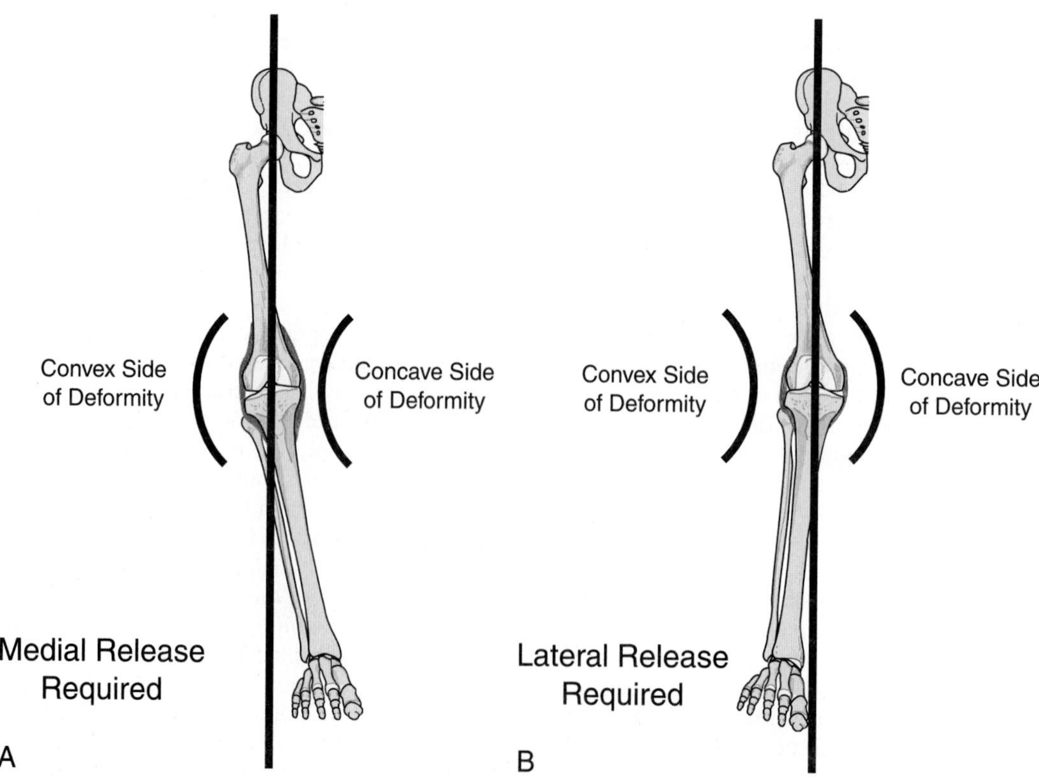

FIGURE 4-24 ■ Diagram illustrating principle of releases for coronal plane deformities in the knee. *A*, Varus deformity. *B*, Valgus deformity.

and the lateral capsule off the tibia should be the initial release. If the lateral compartment remains tight, then release of the iliotibial band (either with a Z-type release of the tendon or release off of Gerdy's tubercle) is recommended if the lateral compartment is tight in extension. If the lateral compartment is tight in flexion, then release of the popliteus tendon is recommended. In many situations where the valgus deformity is large (>15 degrees), both the iliotibial band and popliteal tendon need to be released. For severe valgus deformities, balancing may require release of the lateral collateral ligament (LCL), and if this is done, then one should strongly consider the use of a constrained-type prosthetic design. Correction of significant valgus deformity places the peroneal nerve on stretch. The deformity *most often* associated with a peroneal nerve palsy is combined valgus deformity with flexion contracture. Correction of both deformities places the nerve on significant stretch. If a postoperative peroneal nerve palsy is noted, initial treatment should be release of all compressive dressings and flexion of the knee.

b. Sagittal Plane. In this plane, balancing becomes more sophisticated. In the sagittal plane, the knee has two radii of curvatures; one for the patellofemoral articulation and one for the remaining weight-bearing portion of the knee. The knee, like the hand metacarpal, acts as a modified cam. Stability, in extension and flexion, is provided by different parts of the collateral ligament structures. Balancing in the sagittal plane may require soft-tissue releases but may also require additional bone resection to achieve the correct balance. The goal in sagittal plane balancing is to obtain a gap in extension equal to the gap in flexion. By achieving this goal, the tibial insert, when placed, will be stable throughout the arc of motion. The general rule to follow when balancing the knee in the sagittal plane is as follows: If the gap problem is symmetric (i.e., same problem in flexion and extension), adjust the tibia; if the gap problem is asymmetric (i.e., different problem in flexion and extension), adjust the femur.

The six scenarios for knee balancing are illustrated in Table 4-6.

B. Prosthetic Design—Current total knee prosthetic designs are of three types: unconstrained, constrained nonhinged, and constrained hinged. There are two design types in the unconstrained category, the posterior-cruciate-retaining and posterior-cruciate-substituting (often referred to as posterior stabilized) implants.

Table 4-6. SAGITTAL PLANE BALANCING TOTAL KNEE REPLACEMENT

SCENARIO	PROBLEM	SOLUTIONS
Tight in extension (contracture) Tight in flexion (will not bend fully)	Symmetric gap Did not cut enough tibial bone	(1) Cut more proximal tibia
Loose in extension (recurvatum) Loose in flexion (large drawer test)	Symmetric gap Cut too much tibia	(1) Use thick poly insert (2) Metallic tibial augmentation
Extension good Flexion loose (large drawer test)	Asymmetrical gap Cut too much posterior femur	(1) Increase size of femoral component from anterior to posterior (i.e., go up to next size) (2) Fill up posterior gap with cement or metal augmentation
Extension tight (contracture) Flexion good	Asymmetric gap Did not cut enough distal femur or did not release enough posterior capsule	(1) Release posterior capsule (2) Take off more distal femur bone (1-2 mm at a time)
Extension good Flexion tight (will not bend fully)	Asymmetric gap Did not cut enough posterior bone or posterior cruciate ligament (PCL) scarred and too tight (assuming use of a PCL-retaining knee system) No posterior slope in tibial bone cut (i.e., anterior slope)	(1) Decrease size of femoral component from anterior to posterior (i.e., recut to next smaller size) (2) Recess PCL (3) Check posterior slope of tibia and recut if anterior slope
Extension loose (recurvatum) Flexion good	Asymmetric gap Cut too much distal femur or anteroposterior size too big	(1) Distal femoral augmentation (2) Smaller size femur (anteroposterior) that converts to symmetric gap problem (3) Use thicker tibial polyethylene inset and address tight flexion gap

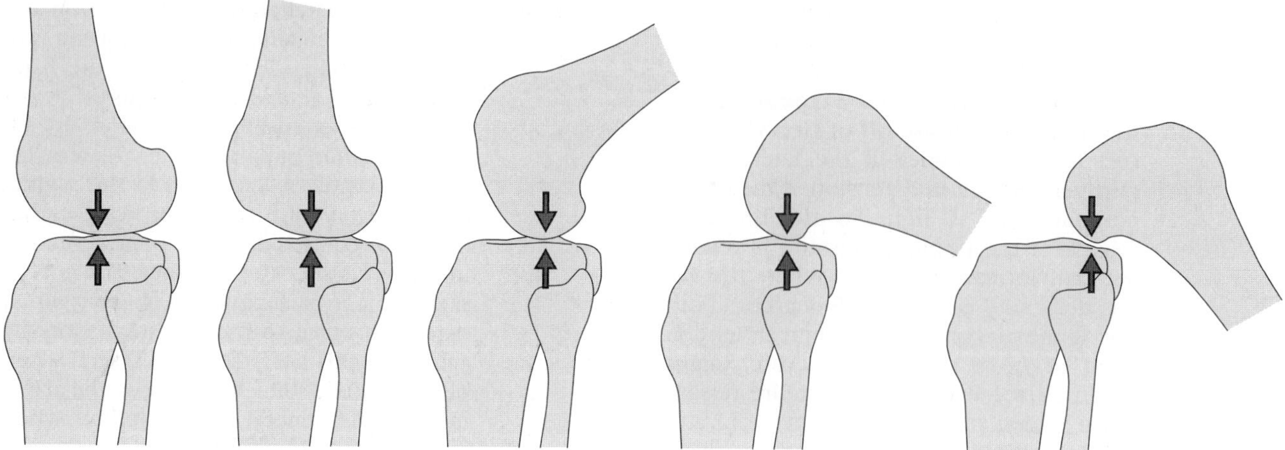

FIGURE 4-25 ■ Femoral rollback is posterior shift of femoral-tibial contact point as knee flexes. Rollback allows femur to clear tibia to provide further flexion.

Initial unconstrained total knee resurfacing designs sacrificed both the anterior cruciate ligament (ACL) and PCL ligaments. A drawback of such designs was limited knee flexion (in the range of 95 degrees) and flexion instability. With knee flexion, the femur could subluxate or dislocate anterior to the tibia.

By preserving the PCL, flexion instability is mitigated because the PCL becomes taut with knee flexion and prevents anterior dislocation of the femur on the tibia (provided adequate knee balancing has been performed). In addition, by preserving the PCL, femoral rollback is produced. Femoral rollback is the posterior shift in the femoral-tibial contact point in the sagittal plane as the knee flexes (Fig. 4-25). The posterior shift in the femoral-tibial contact point allows the posterior femur to flex further without impinging on the posterior tibia. Femoral rollback is controlled by both the ACL and PCL working in concert, but it can still occur without the ACL to some extent. Total knee prosthetic designs that preserve the PCL achieve better knee flexion by allowing femoral rollback. The disadvantage of this design is that femoral rollback occurs without the aid of the ACL, and the consequent rollback is a combination of roll and slide. For rollback to occur, the tibial PE needs to be relatively flat, but this has the detrimental effect of creating high contact stresses. The combination of sliding wear and high contact stresses on the PE can lead to rapid PE wear and failure (see the section on catastrophic wear). To combat this problem, recent PCL-retaining designs contain a more congruent PE insert that allows less rollback. The more congruent articulation reduces the contact stresses on the PE, but it relegates the PCL to a static stabilizer to prevent anterior dislocation of the femur on the tibia. Increased knee flexion is achieved with a posterior offset center of rotation (usually 4–6 mm) and re-creation of the normal posterior tibial slope.

Posterior cruciate-*substituting* implants employ a tibial PE post in the middle of the knee along with a cam situated between the femoral condyles (Fig. 4-26). Depending on the design parameters, the femoral cam will engage against the tibial post at a designated flexion point. At that point, the femur is unable to translate anteriorly, and with further flexion it will mechanically reproduce rollback.

With the knee in the flexed position, the tibial post will prevent the cam from translating anteriorly, thus providing stability. Posterior

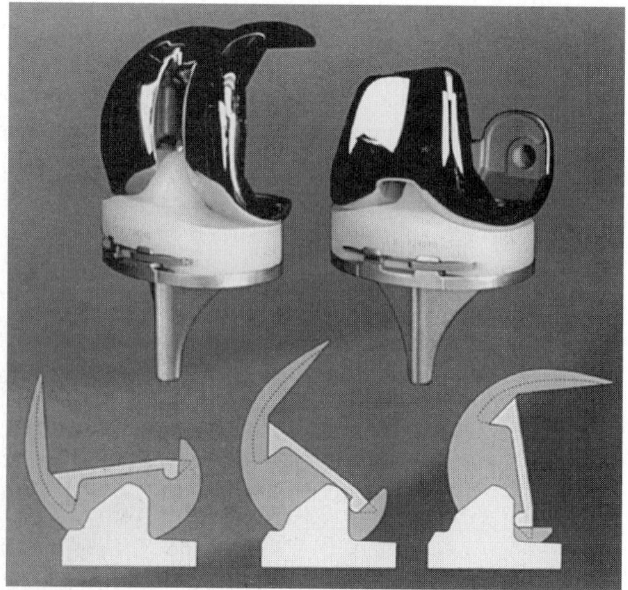

FIGURE 4-26 ■ Posterior-cruciate-substituting (also known as posterior stabilized) knee. Note central polyethylene post and femoral cam device on femur when the knee flexes.

cruciate-substituting designs achieve improved knee flexion and allow mechanical rollback. Because rollback is controlled mechanically, a congruent articulation surface can be used, and this reduces contact stresses on the tibial PE. The disadvantage of the cruciate-substituting design is that knee balancing must be carefully addressed. If the flexion gap is loose, the femur can jump over the tibial post and dislocate (Fig. 4-27). If dislocation occurs, reduction requires sedation or general anesthetic, with the reduction maneuver consisting of knee flexion (at 90 degrees), distraction, and anterior pulling force directed on the tibia. Cam jump can occur with hyperflexion even if the knee is well balanced. With a hyperflexed knee, the femur will impinge on the tibia and lever the femur over the tibial post. Hence if anticipated knee motion after knee replacement surgery is expected to be beyond 130 degrees, a cruciate-retaining design should be considered. A cruciate-substituting design is favored over a cruciate-retaining design in several situations. First, patients with a previous patellectomy should have a cruciate-substituting prosthesis because the weakened extensor force allows for easier anterior femoral dislocation even if the PCL is retained. Second, patients with ***inflammatory arthritis*** can have continued inflammatory changes that will cause late PCL ruptures in total knees that retain the PCL. Third, patients with prior trauma with PCL rupture or attenuation should have a posterior stabilized implant. Finally, the last indication for a cruciate-substituting device is over-release of the PCL during knee ligament balancing. If the tibial articular profile is flat, the knee can translate anteriorly and become unstable. In this situation, conversion to a cruciate-substituting device is preferred.

C. Patellofemoral Articulation—The most common complications in TKR involve abnormal patellar tracking. Avoiding patellar problems in knee replacement is essentially an exercise in Q angle management and understanding the technical aspects that alter the knee joint line. The Q angle is the angle formed by the intersection of the extensor mechanism axis above the patella with the axis of the patellar tendon. The significance of the Q angle in knee replacement surgery is that an increased Q angle is associated with increased lateral patellar subluxation forces. Additionally, most patellofemoral prosthetic designs are not as constraining as the native knee. Thus an increased Q angle can frequently cause patellofemoral maltracking. The goal in TKR is to maintain a normal Q angle with techniques that *do not compromise* mechanical alignment or ligament stability. Several technical rules in TKR should be followed to prevent abnormal patellar tracking. They are summarized in Table 4-7. First, femoral component internal fixation must be avoided. Internal rotation of the femoral component causes lateral patellar tilt and a net increase in Q angle (Fig. 4-28). The preferred

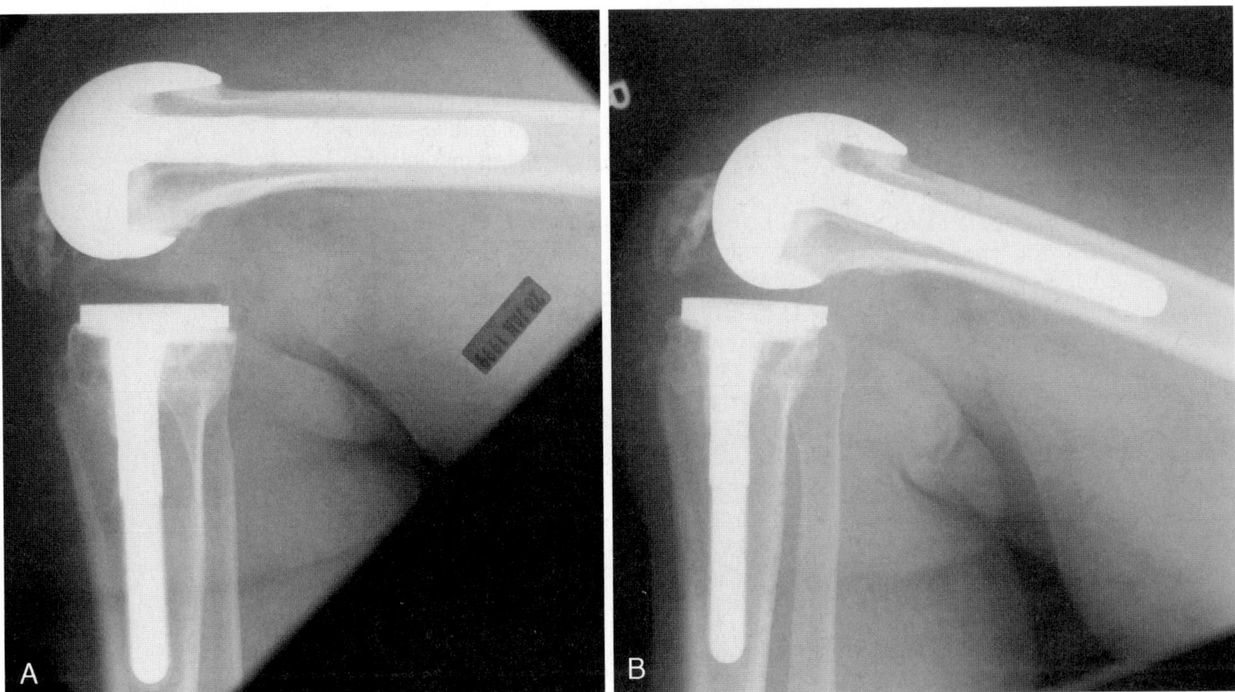

FIGURE 4-27 ■ Femoral cam jump. *A*, Lateral radiograph of femoral cam jump. Femur has hyperflexed, allowing cam to rise above tibial post and dislocate anteriorly. Once in this position, it is very difficult to reduce unless an anesthetic is administered. *B*, Postreduction radiograph of the same knee.

Table 4-7. PREVENTION OF PATELLOFEMORAL MALTRACKING

TECHNICAL ISSUES	GUIDELINE	PROBLEMS	PREFERRED SOLUTION
Femoral component rotation	Do not internally rotate femoral component past neutral axis	Internal rotation of femoral component results in net lateral patellar tilt and increased lateral subluxation	Slight external rotation of femoral component
Femoral component position	Do not medialize femoral component	Increases Q angle	Either central or lateralized position
Tibial component rotation	Do not internally rotate tibial component past medial side of tibial tubercle	Internal rotation of tibial component results in net external rotation of tibial tubercle and increases Q angle	Tibial component centered in area between medial border of tibial tubercle and middle of tibial tubercle
Mechanical alignment of leg	Do not leave leg with net valgus mechanical alignment (i.e., avoid excess valgus)	Excessive valgus alignment increases Q angle	Femoral and tibial bone cuts that restore a *neutral* mechanical alignment of leg
Patella component position	(1) Avoid lateralization of patellar component on patella (2) Avoid inferior position of patellar component on patella	(1) Lateralization of patellar component results in net increase of Q angle (2) Inferior positioning can result in relative patella baja	(1) Patellar component placed in center of patella or in medialized position (2) Patellar component placed in center of patella or in superior position
Joint line position	Avoid bone cuts that raise the joint line	Creates or enhances patella baja	Maintain joint line; lower joint line if possible, when baja deformity present

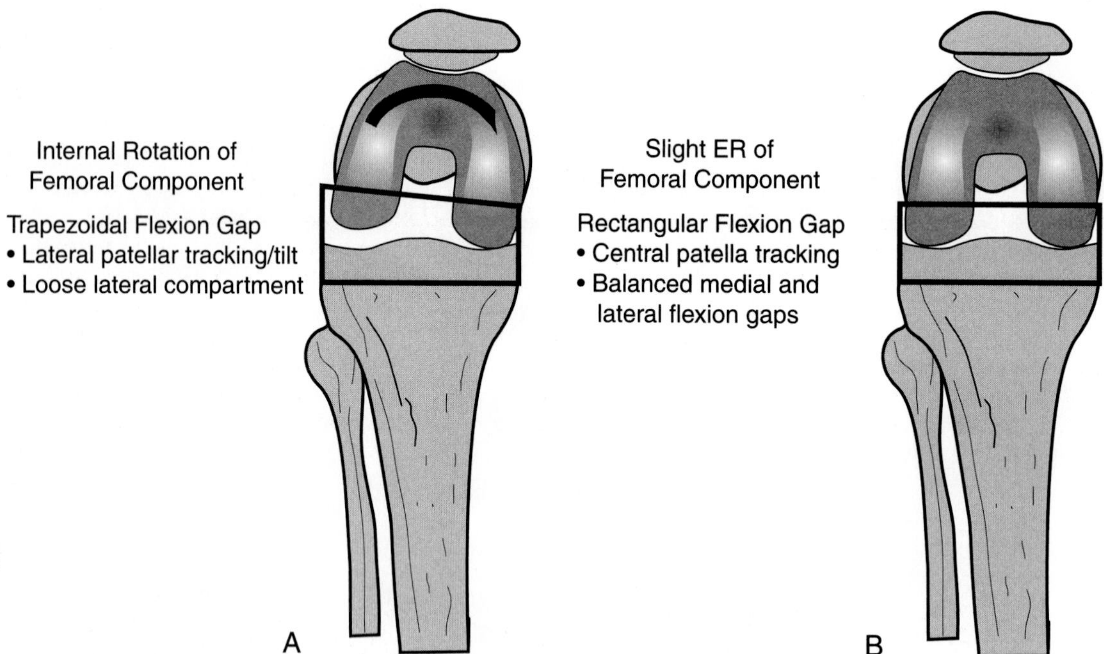

FIGURE 4-28 ■ Femoral component rotation in coronal plane. *A*, Illustration of femoral component that is placed in internal rotation. Internal rotation of femoral component causes lateral flange of femoral component to push patella medial. Result is increased Q angle. Although the patella is neutrally positioned, internal rotation of femoral component gives effect of lateral patellar tilt. In addition, internal rotation of femoral component creates asymmetric flexion gap, making it more difficult to balance the knee. *B*, Femoral component in slight external rotation (ER). This creates symmetric flexion gap, and the trochlear groove matches the patella. Knee is balanced.

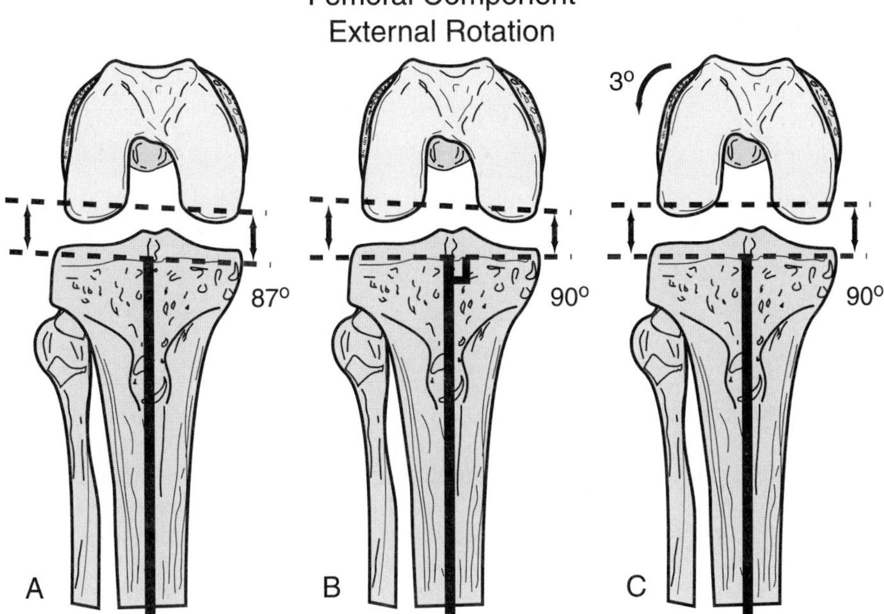

FIGURE 4-29 ■ Diagrams demonstrating rotational alignment of knee in coronal plane in flexion. *A*, Tibia on average has 3 degrees varus tilt. To match this tilt, medial femoral condyle is slightly bigger in dimension than lateral femoral condyle. *B*, Proximal tibia is cut at 90 degrees, perpendicular to the mechanical axis of the tibia. In flexion, this creates an asymmetric flexion gap of the femur when cut parallel to the posterior femoral condyles. *C*, Anteroposterior (AP) cut of femur made in slight external rotation. AP cut matches tibia cut in flexion, creating symmetric flexion gap. Flexion gap is now balanced.

rotational alignment of the femur is slight external rotation to the neutral axis. Normally, the proximal tibia is in slight varus of 3 degrees (Fig. 4-29). In TKR, the tibial is cut at 90 degrees (i.e., perpendicular to the mechanical axis). In order to maintain a symmetric flexion gap, the femoral component must be externally rotated by the same amount to create a symmetric flexion gap. This allows for balanced ligaments in flexion.

Identifying the neutral rotational axis for the femur is not always easy. Occasionally, landmarks can be damaged during the degenerative process. The three generally accepted landmarks defining a *neutral femoral rotational axis* are the anteroposterior axis of the femur, the epicondylar axis, and the posterior condylar axis (Fig. 4-30). The anteroposterior axis of the femur is defined as a line running from the center of the trochlear groove to the top of the intercondylar notch. A line perpendicular to this defines the neutral rotational axis. The epicondylar axis is considered to be slightly externally rotated to the neutral axis, and the femoral component should be placed parallel the epicondylar axis. The other landmark is the posterior condylar axis, where a line made in 3–5 degrees of external rotation to this line defines the neutral axis.

On the tibial side, internal rotation of the tibial component must be avoided. Internal rotation of the tibial component effectively results in relative external rotation of the tibial tubercle. This has the deleterious effect of increasing the Q angle (Fig. 4-31). Anatomic valgus deformities must be corrected back to a normal range (5–7 degrees preferred). The actual goal in TKR is to restore a neutral mechanical alignment. Distal femoral and proximal bone cuts should be made to achieve

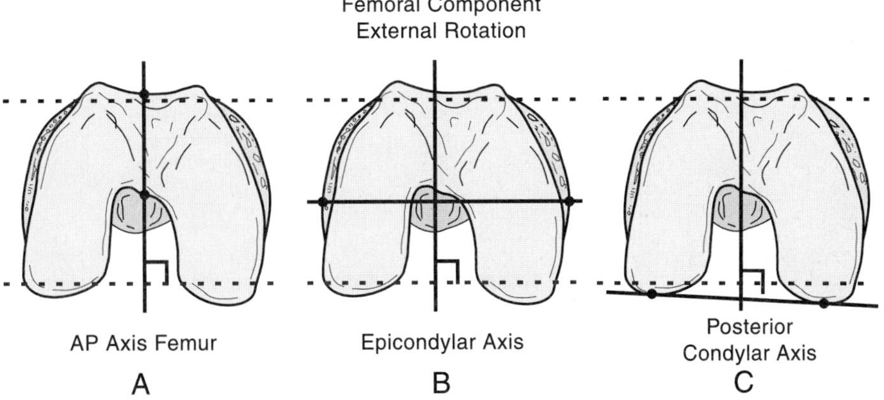

FIGURE 4-30 ■ Determination of femoral component external rotation. *A*, Anteroposterior (AP) axis: defined by center of trochlear groove and intercondylar notch (dots). AP cut is made perpendicular to this axis. *B*, Epicondylar axis: defined by a line connecting centers of medial and lateral epicondylar (dots). AP cut is made parallel to this axis. *C*, Posterior condylar axis: defined by a line connecting bottom of medial and lateral posterior condyles. AP cut is made in 3 degrees of external rotation to this axis line.

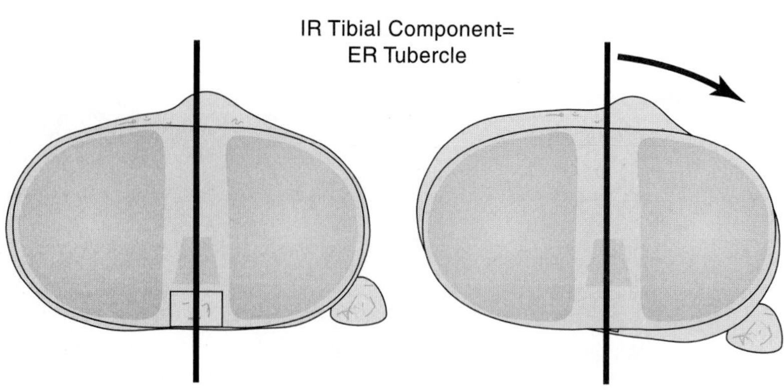

FIGURE 4-31 ■ Demonstration of tibial component internal rotation. Left diagram shows tibial component centered over medial third of tibial tubercle. This is generally considered the preferred position. Right diagram shows internal rotation of tibial component. This causes a net effect of externally rotating tibial tubercle to lateral side, which increases Q angle.

this goal. If excessive valgus remains, there will be an increased Q angle.

When resurfacing the patella, the desired position of the patellar component is central or medialized. A medialized patellar component reduces the Q angle, but it requires the use of a smaller patellar dome (Fig. 4-32). The need for lateral release is less when a small patellar dome is used in a medialized position. Placing a small patellar component in a lateralized position increases the Q angle and lateral subluxation forces. Femoral component position, if it can be adjusted, should be either centered or lateralized. A medialized femoral component places the trochlear groove in a more medial position, which increases the Q angle. Thus this position should be avoided.

Patella baja (or patella infera) is not an infrequent problem encountered in TKR. Patella baja is a condition manifested by a shortened patellar tendon. With patella baja, knee flexion is limited due to patellar impingement on the tibia as the knee flexes. Patella baja is most frequently seen in patients who have had a proximal tibial osteotomy, tibial tubercle shift or transfer, or prior fracture to the proximal tibia. Patella baja is encountered in various degrees. The solutions are limited. First, when performing a TKR, avoid bone cuts that raise the joint line. Raising the joint line will effectively increase the baja deformity. Conversely, lowering the joint line will decrease the deformity. Lowering the joint line can be achieved by using distal femoral augmentation and cutting off more proximal tibia (Fig. 4-33).

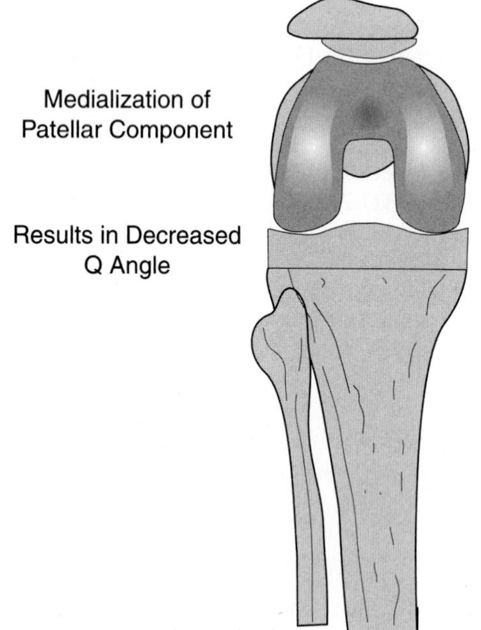

FIGURE 4-32 ■ Medialization of patellar component. With this technique, a small patellar dome is placed on medial side of cut patella (usually centered over trochlear ridge). Because entire patella does not need to be centered in trochlea, the center of the patellar bone is in a lateralized position that reduces Q angle. In addition, lateral retinaculum is more relaxed with patella bone in lateral position.

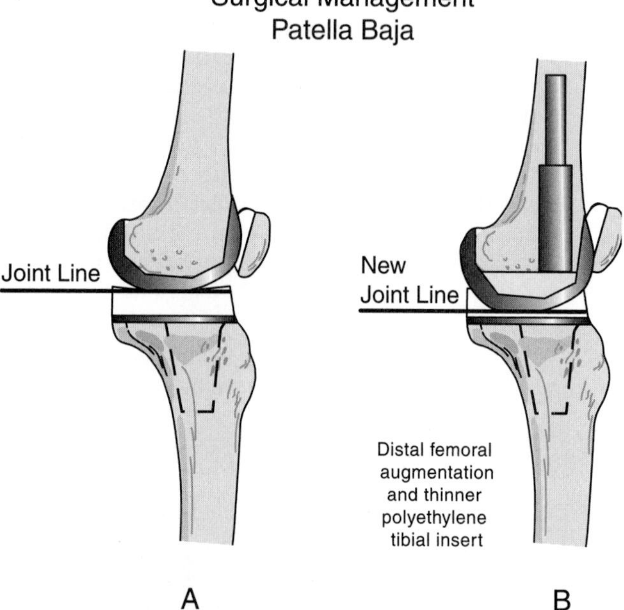

FIGURE 4-33 ■ Diagram illustrating effect of lowering joint line with distal femoral augmentation to improve baja deformity. *A*, Total knee with baja deformity. *B*, Distal femoral augmentation (augments behind femoral component) moves joint line inferiorly. Less tibial polyethylene thickness is required. Baja deformity is improved.

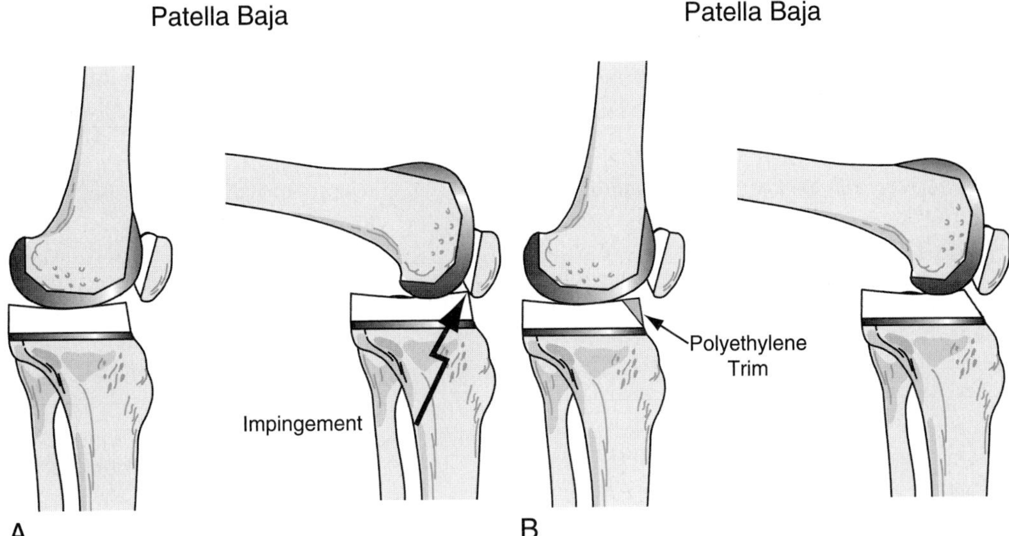

FIGURE 4-34 ■ Diagram showing technique of trimming polyethylene at impingement points in patella baja. *A*, Total knee with baja deformity. Note impingement of inferior pole of patella component with anterior tibial polyethylene. *B*, Trimming of polyethylene to decrease impingement. Trimming is performed with scalpel and should not compromise articulating surfaces or stability. Trimming provides some improvement (usually up to 10 degrees) in flexion range.

Lowering the joint line does not get rid of the deformity entirely, but it does help to provide increased knee flexion. Resurfacing the patella with a small patellar dome placed superiorly can effectively increase patellar tendon length. Inferior bone can be trimmed to prevent impingement. Another useful technique is trimming the anterior tibial PE and patellar PE at the impingement points (Fig. 4-34). This is achieved sharply with a scalpel. It will provide some improved flexion. Only shave PE that does not compromise component stability or patellar tracking. If the baja deformity is severe, one last option is to cut the patella but not resurface. By doing this, there is less patellar impingement, allowing for more knee flexion.

D. Catastrophic Wear: TKR—Catastrophic wear in knee replacement surgery refers to the premature failure of prosthetic implants due to excessive loading, macroscopic failure of PE, and subsequent mechanical loosening (Fig. 4-35). Catastrophic wear does not refer to the long-term effect of submicron and small-micron particle debris generation and associated bony osteolysis. It is a problem of large-scale PE failure resulting from a combination of several factors involved in implant design and biomechanics. The problem is seen primarily in TKR, but depending on the situation and conditions, it can also be seen in prosthetic hip and shoulder replacement. The main issues involved in the phenomenon of catastrophic wear are (1) PE thickness, (2) articular geometry, (3) sagittal plane knee kinematics, (4) PE sterilization, and (5) PE machining.
   1. PE Thickness—PE thickness is of critical importance in the catastrophic wear process. To keep joint contact stresses below the yield strength of UHMWPE, PE thickness must be at least 8 mm. Thinner sections transmit joint stresses to a localized area only, resulting in microscopic and macroscopic PE failure. It is very important to understand that when placing a tibial PE insert into a metal tray, the PE thickness reported represents the total thickness of the metal tray (usually 2-3 mm) plus the PE. Therefore in many instances where 8-10 mm PE inserts are used with a metal base tray, the actual PE thickness at the nadir of the convexity on the articular surface may be as thin as 4-5 mm. Consequently, in many cases where thin PE inserts are used, the yield strength of UHMWPE is exceeded. This is seen most often when thin bone-cut resections are used in younger patients to preserve bone stock for future revision. In this scenario, the young, active patient will cycle the prosthetic

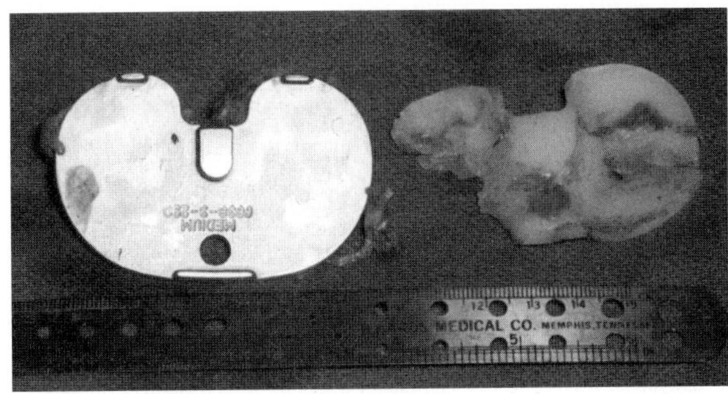

FIGURE 4-35 ■ Photograph of catastrophic wear of polyethylene in a total knee replacement. Note gross fragmentation of tibial polyethylene.

joint at a much higher rate, leading to rapid failure (4–5 years in some instances).

2. Articular Geometry—Another important factor leading to catastrophic failure is articular geometry. A majority of the prosthetic knee implants associated with catastrophic wear have a relatively flat PE articular surface. A flat articular design is disadvantageous in terms of biomechanical loading. With such a design, prosthetic contact areas between the femur and the tibia are low, and contact loads are high. Instead, the goal in prosthetic knee design is to *minimize contact loads*; this is achieved by *maximizing surface contact area*. Newer-generation prosthetic knee designs have improved contact areas by increasing articular congruency. This is achieved by increasing congruency in the coronal and sagittal planes. As a result, instead of seeing a flat PE insert, newer components tend to be more dished in both the coronal and sagittal planes.
3. Sagittal Plane Knee Kinematics—Sagittal plane kinematics played an important role in the design of flat PE inserts. In an effort to improve knee flexion, prosthetic designs used the PCL to provide femoral rollback. Femoral rollback is the posterior shift of the femoral-tibial contact as the knee flexes (Fig. 4-36). Femoral rollback allows the femur to clear the posterior tibia and bend further. In the native knee, femoral rollback is controlled by both the ACL and PCL. Rollback can still occur without an ACL, but fluoroscopic studies observing rollback in PCL-retained TKRs show that the posterior rollback is kinetically displeasing. Instead of a smooth gradual roll, there is a combination of forward sliding, backward sliding, and posterior rolling. In addition, to allow the knee to roll back, a flat PE insert is required. The diskinetic sagittal plane movements seen with PCL-retained implants that have flat PE inserts contribute to the catastrophic wear process. Laboratory studies show that sliding movements (i.e., femoral component translation on the tibia) result in surface and subsurface cracking and significant wear. In contrast, pure rolling movements generated minimal cracking and wear. Therefore newer prosthetic knee designs incorporate less femoral rollback and provide a more congruent articular PE surface. Knee flexion is achieved with other design techniques, such as a posterior center of rotation, utilizing a posterior slope, or by using a posterior cruciate-substituting knee design.
4. PE Sterilization—The last major factor in catastrophic wear involves the sterilization of PE. As previously discussed in the section on osteolysis and PE wear, PE components irradiated in an oxygen environment suffer from PE oxidation. Oxidized PE is mechanically weaker, and the threshold for catastrophic wear is lowered. Excessive loading of oxidized PE can result in rapid PE failure.
5. PE Machining. More recent studies have implicated the *machining process* of PE as a factor leading to PE breakdown. During the machining of PE, cutting tools (lathing or burring tools) create shear forces at the cutting interface that microscopically stretch the PE chains. This effect is most pronounced in the subsurface region of 1–2 mm. In the "sensitized" subsurface region, the PE molecule chains (specifically the amorphous regions) are microscopically stretched and are at an increased energy state. Any oxidation therefore will be more apt to affect this region. As a result, oxidative changes within the machined PE tibial component will show a classical *white band* of oxidation in the subsurface region. This also explains why wear

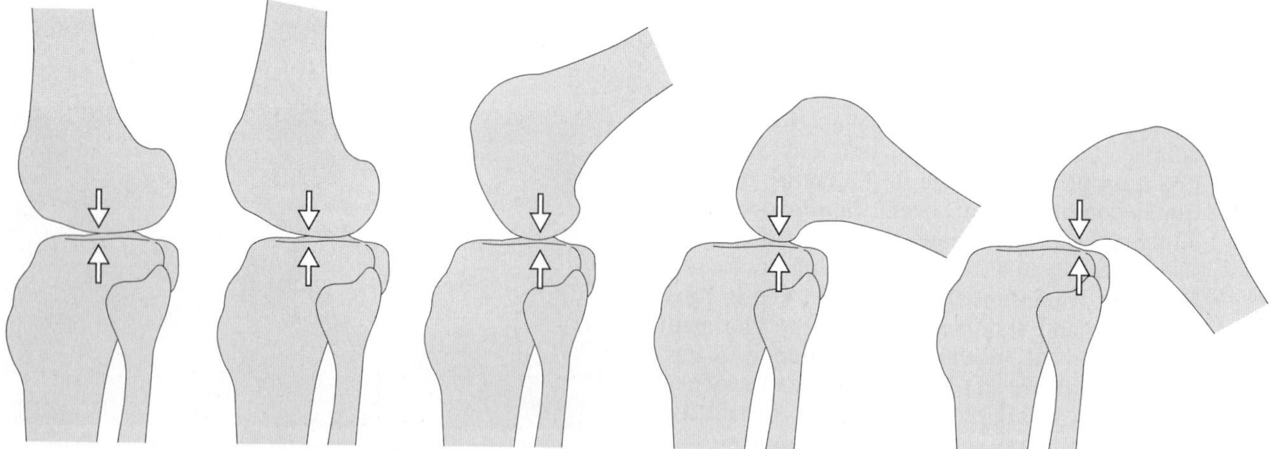

FIGURE 4-36 ■ Femoral rollback is posterior shift of femoral-tibial contact point as knee flexes. Rollback allows femur to clear tibia to provide further flexion.

patterns in total knee tibial bearings consist of subsurface delamination and the associated patterns of pitting and fatigue cracking. The lack of this sensitized region in direct compression molded components may be the reason delamination and subsurface oxidation is rarely observed with this process.

The problem of catastrophic wear is multidimensional. The factors involved and the problems encountered are summarized in Table 4-8. The elimination of only one of the problems will not solve the situation; it will only serve to temporarily mitigate or slow the eventual result. Only with an understanding of all factors involved can there be an effective change in component design and manufacturing to prevent this problem from occurring.

E. Rehabilitation—The single most important factor governing the ultimate flexion range after TKR is preoperative flexion range. As a general rule, postoperative flexion range is equal to preoperative flexion range ±10 degrees. Flexion contractures must be corrected at the time of surgery because fixed contractures usually do not stretch out. On the other hand, the flexion contractures seen postoperatively that are corrected at the time of surgery (while under anesthesia) are usually due to hamstring tightness and spasm. After an anterior arthrotomy, the quadriceps musculature is not firing vigorously, so there is a relative overpull by the hamstring complex. As knee swelling abates, the quadriceps become more active and will counter hamstring overpull. Almost all postoperative knee flexion contractures due to hamstring overpull will stretch out within 6 months. The few that exist after this time may stretch out within 1 year. It is important for patients to be diligent with extension- and flexion-range exercises for up to 3 months postoperatively.

Recent studies have also examined flexion closure of total knee wounds as a means of obviating the need for postoperative continuous passive motion (CPM) devices. Knees closed in flexion tend to recover quicker in the perioperative period and do not need concomitant use of CPM machines.

Manipulation of TKR for arthrofibrosis should be carried out 4–6 weeks postoperatively. The risk of waiting too long for manipulation is that one increases the chance of causing a supracondylar femur fracture. Adhesions in the medial and lateral gutter areas of the knee are the main cause in limiting knee range when arthrofibrosis does occur.

F. Patellar Clunk Syndrome—Patellar clunk syndrome is seen with posterior stabilized total knee implants. A fibrous lump of tissue forms on the posterior surface of the quadriceps tendon just above the superior pole of the patella. This nodule of tissue causes symptoms when it gets caught in the box of the posterior stabilized femoral component as the knee comes from flexion into extension. This usually occurs as the knee reaches 30–45 degrees of flexion. As the

Table 4-8. CATASTROPHIC WEAR IN TOTAL KNEE REPLACEMENT

FACTORS INVOLVED	PROBLEM	SOLUTIONS
Polyethylene (PE) thickness	PE <8 mm thickness PE ≤8 mm thick will exceed yield strength when loaded	Keep thinnest portion of PE above 8 mm Thicker tibial cut All PE tibia (needs to be congruent articulation)
Articular surface design	Flat tibia PE Low-contact surface area High-contact stress load	Congruent articular surface design High-contact surface area Low-contact stress load
Kinematics	Femoral rollback with only posterior cruciate ligament (PCL) (no anterior cruciate ligament) Diskinetic motion in sagittal plane Sliding wear	Minimize rollback with PCL-retained implant design Posterior offset center of rotation for flexion Posterior slope to improve flexion PCL-substituting implant design (Posterior Stabilized Knee)
PE sterilization	Irradiation in air PE oxidation Diminished mechanical properties of polyethylene Subsurface delamination, pitting and fatigue cracking	Irradiation in inert gas or vacuum PE cross-linking Improved wear resistance of PE Alternative bearing surface Ceramic-to-ceramic Metal-to-metal (future prospect)
PE machining	Machining stretches PE chains in subsurface region of 1-2 mm This area more at risk to oxidation Causes subsurface delamination, pitting, and fatigue cracking	Direct compression molding of PE with no machining of articular surface

knee extends further, tension is applied to the entrapped nodule, which subsequently pops out of the box with a palpable and often audible clunk. The reason for the scar formation is not clear. It may occur from a stimulated healing response from cutting the patella and abrading the adjacent quadriceps tissue. Another proposed reason is the use of a small patellar component that fails to lift the quadriceps tendon away from the anterior edge of the intercondylar notch. Recommended treatment is arthroscopic or open débridement of the nodule (Fig. 4-37).

G. Revision TKR—Aseptic failure of a TKR is caused by several factors. These include component loosening, PE wear (catastrophic wear and osteolysis), ligament instability, and patellofemoral maltracking. Tibial component loosening is more common than femoral component loosening.

The major goals of revision knee surgery are (1) extraction of knee components with minimal bone and soft-tissue destruction, (2) restoration of cavitary and segmental bone defects, (3) restoration of the original joint line as best as possible, (4) balanced knee ligaments, and (5) stable knee components.

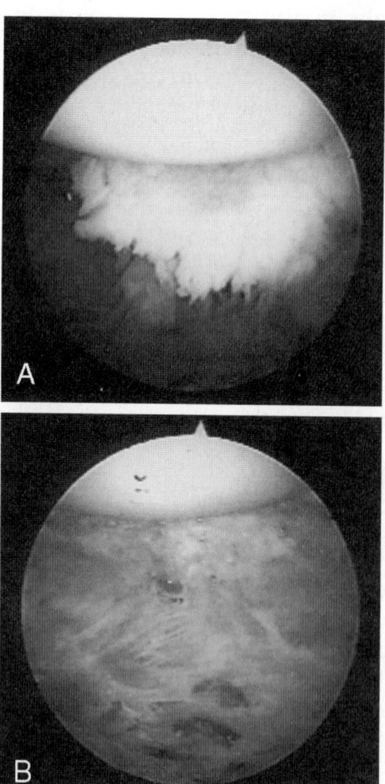

FIGURE 4-37 ■ Arthroscopic photographs of patient with patellar clunk syndrome. *A*, Cephalad view of patella, showing nodule of fibrous tissue hanging down in front of patella. It is this tissue that gets caught in the central box region of the posterior stabilized femoral component. *B*, Same cephalad view after arthroscopic débridement of fibrous nodule. Patellar clunk resolved postoperatively.

The choice of revision knee implants depends on the integrity of the MCL and PCL. If the PCL is attenuated and/or the joint line remains significantly altered, a posterior stabilized implant is recommended. If a PCL-retaining system is used, the option of a posterior stabilized implant should be available at the time of surgery. The integrity of the PCL at the time of revision is often unpredictable.

The next choice in revision TKR implants is the *constrained* nonhinged prosthesis. A constrained nonhinged TKR is an implant that has a large central post that substitutes for MCL or LCL function. The central post is wider and taller than the posterior stabilized design. Remember that a posterior stabilized implant is not a constrained design and does not assist in varus/valgus stability of the knee. The indications for use of a constrained nonhinged TKR are MCL attenuation, LCL attenuation or deficiency, and lastly flexion gap laxity. A knee with a loose flexion gap can be made stable with a tall post. The use of a constrained nonhinged TKR for complete MCL deficiency is controversial. With complete MCL deficiency, all varus loading forces are placed upon the PE post. Consequently, PE post breakage can occur in this situation even with normal (nonexcessive) activity.

The most constrained revision TKR implant is a constrained hinged knee with a rotating platform (see Fig. 4-38). In this design, the femur and tibia are mechanically linked with a connecting bar and bearing. The tibial component is allowed to rotate within a yoke. This allows internal and external rotation during the gait cycle. The rotating platform is needed to reduce the rotational forces that would otherwise be placed on the prosthetic-bone interface. Historically, hinged knee designs that did not have a rotating platform had a very high loosening rate. A constrained hinge knee with a rotating platform should only be used when absolutely necessary. The indications for use of this device are global ligament deficiency (usually trauma or the multiply revised total knee arthroplasty [TKA]), hyperextension instability seen with polio, or resection of the knee for tumor or infection. Relative indications include Charcot arthropathy or complete MCL deficiency (controversial). When using a constrained device for revision TKR (either nonhinged or hinged), medullary stems in the femur and tibia *must* always be used. With the use of constrained implants, the forces at the prosthesis-bone interface are increased. These increased interface forces can be partially ameliorated by the use of diaphyseal stems that can load share in the revision construct.

In many circumstances, the metaphyseal bone in the knee is damaged from mechanical abrasion, osteolysis, or extraction technique. When encountered, these areas should be supported

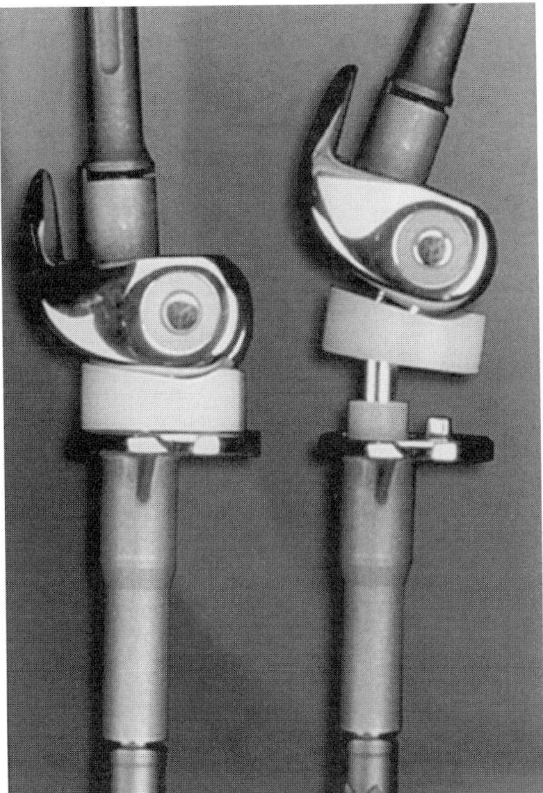

FIGURE 4-38 ■ Photograph of constrained hinged knee with rotating tibial platform. Tibial polyethylene bearing is mechanically linked to femur via large connecting pin. The tibial polyethylene has a distal extension (called a yoke) that extends into metal tibial tray to allow for some internal and external rotation during the knee gait cycle. This relieves some of rotational forces that would otherwise be placed on the prosthesis-bone interface

with medullary stem extensions, which assist with load share. Cavitary defects can be filled with either particulate bone graft or cement. Generally, contained defects 1 cm deep or less can be filled with cement. Segmental deficiencies can be reconstructed with metal augments (wedges or blocks) and/or structural bone grafts. Large segmental deficiencies may require bulk support allografts or modular endoprosthetic devices (Fig. 4-39). Almost all revision TKRs are cemented at the metaphyseal interfaces. In most cases, stem extensions are noncemented and inserted with a press-fit technique. Cementing medullary stems is acceptable.

Reconstruction of the knee after component removal should proceed first with the tibial side. This allows the joint line to be established. A useful guideline in determining the normal joint line is to identify the proximal tip of the fibular head. Generally, the joint line is about 1.5–2 cm above the fibular head. If the contralateral knee is not replaced, a radiograph of the native knee can be used to determine more accurately the distance from fibular head to joint line. Once established, the femur is reconstructed to match the tibia. Balancing is then performed to equalize flexion and extension gaps and to balance medial and lateral gaps. If reconstruction proceeds in this manner, the patellofemoral articulation is usually situated in the appropriate position. Sometimes, patellar baja still occurs and should be addressed accordingly (see section on patellofemoral tracking).

H. Periprosthetic Fracture: Knee—Supracondylar fractures of the femur occur infrequently (less than 1%). The scenario most likely to cause supracondylar fracture is anterior femoral notching in a patient with weak bone (especially rheumatoid arthritis). Supracondylar fracture can also occur as a result of overexuberant manipulation of a total knee implant under anesthesia. Nondisplaced fractures are treated with nonoperative management (cast or cast brace). However, if the prosthesis is mechanically loose, then revision to a long-stem prosthesis is required. For fractures that are displaced, there is no one recommended treatment. Open treatment, no matter what method is chosen, is often difficult and demanding. If the total knee implant is mechanically loose or the fracture disrupts the prosthetic interface, revision with a long-stem prosthesis is required. If the implant is solidly fixed, then an attempt should be made to reduce the fracture and restore anatomic alignment. If the fracture is stable, then treatment with a cast or cast bone is preferred. If the fracture is unstable, the three options for open fixation are (1) supracondylar plate/screw system, (2) supracondylar nail with proximal and distal fixation, and (3) revision TKR with a long medullary stem. Fractures that extend distal to the supracondylar prosthetic flange leave little bone for fixation with either a plate or nail construct. In this situation, revision TKR with a long medullary stem is recommended. Some total knee designs and sizes may not allow passage of a supracondylar nail because of either a closed intercondylar box (seen in posterior stabilized knee designs), or the intercondylar dimension of the available bone is too small for passage of the nail. Comminuted fractures with osteopenic bone (i.e., elderly patients with thin bone) do not do well with plating or nailing. Revision TKR with a long medullary stem is preferred.

Tibia fractures below a total knee implant are uncommon. Nondisplaced fractures are best treated by immobilization and restricted weight-bearing. Displaced fractures are best handled with a long-stem revision prosthesis.

I. Unicompartmental Knee Replacement—A unicompartmental knee replacement is considered an alternative to osteotomy and TKR when degenerative arthritis involves only one compartment. The preservation of cruciate ligaments and the remaining two knee compartments is

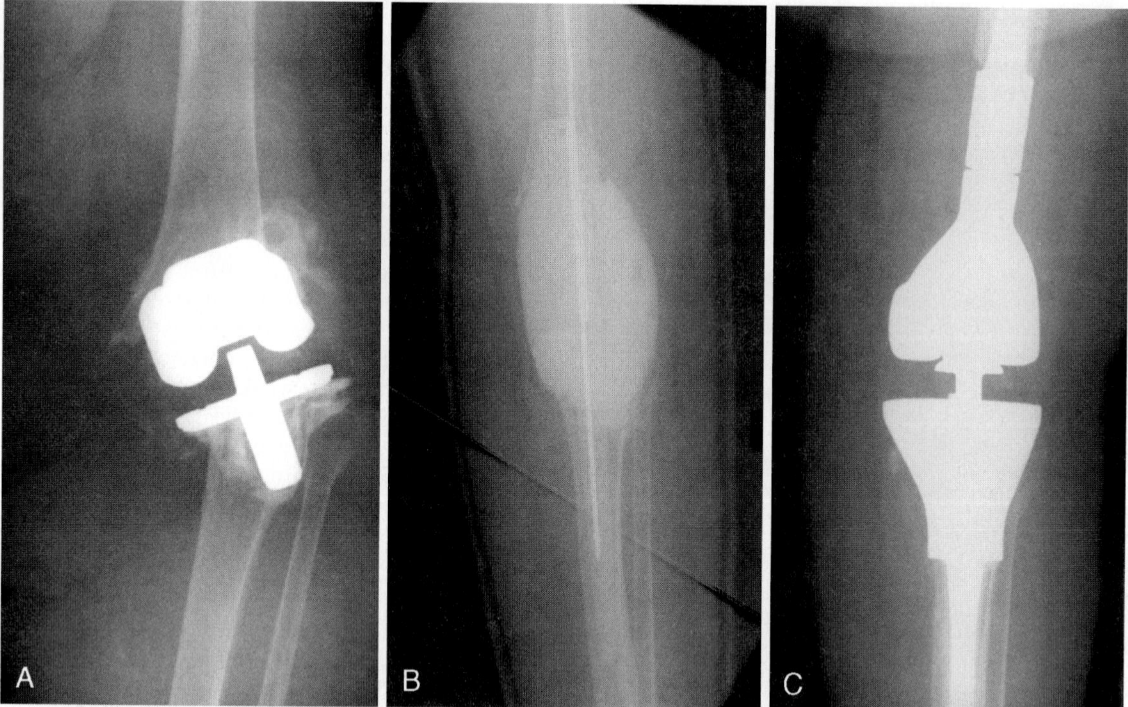

FIGURE 4-39 ■ X-ray photographs of total knee implant requiring endoprosthetic components for reconstruction. *A*, Preoperative x-ray film of an infected total knee with significant bone destruction. *B*, X-ray film of knee after resection arthroplasty and placement of a high-dose antibiotic methylmethacrylate spacer. Patellar tendon was necrotic and was resected. *C*, X-ray film of final reconstruction utilizing endoprosthetic components for reconstruction. Knee articulation is a constrained hinged knee with a rotating tibial platform. Extensor mechanism was reconstructed with a medial gastrocnemius rotational flap with an attached Achilles tendon (half of tendon harvested).

purported to result in more normal knee kinematics than in TKR. Many female patients consider unicompartmental knee replacement an attractive option over osteotomy because it does not produce an angular knee deformity as does an osteotomy. The requirements for unicompartmental knee replacement include (1) preoperatively correctable varus or valgus deformity back to normal alignment, (2) minimum of 90 degrees of flexion, (3) flexion contracture <10 degrees, (4) stress radiographs demonstrating no collapse of the opposite knee compartment, and (5) noninflammatory arthritis.

A fixed varus or valgus deformity preoperatively usually indicates a rigid deformity that cannot be balanced adequately with a unicompartmental replacement. A unicompartmental prosthesis placed in a knee with a residual deformity will be overstressed and will likely fail. The tibial component in a unicompartmental knee replacement is usually thin and is subject to rapid wear. Therefore a unicompartmental replacement should not be used in a high-activity patient or laborer. Heavy weight (over 90 kg) is another contraindication.

V. **Shoulder Replacement Surgery**—Although it has similarities to TKR and THR, total shoulder replacement has its own technical demands that set it apart. First, the range of motion in the shoulder far surpasses the range in either the hip or knee. The success of shoulder replacement surgery is far more dependent on the proper functioning of the soft tissues. Second, the glenoid is far less constrained than the acetabulum, and the forces on the glenoid in shear are significant. This makes the glenoid more prone to mechanical loosening and PE wear.

The two most important factors to take into consideration in shoulder replacement surgery are the condition of the rotator cuff and the amount of glenoid bone stock available for resurfacing. If the rotator cuff is deficient and there is superior migration of the humeral head on preoperative radiographs (Fig. 4-40), glenoid resurfacing is contraindicated. Resurfacing of the glenoid in this circumstance will place excessive stress (in shear) on the superior glenoid and will lead to rapid mechanical loosening and failure. In the situation of a rotator cuff-deficient shoulder with degenerative arthritis, several variations of humeral arthroplasty are recommended. Most common is humeral hemiarthroplasty with a large head that will stay located within the shoulder. A variant of this technique is a bipolar arthroplasty, but this provides no additional benefit to range or function (Fig. 4-41). In either situation, active motion will still be very limited, usually to 45–70 degrees of elevation. A less frequent option is reconstruction of the rotator

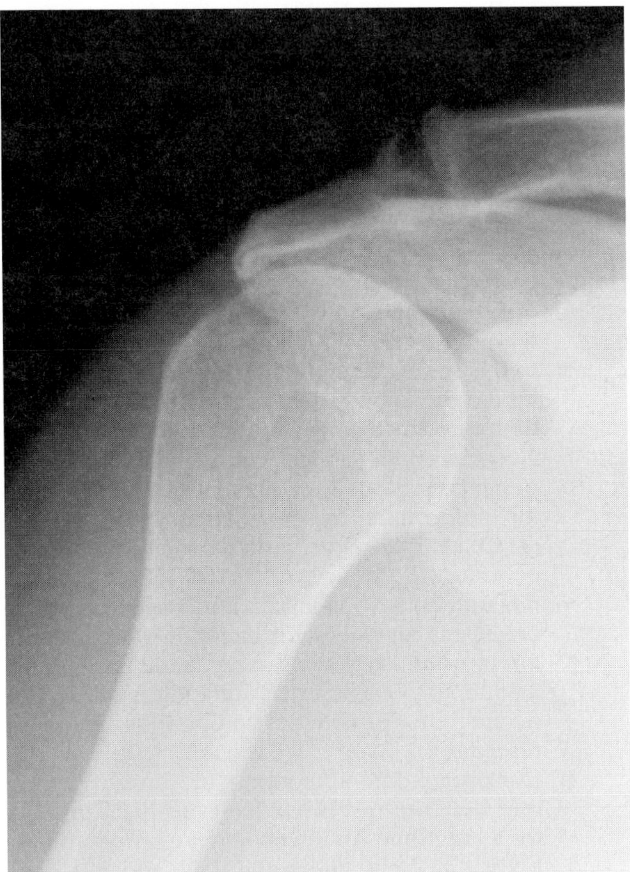

FIGURE 4-40 ■ X-ray photograph of shoulder with chronic rotator cuff deficiency. With absence of rotator cuff, humeral head articulates with undersurface of acromion. Head does not remain centralized with the glenoid fossa.

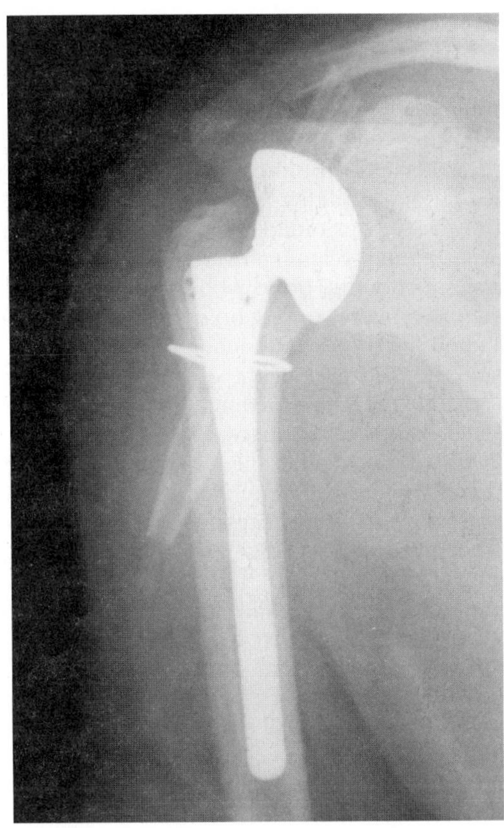

FIGURE 4-41 ■ Six-month postoperative radiograph of bipolar shoulder hemiarthroplasty for comminuted four-part humeral head fracture. At the time of reconstruction, rotator cuff was attenuated.

cuff by superior advancement of the subscapularis and teres musculature, with closure of the superior rotator cuff deficiency. This is combined with humeral head resurfacing, using a humeral head of standard size (i.e., same size as the head resected) or slightly smaller. This technique, initially described by Flatow, may provide in some circumstances improved active range of motion.

The other critical factor when considering shoulder replacement surgery is the integrity of the glenoid. The glenoid fossa is relatively small in size and depth. Mechanical abrasion by the degenerative process may leave little bone and little chance for glenoid resurfacing. A preoperative axillary lateral is an essential part of preoperative evaluation. If the glenoid is eroded down to the coracoid process, glenoid resurfacing is contraindicated. It is also important to assess glenoid version preoperatively. Some suggest using a limited preoperative computed tomography anteversion study to evaluate glenoid version (Fig. 4-42). Patients with osteoarthritis tend to have posterior glenoid erosion and a relative retroversion of the glenoid. This retroversion needs to be corrected intraoperatively to a neutral version.

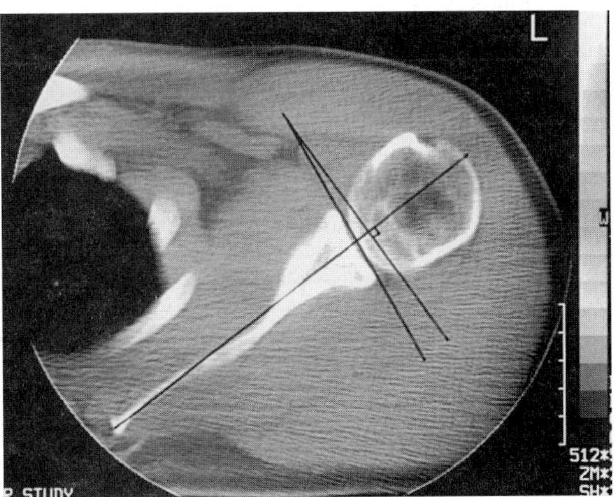

FIGURE 4-42 ■ Computed tomography anteversion study. A limited scan is performed, obtaining a transverse computed tomographic image of shoulder. A line is then drawn from medial tip of scapula to midpoint of glenoid fossa. A line perpendicular to this defines neutral version. A line drawn from anterior glenoid to posterior glenoid defines the patient's glenoid version. This is then compared with neutral version line. In this example, glenoid has 7 degrees of retroversion.

This is most often accomplished with anterior reaming or, less commonly, with posterior augmentation with bone graft.

It is now generally accepted that an all-PE glenoid component should be used if glenoid resurfacing is undertaken. Because the glenoid is relatively small in size and depth, taking away bone during resurfacing arthroplasty is avoided. Preparation for resurfacing usually entails reaming of remaining cartilage and some subchondral bone while glenoid depth is preserved. Keel holes or peg holes are made through the subchondral bone to anchor the prosthesis. As a result, the thickness of the glenoid component used to resurface is small (generally 4–6 mm). If a metal-backed component is used, PE thickness will be significantly reduced and will lead to rapid PE failure.

The choice of humeral stem fixation is similar to that of hip fixation. Successful long-term results can be achieved with cemented stems using modern cement technique (see hip section) or with noncemented porous-coated implants. Porous-coated noncemented stems have a design rationale similar to that of the hip: proximal porous coating to preserve proximal bone stock versus extensive porous coating that has the potential of stress-shielding in the proximal humerus. When considering the choice of humeral implant and fixation, one should take into consideration that the humeral shaft is not as thick and sturdy as the femur. If revision surgery is required, the humeral shaft is more likely to succumb to the effects of osteolysis and mechanical extraction techniques. Therefore a proximal porous stem is favored in this respect. The positioning of the humeral stem should be in retroversion, generally 20–30 degrees. Its position should allow mating with the glenoid. In a situation in which an amount of glenoid retroversion is accepted, less humeral retroversion is required or else the humeral head will dislocate posteriorly.

VI. Prosthetic Joint Infection—Prosthetic joint infection is one of the most devastating complications that can occur in joint replacement surgery. Studies abound as to the correct treatment, but general guidelines are reviewed here. Prosthetic joint infection can be divided into three main categories: (1) Early postoperative infection, (2) hematogenous infection, and (3) chronic infection. Table 4-9 describes the three categories and recommended treatment options.

A. Early Postoperative Infection—With early postoperative infection, the infection is identified within 3 weeks of the joint replacement surgery. In this setting, the infection is usually confined to within the joint space and has not had sufficient time to burrow under the prosthetic-bone interface and hide. Surgical débridement with component retention is recommended. The prognosis for infection-free recovery is good (usually 90% or greater). Modular parts must be removed to débride the fibrin layer that develops between metal and plastic parts. This fibrin layer can harbor organisms for persistent infection. Postoperative intravenous antibiotics are recommended, usually a minimum of 4–6 weeks' duration. If reinfection occurs, the prosthetic components must be resected.

B. Hematogenous Infection—In hematogenous infection, the prosthetic joint has been in place for a long time. An infection develops at another body site (e.g., necrotic gallbladder, sternal wound infection) that results in a hematogenous seeding of the prosthesis. Usually, the afflicted joint becomes painful and swollen soon after the hematogenous event, but the pain and swelling may be masked by other medical treatments, such as antibiotics and steroids. If the infection persists beyond three weeks, it then becomes a chronic infection. Treatment of an acute hematogenous infection is the same as that of an early

Table 4-9. PROSTHETIC JOINT INFECTION CLASSIFICATION AND MANAGEMENT

INFECTION TYPE	DURATION	TREATMENT
Early postoperative infection	Three weeks from initial joint replacement	(1) I&D with retention of components Exchange of modular polyethylene parts Postoperative intravenous (IV) antibiotics (6 weeks) (2) Resection of components if I&D fails
Hematogenous infection	Three weeks from initial hematogenous seeding	(1) I&D with retention of components Exchange of modular polyethylene parts Postoperative IV antibiotics (6 weeks) (2) Resection of components if I&D fails
Chronic infection	>Three weeks from initial joint replacement >Three weeks from initial hematogenous seeding	(1) Two-stage reimplantation with an interval period of IV antibiotics (2) Two-stage arthrodesis with an interval period of IV antibiotics (3) Resection arthroplasty with IV antibiotics postoperatively (4) Amputation

I&D, irrigation and débridement.

postoperative infection. Recurrent infection, if débridement fails, requires surgical extirpation of the prosthetic components.

C. Chronic Infection—In a chronic infection, the infection has been present for more than three weeks. The infection has been persistent and has had time to enter the bone-prosthesis interface and hide. Furthermore, in all cases, the bacteria form a biofilm on the implant. All organisms seen with chronic prosthetic infection develop a biofilm. A biofilm is a polysaccharide layer developed by bacteria that allows bacteria to adhere to prosthetic implants and seal off some of the bacteria colony from immune system attack. Although some of the biofilm can be scrubbed off mechanically, there is no chemical that can be used to safely remove a biofilm. Therefore once an infection is allowed to take hold by existing in the prosthetic-bone interface and forming a biofilm, eradication of the infection requires prosthetic removal along with débridement of infected bone and soft tissue. The bacteria most frequently encountered in chronic prosthetic infection are the coagulase-negative *Staphylococcus* species.

D. Reconstruction of Infected Joint—Once the prosthetic implant has been removed, treatment continues with intravenous antibiotics for 4–6 weeks. Reconstruction of the infected joint thereafter is predicated on a benign clinical examination, a normal serum laboratory analysis (normal Westergren sedimentation rate [WSR] and C-reactive protien [CRP]), and aspiration cultures showing no growth. The type of reconstructive process depends on the overall medical/immune condition of the patient and the condition of the local wound. A patient who is ill with multiple medical problems and a compromised immune system will have a higher likelihood for perioperative complications and reinfection. In this situation, leaving the patient with a resection arthroplasty may be the best solution. If the patient's medical/immune condition is good, the choice for the reconstruction depends on the condition of the local wound.

The condition of the local wound is the most important factor in determining the type of reconstruction after removal of an infected total joint. With chronic infection, soft tissue and bony tissues are affected by the destructive inflammatory process. This causes bone defects, ligament/tendon loss or attenuation, and muscle loss and/or scarring. If significant soft-tissue destruction has occurred and anticipated function of the joint is going to be poor, then a fusion may be a better reconstructive solution. Amputation is reserved for those patients who are very ill or who have severe soft-tissue destruction where neither a fusion nor reconstructive salvage will help.

Reimplantation arthroplasty is utilized if joint function can be adequately preserved. If soft-tissue deficits are present, a local muscle transfer can be rotated to cover the defect and allow for a tension-free closure. Bone defects can be accommodated with modular revision implants or, in some cases, with modular oncologic implants. Bulk-support allografts are an acceptable alternative for large bone defects. The disadvantage of using an allograft for reconstruction is that the surrounding tissues (damaged by the infection) may have an attenuated blood supply, and the graft may not heal and incorporate. Furthermore, if the allograft is placed in a superficial position (e.g., proximal tibia), the allograft can become easily infected from a minor wound dehiscence or from prolonged drainage. Once the allograft is colonized, eradication of the infection is nearly impossible because the allograft is a dead porous structure in which bacteria can easily hide. In contrast, deficits filled by metallic augmentation have only an outer surface for bacteria to adhere to. If colonization does occur, it can be treated successfully with early irrigation and débridement, before a biofilm is allowed to form.

Antibiotic-loaded cement (PMMA) spacers for prosthetic joint infection have been used to preserve the soft-tissue envelope during the period the prosthetic joint has been resected. The elution of antibiotics from methylmethacrylate depends on porosity of the cement, surface area, and antibiotic concentration. Increased porosity allows for better elution of antibiotics. Some PMMA powders have a larger monomer and, in the solid form, they are more porous. Moreover, the addition of large quantities of antibiotics increases porosity even further. Antibiotic beads have a larger surface area than a block and elute more antibiotics. Higher doses of antibiotics in the cement allow for higher antibiotic elution and longer elution time. Antibiotics that are to be used in PMMA must be heat stable as the curing process of PMMA generates high temperature sufficient to deactivate antibiotics. The common antibiotics used with PMMA for prosthetic joint infection are vancomycin, tobramycin, and gentamicin.

VII. Osteotomy

A. Hip Osteotomy—In regard to hip dysplasia, rotational pelvic osteotomy is the preferred reconstruction choice if the hip dysplasia primarily involves poor development of the acetabulum. Prerequisites for pelvic rotational osteotomy include the presence of moderate- to high-grade dysplasia, good residual joint space thickness, absence of femoral head deformity, and absence of angular femoral head-neck deformity in the coronal plane (i.e., coxa valga). Table 4-10 reviews the choices of pelvic osteotomies. For adults with dysplasia, the preferred pelvic osteotomy is the periacetabular (Ganz and colleagues) osteotomy. This osteotomy provides a multiplanar correction, and the acetabulum can

Table 4-10. REVIEW OF PELVIC OSTEOTOMIES

PROCEDURE	OSTEOTOMY DESCRIPTION	REQUIREMENTS	COMMENTS
Salter	Innominate (open wedge)	• Congruous acetabular dysplasia • CE angle >12-15 degrees • Anterior and lateral redirection of acetabulum	• Does not always provide good lateral coverage • Used primarily in early youth
Double or triple innominate	Innominate and pubis or innominate and both rami	• CE angle 0-15 degrees • Congruous acetabular dysplasia	• For more advanced dysplasia • Preserves triradiate cartilage • Used primarily in youth
Spherical acetabular osteotomy	Acetabular Subchondral	• Almost any CE angle • Must have closed triradiate cartilage (compromises vascular supply to area) • Congruous acetabular dysplasia	• Medialization of acetabular segment complex and difficult • Capsulotomy contraindicated • Complications of osteonecrosis and intra-articular penetration frequent
Periacetabular osteotomy (Ganz et al.)	Periacetabular	• Almost any CE angle • Congruous acetabular dysplasia	• Capsulotomy is safe (allows look for labral tears) • Medialization of acetabulum is easy • Minimal fixation required; only 2-4 screws • Preferred osteotomy in adult
Chiari's osteotomy	Curved innominate slides iliac shelf over uncovered femoral head and capsule; interposed capsule undergoes metaplasia into cartilage material	• Unstable aspherical joint	• Salvage osteotomy only • Leaves anterior acetabulum uncovered • Abductor lurch common after Chiari's unless trochanteric advancement is performed

CE, center-edge.

be medialized. This allows re-creation of a normal hip center of rotation.

The use of femoral intertrochanteric osteotomy should be considered in young patients with arthritic afflictions where hip replacement surgery will result in premature failure due to osteolysis and early loosening. Situations in which femoral osteotomy are useful include certain cases of hip dysplasia, osteonecrosis of the femoral head, femoral head deformities from slip of the capital femoral epiphysis, lateral hip impingement in Perthes' disease, and femoral neck nonunion.

Femoral intertrochanteric varus osteotomy is utilized concomitantly with pelvic rotational osteotomy when there is a prominent coxa valga deformity. Another indication for femoral intertrochanteric osteotomy is management of osteonecrosis of the hip. Defining the extent of the necrotic sector is the dominant variable in predicting outcome for osteotomy. Success is inversely related to the size of the necrotic sector. From numerous studies, it is clear that intertrochanteric osteotomy will fail if more than 50% of the femoral head is involved at the time of surgery. The type of intertrochanteric rotational osteotomy depends on the location of the necrotic lesion within the femoral head. The principle is to rotate the femoral head so that there is viable bone and cartilage articulating with the superior weight-bearing portion of the acetabulum. Therefore an intact lateral portion of the femoral head is a prerequisite for varus osteotomy. Conversely, an intact medial femoral head is required for valgus osteotomy. A flexion osteotomy is used in those patients with anterior involvement in the sagittal plane. Conversely, an extension osteotomy can be used in those patients with posterior involvement in the sagittal plane. Biplanar corrections are often required (e.g., flexion-valgus intertrochanteric osteotomy).

In certain cases of post-Perthes' adult arthritis, lateral hip impingement occurs, causing pain. In this problem, radiographs show a superior head osteophyte, which impinges against the lateral acetabulum with hip abduction. In this situation, a pure valgus intertrochanteric osteotomy is effective in alleviating the impingement. This is preferable to femoral head cheilectomy or partial femoral head excision.

In the case of slipped capital femoral epiphysis deformities, a valgus-flexion derotational intertrochanteric osteotomy provides a high incidence of success with pain relief and near-normal restoration of biomechanical function. This technique is effective and safe in most deformities and is preferable to the risks incurred with intra-articular femoral neck osteotomies.

The disadvantage of proximal hip osteotomy is the potentially more difficult stem insertion when converting to THR. This is due to the effects of displacement, rotation, and angulation. Careful preoperative planning is necessary to ensure that the chosen osteotomy will not greatly interfere with future hip replacement surgery. Of particular note, flexion osteotomy should not be performed with anterior closing wedges. Such wedges predispose to significant displacement of the distal fragment and compromise future femoral stem insertion. Instead, gaps created by the osteotomy can be easily filled with bone graft and heal with predictable success.

B. Knee Osteotomy—In degenerative arthritis of the knee, varus or valgus deformities are common. This causes an abnormal distribution of weight-bearing stresses through the joint. These deformities concentrate stress either medially or laterally, and the degenerative changes in that compartment are accelerated. The biomechanical goal of a knee osteotomy is to unload the involved joint compartment by correcting the malalignment. Generally, in the knee joint, varus deformity with medial compartment degenerative arthritis is treated with a valgus-producing proximal tibial osteotomy. Valgus deformity with lateral compartment degenerative arthritis is treated with a varus-producing distal femoral supracondylar osteotomy.

Indications for proximal tibial valgus-producing osteotomy are (1) pain and disability resulting from degenerative arthritis that significantly interface with work and recreation, (2) evidence on weight-bearing radiographs of degenerative arthritis confined to one compartment, (3) the ability of the patient to be compliant postoperatively with partial weight-bearing and motivation to carry out a rehabilitation program, and (4) good vascular status without serious arterial insufficiency.

Contraindications to proximal tibial valgus osteotomy are (1) narrowing of lateral compartment cartilage space on stress radiographs, (2) lateral tibial subluxation of more than 1 cm, (3) medial compartment bone loss of more than 2–3 mm, (4) flexion contracture of more than 15 degrees, (5) knee flexion less than 90 degrees, (6) more than 20 degrees of correction needed, and (7) inflammatory arthritis (e.g., rheumatoid arthritis).

In addition, a relative contraindication is a knee that shows a varus thrust. Best results are achieved when overcorrection to a valgus alignment of 8–10 degrees is achieved and the patient is not overweight. Patients with both risk factors—undercorrection and overweight—had a prevalence of 60% failure after 3 years. The major complications of proximal tibial osteotomy include recurrence of deformity, loss of the normal posterior slope of the tibia, and patella baja. Surgical technique should avoid significant translation of osteotomy fragments to prevent further complications during subsequent TKR. In addition, surgical technique should maintain normal posterior slope of the knee.

The goal with distal varus-producing femoral osteotomy is to produce a horizontal joint line and a tibiofemoral angle of 0 degrees (i.e., anatomic alignment of 0 degrees). The single most common complication in converting to a TKR after supracondylar osteotomy is inability to restore the desired anatomic valgus alignment.

For valgus deformities, a proximal tibial varus-producing osteotomy can be done if the valgus deformity is less than 12 degrees. However, when the valgus deformity is more than 12 degrees, the plane of the joint line deviates significantly from horizontal, and a distal femoral osteotomy is preferred.

VIII. Arthrodesis

A. Hip Arthrodesis—Arthrodesis of the hip is generally reserved for young active patients who are, or plan to be, in a heavy labor occupation and suffer from advanced degenerative arthritis. Hip replacement surgery in these patients will fail rapidly due to excessive stresses placed on the THR construct. Arthrodesis of the hip should be considered an alternative treatment to joint replacement in patients younger than 35 years of age with severe, usually post-traumatic arthritis. The absolute contraindication to hip arthrodesis is active infection of the joint. Relative contraindications include degenerative changes in the lumbosacral spine, contralateral hip, or ipsilateral knee. Another relative contraindication is poor bone stock, from either severe osteoporosis or loss of bone stock. Careful patient selection is important. Hip fusion increases stresses in the lumbar spine, contralateral hip, and ipsilateral knee, and it requires greater energy expenditure for ambulation. Therefore hip fusion should be attempted only in young healthy patients. After hip arthrodesis, degenerative changes develop in adjacent joints 15–25 years after surgery. The most commonly affected joints involved are, in decreasing order, lumbar spine (55–100%), ipsilateral knee and contralateral knee (45–68%), and contralateral hip (25–63%).

Regardless of the technique, the hip should be fused in approximately 30 degrees of flexion, 0–5 degrees of adduction, and 0–15 degrees of external rotation. Abduction is to be avoided because it creates a pelvic obliquity. Internal rotation should also be avoided. The surgical technique for hip arthrodesis is important if later conversion to THR is desired. If lateral plating of the hip and ileum is chosen employing a cobra plate, one should strongly consider a trochanteric osteotomy and elevation of the abductor mechanism to protect it for later use. Once the cobra plate is placed, the trochanter can be placed back down and secured. This technique ensures optional preservation of the abductors for future use with hip replacement surgery. The other technique for hip fusion is anterior plating of the femur with the fusion plate taken into the pelvis, across the anterior column of the pelvis, and superiorly towards the sacroiliac joint. The surgical approach for this technique is the extended Smith-Peterson approach. Through this anterior approach, the femoral head and acetabulum can still be prepared for hip arthrodesis but does not violate the abductor mechanism.

Conversion of a hip arthrodesis to a THR is a difficult task and is associated with a high complication rate. The main indications for conversion are severe, persistent low back pain or pseudoarthrosis after unsuccessful fusion that is sufficiently painful. Another less compelling indication is ipsilateral knee pain. If hip replacement is to be considered, it is important to know whether abductor function is present. Absent abductor function is a contraindication for conversion. The failure rate of THR converted from hip arthrodesis is high, 33% at 10 years. Reasons for failure include loosening, infection, and recurrent dislocation.

B. Knee Arthrodesis—The indications for knee arthrodesis are similar to those for hip arthrodesis. Other indications from primary arthrodesis include (1) painful ankylosis after infection, tuberculosis, or trauma; (2) neuropathic arthropathy; or (3) resection of malignant lesions about the knee.

Currently, the most frequent indication for knee arthrodesis is salvage of a failed TKA. Intramedullary nailing is the preferred technique for arthrodesis when extensive bone loss (seen after failed total knee implant or tumor resection) does not allow compression to be exerted across broad areas of cancellous bone. Union rates in this scenario are much higher (up to 100%) with medullary rod fixation than with external fixation (38%). Bone graft can be used to augment arthrodesis when bone loss is encountered. For primary arthrodesis, the desired position is 5–8 degrees valgus, 0–10 degrees external rotation (to match the other foot), and 0–15 degrees of flexion.

C. Shoulder Arthrodesis—Specific indications for shoulder arthrodesis are (1) painful ankylosis after infection, (2) stabilization in paralytic disorders, (3) post-traumatic brachial plexus palsy, (4) stabilization after massive unreconstructable rotator cuff tears with arthropathy, (5) salvage of failed shoulder replacement, (6) degenerative arthritis in patients not suited for shoulder replacement, (7) stabilization after resection of neoplastic lesions, and (8) recurrent shoulder dislocations.

The recommended position of shoulder arthrodesis is 30-30-30:20-30 degrees of abduction, 20–30 degrees of flexion, and 20–30 degrees of internal rotation. The position of *rotation is the most critical* factor in obtaining optimal function. Shoulder fusion is contraindicated in a patient with an ipsilateral elbow fusion.

IX. **Osteonecrosis**—Osteonecrosis (ON) can occur in many sites, but it has been in the hip where it has received the most attention. Jones and colleagues have shown that the final common pathway involved in ON is an intravascular coagulation. The coagulopathy involves an intraosseous microcirculation coagulation, leading to generalized venous thrombosis and retrograde arterial occlusion. A list of risk factors for ON is shown in Table 4-11. It is now believed that patients with idiopathic ON may suffer from a hypercoagulability disorder and should undergo a hematologic evaluation. A list of recent factors implicated in hypercoagulable states is shown in Table 4-12.

The accepted evaluation and rating system for ON of the hip is the Steinberg classification, modified from Ficat. The classification is listed in Table 4-13. Six stages are defined. Each stage is modified, based on the quantity of head involvement. Head involvement is calculated by multiplying the percentage head involvement on coronal anteroposterior view by the percentage head involvement on sagittal lateral view. For example, a patient with 25% volume involvement has 50% involvement on anteroposterior view and 50% head involvement on lateral view.

Table 4-11. RISK FACTORS FOR OSTEONECROSIS

Alcoholism Antiphospholipid antibody syndrome Dysbaric disorders Endotoxic (Shwartzman) reactions • Systemic bacterial infections Gaucher's disease Hemoglobinopathies • Sickle cell disease Hypercoagulable states Hypercortisolism • Endogenous (Cushing's syndrome) • Exogenous Hyperlipidemia disorders • Type II and type IV hyperlipidemia Hypersensitivity reactions • Allograft organ rejection • Anaphylactic shock Inflammatory conditions • Systemic lupus erythematosus	• Inflammatory bowel disease Malignancy • Metastatic carcinoma • Acute promylelocytic or lymphoid leukemia Pregnancy Radiation therapy Traumatic • Femoral head dislocation • Intracapsular hip fracture Viral infections • HIV • Hepatitis • Cytomegalovirus • Rubella • Rubeola • Varicella

Table 4-12. HEMATOLOGIC FACTORS INVOLVED IN HYPERCOAGULABLE STATES

FACTOR	PROBLEM
Protein C	Deficiency
Protein S	Deficiency
Antithrombin III	Deficiency
Lupus anticoagulant	Presence
Factor V Leiden	Presence
Activated protein C resistance (APCR)	Presence
Prothrombin G 20210 A mutation	Presence
Homocysteine	Excess
Lipoprotein a	Excess
Anticardiolipin antibody	Excess
Factor VIII, IX, or XI	Excess
Clonal increase in platelet count seen in myeloproliferative disorders	Excess

The treatment options for ON include observation, core decompression, vascularized fibular strut grafting, femoral head rotational osteotomy, and hip arthroplasty. Core decompression is generally reserved for early stages of ON *before* subchondral collapse is seen. Core decompression is effective in relieving *intraosseous hypertension*, which is seen in all stages of ON. Reducing intraosseous hypertension has the clinical effect of reducing pain.

Table 4-13. STAGING SYSTEM FOR OSTEONECROSIS OF THE HIP

STAGE	GRADE	CRITERIA
0		X-ray, MRI, and bone scan normal
I		Normal x-ray, abnormal MRI and/or bone scan
II		Abnormal x-ray showing cystic or sclerotic changes in femoral head
III		Subchondral collapse producing *crescent sign*
IV		Flattening of femoral head
V		Joint narrowing with or without acetabular involvement
VI		Advanced degenerative changes
		Quantification of Extent of Involvement
I & II	A	<15% *volume* head involvement on x-ray or MRI
	B	15-30%
	C	>30%
III	A	Subchondral collapse (crescent) beneath <15% of articular surface
	B	Crescent beneath 15-30%
	C	Crescent beneath >30%
IV	A	<15% surface collapse *and* <2 cm depression
	B	15-30% collapse or 2-4 mm depression
	C	>30% collapse or >4 mm depression
V	A	<15% femoral head involvement (same criteria as above)
	B	15-30% of acetabular involvement
	C	>30% involvement

Additionally, a core decompression creates an intraosseous wound that stimulates vascular neogenesis and may allow healing of the infarcted area. Core decompression, even in the early stages, still may not prevent subsequent collapse. Generally, poor results are seen with core decompression in steroid-induced ON. Rotational osteotomy has a role in relatively small-sized lesions whereby the infarcted region can be rotated out of the main weight-bearing region of the hip. The osteotomy selected depends on the location of the lesion and may require either a valgus-producing rotational osteotomy or a varus-producing rotational osteotomy. The osteotomy is in the coronal plane, and extension or flexion correction is in the sagittal plane. Hungerford recommends that osteotomy is to be considered only when the arc of involvement is less than 50%. Lesions larger than this generally have poor results.

Vascularized fibular strut grafting is a relatively new concept in treating ON, which has been championed most recently by Urbaniak. What is most heard about the procedure is the core decompression and insertion of the vascularized fibular strut grafting, but this is only one component. A very important part of the procedure involves the surgical extirpation of the necrotic bone through a large central core hole, followed by autogenous bone grafting (usually taken from the greater trochanter) of the necrotic segment. Curettage of the necrotic segment is taken all the way to subchondral bone. The fibular strut is placed up against subchondral bone, which then heals. This prevents subchondral collapse as the rest of the autogenous bone graft heals. Vascularized fibular strut grafting is generally recommended for earlier stages of ON, but it has been shown to be effective even if some subchondral collapse has occurred. Sometimes, the subchondral bone can even be tapped up to a more congruent position. Vascularized fibular strut grafting is contraindicated when there is "whole head" involvement.

Hip arthroplasty is recommended in advanced stages of ON when degenerative arthritis is present or femoral head collapse is advanced. The choice of hemiarthroplasty versus THR depends on activity level, physiologic age, patient compliance, and preexisting arthritis. Young, active patients tend to do less well with hemiarthroplasty due to rapid wear of the acetabular articular cartilage and the development of pain, particularly in the groin. In contrast, an elderly patient whose ON results from chronic alcohol use and who would be poorly compliant with THR precautions may be best suited with hemiarthroplasty. Patients with radiographic evidence of acetabular degenerative changes should have a THR. Hip fusion should be considered in a very young patient who is (or plans to be) in a heavy labor occupation. Additional autogenous bone grafting is often required, because the necrotic femoral head is collapsed. The results of hip fusion for ON are less favorable than cases for degenerative arthritis without ON.

Selected Bibliography

Arima, J., Whiteside, L.A., McCarthy, D.S., et al.: Femoral rotational alignment, based on the anteroposterior axis, in total knee arthroplasty in a valgus knee. J. Bone Joint Surg. [Am.] 77:1331, 1995.

Barrack, R.L., Mulroy, R.D., and Harris, W.W.H.: Improved cementing techniques and femoral component loosening in young patients with hip arthroplasty: A 12-year radiographic review. J. Bone Joint Surg. [Br.] 74:385, 1992.

Beals, R.K., and Tower, S.S.: Periprosthetic fractures of the femur. Clin. Orthop. 327:238, 1996.

Bloebaum, R.D., Rubman, M.H., and Hofmann, A.A.: Bone ingrowth into porous-coated tibial components implanted with autograft bone chips: Analysis of ten consecutively retrieved implants. J. Arthroplasty 7:483, 1992.

Blunn, G.W., Joshi, A.B., Walker, P.S., et al.: Wear in retrieved condylar knee arthroplasties, a comparison of wear in different designs of 280 retrieved condylar knee prostheses. J. Arthroplasty 12(3):281, 1997.

Bobyn, J.D., Pilliar, R.M., Cameron, H.U., et al.: The effect of porous surface configuration on the tensile strength of fixation of implants by bone ingrowth. Clin. Orthop. 149:291, 1980.

Bono, J.V., Sanford, L., and Toussaint, J.T.: Severe polyethylene wear in total hip arthroplasty: Observations from retrieved AML PLUS hip implants with an ACS polyethylene liner. J. Arthroplasty 9:119, 1994.

Brooker, A.F., Bowerman, J.W., Robinson, R.H., et al.: Ectopic ossification following total hip replacement: Incidence and a method of classification. J. Bone Joint Surg. [Am.] 55:1629, 1973.

Burke, D.W., Gates, E.I., and Harris, W.H.: Centrifugation as a method of improving tensile and fatigue properties of acrylic bone cement. J. Bone Joint Surg. [Am.] 66:1265, 1984.

Canale, S.T.: Campbell's Operative Orthopaedics, 9th ed. St. Louis, C.V. Mosby, 1998.

Cappello, W.N.: Femoral component fixation in the 1990s: Hydroxyapatite in total hip arthroplasty: Five-year clinical experience. Orthopedics 17:781, 1994.

Cella, J.P., Salvati, E.A., and Sculco, T.P.: Indomethacin for the prevention of heterotopic ossification following total hip arthroplasty: Effectiveness, contraindications and adverse effects. J. Arthroplasty 3:229, 1988.

Chandler, H.P., Reineck, F.T., Wixson, R.L., et al.: Total hip replacement in patients younger than thirty years old: A five-year follow-up study. J. Bone Joint Surg. [Am.] 63:1426, 1981.

Chen, F., Mont, M.A., and Bachner, R.S.: Management of ipsilateral supracondylar femur fractures following total knee arthroplasty. J. Arthroplasty 9:521, 1994.

Cofield, R.H., and Briggs, B.T.: Glenohumeral arthrodesis: Operative and long-term functional results. J. Bone Joint Surg. [Am.] 61:668, 1979.

Collier, J., Mayor, M.B., McNamara, J.L., et al.: Analysis of the failure of 122 polyethylene inserts from uncemented tibial knee components. Clin. Orthop. 273:232, 1991.

Cook, S.D., Barrack, R.L., Thomas, K.A., et al.: Quantitative analysis of tissue growth into human porous total hip components. J. Arthroplasty 3:249, 1988.

Dall, D.M., and Miles, A.W.: Reattachment of the greater trochanter: The use of the trochanter cable-grip system. J. Bone Joint Surg. [Br.] 65:55, 1983.

D'Antonio, J., McCarthy, J.C., Bargar, W.L., et al.: Classification of femoral abnormalities in total hip arthroplasty. Clin. Orthop. 296:133, 1993.

David, A., Eitemuller, J., Muhr, G., et al.: Mechanical and histological evaluation of hydroxyapatite-coated, titanium-coated, and grit-blasted surfaces under weight-bearing conditions. Arch. Orthop. Trauma Surg. 114:112, 1995.

Delaunay, S., Dussault, R.G., Kaplan, P.A., et al.: Radiographic measurements of dysplastic adult hips. Skeletal Radiol. 26:75, 1997.

DeLee, J.G., and Charnley, J.: Radiologic demarcation of cemented sockets in total hip replacement. Clin. Orthop. 121:20, 1976.

Ebramzadeh, E., Sarmiento, A., McKellop, H., et al.: The cement mantle in total hip arthroplasty: Analysis of long-term radiographic results. J. Bone Joint Surg. [Am.] 76:77, 1994.

Emerson, R.H., Head, W.C., and Peters, P.C.: Soft-tissue balance and alignment in medial unicompartmental knee arthroplasty. J. Bone Joint Surg. [Br.] 74:807, 1992.

Emerson, R.H., Malinin, T.I., Cuellar, A.D., et al.: Cortical allografts in the reconstruction of the femur in revision total hip arthroplasty: A basic science and clinical study. Clin. Orthop. 285:35, 1992.

Engh, C.A., and Bobyn, J.D.: The influence of stem size and extent of porous coating on femoral bone resorption after primary cementless hip arthroplasty. Clin. Orthop. 231:7, 1988.

Engh, C.A., Bobyn, J.D., and Glassman, A.H.: Porous-coated hip replacement: The factors governing bone ingrowth, stress shielding, and clinical results. J. Bone Joint Surg. [Br.] 69:45, 1987.

Engh, C.A., Glassman, A.H., Griffin, W.L., et al.: Results of cementless revision for failed cemented total hip arthroplasty. Clin. Orthop. 235:91, 1988.

Engh, C.A., Glassman, A.H., and Suthers, K.E.: The case for porous-coated hip implants. Clin. Orthop. 261:63, 1990.

Estok, D.M., and Harris, W.H.: Long-term results of cemented femoral revision surgery using second-generation techniques: An average 11.7 year follow-up evaluation. Clin. Orthop. 299:190, 1994.

Eyerer, P., Ellwanger, Madler, H., et al.: Polyethylene. In Williams, D., ed.: Concise Encyclopedia of Medical and Dental Biomaterials, 1st ed. 1990, Pergamon Press, Oxford, pp. 271–279.

Faris, P.M., Herbst, S.A., Ritter, M.A., et al.: The effect of preoperative knee deformity on the initial results of cruciate-retaining total knee arthroplasty. J. Arthroplasty 7:527, 1992.

Feighan, J.E., Goldberg, V.M., Davy, D., et al.: The influence of surface blasting on the incorporation of titanium-alloy implants in a rabbit intramedullary model. J. Bone Joint Surg. [Am.] 77:1380, 1995.

Foglar, C., and Lindsey, R.W.: C-reactive protein in orthopaedics. Orthopedics 21:687, 1998.

Furman, B.D., Awad, J.N., Li, S., et al.: Material and performance differences between retrieved machined and molded Insall/Burstein type total knee arthroplasties, 43rd Annual ORS, Feb. 9–13, 1997, San Francisco, CA, Paper 643.

Furman, B.D., Ritter, M.A., Li, S., et al.: Effect of resin type and manufacturing method on UHMWPE oxidation and quality at long aging and implant times, 43rd Annual ORS, Feb. 9–13, 1997, San Francisco, CA, Paper 92.

Ganz, R., Klaue, K., Vinh, T.S., et al.: A new periacetabular osteotomy for the treatment of hip dysplasias. Clin. Orthop. 232:26, 1988.

Gillis, A., Furman, B., Li, S., et al.: Oxidation of in vivo vs shelf aged gamma sterilized total knee replacements, Society for Biomaterials 23rd Annual Meeting, April 30–May 4, 1997, New Orleans, LA, Paper 73.

Greene, N., Holtom, P.D., Warren, C.A., et al.: In vitro elution of tobramycin and vancomycin polymethylmethacrylate beads and spacers from Simplex and Palacos. Am. J. Orthop. 27:201, 1998.

Gristina, A.G., and Costerton, J.W.: Bacterial adherence to biomaterials and tissue: The significance of its role in clinical sepsis. J. Bone Joint Surg. [Am.] 67:264, 1985.

Gruen, T.A., McNeice, G.M., Amstutz, H.C.: "Modes of failure" of cemented stem-type femoral components: A radiographic analysis of loosening. Clin. Orthop. 141:17, 1979.

Gsell, R., Johnson, T., Taylor, G., et al.: Zimmer Polyethylene Overview, Zimmer Technical Report, 1997.

Hawkins, R.J., and Neer, C.S., II: A functional analysis of shoulder fusions. Clin. Orthop. 223:65, 1987.

Healy, W.L., Lo, T.C.M., DeSimone, A.A., et al.: Single-dose irradiation for the prevention of heterotopic ossification after total hip arthroplasty. J. Bone Joint Surg. [Am.] 77:590, 1995.

Hedley, A.K., Mead, L.P., and Hendren, D.H.: The prevention of heterotopic bone formation following total hip arthroplasty using 600 rad in a single dose. J. Arthroplasty 4:319, 1989.

Higgins, J.C., and Roesener, D.R.: Evaluation of free radical reduction treatments for UHMWPE. Forty-second Annual Meeting of the ORS, Feb. 19–22, 1996, Atlanta, GA, Paper 485.

Hofmann, A.A., Bloebaum, R.D., Rubman, J.H., et al.: Microscopic analysis of autograft bone applied at the interface of porous-coated devices in human cancellous bone. Int. Orthop. 16:349, 1992.

Holtom, P.D., Warren, C.A., Green, N.W., et al.: Relation of surface area to in vitro elution characteristics of vancomycin-impregnated polymethylmethacrylate spacers. Am. J. Orthop. 27:207, 1998.

Hozack, W.J., Rothman, R.H., Booth, R.E., Jr., et al.: The patellar clunk syndrome: A complication of posterior stabilized total knee arthroplasty. Clin. Orthop. 241:203, 1989.

Hubbard, N.T.: The Effects of Manufacturing Techniques and Calcium Stearate on the Oxidation of UHMWPE, Perplas Medical Technical Report, *** 1997.

Huiskes, R.: Biomechanical aspects of hydroxyapatite coatings on femoral hip prosthesis. In Manley, M.T., ed.: Hydroxyapatite Coatings in Orthopaedic Surgery. New York, Raven Press, 1993.

Jones, J.P., Steinberg, M.E., Hungerford, D.S., et al.: Avascular necrosis: Pathogenesis, diagnosis, and treatment. AAOS Instr. Course Lect. 309, San Francisco, 1997.

Jonsson, E., Lidgren, L., and Rydholm, U.: Position of shoulder arthrodesis measured with moiré photography. Clin. Orthop. 238:117, 1989.

Kaplan, S.J., Thomas, W.H., and Poss, R.: Trochanteric advancement form recurrent dislocation after total hip arthroplasty. J. Arthroplasty 2:119, 1987.

Kjaersgaard-Andersen, P., and Ritter, M.A.: Short-term treatment with non-steroidal anti-inflammatory medications to prevent heterotopic bone formation after total hip arthroplasty: A preliminary report. Clin. Orthop. 279:157, 1992.

Klapperich, C., Komvopoulos, K., and Pruitt, L.: Tribological properties and molecular evolution of UHMWPE, Transactions of the ASME, Journal of Tribology 12:394, 1999.

Kumar, P.J., McPherson, E.J., Dorr, L.D., et al.: Rehabilitation after total knee arthroplasty: A comparison of two rehabilitation techniques. Clin. Orthop. 331:93, 1996.

Landy, M.M., Walker, P.S.: Wear of ultra-high-molecular-weight polyethylene components of 90 retrieved knee prostheses. J. Arthroplasty (Suppl.) S73–S85, 1988.

Laskin, R.S., Rieger, M., Schob, C., et al.: The posterior stabilized total knee prosthesis in the knee with severe fixed deformity. J. Knee Surg. 1:199, 1988.

Lewonowski, K., Dorr, L.D., McPherson, E.J., et al.: Medialization of the patella in total knee arthroplasty. J. Arthroplasty 12:161, 1997.

Livermore, J., Ilstrup, D., and Morrey, B.: Effect of femoral head size on wear of the polyethylene acetabular component. J. Bone Joint Surg. [Am.] 72:518, 1990.

Li, S., Chang, J.D., Salvati, E., et al.: Nonconsolidated Polyethylene Particles and Oxidation in Charnley Acetabular Cups, CORR, No. 319, pp. 54–63, 1995.

Lombardi, A.V., Mallory, T.H., Vaughn, B.K., et al.: Dislocation following primary posterior-stabilized total knee arthroplasty. J. Arthroplasty 8:633, 1993.

Mantas, J.P., Bloebaum, R.D., Skedros, J.G., et al.: Implications of reference axes used for rotational alignment of the femoral component in primary and revision knee arthroplasty. J. Arthroplasty 7:531, 1992.

McKellop, H.A., Shen, F.W., Campbell, P., et al.: Effect of sterilization method and other modifications on the wear resistance of UHMWPE acetabular cups. Polyethylene Wear in Orthopaedic Implants Workshop, Society for Biomaterials 23rd Annual Meeting, April 30–May 4, 1997, New Orleans, LA.

McPherson, E.J., Patzakis, M.J., Gross, J.E., et al.: Infected total knee arthroplasty: Two-stage reimplantation with a gastrocnemius rotational flap. Clin. Orthop. 341:73, 1997.

McPherson, E.J., Tontz, W., Patzakis, M.J., et al.: Outcome of infected total knee utilizing a staging system for prosthetic joint infection. Am. J. Orthop. 28:161, 1999.

McPherson, E.J., Woodson, C., Holtom, P., et al.: Periprosthetic total hip infection: outcomes using a staging system. Clin. Orthop. 403:8-15, 2002.

Nashed, R.S., Becker, D.A., and Gustilo, R.B.: Are cementless acetabular components the cause of excess wear and osteolysis in total hip arthroplasty? Clin. Orthop. 317:19, 1995.

National Institutes of Health: Total hip replacement. NIH Consensus Conference, Sept. 2–14, 12:1, 1994.

National Institutes of Health: Total hip replacement. NIH Consensus Conference. J.A.M.A. 273:1950, 1995.

Nelissen, R.G.H.H., Bauer, T.W., Weidenhielm, R.A., et al.: Revision hip arthroplasty with the use of cement and impaction grafting. J. Bone Joint Surg. [Am.] 77:412, 1995.

Oh, I., Bourne, R.B., and Harris, W.H.: The femoral cement compactor: An improvement in cementing technique in total hip replacement. J. Bone Joint Surg. [Am.] 65:1335, 1983.

Otani, T., Whiteside, L.A., and White, S.E.: The effect of axial and torsional loading on strain distribution in the proximal femur as related to cementless total hip arthroplasty. Clin. Orthop. 292:376, 1993.

Padgett, D.E., Kull, L., Rosenberg, A., et al.: Revision of the acetabular component without cement after total hip arthroplasty. J. Bone Joint Surg. [Am.] 75:663, 1993.

Pak, J.H., Paprosky, W.G., Jablonsky, W.S., et al.: Femoral strut allografts in cementless revision total hip arthroplasty. Clin. Orthop. 295:172, 1993.

Paprosky, W.G., Perona, P.G., and Lawrence, J.M.: Acetabular defect classification on surgical reconstruction in revision arthroplasty. J. Arthroplasty 9:33, 1994.

Peters, C.L., Rivero, D.P., Kull, L.R., et al.: Revision total hip arthroplasty without cement: Subsidence of proximally porous-coated femoral components. J. Bone Joint Surg. [Am.] 77:1217, 1995.

Poggie, R.A., Takeuchi, M.T., and Averill, R.: Effects of resin type, consolidation method and sterilization on UHMWPE, Society for Biomaterials 23rd Annual Meeting, April 30–May 4, 1997, New Orleans, LA, p. 216.

Poilvache, P.L., Insall, J.N., Scuderi, G.R., et al.: Rotational landmarks and sizing of the distal femur in total knee arthroplasty. Clin. Orthop. 331:35, 1996.

Possai, K.W., Dorr, L.D., and McPherson, E.J.: Metal rings for deficient acetabular bone in total hip replacement. Instr. Course Lect. 45:161, 1996.

Ranawat, C.S., Peters, L.E., and Umlas, M.E.: Fixation of the acetabular component. Clin. Orthop. 334:207, 1997.

Ranard, G., Higgins, J., and Schroeder, D.: Density and thermal analysis of molded and machined UHMWPE tibial bearings. Transactions of the 24th Annual Meeting of the Society For Biomaterials, April 22–26, 1998, San Diego, CA, Paper 497.

Ritter, M.A., Faris, P.M., and Keating, E.M.: Posterior cruciate ligament balancing during total knee arthroplasty. J. Arthroplasty 3:323, 1988.

Ritter, M.A., Worland, R., Meding, J.B., et al.: Flat-on-Flat, Nonconstrained Compression Molded Polyethylene Total Knee Replacement, CORR No. 321, December 1995, pp. 79–85.

Ronk, R., Higgins, J., Kinsel, A.: Method for detecting non-consolidation in UHMWPE. Transactions of 10th Annual ISTA Meeting Sept. 25–27, 1997, San Diego, CA, pp. 64–65.

Rowe, C.R.: Arthrodesis of the shoulder used in treating painful conditions. Clin. Orthop. 173:92, 1983.

Santore, R.F., and Murphy, S.B.: Osteotomies about the hip for the prevention and treatment of osteoarthrosis. AAOS Instr. Course Lect. 115. San Francisco, 1997.

Schmalzried, T.P., Jasty, M., and Harris, W.H.: Periprosthetic bone loss in total hip arthroplasty: Polyethylene wear debris and the concept of the effective joint space. J. Bone Joint Surg. [Am.] 74:849, 1992.

Schroeder, D.W., and Pozorski, K.M.: Hip simulator wear testing of isostatically molded UHMWPE, effect of ETO and gamma irradiation. Forty-second Annual Meeting of the ORS, Feb. 19–22, 1996, Atlanta.

Schulte, K.R., Callaghaan, J.J., Kelley, S.S., et al.: The outcome of Charnley total hip arthroplasty with cement after a minimum of twenty year follow-up. J. Bone Joint Surg. [Am.] 75:961, 1993.

Scott, R.D., Cobb, A.G., McQueary, F.G., et al.: Unicompartmental knee arthroplasty: 8 to 12 year follow-up with survivorship analysis. Clin. Orthop. 271:96, 1991.

Scully, S.P., Aaron, R.K., and Urbaniak, J.R.: Survival analysis of hips treated with core decompression or vascularized fibular grafting because of avascular necrosis. J. Bone Joint Surg. [Am.] 80:1270, 1998.

Serekian, P.: Process application of hydroxyapatite coatings. In Manley, M.T., ed.: Hydroxyapatite Coatings in Orthopaedic Surgery. New York, Raven Press, 1993.

Sommerich, R., Flynn, T., Zalenski, E., et al.: The effects of sterilization on contact area and wear rate of UHMWPE. Forty-second Annual Meeting of the ORS, Feb. 19–22, 1996, Atlanta.

Steinberg, M.E., Hayken, G.D., and Steinberg, D.R.: A quantitative system for staging avascular necrosis. J. Bone Joint Surg. [Br.] 77:34, 1995.

Stern, S.H., Becker, M.W., and Insall, J.N.: Unicondylar knee arthroplasty: An evaluation of selection criteria. Clin. Orthop. 286:143, 1993.

Stiehl, J.B., Komistek, R.D., Dennis, D.A., et al.: Fluoroscopic analysis of kinematics after posterior-cruciate-retaining knee arthroplasty. J. Bone Joint Surg. [Br.] 77:884, 1995.

St. John, K.R., Tackeichi, M.J., and Poggie, R.A.: Effects of radiation dose and packaging condition on the oxidation of UHMWPE. Society for Biomaterials 23rd Annual Meeting, April 30–May 4, 1997, New Orleans, LA, Paper 46.

Streicher, R. M., and Schaffner, S.: Significance of the sterilization method and long-term aging on the in vivo wear rate of UHMWPE. Forty-second Annual Meeting of the ORS, Feb. 19–22, 1996, Atlanta.

Sun, D.C., Wang, A., Dumbleton, J.H., et al.: Development of Stabilized UHMWPE Implants with Improved Oxidation Resistance via Crosslinking. Scientific Exhibition, 63rd Annual AAOS Feb. 22–26, 1996, Atlanta.

Tanner, M.G., Hoernschemeyer, D.G., and Whiteside, L.A.: Polyethylene quality variations in currently available bar stock. Sixty-fourth Annual Meeting of the AAOS, Feb 13–17, 1997.

Tsukayama, D.T., Estrada, R., and Gustilo, R.B.: Infection after total hip arthroplasty. J. Bone Joint Surg. [Am.] 78:512, 1996.

Vince, K.G., and McPherson, E.J.: The patella in total knee arthroplasty. Orthop. Clin. North Am. 23:675, 1992.

Wang, A., Essner, A., Dumbleton, J.H., et al.: Wear mechanisms and wear testing of ultra-high molecular weight polyethylene in total joint arthroplasty. Polyethylene Wear in Orthopaedic Implants Workshop, Society for Biomaterials 23rd Annual Meeting, April 30–May 4, 1997, New Orleans.

Wasielewski, R.C., Cooperstein, L.A., Kruger, M.P., et al.: Acetabular anatomy and the transacetabular fixation of screws in total hip arthroplasty. J. Bone Joint Surg. [Am.] 72:501, 1990.

Wilson, P.D., Jr., and Gordon, S.L., eds.: NIH Consensus Development Conference: Total hip joint replacement. Bethesda, MD, March 1982. J. Orthop. Res. 1:189, 1983.

Wong, M., Eulenberger, J., Schenk, R., et al.: Effect of surface topology on the osteointegration of implant materials in trabecular bone. J. Bio. Mat. Res. 29:1567, 1995.

Wroblewski, B.M., Lynch, M., Atkinson, J.R., et al.: External wear of the polyethylene socket in cemented total hip arthroplasty. J. Bone Joint Surg. [Br.] 69:61, 1987.

Wroblewski, B.M., and Siney, P.D.: Charnley low-friction arthroplasty of the hip: Long-term results. Clin. Orthop. 292:191, 1993.

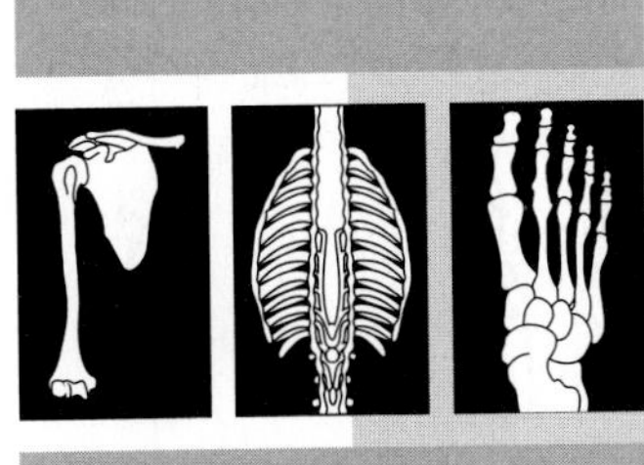

5

Disorders of the Foot and Ankle

E. GREER RICHARDSON

This chapter provides a review of adult foot and ankle deformities. Pediatric and congenital deformities are covered in Chapter 2, Pediatric Orthopaedics.

I. Anatomy and Biomechanics of the Foot and Ankle

The foot and ankle are complex structures that provide support, shock absorption, balance, adaptation to uneven surfaces, and push-off power and direction during standing and gait. Their anatomy and biomechanics are equally complex, and this brief review is not a substitute for a thorough discussion, such as that available in numerous anatomy texts.

A. The Gait Cycle—The normal walking, or gait, cycle consists of stance and swing phases. **Stance phase** occurs when the foot is in contact with the ground from heel strike to toe-off, and constitutes approximately 62% of the gait cycle (Fig. 5-1). **Swing phase** occurs when the foot is off the ground from toe-off to the next heel strike and constitutes 38% of the cycle. The stance phase includes three intervals: the initial period of double limb support, the intermediate period, and the second period of double limb support. **Ground reaction forces for walking reach approximately 1.5 times body weight**. The weight-bearing phase of the gait cycle for each leg is divided into multiple parts: heel strike, foot flat, heel off, and toe off. The running cycle has a float phase, during which neither limb is on the ground, and forces generated increase to almost three times body weight. During the gait cycle, the foot changes from a flexible structure at heel strike to a rigid structure at toe-off. The mechanisms that bring about this conversion are (1) tightening of the plantar aponeurosis, (2) progressive external rotation of the lower extremity, which begins at the pelvis and is passed distally across the ankle joint into the subtalar joint, and (3) stabilization of the transverse tarsal joint, which results from progressive inversion of the subtalar joint.

B. Motions of the Foot and Ankle—The names for various motions about the foot and ankle can be confusing and often are used interchangeably. The commonly accepted terms are shown in Table 5-1.

C. Ankle Axes of Rotation—The ankle axis of movement can be clinically estimated by palpation of the tips of the medial and lateral malleoli (Fig. 5-2); however, this is a simplification of the actual motion. In the horizontal plane, the ankle axis projects from anteromedial to posterolateral; in the coronal plane, from medial cephalad to lateral caudad, with variations between ankles ranging from 74–94 degrees (mean 82 degrees ± 4 degrees) from the vertical axis of the tibia (Fig. 5-3). An in vivo radiographic study of active ankle motion revealed that no single joint axis is present, but rather **ankle movement is described by instant centers of rotation that vary with joint position**. In normal ankles, joint distraction was noted with plantar flexion, sliding movement throughout the midrange, and compression (jamming) at maximal dorsiflexion. The ankle joint axis also has been found to change throughout the range of motion, with different axes for ankles in positions of dorsiflexion and plantar flexion.

D. Musculotendinous Structures During Gait—The anterior compartment of the leg contracts eccentrically (controlled dorsiflexion) at heel strike, lengthening while the gastrocnemius-soleus is quiescent. The gastrocnemius-soleus complex is contracting eccentrically at foot flat, and the anterior tibialis is quiet. The strong gastrocnemius-soleus complex contracts concentrically at heel rise/push-off, and the tibialis anterior (anterior compartment) is quiescent. From heel strike to foot flat there is progressive eversion of the subtalar joint, which unlocks the transverse tarsal joint and

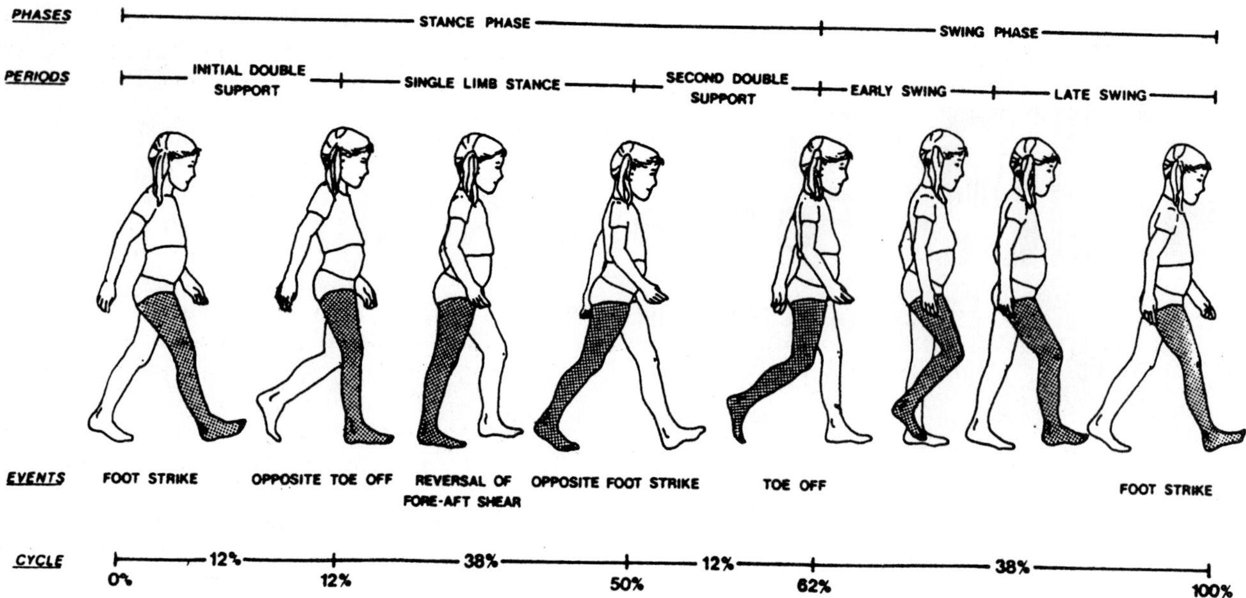

FIGURE 5-1 ■ Typical normal gait cycle, with the phases, period, and events of gait shown. (From Sutherland, D.H., Olsen, R.A., Biden, E.N., Wyatt, M.P.: The development of mature walking. London, MacKeith Press, 1988.)

causes internal rotation of the tibia. The opposite occurs during heel rise. **The plantar aponeurosis originates on the plantar medial aspect of the calcaneus and passes distally, inserting into the base of the flexor mechanism of the toes. It functions as a windlass mechanism, increasing the arch height as the toes dorsiflex during toe off, and is a major support of the medial longitudinal arch.** This is a passive function, which aids hindfoot inversion during heel rise. The main invertor of the subtalar joint during heel rise is the posterior tibial tendon, which initiates subtalar inversion.

II. Physical Examination of the Foot And Ankle—A complete examination includes observation of both extremities below the knee and observation of the gait cycle. The foot should be examined with the patient both standing and sitting.

A. Neurovascular Examination, Muscle Strength, Tendon Competence—A neurovascular examination is mandatory. Pain in the foot or ankle can be caused by neurologic pathology, such as peripheral neuropathy or peripheral nerve entrapment, or spinal pathology, such as a herniated nucleus pulposus. Sensory examination should include

Table 5-1. MOTIONS OF THE FOOT AND ANKLE

Ankle joint	• Dorsiflexion • Plantar flexion
Heel (subtalar joint)	• Inversion (varus)—medially • Eversion (valgus)—laterally
Transverse tarsal joint (talonavicular and calcaneocuboid joints)	• Adduction • Abduction
Combined	• Pronation—dorsiflexion of ankle joint + eversion of subtalar joint + abduction of transverse tarsal joint • Supination—plantar flexion of ankle joint + inversion of subtalar joint + adduction of transverse tarsal joint

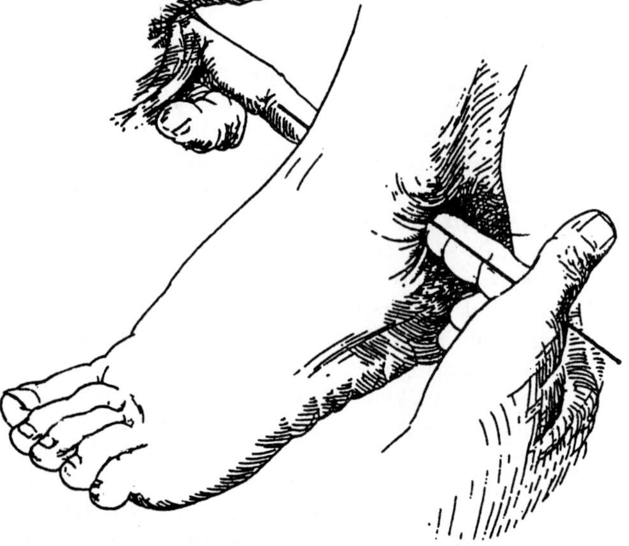

FIGURE 5-2 ■ The ankle axis of movement can be clinically estimated by palpating the tips of the medial and lateral malleoli. (From Mann, R.A.: Biomechanics of the foot and ankle. In Mann, R.A., and Coughlin, M.J., eds.: Surgery of the Foot and Ankle, 6th ed. St. Louis, C.V. Mosby, 1993, p. 17.)

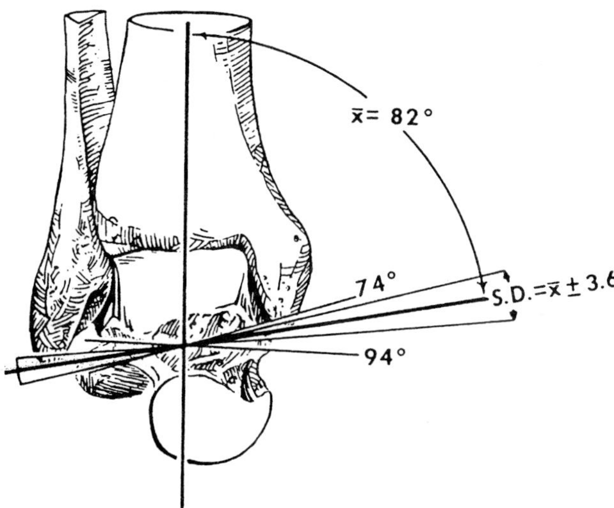

FIGURE 5-3 ■ Ankle-joint axis in the coronal plane projects from medial cephalad to lateral caudad, with variation between ankles ranging from 74–94 degrees from the vertical axis of the tibia. (From Inman, V.T.: The Joints of the Ankle. Baltimore, Williams & Wilkins, 1976, p. 27.)

the deep and superficial peroneal, saphenous, and sural distributions on the dorsal, medial, and lateral surfaces and the medial and lateral plantar branches of the posterior tibial nerve (PTN) distributions plantarward. The plantar intrinsic muscles are innervated by the lateral and medial plantar nerve. When these nerve branches are injured, flexion of the metatarsophalangeal (MTP) joint is weak or absent, and with injury to the deep peroneal nerve (DPN), the function of the extensor digitorum brevis is weak or absent. Vascular evaluation should include palpation of the dorsalis pedis and posterior tibial pulses. A formal vascular evaluation that includes toe pressures and arterial Doppler examination is necessary if pulses are not palpable or healing potential is questionable.

Active and passive ankle dorsiflexion, plantar flexion, inversion, and eversion should be checked. Bilateral inspection and comparison of motion and strength are helpful. It is important to check the posterior tibial muscle for inversion strength from an everted position. The ankle should be plantar flexed to avoid recruitment of the tibialis anterior. When the ankle is in neutral or inverted, the anterior tibial muscle can function as an inverter along with the posterior tibial muscle. From an everted position, only the posterior tibial tendon functions as an inverter. The ability to initiate heel rise from the stance position is accomplished by the posterior tibial tendon. Hindfoot inversion should occur if the tendon is functional.

B. **Joint Motion**—Ankle dorsiflexion and plantar flexion (range 20 degrees dorsiflexion to 40 degrees plantar flexion), subtalar inversion and eversion (range 5–20 degrees), and transverse tarsal motion should be checked. Midfoot motion (flexion, abduction) is assessed at the tarsometatarsal joints, specifically the first tarsometatarsal joint. The MTP joints are tested first for motion, tenderness, or swelling, with careful palpation of the interdigital spaces. The MTP joints are tested for stability with the modified drawer sign. Deviation of a second or third toe with weight bearing indicates collateral ligament (usually lateral) or plantar plate insufficiency, or both.

C. **Palpation/Stability**—The anterolateral and medial ankle ligaments are palpated. **Inversion of the ankle in dorsiflexion will stress the calcaneofibular ligament, and an anterior drawer test with the ankle in plantar flexion places stress on the anterior talofibular ligament.** Percussion over the tarsal tunnel may elicit a Tinel's sign suggestive of PTN irritation. The course of all tendon units should be palpated at rest and as they contract. The Achilles tendon is palpated along its course and insertion to detect any nodules or thickening.

D. **Radiographic Examination**—Plain-film radiography is the mainstay for evaluation of the structure and function of the foot and ankle. Routine weight-bearing views (Table 5-2 and Fig. 5-4) and oblique non–weight-bearing views (Fig. 5-5) are recommended.

Special views may be necessary for evaluation of the phalanges, sesamoid bones, and hindfoot. A routine ankle series usually includes anteroposterior (AP), lateral, and mortise views. The lateral view should include the proximal metatarsals to detect a fracture of the fifth metatarsal metaphyseal-diaphyseal junction (Jones fracture) or

Table 5-2. RADIOGRAPHIC EVALUATION OF FOOT AND ANKLE

Anteroposterior view	Evaluation of tibiotalar joint, distal tibia and fibula peripheral borders of tarsals, and talar dome
Lateral view	Assessment of effusion, talocalcaneal relationships, tibiofibular integrity, and tibiotalar joint congruity
Oblique views (internal—plantar flexion, 45 degrees internal rotation; external—plantar flexion + 45 degrees external rotation)	Additional information about ankle mortise, talar dome, and malleoli
Mortise view	Best information about mortise integrity and talar dome

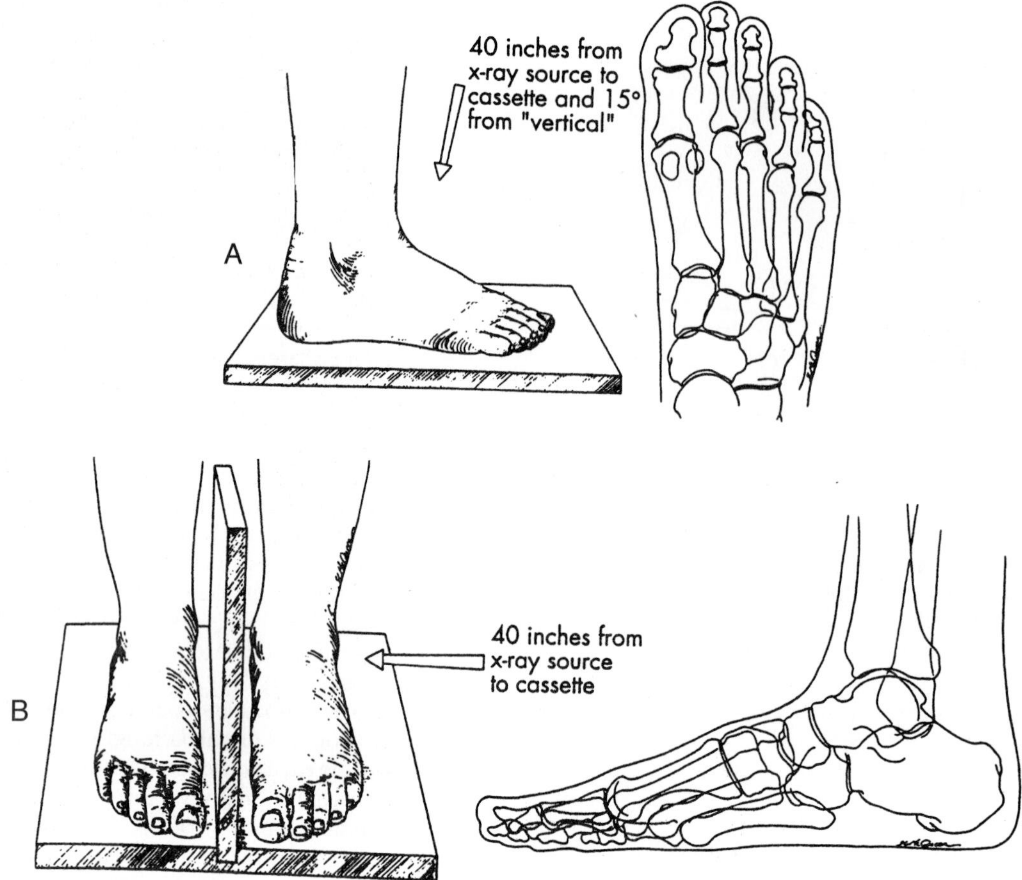

FIGURE 5-4 ■ Radiographic views of the foot. *A*, Weight-bearing dorsoplantar view. *B*, Weight-bearing lateral view. (From Richardson, E.G.: Disorders of hallux. In Canale, S.T., ed.: Campbell's Operative Orthopaedics, 10th ed. St. Louis, C.V. Mosby, 2003, p. 3921.)

an avulsion of its base by the peroneus brevis tendon. Weight-bearing AP and lateral views can be obtained to evaluate structural changes in the ankle joint. Stress views are used to evaluate ligamentous stability in patients with suspected soft-tissue injuries. Varus, valgus, and anterior drawer stress views are the most commonly used; flexion, extension, and subtalar inversion stress views have been described. Bone scanning is helpful for early identification of stress fractures. Computed tomography (CT) scanning is primarily used for evaluation of foot and ankle fractures, especially

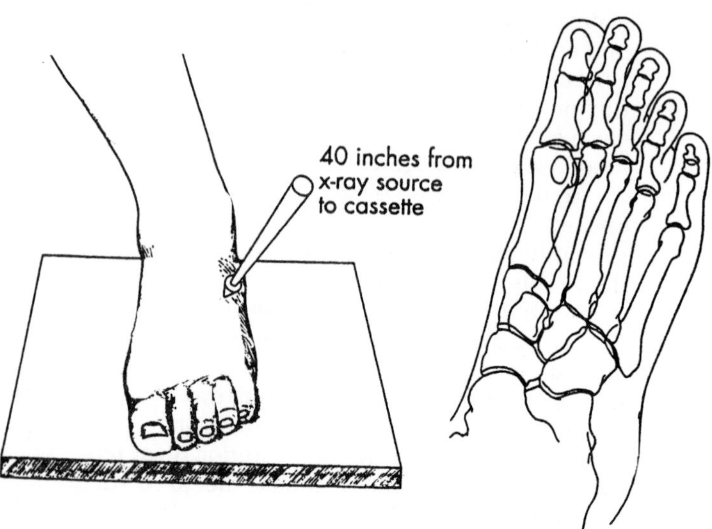

FIGURE 5-5 ■ Non–weight-bearing lateral oblique radiographic view. (From Richardson, E.G.: Disorders of hallux. In Canale, S.T., ed.: Campbell's Operative Orthopaedics, 10th ed. St. Louis, C.V. Mosby, 2003, p. 3921.)

fractures of the calcaneus, talus, midfoot, and navicular in the foot and triplane, Tillaux, pilon, and trimalleolar fractures in the ankle, but it is also helpful in diagnosing middle-facet tarsal coalition. Magnetic resonance imaging (MRI) generally is better for evaluation of neoplasms, infections, foreign bodies, osteochondral lesions, tendinous injuries, osteonecrosis, arthritis, and congenital anomalies.

III. Hallux Valgus

A. Adult Hallux Valgus. Hallux valgus (lateral deviation of the great toe) is not a single deformity but a complex deformity of the first ray that frequently is accompanied by deformity and symptoms in the lesser toes (Fig. 5-6). Factors influencing the development of hallux valgus include genetic predisposition, inappropriate footwear, and certain anatomic and structural abnormalities: pronated flatfeet, abnormal insertion of the tibialis posterior tendon, increased obliquity of the first metatarsomedial-cuneiform joint, an abnormally long first ray, incongruous articular surfaces of the first MTP joint, and excessive valgus tilt of the articular surface of the first MT head and proximal phalangeal articular surface may contribute singly or in combination to the deformity (Fig. 5-7).

B. Pathophysiology—An increased valgus angle of the first MTP joint (hallux valgus angle [HVA] of more than 15 degrees) will not result in pronation of the great toe until it is excessive (approximately 30–35 degrees). When present, this abnormal rotation moves the abductor hallucis, which is normally slightly plantar to the flexion-extension axis of the first MTP joint, farther plantarward (Fig. 5-8), leaving the medial capsular ligament as the only restraining medial structure. The adductor hallucis, which is

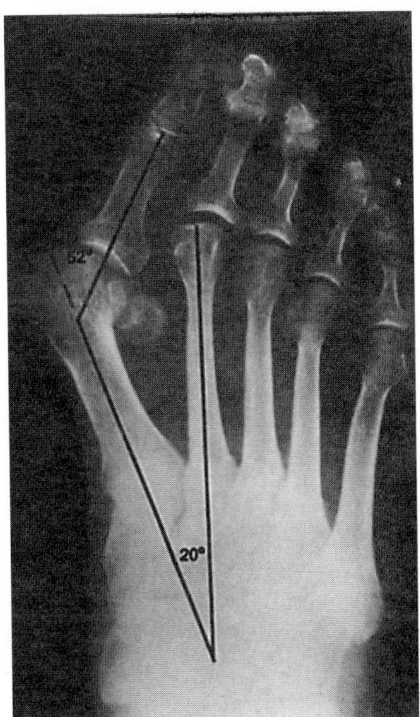

FIGURE 5-7 ■ Hallux valgus complex. Note increast in intermetatarsal angle, lateral dislocation of sesamoids, subluxation of first MTP joint (leaving MT head uncovered), and pronation of great toe associated with marked hallux valgus. (From Richardson, E.G.: Disorders of hallux. In Canale, S.T., ed.: Campbell's Operative Orthopaedics, 10th ed. St. Louis, C.V. Mosby, 2003, p. 3921.)

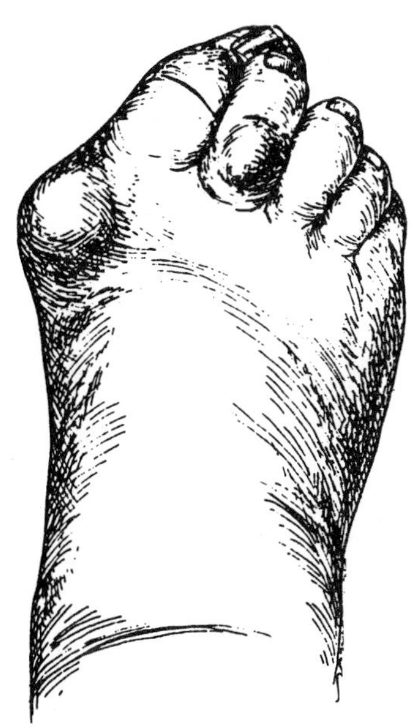

FIGURE 5-6 ■ Multiple components of hallux valgus and associated deformities. (From Richardson, E.G.: Disorders of hallux. In Canale, S.T., ed.: Campbell's Operative Orthopaedics, 10th ed. St. Louis, C.V. Mosby, 2003, p. 3916.)

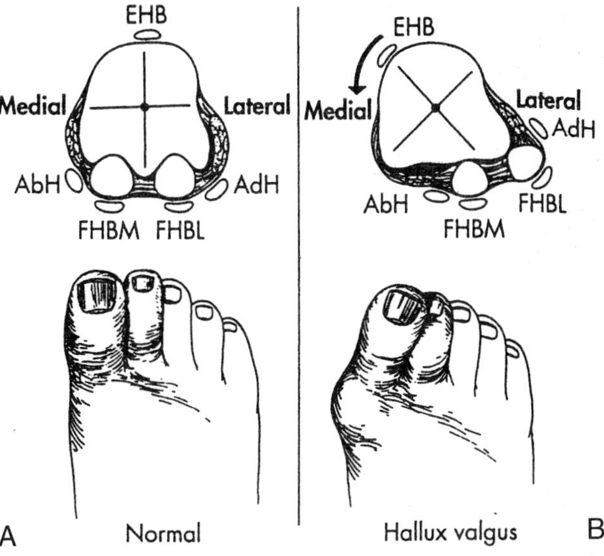

FIGURE 5-8 ■ Pronation of hallux. *A*, Normal. *B*, Note plantar shift of abductor hallucis (AbH) and lateral shift of sesamoids with associated intrinsic muscles of hallux. AdH, adductor hallucis; EHB, extensor hallucis brevis; FHBM, flexor hallucis brevis muscle; FHBL, flexor hallucis brevis ligament. (From Miller, J.: Acquired hallux varus: a preventable and correctable disorder. J. Bone Joint Surg. 57-A:183, 1975.)

unopposed by the abductor hallucis, pulls the great toe farther into valgus, stretching the medial capsular ligament (particularly the capsulosesamoid portion), attenuating this structure, and allowing the MT head to drift medially from the sesamoids. In addition, the flexor hallucis brevis, flexor hallucis longus (FHL), adductor hallucis, and extensor hallucis longus increase the valgus moment at the MTP joint, further deforming the first ray. The sesamoid ridge on the plantar surface of the first MT head (the crista) flattens because of pressure from the tibial sesamoid. With this restraint lost, the fibular sesamoid displaces partially or completely into the first intermetatarsal space. Once the sesamoid bones are subluxated from their facets, the deformity almost always increases, although it may require months to years to do so.

C. **Evaluation of the Adult Foot with Hallux Valgus**. In addition to a careful clinical examination, several radiographic angles are helpful in determining the severity of hallux valgus deformity and in choosing appropriate treatment (Table 5-3).

Other radiographic findings that help determine appropriate treatment include the relative lengths of the first and second metatarsal, the congruency of the joint, the shape of the metatarsal head, and the presence of arthritic changes or pes planus deformity. The importance of the position of the tibial sesamoid has become more apparent, and the grade of displacement of this sesamoid is determined relative to a line that bisects the long axis of the first metatarsal shaft: grade 0, no displacement; grade 1, less than 50% overlap of the reference line; grade 2, more than 50% overlap of the reference line; and grade 3, complete displacement beyond the reference line (Fig. 5-9).

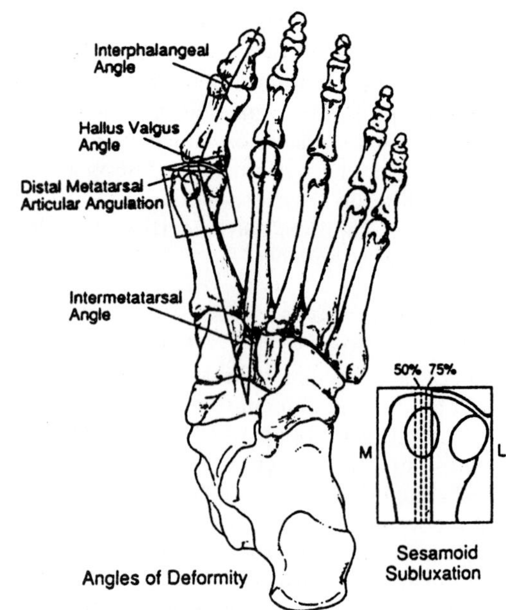

FIGURE 5-9 ■ Angles of deformity. Tibial sesamoid is considered medial if 75% of its width is medial to the central line; lateral, if 75% is lateral to central line. Otherwise, the sesamoid is considered to be centrally located. (From Pedowitz, W.: Bunion deformity. In Pfeffer, G., Frey, C., eds.: Current Practice in Foot and Ankle Surgery. New York, McGraw Hill, 1993.)

D. **Conservative Treatment**—Initially, most patients can be treated nonoperatively with appropriate shoe modifications, exercises, and activity adjustments. Some hallux valgus deformities can be well treated with wide-laced (high toe box) shoes. If concurrent hammer toe or crossover-toe deformities exist, extra-depth shoes may be helpful. Stretching the leather over the bunion region can also be beneficial.

Table 5-3. IMPORTANT RADIOGRAPHIC ANGLES IN EVALUATION OF HALLUX VALGUS

Angle	Location	Importance	Normal
Hallux valgus interphalangeus	Between long axes of first proximal phalanx and first distal phalanx, bisecting their diaphysis	Identifies degree of deformity at the IP joint	<8 degrees
Hallux valgus	Between long axes of first proximal phalanx and first metatarsal, bisecting their diaphysis	Identifies degree of deformity at the MTP joint	<15 degrees
Metatarsus primus varus	Between long axes of first metatarsal and first cuneiform	Identifies obliquity versus subluxation of MTC joint	<25 degrees
First intermetatarsal (Hardy and Clapham)	Between long axes of first and second metatarsal, bisecting shafts of first and second metatarsals	Not influenced by overresection of medial eminence. Not accurate for postoperative evaluation of distal osteotomies	<10 degrees
Distal metatarsal articular	Angle of line bisecting MT shaft with line through base of distal articular cartilage cap	Offset of angle is predisposing factor in development of hallux valgus	<15 degrees
Phalangeal articular	Articular angle of base of proximal phalanx in relation to longitudinal axis	Offset of angle is predisposing factor in development of hallux valgus	7–10 degrees

E. Surgical Treatment— Surgery is appropriate for painful deformities that are not improved with conservative measures, but no procedure should be recommended until the entire foot, not just the first ray, is thoroughly examined clinically while the patient is standing, sitting, supine, and prone. Particular attention should be given to the remainder of the forefoot, and corns, calluses, warts, interdigital neuromas, bunionettes, hammer toes, and claw toes should be identified. Although the pain and deformity may be relieved after correction of the hallux valgus, the result can be compromised if symptoms in the lesser toes or the metatarsals remain. This should be explained carefully to the patient before surgery to avoid false expectations and disappointment. Finally, the midfoot and hindfoot must be examined carefully before making treatment recommendations for forefoot surgery.

Any procedure chosen must taken into account the following structural components:

1. Valgus deviation of the great toe (hallux valgus)
2. Varus deviation of the first metatarsal
3. Pronation of the hallux, first metatarsal, or both
4. Hallux valgus interphalangeus
5. Arthritis and limitation of motion of the first MTP joint
6. Length of the first metatarsal relative to lesser metatarsals
7. Excessive mobility or obliquity of the first metatarso-medial-cuneiform joint
8. The medial eminence (bunion)
9. The location of the sesamoid apparatus
10. Intrinsic and extrinsic muscle-tendon balance and synchrony

Inadequate vascularity or sensibility should be investigated thoroughly before hallux valgus surgery is considered. In addition, the position of the articular surface of the metatarsal head in relation to the longitudinal axis of the first metatarsal should be determined.

With more than 130 procedures described for the treatment of hallux valgus, it is not possible to discuss them all. Often soft-tissue and bony procedures must be combined to obtain adequate correction. **Treatment algorithms** (Table 5-4) provide guidelines for deciding which procedures are appropriate.

1. **Soft-Tissue Procedures**
   The usual candidate for soft-tissue correction of the hallux valgus complex is a 30- to 50-year-old woman with clinical symptoms and an HVA of 15–25 degrees, intermetatarsal angle (IMA) of less than 13 degrees, valgus of the interphalangeal (IP) joint of less than 15 degrees, no degenerative changes at the MTP joint, and a history of failure of conservative management. The modified McBride procedure is basically a combination of the procedures described by Silver in 1923 and McBride in 1928 and later modified by DuVries and popularized by Mann. The results of this procedure are successful in properly selected patients (Fig. 5-10).
2. **Combined Soft-Tissue and Bony Procedures**
   Metatarsal Osteotomy
   The **chevron** (Fig. 5-11) and **biplanar chevron** (Fig. 5-12) osteotomies are mostly intracapsular, distal metatarsal osteotomies, most often used to correct mild to moderate hallux valgus deformities. A symptomatic patient with an IMA angle of 13 degrees or less and an HVA of less than 30 degrees is the best candidate. If there is an anatomically inherent increased valgus posture (set angle) to the first metatarsal articular surface (distal metatarsal articular angle [DMAA] of more than 15 degrees), correction in both the axial and frontal planes is possible.

   The **Mitchell osteotomy** (distal) is extracapsular. Because of its more proximal location in the distal metatarsal it can correct larger deformities. The medial eminence is excised, and a step-cut osteotomy is made approximately 1.5–2 cm proximal to the medial border of the articular surface of the first metatarsal head (Fig. 5-13). This procedure is

Table 5-4. HALLUX VALGUS TREATMENT ALGORITHMS

Hallux valgus <25 degrees	
Congruent joint	Chevron osteotomy Mitchell osteotomy
Incongruent joint (subluxation)	Distal soft-tissue realignment Chevron osteotomy Mitchell osteotomy
Hallux valgus 25–40 degrees	
Congruent joint	Chevron osteotomy + Akin procedure Mitchell osteotomy
Incongruent joint	Distal soft-tissue realignment + proximal osteotomy Mitchell osteotomy
Severe hallux valgus 25–40 degrees	
Congruent joint	Double osteotomy Akin + chevron osteotomy Akin + first MT osteotomy Akin + first cuneiform opening-wedge osteotomy
Incongruent joint	Distal soft-tissue realignment + proximal osteotomy First MT crescentic osteotomy First cuneiform opening-wedge osteotomy
Hypermobile first metatarsocuneiform	Distal soft-tissue realignment + fusion of first metatarsocuneiform joint

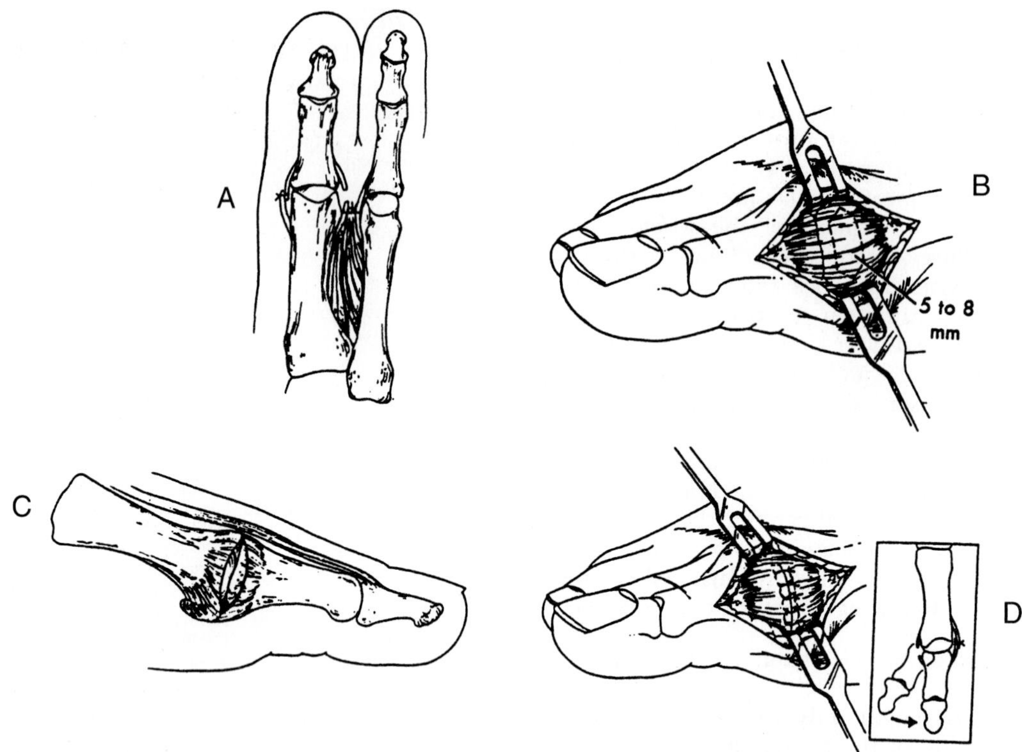

FIGURE 5-10 ■ Modified McBride bunionectomy (DuVries, Mann). *A*, Medial capsule of second MTP joint is sutured to lateral capsule of first MTP joint with interposition of released adductor hallucis. *B*, Medial capsular resection. *C*, Configuration after capsule resection. *D*, After capsular imbrication, hallux should rest in neutral position or not exceed 5 degrees of varus. (From Richardson, E.G.: Disorders of hallux. In Canale, S.T., ed.: Campbell's Operative Orthopaedics, 10th ed. St. Louis, C.V. Mosby, 2003, p. 3930.)

indicated in a patient with moderate hallux valgus deformity (HVA less than 35 degrees and IMA less than 15 degrees).

The **scarf, Ludloff, and Mau osteotomies** are made in the metatarsal shaft. The Ludloff and Mau osteotomies are oblique osteotomies (Fig. 5-14*A* and *B*) and the scarf is a step-cut osteotomy (Fig. 5-14*C*). Primary indications for these osteotomies include an increased IMA (14–18 degrees), a normal or increased DMAA, adequate bone stock, and symptomatic hallux valgus deformity.

Proximal crescentic or chevron (broomstick) osteotomy is combined with medial eminence removal and first web space lateral capsular and adductor tendon release. The configuration of the osteotomy may be dorsal semicircular (Fig. 5-14*D*) or lateral V-shaped (Fig. 5-14*E*). These are technically demanding procedures—crescentic osteotomy requires three incisions and chevron osteotomy one or two—but they can correct severe hallux valgus deformity (IMA of 20 degrees and HVA of 50 degrees).

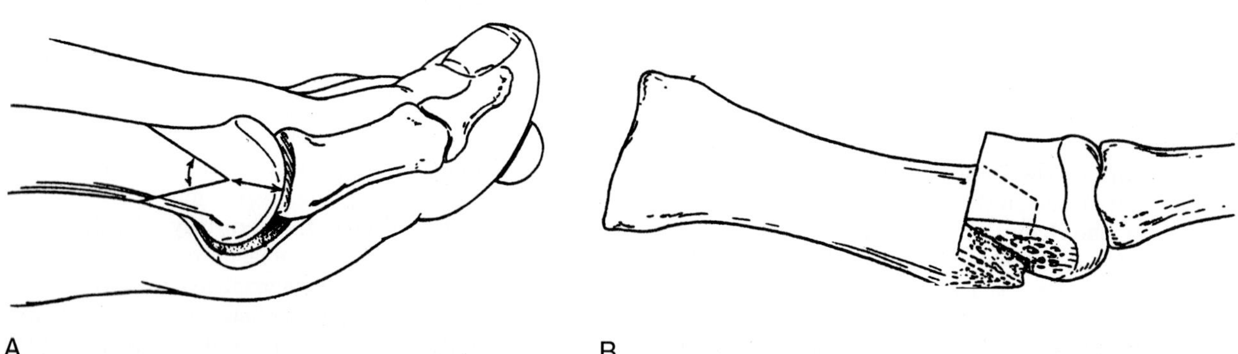

FIGURE 5-11 ■ Chevron osteotomy. *A*, Position of saw cuts. *B*, Lateral transposition of metatarsal head. (From Myerson, M.S.: Hallux valgus. In Myerson, M.S., ed.: Foot and Ankle Disorders. Philadelphia, WB Saunders, 2000, p. 239.)

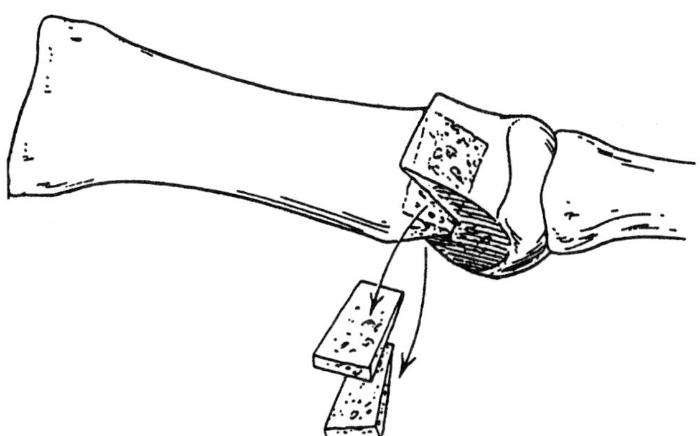

FIGURE 5-12 ■ Biplanar osteotomy adds medially based wedge excision to chevron osteotomy. (From Myerson, M.S.: Hallux valgus. In Myerson, M.S., ed.: Foot and Ankle Disorders. Philadelphia, WB Saunders, 2000, p. 239.)

A chevron osteotomy can be combined with an **Akin (proximal phalangeal) osteotomy** and medial eminence removal to obtain slightly more correction than possible with a chevron osteotomy alone. This is especially true if the articular base of the proximal phalanx has a lateral slope or there is a hallux valgus interphalangeus associated with the valgus deformity at the MTP joint. The IMA should still be 13 degrees or less, but the HVA can be as high as 35 degrees. This procedure (chevron-Akin double osteotomy) adds significant cosmetic improvement in selected patients (Fig. 5-15).

Resection arthroplasty, as described by Keller and Hamilton, involves medial eminence removal, resection of the base of the proximal phalanx, stabilization of the shortened hallux on the first metatarsal (usually with one or two pins), and medial capsulorraphy. The modification by Hamilton is a capsulo-tendinous interposition within the resection joint. It will correct moderate to severe valgus of the hallux (HVA 30–45 degrees) and mild to moderate IMA (less than 14 degrees). It is indicated

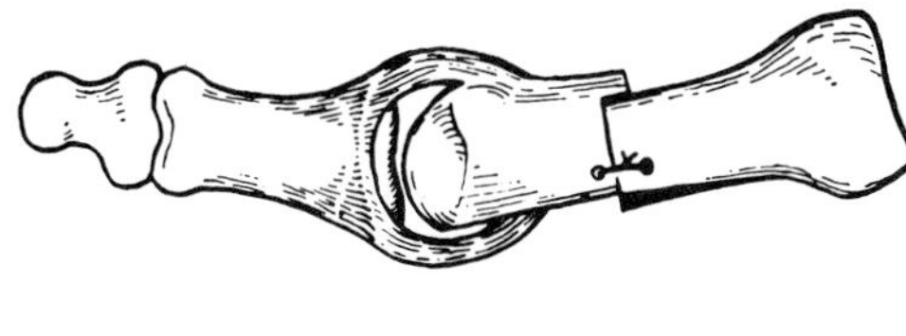

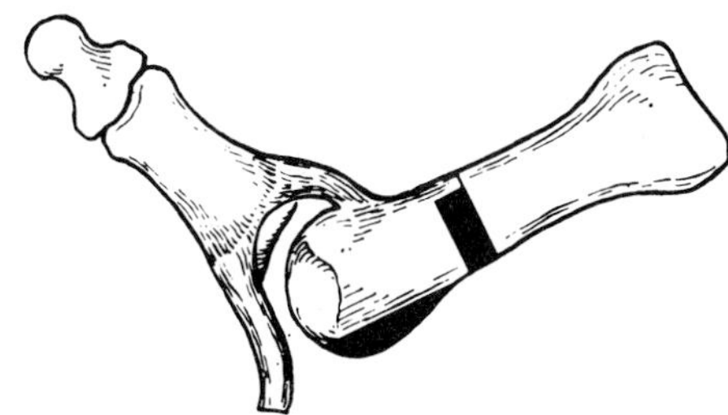

FIGURE 5-13 ■ Mitchell osteotomy. Medial eminence is removed in line with medial aspect of metatarsal. Distal cut is then made in metatarsal and osteotomy is laterally displaced. Degree of lateral displacement depends on magnitude of deformity. (From Mann, R.A., Coughlin, M.J.: The Video Textbook of Foot and Ankle Surgery. St. Louis, Medical Video Productions, 1991.)

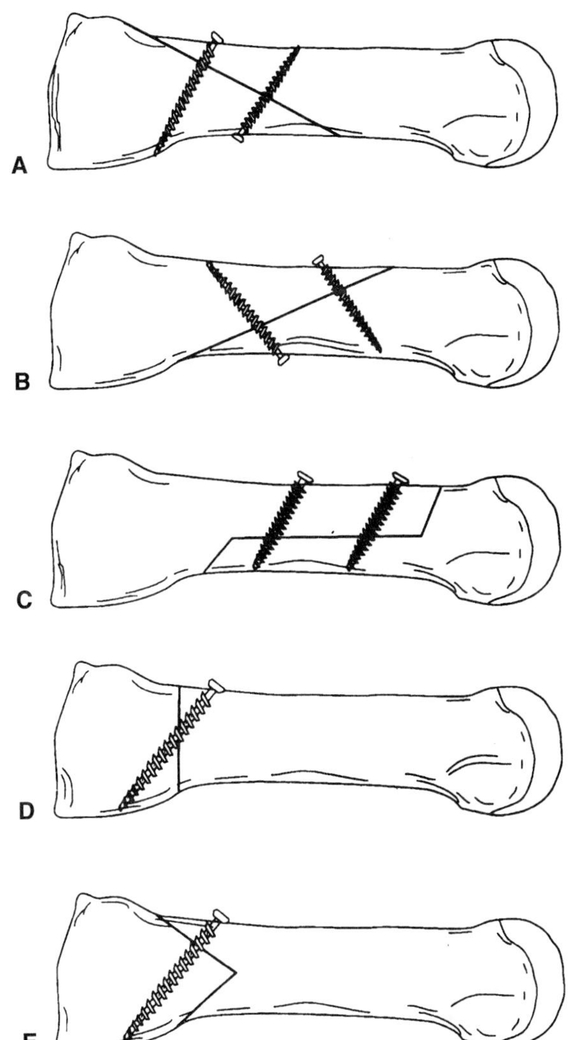

FIGURE 5-14 ■ Proximal metatarsal osteotomies. *A*, Oblique shaft (Ludloff). *B*, Reverse oblique shaft (Mau). *C*, Rotational Z (scarf). *D*, Crescentic. *E*, Proximal chevron. (From Nyska, M., Trnka, H-J., Parks, B.G., Myerson, M.S.: Proximal metatarsal osteotomies: a comparative geometric analysis conducted on sawbone models. Foot Ankle Int. 23:938–945, 2002.)

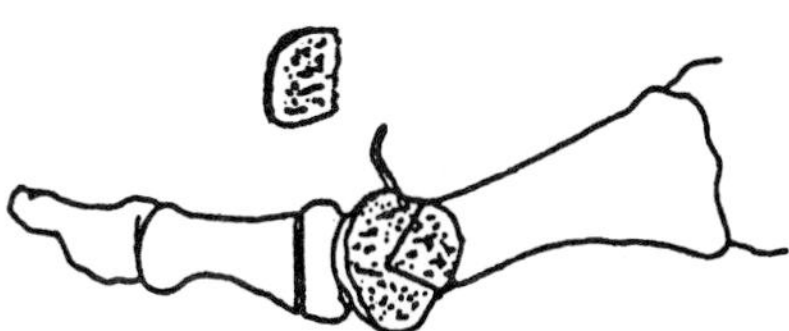

FIGURE 5-15 ■ Akin osteotomy parallels concavity at base of MT, where 1-mm wedge of bone is removed. (From Mitchell, L.A., Baxter, D.E.: A chevron-Akin double osteotomy for correction of hallux valgus. Foot Ankle 12:7, 1991.)

in older patients with reduced functional demands and severe degenerative joint disease of the MTP joint. Silicone rubber interposition arthroplasty is not recommended because of fragmentation of the implant and foreign-body reaction. Metal-plastic prostheses are not recommended because of insufficient wear characteristics and soft-tissue coverage.

MTP arthrodesis is an excellent pain-relief procedure, as well as a moderately successful correction of deformity, in patients with moderate to severe hallux valgus deformity, degenerative arthritis of the first MTP joint with articular symptoms, and reduced range of motion of the first MTP joint, particularly if painful callosities are present beneath one or more lesser metatarsal heads. The IMA may spontaneously reduce 4–5 degrees after arthrodesis, and at least 3-degrees reduction of this angle should routinely occur. Metatarsalgia from lesser metatarsal head overload usually is greatly improved.

***First metatarsocuneiform arthrodesis* (Lapidus procedure)** is recommended for patients with moderate to severe hallux valgus deformity, a hypermobile first ray, a markedly medially slanted articular surface at the first MTC joint, and cortical hypertrophy of the second metatarsal indicative of second metatarsal overload. It can correct deformities of up to 20 degrees IMA and approximately 50 degrees HVA. Medial eminence removal and first web space release of the adductor and lateral capsule are added to the arthrodesis. This requires three skin incisions, as does the proximal (dorsal) metatarsal osteotomy. It is a technically demanding procedure and is not used as often as are various metatarsal osteotomies.

3. Complications of Hallux Valgus Surgery

As with any surgical procedure, complications after hallux valgus surgery can include delayed wound healing, infection, vasomotor disturbances, and even thrombophlebitis. Some complications are more procedure specific.

Soft-tissue procedures. The major complication of simple bunionectomy (Silver procedure) and the modified McBride procedure is recurrence of the hallux valgus deformity. This most often is due to an attempt at correcting too great a deformity. The second most frequent complication after the modified McBride procedure is hallux varus. This is caused by overplication of the medial capsule combined with excessive removal of bone during medial eminence resection. Hallux varus is not as common after the McBride procedure since excision of the fibular sesamoid, which was a part of the original technique, has been abandoned.

Metatarsal Osteotomy

Chevron osteotomy. A common complication after chevron osteotomy is recurrence of the hallux valgus deformity caused by an attempt at correction of too great a deformity. The second most frequent complication is malunion, especially dorsal malunion, with resultant transfer metatarsalgia. Although shortening and varus or valgus malunion can occur, they are not as common since internal fixation has become standard. Avascular necrosis of the capital fragment (distal head) is rarer than once reported (up to 20%), but if extensive necrosis occurs, salvage is not difficult, usually requiring an arthrodesis with or without interposition bone graft to maintain length. Nonunion is rare.

Mitchell osteotomy. The most common complication within the first 3–5 years after this osteotomy is malunion, which can produce both shortening and dorsiflexion with transfer metatarsalgia. Long-term follow-up (more than 10 years) has shown recurrence of the hallux valgus deformity to be as common or more common than malunion.

Shaft osteotomies (Ludloff, scarf, Mau). The most common complication of shaft osteotomies is malunion with transfer metatarsalgia. However, delayed union, nonunion, recurrence of the hallux valgus deformity, and hallux varus have been reported. These osteotomies carry the highest complication rates overall of any of the procedures for hallux valgus, testifying to their technical difficulty.

Proximal metatarsal osteotomy. Hallux varus is the most common complication (11–13%) after crescentic proximal metatarsal osteotomy, with dorsiflexion malunion and recurrence of the hallux valgus deformity not far behind. Nonunion is rare.

Chevron-Akin double osteotomy. Because these osteotomies are done on both sides of the MTP joint, loss of motion at that joint is common, although rarely clinically important. Recurrence of deformity probably is the most important clinical complication. Malunion (metatarsal) and delayed union (phalanx) are less common complications.

Resection arthroplasty (Keller, Hamilton). Recurrence of deformity is the most common complication; however, the complication that elicits the most complaints clinically is transfer metatarsalgia. Other reported complications include stress fractures of the lesser metatarsals from insufficient first-ray load-sharing, hallux varus, and development of a hammer toe deformity of the second or third digit from recruitment of those digits in terminal stance and toe-off phases of the ambulation cycle.

Arthrodesis. Nonunion and malunion are equally troublesome complications of arthrodesis. These occur, however, in fewer than 10–15% of patients. With a nonunion, the deformity may recur, along with articular and periarticular pain. With malunion, especially dorsiflexion malunion, shoe wear is a difficulty and transfer metatarsalgia may occur or recur.

F. Juvenile and Adolescent Hallux Valgus

Several factors separate these patients from adult patients with hallux valgus deformity.

1. Pain, either at the MTP joint or beneath the lesser metatarsal heads, may not be the primary complaint.
2. A bunion secondary to medial eminence and bursal hypertrophy may be a minor part of the deformity.
3. Varus of the first metatarsal with a widened IMA is almost always present.
4. The DMAA is increased.
5. Hypermobile flatfoot with pronation of the foot during weight bearing frequently is associated with the deformity (Coughlin's data do not support this).
6. Recurrence of the hallux valgus deformity is more frequent, especially with flatfoot deformity.
7. Hallux valgus interphalangeus may be prominent yet easily overlooked and may cause unsatisfactory correction of the deformity.
8. The family history frequently is positive for hallux valgus.
9. Soft-tissue procedures alone are unlikely to result in permanent correction.
10. Osteotomy, single or double, of the first metatarsal is almost always necessary to obtain and maintain correction.

1. Surgical Treatment

The most difficult combination of deformities to correct is hypermobile flatfoot, metatarsus primus varus, and hallux valgus accompanied by an increased DMAA (more than 15–20 degrees).

Chevron distal first metatarsal osteotomy. Only **mild hallux valgus deformities** in adolescents are correctable with this osteotomy. An HVA of less than 25 degrees and IMA of less than 13 degrees respond best. The most appealing benefit of this osteotomy is its ability to correct an excessive DMAA (often present in adolescent hallux valgus) if a small (1–3 mm) wedge is removed medially, converting the osteotomy into biplanar correction by becoming not only a **transpositional** but also an **angular** osteotomy (Milch).

Mitchell osteotomy. Although good corrections of mild to moderate deformities have been reported with this osteotomy. Shortening of the first metatarsal and failure to maintain enduring correction have decreased its utility.

Proximal first metatarsal osteotomy. Both moderate (IMA of 13–15 degrees and HVA of 30–34 degrees) and severe (IMA of more than 15 degrees and HVA of more than 35 degrees) deformities can be corrected with this osteotomy. Dome-shaped (crescentic), chevron, step-cut, and opening and closing-wedge configurations can be used. The most commonly used proximal metatarsal osteotomy is the dome-shaped or crescentic osteotomy done **after physeal closure.** Internal fixation must be used to stabilize the osteotomy and avoid a malunion. A proximal osteotomy should **not** shorten or lengthen the metatarsal.

Double first metatarsal osteotomy (Fig. 5-16). This procedure is useful when the IMA is 13–14 degrees or more and the DMAA is excessive, particularly 20 degrees or more. The distal osteotomy must be a closing wedge (1.3 mm) to correct the abnormal DMAA and in **severe** deformity also can be a transpositional (chevron) osteotomy to add correction of an IMA of 16 degrees or more. Adding this transpositional component distally relieves part of the burden of IMA correction on the proximal osteotomy, decreasing the possibility of hallux varus caused by over-correction of the IMA with the basilar osteotomy.

First cuneiform osteotomy. This osteotomy is recommended to correct **severe** deformity in patients with generalized ligamentous laxity (usually adolescent girls) and particularly a hypermobile first ray in a hypermobile flatfoot. This is an **opening**-wedge

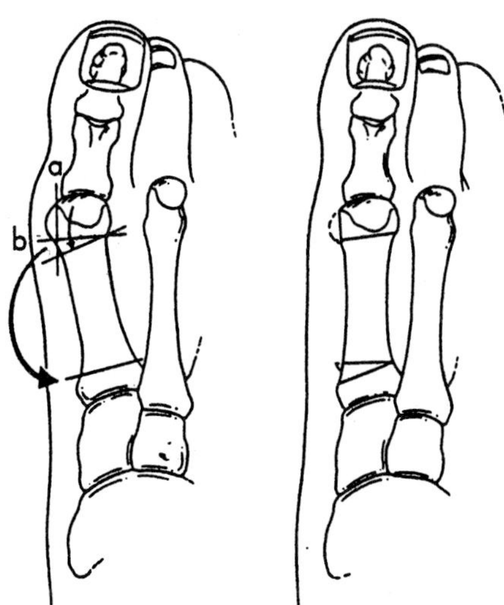

FIGURE 5-16 ■ Double first metatarsal osteotomies. (From Richardson, E.G.: Disorders of hallux. In Canale, S.T., ed.: Campbell's Operative Orthopaedics, 10th ed. St. Louis, C.V. Mosby, 2003, p. 3972.)

osteotomy requiring often a 1-cm tricortical iliac crest graft (allograft can be used). An indication for this osteotomy, in addition to a hypermobile first ray, is a severe deformity in an adolescent with open physes, because the proximal first metatarsal physis is not vulnerable as with a proximal metatarsal osteotomy. In addition, this osteotomy can be augmented with a distal first metatarsal osteotomy as well as an Akin (proximal phalangeal medial closing wedge) osteotomy. This triple osteotomy (Coughlin) should be reserved for only the most severe adolescent hallux valgus deformity with a hypermobile first ray.

2. **Complications of Surgery for Adolescent Hallux Valgus**

The most common complication is **recurrence** of deformity, particularly if done in a skeletally immature foot. **Malunion**, especially if associated with shortening or dorsiflexion of the distal fragment, shifts weight bearing to the lesser metatarsals and may result in a patient with only mild preoperative symptoms (even with a severe deformity) becoming much more symptomatic postoperatively.

IV. Sesamoid Injuries of the Hallux

The hallucal sesamoids, although small and seemingly insignificant, play an important role in the function of the great toe by **absorbing weight-bearing pressure, reducing friction, and protecting tendons**. However, the functional complexity and anatomic location of these small bones make them vulnerable to injury from shear and loading forces (Table 5-5).

The **tibial sesamoid is the more commonly injured** of the two because of its central location beneath the first metatarsal head. Hyperextension and axial loading are the most common mechanism of injury resulting in fracture (or sprain of the capsulo-ligamentous complex). A **bipartite tibial sesamoid** is present in about 10% of the population and in 25% of these the condition is bilateral. This congenital condition must be differentiated from a sesamoid fracture. The fibular sesamoid rarely is bipartite.

Table 5-5. CONDITIONS AFFECTING THE HALLUCAL SESAMOIDS

Fracture (acute, stress)
Dislocation
Inflammation (sesamoiditis)
Traumatic
Infectious
Arthritic
Chondromalacia
Flexor hallucis brevis tendinitis
Osteochondritis dissecans

A patient with a sesamoid injury may complain of generalized pain around the big toe or may describe pain after a sudden stop or snap during running. Usually, however, patients complain of pain as the hallux extends in the terminal part of the stance phase of gait. If the first metatarsal is plantar flexed, an intractable plantar keratosis may have developed. Neuritic symptoms and numbness also may occur if a digital nerve is compressed by edema, inflammation, or displacement of a bipartite or fractured sesamoid.

Although traumatic injuries usually can be diagnosed easily, other pathologic conditions may be overlooked. Careful physical and radiographic examinations are necessary to determine the cause of pain and allow a recommendation of the optimal treatment. Routine AP and oblique radiographs may be helpful; the medial oblique (sesamoid view) is helpful for evaluating the tibial sesamoid, and the axial sesamoid view (Fig. 5-17) should be obtained if a pathological condition of the fibular sesamoid is suspected. Bone scanning helps determine if a bipartite sesamoid is present and may help identify MTP joint and sesamoid pathology not visible on radiographs. Initial treatment generally includes

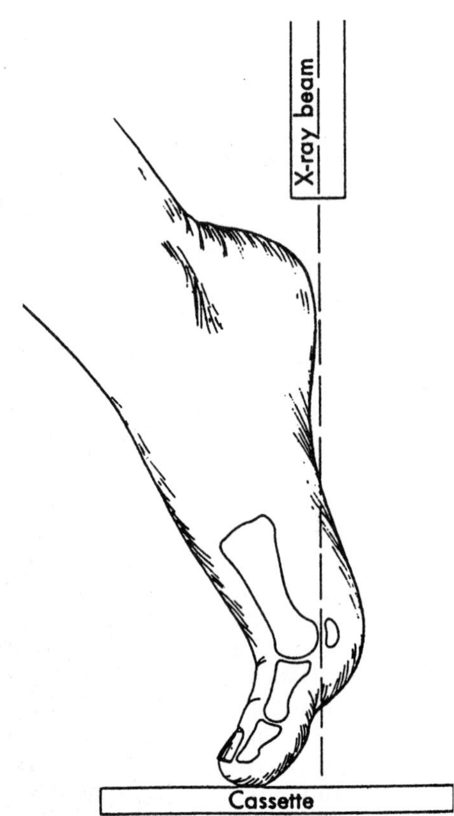

FIGURE 5-17 ■ Axial sesamoid view obtained with patient up on toes. (From Richardson, E.G.: Disorders of hallux. From Canale, S.T., ed.: Campbell's Operative Orthopaedics, 10th ed. St. Louis, C.V. Mosby, 2003, p. 4007.)

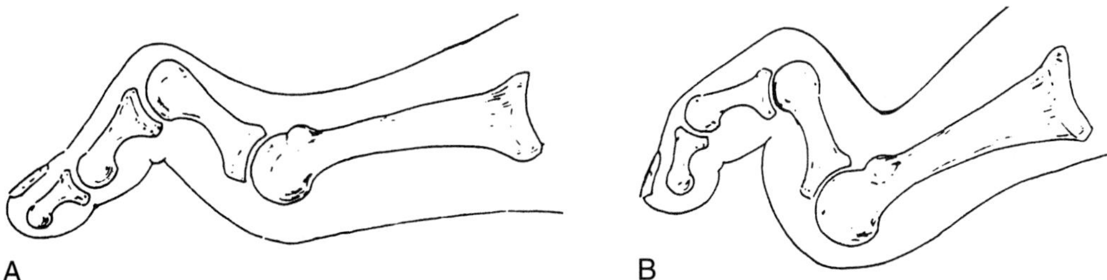

FIGURE 5-18 ■ Hammer toe (*A*) and claw toe (*B*) deformities.

nonsteroidal anti-inflammatory drugs (NSAIDs), modification of activity, full-length shoe orthoses with a metatarsal pad and a relief beneath the first metatarsal head, a metatarsal bar on the sole of the shoe, or cast immobilization. If symptoms are not improved after several months, surgical treatment is indicated. Surgical treatment may include partial or complete resection of the sesamoid, shaving of a prominent tibial sesamoid, or autogenous bone grafting for nonunion. Excision of both sesamoids should be avoided if possible.

V. Lesser-Toe Deformities

Mallet toe (distal interphalangeal [DIP] joint), hammer toe (proximal interphalangeal [PIP] joint), and **claw toe** (MTP joint) are the most common lesser-toe deformities, with hammer toe deformity being the most common. With any of these pathological entities, the differentiation between flexible (passively correctable) and fixed (not passively correctable) deformity greatly influences the choice of surgical procedure. A crossing of the second toe over (dorsal to) the hallux is not truly a hammer or claw toe deformity; for lack of a better term, this is simply called cross-over-toe deformity.

A. Hammer Toe and Claw Toe Deformities

Hammer toe and claw toe deformities (Fig. 5-18) are differentiated from each other by the fact that in a claw toe deformity MTP joint hyperextension is the **primary** pathology, with any opposite deformity (flexion) at the PIP or DIP joint secondary to chronic extension of the MTP joint. **The extensor digitorum longus tendon can extend the PIP and DIP joints only if the MTP joint is in a neutral or slightly flexed position.** This is one reason high-heeled shoes (which hold the toes in chronic extension) allow the long flexor tendon to overpull at the PIP and DIP joints unopposed by the long toe extensors. If all four lesser toes have claw deformities (MPT extension and PIP flexion), a neurologic abnormality should be suspected. If claw toe deformity is present in only the second toe, or occasionally the second and third toes, a neuromuscular cause is less likely.

Synovitis of the second MTP joint is the most common inciting event in the etiology of a claw or hammer toe deformity. This usually is from overuse, which may be due to an excessively long second metatarsal (4 mm or more of the second metatarsal head projects distal to the first metatarsal head), a varus of the first metatarsal that places increased load on the second MTP joint (especially the plantar plate), a hypermobile first ray, or chronic buckling of the PIP joint in high-heeled, tight toe-box shoes. This type of shoe forces the MTP joint into chronic hyperextension, with repetitive injury to the plantar plate and eventually attritional insufficiency. Once this occurs, the base of the proximal phalanx translates dorsally, carrying the interossei and lumbrical tendons with it. Once the flexion moment arm of the intrinsic muscle-tendon units pass dorsal to the instant centers of rotation of the metatarsal head, **no primary flexion force on the MTP remains** (Fig. 5-19).

B. Cross-Over-Toe Deformity

In **cross-over-toe deformity** there may be deformity of the PIP joint if the plantar plate becomes

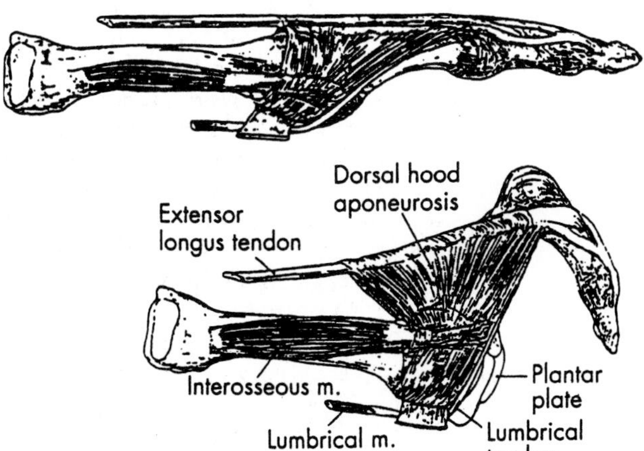

FIGURE 5-19 ■ Anatomy of extrinsic and intrinsic musculature of MTP joint. (From Myerson, M.: Claw toes, cross-over deformity, and instability of the second metatarsophalangeal joint. In Myerson, M., ed.: Current Therapy in Foot and Ankle Surgery. St. Louis, C.V. Mosby, 1993.)

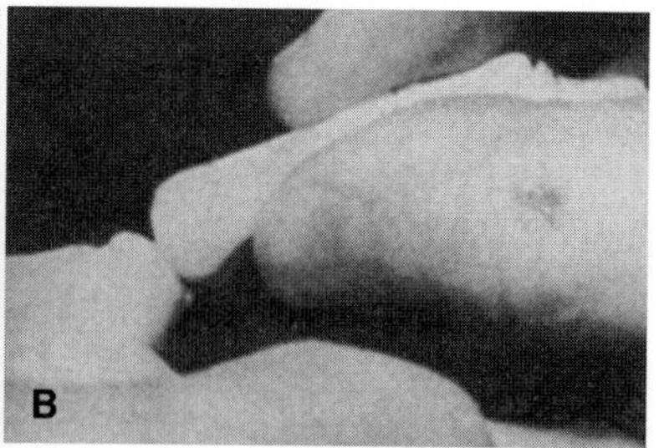

FIGURE 5-20 ■ Lachman test of metatarsophalangeal joint stability. *A*, Starting position. *B*, Positive Lachman test. (From Thompson, F.M., Hamilton, W.G.: Problems of the second metatarsophalangeal joint. Orthopedics 10:83, 1987.)

incompetent early in the pathologic process, causing **dorsal instability** of the joint. The second ray has two dorsal interossei, but no plantar interosseous muscle-tendon unit. The lumbrical is on the medial side of the joint and has an unopposed medial or adduction moment at the second MTP joint. This imbalance promotes attritional rupture of the lateral capsuloligamentous restraints, and the second toe begins deviating medially. The dorsomedial subluxation now is unopposed and grows progressively worse (Fig. 5-20).

C. **Mallet Toe Deformity**

Mallet toe deformity (DIP joint) may occur as an isolated lesser-toe deformity (usually second or third toe) or in conjunction with a claw toe deformity. Congenital mallet toe deformity is not uncommon and often is associated with not only flexion but also lateral deviation at the DIP joint.

Table 5-6. TOE DEFORMITIES TREATMENT

DEFORMITY	TREATMENT	COMMENTS
Hammer toe, without fixed flexion contracture at MTP joint	Transfer of FDL dorsally over midshaft of proximal phalanx	If active flexion less than 10–15 degrees, add EDL lengthening or tenotomy
Hammer toe, with fixed flexion contracture	Resection of head and neck of proximal phalanx + EDB tenotomy + EDL lengthening	
Claw toe without fixed contracture at MTP or PIP joint	EDB tenotomy + EDL lengthening + flexor-to-extensor transfer	
Claw toe with fixed contracture	EDB tenotomy + EDL lengthening + ***complete capsulectomy*** at the MTP joint + resection of head and neck of proximal phalanx	For more correction, oblique shortening MT osteotomy (usually of the second MT) can be added and stabilized with internal fixation (Weil osteotomy)
Claw toe of all four lesser toes	Resection of PIP joint + MTP joint capsulotomy with tendon release and lengthening + distal MT shortening osteotomy	Occasionally partial MT head resection arthroplasty + MT plantar condylectomies
Crossover toe	MTP joint medial capsular release + lateral capsular imbrication + EDB tenotomy + EDL lengthening	With mild or moderate subluxation, add flexor-to-extensor transfer; with severe subluxation or dislocation, add bony procedures such as distal MT shortening (Weil) osteotomy or resection of head and neck of proximal phalanx, or both
Fifth-toe hard corn	Resection of head and neck of proximal phalanx	
Congenital varus with overlapping of fifth toe	Ruiz-Mora procedure (Fig. 5-21).	Variable, often disappointing results
Interdigital corns	Resection of head and neck of proximal phalanx of fifth toe (preferred) or lateral condyle of base of fourth toe	Removal of corners of condyle usually disappointing
Intractable plantar keratosis (IPK)	Excision of plantar condyles of involved MT head(s)	Transfer callus may develop
Bunionette (tailor's bunion) of fifth toe	Initially, wide-toe box shoes and various over-the-counter pads; surgery for persistent symptoms	Surgical treatment requires removal of plantar aspect of fifth MT head in addition to lateral flare (Fig. 5-22)

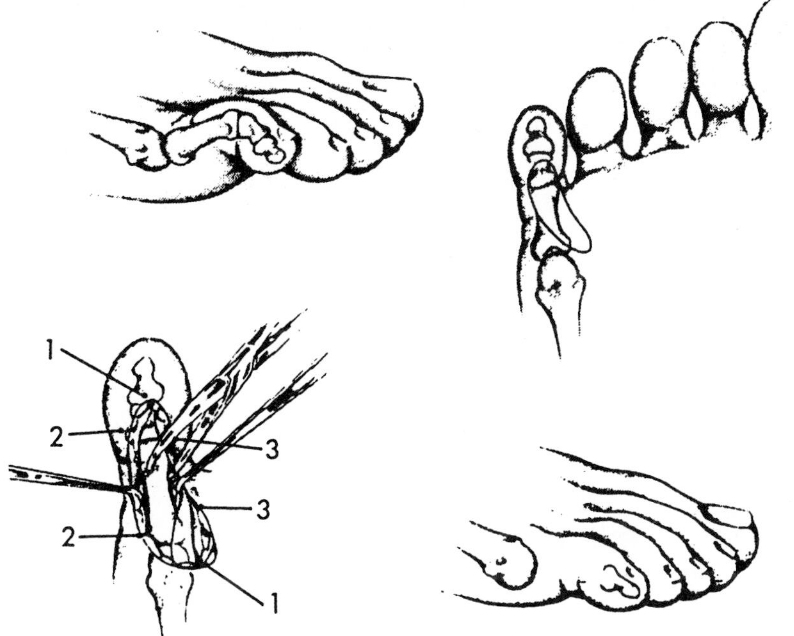

FIGURE 5-21 ■ Ruiz-Mora operation to correct congenital contracture of fifth toe *(A)*. *B*, Ellipse of skin is excised from plantar surface of toe and foot. *C*, Proximal phalanx of toe is excised. In closing skin, point 1 is sutured to point 1, 2 to 2, and 3 to 3. *D*, Appearance of toe after surgery. (From Beaty, J.H.: Congenital anomalies of lower extremity. In Crenshaw, A.H., ed.: Campbell's Operative Orthopaedics, 7th ed. St. Louis, C.V. Mosby, 1987, p. 2628.)

Surgical treatment of these **lesser-toe deformities** may require both soft-tissue and bony procedures (Table 5-6 and Figs. 5-21 and 5-22).

D. **Interdigital (Morton) Neuroma**

1. ***Anatomy and pathophysiology.*** Describing this condition as a "neuroma" is actually incorrect. The haphazard proliferation of axons seen in a traumatic neuroma is not present. The enlargement of the nerve is caused by deposition of collagenous and hyaline material. The pathologic process is probably degenerative rather than proliferative, with repetitive trauma to the nerve from the transverse intermetatarsal ligament (especially in shoes that cause MTP joint extension, which displaces the nerve distally), but this has not been definitively established. Repetitive microtrauma, perineural fibrosis, ischemia from vasonervorum constriction or occlusion, and endoneural edema probably are ultimately responsible for the symptoms of interdigital neuroma. Microscopic pathological findings are (1) perineural fibrosis (most often noted in pathology reports from surgical specimens), (2) thickened and hyalanized walls or arterioles, (3) demyelinization and degeneration of nerve fibers, (4) endoneural edema, (5) absence of inflammatory changes, and (6) frequent bursal tissue accompanying the specimen (Fig. 5-23). The common digital nerve to the third web space normally is slightly enlarged. The most medial branch of the lateral plantar nerve (LPN) merges with the most lateral branch of the medial plantar nerve (MPN) just proximal to the deep transverse intermetatarsal ligament. At that juncture the two nerve branches begin sharing a common perineurium. This anatomic peculiarity does not exist in the other web spaces. This may explain why interdigital neuroma (IDN) is more often diagnosed in the third web space. Although IDNs are found with equal frequency in the second and third web spaces in pathologic specimens from elderly patients, clinical symptoms of IDN occur in the third space in approximately 80% of patients.

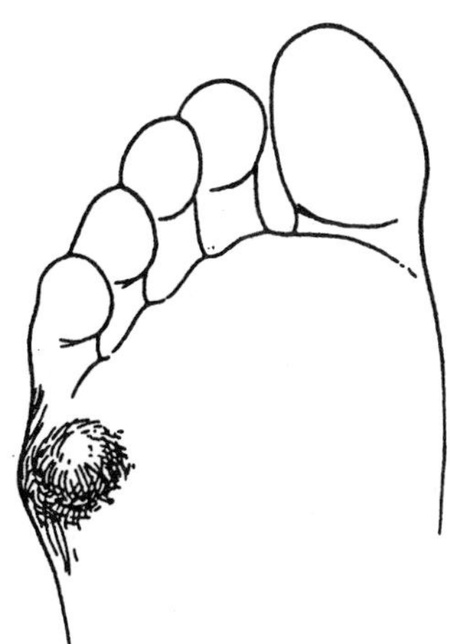

FIGURE 5-22 ■ Callus beneath fifth metatarsal head. If extension deformity is present at fifth metatarsophalangeal joint, painful callus may develop beneath fifth metatarsal head. (From Murphy, G.A.: Lesser toe abnormalities. In Canale, S.T., ed.: Campbell's Operative Orthopaedics, 10th ed. St. Louis, C.V. Mosby, 2003, p. 4074.)

2. **Physical Examination**

IDN is most frequent in females (eight or nine times more often than males), especially in

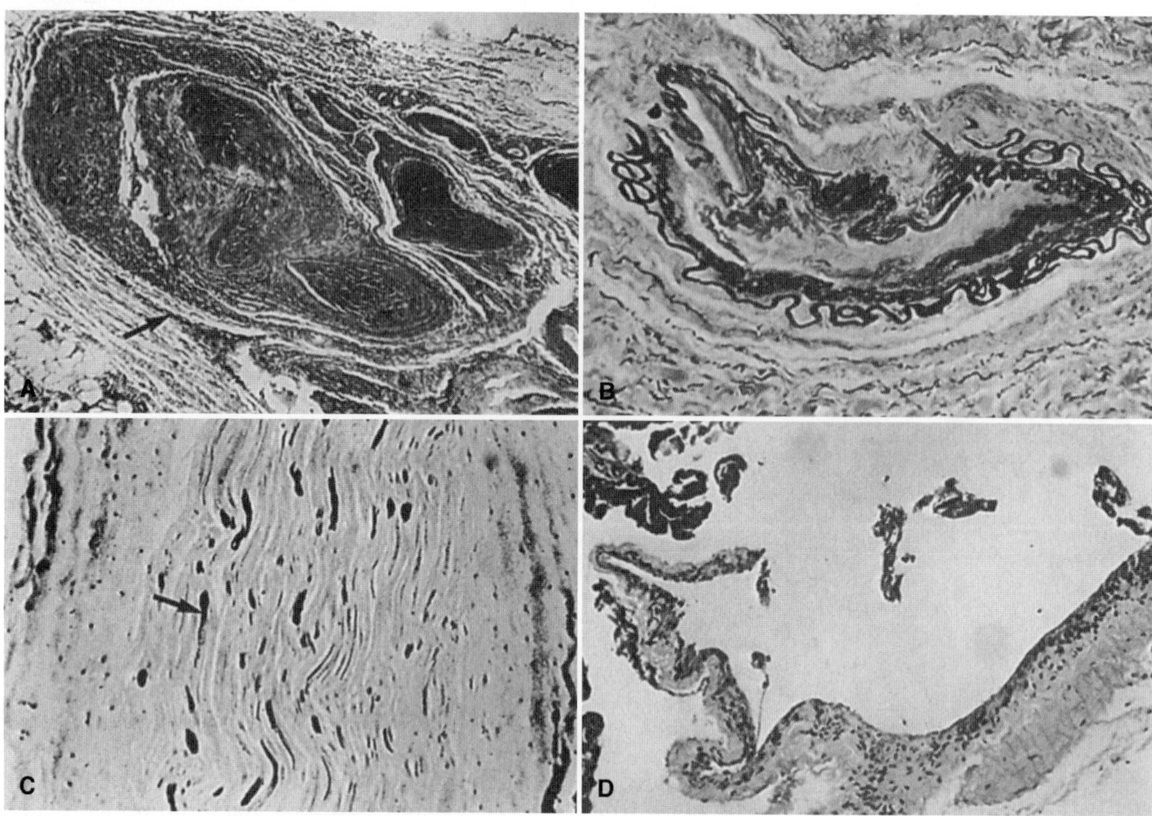

FIGURE 5-23 ■ Pathologic finding of interdigital neuroma. *A*, Interdigital nerve is greatly thickened by perineural fibrous tissue *(arrow)* (hematoxylin and eosin stain). *B*, Vessels in region often show degenerative changes such as fraying and duplication of internal elastic lamina *(arrow)* (Verhoeff–van Gieson stain). *C*, Some axons are missing and others show degenerative changes *(arrow)* (Bielschowsky stain). *D*, Small bursa may be found in the region (hematoxylin and eosin stain). (From Richardson, E.G.: Neurogenic disorders. In Canale, S.T., ed.: Campbell's Operative Orthopaedics, 10th ed. St. Louis, C.V. Mosby, 2003, p. 3921.)

those who wear shoes with a constricting toe box and elevated heels. Symptoms may be localized to paresthesia or dysesthesia in the two adjacent toes (usually third and fourth toes), but often are vague, diffuse discomfort in the forefoot, midfoot, and lower leg. In describing the pain, patients often will indicate the dorsal surface of the foot, even though the pathology is plantar. Pain often is relieved by removing the shoe and massaging the foot. Observing the patient massaging the area of the foot that gives relief sometimes is the only way symptoms can be localized. By far the most common physical finding is tenderness in the web space (usually the third); this tenderness in the web space may be increased by palpation while displacing the metatarsals toward one another by forefoot compression. Firmly palpating the distal intermetatarsal and web spaces with the patient standing is the best way to rule out IDN. Objective signs of decreased sensibility in a web space are uncommon, but do occur and should be evaluated because they help confirm the diagnosis.

3. **Treatment**

Nonoperative treatment includes a wide toe box shoe with a firm sole, a metatarsal pad (inside shoe) or bar (sole of shoe), and occasionally a steroid injection. If this fails to relieve symptoms, resection of the neuroma 2–3 cm proximal to the deep transverse intermetatarsal ligament through a dorsal incision is recommended. Displacing and burying the proximal neural stump within the intrinsic muscles also is recommended. Resection of a nerve that appears anatomically normal during surgery is controversial. Simply releasing the deep transverse intermetatarsal ligament is recommended by some, but even normal-appearing resected nerves return with the diagnosis of perineural fibrosis, endoneural edema, demyelinization of some of the nerve fibers, and occasionally arteriolar wall hyalinization. When a patient has been followed long enough and examined repeatedly, as well as failed nonoperative treatment, simply releasing the deep transverse metatarsal ligament may not be sufficient to relieve symptoms. Particularly troublesome is to re-explore the operated area only to find the deep transverse intermetatarsal ligament as thick as, if not thicker than, it was found initially. This controversy is not presently resolved. Surgical resection of IDN produces 80–85% good to excellent results.

4. ***Recurrent IDN*** is a glioma or bulbous enlargement of the neural stump (stump neuroma), most often due to inadequate proximal resection of the nerve. However, there are patients who have had adequate proximal resection only to continue with pain in the area of the neuroma stump even placed well into the arch and away from any weight-bearing area. In this clinical setting, careful palpation of the PTN and its branches distal to the flexor retinaculum is essential. These symptoms may represent an "irritable" PTN and no diagnosis beyond this can be found in spite of an extensive work-up. However, if the recurrent symptoms are very localized and reproducible and all nonoperative treatment has failed to relieve the patient's localized symptoms, then a traction neuritis resulting from neural stump adherence to adjacent bony and soft tissue can be assumed. This stump neuroma can be excised through another dorsal incision or through a plantar incision placed between the appropriate metatarsal heads (preoperatively the patient should palpate the metatarsal heads between which the incision will be placed to clarify that the initial firm fibrous reaction that slowly resolves is not the metatarsal head and is not due to the incision). A plantar incision allows access to a very proximal location in which to place the resected neuroma stump. However, the dorsal incision also allows adequate resection if it is extended into the proximal aspect of the intermetatarsal space and the metatarsals are spread well apart during the dissection. The success rate after excision of a recurrent or stump neuroma is 65–75%, compared with the 80–85% success rate after initial excision.

VI. Neurologic Disorders

A. Tarsal Tunnel Syndrome (TTS)

From the medial malleolus to the adjacent surface of the calcaneus, a dense, fibrous, unyielding structure, the flexor retinaculum (laciniate ligament), covers the contents of the tarsal tunnel. The tendons of the long toe flexors (FHL and flexor digitorum longus [FDL]) and the primary invertors of the ankle (the tibialis posterior tendon) accompany the posterior tibial neurovascular bundle. Fibrous septa from the deep surface of the retinaculum to the calcaneus create separate compartments for the tendons and neurovascular bundle. Any structure within this "tunnel" or any structure exterior and adjacent to this tunnel can cause TTS.

The symptoms of TTS may be vague and misleading, with pain reported either proximal to the flexor retinaculum or distally into one or more toes, the medial or lateral aspect of the foot, and occasionally even the dorsum of the foot. The symptoms can be exacerbated by activity, but not uncommonly the patient will state that pain is greatest at night or at rest or even with elevating or lowering the extremity. Any patient with symptoms of an IDN must be examined for PTN tenderness beneath the flexor retinaculum. If tenderness over the PTN is present, excision of the neuroma should be considered and the nerve should be evaluated clinically and electromyographically.

Physical examination should include palpation of the PTN within the tarsal tunnel and immediately proximal and distal to it; this often elicits tenderness. The contralateral limb should be compared with the symptomatic one for any abnormal contouring (edema, a mass, varicosities) and any differences in sweating patterns, skin dryness and scaling, especially along the distribution of the medial or lateral plantar nerve. Subtalar motion should be evaluated and a middle facet coalition suspected if TTS coexists with limitation of subtalar motion.

The **history often is the most useful diagnostic aid.** When positive history and physical examination findings are combined with positive electromyographic studies, the diagnosis of TTS should be evident in over 90% of patients. The **etiology** of TTS, however, is not obvious even after the diagnosis is reasonably certain. In most patients with signs and symptoms of TTS no definitive cause can be identified (idiopathic TTS). The most common causes of constriction of the PTN within or adjacent to the taesal tunnel are ganglia of tendon sheaths or from the subtalar joint, traumatic or inflammatory tenosynovitis, perineural fibrosis from severe hindfoot or ankle trauma with or without bony encroachment, and varicosities. Accessory muscles within the taesal tunnel (accessory FDL, soleus), middle facet tarsal coalition with reduced subtalar motion and fixed valgus position of the hindfoot, and tumors of the nerve sheath are additional objective causes of TTS.

1. ***Treatment.*** Patients with space-occupying lesions, previous hindfoot trauma, fixed hindfoot deformity (valgus), positive electromyographic findings (distal motor latencies of 7.0 msec or more, prolonged sensory latencies more than 2.3 msec, decreased amplitude of motor action potentials in the abductor hallucis or abductor digiti minimi muscles), and reproducible positive physical findings are the best candidates for surgery. However, **the diagnosis of TTS remains a clinical one**, and

treatment should be ultimately based on the history and physical examination. Repeated examinations before surgical release are helpful. An MRI may be helpful to rule out an accessory muscle or soft-tissue tumor.

Shoe modifications (medial sole, heel wedge, or both), immobilization in a walking cast, and possibly anti-inflammatory medications have been suggested, but these generally are ineffective and once the diagnosis is established, surgery is indicated. It is very important in the surgical technique to release not only the flexor retinaculum but also the deep investing fascia of the lower leg, which is contiguous with the proximal border of the retinaculum (3-4 cm proximally), and the superficial and deep fascia of the abductor hallucis where the PTN passes beneath this muscle. Because the PTN divides into the medial and lateral plantar nerves beneath the flexor retinaculum in over 90% of patients, both branches of this nerve must be traced beneath the abductor hallucis muscle-tendon unit and released from any constriction (Figs. 5-24 and 5-25).

2. ***Recurrence.*** The most common etiology of recurrence of TTS symptoms after surgery is an inadequate release. Because the additional fibrous reaction after repeat release often produces symptoms as severe as or more severe than those before surgery, **repeat tarsal tunnel release generally is not recommended unless a space-occupying lesion recurs or develops** after an adequate release of the flexor retinaculum and adjacent fibrous structures.

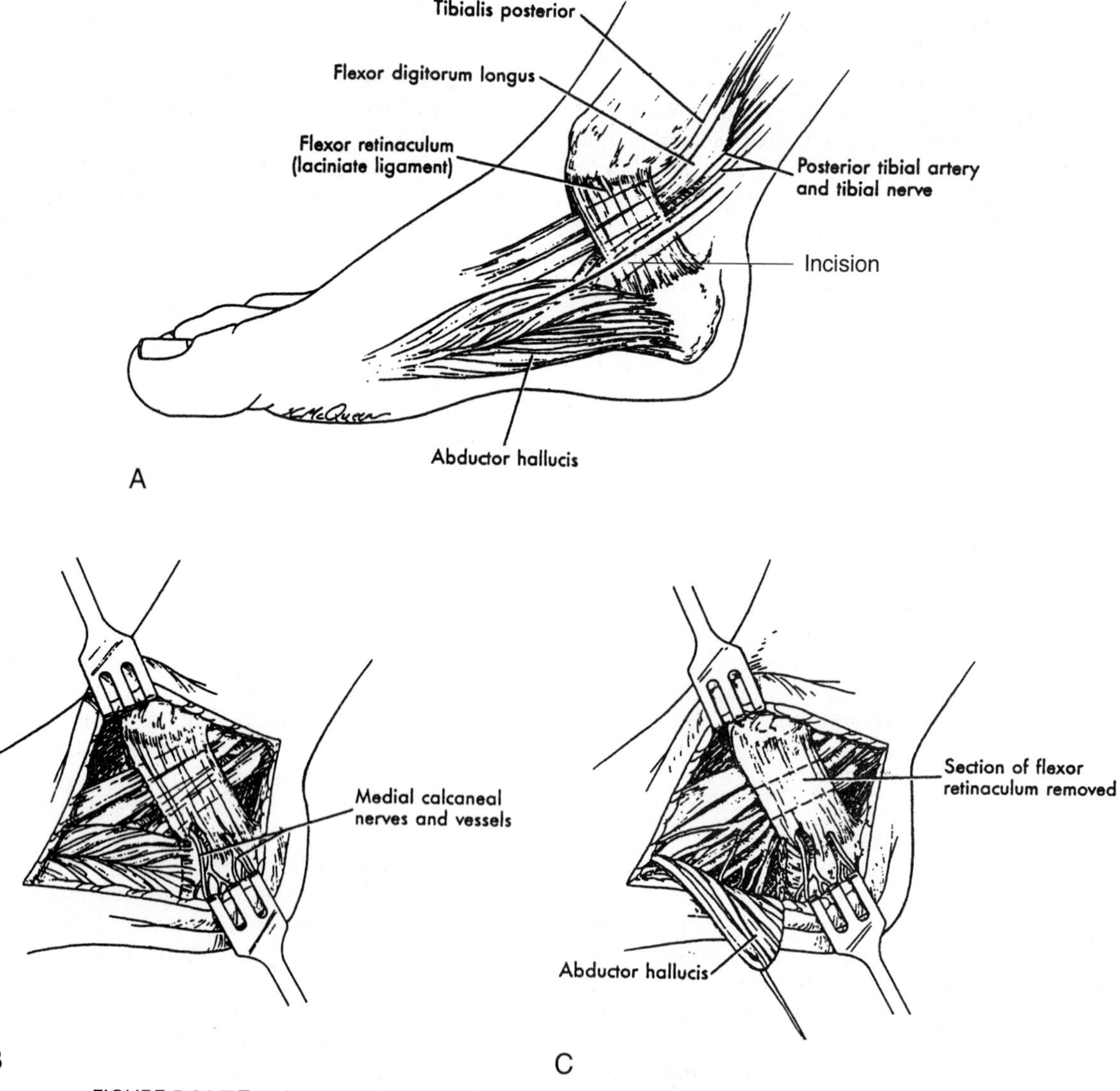

FIGURE 5-24 ■ Tarsal tunnel release. *A,* Skin incision. *B,* Note branches of medial calcaneal nerve and artery penetrating the retinaculum. Broken line indicates incision for reflecting abductor hallucis muscle. *C,* Abductor hallucis is reflected plantarward, and section of flexor retinaculum to be removed is outlined. (From Richardson, E.G.: Neurogenic disorders. In Canale, S.T., ed.: Campbell's Operative Orthopaedics, 10th ed. St. Louis, C.V. Mosby, 2003, p. 4132.)

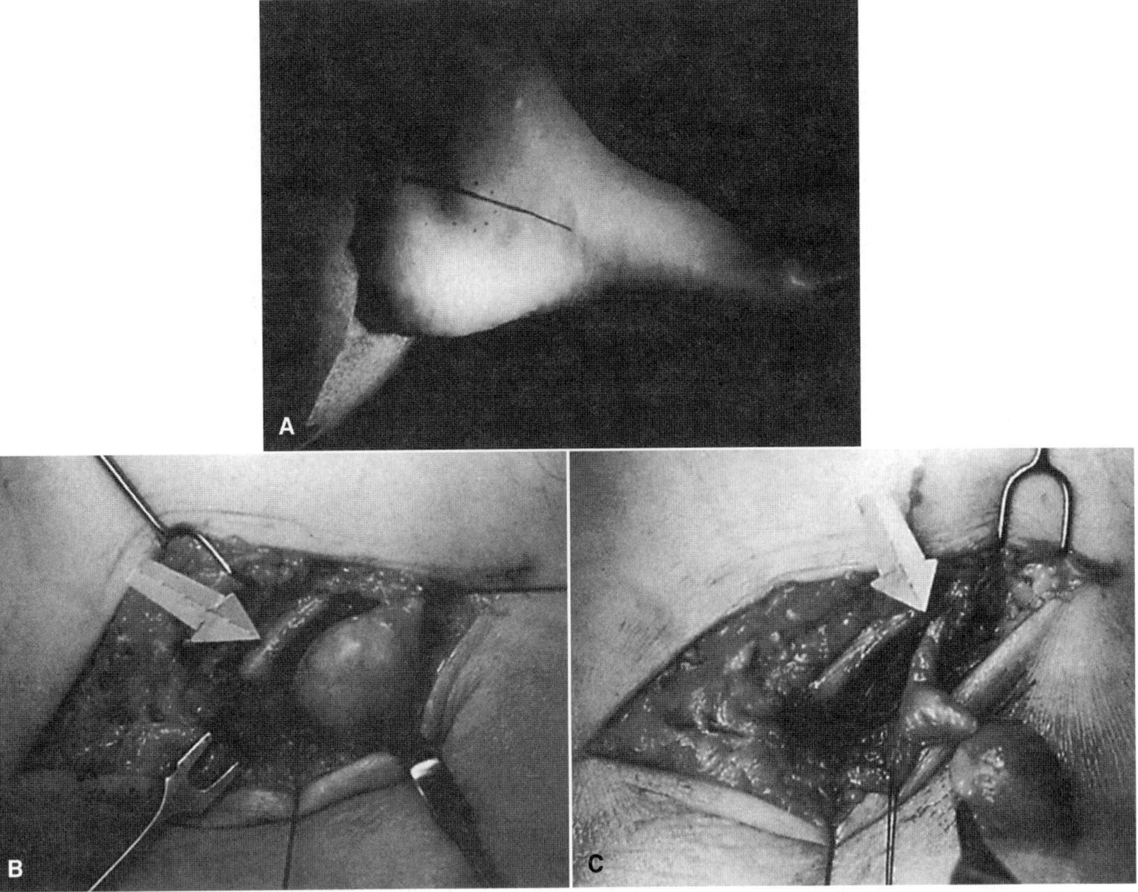

FIGURE 5-25 ■ *A*, Incision for release of tarsal tunnel. Note fullness outlined by dots. *B* and *C*, *Arrow* points to lateral plantar nerve. Tumor involves medial calcaneal branch of nerve. Tumor was resected leaving most of this branch intact. (From Richardson, E.G.: Neurogenic disorders. In Canale, S.T., ed.: Campbell's Operative Orthopaedics, 10th ed. St. Louis, C.V. Mosby, 2003, p. 4133.)

B. Anterior Tarsal Tunnel Syndrome (DPN Entrapment)

Impingement of the DPN by the distal margin of the inferior extensor retinaculum (IER) is most often diagnosed in patients with dorsal osteophytes over the apex of the medial longitudinal arch. The osteophyte and often a ganglion cyst from degenerative and attritional capsuloligamentous injury trap the nerve between the retinaculum (serving as a pulley for the external tendons) and the osteophyte and/or ganglion. Additional sources of entrapment are tightly laced shoes (especially jogging shoes and ski boots) and anterior osteophytes off the navicular, talus, or tibia more proximal and beneath the "superior roof" of the IER. Athletes who have experienced multiple ankle sprains with traumatic osteophyte formation are more likely to have proximal entrapment, and patients with degenerative arthritic changes are likely to have more distal entrapment by the IER (Fig. 5-26).

1. ***Examination.*** The most common symptoms are dysesthesias and paresthesias on the dorsum of the foot radiating into the first web space because of DPN irritation. A positive Tinel's sign and decreased sensation in the first web space may be present; however, just as frequently the symptoms are vague dorsal foot pain or even distal anterior leg pain, with or without relation to activity. Consequently, palpation (rolling the nerve) and percussion should be done, and both feet should be inspected and compared to identify any differences in dorsal midfoot prominence (convexity). DPN impingement on the dorsum of the midfoot probably is more common than appreciated.
2. ***Treatment.*** A well-padded tongue of a shoe that is loosely laced may be all that is required. If this is not successful, a full-length rocker-sole steel shank approximately $\frac{1}{16}$-inch wide often relieves symptoms, especially in patients with midfoot degenerative arthritic

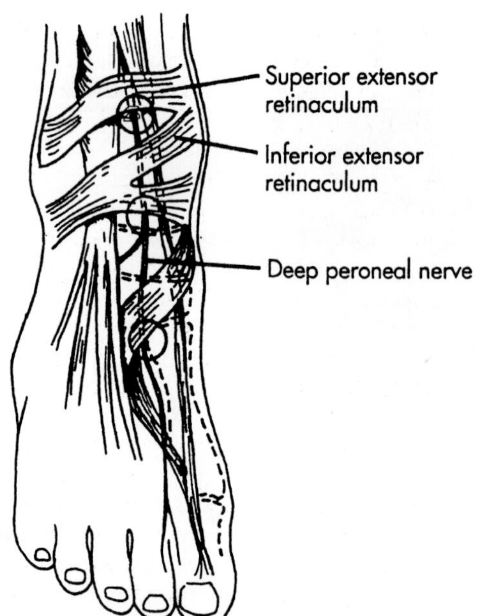

FIGURE 5-26 ■ Deep peroneal nerve entrapment. Circles denote areas of impingement. (From Mann, R.A.: Diseases of the nerves. In Coughlin, M.J., Mann, R.A., eds.: Surgery of the Foot and Ankle, 7th ed. St. Louis, C.V. Mosby, 1999, p. 521.)

osteophytes or cysts. If surgery is required, the patient must know the recuperation is prolonged and paresthesias and even dysesthesias may persist for weeks or months. It is imperative that no vasomotor (reflex sympathetic dystrophy) symptoms or signs are present preoperatively because they will be exacerbated by surgery. Surgical technique should include locating the DPN distally, just lateral to the extensor hallucis brevis (EHB) tendon, and tracing it proximally, while releasing all fascial and retinacular restraints about the nerve. Also included are removal of any osteophytes or ganglion cysts and any dorsal capsuloligamentous tissue that may have contributed to the ganglion. Enough bone should be removed dorsally to reduce the area of entrapment to a slight concavity instead of a convexity. Meticulous hemostasis and immobilization in a short-leg boot or cast are recommended.

C. Upper Motor Neuron Injury

In a patient with a cerebrovascular accident (CVA), an equinovarus deformity of the ankle and foot frequently develops. Early splinting and therapy are indicated. If the deformity is such that a locked ankle-foot orthosis (AFO) cannot be fitted, an Achilles tendon lengthening is indicated. Surgery should not be done until at least 6 months after injury, and in patients with head injuries and severe spasticity, 12–18 months should be allowed for maximal recovery before tenotomies, tendon lengthenings, or fascial releases are done.

If a tendo Achilles lengthening (TAL) does not allow satisfactory bracing of an equinovarus deformity, a split anterior tibial tendon transfer to the lateral aspect of the midfoot is indicated. The posterior tibial tendon, although the strongest inverter of the hindfoot, rarely is over-reactive in the stance phase of gait; if this occurs, however, it should be transferred through the interosseous membrane and attached to the midfoot. Transfer of the posterior tibial tendon and split anterior tibial transfer (SPLATT) should not be done simultaneously. The muscle-tendon units that can contribute to an equinovarus deformity are the gastrocsoleus, posterior tibial, FDL, and FHL. Although the anterior tibial tendon is an ankle dorsiflexor, as well as an inverter, if the ankle is forced into equinus by spasticity or contracture following an upper motor neuron injury, it can be a major contributor to the varus component of the equinovarus deformity.

D. Charcot-Marie-Tooth Disease (Peroneal Muscular Atrophy, Hereditary Motor Sensory Neuropathy)

Charcot-Marie-Tooth (CMT) disease is the most common inherited neuropathy, affecting approximately 1 in every 2500 people. There are many genetic variants of CMT disease and more are described as diagnostic tools become more sophisticated. In the autosomal dominant form of CMT disease there is a duplication of chromosome 17. An abnormal myelin protein is the basis of CMT degenerative neuropathy. Males are more commonly affected, but the disease usually is more severe in females. The earlier the onset, the more severe the neurologic findings, and the autosomal recessive presents earliest, usually at less than 10 years of age. Sex-linked recessive inheritance usually presents in the second decade, and the autosomal dominant in the third decade. Sensory deficit is variable and may manifest as proprioceptive loss more than pure sensory deficit. However, when sensory loss is severe, recurrent ulceration, deep infection, and even neuropathic arthropathy can mimic diabetic neurologic loss.

1. ***Examination.*** Patients complain of deformity and awkward gait more often than pain. These complaints are manifestations of the common findings on physical examination. The physical examination reveals a symmetrical elevation of the arches, a plantar flexed first ray, hindfoot varus, claw toes, decreased ankle jerks, and a flatfoot or toe-heel gait (marionette gait). In addition, the extensor digitorum brevis and EHB are atrophied. The patient's thighs appear normal size, but the lower legs appear smaller than normal. Prominent and tender callosities may be present beneath the metatarsal heads because of the cavus deformity associated with claw toes and distal migration of the forefoot pad.

The toe extensors are recruited in the swing phase of gait as ankle dorsiflexors because of a weak tibialis anterior. Ankle eversion is weak due to peroneus brevis atrophy, but the peroneus longus function remains strong. It is this imbalance from a weakened tibial is anterior compared with the peroneus longus that contributes to the plantar flexed first metatarsal. With the first metatarsal plantar flexed and the forefoot pronated (valgus), the hindfoot supinates, compensatory hindfoot varus develops, and the distal tibia and fibula externally rotate. Once the spectrum of linked deformities develops, it is a matter of time until they become fixed. It is this differentiation between fixed (cannot be passively corrected) and flexible (passively correctable) deformities that has such profound effect on the treatment plan. The Coleman block test (Fig. 5-27) can be used to determine if a hindfoot varus deformity is fixed or flexible.

2. ***Treatment***. In an adolescent with closed physes and a supple deformity, surgical rather than brace management currently is recommended because of the progressive pattern of this disease. Once fixed deformity develops, surgical correction may require arthrodesis rather than osteotomy. If brace management is chosen, a locked-ankle short-leg (AFO) with an outside (varus correcting or lateral) T-strap is recommended. A rocker sole also aids the gait and decreases energy expended.

   Surgical treatment involves (1) release of the plantar fascia, (2) closing-wedge dorsiflexion osteotomy of the first metatarsal (occasionally including the second metatarsal in older patients), (3) calcaneal sliding and closing-wedge osteotomy, (4) transfer of the peroneus longus into the peroneus brevis at the level of the distal fibula, and (5) frequently a TAL. Fixed deformities usually require a triple arthrodesis for hindfoot correction with transfer of the posterior tibial tendon through the interosseous membrane and a TAL. A plantar fascia release, dorsiflexion osteotomy of the first or second metatarsal or both, and correction of the claw toe deformities might also be required. If this many procedures are required to correct multiple fixed deformities, they should be staged. The clawed hallux can be surgically treated with a Jones procedure (arthrodesis of the interphalangeal joint and transfer of the extensor hallucis longus to the first metatarsal). Clawing of the lesser toes is improved by flexor-to-extensor transfers and extensor tendon lengthening or tenotomy if flexible or capsulotomies of the MTP joints, extensor tendon lengthenings, and resection of the head and neck of the proximal phalanges if fixed. The younger the patient the more important it is to try soft-tissue releases, tendon transfers, and osteotomies to avoid degenerative arthritic changes in joints adjacent to those that have been arthrodesed. Even in *mild* fixed deformities, every effort should be made to preserve cartilage unless the deformities cannot be corrected without arthrodesis.

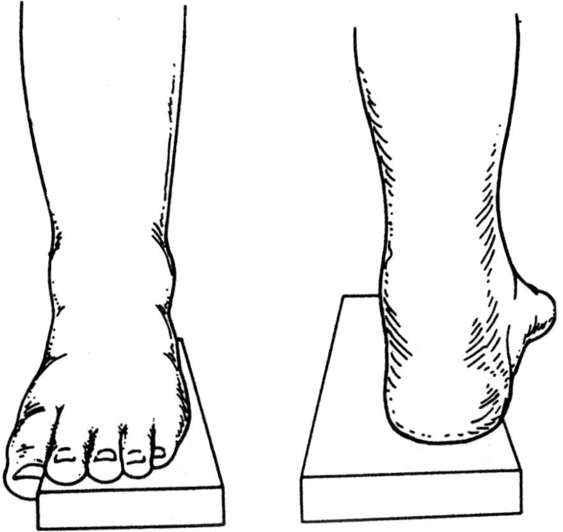

FIGURE 5-27 ■ Lateral block test. Plantar-flexed first metatarsal is allowed to hang free from block; supple hind part of foot then corrects. (From Paulos, L., Coleman, S.S., Samuelson, K.M.: Pes cavovarus: review of a surgical approach using selective soft-tissue procedures. J. Bone Joint Surg. 62-A:942, 1980.)

E. Post-Polio Syndrome

This is a most distressing problem to patients who usually had their attack of polio four or five decades earlier. They have managed by overuse of remaining muscles to function reasonably well, and at times the examiner is amazed that the patients have functioned at the level they have. To tell them that the brace they wore decades ago may need modification and reinstitution is emotionally trying or even devastating. The most likely etiology of symptoms is simply aging plus overuse of compensatory muscles. Reactivation of the virus has been suggested, but no sound evidence supports a viral etiology. The treatment is almost always nonoperative, with activity modification and appropriate orthotic management. Occasionally, selected arthrodeses are needed for stability and to correct fixed deformity to make the foot braceable.

VII. Inflammatory Arthritis

A. Rheumatoid Arthritis (RA)

In approximately 17% of patients with RA, the first symptoms of their disease are in their feet. Usually the inflammatory process involves both feet, although the resulting deformities may not be symmetrical depending on the weight-bearing pattern of the patient, as well as the extent of synovitis in particular joints. Eventually 85–90% of patients with long-standing RA have at least minor forefoot involvement. The inciting pathologic event is **synovitis** followed by release of proteineases and collagenases, which impair periarticular capsuloligamentous integrity, as well as destroy hyaline cartilage. The MTP joints are most often involved initially. With continued synovitis, instability develops and weight-bearing forces subluxate the base of the proximal phalanges dorsally on the metatarsal heads. The intrinsic-extrinsic muscle-tendon balance is lost, and claw toe deformity develops. With the plantar forefoot pad displaced distally by the hyperextended toes, large bursae develop beneath the metatarsal heads. Pain beneath the metatarsal head with weight bearing and pain over the dorsum of the PIP joints from the chronic flexion posture, which causes impingement of the toes in the toe box of the shoe, are usually what prompts the patient to seek medical attention. Hallux valgus usually is present, but most often is not the major complaint of the patient concerning the forefoot (Fig. 5-28).

The midfoot is not commonly involved with RA, but, if it is, the talonavicular and naviculocuneiform articulations are the most often affected. This results in collapse of the medial longitudinal arch and pronation or valgus, or both, of the forefoot on the midfoot and hindfoot.

The hindfoot most often develops a valgus deformity due to disruption of the talocalcaneal interosseous ligament. This ligament has a synovial covering and the rheumatoid synovitic process weakens this important stabilizer of the subtalar joint. Weight bearing forces the calcaneus into valgus and the subtalar joint, followed by the midtarsal joint, subluxates, resulting in the typical deformities of hindfoot valgus, midfoot-forefoot abduction, and collapse of the medial longitudinal arch (Fig. 5-29). Chronic hindfoot valgus results in shortening of the Achilles tendon.

The role that an insufficient posterior tibial tendon plays in the development of these deformities is uncertain, but it too may become involved in the rheumatoid inflammatory process and, because of lengthening, loss of excursion, or rupture, no longer can contribute to the integrity of the medial longitudinal arch. It should always be examined, as should the ankle joints. A weight-bearing AP radiograph of both ankles, preferably on the same cassette for detection of subtle differences, should be obtained to be certain that valgus instability of the ankle joint has not contributed to the hindfoot valgus. Finally, if there are angular deformities at the hip or knee, it is best that they be corrected before realignment of the hindfoot and ankle (Fig. 5-30).

Treatment. Extra-depth shoes with deep toe boxes and padded heel counters, as well as soft but supportive insoles, are used for forefoot and midfoot involvement. If hindfoot deformity is marked, a locked or limited-motion AFO with a valgus correcting T-strap is added. This may be all the patient needs.

Surgical treatment is most often directed to the forefoot deformities. If the interphalangeal joint of the hallux is not unstable, the most useful procedure for the hallux is an arthrodesis of the MTP joint in 15 degrees valgus in the frontal plane, 10 degrees extension in the sagittal plane

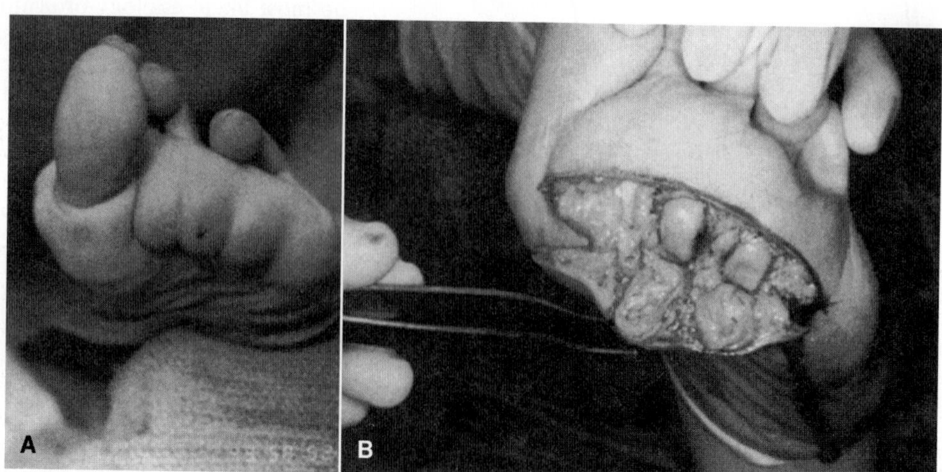

FIGURE 5-28 ■ Rheumatoid arthritis of forefoot. *A*, Intraoperative photograph. *B*, Note large metatarsal head bursae on skin flap and dislocated metatarsal heads. (From Richardson, E.G.: Rheumatoid foot. In Canale, S.T., ed.: Campbell's Operative Orthopaedics, 10th ed. St. Louis, C.V. Mosby, 2003, p. 4096.)

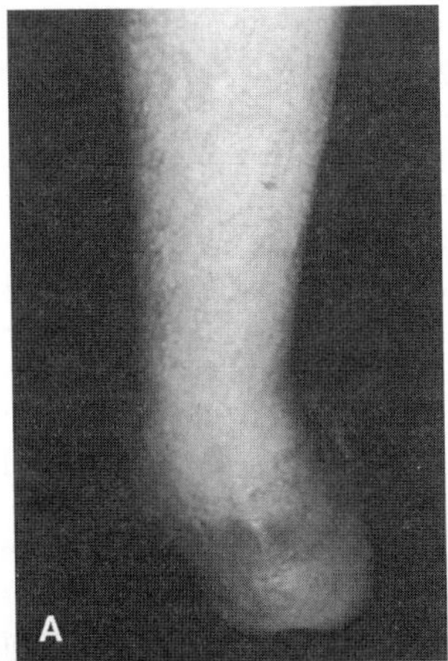

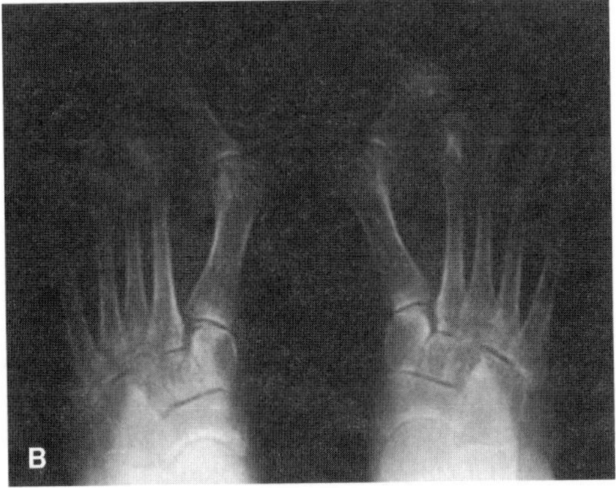

FIGURE 5-29 ■ *A*, Heel valgus and foot pronation secondary to rheumatoid arthritis. With time the forefoot deformity may become fixed. If subtalar and midtarsal joints are reduced surgically, forefoot is actually in pronounced supination relative to hindfoot. This may make it difficult to plantar flex the first ray enough to produce a plantigrade foot during weight bearing. *B*, Note multiple dislocations of MTP joints. (From Richardson, E.G.: Rheumatoid foot. In Canale, S.T., ed.: Campbell's Operative Orthopaedics, 10th ed. St. Louis, C.V. Mosby, 2003, p. 4090.)

(to the sole of the foot or 20 degrees to the first metatarsal), and neutral rotation in the axial plane. For the lesser toes, resection of the metatarsal heads at the neck-shaft level and correction of the PIP joint deformity by resection of the head and neck of each proximal phalanx are most often recommended. Forefoot surgery in a patient with RA and long-standing, severe symptoms and deformity can be one of the most rewarding procedures in orthopaedics. If the interphalangeal joint of the hallux is unstable, arthrodesis of this joint and resection of the base of the proximal phalanx is recommended, although recurrent hallux valgus is the rule rather than the exception. The most common midfoot procedure is an arthrodesis of the talonavicular joint, which can improve the collapsed arch. When the talonavicular arthrodesis is combined with a calcaneo-cuboid arthrodesis, the patient may gain a stable, painless midfoot. A percutaneous TAL adds to the success of this procedure.

For fixed hindfoot deformities (usually valgus), a triple arthrodesis is necessary, along with a TAL. The most difficult problem is the combination of ankle, hindfoot, and midfoot joint destruction and deformity. Total ankle arthroplasty and limited peritalar staged arthrodeses currently are recommended, although data from longer than a 5–10 year follow-up is not available from multiple centers with similar patient cohorts. If the midfoot is relatively spared both clinically and radiographically and both the ankle and subtalar joints are symptomatic, arthrodesis of the ankle and subtalar joints is an acceptable salvage procedure that may markedly relieve the patient's symptoms and improve function.

B. **Crystalline-Induced Arthropathies (Gout or Pseudogout).** Gout and pseudogout are crystalline deposition diseases. Gout may be induced

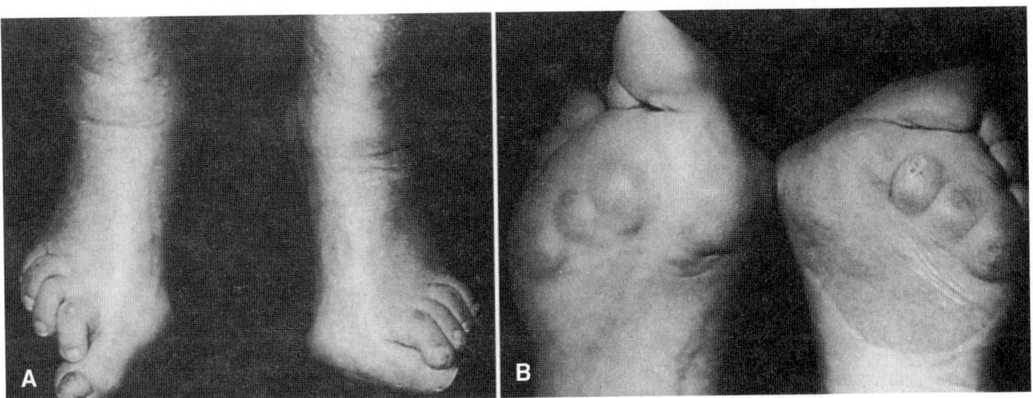

FIGURE 5-30 ■ *A* and *B*, Multiple deformities of rheumatoid arthritis. (From Richardson, E.G.: Rheumatoid foot. In Canale, S.T., ed.: Campbell's Operative Orthopaedics, 10th ed. St. Louis, C.V. Mosby, 2003, p. 4088.)

by certain medications that increase serum uric acid, localized trauma, alcohol, or purine-rich foods, as well as by the postsurgical state. Gout is a disease of abnormal purine metabolism resulting in precipitation and deposition of monosodium urate crystals into synovial-lined joints. The deposition of these needle-shaped crystals into the joint fluid induces a severe inflammatory response. The attack is sudden and very painful, with intense signs of inflammation (redness, swelling, warmth, tenderness). The great toe MTP joint is most often involved (50–75% of initial attacks), and over a chronic course, 90% of patients with gouty attacks will have one or more episodes involving the hallux MTP joint (podagra). Men are more commonly afflicted than women, and characteristic radiographic signs are inordinate soft-tissue enlargement about the MTP joint and bony erosions at a distance from the joint articular surface, as well as erosions on both sides of the joint. However, in the chronic condition, after a number of attacks and large deposits of gouty residue (tophi), extensive articular and periarticular destruction can occur.

The diagnosis of gouty arthropathy usually is a clinical one, with a characteristic history ("Not even a sheet could touch it.") and physical findings. However, pathognomonic signs are needle-shaped monosodium urate crystals, which under polarized light are strongly negatively birefringent. The serum uric acid may or may not be elevated. Treatment of an acute attack usually is with indomethicin or colchicine. If chronic gouty attacks have destroyed the joint or deposited large quantities of tophi, an arthrodesis or removal of quantities of tophaceous debris, or both, may be required.

Pseudogout (chondrocalcinosis) commonly affects the knee, but may present in an articulation of the foot or ankle. It, too, may have a severe initial inflammatory response due to deposition of calcium pyrophosphate dihydrate (CPPD) crystals in or about a joint. Pseudogout usually is articular with less periarticular soft-tissue involvement than gout, although inflammatory signs may be striking. The diagnosis is confirmed by joint aspiration, which reveals weakly positive birefringent crystals under polarized light microscopy. These crystals may have varied shapes. The lesser MTP joints can be affected, as well as the talonavicular and subtalar joints. The joints usually are not involved in gout. On radiographs, intra-articular calcifications often are seen, which are **not** characteristic of gout. With recurrent attacks over a long period, joint destruction can occur, but this is rare. Treatment is with rest, oral NSAIDs for the acute chemical synovitis and protected weight bearing.

C. Seronegative Spondyloarthropathies (SNSA)

These inflammatory arthritides are distinguished from RA clinically by a higher incidence of involvement of entheses (i.e., the interface between collagen and bone where ligament, tendon, and capsular tissues insert into bone). A predilection for involvement of this transitional tissue is found in psoriatic arthritis, ankylosing spondylitis, and Reiter syndrome. These arthritides also may destroy articular cartilage but characteristically are more destructive toward collagen and fibrocartilage. Osteopenia is rare in these entities, and in contrast to RA, they often present in the foot as plantar fasciitis or Achilles tendinitis. Although inflammatory arthritis associated with inflammatory bowel disease may present as arthralgia or arthritis, it too can present as an enthesopathy. Certainly, any young adult male with unilateral or bilateral plantar fasciitis or Achilles tendinitis, particularly with calcaneal exostoses (bone spurs), should be examined and appropriate serologic studies done to rule out Reiter syndrome, ankylosing spondylitis, psoriatic arthropathy, or enthesopathy associated with inflammatory bowel disease.

1. Psoriatic Arthropathy

A patient with **psoriatic arthropathy** may have "dactylitis" of a lesser toe. This inflammatory process involves bone, periosteum, capsuloligamentous tissue, and tendons. The descriptive term for erythema and cylindrical enlargement of a single digit of the foot in a patient with psoriasis is "sausage toe." Among patients with psoriasis, approximately 10–20% will develop arthritis and 1–2% will have severe foot involvement. The earlier the onset of the psoriasis, the more likely arthritis or dactylitis will develop.

The peak age for patients seeking treatment for arthritides and/or enthesitis is between 20 and 40 years of age, and gender distribution is almost equal. Arthritis mutilans (severe destruction of synovial joints) is rare, frequently beginning in the DIP joints of digits of the hand and feet and producing a "pencil-in-cup" radiographic appearance. Nail pitting is common. Even with the absence of skin lesions (in 10–20% of patients with psoriatic arthritis, the arthritis precedes the skin lesions), a patient with dactylitis and nail pitting should be followed for the possible development of psoriasis. The oral agents used for treatment are NSAIDs for mild symptoms, methotrexate for severe psoriasis and arthritis, and sulfasalazine for patients with spondylitis. The strongest radiographic sign of psoriatic arthritis is erosive arthritis of the DIP joint(s) with osteolysis and shortening of the digits. Surgery of the feet rarely is required in patients with psoriatic arthritis, but the indications and procedures are similar to those for RA.

2. Reiter Syndrome

Patients with **Reiter syndrome** (reactive arthritis) usually have a gastrointestinal or urologic infection associated with or preceding the onset of arthritis. HLA-B27 antigen is strongly associated with Reiter syndrome (approximately 95%). The triad of uveitis, arthritis, and urethritis is infrequent, but Achilles tendinitis, retrocalcaneal bursitis, plantar fasciitis, and dactylitis frequently are present in patients with Reiter syndrome. Fluoroquinolone antibiotics such as ciprofloxacin hydrochloride (Cipro) and ofloxacin (Floxin) often are used to treat the inciting bacterial agent (*Chlamydia trachomatis* in urogenital infection). However, this group of antibiotics can exacerbate the Achilles tendinitis or plantar fasciitis and should be discontinued if the patient has either of these conditions, unless no other treatment is available. Orthopaedic surgery rarely is required.

D. **Ankylosing spondylitis** rarely initially presents in the foot; however, if it does, most commonly it is as plantar fasciitis or Achilles insertional tendinitis. The heel pain may be severe and so resistant to treatment that local radiotherapy is used. Particularly suggestive of ankylosing spondylitis are bony erosions at the plantar fascial origin in a young adult male with back pain and stiffness. HLA-B27 antigen is present in over 90% of these patients and males are affected five times more commonly than females. Surgery in the foot rarely is needed, but consists of plantar fascia release or débridement of part of the insertion of the Achilles tendon with removal of any impinging bone from the calcaneal tuberosity.

E. **Arthritis associated with Lyme disease** is the most common vector-borne illness in the United States, with three endemic areas: the Northeast, Midwest (particularly Wisconsin and Minnesota), and far West (particularly the Northwest). The *Ioxodes* tick genus transmits the disease. The most common hosts are deer, and the most common reservoirs are field mice and wood rats. The infectious organism transmitted by the tick is a spirochete *B. burgdoferi*, which is identified serologically by a specific immunoglobulin G (IgG) response. The serologic response does not occur for 6–8 months after inoculation and may not peak for many months.

The pathognomonic presentation of Lyme disease is erythema migrans, which is a round, red patch at the site of a tick bite that gradually enlarges and becomes clear in the center. It is quite large, often more than 5 cm in diameter. Two thirds of patients with Lyme disease experience erythema migrans. Symptoms may be vague and nonspecific, with flu-like complaints, including arthralgias. If the arthralgias continue for a prolonged period, an orthopaedist often is consulted. In the foot and ankle (the knee is the most commonly involved joint), the most common signs are a deep, diffuse aching and a clinical picture of an inflammatory tendonitis. Factors that should alert the orthopaedist to the possibility of Lyme disease are the chronicity and nonspecificity of the disease in an endemic area or in a patient who has recently (even months before examination) been in the woods of an endemic area.

Radiographs usually are normal, and physical examination may find little abnormality. Treatment is with a penicillin-derivative antibiotic, usually amoxicillin, or a tetracycline derivative (doxycycline) if the patient has an allergy to penicillin. Antibiotic treatment usually is curative, but articular destruction may occur in a small percentage of patients with Lyme disease.

VIII. Osteoarthritis

Osteoarthritis, or degenerative joint disease (DJD), more commonly involves the knees and hips rather than the ankle. The exact reason is unknown; however, osteoarthritis or degenerative arthritis commonly involves the naviculocuneiform, intercuneiform, and metatarsocuneiform joints as well as the first MTP joint. Isolated osteoarthritic destruction of the talonavicular joint certainly occurs, as does isolated involvement of the subtalar joint, but much less commonly than the midfoot joints distal to the midtarsal joints. Presumably the limited motion (2–4 degrees) in the naviculocuneiform, intercuneiform, and metatarsocuneiform joints and the large repetitive forces absorbed in these joints account for the frequency of their involvement in osteoarthritis. The arthritic process can place additional strains on capsular, ligamentous, and tendinous supports and restraints with resultant collapse deformity resembling posterior tibial insufficiency or post-traumatic Lisfranc injury (Fig. 5-31).

Initial treatment should be orthotic support, including bracing if the patient agrees. If this fails, limited arthrodeses, preferably with bone graft and always with internal fixation, is indicated. The medial (first ray) or central (second and third rays) column, or both, are most often involved and can be successfully treated with surgery. The mobile lateral column (fourth and fifth metatarsals and cuboid joints) should **not** be arthrodesed. Partial resection arthroplasty, with or without a collagen (tendon) spacer, in these lateral joints is reasonable.

Degenerative arthritis of the first MTP joint often results in ***hallux rigidus,*** in which motion of the joint is limited to varying degrees. A number of causative factors have been suggested, including trauma, repeated microtrauma, osteochondral fractures (particularly in adolescent and young adult athletes), hyperextension of the first metatarsal, an abnormally long first metatarsal, and severe foot pronation; however, in adults, hallux rigidus is most often caused by degenerative arthritis. Patients complain of tenderness over the dorsum

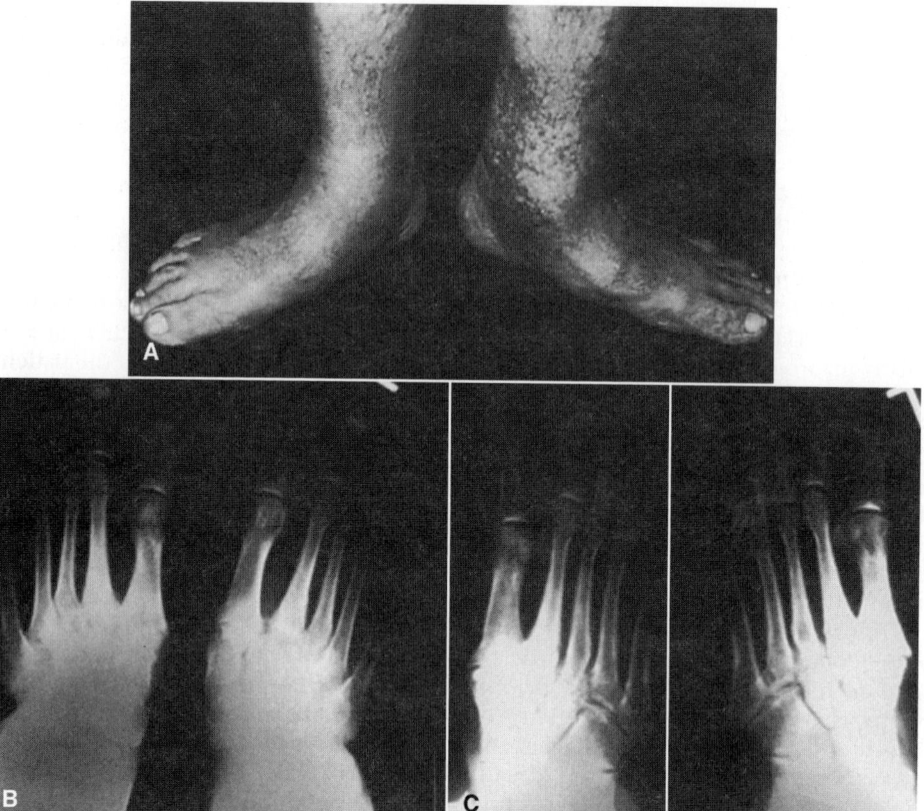

FIGURE 5-31 ■ *A*, Arch collapse caused by degenerative arthritis at Lisfranc articulations. *B* and *C*, AP and oblique radiographs of another patient with similar clinical findings demonstrating degenerative arthritic changes at Lisfranc joints and resultant collapse deformity at these articulations. This probably represents erosive osteoarthritis with secondary enthesopathy and weakening of plantar metatarsal cuneiform, metatarsal cuboid, and intermetatarsal basilar ligaments. (From Murphy, G.A.: Disorders of tendons and fascia In Canale, S.T., ed.: Campbell's Operative Orthopaedics, 10th ed. St. Louis, C.V. Mosby, 2003, p. 4196.)

of the first MTP joint and limited dorsiflexion. The earliest radiographic sign may be a small depression in the dome of the metatarsal head (Fig. 5-32). When the hallux is extended, abutment of the proximal phalanx against this lesion in the articular cartilage produces pain and instinctive flexion of the joint, thereby limiting extension. As the disease worsens, an osteophyte at the dorsal articular margin of the metatarsal head presents a mechanical block to extension. The severity of hallux rigidus is determined by radiographic appearance: grade I, mild to moderate osteophyte formation with joint space preservation; grade II, moderate osteophyte formation with joint space narrowing and subchondral sclerosis; and grade III, marked osteophyte formation and diminished joint space, including the inferior portion. Most patients with grade I and II changes can be treated with cheilectomy (removal of the proliferative bone from around the metatarsal head), which removes the buttress preventing dorsiflexion of the proximal phalanx on the metatarsal head (Fig. 5-33); some authors have reported that adding an extension osteotomy of the proximal phalanx improves patient satisfaction. Patients with grade III changes usually require arthrodesis or Keller resection arthroplasty.

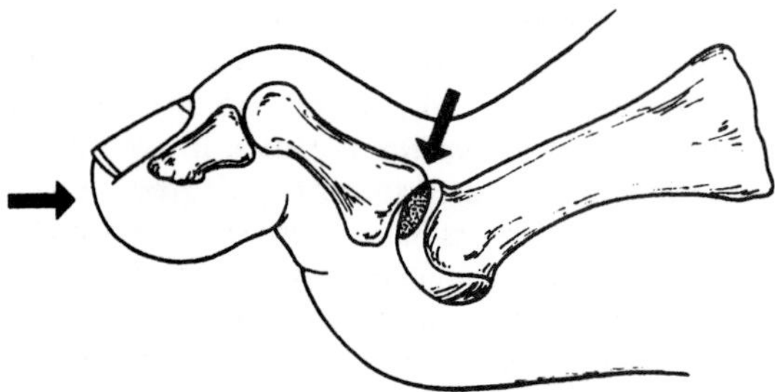

FIGURE 5-32 ■ Location of chondral or osteochondral lesion produced by forceful extension and impaction of metatarsal head. (From McMaster, M.J.: The pathogenesis of hallux rigidus. J. Bone Joint Surg. 60-B:82, 1978.)

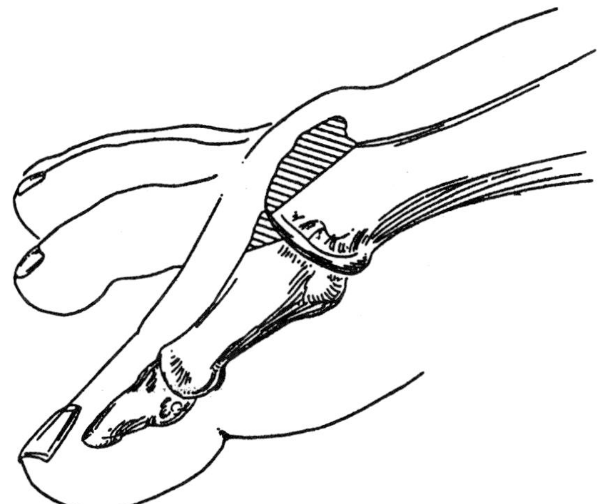

FIGURE 5-33 ■ Line of resection for cheilectomy. (From Pfeffer, G.B.: Cheilectomy. In Johnson, K.A., ed.: Master techniques in orthopaedic surgery: the foot and ankle. New York, Raven, 1994.)

IX. Pes Planus and Pes Cavus Deformities in Adults

Pes planus in adults is best described as congenital or acquired, flexible or rigid, and symptomatic or nonsymptomatic. Rigid pes calcaneovalgus deformity, with or without tarsal coalition, is discussed in Chapter 2, Pediatric Orthopaedics.

A. Flexible Pes Planus Deformity

Flexible pes planus deformity (arch reconstitutes with non-weight-bearing) in adults usually can be successfully treated by the use of a shoe with a supportive arch or molded arch support, or both. However, the examiner must carefully evaluate the ease or difficulty of passive reduction of the midtarsal joint (talonavicular, calcaneocuboid) and passive correction of the forefoot in the axial plane (correction of supination or forefoot varus). Also important is the tightness of the gastrocnemius-soleus complex through the Achilles tendon with the subtalar and midtarsal joints in "subtalar neutral" position; stretching of the gastrocnemius-soleus-Achilles-muscle-tendon unit may be necessary after correction of hindfoot valgus.

B. Rigid Pes Planus Deformity

Rigid pes planus in adults may result from longstanding congenital pes planus which, over many years, becomes less and less flexible. It is a spectrum, but once the subtalar neutral, midtarsal neutral position can no longer be passively reached and forefoot rotation cannot be corrected (pronated) past neutral or into a plantigrade position, then rigid pes planus is present. Frequently, an undiagnosed tarsal coalition, particularly of the middle facet, will render the hindfoot rigid and the midfoot semirigid. The patient complains of foot fatigue, periarticular pain at the talocalcaneal joint, and aching deep in the sinus tarsi and in the talo-fibulo-calcaneal "joint." The more rigid the deformity, the more difficult the treatment. Medial sole and heel wedges (1/8–3/16 inches) in work and recreation shoes, semirigid molded insoles, and gastrocnemius-soleus stretching exercises are recommended. Occasionally, pain becomes so severe that peroneal muscle "spasm" develops from pulling against a rigid valgus hindfoot while the peroneal muscles rest in a chronically shortened position. The combination of peroneal muscle and heel cord tightness with sinus tarsi, perisubtalar, and lateral gutter pain at the talo-fibulo-calcaneal articulation can cause symptoms so severe that a double-upright brace with a locked ankle, inside T-strap, and rigid rocker sole (or similar AFO) is required to relieve pain. When this is unsuccessful, an arthrodesis of the subtalar joint or even a triple arthrodesis (if the midtarsal joint deformity is rigid or semirigid) may be required. In an adult with a fixed pes planus deformity, resecting a tarsal coalition probably will not provide long-term relief of symptoms.

C. Acquired Pes Planus Deformity

Acquired pes planus deformity in adults is most often caused by posterior tibial tendon insufficiency. With progressive loss of function of this vital hindfoot inverter muscle-tendon unit, progressive hindfoot valgus occurs and midtarsal abduction and forefoot supination (varus) deformities develop. As in congenital flexible pes planus, which may progress to varying degrees of rigidity in adults, acquired deformity from posterior tibial tendon insufficiency can progress to varying degrees of fixed posture. While flexible, the deformities can be treated with the same methods as congenital pes planus deformity; however, more surgical options are available for the treatment of acquired pes planus in adults (see the section on tendon pathology).

D. Pes Cavus Deformity

Pes cavus deformity (high-arched, symptomatic foot) often occurs in patients with a family history of similar deformities, suggesting the diagnosis of a **hereditary motor-sensory neuropathy** (HMSN). CMT disease (peroneal muscle atrophy) is the most common inherited neuropathy, affecting 1 in 2500 people. There are, however, many types of HMSN and more are being described.

E. CMT Disease

CMT disease is broadly classified as hypertrophic (type I) or neuronal (type II), with many subgroups in each type. This is a pathologic typing indicating either thickened nerves with abnormal and excessive fatty myelin (type I) or loss and atrophy of neuronal axons (type II). These pathologic changes "die back" to the anterior horn cells, with degeneration of the posterior columns and nerve roots.

Type II (neuronal) CMT disease has an autosomal recessive inheritance and an onset between 5 and 15 years of age. It predominantly affects males (3:2) and causes progressive weakness and atrophy of the legs below the knees, giving a "stork leg" appearance. The cavus deformity progresses to cavovarus and claw toes faster than in type I CMT disease.

Type I (hypertrophic) CMT disease has an autosomal dominant inheritance and a later onset (20–30 years of age) and causes less severe deformity in the lower extremities, although hand weakness is more severe than in type II CMT disease, often resulting in difficulty writing, turning door knobs, gripping firmly, and opposing the thumb to the fingers.

Electrodiagnostic studies in type I CMT disease show marked decrease in motor nerve conduction velocity, whereas type II CMT disease has normal or mildly decreased motor nerve conduction. Physical findings vary markedly, even among members of the same family with the same type of disease. One family member may be mildly affected with minimal functional impairment, whereas profound physical impairment may be present in a close relative.

The first muscles to atrophy are the intrinsic muscles of the foot, followed by the peroneus brevis muscle. Surprisingly, the peroneus longus muscle is spared until late in the course of the disease. Atrophy of these muscles is followed by weakness in the toe extensors and tibialis anterior, resulting in a drop foot and marionette gait. The ankle jerk reflex usually is absent, although the knee jerk reflex remains intact. Proprioceptive and sensory loss occur to varying degrees, but when this loss is pronounced, physical impairment increases markedly. Patients usually remain ambulatory, albeit often with difficulty. Mental function is not impaired, and pregnancy before age 30 may markedly exacerbate progression of the physical impairment. Scoliosis, although frequently present to a minimal degree, rarely requires treatment (10–15% of cases).

A patient with CMT disease usually has an awkward gait, painful callosities beneath the metatarsal heads from the clawed toes, and less frequently, ankle instability. The physical examination must document flexibility of all components of the deformity, including hindfoot varus (Coleman block test, see Fig. 5-27), midfoot adduction, and forefoot pronation (valgus). In addition, the first ray often is plantar flexed early in the course of the disease (Fig. 5-34) due to a strong peroneus longus and weakened tibialis anterior, and the correctability of the deformity, as well as the clawing of the toes, must be documented. Sensory and proprioceptive function also must be evaluated.

Treatment recommendations vary, but in general in severely affected younger patients, surgical treatment is more aggressive. The hindfoot varus is treated by a closing-wedge osteotomy, with or without lateral translation of the tuberosity fragment, if the varus heel is not correctable on the Coleman block test. If the varus hindfoot is correctable, then a combination of procedures can be used to correct the cavovarus deformity and reduce the calcaneal pitch (Fig. 5-35): plantar

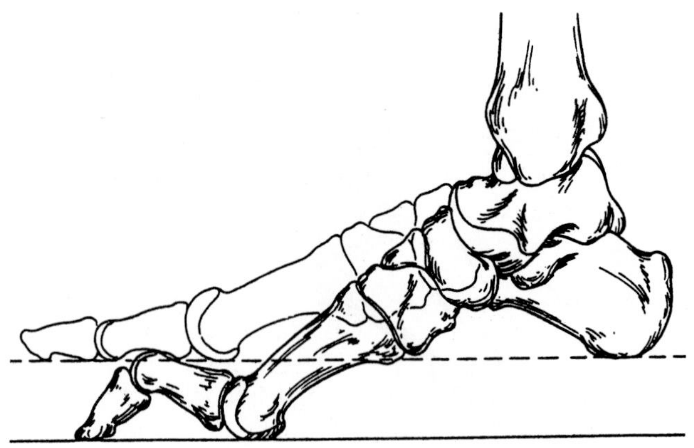

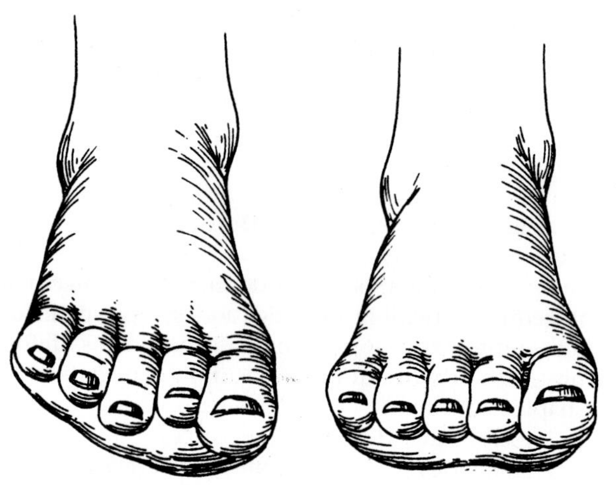

FIGURE 5-34 ■ Lateral and frontal views of plantar flexed first ray as seen in Charcot-Marie-Tooth disease. (From Murphy, G.A.: Disorders of tendons and fascia. In Canale, S.T., ed.: Campbell's Operative Orthopaedics, 10th ed. St. Louis, C.V. Mosby, 2003, p. 4144.)

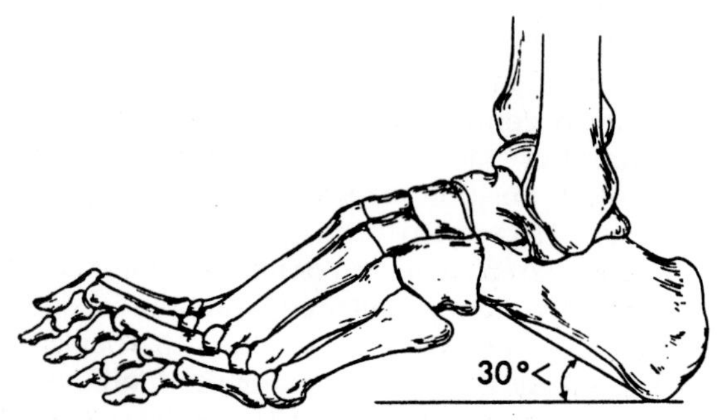

FIGURE 5-35 ■ Calcaneal pitch angle. (From Murphy, G.A.: Disorders of tendons and fascia. In Canale, S.T., ed.: Campbell's Operative Orthopaedics, 10th ed. St. Louis, C.V. Mosby, 2003, p. 4146.)

fascia release, elevation of the first metatarsal by basilar closing-wedge osteotomy, transfer of the peroneus longus to the peroneus brevis at the ankle joint, and correction of the clawed toes. If ankle equinus is not correctable past neutral position, TAL usually is required. Surgery in the second or third decade of life will aid in balancing the foot without arthrodesis, but the patient may still need an AFO.

Brace and shoe wear management may be all that is required to maintain a plantigrade foot if the deformities are passively correctable. This is especially important in laborers or workers who stand most of the day because extensive reconstructive surgery may correct deformity but not allow prolonged standing and walking. If a double upright locked ankle brace is used for durability, the T-strap must be on the outside of the shoe (varus correction).

Fixed varus deformity with fixed cavus, cavovarus, or equino-cavovarus deformities in adults requires a hindfoot stabilization procedure, such as triple arthrodesis, and transfer of the tibialis posterior through the interosseous membrane to the dorsolateral midfoot. TAL and staged procedures may be required to correct the plantar flexed first (and often second) metatarsals and the claw toe deformities. Bracing while the patient is working often is indicated after correction of the deformities to maintain correction and protect the arthrodesed joints. A full-length metal rocker sole in a work boot that is attached to the brace is useful for this protection.

X. Tendon Pathology

A. Posterior Tibial Tendon Insufficiency (PTTI)

PTTI should be suspected in an overweight, middle-aged patient with a life-long history of pes planus who complains of pain and a "weak foot." Patients usually report a gradual onset of pain at the medial ankle, hindfoot, and midfoot, accompanied by further loss of the longitudinal arch and a "turning out of the foot," representing a valgus heel and abducted midfoot. Approximately 20% of patients recall an acute injury followed by immediate or gradual worsening of the pre-existing pes planus deformity.

Physical examination commonly reveals tenderness just posterior to the tip of the medial malleolus, extending to the tuberosity of the tarsal navicular, an area of 2–3 cm where decreased vascularity has been confirmed by vascular injection studies. It is this zone where the tendon most commonly begins its attenuation and finally ruptures. The heel of the affected foot rests in more valgus when the patient stands than does the contralateral foot, and the midfoot is in abduction. With the patient standing, facing away from the examiner, with the feet straight ahead, the fourth and fifth toes of the affected foot can be seen ("too many toes" sign). With the patient non-weight-bearing and the hindfoot and midfoot brought to subtalar and midtarsal congruency, the forefoot is markedly supinated (forefoot varus). It is from this position that the Achilles tendon should be examined for tightness. Finally, all components of the deformity resulting from PTTI must be evaluated for any fixed components. Plain radiographs in the weight-bearing position are essential to augment the physical examination and to plan any surgery that may be required. In a young patient, especially a young male, with minimal if any pes planus in either foot, a sero-negative spondyloarthropathy or other inflammatory enthesopathy or arthropathy must be considered.

The choice of treatment for PTTI is aided by a classification system that emphasizes stages of pathology (Table 5-7).

B. Peroneal Tendon Insufficiency (PTI)

(Peroneal tendon subluxation is discussed in Chapter 3, Sports Medicine.

Tears of the peroneal tendons, one or both, may result acutely from violent dorsiflexion, eversion of the plantar flexed, inverted foot. However, most peroneal tendon pathology in nonathletic adults is due to a degenerative process with repetitive, mild trauma over a prolonged period. Any loss of normal heel valgus even at heel neutral position places the peroneal tendons, particularly the peroneus longus, at risk similar to excessive heel valgus placing the posterior tibial tendon at risk of injury from mild but repetitive trauma.

As with PTTI, a classification scheme is helpful in making treatment decisions for PTI (Table 5-8).

C. Anterior Tibial (AT) Tendon Injuries

Tenosynovitis of the anterior tibial tendon occurs most often in young to middle-aged patients who have an inflammatory arthritis. Pain, tenderness, and swelling usually are at the ankle joint level. Treatment is immobilization in a walking cast or removable walking boot and NSAIDs.

Tear or rupture of the anterior tibial tendon is most common in elderly patients who complain of poorly localized dorsal foot and ankle pain. Unless a complete rupture has produced a dropfoot, steppage gait, the diagnosis often is difficult. Thorough physical examination will reveal severe tenderness at the medial cuneiform–first metatarsal area of tendon insertion. If complete rupture has occurred distally, this tenderness is absent, but a tender mass can be palpated at the ankle joint level because of proximal retraction of the ruptured tendon. Incomplete tears are treated by immobilization in a walking cast for 6 weeks. If symptoms persist, an AFO is fabricated and worn for 4–6 months or until all symptoms have resolved. Complete ruptures are difficult to treat because of the age of the patients, many of whom are in their 70s or 80s, and the degeneration of the tendon, which has avulsed from bone. A short-leg walking cast is worn for 6–8 weeks while a molded AFO is being fabricated. The AFO is worn

Table 5-7. POSTERIOR TIBIAL TENDON INSUFFICIENCY CLASSIFICATION

STAGE	DESCRIPTION	TREATMENT
I	• Tenosynovitis without increased deformity compared with opposite side • Swelling and tenderness along course of tendon from medial malleolus toward navicular tuberosity • Patient able to invert foot actively on double-leg toe raise test and able to perform single-leg toe raise	Immobilization in a walking cast and NSAIDs are used for 3–4 months before tenosynovectomy is recommended. Results of both treatments are good, but a trial of nonsurgical treatment is recommended initially.
II	• Patient unable to perform single-leg toe raise due to loss of function of posterior tibial tendon; inversion against resistance difficult or impossible • Hindfoot remains flexible, and with hindfoot in neutral, forefoot can be brought into neutral • Mild lateral or sinus tarsi impingement pain • Collapse deformity disrupting Meary's line or talo-first metatarsal line on weight-bearing radiograph common	Bracing and appropriate molded insoles that are posted medially may relieve symptoms but will not correct deformity. If no improvement after 3–6 months, surgery is recommended. A calcaneal sliding osteotomy through the calcaneal tuberosity to correct part of the heel valgus or a lateral calcaneal lengthening osteotomy (Evans procedure) to correct larger degree of heel valgus, and transfer of the FDL tendon to the navicular tuberosity are recommended. Percutaneous TAL and débridement of part or all of the PTT may also be required.
III	• Fixed valgus hindfoot deformity with forefoot abduction • Degenerative changes in subtalar joint and midfoot on radiograph • Significant lateral sinus tarsi pain	Because of fixed deformity and degenerative changes, hindfoot fusion is recommended (usually with TAL). Subtalar arthrodesis alone often does not correct enough deformity to satisfy the patient. A midtarsal (talonavicular, calcaneocuboid) or triple arthrodesis is preferred.

Table 5-8. PERONEAL TENDON INSUFFICIENCY CLASSIFICATION

TYPE	DESCRIPTION	TREATMENT
I	• Peroneal tendonitis without subluxation or tear • Middle-aged, often athletic, patients who commonly participate in acceleration-deceleration sports or are distance runners • Pain beneath superior peroneal retinaculum (SPR), exacerbated by forceful eversion • Tender to palpation at SPR • Mild to moderate swelling • No structural abnormality • Pain not reproduced by forceful plantar flexion of first ray against resistance or forceful dorsiflexion and eversion of ankle	Nonoperative in walking cast or removable boot for 6–12 weeks (removed only for bathing); anti-inflammatory agents also may be used. AFO is worn until symptoms and signs of inflammation have resolved. Occasionally, tenosynovectomy is required, but inflammatory arthritic process should be ruled out before surgery.
II	• Similar to type I but involves subluxation of peroneal tendons due to incompetent SPR • Patients usually younger than those with type I pathology and very athletic • Incomplete, intrasubstance tear of tendon (usually peroneus brevis) may be present or fraying of tendon border where it passes over long ridge of peroneal groove	Treatment includes repair of the SPR, deepening of the fibular groove, and repair of any longitudinal tears of one or both tendons (see Chapter 3, Sports Medicine).
III	• Complete or incomplete rupture of one or both tendons following prolonged degenerative process • If peroneus longus is ruptured and brevis is intact, rupture usually is at cuboid groove within or at proximal edge of the sesamoid (ossified in approximately 15%) • Fixed heel varus common, especially with complete rupture of both peroneal tendons	Repair of complete rupture of peroneus longus tendon is very difficult due to the degenerative condition of the tendon and its location at the lateral-plantar border of the foot. Preferred surgical treatment is excision of the degenerative tendon and side-to-side suture of the peroneus longus to brevis proximal to the SPR. If both tendons are ruptured, every attempt is made to salvage at least one tendon in continuity, preferably the peroneus brevis. In addition, a lateral calcaneal closing-wedge sliding osteotomy through the tuberosity may be needed to correct heel varus. If both tendons are ruptured and the ankle is unstable, a Bröstrom repair of the lateral ligaments, calcaneal osteotomy, and tendon repair may be required. If patient is not a good surgical candidate, a double upright AFO with an outside (valgus correcting) T-strap and locked or limited ankle motion may control symptoms sufficiently for work and limited recreation.

for an additional 6 months, after which the patient usually wears it only when needed, such as for distance walking. A cortisone injection at the site of the insertion of the anterior tibial tendon may dramatically relieve symptoms, but as with other tendon entheses, it may contribute to tendon rupture.

D. FHL Tendon Injuries

The presenting symptom of tenosynovitis, stenosing tenosynovitis, or nodular tendinosis of the FHL is posterior ankle pain, poorly localized and worsened by certain ankle positions (especially acute plantar flexion) and occasionally associated with triggering of the hallucal interphalangeal (ID) joint. Tenosynovitis of the FHL is most often caused by repetitive trauma, and dancers are particularly vulnerable to this injury; even in this athletic subgroup, however, it is rare. Physical examination reveals marked tenderness in the area of the posterior tubercle of the talus. If a nodule is present in the FHL tendon, full extension of the hallucal IP joint with the ankle dorsiflexed may be difficult or impossible because the nodular tendon cannot pass beneath the constricting pulley connecting the medial and lateral tubercles of the posterior process of the talus.

Laceration of the FHL proximal to the MTP joint in young patients should be repaired if the patient cannot flex or stabilize the MTP joint by the remaining flexor hallucis brevis. However, the repair is anatomically demanding because of the tendon's retraction into the midfoot and the vulnerability of the most medial branch of the medial plantar nerve (Fig. 5-36). In addition, if the tendon cannot be repaired far enough proximally so that the suture area avoids the pulley at the MTP joint of the hallux, it is better left unrepaired. After tendon repair, a short-leg walking cast is worn for 4–6 weeks, followed by a removable walking boot until MTP and IP joint motion returns. Repairing the tendon within the pulley system of the hallux proper is not recommended.

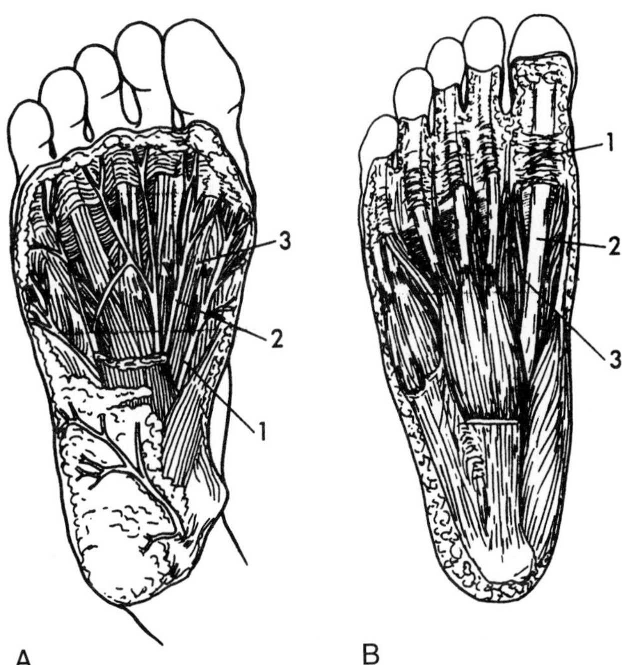

FIGURE 5-36 ■ *A, 1,* Medial proper branch of medial plantar nerve of tibial side of hallux; *2,* common digital branch of medial plantar nerve to first web; *3,* flexor hallucis longus (FHL) tendon. *B, 1,* Pulley of FHL at first MTP joint; *2,* FHL; *3,* lateral head of flexor hallucis brevis. (From Sarrafin, S.K.: Anatomy of the foot and ankle: descriptive, topographic, functional. Philadelphia, JB Lippincott, 1983.)

XI. Heel Pain

A. Plantar Fasciitis

The typical patient with plantar fasciitis is an overweight 40- to-70-year-old with severe plantar heel pain on first ambulating in the morning and localized tenderness at the plantar medial tuberosity of the calcaneus. In half of these patients, a traction osteophyte (heel spur) is apparent on radiographs, and in approximately a third it is bilateral. Plantar fasciitis is most likely a degenerative process, with microtears of the plantar fascial origin. Over an extended period, if the traumatic inflammatory reaction is not treated, fibrous, cartilaginous, and finally bony phases of repair occur, resulting in the traction osteophyte. In a small subgroup of patients with plantar fasciitis (5–10%), there is concomitant entrapment of the first branch of the lateral plantar nerve, which innervates the abductor digiti minimi. These patients have point tenderness over the proximal origin of the abductor hallucis medially where the lateral plantar nerve passes deep to this muscle's deep fascia of origin. Whether this "entrapment" is fibrous or from adjacent inflammatory reaction of the injured plantar fascia is difficult to ascertain.

Treatment of plantar fasciitis is nonoperative for 6–12 months, using stretching and massage of the plantar fascia origin and Achilles tendon, cushioned heel inserts, night splints, or walking casts. If surgery is required, only the medial third of the plantar fascia is released in order to not weaken the medial longitudinal arch and thereby overload the lateral column of the foot. This complication can cause prolonged (12–24 months) dorsolateral foot pain in the area of the cuboid, lateral cuneiforms, and bases of the fourth and fifth metatarsals that is far worse for the patient than the original plantar fascia symptoms. If nerve entrapment is part of the symptomatology, release of the deep fascia of the abductor hallucis muscle is necessary (Fig. 5-37).

B. Central Heel Pain

This pain is localized in the central portion of the heel pad and in layman's terms is called

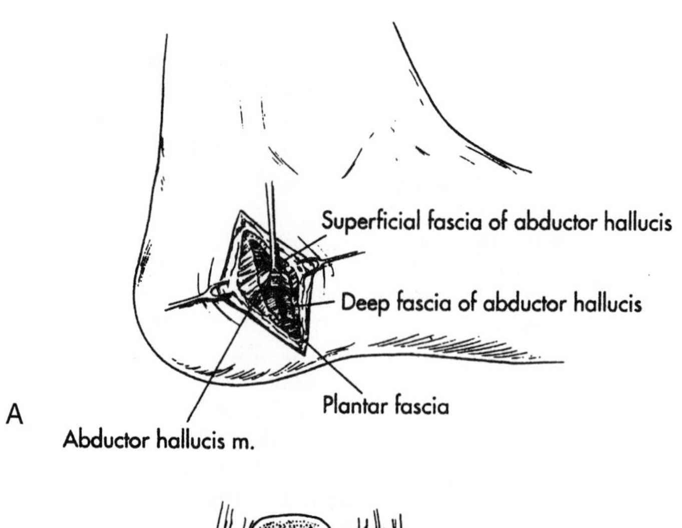

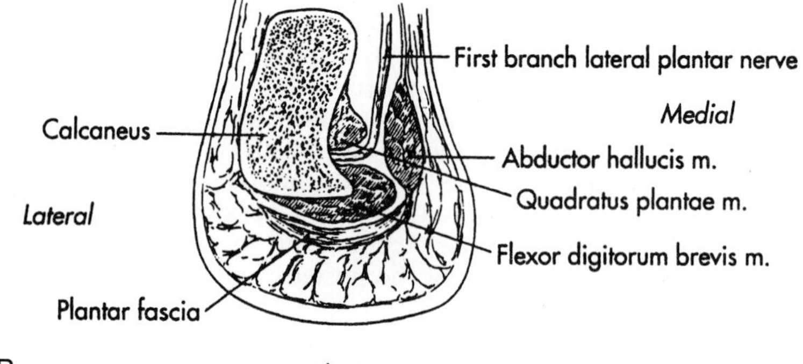

FIGURE 5-37 ■ Plantar fascia and nerve release. *A*, Abductor hallucis muscle is reflected proximally. *B*, Cross-sectional anatomy of heel along course branch of lateral plantar nerve. (From Schon, L.C.: Tarsal tunnel release. In Myerson, M., ed.: Current Therapy in Foot and Ankle Surgery. St. Louis, C.V. Mosby, 1993.)

a "stone bruise." It most likely represents a mild to moderate traumatic periostitis associated with an atrophic heel pad and reduced cushioning in older patients. In young or middle-aged patients, with or without a palpable bursa or nodule, an inflammatory arthritis must be ruled out. Rheumatoid arthritis, ankylosing spondylitis, Reiter syndrome, and arthritis associated with inflammatory bowel disease must be ruled out. Treatment of acute symptoms is pressure relief with cushioned insoles and possibly a well-padded cast for several weeks. Long-term, the patient will need shoes with crepe or crepe-like soles and continued use of cushioned heel pads.

C. **Posterior Heel Pain (Retrocalcaneal Bursitis, Haglund Deformity, Insertional Achilles Tendinitis)**

1. ***Retrocalcaneal bursitis*** and ***Haglund deformity*** are more common in young to early middle-aged patients with swelling and tenderness just anterior to the Achilles tendon, 2–3 cm proximal to its insertion, and often associated with a proximal superior aspect of the calcaneal tuberosity superolaterally (Fig. 5-38). Nonoperative treatment with rest, immobilization, physical therapy modalities, and anti-inflammatory agents usually is successful. Occasionally, the prominent aspect of the tuberosity needs to be excised, along with the retrocalcaneal bursa.
2. ***Insertional Achilles tendonitis*** **(IAT)** usually occurs in an older middle-aged or elderly patient with a tight heel cord. It represents repetitive microtrauma at the enthesis and progressive inflammatory stages of fibrosis followed by cartilaginous and then osseous metaplasia. The examiner and patient may meet at any point along this spectrum. In the mild to moderate condition without extensive bony transformation of the tendon at the enthesis, nonoperative treatment consisting of a combination of rest, stretching of the gastrocsoleus muscle-tendon unit, night splints or a cast, and a small heel lift inside the shoe usually relieve symptoms. If not, 6–9 months in a locked-ankle AFO should be successful.

   In a patient with more extensive involvement of the Achilles tendon insertion (more than half the insertion width), nonoperative treatment is less successful, but should be considered, especially the use of an AFO with a locked ankle for several months. If this fails, excision of the diseased tendon and removal of the superior aspect of the calcaneal tuberosity are indicated. If more than half of the

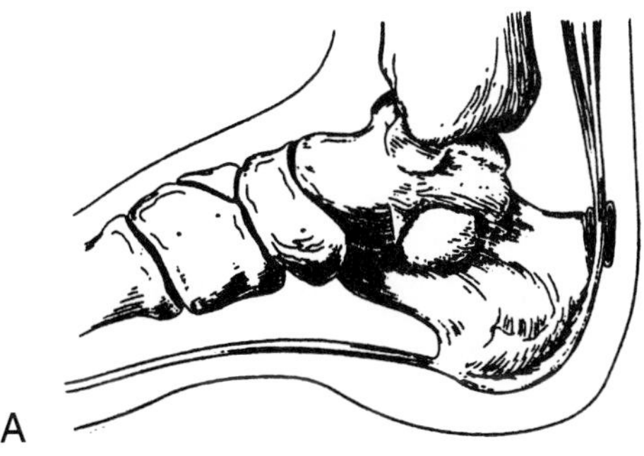

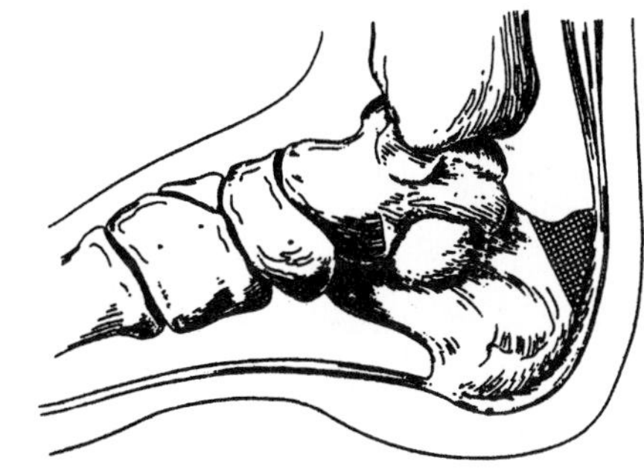

FIGURE 5-38 ■ *A*, Calcaneus with retrocalcaneal and superficial calcaneal tendon bursae before ostectomy. *B*, Large portion of calcaneus needs to be removed or symptoms will recur. (From Frey, C., and Pfeffer, G.B.: Surgical management of Haglund's deformity. In Myerson, M., ed.: Current Therapy in Foot and Ankle Surgery. St. Louis, C.V. Mosby, 1993.)

tendon insertion must be removed, augmentation by the FHL tendon is recommended.

XII. The Diabetic Foot

A. Pathophysiology

Neuropathy, angiopathy, retinopathy, and myelopathy, alone or in combination and in varying degrees of severity, determine the clinical findings and therefore the treatment alternatives for the diabetic foot. However, it is **neuropathy** that most profoundly influences the clinical course in diabetic foot pathology. The neuropathy may be mild and minimally alter the course of care, but when somatosensory and autonomic involvement is present, severe clinical sequelae are common. Fewer than a third of patients with diabetic plantar foot ulcers have decreased arterial flow to the foot. The ulcers are from repetitive stresses, both shear and axial loading forces, that damage the superficial skin layer. Yet the patient cannot perceive injury and progressive tissue destruction occurs. Combined with the absence of normal moisture and glandular skin elements lubricating the skin due to autonomic nerve damage, the diabetic neuropathy places the foot, particularly the plantar surface, at grave risk for ulceration, deep infection, and amputation.

B. Diabetic Ulceration

To predict healing of a diabetic foot ulcer, pulse volume recordings, transcutaneous oxygen pressures, and Doppler flow pressures are all useful. The ischemic index also is useful and represents the ratio of ankle to brachial pressures. A ratio of 0.6, an absolute ankle pressure of 70 mm Hg or more, and an absolute toe pressure of 40 mm Hg or more are strong indicators that a diabetic ulcer without extensive osteomyelitis or a limited foot amputation should heal. If there is calcification of the arterial tree about the ankle, these pressures can be falsely raised and decrease the reliability of the ischemic index. In that case, the combination of the ischemic index and transcutaneous oxygen pressures is helpful. The "gray zone" for predictability of ulcer healing with the ischemic index is 0.5–0.6 and of the transcutaneous oxygen tension 30–40 mm Hg. If the transcutaneous oxygen is more than 40 mm Hg, the ulcer should heal.

The overlapping degrees of underlying pathologic conditions (ischemia, neuropathy, infection) preclude treatment standardization. In caring for the ulcerated diabetic foot, an appropriate treatment plan depends on the determination of whether the ulcer is primarily **neurotrophic** or **ischemic**, whether it is localized or a deep abscess with multiple tissue plane involvement, and whether osteomyelitis or pyarthrosis, or both, are present.

The Wagner classification of diabetic ulcers is helpful to plan treatment, although variations in treatment must be adapted to individual patients (Table 5-9).

C. Neuropathic Arthropathy (Charcot Foot)

A classification and staging system based on radiographic findings is useful in evaluation and treatment of Charcot arthropathy. In stages I, II, and III, radiographic diagnosis is straightforward even on plain films. Osteopenia, joint subluxation or dislocation, and bony fragmentation are seen early, followed by bony malunion and varying degrees of sclerosis. What is difficult diagnostically is differentiating osteomyelitis from Charcot bony changes or determining if both are present. Currently, a white blood cell–labeled scintigraphy (technetium-indium) with MRI correlation is the most likely study to aid this differentiation with both sensitivity and specificity. In stages 0 and I, infection often is diagnosed when, in fact, the clinical picture represents profound autonomic neuropathy. Particularly if an ulcer is present, deep infection is assumed and must be ruled out. This differentiation is very difficult, but in most patients with neuropathic arthropathy deep infection (osteomyelitis) is either absent or quite localized in exposed bony prominences, which are easily excised (Table 5-10).

Table 5-9. WAGNER CLASSIFICATION OF DIABETIC ULCERS

GRADE	DESCRIPTION	TREATMENT
Grade 0	Skin intact but bony deformities produce a "foot at risk"	Extra-depth shoes, custom-molded pressure relief insoles, serial examinations
Grade 1	Localized, superficial ulcer	Débridement of the ulcer in the office. A total contact cast is recommended if palpable or strongly positive Doppler pulses and wound margins that bleed well with local débridement are present. The risk of loss of a vascularly compromised foot in an occlusive cast must be weighed against the risk of leaving the ulcer. The patient and physician make this decision together. The potential for healing even large, full-thickness ulcers is so high using total contact casting that some degree of ischemia is acceptable. Also, the extent of possible tracking of the ulcer is important to document (Fig. 5-39). Initially, the cast is changed weekly, then biweekly until healing occurs. This usually can be done in the office
Grade 2	Deep ulcer to tendon, bone, ligament, or joint	This usually requires formal débridement in the operating room, followed by a total-contact cast
Grade 3	Deep abscess, osteomyelitis	If area of osteomyelitis can be locally débrided (with profound neuropathy this may be done in the office) and adequate bleeding is present, a total-contact cast is indicated. The cast is changed weekly or more often if drainage is initially extensive
Grade 4	Gangrene of toes or forefoot	Because ischemia is present, vascular surgery consultation is required to decide if arterial vascular reconstruction is possible. If increased arterial flow can be established, the ulcer or a more limited partial foot amputation may heal
Grade 5	Gangrene of entire foot	Major amputation; arterial bypass surgery may allow a below-knee amputation to heal

Initial treatment usually is nonoperative, although early surgical treatment to restore alignment, relieve bony prominences that threaten ulceration, and stabilize the affected joints with internal fixation and selected arthrodeses currently has its proponents. However, most orthopaedists who care for large numbers of patients with diabetic foot problems limit surgery of the neuropathic foot to:

1. Removing bony prominences under ulceration or pre-ulcerative lesions
2. TAL
3. Selected arthrodeses following the consolidative stage of Charcot arthropathy in feet that are unbraceable due to the deformity.

Limited or partial foot amputation when vascularity allows is the goal in diabetic, ulcerated feet. The loss of three lateral rays, two medial rays, or one or two central rays still provides a functional, braceable foot, which is preferable to a below-knee amputation. Lisfranc and Chopart amputation (Fig. 5-40) with TAL also are functional partial foot amputations. Although the Syme amputation still has use, it probably should be limited to the younger

Table 5-10. CHARCOT ARTHROPATHY STAGES

STAGE	DESCRIPTION	INITIAL TREATMENT
0	• Unilateral edema, erythema, and associated warmth • No break in skin integrity • Radiographs negative or show local osteoporosis	Cast immobilization, non-weight-bearing, assuming arterial flow is adequate. Arterial flow is almost always good in patients with Charcot arthropathy and, in fact, contributes through the autonomic neuropathy to the profound bone absorption frequently seen in the earliest phases.
I	• Unilateral edema, erythema, and warmth • Radiographs show osseous destruction, joint dislocation or subluxation	
II	• Decreased local edema, erythema, and warmth • Radiographs show coalescence of small fracture fragments and absorption of fine bone debris	Weight-bearing immobilization until tissue homeostasis is evident; then AFO with locked or limited motion ankle and appropriate shoes with molded insoles. Eventually the AFO can be used on a limited basis.
III	• No or minimal edema, erythema, or warmth • Radiographs show consolidation and remodeling of fracture fragments	

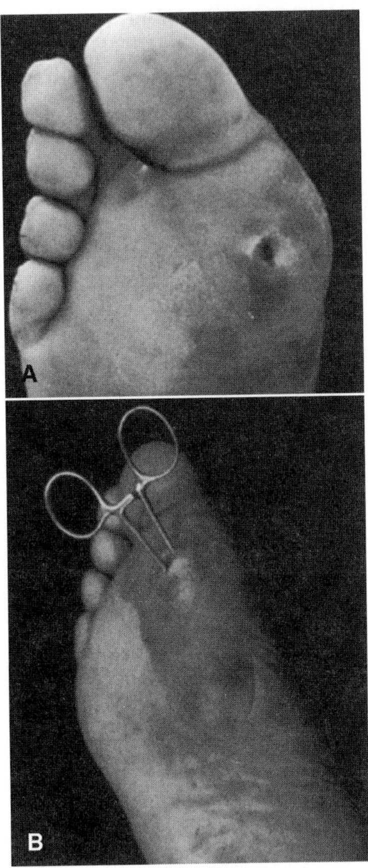

FIGURE 5-39 ■ Diabetic abscess. *A*, Note discoloration proximal to abscess beneath first metatarsal head. *B*, Depth of abscess is remarkable. (From Richardson, E.G.: Diabetic foot. In Canale, S.T., ed.: Campbell's Operative Orthopaedics, 10th ed. St. Louis, C.V. Mosby, 2003, p. 4116.)

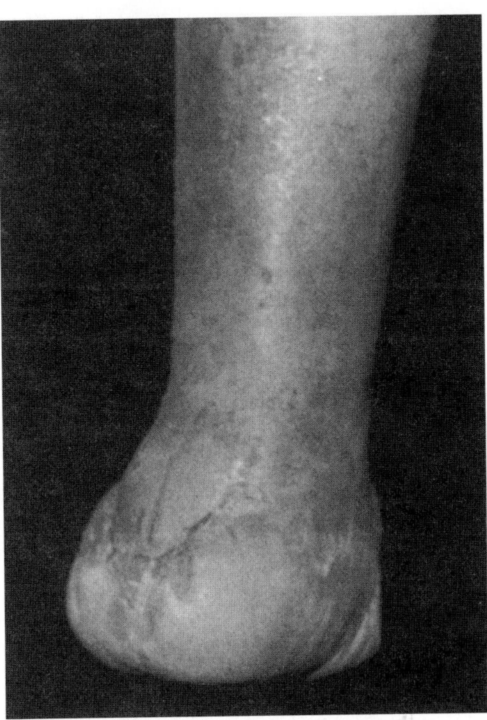

FIGURE 5-40 ■ Chopart amputation with percutaneous lengthening of calcaneal tendon for extensive midfoot and forefoot infection in diabetic foot. Vascular supply was good but profound neuropathy was present. (From Richardson, E.G.: Diabetic foot. In Canale, S.T., ed.: Campbell's Operative Orthopaedics, 10th ed. St. Louis, C.V. Mosby, 2003, p. 4126.)

patient with excellent pulses at the ankle, sufficient skin for closure, and an environment where a skilled prosthetist is available.

XIII. Fractures and Dislocations of the Foot

A. Calcaneal Fractures

Fractures are generally divided into articular and exarticular fractures. Either kind can be displaced or nondisplaced, open or closed, which markedly affects clinical outcome.

1. ***Extra-articular calcaneal fractures*** are tuberosity avulsion fractures caused by forceful Achilles tendon contraction, anterior process fractures from avulsion by the bifurcate ligament, and beak fractures of the tuberosity of the calcaneus that do not involve the Achilles tendon. These fractures can be treated nonoperatively with cast immobilization unless displaced. If a tuberosity beak fracture or anterior process fracture is displaced more than 1 cm and the fragment is large enough to support internal fixation, the fragment should be replaced and fixed. If the fragment is displaced more than 1 cm but is too small for internal fixation, it should be excised (Fig. 5-41).
2. ***Articular calcaneal fractures***. Isolated sustentaculum fractures without posterior facet involvement are rare; however, persistent medial hindfoot pain after an injury which should have clinical resolution should be evaluated by CT scanning for this injury. Rarely will open reduction and internal fixation be required.
3. ***Posterior facet fractures***. Approximately 75% of all fractures of the calcaneus are posterior facet fractures, and most of these have

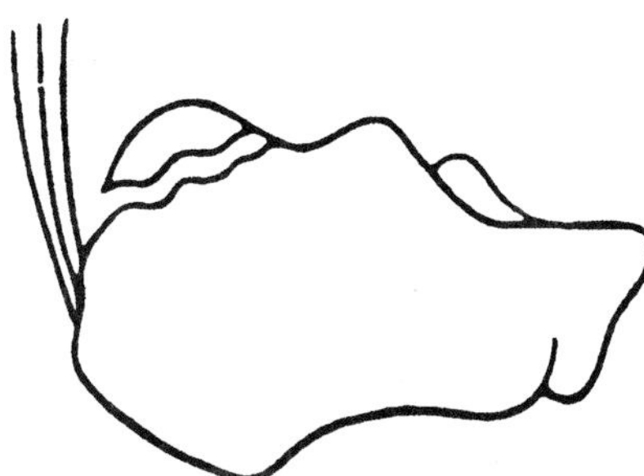

FIGURE 5-41 ■ *A*, Beak fracture does not involve calcaneal tendon and can be treated nonoperatively if less than 1 cm of displacement is present. (From Lowery, R.B., Calhoun, J.H.: Fractures of the calcaneus. 1. Anatomy, injury, mechanism, and classification. Foot Ankle 17:360, 1996.)

some degree of displacement. Displacement of a posterior facet fracture of more than 2–3 mm is an indication for open reduction and internal fixation (ORIF). The classification system of Sanders (Fig. 5-42), based on CT scanning, is the most widely used, although the Essex-Lopresti (Fig. 5-43), based on radiographic appearance, also is helpful. Axial loading and shear forces account for the mechanism of injury, and one or more fragments of the posterior facet are impacted into the body of the calcaneus. This reduces or reverses the Böhler angle (Fig. 5-44), which normally is 25–40 degrees,

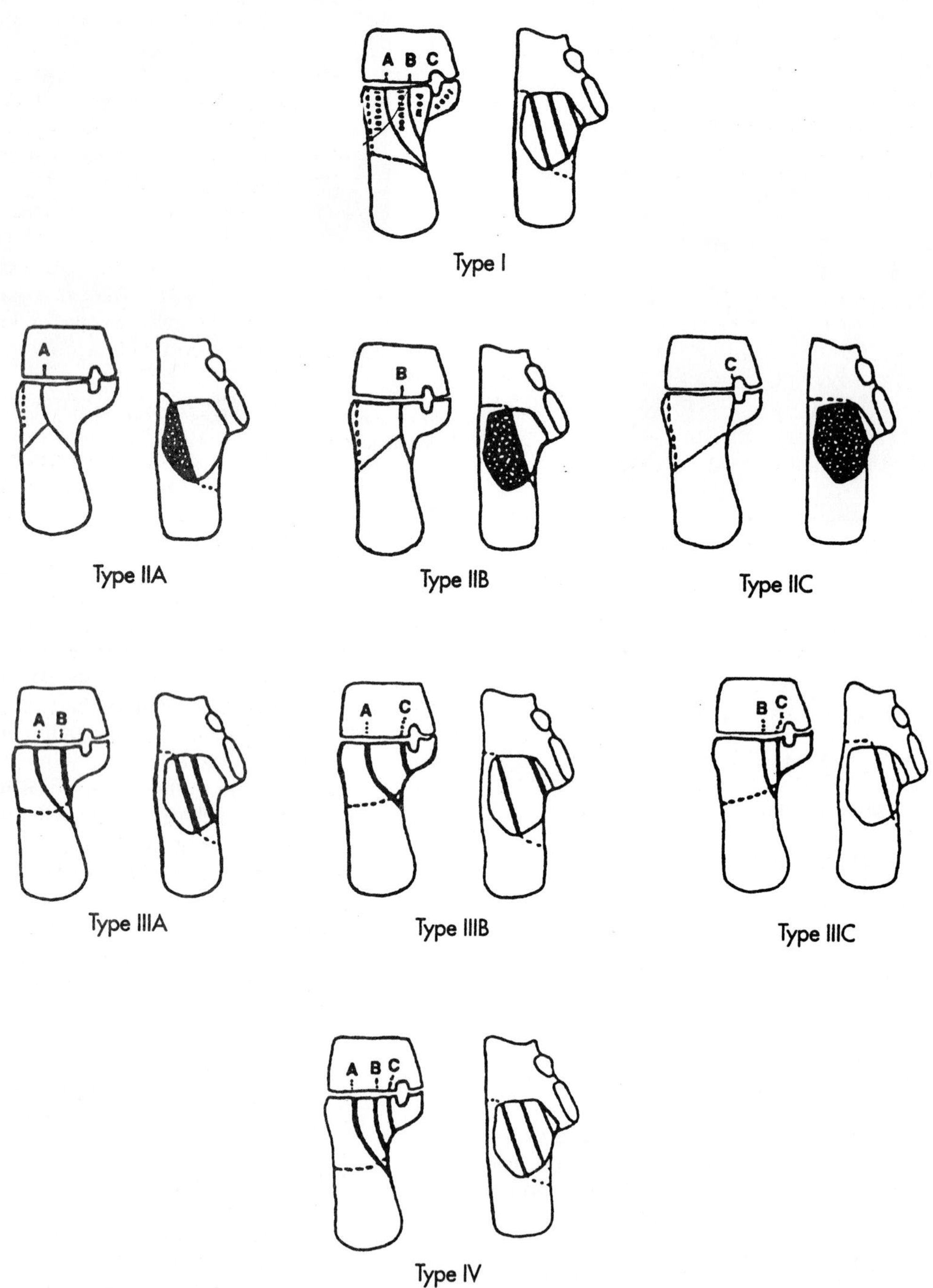

FIGURE 5-42 ■ Computed tomography scan classification of intra-articular calcaneal fractures. (From Sanders, R., Fortin, P., DiPasquale, T., Walling, A.: Operative treatment in 120 displaced intra-articular calcaneal fractures: results using a prognostic computed tomography scan classification. Clin. Orthop. 290:87, 1993.)

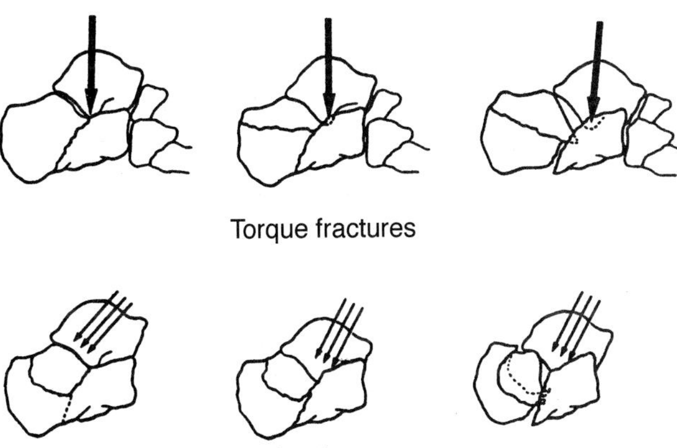

FIGURE 5-43 ■ Essex-Lopresti classification of calcaneal fractures. (From Murphy, G.A.: Fractures and dislocations of foot. In Canale, S.T., ed.: Campbell's Operative Orthopaedics, 10th ed. St. Louis, C.V. Mosby, 2003, p. 4233.)

and "bursts" the lateral wall of the calcaneus laterally beneath the fibula. This multiplane disruption of the posterior facet can result in calcaneofibular abutment, peroneal tendon encroachment, articular pain, heel pad crush symptoms, and shoe-wear difficulty from a shortened, widened, and flattened calcaneus.

Routine plain films (AP, lateral, oblique, and axial os calcis views) are helpful to evaluate the Böhler angle and the degree of calcaneal shortening. CT scanning in the coronal plane (posterior and middle facets) and axial plane (calcaneocuboid joint involvement and tuberosity displacement) is very helpful for evaluating this multiplane injury as well as for preoperative planning. If CT scanning is not available, a Broden oblique view of the ankle is helpful to evaluate posterior facet displacement.

The prognosis for articular fractures of the calcaneus treated by either nonoperative or operative methods is guarded, and operative

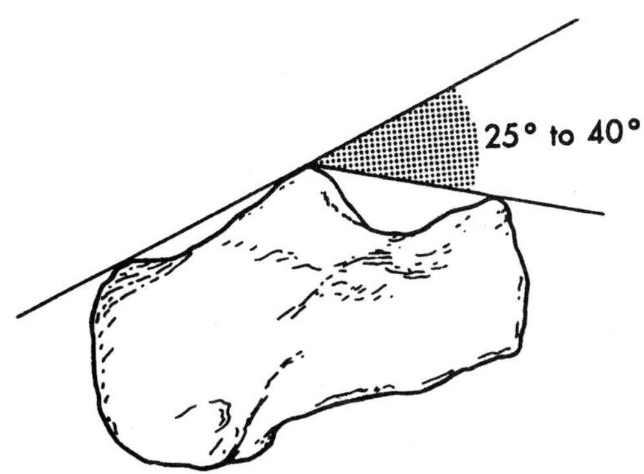

FIGURE 5-44 ■ Böhler angle. (From Murphy, G.A.: Fractures and dislocations of foot. In Canale, S.T., ed.: Campbell's Operative Orthopaedics, 10th ed. St. Louis, C.V. Mosby, 2003, p. 4233.)

management is controversial in patients who smoke or who are more than 50–60 years old. Sanders, however, does not believe age should be a factor and reported approximately 75–80% good to excellent results in types II and III articular fractures treated with ORIF. The recommended treatment of type I fractures is non-weight bearing for 4–6 weeks and early motion after a short period of immobilization (2–3 weeks) for soft-tissue stabilization. Type IV fractures are very comminuted and severely displaced and have a poor prognosis regardless of treatment. Restoration of calcaneal anatomy and primary arthrodesis of the posterior facet with bone grafting, if needed, is gaining popularity but is a technically demanding procedure.

B. Fractures of the Talus

The classification system devised by Hawkins, and modified by Canale and Kelley, is most commonly used to evaluate talar neck fractures. Other fractures of the talus are talar head fractures, lateral process fractures (skate boarder's fracture), posteromedial tuberosity fractures, and posterior process fractures. Lateral process and medial tuberosity fractures are articular. Posterior process fractures usually are not articular unless quite large. Fractures of the body of the talus carry a high risk of avascular necrosis if displaced and some risk even if nondisplaced. Types II, III, and IV talar neck fractures also have high incidences of avascular necrosis.

The prognosis for fractures of the talus is directly related to the degree of injury to its unique blood supply. The **artery of the tarsal canal** from the tibialis posterior is the primary blood supply to the talar body. Branches of the **dorsalis pedis** and **peroneal arteries** supply the talar head and neck and a limited portion of the talar body retrograde through the talar neck. Avascular necrosis of the talar body following displaced talar neck or talar body fractures is directly related to the degree of injury to these three arterial and vascular leashes supplying the talus, as well as to the limited arterial supply to the medial and inferior talar body through the deep deltoid ligament.

The mechanism of injury of talar neck fractures is dorsiflexion or inversion, or both, causing a shear fracture. The force required to fracture the talus is approximately twice the force required to fracture the calcaneus or navicular. **Complications of talar neck fractures are related to the degree of displacement.** Classification is helpful for predicting complications and clinical outcomes, as well as for treatment planning (Table 5-11).

Avascular necrosis after type I talar neck fractures is believed to be due to undiagnosed subluxation of the subtalar or tibiotalar joint or occult talar body fracture. The **Hawkins sign**

Table 5-11. CLASSIFICATION OF TALAR NECK FRACTURES

TYPE	DESCRIPTION	TREATMENT	COMPLICATIONS
I	Nondisplaced talar neck fracture	Non–weight-bearing cast until union (usually 6–8 weeks)	• Avascular necrosis (AVN) 13% (Fractures that develop AVN may have reduced spontaneously)
II	Displaced talar neck fracture with subluxation or dislocation of subtalar joint, but intact ankle mortise	Occasionally, closed reduction and internal fixation in sagittal plane with fluoroscopy; usually ORIF	• AVN 30–45% • Post-traumatic arthritis subtalar joint 40–90%
III	Displaced talar neck fracture with dislocation of talar body from ankle mortise	ORIF	• AVN 90–100% • Post-traumatic arthritis subtalar and tibiotalar joints 40–90% • Nonunion 13% • Malunion 27%
IV	Displaced talar neck fracture with dislocation of talar body from ankle mortise and subluxation or dislocation of talonavicular joint	ORIF	• AVN 90–100% • Post-traumatic arthritis subtalar and tibiotalar joints 40–90% • Nonunion 13% • Malunion 27%

is useful as a prognostic indicator for displaced talar neck fractures. A subchondral radiolucency present in the talar dome on an AP radiograph 6–8 weeks after a talar neck fracture suggests blood supply to this region. The current use of MRI to detect avascular necrosis of the talar body gives more precise information regarding the presence and extent of avascular necrosis, but its usefulness postoperatively often is limited by the metal used for internal fixation.

1. ***Talar body fractures*** (10–25% of talar fractures)
   Nondisplaced fractures of the talar body are difficult to detect. Any patient not recovering from a presumed ankle sprain in a timely fashion should have a CT scan to rule out talar body fracture. The force required to fracture the talar body is great, and complications such as avascular necrosis and post-traumatic arthritis of the subtalar or tibiotalar joint are frequent. Avascular necrosis occurs after up to 25% of nondisplaced coronal shear fractures and after 40–50% of displaced fractures. If the talar body is extruded from the ankle mortise and associated with even a minimally displaced fracture, avascular necrosis develops in 90–100% of cases. In horizontal or axial shear fractures of the talar body, even nondisplaced, the incidence of avascular necrosis of the talar dome is almost 100% because the fragment is separated from all blood supply, as opposed to sagittal and coronal (frontal) talar body fractures, which may leave a portion of the blood supply intact.

   Talar body fractures with more than 2 mm of displacement are treated with ORIF. Occasionally, this will require a medial malleolar osteotomy, especially with mid-body fractures. If malleolar osteotomy is required to adequately expose and fix the fracture, it is imperative that the blood supply to the talar body through the deep deltoid ligament be preserved. Nondisplaced fractures can be treated with a non-weight-bearing cast for 6–8 weeks, but delayed union and avascular necrosis are common even with these nondisplaced fractures and the patient and family must be informed of this.
2. ***Talar process fractures (lateral, posterior, and posteromedial)***
   These fractures are best seen with CT scanning. Treatment in a non-weight-bearing cast for 6–10 weeks usually is sufficient. If the fragments are displaced enough that the likelihood of union is remote, excision is recommended unless the fragment is large enough for internal fixation. Lateral process fractures are most common because of the popularity of snowboarding and skateboarding. Fractures of the posteromedial talar tubercle are especially difficult to diagnosis, and any persistence of localized tenderness of the talus just posterior to the middle facet should be evaluated by CT scan.

   Osteochondral fractures of the talus are discussed in Chapter 3, Sports Medicine.

   Subtalar dislocations, navicular and cuboid fractures, Lisfranc joint injuries, and metatarsal and phalangeal fractures are discussed in Chapter 10, Adult Trauma.

C. **Fractures of the Tarsal Bones**
   Five relatively small bones create a stable connection between the more mobile hindfoot and forefoot: the navicular, the cuboid, and three cuneiform bones (Fig. 5-45). Isolated injuries to individual tarsal bones are infrequent; most often surrounding soft tissues and other bones and joints also are injured. Whether the injury is isolated or combined, early accurate

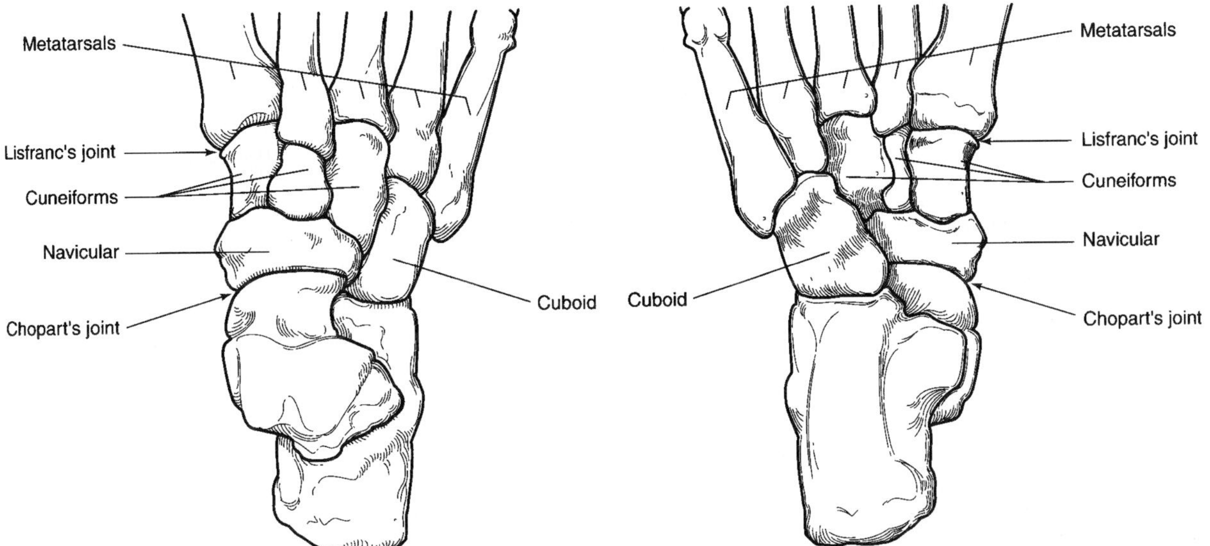

FIGURE 5-45 ■ Bony anatomy of the midfoot: dorsal view *(left)* and plantar view *(right)*. (From Early, J.S.: Fractures and dislocations of the midfoot and forefoot. In Bucholz, R.W., and Heckman, J.D., eds.: Rockwood and Green's Fractures in Adults, 5th ed. Philadelphia, Lippincott Williams & Wilkins, 2001, p. 2183.)

diagnosis is essential to proper treatment. Goals of treatment include maintenance of the relative lengths of the medial and lateral columns of the foot and preservation of the function of the talonavicular joint. Prolonged non–weight-bearing or protected weight-bearing may be required for adequate healing of ligaments and other soft-tissue structures.

1. ***Cuboid fractures.*** Fracture and dislocations involving the cuboid bone are uncommon. They can be caused by direct crushing injuries, indirect twisting or impaction forces, or repetitive stresses. The classic indirect cuboid injury is a "nutcracker" fracture. When the forefoot is violently everted on the hindfoot, the cuboid bone is pinched between the anterior aspect of the calcaneus and the bases of the fourth and fifth metatarsals, often resulting in a displaced fracture of the cuboid with involvement of the calcaneocuboid joint, the cuboid-metatarsal articulation, or both. Cuboid fractures often are overlooked because of their rarity and because they may not be apparent on standard AP and lateral radiographs; they are best seen on a 30 degree medial oblique view. Tenderness and swelling over the lateral midfoot with pain to palpation in this area are the usual presenting signs. Patients with cuboid fractures usually are unable to bear weight on the injured extremity. Because the cuboid has a central role in maintaining the integrity of the lateral column of the foot, displaced fractures should be reduced anatomically to avoid persistent dysfunction. Satisfactory results generally can be obtained with open anatomic reduction and internal fixation and bone grafting when needed.

   Cuboid stress fractures have been reported, but are rare. Most reported cuboid stress fractures have been in athletes, especially runners, with a marked increase in training or competition. Cuboid stress fractures may follow lengthening of the plantar fascia from traumatic tears or surgical release, possibly because this weakens the support of the medial longitudinal arch provided by the plantar fascia. Tenderness of the cuboid bone may be mistaken for peroneal tendonitis. Bone scan or MRI helps identify the stress fracture. Treatment is as for other stress fractures in the foot: relative immobilization and activity modification, followed by gradual return to full activities.

   Cuboid dislocations also are uncommon, but can occur in falls from heights or with a violent twisting mechanism. Physical examination finds a swollen, painful lateral midfoot with a palpable deformity corresponding to the dislocated cuboid bone. The dislocation can be identified best on an oblique radiographic view and its direction best determined on a lateral view. Obtaining and maintaining anatomic reduction are essential. Closed reduction can be attempted, but open reduction usually is required.

   Cuboid subluxations are most common in professional dancers with hypermobile joints. The diagnosis is difficult and should be suspected in this group of athletes. Radiographs usually are negative. Passive movement of the foot from plantar-flexion inversion to dorsiflexion eversion may produce a palpable click at the calcaneocuboid joint. Bone scanning may be helpful to identify the subluxation.

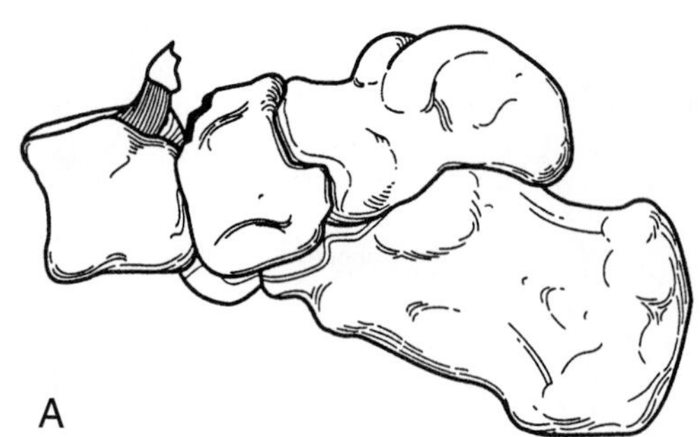

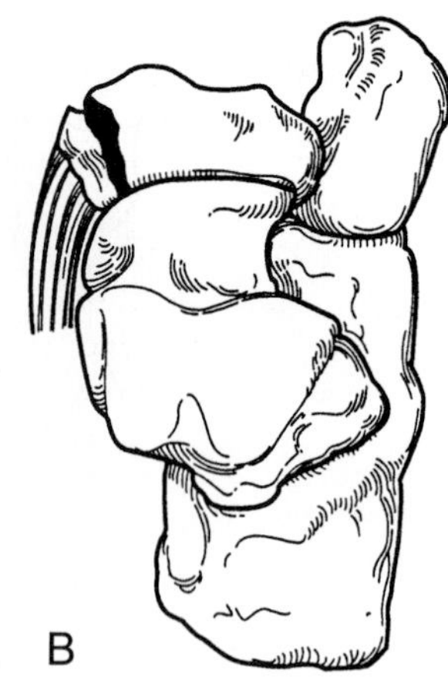

FIGURE 5-46 ■ *A*, Avulsion-type navicular fracture can involve either talonavicular or naviculocuneiform ligaments. *B*, Tuberosity fractures usually are traction-type injuries with disruption of the posterior tibial tendon insertion without joint disruption. (From Early, J.S.: Fractures and dislocations of the midfoot and forefoot. In Bucholz, R.W., Heckman, J.D., eds.: Rockwood and Green's Fractures in Adults, 5th ed. Philadelphia, Lippincott Williams & Wilkins, 2001, p. 2185.)

2. ***Navicular fractures.*** Fractures of the navicular bone can range from mild avulsion fractures to comminuted fracture-dislocations. Because of its importance in naviculotalar articulation and in maintaining the medial column of the foot, navicular injuries can be debilitating.

   Avulsion fractures (Fig. 5-46*A*) are the most common navicular fractures, and patients typically describe a painful twisting of the midfoot. The area over the navicular bone is swollen and painful, and walking is difficult or impossible. Because of the associated ligamentous injuries, pain may be out of proportion to the bony injury visible on radiographs. Most avulsion navicular fractures can be treated conservatively, but a lengthy period (8–12 weeks) of non-weight-bearing and restricted weight bearing may be required, and full recovery may require up to 6 months. Operative treatment is indicated for reattachment of an avulsion of the posterior tibial tendon insertion.

   Fractures of the navicular body (Fig. 5-46*B*) are not as common as avulsion fractures but can be much more serious. The force required to fracture the navicular body often causes subluxation or dislocation and other injuries to the midfoot. The usual mechanism of injury is application of an indirect axial load; crush injuries are associated with severe soft-tissue disruption and other midtarsal fractures. The fracture usually can be identified on standard AP, lateral, and oblique views of the foot, and CT scanning is helpful to determine the extent of the injury. Undisplaced navicular body fractures can be treated with immobilization, but displaced fractures generally require operative treatment. Sangeorzan and colleagues classified navicular body fractures into three distinct patterns: type I, transverse fracture line; type II, dorsolateral to plantar medial fracture line with forefoot adduction; and type III, central or lateral comminution with forefoot abduction (Fig. 5-47).

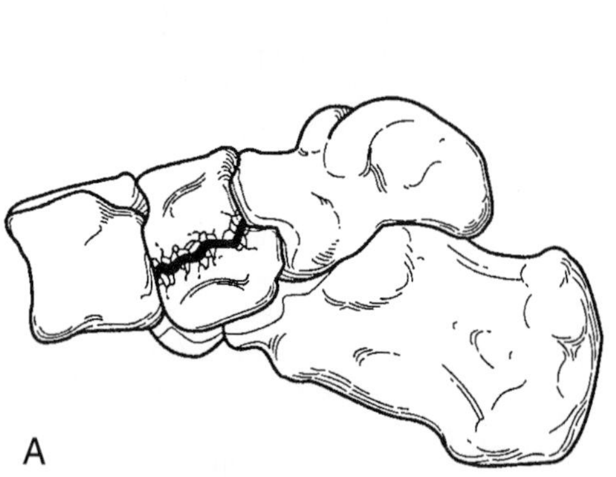

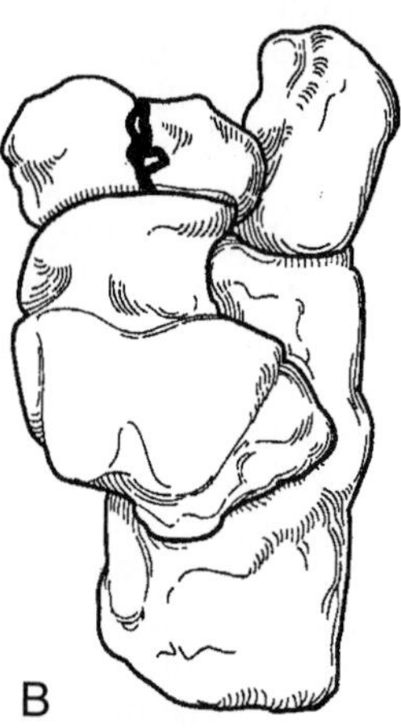

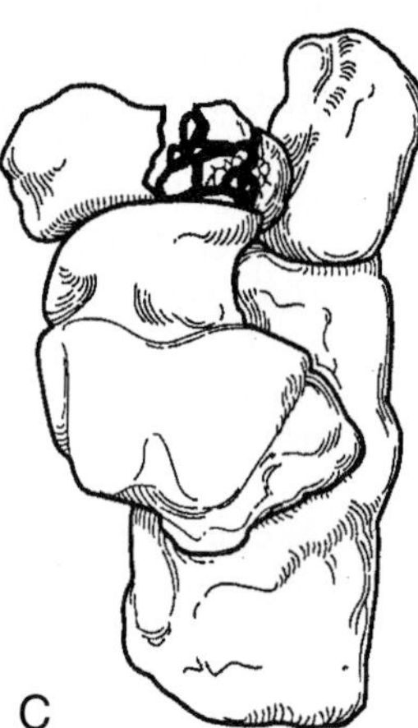

FIGURE 5-47 ■ *A*, Type I navicular body fracture splits navicular into dorsal and plantar segments. *B*, Type II body fractures create medial and lateral segments; fracture usually follows either of the two intercuneiform joint lines. Stress fractures usually are of this type. *C*, Type III body fractures have comminution of the fragments and marked displacement of the medial and lateral poles. (From Early, J.S.: Fractures and dislocations of the midfoot and forefoot. In Bucholz, R.W., Heckman, J.D., eds.: Rockwood and Green's Fractures in Adults, 5th ed. Philadelphia, Lippincott Williams & Wilkins, 2001, p. 2185.)

Regardless of type, anatomic or "satisfactory" reduction is required; satisfactory reduction is defined as restoration of at least 60% of the talonavicular joint surface as seen on AP and lateral radiographs.

Navicular stress fractures are most common in athletes whose sports require sudden changes in direction or explosive movements (such as sprinters, hurdlers, high jumpers, and basketball players); they are infrequent in the general population. The typical history is of an insidious onset of midfoot pain that is worse after athletic activity and better after rest. Symptoms may be vague and even misleadingly benign considering the seriousness of this injury. Vague midfoot pain without significant trauma should suggest a stress fracture of the navicular. Point tenderness usually is present over the lateral half of the navicular bone. The fracture may not be visible on plain radiographs because the characteristic fracture pattern is almost vertical and many are undisplaced and incomplete. Bone scanning shows an area of increased uptake in the area of the navicular stress fracture, and CT scanning confirms the diagnosis and identifies the fracture pattern. Initial treatment is conservative, with immobilization in a short-leg walking cast for at least 6 weeks, followed by a gradual return to activities. Operative treatment may be indicated for complete or comminuted fractures or delayed union or nonunion of incomplete fractures. Bone grafting may be required for nonunion.

3. ***Fractures of the cuneiform bones.*** Fractures and dislocations involving the cuneiform bones are relatively uncommon; isolated fractures or dislocations have been reported, but most occur in association with other midfoot injuries. Of the three cuneiform bones, the medial is the most commonly injured. Displaced or unstable medial cuneiform injuries require anatomic reduction and stable fixation.

D. Fracture-Dislocations of the Tarsometatarsal Articulation (Lisfranc Joint)

Injuries to the Lisfranc joint can range from mild sprains or subtle subluxations to widely displaced, debilitating injuries. Most injuries to the Lisfranc joint are caused by indirect rotational forces. Usually a force is applied along the longitudinal axis of a foot that is in slight equinus and has the metatarsals planted firmly on the ground distally (Fig. 5-48). Direct injuries, caused by a crushing force applied directly to the joint as in a fall from a height or motor vehicle collision, often are associated with

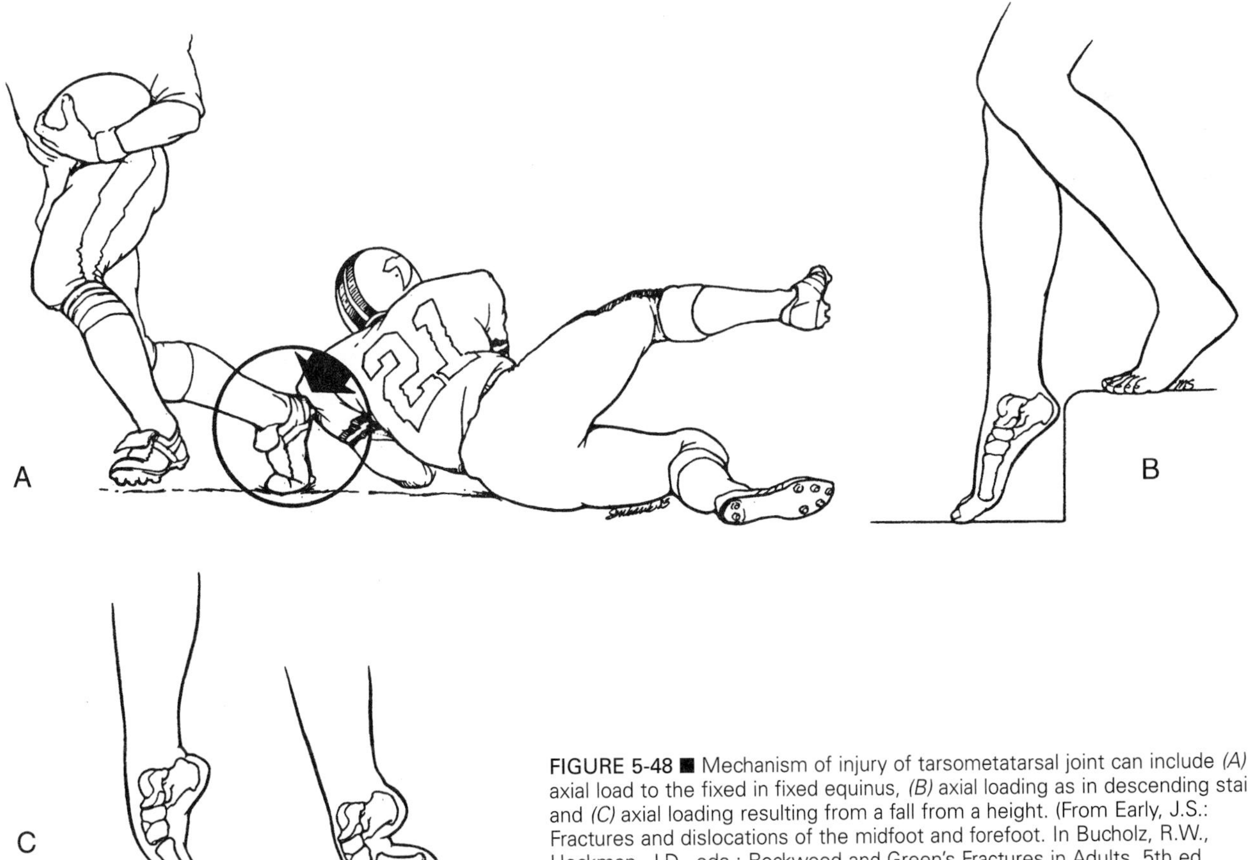

FIGURE 5-48 ■ Mechanism of injury of tarsometatarsal joint can include *(A)* axial load to the fixed in fixed equinus, *(B)* axial loading as in descending stairs, and *(C)* axial loading resulting from a fall from a height. (From Early, J.S.: Fractures and dislocations of the midfoot and forefoot. In Bucholz, R.W., Heckman, J.D., eds.: Rockwood and Green's Fractures in Adults, 5th ed. Philadelphia, Lippincott Williams & Wilkins, 2001, p. 2204.)

fracture comminution, soft-tissue injury, and compartment syndrome. The pattern of injury varies according to the point of application of the force and the amount of force applied. Fractures of the cuneiforms, cuboid, and metatarsals (most often the second) are common with these injuries, as are ligamentous disruptions.

Diagnosis

Careful physical examination is essential to accurate diagnosis. Pain anywhere over the tarsometatarsal joint complex is suggestive of an isolated injury. Pain in the midfoot with attempted single-limb heel rise also suggests a Lisfranc injury. Passive dorsiflexion and plantarflexion of individual metatarsal elicits pain at the proximal articulations. Plantar ecchymosis suggests ligamentous injury.

Radiographic examination evaluates the stability of the joint and determines the presence of associated injuries. If possible, weight-bearing AP, lateral, and 30 degree oblique views should be obtained. If the patient is unable to bear weight because of pain or other injuries, non–weight-bearing views are helpful preliminary studies. Disruption of the normal in-line arrangement between the metatarsal base and the opposing tarsal bone on any of the three views is indicative of a Lisfranc injury. The AP view allows evaluation of the lateral border of the first cuneiform with the first metatarsal base and the medial border of the second metatarsal base with the second cuneiform. The 30 degree oblique view shows the alignment of the medial border of the third metatarsal with the lateral cuneiform and the medial border of the fourth metatarsal base with the medial border of the cuboid. The lateral view allows a rough assessment of the dorsum of the second metatarsal with the middle cuneiform. The position of the second metatarsal on the AP view and the position of the fourth metatarsal on the oblique view are the most consistent indicators of an unstable injury. A small avulsion fracture off the base of either the medial cuneiform bone or the second metatarsal may be visible ("fleck sign"). If necessary to confirm the diagnosis, stress views can be obtained, usually with the use of an ankle block to minimize pain and muscle guarding. CT scanning and MRI can help evaluate the plantar bony structures and determine the amount of comminution.

Classification

Several classification systems have been proposed for Lisfranc injuries. The system described by Quenu and Kuss divides these injuries into three types based on the resultant pattern (Fig. 5-49). The more recent Orthopaedic Trauma Association (OTA) classification also classifies these injuries by the resulting deformity (Fig. 5-50).

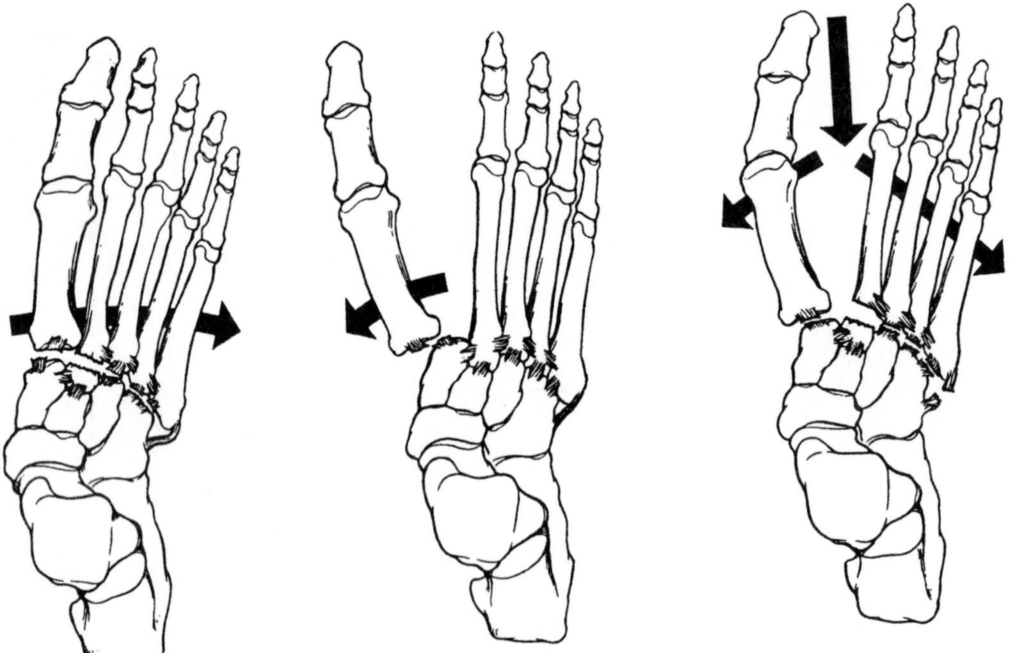

FIGURE 5-49 ■ Classification of tarsometatarsal injuries described by Quenu and Kuss: homolateral, partial, divergent. Further subdivisions are used to identify the direction of the dislocation in the homolateral pattern (medial or lateral) and the partial dislocation (first or lesser). (From Early, J.S.: Fractures and dislocations of the midfoot and forefoot. In Bucholz, R.W., and Heckman, J.D., eds.: Rockwood and Green's Fractures in Adults, 5th ed. Philadelphia, Lippincott Williams & Wilkins, 2001, p. 2207.)

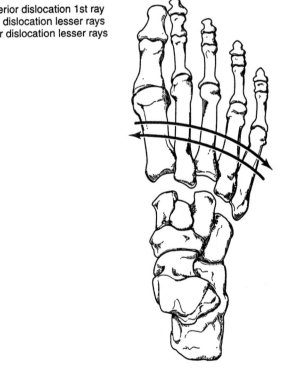

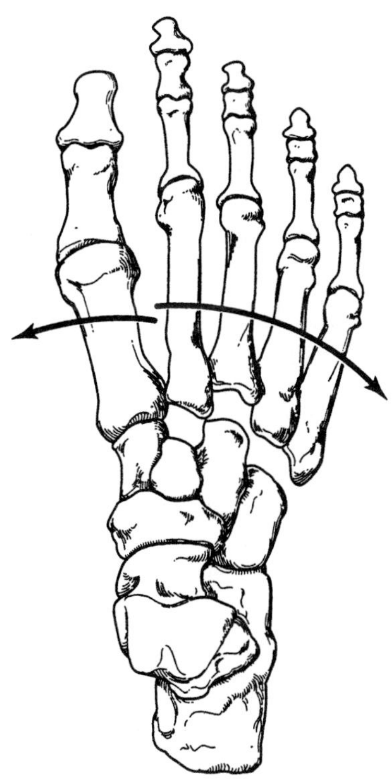

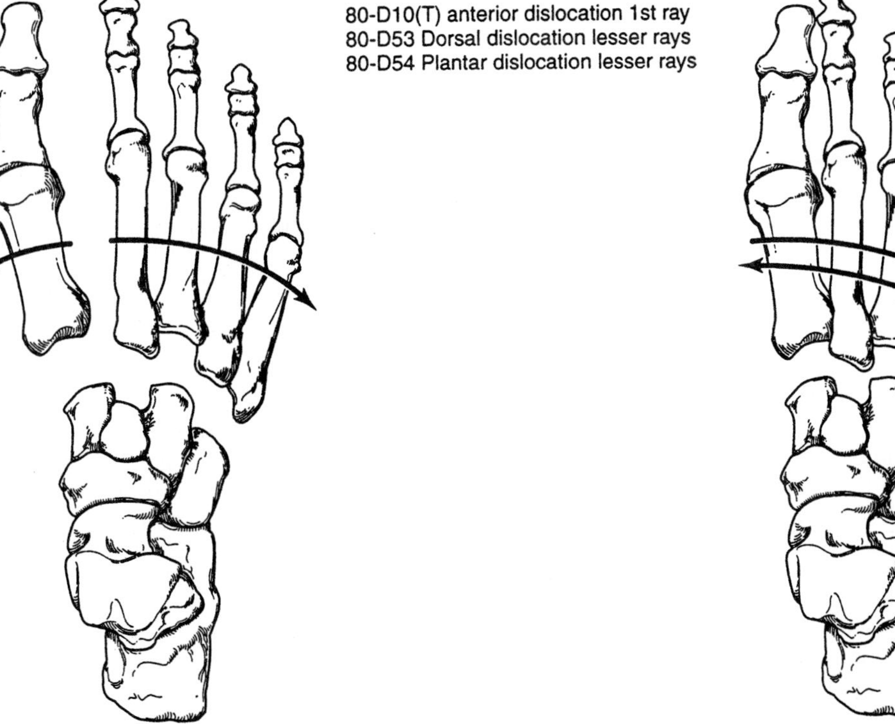

FIGURE 5-50 ■ Classification of the Orthopaedic Trauma Association (OTA) for tarsometatarsal injuries. (From J. Orthop. Trauma 10 (Suppl.) 1:150, 1996.)

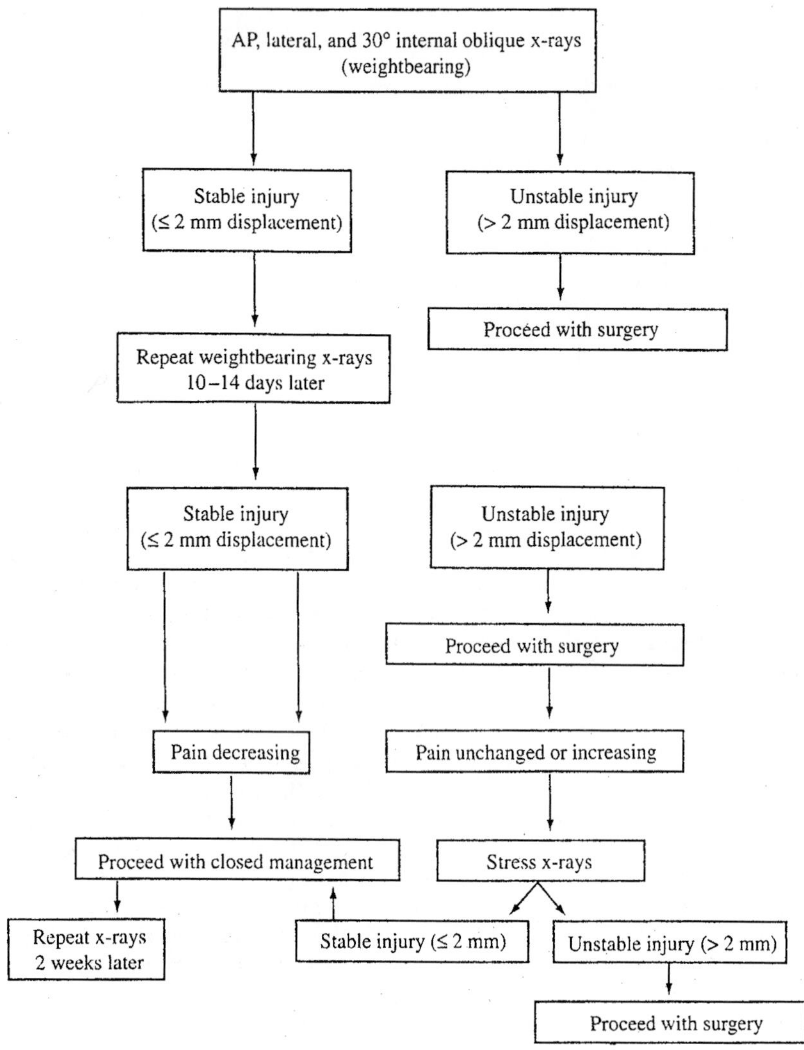

FIGURE 5-51 ■ Algorithm for treatment of tarsometatarsal injuries based on radiographic evaluation. (From Chiodo, C.P., Myerson, M.S.: Developments and advances in the diagnosis and treatment of injuries to the tarsometatarsal joint. Orthop. Clin. North Am. 32:11–20, 2001.)

Treatment (Fig. 5-51)

Closed treatment of tarsometatarsal injuries generally is indicated when the tarsometatarsal joint is displaced less than 2 mm in any plane and there is no evidence of joint line instability on weight-bearing or stress views. Patients who present with painful weight-bearing, pain with metatarsal motion, and tenderness to palpation but no clinical or radiographic signs of instability should be considered to have midfoot "sprains," and should be treated with rest, ice, compression, and elevation initially, then with immobilization in a short-leg walking cast for approximately 6 weeks, followed by a weight-bearing cast for another 4–6 weeks.

Any instability in this joint requires anatomic reduction. Presently, instability is defined as more than 2-mm shift in normal joint position. Most Lisfranc dislocations can be reduced closed with gentle axial traction. Cannulated or standard 4-mm cancellous screws can be inserted under image control to maintain reduction (Fig. 5-52). If closed reduction is inadequate or severe comminution is present, open reduction is preferred, especially in partial or divergent injury patterns.

Compartment syndrome usually occurs only with high-energy Lisfranc fracture-dislocation, but should be considered whenever there is severe swelling. Compartmental pressure measurement should be attempted; however, if individual compartments cannot be evaluated, clinical suspicion is enough to warrant decompression. A long medial incision can be used to decompress the abductor hallucis and deep compartments of the foot, including the calcaneal compartment. Two incisions, one between the second and third and one between the fourth and fifth metatarsals, are used for the dorsal intrinsic compartments.

E. Fractures of the Metatarsals

Fractures of the metatarsals are caused by direct or indirect forces. Acute direct forces occur

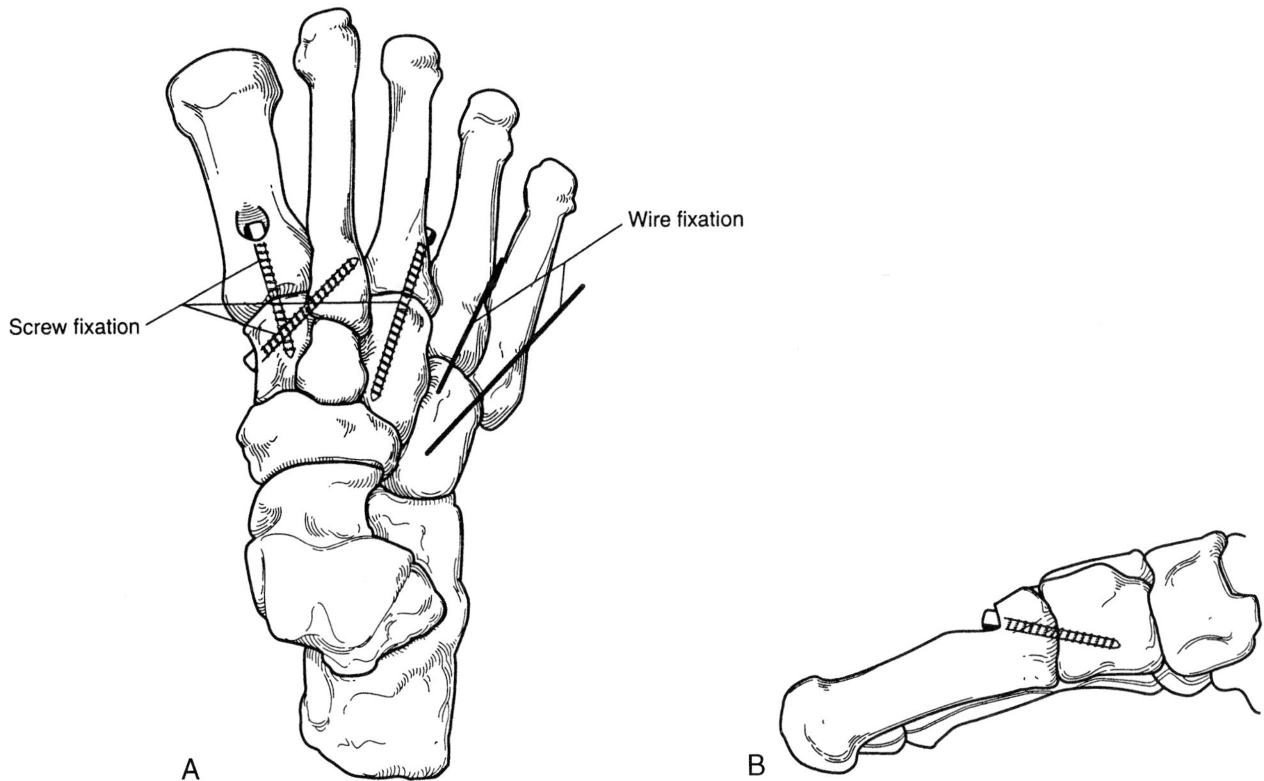

FIGURE 5-52 ■ Fixation of tarsometatarsal injuries. *A*, 3.5-mm screws are used to stabilize medial column; the usual procedure restores the position of the second metatarsal first, followed by the third and then the first. If necessary, the lateral column can be stabilized with percutaneous Kirschner wires. *B*, Longitudinal cross-section shows recommended notching of metatarsal base to avoid fracturing the cortex. (From Early, J.S.: Fractures and dislocations of the midfoot and forefoot. In Bucholz, R.W., Heckman, J.D., eds.: Rockwood and Green's Fractures in Adults, 5th ed. Philadelphia, Lippincott Williams & Wilkins, 2001, p. 2213.)

most commonly as a result of crushing-type injuries, such as heavy object falling onto the dorsum of the foot, producing transverse or comminuted fracture patterns, often of adjacent metatarsals, with varying degrees of skin injury. Chronic direct forces produce stress fractures, most commonly of the diaphyses of the second and third metatarsals. Indirect forces occur when the forefoot is held fixed and the leg or foot is twisted, producing an oblique metatarsal fracture pattern with soft-tissue swelling.

Metatarsal fractures may produce pain, swelling, ecchymosis, deformity, inability to bear weight, pain with passive motion, and crepitus. Initial radiographic evaluation should include simulated weight-bearing AP and lateral views and oblique views. Bone scans are helpful to identify stress fractures. Anatomically, the metatarsals fall into three distinct groups: the first and fifth metatarsals because of their locations and unique functions, and the three central metatarsals because of the interconnectivity.

1. ***Fractures of the metatarsal base.*** Injuries to the metatarsal bases occur primarily through metaphyseal bone and heal rapidly (within 6 weeks). Oblique fractures heal more rapidly than transverse or comminuted fractures. When multiple metatarsals are fractured, a Lisfranc injury must be ruled out.
2. ***Fractures of the metatarsal shaft.*** The ***first metatarsal*** is wider and shorter than the four lesser metatarsals. The lack of interconnecting ligaments between the first and second metatarsal bones allows independent motion of the hallux. The first metatarsal head supports two sesamoid bones that provide two of the six contact points of the foot, meaning that the first ray supports a third of the forefoot weight at any one time. It is important to maintain the normal position of the first ray in relation to the foot. As seen on stress radiographs, manual displacement of the position of the first metatarsal through the joint or fracture indicates an instability that requires fixation. If no instability is present, isolated first metatarsal fractures can be treated in a short-leg cast for 4–6 weeks. Any evidence of instability or loss of normal position of

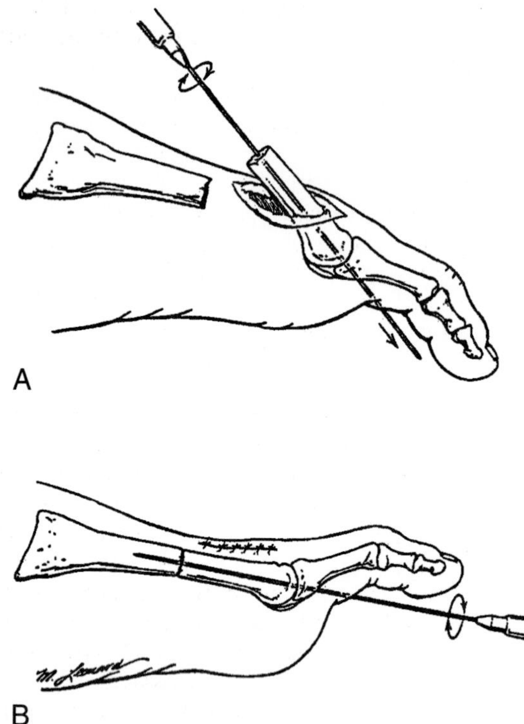

FIGURE 5-53 ■ *A*, Kirschner wire is inserted retrograde into metatarsal shaft with minimal dorsiflexion of the metatarsophalangeal joint to avoid impaling the plantar plate. *B*, Kirschner wire is then advanced antegrade across the fracture. (From Thordarson, D.B.: Fractures of the midfoot and forefoot. In Myerson, M.S., ed.: Foot and Ankle Disorders. Philadelphia, WB Saunders, 2000, p. 1288.)

the metatarsal head requires operative stabilization. The method of fixation depends on the configuration of the fracture and may include closed reduction and percutaneous smooth wire fixation (Fig. 5-53) or open reduction and screw or plate-and-screw fixation. External fixation may be indicated for severely comminuted fractures with inadequate intact bone to allow lag screw fixation or to support a one-third tubular plate.

Fractures of the ***central metatarsals*** are more common than those of the first metatarsal and can be isolated injuries or part of a more complex injury pattern. Almost all isolated individual central metatarsal fractures can be treated closed. Generally accepted criteria for in situ management in a hard-sole or stiff-sole shoe are less than 10 degrees of angulation along the long axis of the shaft and less than 4-mm translation of the shaft. Sagittal plane displacement of a metatarsal head in either extension or plantar flexion or excessive shortening of a metatarsal will lead to metatarsalgia and chronic forefoot pain, and closed reduction and percutaneous pinning are indicated. Occasionally, severe displacement requires ORIF.

Most injuries of the ***fifth metatarsal*** occur in athletic or dance activities. Fifth metatarsal fractures often are described as "Jones fractures," because of his description of fractures of the fifth metatarsal in four dancers. However, more recent descriptions include three types of fractures in the fifth metatarsal (Fig. 5-54). *Avulsion fractures* at the base of the fifth metatarsal (zone 1) are the most common and usually occur from an indirect load that causes tension on the lateral band of the plantar fascia. The size of the avulsed fragment varies from a small fleck of bone to almost the whole tuberosity. Almost all tuberosity avulsion fractures can be treated in a hard-sole shoe or walking cast until pain subsides. Rarely, a displaced or intra-articular tuberosity avulsion fracture with extensive articular step-off requires open reduction and internal fixation with a screw or Kirschner wires.

Injuries in zone 2 are *true Jones fractures* and are acute injuries believed to be caused by application of a large adduction force to the forefoot with the ankle plantar flexed. If the force is of sufficient magnitude, a transverse or short oblique fracture results at the junction of the metaphysis and the diaphysis, entering the fourth-fifth metatarsal joint. The recommended treatment of acute nondisplaced Jones fractures is immobilization in a non-weight-bearing short-leg cast for 6–8 weeks. If healing is not adequate after 6–8 weeks, protection can be continued or intramedullary screw fixation with bone grafting can be done. In high-performance athletes, early operative intervention may be warranted to allow rapid return to sports.

Proximal diaphyseal stress fractures (zone 3) occur mainly in athletes and occur in the proximal 1.5 cm of the diaphyseal shaft of the metatarsal. Repetitive cyclic loads such as those produced by high-level athletic activity appear to be the underlying

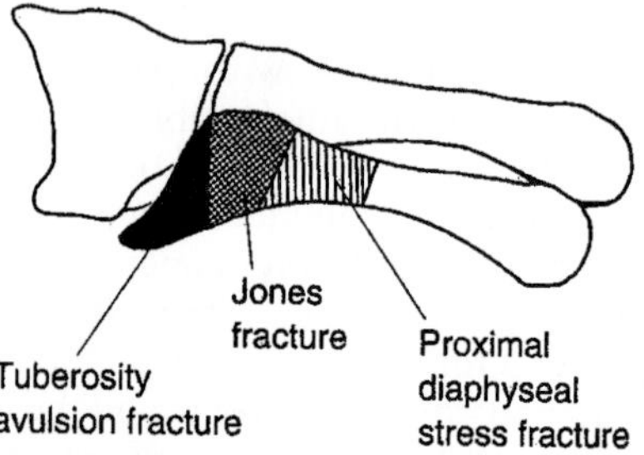

FIGURE 5-54 ■ Fracture zones of proximal fifth metatarsal fractures. (From Lawrence, S.T., Botte, M.J.: Jones fractures and related fractures of the proximal fifth metatarsal, Foot Ankle Int. 14:358–365, 1993.)

mechanism for these injuries. Tensile forces result in microfractures at the lateral cortex and continued loading propagates the fracture medially. *Dancer's fractures* are spiral, oblique fractures that progress from distal-lateral to proximal-medial and are caused by a rotational force applied to the foot while axially loaded in a plantar flexed position, usually by rolling over the outer border of the foot. Torg and colleagues described a radiographic continuum of fifth metatarsal stress fractures that included three types. Acute fractures are characterized by a fracture line with sharp margins, without widening or radiolucency, and minimal cortical hypertrophy or evidence of periosteal reaction. A delayed union is characterized by a previous injury or fracture, a fracture line that involves both cortices and displaced associated periosteal new bone, a widened fracture line with adjacent radiolucency resulting from bone resorption, and evidence of intramedullary sclerosis. Nonunions are identified by a history of repetitive trauma and recurrent symptoms, a wide fracture line with periosteal new bone and radiolucency, and complete obliteration of the medullary canal by sclerotic bone at the fracture site.

Acute diaphyseal stress fractures (Torg type I) can be treated with non-weight-bearing immobilization for 6–8 weeks. Delayed unions (type II) and nonunions (type III) usually require operative treatment with closed axial intramedullary-screw fixation, tricortical-inlay bone grafting, or a combination of the two techniques. Recent studies have reported good results with the use of electrical stimulation in the treatment of small series of delayed unions and nonunions of the proximal fifth metatarsal.

F. MTP Joint Injuries

Injury to the first MTP joint complex is common in sports injuries and can range from a minor sprain to frank dislocation or disruption of the complex. Mechanisms of injury described include hyperdorsiflexion (turf toe), plantar flexion (sand toe), and valgus and varus stresses; simultaneous axial loading of the joint occurs with all of these. Careful physical examination is necessary for accurate diagnosis. Pain with weight-bearing or exertional activities may be the only sign of a mild, isolated injury. The loss of the normal parabolic cascade of the toes is suggestive of injury to the MTP joint. The range of joint motion and stability in all planes should be compared with the contralateral joint to identify subtle differences. Acute instability in any plane indicates a significant injury. The dorsoplantar translation test (Fig. 5-55) is useful for evaluating stability. Increased translation relative to the contralateral side indicates instability of the capsuloligamentous complex. Radiographs should include weight-bearing AP and lateral views, medial and lateral oblique views, and sesamoid views. Sprains of the MTP joint can be treated with rest and immobilization depending on the severity of the sprain. Stiff-soled shoes or rigid inserts can be used to minimize capsular stretch. Operative treatment rarely is required except for intra-articular fractures or significant instability. Acute dislocations should be immediately reduced with gravity traction. Easy reduction indicates an injury to the plantar plate and an unstable joint; if the plantar plate is intact, closed reduction usually is not possible. With either an unstable joint or

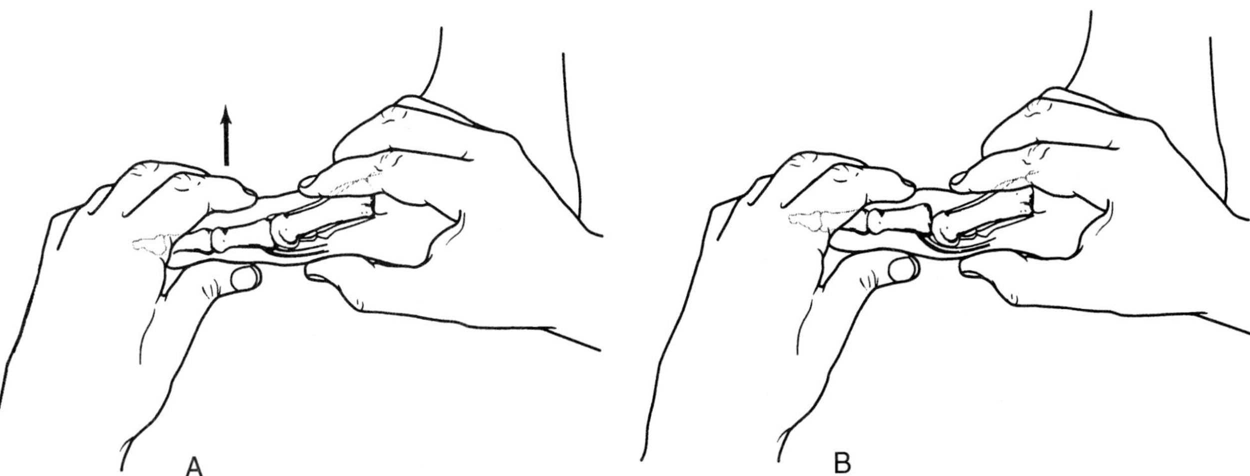

FIGURE 5-55 ■ Test of stability of the metatarsophalangeal joint. *A*, Position of hands to test dorsoplantar stability of plantar complex. *B*, Direction of motion. (From Early, J.S.: Fractures and dislocations of the midfoot and forefoot. In Bucholz, R.W., Heckman, J.D., eds.: Rockwood and Green's Fractures in Adults, 5th ed. Philadelphia, Lippincott Williams & Wilkins, 2001, p. 2230.)

an irreducible dislocation, operative treatment is necessary to restore stability and function.

The ***sesamoids*** are part of the capsuloligamentous structure of the first MTP joint, where they function as shock absorbers and as a fulcrum to support the weight-bearing function of the hallux. Located on either side of the FHL, they form a bony tunnel to protect the tendon. Injuries to the sesamoids can range from sesamoiditis to stress fracture and acute fracture. Acute injuries can be caused by a fall from a height or by landing from a jump, as in ballet dancers, as well as by the hyperpronation and axial loading mechanism that results in MTP joint dislocation. Repetitive loading can result in stress fractures. The medial sesamoid is more often injured than the lateral sesamoid.

The presenting symptom usually is localized pain on the plantar aspect of the joint directly over the involved sesamoid. A soft-tissue callus over the sesamoid indicates a chronic injury. AP and lateral radiographs should be obtained, but sesamoid views (see Fig. 5-17) are most helpful. Partite sesamoids are present in up to 30% of the population and should not be mistaken for fracture; the edges of a partite sesamoid are smooth and sclerotic, whereas fracture margins are rough and irregular. CT and MRI can be helpful in identifying sesamoid injury.

Initial treatment of any isolated, stable injury of the sesamoids is immobilization for 4-6 weeks, followed by use of a stiff-sole shoe for another 4-6 weeks. Complete relief of symptoms can take up to 6 months. If symptoms persist, excision of the sesamoid or bone grafting of the ununited defect should be considered. If the articular surface of the sesamoid is intact, bone grafting is the best treatment option. Excision of sesamoid can lead to an imbalance in the dynamic mechanism of the MTP joint that can result in transfer metatarsalgia, hallux varus or valgus deformities, or cock-up toe deformities.

G. Phalangeal Fractures

Phalangeal fractures are the most common injuries to the forefoot; the proximal phalanx of the fifth toe is the one most often involved. Phalangeal fractures usually are caused by a stubbing mechanism (axial loading with varus or valgus force) or by a heavy load dropped onto the foot. Presenting symptoms are pain, ecchymosis, and swelling. All nondisplaced phalangeal fractures, with or without articular involvement, can be treated with stiff-soled shoes and protected weight-bearing. "Buddy taping" of the injured toe to an adjacent toe may improve pain relief and help stabilize potentially unstable fractures. Fractures with clinical deformity require reduction; closed reduction with gravity traction and axial realignment usually is possible and the reduction usually is stable. Operative treatment rarely is required for gross instability or intra-articular discontinuity.

Selected Bibliography

ANATOMY AND BIOMECHANICS

Hunt, A.E., Smith, R.M., Torode, M.: Extrinsic muscle activity, foot motion and ankle joint moments during the stance phase of walking. Foot Ankle Int. 22:31-41, 2001.

Salathe, E.P., Arangio, G.A.: A biomechanical model of the foot: the role of muscles, tendons, and ligaments. J. Biomech. Eng. 124:281-287, 2002.

PHYSICAL EXAMINATION

Chambers, H.G., Sutherland, D.H.: A practical guide to gait analysis. J. Am. Acad. Orthop. Surg. 10:222-231, 2002.

HALLUX VALGUS

Aronson, J., Nguyen, L.L., Aronson, E.A.: Early results of the modified Peterson bunion procedure for adolescent hallux valgus. J. Pediatr. Orthop. 21:65-69, 2001.

Coughlin, M.J., Saltzman, C.L., Nunley, J.A., II: Angular measurements in the evaluation of hallux valgus deformities: a report of the ad hoc committee of the American Orthopaedic Foot & Ankle Society on angular measurements. Foot Ankle Int. 23:68-74, 2002.

Donley, B.G., Vaughn, R.A., Stephenson, K.A., Richardson, E.G.: Keller resection arthroplasty for treatment of hallux valgus deformity: increased correction with fibular sesamoidectomy. Foot Ankle Int. 23:699-703, 2002.

Richardson, E.G.: Complications after hallux valgus surgery. Instr. Course. Lect. 48:331-342, 1999.

Richardson, E.G., Donley, B.G.: Disorders of hallux. In Canale, S.T., ed.: Campbell's Operative Orthopaedics, 10th ed. St. Louis, C.V. Mosby, 2003.

Thordarson, D.B., Rudicel, S.A., Ebramzadeh E., Gill, L.H.: Outcome study of hallux valgus surgery—an AOFAS multi-center study. Foot Ankle Int. 22:956-959, 2001.

Veri, J.P., Pirani, S.P., Claridge, R.: Crescentic proximal metatarsal osteotomy for moderate to severe hallux valgus: a mean 12.2 year follow-up study. Foot Ankle Int. 22:817-822, 2001.

SESAMOID INJURIES

Richardson, E.G.: Hallucal sesamoid pain: causes and surgical treatment. J. Am. Acad. Orthop. Surg. 7:270-278, 1999.

LESSER-TOE DEFORMITIES

Coughlin, M.J., Dorris, J., Polk, E.: Operative repair of the fixed hammertoe deformity. Foot Ankle 21:94-104, 2000.

Femino, J.E., Mueller, K.: Complications of lesser toe surgery. Clin. Orthop. 391:72-88, 2001.

Murphy, G.A.: Mallet toe deformity. Foot Ankle Clin. 3:279, 1998.

Murphy, G.A.: Lesser toe abnormalities. In Canale, S.T., ed.: Campbell's Operative Orthopaedics, 10th ed. St. Louis, C.V. Mosby, 2003.

Richardson, E.G.: Lesser toe deformities: an overview. Foot Ankle Clin. 3:195-198, 1998.

NEUROGENIC DISORDERS

Coughlin, M.J., Pinsonneault, T.: Operative treatment of interdigital neuroma. A long-term follow-up study. J. Bone Joint Surg. [Am.] 83:1321-1328, 2001.

Richardson, E.G.: Neurogenic disorders. In Canale, S.T., ed.: Campbell's Operative Orthopaedics, 10th ed. St. Louis, C.V. Mosby, 2003.

INFLAMMATORY ARTHRITIS

Coughlin, M.J.: Rheumatoid forefoot reconstruction. A long-term follow-up study. J. Bone Joint Surg. [Am.] 82:322-341, 2000.

Easley, M.E., Trnka, H.J., Schon, L.C., Myerson, M.S.: Isolated subtalar arthrodesis. J. Bone Joint Surg. [Am.] 82:613-624, 2000.

Hamalainen M., Raunio, P.: Long-term follow-up of rheumatoid forefoot surgery. Clin. Orthop. 340:34-38, 1997.

Richardson, E.G.: Rheumatoid foot. In Canale, S.T., ed.: Campbell's Operative Orthopaedics, 10th ed. St. Louis, C.V. Mosby, 2003.

OSTEOARTHRITIS

Brage, M.: Degenerative joint disease of the midfoot. Foot Ankle Clin. 4:355–368, 1999.

Ishikawa, S.N., Abidi, A.: Degenerative disease of the hindfoot. Foot Ankle Clin. 4:369–394, 1999.

Shereff, M.J., Baumhauer, J.F.: Hallux rigidus and osteoarthrosis of the first metatarsophalangeal joint. J. Bone Joint Surg. [Am.] 80:898–908, 1998.

PES PLANUS AND PES CAVUS

Giannini, S., Ceccarelli, F., Benedetti, M.G., et al.: Surgical treatment of adult idiopathic cavus foot with plantar fasciotomy, naviculocuneiform arthrodesis, and cuboid osteotomy: A review of thirty-nine cases. J. Bone Joint Surg. [Am.] 84 (Suppl.) 2:62–69, 2002.

Malicky, E.S., Crary, J.L., Houghton, M.J., et al.: Talocalcaneal and subfibular impingement in symptomatic flatfoot in adults. J. Bone Joint Surg. [Am.] 84:2005–2009, 2002.

McCormack, A.P., Ching, R.P., Sangeorzan, B.J.: Biomechanics of procedures used in adult flatfoot deformity. Foot Ankle Clin. 6:15–23, 2001.

Murphy, G.A.: Pes planus. In Canale, S.T., ed.: Campbell's Operative Orthopaedics, 10th ed. St. Louis, C.V. Mosby, 2003.

TENDON PATHOLOGY

Coetzee, J.C., Hansen, S.T.: Surgical management of severe deformity resulting from posterior tibial tendon dysfunction. Foot Ankle Int. 22:944–949, 2001.

Cohen, B.E., Johnson, J.E.: Subtalar arthrodesis for treatment of posterior tibial tendon insufficiency. Foot Ankle Clin. 6:121–128, 2001.

Crates, J., Richardson, E.G.: Treatment of stage I posterior tibial tendon dysfunction with medial soft-tissue procedures. Clin. Orthop. 365:46–49, 1999.

Hockenbury, R.T., Sammarco, G.J.: Medial sliding calcaneal osteotomy with flexor hallucis longus transfer for the treatment of posterior tibial tendon insufficiency. Foot Ankle Clin. 6:569–581, 2001.

Johnson, J.E., Cohen, B.E., DeGiovanni, B.F., Lamdan, R.: Subtalar arthrodesis with flexor digitorum longus transfer and spring ligament repair for treatment of posterior tibial tendon insufficiency. Foot Ankle Int. 21:722–729, 2000.

Murphy, G.A.: Disorders of tendons and fascia. In Canale, S.T., ed.: Campbell's Operative Orthopaedics, 10th ed. St. Louis, C.V. Mosby, 2003.

Schepsis, A.A., Jones, H., Haas, L.A.: Achilles tendon disorders in athletes. Am. J. Sports Med. 30:287–305, 2002.

HEEL PAIN

Pfeffer, G.B.: Plantar heel pain. Instr. Course. Lect. 50:521–531, 2001.

Schneider, W., Niehus, W., Knahr, K.: Haglund's syndrome: disappointing results following surgery—a clinical and radiographic analysis. Foot Ankle Int. 21:26–30, 2000.

Watson, T.S., Anderson, R.B., Davis, W.H., Kiebzak, G.M.: Distal tarsal tunnel release with partial plantar fasciotomy for chronic heel pain: an outcome analysis. Foot Ankle Int. 23:530–537, 2002.

DIABETIC FOOT

Guyton, G.P., Saltzman, C.L.: The diabetic foot: basic mechanisms of disease. Instr. Course. Lect. 51:169–181, 2002.

Myerson, M.S., Alvarez, R.G., Lam, P.W.: Tibiocalcaneal arthrodesis for the management of severe ankle and hindfoot deformities. Foot Ankle Int. 21:643–650, 2000.

Robertson, D.D., Mueller, M.J., Smith, K.E., et al.: Structural changes in the forefoot of individuals with diabetes and a prior plantar ulcer. J. Bone Joint Surg. [Am.] 84:1395–1404, 2002.

Simon, S.R., Tejwani, S.G., Wilson, D.L., et al.: Arthrodesis as an early alternative to nonoperative management of Charcot arthropathy of the diabetic foot. J. Bone Joint Surg. [Am.] 82:939–950, 2000.

FRACTURES AND DISLOCATIONS

Aktuglu, K., Aydogan, U.: The functional outcome of displaced intra-articular calcaneal fractures: a comparison between isolated cases and polytrauma patients. Foot Ankle Int. 23:314–318, 2002.

Armagan, O.E., Shereff, M.J.: Injuries to the toes and metatarsals. Orthop. Clin. North Am. 32:1–10, 2001.

Biedert, R., Hintermann, B.: Stress fractures of the medial great toe sesamoids in athletes. Foot Ankle Int. 24:137–141, 2003.

Buckley, R., Tough, S., McCormack, R., et al.: Operative compared with nonoperative treatment of displaced intraarticular calcaneal fractures: a prospective, randomized, controlled multicenter trial. J. Bone Joint Surg. [Am.] 84:1733–1744, 2002.

Chiodo, C.P., Myerson, M.S.: Developments and advances in the diagnosis and treatment of injuries to the tarsometatarsal joint. Orthop. Clin. North Am. 32:11–20, 2001.

Coris, E.E., Lombardo, J.A.: Tarsal navicular stress fractures. Am. Fam. Physician 67:85–90, 2003.

Larson, C.M., Almekinders, L.C., Taft, T.N., Garrett, W.E.: Intramedullary screw fixation of Jones fractures. Analysis of failure. Am. J. Sports Med. 30:55–60, 2002.

Murphy, G.A.: Fractures and dislocations of the foot. In Canale, S.T., ed.: Campbell's Operative Orthopaedics, 10th ed. St. Louis, C.V. Mosby, 2003.

Nunley, J.A.: Fractures of the base of the fifth metatarsal: the Jones fracture. Orthop. Clin. North Am. 32:171–180, 2001.

Nunley, J.A., Vertullo, C.F.: Classification, investigation, and management of midfoot sprains: Lisfranc injuries in the athlete. Am. J. Sports Med. 30:871–878, 2002.

Pinney, S.J., Sangeorzan, B.J.: Fractures of the tarsal bones. Orthop. Clin. North Am. 32:21–33, 2001.

Quénu, E., Küss, G.: Étude sue les luxations du metatarse (luxations metatarsotarsiennes) du diastasis entre le 1er et le 2e metatarsien. Bev Chir 39: 2811-1290, 1909.

Randle, J.A., Kreder, H.J., Stephen, D., et al.: Should calcaneal fractures be treated surgically? A meta-analysis. Clin. Orthop. 377:217–227, 2000.

Richardson, E.G.: Hallucal sesamoid pain: causes and surgical management. J. Am. Acad. Orthop. Surg. 7:270–278, 1999.

Richter, M., Wippermann, B., Krettek, C., Schratt, H.E., Hufner, T., Therman, H.: Fractures and fracture dislocations of the midfoot: occurrence, causes, and long-term results. Foot Ankle Int. 22:392–398, 2001.

Rosenberg, G.A., Sferra, J.J.: Treatment strategies for acute fractures and nonunions of the proximal fifth metatarsal. J. Am. Acad. Orthop. Surg. 8:332–338, 2000.

Torg, J.S., Balduini, F.C., Zelko, R.R., et al.: Fractures of the base of the fifth metatarsal distal to the tuberosity. Classification and guidelines for non-surgical and surgical management. J. Bone. Joint. Surg. 661-1A: 209–214, 1984.

Zmurko, M.G., Karges, D.E.: Functional outcome of patients following open reduction and internal fixation for bilateral calcaneus fractures. Foot Ankle Int. 23:917–921, 2002.

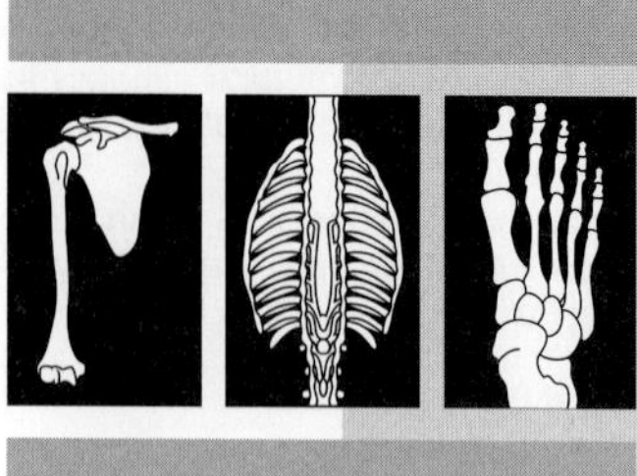

6 Hand and Microsurgery

RICHARD F. HOWARD

I. Anatomy and Pathophysiology (see also Chapter 11, Anatomy)

COMP	TENDON	ASSOCIATED PATHOLOGIC CONDITIONS
1	EPB/APL	De Quervain's tenosynovitis
2	ECRL/ECRB	Intersection syndrome
3	EPL	Drummer's wrist and traumatic rupture with distal radius fracture
4	EIP/EDC	Extensor tenosynovitis
5	EDM	Vaughn-Jackson syndrome (ischemic rupture in rheumatics)
6	ECU	Snapping ECU (unstable ECU subsheath)

A. Joint Flexion and Extension

JOINT	FLEXION	EXTENSION IO
MCP	IO, lumbricals	EDC (sagittal bands)
PIP	FDS, FDP	Lumbricals (lateral bands) EDC (central slip)
DIP	FDP	EDC (terminal tendon) ORL (Landsmeer's ligament)

B. Relationships

1. The extensor indicis proprius (EIP), extensor digiti minimi (EDM), and extensor pollicis longus (EPL) are all ulnar to the extensor digitorum communis (EDC) and extensor pollicis brevis (EPB). The extensor carpi radialis brevis (ECRB) (central wrist extensor) is also ulnar to the extensor carpi radialis longus (ECRL) at the level of the wrist (Fig. 6-1).
2. Digital cutaneous ligaments—Cleland's ligament: dorsal (**c**eiling). **G**rayson's ligament: volar (**g**round); stabilizes the neurovascular bundle with finger flexion and extension (Fig. 6-2).
3. There are four dorsal **interosseous (IO)** abductors (DAB) with insertions on the index finger, long finger (both ways; radial and ulnar), and ring finger. There are three palmar adductors that adduct the index finger, ring finger, and small finger. These muscles also flex the metacarpophalangeal (MCP) and contribute to proximal interphalangeal (PIP) extension through the lateral bands (Figs. 6-3 and 6-4).
4. The **lumbrical muscles** originate on a tendon flexor digitorum profundus (FDP) and insert on a tendon (*radial lateral band of the extensor expansion*). The lumbrical tendons pass volar to the transverse metacarpal ligament. The radial two lumbricals are innervated by the median nerve and the ulnar two by the ulnar nerve. The ulnar-innervated lumbricals are bipennate, and the median innervated lumbricals are unipennate (Fig. 6-5).
5. The thenar and hypothenar abductors are superficial; the opponens muscles are deep. The flexor pollicis brevis has dual innervation: the median nerve innervates the superficial head and the ulnar nerve innervates the deep head. This branch of the ulnar nerve is its terminal branch. The remainder of the thenar muscles are innervated by the median nerve alone. The hypothenar muscles are innervated by the ulnar nerve. *The abductor pollicis brevis is primarily responsible for palmar abduction of the thumb.*
6. The superficial arch is distal, and the ulnar artery is its predominant supply. The deep arch is proximal and is primarily fed by the deep branch of the radial artery. The classic complete (codominant) arch is present in only a third of patients—hence the importance of the Allen test. *The deep branch of the radial artery becomes the deep arch as it passes between the two heads of the first dorsal interosseous muscle.* The princeps pollicis artery is the continuation of the deep branch of the radial artery after it gives off the branch to the deep arch. This then bifurcates into the thumb digital arteries after giving off the branch to the radial side of the index finger (radialis indicis). There are three common digital arteries in the second

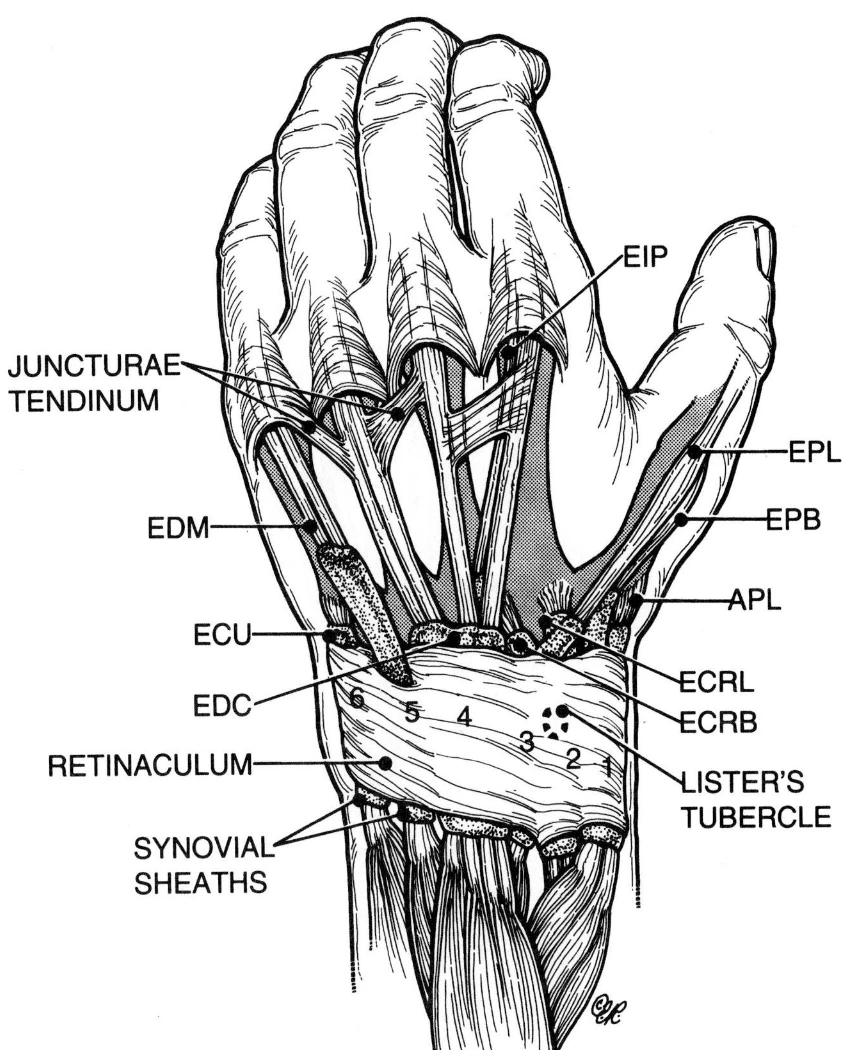

FIGURE 6-1 ■ Dorsal compartments of the wrist and extensor tendons. The fist compartment contains the abductor pollicis longus (APL) and extensor pollicis brevis (EPB); the second, the radial wrist extensors, extensor carpi radialis longus (ECRL), and extensor carpi radialis brevis (ECRB); the third, the extensor pollicis longus (EPL); the fourth, the extensor digitorum communis (EDC) to the fingers and the extensor indicis proprius (EIP); the fifth, the extensor digiti minimi (EDM); and the sixth, the extensor carpi ulnaris (ECU). (From Doyle, J.R.: Extensor tendons—Acute injuries. In Green, D.P., Hotchkiss, R.M., Pederson, W.C., eds., Green's Operative Hand Surgery, 4th ed., New York, Churchill Livingstone, 1998, p. 1951.)

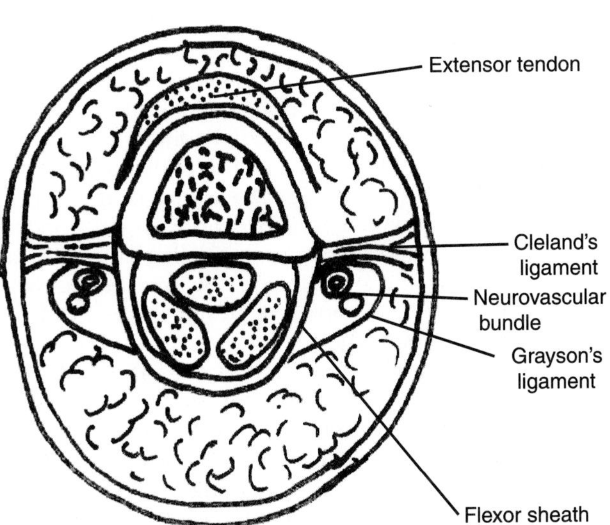

FIGURE 6-2 ■ Cross-section of the finger. The neurovascular bundle is contained by Cleland's ligament dorsally and Grayson's ligament palmarly.

through the fourth web spaces that bifurcate into the proper digital arteries. The digital artery to the ulnar side of the small finger is the first branch off the superficial arch. Arteries are volar to the nerve in the palm and dorsal in the digit (Fig. 6-6).

7. There are nine flexor tendons and one nerve (median nerve) in the carpal tunnel. The flexor pollicis longus is the most radial structure. The palmar cutaneous branch of the median nerve usually lies between the palmaris longus and the flexor carpi radialis at the level of the wrist flexion crease. The usual pattern of the recurrent motor branch of the median nerve is extraligamentous branching and recurrent innervation (50%). Other relatively common patterns include subligamentous branching with recurrent innervation (30%) and transligamentous branching and innervation (20%). Other variations are extremely rare (Fig. 6-7).

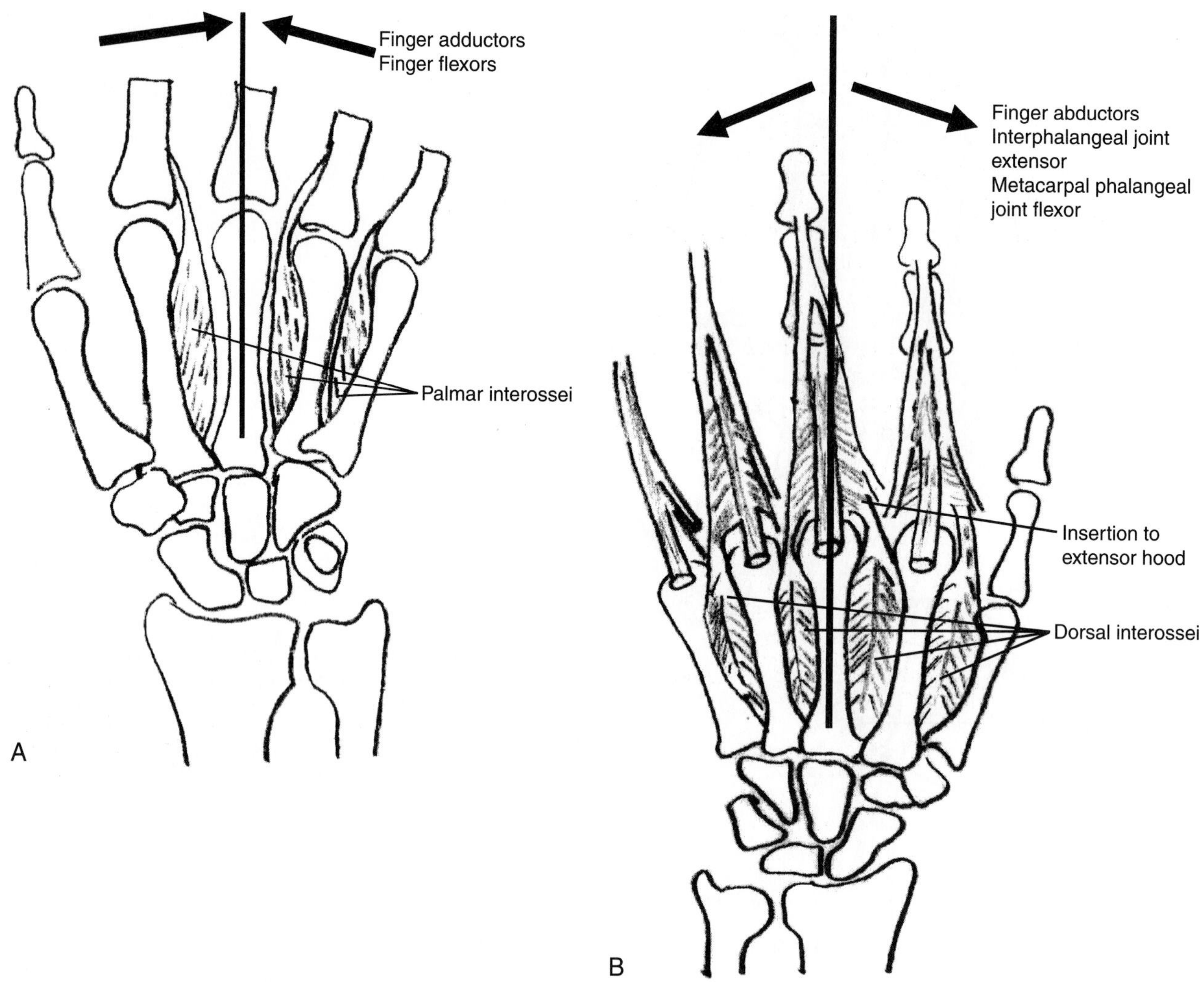

FIGURE 6-3 ■ *A.* Palmar interossei muscles. The tendons pass volar to the axis of rotation of the metacarpophalangeal joint, and are flexors and adductors of the MP joint. *B.* Dorsal interossei. These ulnar innervated muscles adduct and flex the metacarpalphalangeal joints and extend the interphalangeal joints.

8. Flexor Pulley System—Cruciate pulleys: number three at the level of the joints; they primarily facilitate sheath collapse and expansion during digital motion. Annular pulleys: number five located between the joints. *A2 and A4 are critical to preserve* so as to prevent bowstringing of the tendons with digital flexion (these are the ones that derive their origin from bone proximal and middle phalanx, respectively) (Fig. 6-8).
9. The Oblique Retinacular Ligament (of Landsmeer) (Fig. 6-9)—Originates from the periosteum of the proximal phalanx and the A2 and C1 pulleys. It inserts into the terminal tendon. *It functions to link PIP and distal interphalangeal joint (DIP) extension.* As the PIP joint extends, the volarly positioned ligament at this joint tightens. As it tightens, it pulls on the terminal tendon because it is positioned dorsally at the level of the DIP joint.
10. Small Finger Variations—Flexor digitorum superficialis (FDS) is absent in a third of the population; that is why comparison with the opposite side is important when evaluating for an FDS laceration in a small finger. EDC may be absent in half, and extension is achieved via the EDM.

C. Pathophysiology

1. Intrinsic Minus or Claw Hand—This condition is secondary to ulnar/median nerve palsy or Volkmann's ischemic contracture. Musculotendinous weakness or tightness leads to an imbalance of forces, yielding MCP hyperextension and interphalangeal (IP) joint flexion (Fig. 6-10). This characteristic posture results in deformity with loss of ability to perform

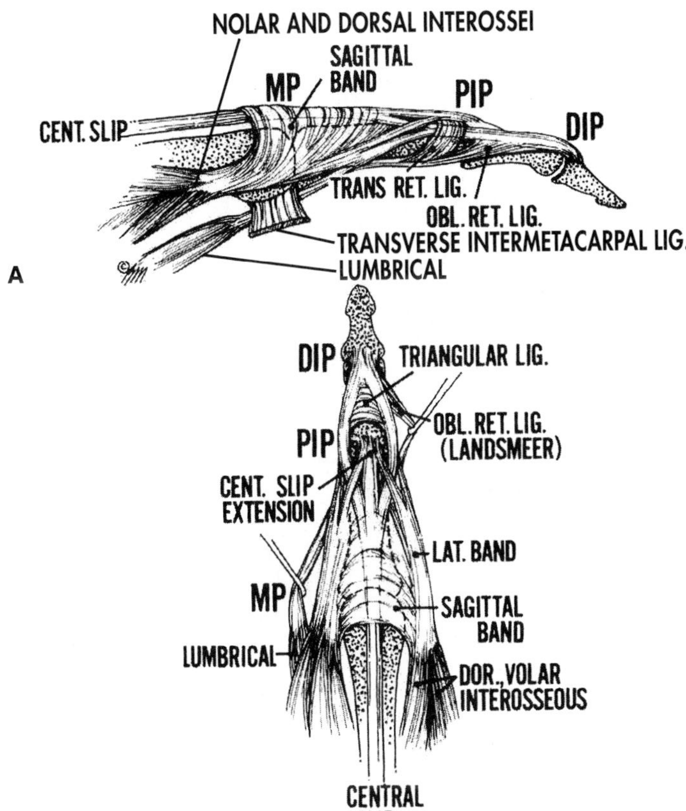

FIGURE 6-4 ■ Dorsal and lateral views of the extensor mechanism. The lumbrical tendon passes volar to the transverse metacarpal ligament, and the interossei tendons pass dorsal to the ligament. (From Doyle, J.R.: Extensor tendons—Acute injuries. In Green, D.P., Hotchkiss, R.M., Pederson, W.C., eds., Green's Operative Hand Surgery, 4th ed. Churchill Livingstone, New York, 1998, p. 1953.)

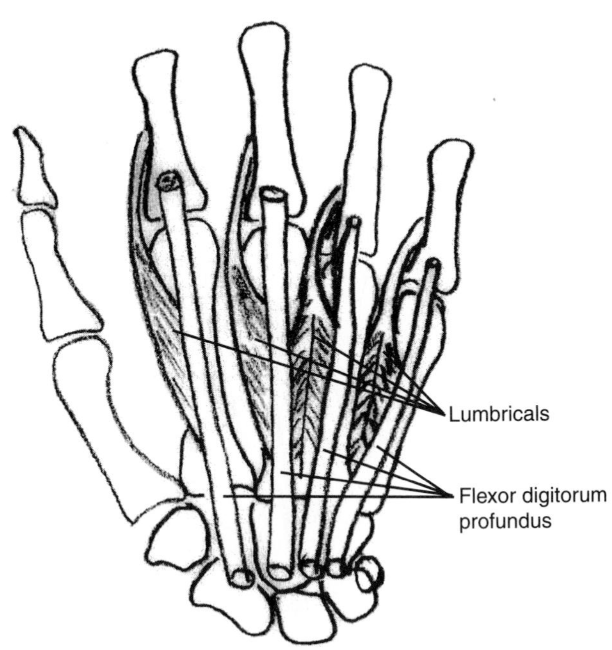

FIGURE 6-5 ■ Lumbrical muscles. The muscles originate from the flexor digitorum profundus and insert to the lateral band. The ulnar two lumbricals are bipennate, and the radial two are unipennate.

prehensile grasp and diminished grip and pinch strength. Operative treatment is directed at preventing MCP joint (MCPJ) hyperextension either by a passive tenodesis or an active tendon transfer.

2. Intrinsic Plus Hand—This is caused by intrinsic tightness or spasticity. This is generally a result of trauma or distal joint malalignment, as occurs in rheumatoid arthritis (RA). The Bunnell test differentiates intrinsic from extrinsic tightness. A positive test result for intrinsic tightness is demonstrated when there is less PIP flexion with MCPJs hyperextended (which puts the volarly oriented intrinsics on stretch), compared with when MCPJs are flexed (which puts the dorsally oriented extrinsics on stretch) (Fig. 6-11). The intrinsic plus position is characterized by MCPJ flexion and interphalangeal joint (IPJ) extension. Depending on the degree of tightness, passive stretching exercises are indicated. Otherwise, operative treatment is directed at loosening the intrinsics, either by a distal release when the deformity is severe, involving both the MCPJs and IPJs, or when the intrinsic muscles are fibrotic and dysfunctional,

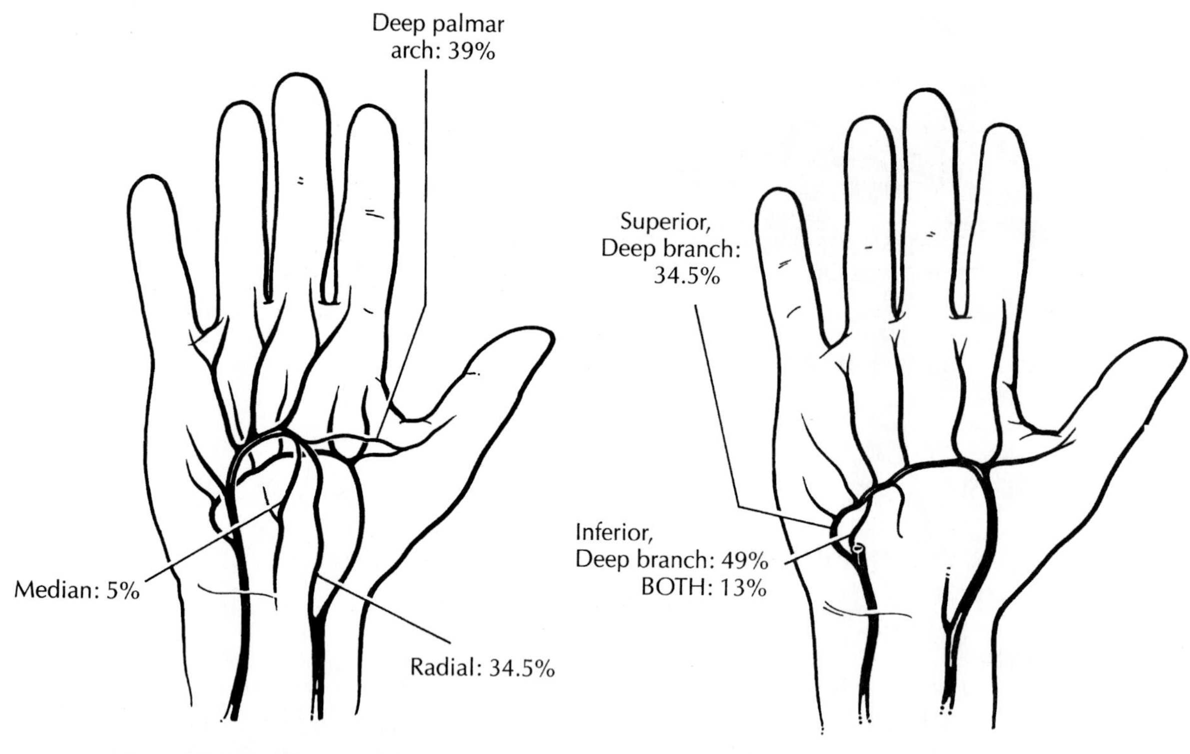

FIGURE 6-6 ■ The superficial palmar arch is completed by branches from the deep palmar arch, radial artery, or median artery in 78.5% of the patients; the remaining 21.5% are incomplete. The deep palmar arch is completed by the superior branch of the ulnar artery, the inferior branch of the ulnar artery, or both in 98.5% of patients. (From Koman, L.A. et al: Vascular disorders. In Green's Operative Hand Surgery, 4th ed. New York, Churchill Livingstone, 1998, p. 2255.)

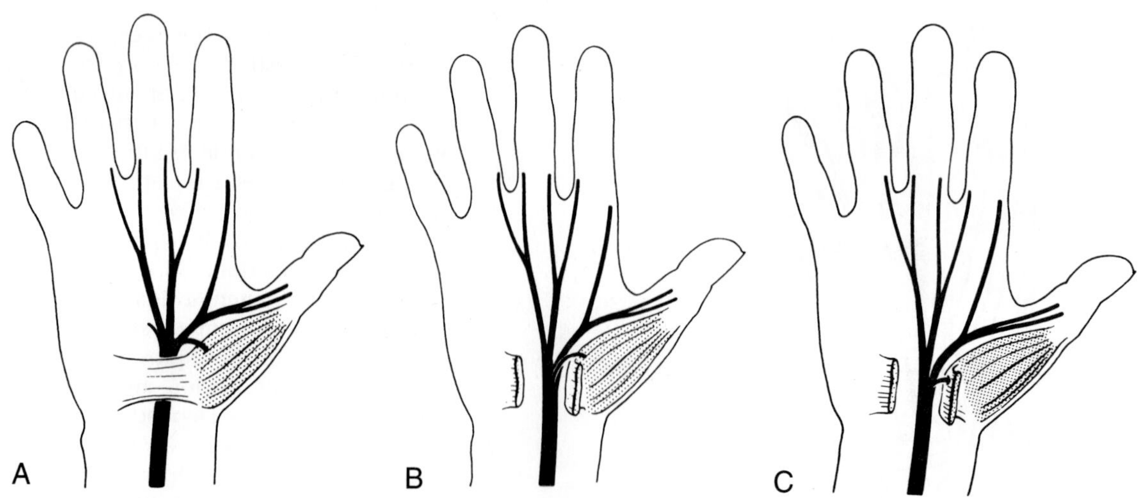

FIGURE 6-7 ■ Variations in the median nerve anatomy in the carpal tunnel. *A*, Extraligamentous and recurrent, the most common. *B*, Subligamentous branching of a recurrent median nerve. *C*, Transligamentous course of the recurrent branch of the median nerve. (From Lanz, U.: Anatomic variations of the median nerve in the carpal tunnel. J. Hand Surg. 2A:44-53, 1977.)

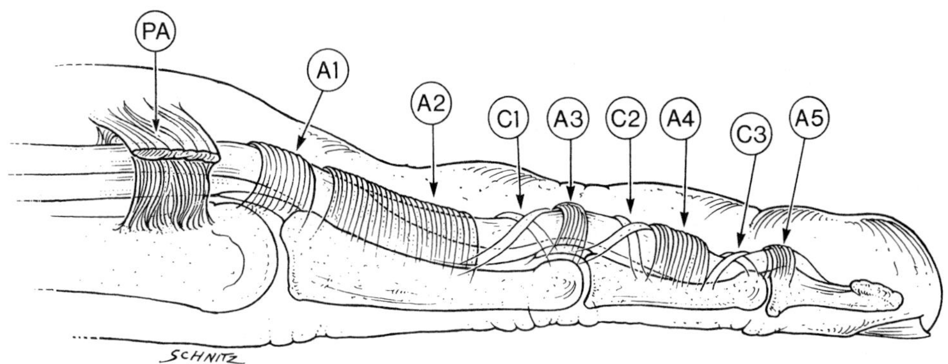

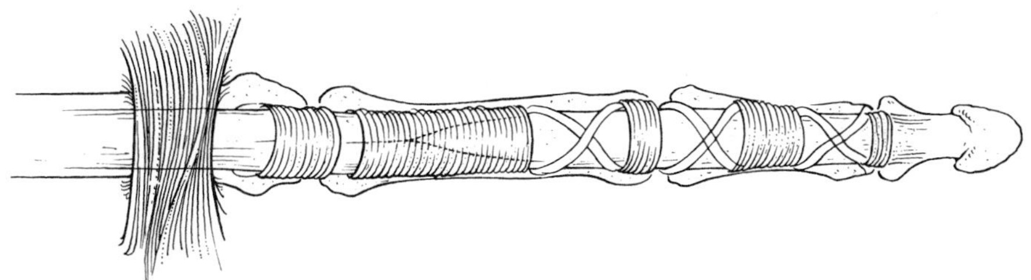

FIGURE 6-8 ■ Lateral *(top)* and palmar *(bottom)* views of a finger depict the digital flexor sheath. A1, A3, A5 pulleys originate from the volar plate. The A2 and A4 pulleys originate from bone and are the critical pulleys required for normal finger flexion. (From J.W. Strickland: Flexor tendons- acute injuries. In Green, D.P., ed., Operative Hand Surgery, 4th ed., Churchill Livingstone, New York, 1999, p. 1853.)

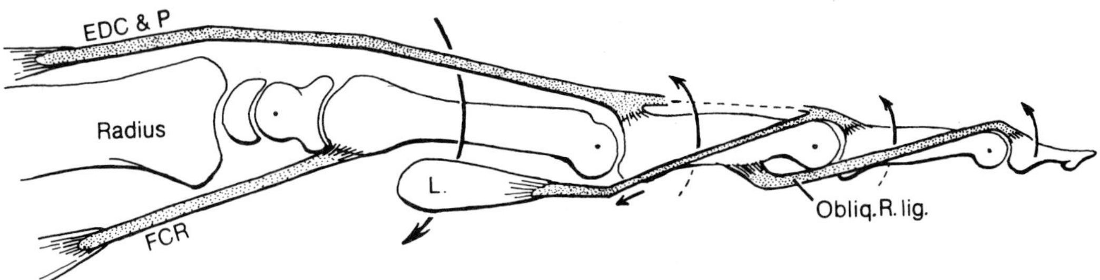

FIGURE 6-9 ■ As the wrist is flexed by the flexor carpi radialis (FCR) and the flexor carpi ulnaris, tone is increased in the extensor digitorum communis and proprius systems (EDC and P), thus passively bringing the metacarpophalangeal joint into extension. Extension of the metacarpophalangeal joint increases the tone in the intrinsic system, thereby extending the interphalangeal joints through the lateral bands and oblique retinacular ligament (Obliq.R. lig.). (From Green, D.P., Hotchkiss, R.M., Pederson, W.C., and Lampert, R., eds.: Green's Operative Hand Surgery, 4th ed. New York, Churchill Livingstone, 1999. Adapted from Littler, J.W., Burton, R.I., and Eaton, R.G.: The dynamics of digital extension. AAOS Sound Slide Program 467, 468, 1976.)

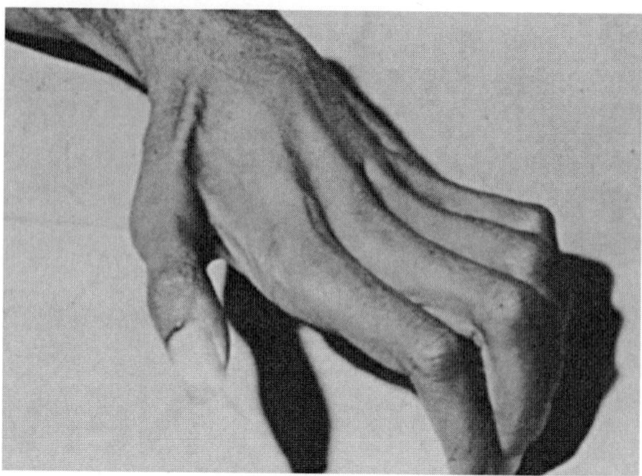

FIGURE 6-10 ■ A combined median-ulnar palsy with intrinsic motor atrophy and atrophy of the volar pulps of the digits. There is a flat transverse palmar arch and clawing of the fingers. An adduction contracture has developed in the thumb. (From Green, D.P., Hotchkiss, R.N., Pederson, W.C., and Lampert, R., eds.: Green's Operative Hand Surgery, 4th ed. New York, Churchill Livingstone, 1998.)

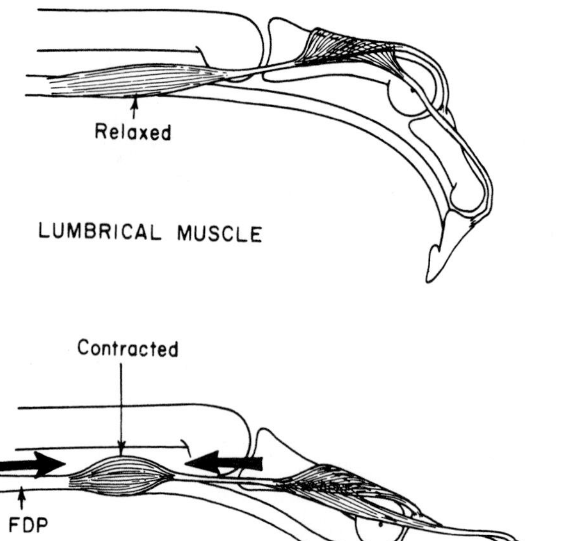

FIGURE 6-12 ■ Lumbrical function. When the lumbrical is relaxed and the flexor digitorum profundus (FDP) tendon contracts, the interphalangeal joints flex *(top)*. When the lumbrical contracts and the FDP relaxes, the interphalangeal joints extend (bottom). (From Smith, R.: Intrinsic contractures. In Green, D.P., Hotchkiss, R.N., and Pederson, W.C., Lampert, R., eds.: Green's Operative Hand Surgery, 4th ed. New York, Churchill Livingstone, 1999, p. 607.)

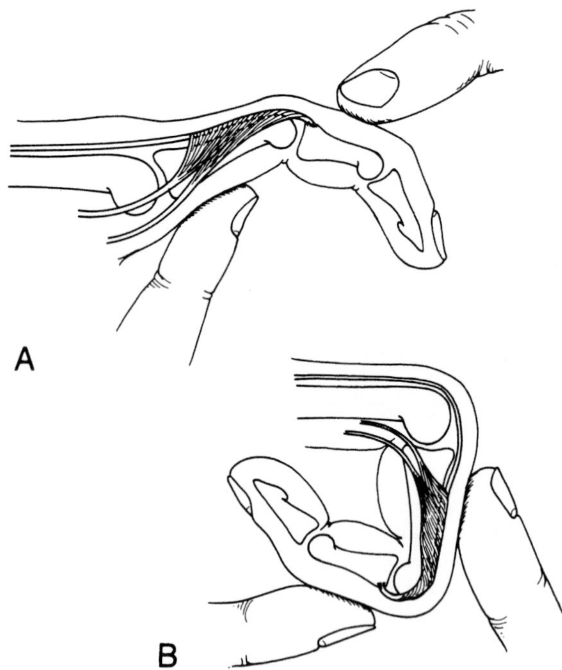

FIGURE 6-11 ■ Intrinsic tightness test. In most cases of intrinsic tightness there is less flexion of the proximal interphalangeal joint when the metacarpophalangeal (MCP) joint is held extended *(A)* than when the MCP joint is flexed *(B)*. (From Smith, R.: Intrinsic contractures. In Green, D.P., Hotchkiss, R.N., and Pederson, W.C., Lampert, R., eds.: Green's Operative Hand Surgery, 4th ed. New York, Churchill Livingstone, 1999, p. 607.)

or by a proximal muscle slide when the intrinsics are spastic or have remaining useful function.

3. Lumbrical Plus Finger—This disorder is characterized by paradoxic extension of the IPJs while attempting to flex the finger. It is most often caused by laceration of the FDP tendon distal to the lumbrical origin. When the FDP contracts to flex the finger, it pulls on the lumbrical, which inserts on the radial lateral band of the extensor expansion. Therefore the IP joints paradoxically extend (Fig. 6-12). This problem is treated by release of the lumbrical tendon in the finger or by repair of the FDP to its insertion under correct tension.
4. Swan neck deformity is characterized by hyperextension of the PIP joint and flexion of the DIP joint (Fig. 6-13). It is caused by an imbalance of forces at the PIP joint and a lax volar plate. Improper balance results from MCPJ volar subluxation (as occurs in rheumatoid patients), mallet finger, laceration or transfer of FDS, and intrinsic contracture. As the PIP joint hyperextends, transverse retinacular ligaments tether the conjoined lateral bands, restricting their excursion and effect on the distal IPJ. Double-ring splints can be used to prevent hyperextension of the PIP joint. Operative treatment options include FDS tenodesis, spiral oblique retinacular ligament

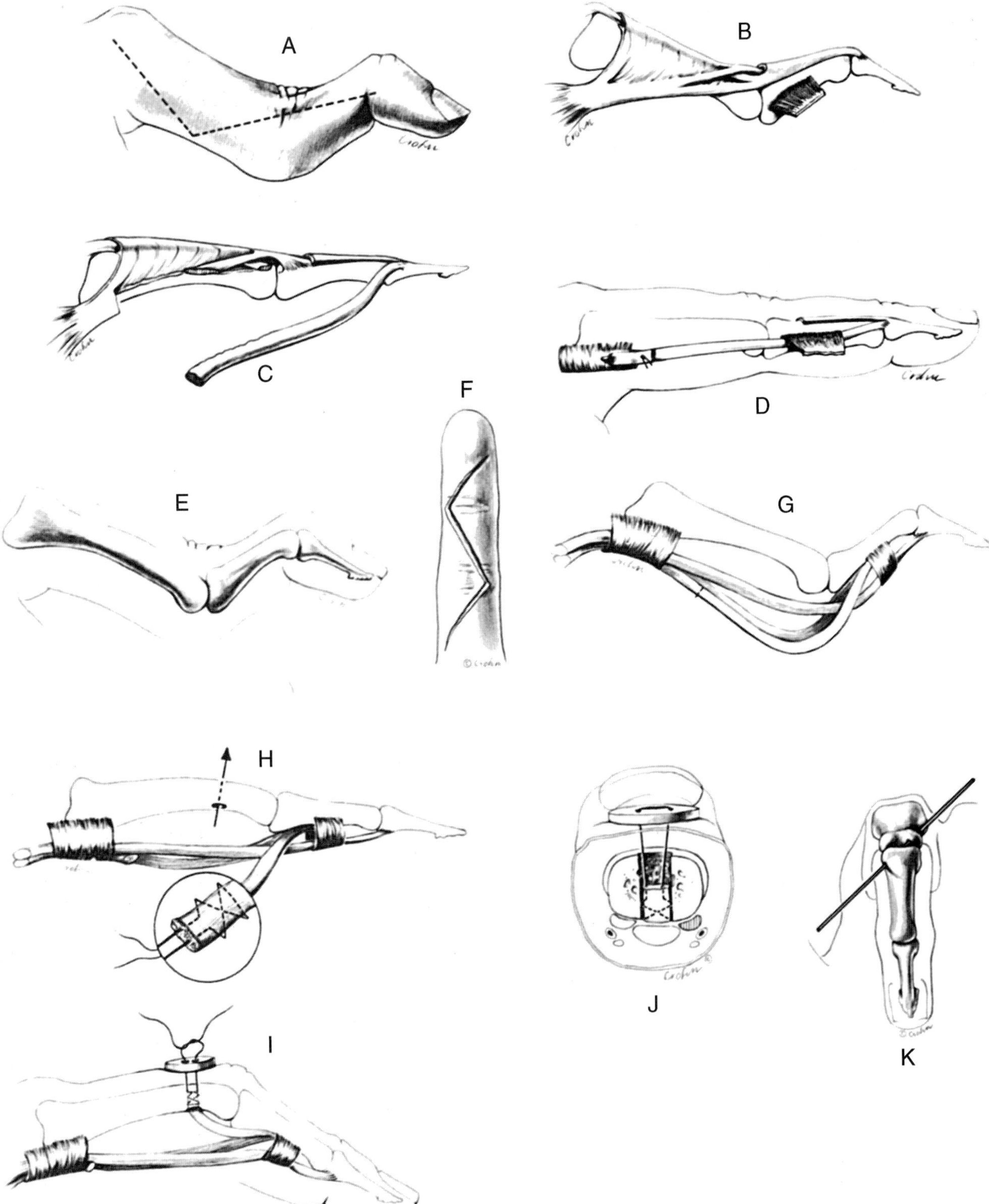

FIGURE 6-13 ■ *A–D,* Littler oblique retinacular ligament reconstruction. *E–K,* Littler superficialis tenodesis. (From Green, D.P., Hotchkiss, R.M., Pederson, W.C., and Lampert, R., eds.: Green's Operative Hand Surgery, 4th ed. New York, Churchill Livingstone, 1998. Parts *A–D* adapted from Littler, J.W.: The finger extensor mechanism. Surg. Clin. North Am. 47:415–432, 1967; Parts *E–K* adapted from Burton, R.I.: The hand. In Goldstein, L.A., and Dickerson, R.C., eds.: Atlas of Orthopaedic Surgery, 2nd ed. St. Louis, C.V. Mosby, 1981, pp. 137–170.)

reconstruction, or proximal Fowler (central slip) tenotomy.

5. Boutonnière deformity is characterized by PIP flexion and DIP hyperextension (Fig. 6-14). It is caused by central slip rupture or attenuation (secondary to capsular distension as in RA), laceration, or traumatic disruption. Volar subluxation of the lateral bands due to incompetence or disruption of the triangular ligament leads to increasing deformity as the lateral bands become a flexor of the PIP, with the majority of their forces being transmitted to the DIP joint, resulting in hyperextension of the DIP. The Elson test is most reliable in diagnosing an acute boutonnière before deformity is evident. A positive Elson test (indicating central slip rupture) is present when the PIP joint is bent 90 degrees over the edge of a table, and with resisted middle phalanx extension the DIP joint goes into rigid extension because all the forces are distributed to the terminal tendon through the intact lateral bands. A negative test result is demonstrated when the distal interphalangeal joint (DIPJ) remains floppy with this maneuver. If recognized before contractures develop and in the acute healing phase, an extension splint that allows active DIP flexion exercises is effective. Treatment with splints

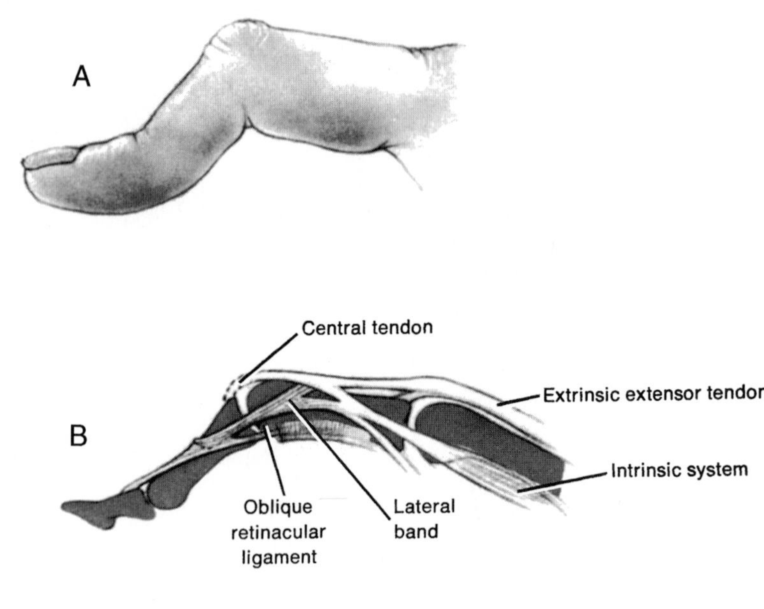

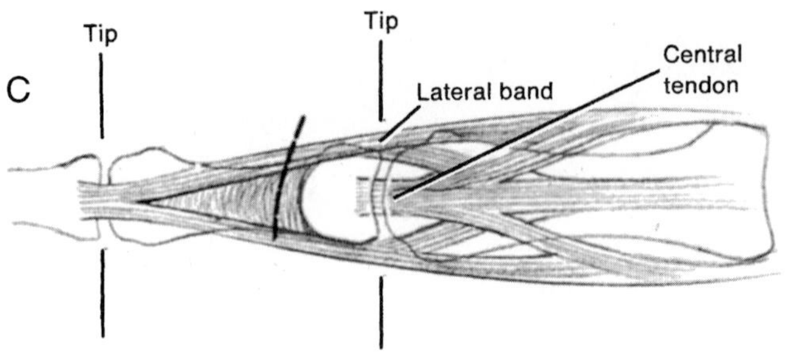

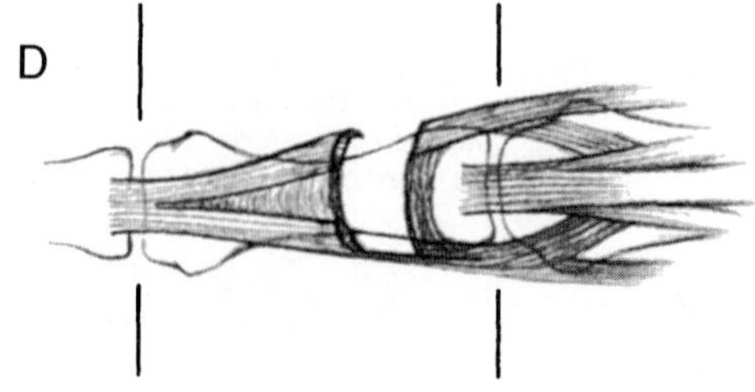

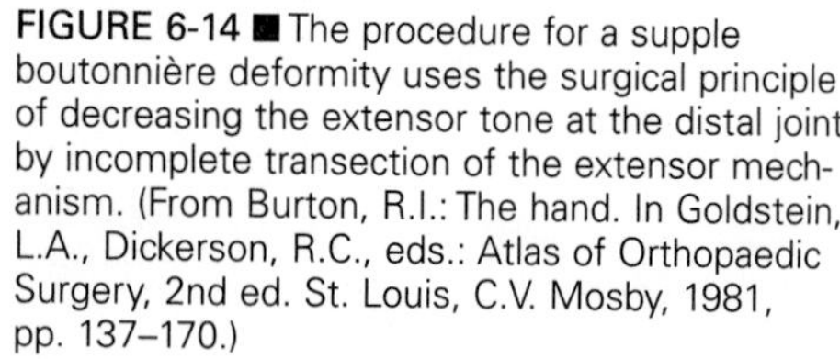

FIGURE 6-14 ■ The procedure for a supple boutonnière deformity uses the surgical principle of decreasing the extensor tone at the distal joint by incomplete transection of the extensor mechanism. (From Burton, R.I.: The hand. In Goldstein, L.A., Dickerson, R.C., eds.: Atlas of Orthopaedic Surgery, 2nd ed. St. Louis, C.V. Mosby, 1981, pp. 137–170.)

Table 6-1. NERVE COMPRESSION PHASES

PHASE	SYMPTOMS	NCV	EMG	PATHOLOGY	TREATMENT
Early	Intermittent	Normal or ↑ sensory latency	Normal	Edema	Nonoperative
Intermediate	Constant	+	±	Edema	Surgery
Late	Sensory and motor deficit	+	+	Fibrosis and axonal loss	Surgery-less predictable outcome

EMG, electromyography; NCV, nerve conduction velocity.

may be effective as late as 4 weeks after injury. Chronic cases are treated with a distal Fowler (terminal tendon) tenotomy or a secondary tendon reconstruction (Tendon graft, Littler, Matev), but only after passive joint motion is restored. After terminal tendon tenotomy, DIP extension is provided by the oblique retinacular ligament (ORL). The pseudoboutonnière deformity refers to PIP joint flexion contracture in the absence of DIP hyperextension. The pseudoboutonnière finger flexes at the DIP in the fist position, whereas the boutonnière finger does not.

6. The quadrigia effect involves an active flexion lag in fingers adjacent to a digit with an injured, adhesed, or improperly repaired FDP tendon. It results from the tethering of the normal FDP tendons by the injured or repaired FDP, because they all share a common muscle belly. As the injured digit reaches its maximum flexion, the FDP tendons in adjacent digits can have no further proximal excursion because all forces of the common muscle belly are being expended on the injured and tethered digit. It is treated by correcting the problem in the injured digit. Similarly, PIP joint stiffness in one finger may prevent flexion of adjacent digits.

II. Compressive Neuropathies

A. Introduction

1. Phases of Compressive Neuropathy—Compression neuropathy is characterized by phases of disease (Table 6-1). Appropriate treatment depends on the phase of the disease. Decisions are guided by physical examination and electromyography (EMG) and nerve conduction velocity (NCV) studies.
2. Double Crush Phenomenon—Normal axon function is dependent on factors synthesized in the nerve cell body. Blockage of axonal transport at one point makes the entire axon more susceptible to compression elsewhere. Outcome of surgical decompression may be disappointing unless all points of compression are addressed. It is logical to start with less complex distal releases first.
3. Etiology of Compressive Neuropathy (Table 6-2)
4. Sensory Testing—**Threshold Tests**: Semmes-Weinstein monofilament or vibration measures a single nerve fiber innervating a receptor or group of receptors. This test is good for subtle changes as occur in compressive neuropathy with gradual nerve-fiber loss (Semmes-Weinstein monofilament: slowly adapting vibration test: quickly adapting fibers). *Threshold tests are the most sensitive measure of abnormal sensory nerve function.* **Innervation density test**: Static and moving two-point discrimination (S2PD and M2PD) measures multiple overlapping receptive fields and requires overlapping of different sensory units and complex cortical integration. This test is good for assessing functional nerve regeneration after nerve repair. (S2PD: slowly adapting fibers; M2PD: quickly adapting fibers.) During sensory nerve regeneration M2PD precedes S2PD (Table 6-3).

Table 6-2. NERVE COMPRESSION ETIOLOGY

SYSTEMIC	INFLAMMATORY	FLUID IMBALANCE	ANATOMY	MASS
Diabetes	RA	Pregnancy	Synovial fibrosis	Ganglion
Alcoholism	Infection	Obesity	Lumbrical encroachment	Lipoma
Renal failure	Gout		Anomalous tendon	Hematoma
Raynaud's	Tenosynovitis		Median artery	
			Fracture deformity	

RA, rheumatoid arthritis.

Table 6-3. SEQUENTIAL ORDER OF SENSORY NERVE FUNCTIONAL RECOVERY

1. Anesthesia
2. Pressure (proprioception)
3. Pain (protective)
4. Moving touch
5. Moving two-point discrimination
6. Static two-point discrimination
7. Threshold tests (monofilaments and vibration)

5. Electrical testing (EMG and NCV)—The results are often the only objective evidence of a neuropathic condition (operator dependent). Ambient room temperature affects results and should be reported in the study. The NCV portion is the best adjunctive test to confirm the diagnosis. It is useful in patients with secondary gain issues. The test is ***not needed to establish the diagnosis.*** The outcome does not correlate with positive or negative findings. Demyelination interrupts normal saltatory conduction, resulting in increased latency (slowing) of NCVs. The number of axons carrying a signal is roughly proportional to the amplitude of the action potential. Sensory fibers are smaller and have less myelin than motor fibers, thus sensory NCVs are prolonged earlier in the disease process than motor NCVs. As axons cease to function, the sensory nerve action potential (SNAP) decreases in amplitude. As the disease progresses to moderate or severe phases, functioning motor axons decrease in number, and the compound motor action potentials (CMAP) decrease in amplitude (Table 6-4).
6. The evaluation and management of compression neuropathy requires a detailed knowledge of nerve anatomy (Table 6-5). Cervical radiculopathy or proximal nerve entrapment may coexist with distal nerve compression in the double crush syndrome (Fig. 6-15).

B. Median Nerve

1. Carpal Tunnel Syndrome (CTS) is the most common compressive neuropathy in the upper extremity. The most sensitive provocative test is the carpal tunnel compression test (Durkin's test). EMG/NCV: distal sensory latencies >3.2 ms or motor latencies >4.2 ms are abnormal. Normal conduction velocity, which is less specific than latencies, is 52 m/sec. Synovium in idiopathic CTS is characterized by edema, ***fibrous,*** and scattered lymphocytes. Special stains will reveal amyloid deposits in some cases. This pathologic synovium is the most frequent cause of idiopathic CTS. Nonoperative treatment includes night splints, avoiding aggravating activity, and nonsteroidal anti-inflammatory drugs (NSAIDs). Steroid injections yield transient relief in 80% of patients; 22% of patients are symptom free at 12 months and 40% symptom free when <1 year symptoms, normal (nl) 2PD, 1–2 ms prolongation sensory/motor latencies, no denervation

Table 6-4. EMG FINDINGS IN VARIOUS NERVE DISORDERS

FINDING	ROOT LESION	PLEXUS LESION	FOCAL LESION	AXONAL POLYNEUROPATHY	DEMYELINATING POLYNEUROPATHY
MAP	±↓	↓	±↓	diffuse ↓	±↓
SNAP	nl	↓	±↓	diffuse ↓	±↓
Distal latency	nl	nl	↑	nl	↑
Conduction velocity	nl	nl	↓ focal	nl	↑ diffuse
Fibrillation	+ acute	+ acute	± severe	+	±
Polyphasics	+ chronic	+ chronic	± severe	+	±

Modified from Robinson, L.R.: The role of neurophysiologic evaluation in diagnosis. J. Am. Acad. Ortho. Surg. 8(3):195, 2000.
EMG, electromyography; MAP, motor action potential; SNAP, sensory nerve action potential; nl, normal.

Table 6-5. COMPRESSION NEUROPATHY

PHASE	PATHOLOGY	SYMPTOMS	NCV SENSORY	NCV MOTOR	EMG	TREATMENT
Mild	Edema	Intermittent	±	−	−	Splints
Moderate	Demyelinated	Constant	+	+	−	Surgery
Severe	Axonal loss and fibrosis	Constant with sensory and/or motor loss	+	+	+	Surgery yields inconsistent results

NCV, nerve conduction velocity; EMG, electromyography.

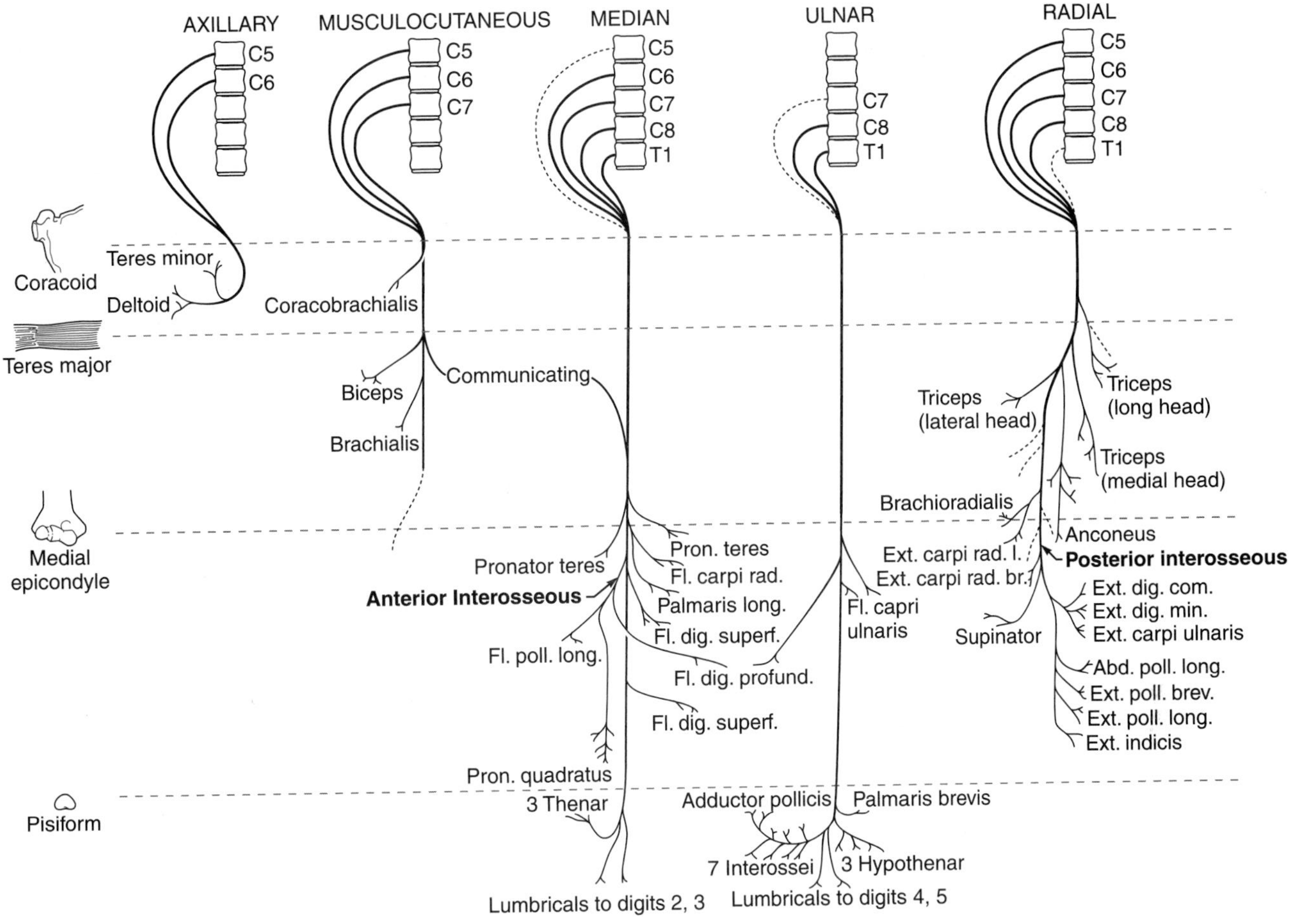

FIGURE 6-15 ■ Motor innervation of the upper extremity. (From Swanson, A.B., DeGroot, G.: Evaluation of permanent impairment in the hand and upper extremity. In Doege, T.C., ed.: Guides to the Evaluation of Permanent Impairment, 4th ed. Chicago, American Medical Association, 1993.)

potentials or atrophy. The **most common complication of endoscopic carpal tunnel release (ECTR) is incomplete division of the transverse carpal ligament**. This procedure is associated with a transient acceleration in rehabilitation (about 2 weeks). Pilar pain has not been improved, and palmar pain has not been eliminated. Long-term results of ECTR and open CTR are equivalent. *Complication rates are most closely associated with the experience of the operating surgeon, rather than the operative technique.* After standard open release, grip strength returns to preoperative level in 3 months and pinch strength returns in 6 weeks. Lengthened repair of the transverse carpal ligament is only necessary if concomitant flexor tendon repair is done, requiring immobilization with the wrist in flexion. Results of CTR are not improved by internal neurolysis, tenosynovectomy, or antebrachial fascia release. Concomitant release of Guyon's canal is not necessary because it is decompressed with CTR. Only 25% of patients will have complete relief of symptoms after repeat CTR; 25–40% will have no relief; the rest will have some improvement. Success of redo CTR is no greater when incomplete release of the transverse carpal ligament is found. Indicators of successful redo CTRs are: nocturnal symptoms, short incisions, and relief of symptoms after steroid injection.

2. Pronator Syndrome—Sites of compression: supracondylar process, ligament of Struthers, bicipital aponeurosis, deep head of the pronator teres, and the origin of the FDS (Fig. 6-16). The supracondylar process occurs in 1% of the population. The ligament of Struthers travels from the tip of the process to the medial epicondyle. This can precipitate both median and ulnar nerve symptoms. The brachial artery or, if split high, the ulnar artery and median nerve are under the ligament; therefore forearm claudication brought on by elbow extension with forearm supination can occur. Differences from CTS include sensory disturbance over the distribution of the palmar cutaneous

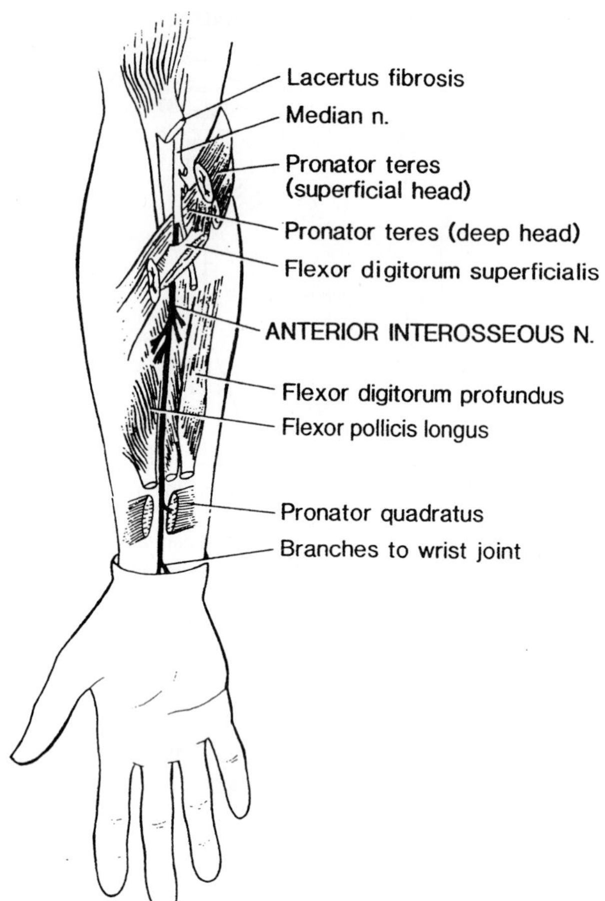

FIGURE 6-16 ■ Schematic anatomy of the anterior interosseous nerve. (From Chidgey, L.K., and Szabo, R.M.: Anterior interosseous nerve compression syndrome. In Szabo, R.M., ed.: Nerve Compression Syndrome—Diagnosis and Treatment. Thorofare, NJ, Slack, 1989, pp. 153–162.)

branch of median nerve, anterior proximal forearm pain, Tinel's proximal anterior forearm, usually no night symptoms. Provocative tests for specific sites of compression are: resisted elbow flexion with forearm supination (bicipital aponeurosis), resisted forearm pronation with elbow extended (two heads of pronator teres [PT]), and isolated long finger PIP joint flexion (FDS origin). An elbow x-ray study is a mandatory preoperative examination. EMG and NCV may be helpful, but are usually normal. This condition usually responds to a nonoperative approach of rest splinting and NSAIDs (3–6 months). Failing this, a global decompression of all potential sites of compression yields a variable treatment outcome, with relief of symptoms in 80% of patients in most studies.

3. Anterior Interosseous Nerve (AIN) Compressive Neuropathy—This syndrome involves **motor loss without sensory involvement**. AIN-innervated muscles: radial two FDP, flexor pollicus longus (FPL), pronator quadratus (PQ) plus or minus anterior forearm pain (see Fig. 6-16). The FDP and FPL are tested by asking the patient to make the "A OK" sign *(precision tip-to-tip pinch)*. PQ involvement is tested by resisted pronation with the elbow maximally flexed. Bilateral AIN palsy may indicate Parsonage-Turner syndrome (viral brachial neuritis), especially if motor loss was preceded by intense pain in the shoulder region. EMG/NCV is helpful in confirming the diag-nosis. It is important to rule out a tendon disruption if only one finger is weak (Mannerfelt-Norman syndrome: FPL rupture). Sources of compression include fibrous bands within the pronator teres, FDS arcade, edge of the lacertus fibrosus, enlarged bicipital bursa, and Gantzer's muscle (accessory head of the FPL). Nonoperative treatment involves observation and elbow splinting in 90 degrees of flexion (8–12 weeks). Surgical decompression is recommended failing a trial of nonoperative management; results are generally satisfactory if done within 3–6 months from the onset of symptoms. The vast majority recover without surgery.

C. Ulnar Nerve

1. Cubital tunnel syndrome is most often due to compression of the ulnar nerve between the two heads of the flexor carpi ulnaris (FCU). Other potential sites of compression include the arcade of Struthers (the hiatus in the medial intermuscular septum), Osborne's ligament (from the medial epicondyle to the olecranon, fibers within the FCU, and the anconeus epitrochlearis muscle (Fig. 6-17). Other sources of compression include tumors, ganglions, cubitus valgus, bony spurs, and a medial epicondyle nonunion. Symptoms include paresthesias over small finger and ulnar half of the ring finger and ulnar dorsal hand, weakness of the intrinsics with a positive Froment's sign (FPL compensating for paralyzed thumb adductor) or Jeanne's sign (compensatory hyperextension of thumb metacarpal phalanseal [MP] joint) and/or weakness of the ulnar two FDPs (Pollock's test) can also be seen. Examination findings include a positive Tinel's sign over the cubital tunnel and positive elbow flexion test result (60 seconds). EMG/NCV is helpful in establishing the diagnosis. Nonoperative treatment includes NSAIDs, activity modifications, and night-time 45-degree extension splint (effective in 50% of cases). A number of surgical procedures are used for this disorder, including release of the cubital tunnel retinaculum, medial epicondylectomy, or anterior transposition (subcutaneous, submuscular, intramuscular). Generally, any technique yields 80–90% good results when symptoms are intermittent and denervation has not occurred. Better results

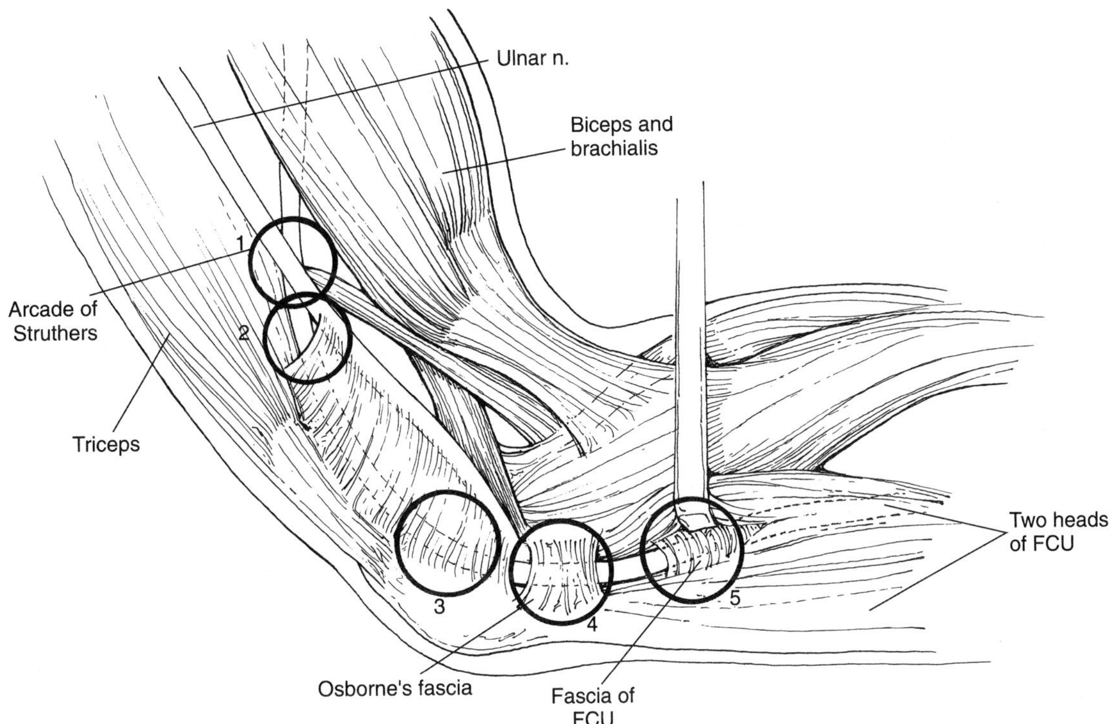

FIGURE 6-17 ■ Sites of ulnar nerve entrapment. The nerve may be entrapped by (1) the arcade of Struthers, (2) the medial intermuscular septum, (3) the distal transverse fibers of the arcade of Struthers, (4) Osborne's ligament, and (5) the fascia of the flexor carpi ulnaris (FCU) and fascial bands within the FCU. (From Miller, M.D., Howard, R.F., Plancher, K.: Surgical Atlas of Sports Medicine, WB Saunders, 2003, p. 402.)

with fewer recurrences are seen with anterior submuscular transposition in cases with moderate (continuous symptoms) and severe (evidence of denervation) compression. **Poor prognosis correlates most closely with intrinsic atrophy.**

2. Ulnar Tunnel Syndrome—This is due to ulnar nerve compression in Guyon's canal. The roof of the tunnel is the volar carpal ligament. The floor is the transverse carpal ligament and the pisohamate ligament. The ulnar wall is the hook of hamate, and the radial wall is the pisiform and abductor digiti minimi (ADM) muscle belly. Symptoms may be pure motor, pure sensory, or mixed based on location of compression within the tunnel. Pain is more infrequent when compared with CTS. Causative factors include ganglia from the triquetrohamate joint (80% nontraumatic cases), nonunited hook of hamate fracture, ulnar artery thrombosis, anomalous muscle, and palmaris brevis hypertrophy. The ulnar tunnel is divided into three zones (Fig. 6-18).
   a. Zone 1: proximal to bifurcation of the nerve and associated with mixed motor sensory symptoms.

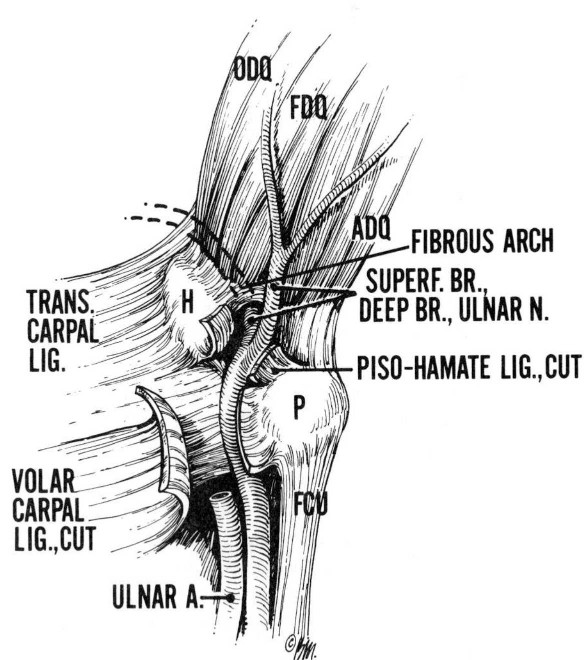

FIGURE 6-18 ■ The ulnar nerve courses through Guyon's canal between the volar carpal ligament and the transverse carpal ligament. P, pisiform; H, hamate. (From Green, D.P., Hotchkiss, R.M., Pederson, W.C., eds.: Green's Operative Hand Surgery, 4th ed. New York, Churchill Livingstone, 1998.)

b. Zone 2: surrounds deep motor branch and has motor symptoms only. Ganglia and hook-of-hamate pathology are the most likely cause in zones 1 and 2.
c. Zone 3: surrounds superficial sensory branch and has sensory symptoms only. *Thrombosis of the ulnar artery is the most likely cause in zone 3.*
d. Treatment: identifying the cause is the key to treatment. Computed tomography (CT) for hook-of-hamate fracture, magnetic resonance imaging (MRI) for ganglion cyst, Doppler ultrasound for ulnar artery thrombosis. Nonoperative treatment if warranted includes avoiding aggravating activities, splints, and NSAIDs. Operative treatment involves treating the underlying cause and decompressing the area of entrapment.

D. Radial Nerve

1. Arm—Although rare, the radial nerve can be compressed by a fibrous arch from the lateral head of the triceps (also remember the Holstein-Lewis fracture pattern at the junction of the middle and distal third of radius). Clinical findings include weakness of posterior interosseous nerve (PIN) and proximally innervated muscles (Henry's mobile wad). Also, radial sensory symptoms may be present. EMG and NCV are very helpful. Observation for up to 3 months is warranted; if no recovery, surgical decompression is indicated.
2. Posterior Interosseous Nerve Compression Syndrome—Symptoms include pain at the lateral elbow and weakness and ulnar drift with wrist extension (ECRL innervated higher than the PIN takeoff). This nerve carries no sensory fibers for cutaneous innervation; however, it does carry sensory fibers from the dorsal wrist capsule. The PIN innervates the ECRB, supinator, EIP, ECU, EDC, EDM, APL, EPB, and EPL (Fig. 6-19). EMG is usually diagnostic. Anatomic sites of compression include thickened fascia at radiocapitellar joint, radial artery recurrent leash of Henry, edge of ECRB, arcade of Frohse, and distal edge of the supinator (Fig. 6-10). Unusual causes include chronic radial head dislocation, fractured radial head or neck, rheumatoid synovitis of the radiocapitellar joint, or mass (lipoma, ganglion) at the elbow. In a rheumatoid patient PIN palsy must be differentiated from extensor tendon rupture; a normal tenodesis test confirms the diagnosis of PIN palsy. PIN compression is treated by avoiding aggravating activities, and with NSAIDs. If this fails to provide recovery in 3 months, surgical decompression is warranted. Surgical decompression provides good-to-excellent results for 85% of patients.
3. Radial Tunnel Syndrome *is a pain-only problem without motor or sensory dysfunction*. It involves the same nerve as PIN syndrome, same sights of entrapment, but a different presentation and a different response to treatment. Provocative tests include long finger extension test (positive result if pressure over P1 of the long finger reproduces pain at the edge of the ECRB) and the resisted supination test. **EMG/NCV is not helpful in this condition**. The chief differential is lateral epicondylitis (coexists in 5% of patients). In radial tunnel syndrome the maximum tenderness is distal to the radial head in a line from the lateral epicondyle through the radial head to a point 2–3 cm more distal over the radial tunnel. A long nonoperative approach is warranted (1 year) as well as activity modification, temporary splinting, NSAIDs, and other modalities of therapy. Operative release is often disappointing, with only 50–80% good-to-excellent results reported and maximal recovery not until 9–18 months after surgery.
4. Wartenberg's Syndrome (cheiralgia paresthetica) is a compressive neuropathy of the sensory branch of the radial nerve. It is compressed between the brachioradialis (BR) and

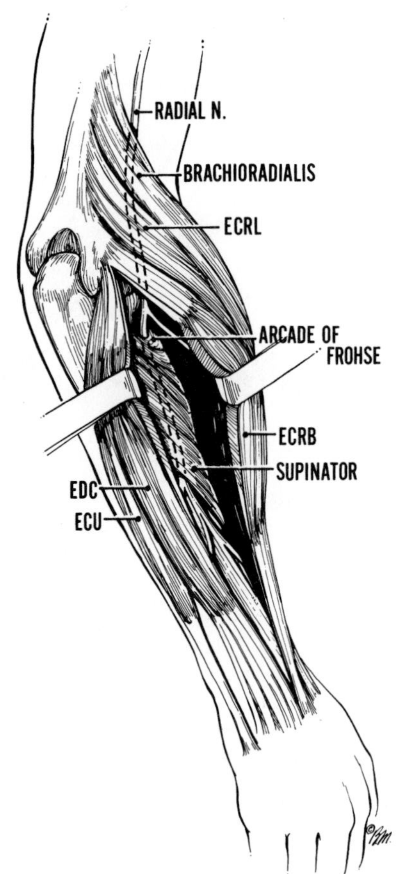

FIGURE 6-19 ■ Extension of the posterior Thompson approach to the radial tunnel. (From Green, D.P., Hotchkiss, R.M., Pederson, W.C., eds.: Green's Operative Hand Surgery, 4th ed. New York, Churchill Livingstone, 1998.)

ECRL with forearm pronation (by a scissor-like action between the tendons). Symptoms include pain, numbness, and paresthesias over radiodorsal hand. The provocative tests include forceful forearm pronation (60 seconds) and a positive Tinel's sign over the nerve. This condition is treated by rest, NSAIDs, avoiding aggravating activities, and wrist splints. Surgical decompression is warranted if a 6-month trial nonoperative treatment fails.

E. Other Compressive Neuropathies

1. Suprascapular Nerve Entrapment Syndrome (SNES) presents with acute onset of deep, diffuse, posterolateral shoulder pain. It occurs after trauma or aggressive athletic activity. The most consistent finding is pain with palpation over suprascapular notch. EMG/NCV is very helpful in establishing the diagnosis. Spinati muscle atrophy is also common, usually because of a delay in diagnosis. MRI may be helpful in cases where a ganglion is compressing the nerve. The current trend is toward early surgical decompression through the posterior approach. In some cases only the infraspinatus is involved. Isolated infraspinatus atrophy is most often secondary a ganglion at the spinoglenoid notch. Spinoglenoid notch ganglions are associated with glenoid labrum tears in almost 100% of cases.
2. Thoracic Outlet Syndrome—There are two types: vascular and neurogenic. The vascular variety involves subclavian artery disease or aneurysm and is easily diagnosed by examination and imaging (angiogram). The neurogenic variety is infrequent and diagnosed by clinical examination alone (EMG/NCV rarely helpful). A cervical spine film should be taken to rule out a cervical rib. Chest radiograph is taken to rule out Pancoast's tumor. The provocative tests (Wright's hyperabduction maneuver, Adson's test, at attention test, elevation test) are rarely helpful because results are often abnormal in normal subjects. Sites of compression include a cervical rib, anterior scalene muscle, congenital fibrous bands, or the sternocleidomastoid muscle. A therapy approach is tried first, focusing on shoulder girdle strengthening and proper posture and relaxation techniques. The favored surgical procedure, if necessary, is a transaxillary first rib resection with 90% good-to-excellent results reported. Complication rates from the procedure are significant.

III. Tendon Injuries

A. **Extensor Tendons**—Description and treatment based on zones (Table 6-6). In general, partial lacerations (<50%) should be treated with early motion. Repair of partial lacerations actually impairs tendon healing and precipitates unnecessary adhesions. Traditionally, extensor tendon repairs have been managed with postoperative immobilization. The current trend is toward early mobilization (at 3 postoperative days) in a dynamic splint, particularly with multiple tendon lacerations beneath the extensor retinaculum or when there are associated injuries. This new trend is applicable to injuries in zones V–VIII. Its usefulness in zones II–IV is less clear, where traditional postoperative immobilization is usually satisfactory.

Table 6-6. TENDON ZONES OF INJURY EXTENSOR

ZONE	FINGER	THUMB
I	DIP joint	IP Joint
II	Middle phalanx	Proximal phalanx
III	PIP joint	MCP joint
IV	Proximal phalanx	Metacarpal
V	MCP joint	CMC joint radial styloid
VI	Metacarpal	
VII	Dorsal wrist retinaculum	
VIII	Distal forearm	
IX	Middle and proximal forearm	

DIP, distal interphalangeal joint; PIP, proximal interphalangeal; MCP, metacarpophalangeal; CMC, carpometacarpal.

1. Zone I (mallet finger) represents a disruption of the terminal tendon. Treatment involves extension splinting for 6 weeks (80% good-to-excellent results reported). Greater complication rates are seen with a dorsal splint, and hyperextension should be avoided. Mallet fingers associated with a fracture are generally treated in an extension splint unless the distal phalanx is volarly subluxated, in which case reduction and pinning of the joint should be done. The chronic mallet finger can be treated as a fresh injury up to 4 weeks after injury. Repair, imbrication, or reconstruction of the terminal tendon (joint then held extended 6–8 weeks) is indicated when the time from injury is more than 4 weeks and the joint is supple, congruent, and without arthritis. If the joint is otherwise, the best option is a DIP fusion. Loss of terminal tendon insertion causes proximal migration of the extensor apparatus with transfer of forces to the PIP joint (PIPJ). If the volar plate is lax or attenuates over time, a swan neck deformity can develop in conjunction with the mallet finger. The favored technique for correction of this problem is a spiral oblique retinacular ligament (SORL) reconstruction. Other options include a sublimis tenodesis or a Fowler central slip tenotomy.
2. Zone II (Finger: Middle Phalanx and Thumb: Proximal Phalanx)—The mechanism of injury usually involves laceration or crush. Insignificant (<50%) disruptions of the tendon are treated with skin and wound care and mobilization at

7–10 days from injury. Significant (>50%) disruptions are treated similarly to mallet finger. Tendon lacerations are sutured and a static extension splint applied for 4–6 weeks.

3. Zone III (Boutonnière Finger PIPJ, Thumb MPJ)—The three components of the acute boutonnière deformity include (1) disruption of the central slip, (2) attenuation of the triangular ligament, and (3) volar migration of the lateral bands. The transverse retinacular ligaments, which originate on the lateral bands and insert on the volar plate, eventually become contracted, thus holding the lateral bands subluxated. Diagnostic tests include the Elson test or evidence of a 15- to 20-degree (or greater) loss of active extension of the PIPJ with the wrist and MPJs fully flexed. Treatment of acute boutonnière involves splinting the PIPJ in full extension for 6 weeks with active DIP joint flexion exercises. Holding the PIP joint in full extension reduces the separation of the ends of the central slip. Active flexion of the DIP joint draws the lateral bands distally and dorsally, further coapting the disrupted tendon ends. Indications for operative intervention include a displaced avulsion fracture or an open wound requiring irrigation and débridement (I&D) anyway. When there is loss of tendon substance, this is managed by free tendon graft or a flap of the extensor mechanism turned distally like an Achilles tendon repair. Treatment of a chronic boutonnière deformity is best done after the joint has full passive mobility. If this cannot be accomplished with therapy and splints, it may need to be done in a two-stage surgical procedure, with the first stage being a joint release. Options include a soft-tissue release (distal Fowler tenotomy: release of the extensor mechanism at the junction of the middle and proximal thirds of the middle phalanx, which leaves the oblique retinacular ligament [ORL] intact; the lateral bands slide proximally, increasing extensor tone at the PIPJ and the intact ORL, which provides extensor tone at DIPJ) or a secondary tendon reconstruction such as excision of scar tissue and direct repair of central slip or V-Y advancement, free tendon graft, lateral band transfer procedure (Littler [ulnar lateral band through radial lateral band to P2] or Matev [ulnar lateral band transferred to distal stump radial lateral band, proximal stump radial lateral band brought through central slip and anchored at the dorsal base of P2] (Fig. 6-20).
4. Zone IV (Proximal Phalanx of Finger and Thumb MC)—These are managed similarly to zone II injuries. Partial laceration in this region is common and should not be repaired if less than 50% of the tendon. Tendon adhesions cause functional loss due to flexion loss, rather than extensor lag. Tenolysis is more often required at this level. Tenolysis improves flexion, but extensor lag often persists.

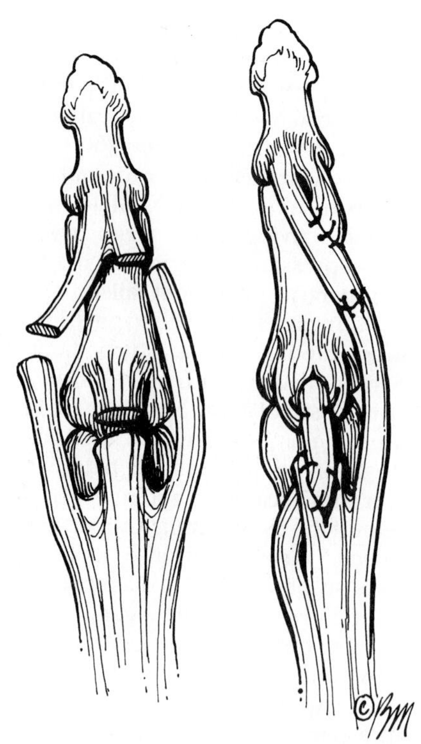

FIGURE 6-20 ■ Matev reconstruction of the central slip. The radial lateral band is incised over the middle phalanx, then freed and brought through the central tendon at the proximal interphalangeal joint, inserting it into the base of the middle phalanx. The ulnar lateral tendon is then advanced into the distal portion of the radial lateral tendon and remnant of central tendon at the distal interphalangeal joint. (From Green, D.P.: Operative Hand Surgery, 3rd ed. New York, Churchill Livingstone, 1993. Adapted from Swanson, A.B.: Flexible Implant Resection Arthroplasty in the Hand and Extremities. St. Louis, C.V. Mosby, 1973.)

5. Zone III and IV (Thumb)—The EPB and EPL are easily distinguishable at this level. Significant disruptions (>50%) are repaired with a core suture. Postoperatively it is splinted with the wrist and MPJ in extension for 3–4 weeks, then mobilization is started.
6. Zone V (MP Joint)—Beware of human bite wounds at this level. Lacerations involving >50% of the tendon substance should be repaired. Early mobilization in a dynamic extension outrigger splint is encouraged by some authors. Immobilization for 3–4 weeks with wrist extended 30–40 degrees and MPs flexed to 45 degrees yields results similar to dynamic extension programs.
7. Traumatic Dislocation of the Extensor Tendon (Sagittal Band Rupture)—This is seen after laceration or forceful resisted flexion or extension injuries. *The long finger is the most commonly involved digit.* If diagnosed early (within a week) it may be treated with extension splint for 6 weeks. If diagnosis is delayed,

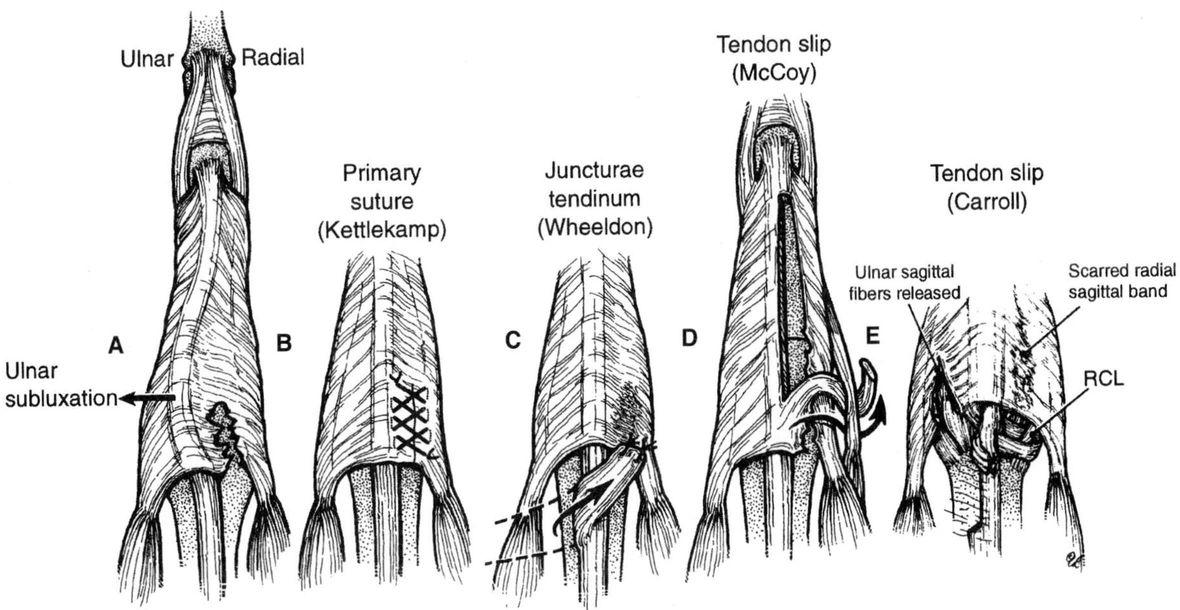

FIGURE 6-21 ■ Sagittal band reconstruction. (From Doyle, J.R.: Extensor tendons—Acute injuries. In Operative Hand Surgery, Green Ed, 4th ed., p. 1979.)

direct repair is indicated. If the sagittal band cannot be mobilized for direct repair, an extrinsic extensor centralization procedure is done (Fig. 6-21).

8. Zone VI (Metacarpal)—Significant lacerations (>50%) are repaired with core suture, and dynamic splint mobilization is started early. As with zone V, results of delayed mobilization in wrist extension are similar to dynamic extension programs. There is an excellent prognosis for tendon repairs at this level if no fracture or crush injury is involved.
9. Zone VII (Wrist)—Lacerations at this level are associated with damage to the extensor retinaculum. Repair of significant lacerations with a core suture technique is advised. It is no longer recommended to excise portions of the extensor retinaculum over the repair sites; instead, early dynamic splint mobilization is advised. Static splinting is not advisable at this level.
10. Zone VIII (Distal Forearm)—These disruptions are at the level of the musculotendinous junction. The tendons obviously hold suture well, but sutures in muscle risk ischemia and failure. Remember that tendons originate from a fibrous septa that runs several centimeters within the muscle belly. This is the tissue that will hold a stitch. Postoperatively, static immobilization of the wrist in extension (40–45 degrees) and the MPJs in flexion (15–20 degrees) for 3–4 weeks is required.
11. Zone IX (Proximal Forearm)—These disruptions are often secondary to penetrating trauma and are associated with neurovascular injury, which adversely affects the prognosis. Repair is done with figure-of-eight Vicryl or tendon grafts placed through the epimysium. After repair, the elbow and wrist are immobilized for 4 weeks in flexion and extension, respectively.

B. **Flexor Tendons**—Description and treatment based on zones (Fig. 6-22). Tendon healing is divided into three phases: (1) inflammatory, (2) fibroblastic, and (3) remodeling (Table 6-7). **Tendon repairs are the weakest between postoperative days 6 and 12.** Tendon structure compared with ligament: *Tendons have more collagen and are less viscoelastic.* They have more organized collagen strands and deform less under an applied load. Both fail in a nonlinear fashion.
   1. Zone I (Distal to FDS Insertion)—Only FDP injured, direct repair is advocated. Profundus advancement of 1 cm or greater carries a risk of flexion contracture or inducing a quadrigia effect. Early patient-assisted passive range of motion (ROM) (Duran program) or Kleinert's protocol (dynamic splint-assisted passive ROM) is preferred at this level. The primary complication at this level is flexion contracture of the DIPJ. Injury at this zone can also be a result of an avulsion injury ("rugger jersey" finger) (Table 6-8). In this situation the tendon is reinserted by pull-out suture technique, with the suture tied over a dorsal button.
   2. Zone II (Within the Finger Flexor Retinaculum)—Also known as "no man's land," because for years repair of both tendons

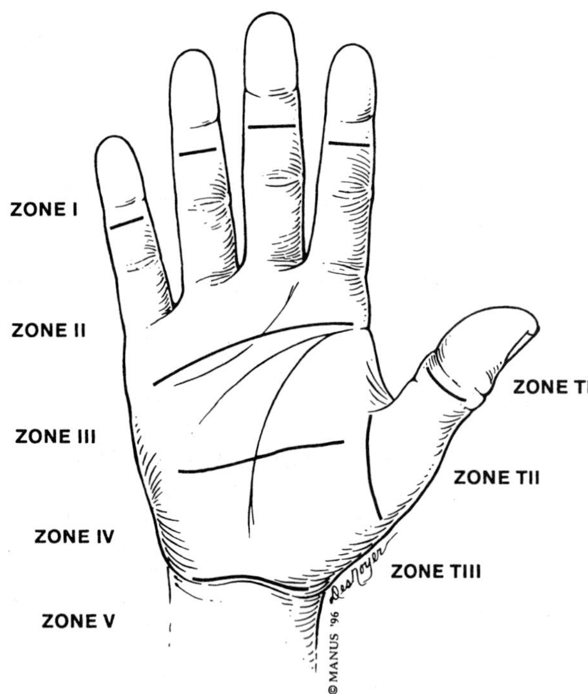

FIGURE 6-22 ■ Zones of tendon injury. (From Green, D.H., Hotchkiss, R.M., Pederson, W.C., and Lampert, R., eds.: Green's Operative Hand Surgery, 4th ed. New York, Churchill Livingstone, 1998.)

was thought to be fruitless. At this level both tendons (FDS/FDP) are injured. Repair of both tendons is now advocated, followed by an early mobilization program (Kleinert, Duran). The tendon laceration may be at a different level than the skin laceration depending on the position of the finger when laceration occurred.

3. Zone III (the Palm)—Concomitant neurovascular injury is likely, which dramatically diminishes the prognosis. Good results from direct repair are usual because of absence of the retinacular structures.
4. Zone IV (the Carpal Tunnel)—Close quarters and synovial sheaths make postoperative adhesions likely. *The transverse carpal ligament should be repaired in a lengthened fashion,* which prevents bowstringing and allows for immobilization of the wrist in flexion.
5. Zone V (Wrist and Forearm)—Repairs in this zone have a favorable prognosis. The results are diminished when there is concomitant neurovascular injury.
6. Thumb—End-to-end repair of the FPL is advocated. It is recommended to work outside of zone III (beneath the thenar muscles) so as to avoid injury to the recurrent motor branch of the median nerve. The oblique pulley is the most important but, if necessary, either the A1 or the oblique pulley may be incised to facilitate repair. One of them should be preserved or bowstringing of the tendon will result. Results of FPL repair differ from the finger. First, early motion rehabilitation protocols do not show significantly better long-term results in the thumb. In addition, FPL repair is associated with 20% rupture rate in some series, considerably higher than the 2–5% rate in the fingers.
7. Suture Technique—Core grasping suture: **Number of grasping loops not as significant as the number of suture strands that**

Table 6-7. TENDON-HEALING PHASES

HEALING PHASE	DAYS	HISTOLOGY	TENSILE STRENGTH	COMMENTS
Inflammatory	0–5	Cellular proliferation	None	Neoangiogenesis
Fibroblastic	5–28	Fibroblastic proliferation, disorganized collagen	Increasing	Fibronectin attracts fibroblasts
Remodeling	>28	Linear collagen organization	Will tolerate controlled active motion	Collagen cross-linking along stress lines stimulated by stress

Table 6-8. LEDDY CLASSIFICATION OF PROFUNDUS AVULSIONS

TYPE	TENDON RETRACTION LEVEL	REPAIR	INTERVAL/TREATMENT
I	Palm	(Disvascular)	7–10 days
II (most common)	PIPJ (held by vinculum longus)		3 mo
III	A4 pulley (held by bony avulsion fragment)	ORIF fragment	
IIIa	Type III but profundus also avulses off fracture fragment	Treatment based on level of tendon retraction	

PIPJ, proximal interphalangeal joint; ORIF, open reduction, internal fixation.

cross the repair site. Loops tend to collapse under load and result in gapping. Strength of the repair has a linear relationship to the number of strands crossing the repair, and repairs most often rupture at the knots. Circumferential epitendinous suture not only improves tendon gliding but also improves the strength of the repair and allows for less *gap formation, which is the initial event in repair failure.* The epitenon suture adds roughly 20% to the tensile strength of the repair. Tensile strength requirements for early active motion rehabilitation protocols require a minimum of a four-strand, and preferably six-strand, repair.

8. Sheath repair remains controversial. It supposedly takes advantage of the synovial pathway for tendon nutrition. However, clinical results with sheath repair are the same as without. Most hand surgeons close the sheath, if possible, but will not go to great lengths to do so.
9. Postoperative controlled mobilization has been the major advance that has improved results of repair in zone II. It limits restrictive adhesions and improves tendon-healing biology. The two typically used protocols are (1) the Kleinert (active extension, dynamic splint assisted passive flexion), although the Mayo synergistic splint is now favored because it incorporates active wrist motion, improving overall tendon excursion; and (2) the Duran (active extension, patient-assisted passive flexion). Both programs essentially employ controlled motion for 6 weeks. Newer protocols modify these basic programs by adding various forms of active motion. Active motion protocols require a minimum four-strand core suture, preferably six-strand.
10. Flexor Tendon Reconstruction—Primary tendon graft is rarely used secondary to improved results with primary repair. A one-stage reconstruction is only advocated if the flexor sheath is pristine and the digit has full passive motion. Otherwise a two-stage procedure is advocated. A temporary silicone tendon implant is used to create a favorable bed for tendon graft. Active implants are available but provide little clinical benefit over the standard passive rod. Stage one is followed by a 3-4-month interval to allow for achieving tissue stability before the biologic tendon graft is placed. Total active motion of 260 degrees is usually achievable; however, flexion contractures are common. Available grafts include the palmaris longus, which is most often used (absent in 15% of upper extremities). The plantaris is an alternative if a longer graft is needed (absent in 19%). Otherwise a long toe extensor can be used. Intrasynovial grafts such as the FDL have less adhesions than extra synovial grafts at 6 weeks; however, clinical result are not significantly different. Extrasynovial grafts remain the mainstay of treatment.
11. Grafting through an Intact Superficialis—If the patient can demonstrate a need, it may be considered (e.g., concert pianist, hand surgeon). Occasionally this is indicated in the small finger, where 34% of people have an incompetent FDS. In general it is avoided, because of the potential complications and resultant PIP contracture. In most cases where DIPJ stability is desired, fusion is preferred.
12. Tenolysis may be indicated when there is a discrepancy between active and passive motion after therapy and the soft tissues have stabilized (usually >3 months). Ideally it should be deferred until all adjacent joints have full passive motion. It is important to preserve critical pulleys (A2 and A4) during tenolysis. Postoperative therapy is extensive.
13. Pulley Reconstruction—Ideally one pulley should be placed proximal and distal to each joint requiring pulley reconstruction. Considerable force is placed on the reconstructed pulley: a force of 3 N on the fingertip generates 107 N on the pulley. Available techniques include triple loop (favored), fibrous rim method, belt loop method, FDS tail method. Distal to the PIP the graft is placed around the extensor tendon, while proximal to the PIP the graft is placed deep to the extensor tendon.

IV. Hand Infections—Can involve any tissue type and a wide variety of pathogens (Table 6-9). Early recognition and appropriate treatment followed by vigorous therapy are the keys to successful treatment.

A. Paronychia/eponychia are the most common infections in the hand. These are infections of the nail fold and are most commonly caused by *Staphylococcus aureus*. It is treated by I&D and partial or total nail plate removal, oral antibiotics, and dressing changes. It is important to preserve the eponychial fold by placing material between the skin and the nail bed after débridement. Chronic cases that failed to respond to oral antibiotics are often secondary to *Candida albicans* and occur more commonly in diabetics. In rare cases marsupilization (excision of dorsal eponychium) may be required.
B. Felon—An infection of the finger tip pulp. It is similarly treated with I&D through midlateral incisions (the "fish-mouth" incision carries a risk of tip necrosis). It is important to break up the septa to adequately decompress the fingertip; otherwise, local compartment syndrome can occur. This is usually treated with intravenous (IV) antibiotics. Incisions are usually placed on the ulnar side except on the thumb and small finger, where they are placed on the radial side.

Table 6-9. HAND INFECTIONS

SOURCE	LOCATION	PATHOGEN	ANTIBIOTIC	COMMENT
Paronychia	Eponychium	*S. aureus*	Dicloxacillin or clindamycin po nafcillin IV	Release eponychial fold May require nail removal
Felon	Pulp space	*S. aureus*	Dicloxacillin or clindamycin po nafcillin IV	Release all septa Volar incision preferred
Human bite	MCP and PIP	*Strep sp.* *S. aureus* *Eikenella corrodens*	Ampicillin/sublactam IV PCN for *E. corrodens*	Tx failure with cephalosporins usually due to *E. corrodens*
Dog and cat bites	Varied	*α-hemolytic Strep (46%)* *Pasteurella multocida (26%)* *S. aureus (13%)* *Anaerobes (41%)*	Ampicillin/sublactam IV or oral amoxicilli-clavulanic acid	Failure of oral Tx common
Necrotizing Fasciitis	Varied	*Clostridia* *Group A β-strep.*	Broad-spectrum triple antibiotic—PCN, clindamycin, gentamicin	32% mortality Amputations frequent
Fungal	Cutaneous	*Candida albicans*	Topical antifungal	Common in diabetics with chronic paronychia
	Nail	*Trichophyton rubrum*	Oral ketoconazol or iatroconazol	Pulse dosing 1 week per month
	Subcutaneous	*Sporothrix schenckii* *Mycoplasm sp.*	Based on culture	

IV, intravenously; MCP, metacarpophalangeal; PIP, proximal interphalangeal; PCN, penicillin; Tx, treatment.

C. Human Bite—This is a potentially serious infection that should be treated with I&D, especially if joints or tendon sheaths are violated. It most commonly involves the third or fourth MCPJs (fist to mouth). The most common organisms isolated are alpha-hemolytic *Streptococcus* and *S. aureus*. The incidence of *Eikenella corrodens* varies from 7% to 29%. Antibiotics of choice include ampicillin/sublactam or amoxicilli-clavulanic acid (Augmentin).

D. Dog and Cat Bites—Also potentially serious injuries often requiring I&D. The frequency of various isolates is as follows: alpha-hemolytic strep (46%), *Pasteurella multocida* (26%), *S. aureus* (13%), anaerobes (41%). The drugs of choice include ampicillin/sublactam or amoxicilliclavulanic acid.

E. Suppurative Flexor Tenosynovitis—An infection of the flexor tendon sheath. The cardinal clinical signs were described by Kanavel: flexed posture, fusiform swelling, pain with passive extension, and flexor sheath tenderness. If recognized early the patient can be admitted and treated with IV antibiotics. If the signs improve within the first 24 hours, surgery may be avoided. Otherwise, the treatment of choice is I&D and IV antibiotics. Many different incisions have been described; however, the principle is thorough irrigation of the involved tendon sheath. Continuous drip irrigation with an indwelling catheter carries a risk for compartment syndrome. The classic "horseshoe abscess" is based on proximal connection of thumb and small finger flexor sheaths in Parona's space (potential space between pronator quadratus and FDP tendons). Spread of infection into deep spaces is as follows: index and thumb to thenar space; long, ring, and small to midpalmar space; small can also spread into the ulnar bursa.

F. Herpetic Whitlow—Occurs with increased frequency in medical/dental personnel. It is a viral infection caused by herpes simplex virus. It presents clinically with pain followed by erythema, which then develops into a small, vesicular rash, which may coalesce to form a bullae. The diagnosis is confirmed by culture (1–5 days) or Tzank smear (less sensitive than culture) The process is self-limited, usually resolving in 3–4 weeks. I&D is not recommended because rates of secondary bacterial infection are high. Treatment with acyclovir may shorten the duration.

G. Deep Potential Space Infections—**Collar button abscess** occurs in the web space between digits. It is treated by I&D with volar and dorsal incisions, which avoid incising the skin in the web, and IV antibiotics. **Midpalmar space infections** are rare. Clinically there is a loss of midline contour of the hand and palmar pain elicited with flexion of the long, ring, and small fingers. It is similarly treated with I&D and IV antibiotics. The **thenar space infection** presents with pain and swelling over the thenar eminence exacerbated by flexion of thumb and index finger. I&D and IV antibiotics are also required. The **hypothenar space infection** is also rare but it is treated the same way.

H. Necrotizing Fasciitis—Results from streptococci infection (gram-negative cocci known as

Meleney's disease) or as a result of clostridia (gram-positive rod). Group A beta-hemolytic streptococci is the most common organism. Suspicion of this condition should be raised in host compromised patients (diabetes, cancer [CA]). It requires emergency radical débridement and broad-spectrum antibiotic coverage started empirically to include penicillin, clindamycin, metronidazole, and an aminoglycoside. Hemodynamic monitoring is a must. Amputation may be necessary because the average mortality rate is 32.2%. Hyperbaric oxygen is helpful when anaerobic organisms are present.

I. Fungal Infection—Serious infections are seen most frequently in host-compromised patients. These infections are divided into three categories: cutaneous, subcutaneous, and deep. **Cutaneous**: Chronic infection of the nail fold most commonly caused by *C. albicans*. It is treated with topical antifungals. Onychomycosis is a destructive, deforming infection of the nail plate most commonly caused by *Trichophyton rubrum*. This is also treated with topical antifungal agents; systemic therapy with griseofulvin or ketoconazole may be necessary. **Subcutaneous:** Most commonly caused by *Sporothrix schenckii*. It follows penetrating injury while handling plants or soil (rose thorn). It starts with a papule at the site of inoculation, with subsequent lesions developing along lymphatic channels. The treatment is potassium iodine supersaturated solution irrigation. **Deep:** Involves three forms: tenosynovial infection, septic arthritis, osteomyelitis. Treatment is based on fungal cultures and involves surgical débridement and an IV antifungal, such as amphotericin B. True pathogens include histoplasmosis, blastomycosis, coccidioidomycosis. Opportunistic infections include aspergillosis, candidiasis, mucormycosis, cryptococcosis.

J. Atypical Mycobacterial Infections—These organisms are widely distributed in the environment but are infrequent human pathogens. The most common infecting organisms include *M. marinum, M. kansasii, M. terrae, M. avium-intracellulare.* Musculoskeletal manifestations involve the wrist and hand in 50% of cases. *M. marinum:* proliferates in fresh and salt water enclosures. *M. avium-intracellulare:* found in soil, water, poultry (most frequently isolated organism in terminal AIDS patients). *M. kansasii* and *M. terrae:* found in soil. The diagnosis is based on biopsy for histopathology. Cultures and sensitivities are a must, and they require special medium at exact temperatures (**32°C**). A chest x-ray (CXR) is mandatory to rule out hematogenous spread. Treatment generally requires surgical débridement and oral antibiotics. Rifampin, ethambutol, or tetracycline is the drug of choice.

K. Hand Infection and Human Immunodeficiency Virus (HIV)—Virulence of organism enhanced by immunocompromised state. The following organisms are frequent isolates: Viral (**herpes simplex,** cytomegalovirus), fungal (candidiasis, *Cryptococcus,* histoplasmosis, aspergillosis), protozoal, mycobacteria. Herpes simplex is the overall most common hand infection in AIDS patients.

V. Vascular Occlusion/Disease

A. Evaluation techniques include the **three-phase bone scan**—Phase I (pictures taken within 2 minutes: extremity arteriogram); Phase II (pictures at 5–10 minutes: soft-tissue images demonstrating cellulitis or synovial inflammation); Phase III (pictures taken at 2–3 hours: these are the bone images; reflex sympathetic dystrophy is demonstrated by a diffusely positive phase III image that does not correlate with positive phase I and II studies; osteomyelitis is also seen in this phase); Phase IV (delayed 24-hour films are useful to differentiate osteomyelitis from adjacent cellulitis if there is a question). **Segmental limb pressures** are done with a blood pressure cuff 1.2 × the diameter of the extremity and a 10-MHz Doppler probe. A difference of 20 mm Hg between arms is abnormal. A difference of 1 mm Hg between fingers is abnormal. The sensitivity of the test is increased if also done after exercise. A **duplex scan** visualizes arterial intimal lesions, true and false aneurysms, and anterior venous (AV) fistulas. **Photoplethysmography** demonstrates arterial insufficiency when there is a loss of the dicrotic notch or a decreased rate of rise in the systolic peak. **Cold stimulation testing** demonstrates autonomic vascular dysfunction because patients with arterial disease require more than 20 minutes to return to pre-exposure temperatures when submersed for 20 seconds in ice water, whereas the usual time is 10 minutes. The **arteriogram** remains the *gold standard* for elucidating the nature and extent of thrombotic and embolic disease. It is invasive with antecedent risks; therefore it is generally considered a preoperative test. **Ultrasound duplex imaging** is emerging as a noninvasive test with near equal sensitivity and specificity in experienced hands.

B. Compartment Syndrome—Caused by increased pressure in a closed fascial space leading to tissue ischemia, death, and fibrosis. Findings include the five *p*'s: pain, pallor, pulselessness, paresthesias, and paralysis. *Pain accentuated with passive stretch is the most sensitive indicator*. Compartment pressures are diagnostic when pressures are 30 mm Hg, indicating that immediate fasciotomy is required (use a lower threshold in hypotensive patients—20 mm Hg). Muscle viability is determined by the four *c*'s: color, consistency, contractility, capacity to bleed.

C. Volkmann's Ischemic Contracture—A post-traumatic wrist, hand, and forearm contracture resulting from death and fibrosis of forearm musculature. *The most severely involved muscles are the FDP and FPL*. Three varieties and their treatment have been described (Table 6-10).

Table 6-10. STAGES OF VOLKMANN'S ISCHEMIC CONTRACTURE

TYPE	AFFECTED MUSCLES	TREATMENT
Mild	Wrist flexors	Dynamic splinting, tendon lengthening
Moderate	Wrist and digital flexors	Excision necrotic muscle, neurolysis (median, ulnar), BR to FPL and ECRL to FDP tendon transfers, distal slide of viable flexors (usually FDS)
Severe	Flexors and extensors	Excision necrotic muscle, neurolysis, tendon transfers; may need functioning free muscle transfer if insufficient motors are available for transfer

BR, brachioradialis; FPL, flexor pollicus longus; ECRL, extensor carpi radialis longus; FDP, flexor digitorum profundus; FDS, flexor digitorum superficialis.

D. **Occlusive Vascular Disease**—Can be caused by arterial trauma, emboli, atherosclerosis, or a variety of systemic diseases. It presents with claudication, paresthesias, and cold intolerance. It tends to be unilateral, whereas vasospastic disease tends to be bilateral.

1. Post-traumatic—Most common in upper extremity is the hypothenar hammer syndrome, which is thrombosis of the ulnar artery at Guyon's canal. The thrombus stimulates sympathetic fibers, inducing vasospasm distally, which further compromises circulation; embolization can also occur and will *most likely affect the ring finger* because of the angle of take-off of the common digital arteries of the third and fourth webs. Options for treatment include resection of the thrombosed segment, effecting a local sympathectomy, or resection and reconstruction (with vein graft). Some advocate intraoperative digital brachial index (DBI) measurements to determine whether reconstruction is necessary. (DBI ≤ 0.7 would be an indication for reconstruction). It has been suggested in the literature that re-establishing circulation may diminish cold intolerance.
2. Embolic Disease—Upper-extremity emboli compose 20% of all arterial emboli; of these 70% are of cardiac origin. Occasionally emboli are derived from the subclavian system as a result of thoracic outlet syndrome. Once recognized, the patient is heparinized, and embolectomy is performed if possible. Heparin is continued for 7–10 days followed by 3 months of warfarin. If the vessels affected are too small for embolectomy, streptokinase and urokinase have been shown to be beneficial, especially if done within 36 hours of occlusion. Tissue-plasminogen activator is currently the favored thrombolytic agent because of its specificity for the clot and long-lasting effect. If the emboli are from a proximal aneurysm, this is treated with resection of the aneurysm and reconstruction of the vessel. Sympathectomy will only relieve vasospasm and not prevent further embolization.
3. **Arteritis and Other Systemic Diseases**
   a. **Thromboangiitis Obliterans** (Buerger's Disease)—A vasculitis seen in smokers that initially involves distal vessels and progresses proximally. The treatment is simple for the doctor and hard for the patient: stop smoking. Ischemic lesions are treated with wound care and amputation, if necessary.
   b. **Giant Cell Arteritis**—Mainly involves arteries of the head and aortic branches in older women. In the upper extremity, involvement of the subclavian and axillary artery is seen. When associated with myalgias and arthralgias, it constitutes the syndrome known as *polymyalgia rheumatica*. Temporal artery biopsy is diagnostic. Treatment is with high-dose steroids and arterial reconstruction if ischemia persists.
   c. **Takayasu's Arteritis**—Also involves the subclavian and axillary artery but is more prevalent in young women. Intimal proliferation is responsible for the arterial stenosis. This condition has variable response to steroids.
   d. **Polyarteritis Nodosa**—A necrotizing arteritis associated with aneurysmal dilations of small vessels. These lesions have a predilection for bifurcations and tend to occur at the level of the bifurcation of the common digital arteries in the upper extremity.
   e. **Connective Tissue Disorders** (Lupus, Scleroderma, RA)—Can cause segmental arterial occlusion from deposition of antigen-antibody complexes in the vascular endothelium. This usually occurs at the level of the digital arteries and presents with ischemia with superimposed vasospastic disease. Treatment involves getting the underlying disease process under control and treating the vasospasm, as described later.
   f. **Atherosclerosis**—Usually involves the subclavian and axillary arteries and is more common on the left side (3:1). Proximal subclavian occlusions can induce a subclavian steal syndrome wherein blood is shunted away from the brain stem by a reversal of flow in the vertebral artery to meet the upper extremity demands. In proximal subclavian occlusions (proximal to vertebral artery), central nervous system symptoms are more common; with distal

Table 6-11. CAUSES OF SECONDARY VASOSPASTIC DISORDER

1. Connective tissue disease: scleroderma (incidence of Raynaud's 80–90%), SLE (incidence 18–26%), dermatomyositis (incidence 30%), RA (incidence 11%)
2. Occlusive arterial disease
3. Neurovascular compression: thoracic outlet syndrome
4. Hematologic abnormalities: cryoproteinemia, polycythemia, paraproteinemia
5. Occupational trauma: percussion and vibratory tool workers
6. Drugs and toxins: sympathomimetics, ergot compounds, beta-adrenergic blockers
7. CNS disease: syringomyelia, poliomyelitis, tumors/infarcts
8. Miscellaneous: RSD, malignant disease

RSD, reflex sympathetic dystrophy.

subclavian occlusions, arm claudication is more common. Digital ischemia is more frequently caused by emboli than by distal plaques. This is treated with extra-anatomic bypass of the subclavian artery.

E. **Vasospastic Disease**—Symptoms include periodic digital ischemia brought on by cold temperatures or other sympathetic stimuli to include emotional stress or pain. Initially fingers blanch (white), followed closely by cyanosis (blue) as deoxygenated blood pools during persistent vasospasm. The final ruborous (red) appearance is associated with vasodilation and is coincident with burning pain and dysesthesias.

1. **Raynaud's**
   a. **Phenomenon:** Episodic digital ischemia with typical color changes and dysesthesias.
   b. **Syndrome:** When Raynaud's phenomenon occurs as a result of a disease (Table 6-11). These patients are generally older than those with Raynaud's disease, trophic changes are usually present, pulses are often absent, the problem is usually asymmetric, and an angiogram often demonstrates a lesion.
   c. **Disease**: Primary vasospastic disorder that is usually seen in young women. In order to make the diagnosis, symptoms and characteristics must satisfy Allen and Brown's criteria: (1) intermittent attacks of discoloration of the acral parts, (2) bilateral involvement, (3) absence of clinical arterial occlusion, (4) gangrene or atrophic changes are rare, (5) symptoms present for 2 years, (6) absence of previous disease to which vascular reactivity can be attributed, (7) a predominance in women.

   Treatment is focused on the underlying disease (if known) and a common-sense approach such as: avoid cold exposure and stop smoking. Medical intervention includes intra-arterial reserpine (*does not help ulcer healing*), calcium channel blockers, or drugs aimed at improving blood elements (aspirin [A.S.A.], dipyridamole [Persantine], pentoxifylline [Trental]). Thermal biofeedback is helpful in 67–92% of patients. Microvascular reconstruction can be helpful if a damaged or occluded area can be identified and the underlying disease can be controlled. Digital sympathectomy can be considered after proving it will be of benefit with pulse volume recordings before and after local sympathetic block.

F. Reflex Sympathetic Dystrophy—Neurologic dysfunction following trauma, prolonged immobilization, surgery, or disease characterized by intense/exaggerated pain, vasomotor disturbance, delayed functional recovery, hyperhidrosis, swelling, osteopenia, and trophic skin changes. It is caused by sustained efferent sympathetic nerve activity perpetuated in a reflex arc. If it is associated with a definable nerve injury it is known as causalgia. The stages have been described by Lankford and Evans (Table 6-12).

   Diagnosis—Four cardinal signs include disproportionate amount of pain, swelling, stiffness, discoloration. Relief with sympathetic blockade is diagnostic. Thermography, radiographs, and a three-phase bone scan are also helpful. *Early diagnosis is critical to successful treatment.* Treatment includes physical therapy (pain-free active ROM, fluidotherapy, transcutaneous electrical nerve simulation). Sympathectomy, either chemical (four blocks of the stellate ganglion) or surgical (if persistent symptoms after four blocks or symptoms >6 months' duration), can be curative. Prevention is the key (avoiding nerve injury, tight dressings, or prolonged immobilization).

Table 6-12. STAGES OF REFLEX SYMPATHETIC DYSTROPHY

STAGE	ONSET (MONTHS)	FINDINGS
Acute	0–3	Pain, swelling, warmth, redness, decreased ROM, normal radiographs, positive three-phase bone scan, hyperhidrosis
Subacute	3–12	Worse pain, cyanosis, dry skin, worse stiffness, atrophy of skin, osteopenia on radiograph
Chronic	>12	Diminished pain, fibrosis, glossy skin that is dry and cool, joint contractures, extreme osteopenia

ROM, range of motion.

G. Frostbite—Rapid rewarming (40°–44°C water baths) is done with analgesia, tetanus prophylaxis, antibiotics, and wound care. Delay amputation until complete demarcation and mummification has occurred. Active and passive ROM and functional splinting are done from the start. Surgical sympathectomy may be required for late persistent vasospastic disease. Anticoagulation, dextran, and intra-arterial reserpine are not useful.

VI. Replantation / Microsurgery

A. Traumatic Amputation

1. Favorable indications for replantation
   a. Almost any part in a child
   b. Multiple digits
   c. Individual digit distal to the FDS insertion
   d. Thumb
   e. Wrist or proximal
2. Unfavorable indications for replantation
   a. Individual finger proximal to FDS insertion
   b. Crushed or mangled parts
   c. Amputations at multiple levels
   d. Arteriosclerotic vessels
   e. Other serious injury or disease
   f. Mentally unstable patients
   g. Signs of severe vessel trauma (red line sign: branch tears along vessel; ribbon sign: elastic recoil from traction media and intima usually separated)
   h. Polytrauma
3. Care of the Amputated Part—Replantation is not recommended if warm ischemia time is >6 hours for level proximal to the carpus or >12 hours for a digit. Cool ischemia times of <12 hours proximal to carpus or <24 hours for a digit; retain the option for replantation. The amputated part should be wrapped in moist gauze (lactated Ringer's solution); this is placed in a sealed plastic bag, which is then placed on regular ice (not dry ice).
4. Operative Sequence of Replantation—(1) bone, (2) extensor tendons, (3) flexor tendons, (4) arteries, (5) nerves, (6) veins, and (7) skin. *For multiple amputations, the structure-by-structure technique is faster and has a higher viability rate.* The priority for digit replantation is thumb, long, ring, small, index.
5. Postoperative Care—Warm room (80°F), adequate hydration, aspirin, dipyridamole, low-molecular-weight dextran 30–40 mL/hr, and heparin, if necessary. There is a higher incidence of postoperative hemorrhage when two anticoagulants are used with aspirin rather than one (53% rate rather than 2% rate). Nicotine, caffeine, and chocolate are not allowed.
6. Monitoring—Close observation of color, capillary refill, and Doppler pulse remains the most reliable method. Pulse oximetry is a reliable monitor; saturation less than 94% indicates potential vascular compromise. Skin surface temperature is a noninvasive, reproducible, and safe method to aid close observation. A drop in temperature >2°C in 1 hour or temperature below 30°C indicates decreased digital perfusion.
7. Arterial Insufficiency—If arterial insufficiency develops: release constricting bandages, place the extremity in a dependent position, consider heparinization, consider stellate ganglion blockade, explore early if these maneuvers do not work. Thrombosis secondary to vasospasm is the most frequent cause for early replant failure. If this happens, revision of the anastomosis will likely be required.
8. Inadequate Venous Outflow—Causes part engorgement, diminished inflow, and eventually, part loss. It is treated with extremity elevation. If this fails to resolve the problem, leeches are tried (they produce the anticoagulant hirudin, which yields 8–12 hours of sustained bleeding; *Aeromonas hydrophila* infection is a risk). If leeches are not available or tolerated by the patient or nursing staff, heparin-soaked pledgets can be used. A last resort is a surgical arteriovenous anastomosis.
9. Complications—First, infection; second, cold intolerance (which can last up to 2 years post replantation). *Smoking causes a more pronounced effect on vasoconstriction in the replanted digit compared with the normal digit.*
10. Results—Successful salvage depends primarily on mechanism of injury and ischemic time. Sharp amputations with cold ischemia <8 hours survive replantation in 94% of cases; however, success drops to 74% if ischemic time is >8 hours. Replanted fingers typically have 50% total active motion, and 2PD of 10 mm.
11. Forearm and Arm Replantations—Muscle necrosis leads to *myoglobinuria, which can precipitate renal failure and threaten the patient's life;* infection is also prevalent because of the difficulty in obtaining a sufficient débridement. Arterial inflow is established early (usually before skeletal stabilization), using shunts, if necessary, to minimize ischemia time. Fasciotomies are always performed. Fastidious débridement and second-look surgery in 72 hours are necessary. Blood loss during the procedure must be closely monitored.

B. Ring Avulsion Injuries—Classified based on the extent of the injury (Urbaniak)

1. Class 1: Circulation adequate, standard bone and soft-tissue treatment.
2. Class 2: Circulation inadequate, vessel repair preserves viability (others have divided 2 into 2A: no additional bone-tendon-nerve injury, and 2B: these additional injuries are present).
3. Class 3: Complete degloving or complete amputation.

Advances in technique with interposition grafts have improved results with replantation of these injuries. In general, class 2B and 3 injuries are better treated with amputation. The most common complication after successful replantation is cold intolerance (30–70% incidence).

C. Fingertip Amputations—The goal is to provide a sensate, durable tip with adequate bony support for the nail. It is generally agreed that when the surface area lost is 1 cm^2 and there is no bone exposed, healing by secondary intention yields a satisfactory result. For many this is the treatment of choice whenever there is no bone exposed. Others argue that wound contraction will draw the nail down over the tip, causing a hook-nail deformity. It is universally agreed that any type of closure that draws the nail bed curving over the tip will lead to a hook-nail deformity, so *tight tip closures should be avoided*. If for some reason healing by secondary intention is judged not to be a satisfactory option, full-thickness skin graft from the hypothenar eminence is a good choice. If bone is exposed, it may be rongeured back so long as the bone loss does not compromise the support of the nail bed. If rongeuring the bone is judged to be a bad choice, a coverage procedure is indicated because exposed bone will impede healing by secondary intention. Straight or dorsally angulated amputations are best covered with a volar V-Y advancement flap (Atasoy) or a double lateral V-Y advancement flap (Kutler) (Fig. 6-23). The volar arterialized advancement flap of Moberg is a reasonable choice in the thumb, but it leads to excessive joint stiffness in a finger. A volarly angled amputation is covered with a cross finger flap, a thenar crease flap, or a thenar H flap. The thenar crease and thenar H flaps can lead to joint contractures in adults because the PIP joint is held in flexion for 2 weeks before the pedicle is divided. These flaps are generally best reserved for young people (<40 years of age). Thenar flaps are preferred over cross finger flaps because they do not scar the dorsum of the adjacent finger. Other more complex flaps such as the second dorsal metacarpal artery island flap (comes with a nerve and is sometimes used for thumb tip coverage) or the homodigital island flap (must prove that both digital arteries are intact before harvesting this flap) are available if the aforementioned choices are judged to be insufficient or less desirable.

D. Microsurgery

1. Wound Classification—It is important to obtain early consultation (first 48 hours) from the reconstructive surgeon who may be assisting with wound management. It is generally accepted that limb salvage is not indicated when a sensate limb is not achievable, when adequate débridement is not achievable, and when a limb with sufficient mobility and stability is not achievable. The single most important procedure is early aggressive wound débridement (ideally within 6 hours of injury). Several classification systems are available that aid in wound assessment and therefore treatment decisions. The mangled-extremity severity score (MESS) provides a guide to determining the expected outcome from a limb salvage attempt by weighing the energy of injury, limb ischemia, hemodynamic status, and the patient's age (Table 6-13). A MESS score >7 is a relative contraindication to limb salvage, whereas a score <4 indicates a limb with a good prognosis if salvaged. However, the current literature suggests this system is not reliable for upper extremity trauma. The Gustilo classification of open fractures (see Chapter 10) remains a useful tool because it emphasizes the condition of the soft-tissue envelope. Wounds that have a compromised soft-tissue envelope are more likely to develop infection (Gustilo types I–IIIA, 12% infection rate; Gustilo types IIIB and IIIC, 56% infection rate) and are also more likely to go on to nonunion.
2. Timing of Wound Coverage—Early coverage of traumatic wounds has the following advantages: lower flap failure rate, effects of fibrosis minimized, easier flap planning and vessel anastomoses, less vascular spasm and the veins are easier to work with, lower infection rates, diminished time of hospitalization, less tissue desiccation, fewer number of overall surgeries to final result. Godina noted an advantage to early soft-tissue coverage in a large series of complex lower-extremity trauma cases. Wounds that were covered in less than 6 days had the fewest complications (0.7%). Those covered between 6 days and 3 months had the highest failure rate (17.5%). Those that were covered after 3 months when the wound had stabilized had an intermediate result (9% failure rate). The rate of infection goes from 0.7% to 17% when wound coverage is delayed past 7 days.
3. The Reconstructive Ladder—The goal is to restore the limb to useful function while diminishing morbidity using the simplest methods that are judged to be appropriate for the wound in question. Primary closure is considered first. If this is not an option, successively more complex methods are considered: delayed primary closure, skin grafting, rotation flap, and finally free-flap coverage.
   a. Primary Wound Closure—Undue tension causes local tissue ischemia and wound dehiscence or compartment syndrome. Wounds that are clean, with minimal bacterial contamination, and that are less than 6 hours old are usually safe to close primarily.
   b. Secondary Wound Closure—Closure by wound granulation and epithelialization.

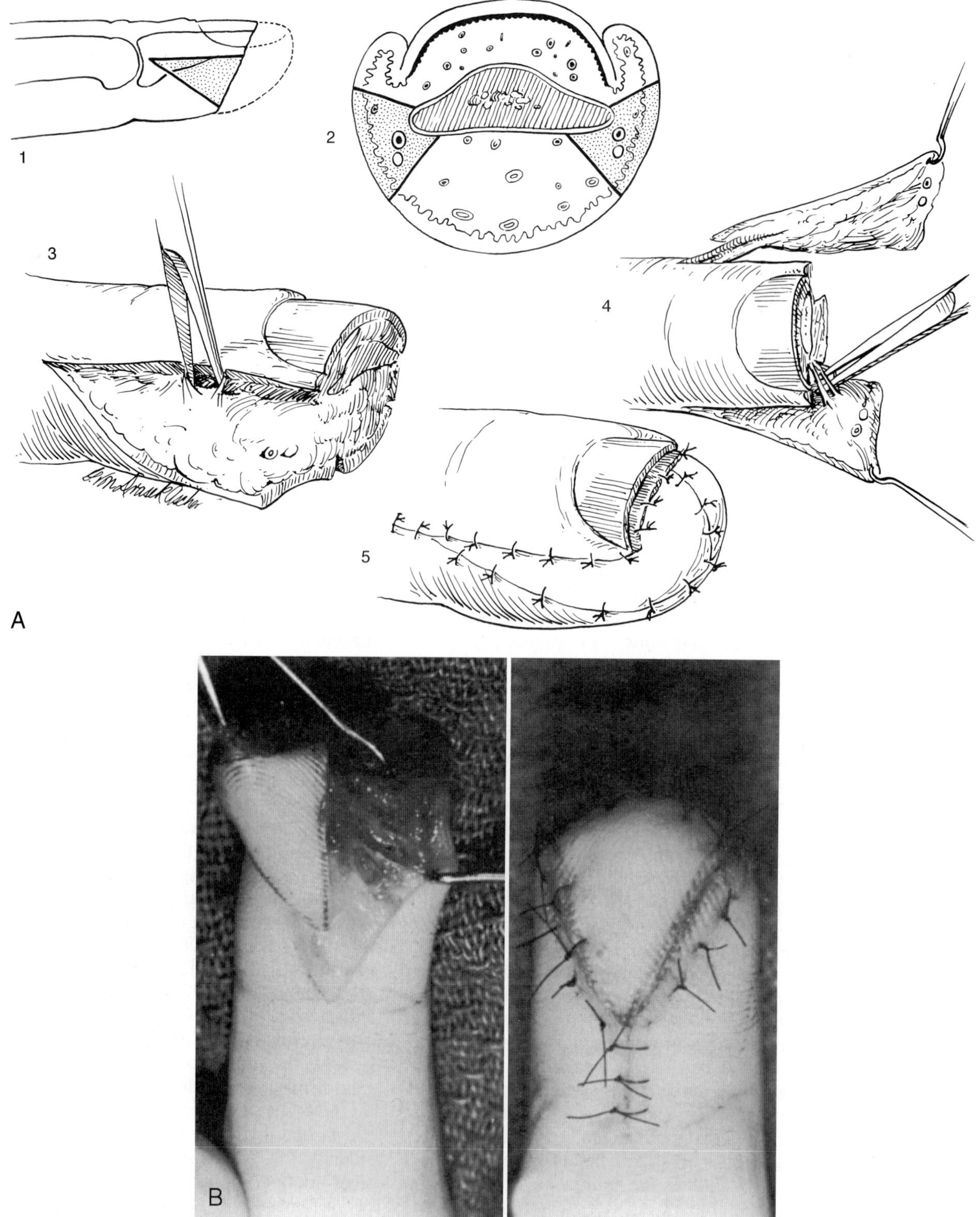

FIGURE 6-23 ■ *A,* Kutler double lateral V-Y advancements. *(1)* The advancement flaps are designed over the neurovascular pedicles and carried right down to the bone *(2)*. The fibrous septa are defined and *(3)* divided, permitting free mobilization *(4)* on the neurovascular pedicles alone. The flaps then advance readily to the midline *(5)*. *B,* The volar V-Y advancement flap. (From Green, D.H., Hotchkiss, R.M., Pederson, W.C., and Lampert, R., eds.: Green's Operative Hand Surgery, 4th ed. New York, Churchill Livingstone, 1998.)

Table 6-13. MANGLED EXTREMITY SEVERITY SCORE

CRITERIA	SCORE
Energy of Injury	
Low	1
Medium	2
High	3
Massive	4
*Ischemia**	
No ischemia	0
Decreased pulses	1
Thready pulses	2
No pulses	3
Shock	
Normal	0
Transient	1
Prolonged	2
Age	
<30 yr	0
30–50 yr	1
>50 yr	2

*Ischemia score doubles when warm ischemia time >6 hours.

This requires regular dressing changes and is associated with contraction over time. The Papino graft (filling the defect with cancellous bone graft) is intended to stimulate this process when bone is exposed. This method poses some danger of late infection when devascularized tissues are present within the wound (such as bone stripped of its periosteum). Granulation can occur over exposed implants, but it takes a very long time.

c. Skin Grafts—Require a well-vascularized bed for them to take. Split-thickness grafts are 0.012–0.025 inches thick. The thinner the graft, the more wound contraction will occur. Donor sites re-epithelialize because dermal papillae are left behind. Once it is re-epithelialized it can be used for skin graft again, if needed. Meshing a split-thickness graft increases the surface area that can be covered and allows for egress of hematoma. Failure of skin grafting is caused by shear, hematoma, and infection. Full-thickness grafts have a higher failure rate than split-thickness grafts, but they yield a better cosmetic result and are generally more durable than split-thickness grafts. *Full-thickness grafts do not contract*, and for that reason are preferable to cover hand defects, except for the dorsum of the hand, where a nonmeshed split-thickness graft yields the best results. Full-thickness grafts regain better sensibility because of more retained sensory receptors.

d. Flap Reconstruction—A flap is a unit of tissue that is supported by blood vessels and is moved from a donor site to a recipient site to cover a defect of tissue. This unit can be composed of one or several tissue types: skin, fascia, muscle, tendon, nerve, and bone. A flap composed of more than one tissue type is called a *composite flap*. Flap reconstruction has some biologic advantages, such as lower secondary infection rates and higher bone union rates. This relates to a flap's ability to improve a portion of the soft-tissue envelope by virtue of the fact that it is vascularized. Increased success of treating osteomyelitis with muscle flaps is attributed to improved tissue perfusion. Flaps are indicated when the wound has exposed tissue such as bone (stripped of its periosteum), tendons (stripped of paratenon), cartilage, or orthopaedic implants that cannot revascularize a skin graft. They are also indicated when a skin graft may impair later reconstruction or be subject to excessive exposure and repeated ulceration. Flaps can be classified by their vascular supply, tissue type, and donor site location and method of transfer.
   (1) Classification according to blood supply
      (a) Axial pattern flaps have a single arteriovenous pedicle (types include peninsular [pedicle and overlying skin] flap, island [pedicle only] flap, free flap).
      (b) Random pattern flaps are supported by the microcirculation with no single arteriovenous system (e.g., Z-plasty, rotation flap).
      (c) Venous flaps involve flow though the venous system only where the distal vein in the flap is hooked up to a donor artery and the proximal vein in the flap is hooked up to a recipient vein.
   (2) Classification according to tissue type
      (a) Cutaneous flaps include skin and subcutaneous tissue (e.g., thenar H flap).
      (b) Fascia or fasciocutaneous flaps include fascia with or without the overlying skin (e.g., radial forearm flap).
      (c) Muscle or musculocutaneous flaps involve perforators supplied via the pedicle that allow harvesting with overlying skin if needed (e.g., latissimus dorsi). If the motor nerve is not preserved, a muscle flap will atrophy to about 50% of its original size.
      (d) Bone and osteocutaneous flaps (e.g., fibula with or without overlying skin).

(e) Composite flaps are composed of several tissue types, allowing for single-stage reconstructions (e.g., free toe transfer, osteocutaneous flap).

(f) Innervated flaps involve a tissue unit with its nerve supply. These can involve a motor nerve (e.g., gracilis flap: motor branch of obturator nerve) or a sensory nerve (e.g., lateral arm flap: posterior cutaneous nerve of the arm).

(3) Classification according to mobilization

(a) Local—Transposition flaps are geometric in their design and can be random pattern (rhomboid flap) or axial pattern (first dorsal metacarpal artery island flap) regarding their blood supply. A Z-plasty is a form of a transposition flap. The lengths of the limbs of a Z-plasty should always be the same. The angles can vary. As the angle increases, so does the lengthening that occurs along the line of the central limb. The commonly used 60-degree angle theoretically yields a 75% lengthening along the line of the central limb. If sufficient skin is not available for one large Z-plasty, they can be done in series. *The longitudinal gain is aggregate, whereas the transverse loss is not.* Rotation flaps are not geometric and are all random pattern regarding their blood supply. (*It is important not to make a random pattern flap longer than the width of the base so as not to exceed the capacity of the microcirculation.*) Advancement flaps advance in a straight line to fill the defect; they can also be either random pattern (V-Y advancement flap) or axial pattern (Moberg's advancement flap).

(b) Distant—Flaps can be transferred either in stages or in a single stage as a free tissue transfer. Flaps transferred in stages are raised from their anatomic location and placed in the defect without dividing the base (groin flap). Neovascularization occurs from the wound bed into the graft. After this (usually at 14–21 days), the pedicle of the flap is divided and inset into the defect. Free flaps are all axial pattern. They are raised on the pedicle, which is then divided and reanastamosed to donor vessels in the same operation. *It is important to remember that the anastomoses should be done out of the zone of injury.*

4. Causes of Flap Failure—The main cause is inadequate arterial blood flow. Often vasospasm is the culprit leading to thrombosis at the anastomosis. Other factors that compromise inflow include hypotension, compression, hematoma, edema, infection, hypothermia, and vasoconstrictive agents, such as nicotine. Outflow problems can also lead to the demise of a flap. In this situation the flap will become engorged with blood as evidenced by a purple discoloration and unusually brisk capillary refill. Eventually, altered hemodynamic pressure differentials can compromise inflow, leading to flap failure.

5. Thumb Reconstruction—*The wrap-around procedure: best duplicates thumb appearance and size.* The great-toe transfer: provides mobility and growth potential, and it is very stable. The second-toe transfer: provides mobility and growth potential, but it is the least stable. The great- and second-toe transfers have the same vascular pedicle: first dorsal metatarsal artery, a branch of the dorsalis pedis, runs superficially in 78% of cases. In 22% of cases it arises deeply from the descending branch of the dorsalis pedis artery to ascend in the first metatarsal space, coursing beneath or through the first dorsal interosseous muscle. Indications include traumatic loss and congenital deficiency. If pollicization of a damaged digit that is not useful in its orthotopic location is an option, this is preferable over toe-to-hand transfer. The wrap-around procedure is preferred when loss is distal to a mobile MCPJ in an adult. The great-toe transfer is otherwise preferred because of its stability. The second-toe transfer is useful when length is needed, requiring the MCPJ and a portion of the second metatarsal. Harvesting the great-toe MCPJ should be avoided. Osteoplastic reconstruction is considered in patients who are not good candidates for microarterial anastomosis if no option for pollicization exists, such as amputation through the carpometacarpal (CMC) joint (Fig. 6-24).

6. Microsurgical Bone Reconstruction—Donor sites include any expendable bone with an identifiable vascular pedicle (most commonly used are the fibula and the anterior iliac crest). The free fibula is based on the peroneal artery pedicle and is useful for diaphyseal reconstruction. The free iliac crest is based on the deep circumflex iliac vessels and is useful for metaphyseal reconstruction. Indications include extensive post-traumatic defects (>6–8 cm, best results), post-tumor intercalary resection, osteomyelitis (worst results), congenital pseudarthrosis of the tibia

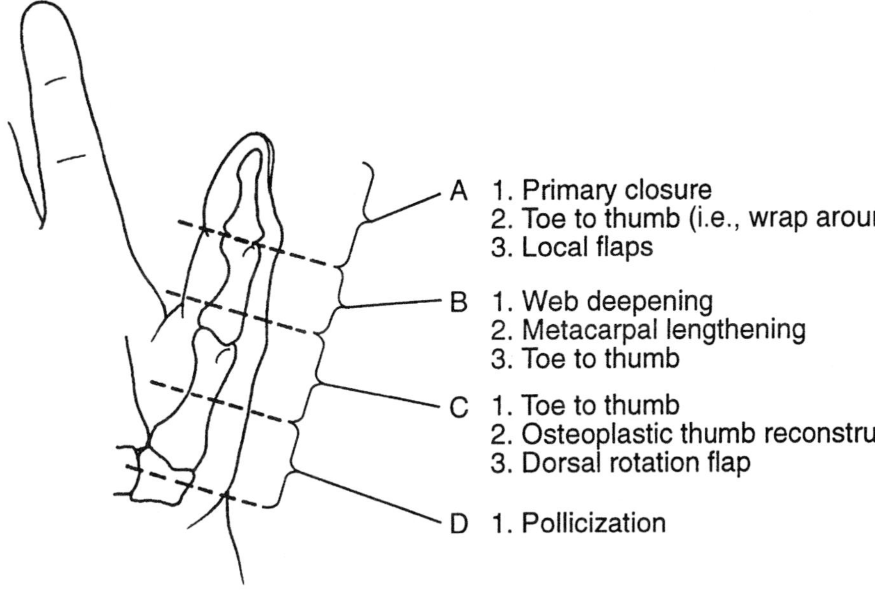

FIGURE 6-24 ■ Thumb reconstruction options based on level of amputation. (From Trumble, T.E.: Principles of Hand Surgery and Therapy. Philadelphia, WB Saunders, 2000, p. 479.)

or ulna, resistant nonunions, failed prior conventional bone graft, postirradiation fractures, allograft nonunion, and avascular necrosis. Success rates average 88% overall. The best results are in nonseptic cases. Adjuvant radiation and chemotherapy adversely effect results. Average time to union is 6 months.

7. Microsurgical Joint Transfer—Remains controversial. Donor sites include the metatarsal phalangeal joint or PIPJ of the second toe. Indications include a destroyed PIPJ or MCPJ in a child with associated epiphyseal plate injury or in young, active persons who are not candidates for conventional arthroplasty. A limited but useful ROM with good lateral stability can usually be achieved (adult, 32 degrees; child, 37 degrees). The chief complication is the limited ROM.
8. Microsurgical Functioning Free Muscle Transfer—The most frequently used donor is the gracilis muscle (nerve; anterior division of obturator vessel; branch of medial femoral circumflex artery). Alternatives associated with success include the latissimus dorsi, pectoralis major, rectus femoris, semitendinosis, and medial gastrocnemius. The chief indication is restoration of active digital flexion in a severe Volkmann's ischemic contracture. Prerequisites include full passive motion of the digits and wrist and a stable wrist joint. Results are markedly better if the intrinsics are intact. Overall, 83% of patients have return of some degree of useful function. Other indications include brachial plexus palsy reconstruction.
9. Defects over the Tibia—A gastrocnemius flap is used for wounds over the proximal third (medial head for medial and midline defects, lateral head for lateral defects). A soleus flap is used for wounds in the middle third of the leg if the soleus is in good condition. Free flaps are generally used for wounds over the distal third of the leg if a fasciocutaneous pedicle flap such as the sural artery island flap is not available. Free flaps are also used for large defects or when the gastrocnemius and soleus are damaged.

VII. Wrist Pain/Instability

A. Introduction—Wrist Evaluation

1. Functional ROM

MOTION	DEGREES
Dorsiflexion	40
Volaflexion	40
Radioulnar deviation arc	40

2. Examination involves bilateral functional assessment, including: ROM, digital flexion/extension lags, sensibility, grip strength, and provocative maneuvers.

PROVOCATIVE MANEUVERS

Eponym	Tests For Instability At:
Watson test	Scapholunate (SL) interval
Regan test	Lunotriquetral (LT) interval
Kleinman test	Dynamic assessment LT instability
Lichtman test	Dynamic assessment of midcarpal instability
TFCC grind	Assessment for TFCC pathology
ECU snap	Assessment for unstable ECU
Piano key sign	DRUJ instability

3. Plain radiographs

INTERVAL	NORMAL ANGLE, GAP, OR RELATIONSHIP
SL angle	30–60 degrees (average 47 degrees)
Capitolunate angle	0–15 degrees
Radiolunate angle	−25 to +10 degrees
SL gap	<3 mm

4. Arthroscopy—Has been shown to be more sensitive and specific than arthrography and as least as sensitive and specific as arthrotomy. Other valuable diagnostic tests include fluoroscopic motion studies (dynamic instability), bone scan (infection, reflex sympathetic dystrophy), MRI (avascular necrosis [AVN], ligament disruptions, tumors), CT scan (fractures, structural abnormalities), and diagnostic injections. Arthrography has fallen out of favor because of its lack of specificity.
5. Kinematics—The proximal carpal row (scaphoid, lunate, and triquetrum) flexes in radial deviation and extends in ulnar deviation. There are two main theories as to why this happens. Radial side theory (Linschied): With radial deviation there is a rotational moment on the scaphoid via forces applied by the radius and the trapezium, which favors flexion. In ulnar deviation the radioscaphocapitate and scaphotrapezial ligaments tighten, lifting the scaphoid into extension. Ulnar side theory (Weber): With radial deviation the triquetrum moves to the dorsoradial facet of the helicoid hamate joint. This flexes the lunate and the scaphoid via forces transmitted through the interosseous ligaments. In ulnar deviation the triquetrum translates to the volar ulnar facet of the hamate, subsequently extending the rest of the proximal carpal row. These concepts are fundamental to understanding pathomechanics of ligament ruptures. The wrist instability diagram (Fig. 6-25) assists in understanding the various instability patterns.

B. Wrist Instability—Classification; this helps to localize the instability based on established patterns recognizable on plain radiographs. The advent of arthroscopy of the wrist and MRI have identified lesser degrees of instability amenable to treatment, usually with less invasive methods than open surgery. Midcarpal joint arthroscopy best demonstrates subtle degrees of instability.
1. CID (Carpal Instability Dissociative)—Disruption of an intercarpal ligament within a carpal row.
   a. Dorsal Intercalated Segment Instability (DISI)—Disruption of the SL ligament or unstable fracture of the scaphoid. Usually there is associated disruption of the volar radiocarpal ligaments. Other causes associated with DISI include Kienbock's disease.

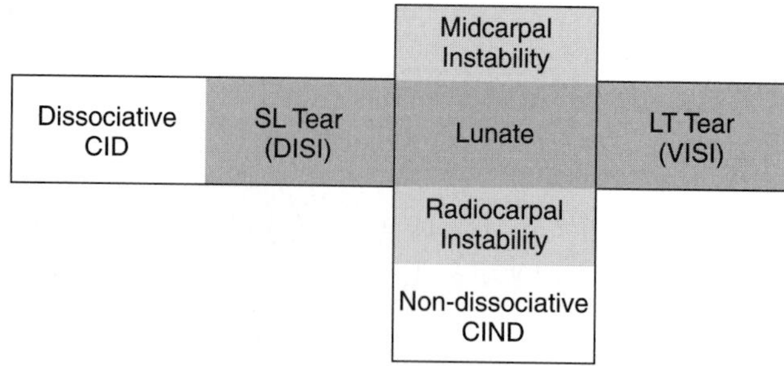

WRIST INSTABILITY DIAGRAM

FIGURE 6-25 ■ Wrist instability. Carpal instability dissociative (CID) results from intercarpal ligament rupture. Scapholunate (SL) rupture results in dorsal intercalated segmental instability (DISI), and lunotriquetral (LT) rupture results in volar intercalated segmental instability (VISI). Carpal instability nondissociative (CIND) results from extrinsic carpal ligament rupture and is either midcarpal or radiocarpal.

Pertinent radiographic findings include an SL gap >3 mm on posteroanterior (PA) view with clenched fist (Terry Thomas's sign). There can be a break in Gilula's arc at the SL interval, although this is not always abnormal. There also may be a cortical ring sign. An SL angle >60 degrees on neutral rotation lateral and an abnormal radiolunate angle (>15 degrees) are also seen. An unstable scaphoid fracture is associated with malalignment in flexion and scaphoid foreshortening—the so-called hump-back deformity. It is seen radiographically by displacement >1 mm, SL angle >60 degrees, capitolunate (CL) angle >15 degrees. Current treatment recommendations for SL instability with DISI are repair of the SL ligament (linkage procedure) if possible (effective up to 17 months from injury in one study). Soft-tissue repair will be successful if the deformity is supple, such that the deformity can be corrected without extensive soft-tissue release. If the ligament is not repairable or the deformity is not supple, a stabilization procedure such as a scaphotrapezialtrapezoidal (triscaphe) (STT) fusion (scapholunocapitate or scaphocapitate are also favored fusions) is advised. Reconstruction of the ligament with a tendon weave is currently not advised because of high incidence of late failure. A number of bone retinaculum reconstructions are currently under investigation. Early reports suggest that they are effective for dynamic instability. A Blatt dorsal capsulodesis is often added to a ligament repair and remains a viable alternative for a chronic instability when ligament repair is not feasible and the wrist is supple. Unstable scaphoid fractures are best treated by open reduction, internal fixation (ORIF).

b. Volar Intercalated Segment Instability (VISI)—Involves disruption of the LT interosseous ligament. A static instability pattern will not be evident unless the dorsal radiocarpal ligament is also disrupted (Viegas S) as well as the ulnocapitate ligament (Trumble T). Pertinent radiographic findings include a break in Gilula's arc on the PA view and a radiolunate or capitolunate angle >15 degrees. Arthroscopy is helpful in establishing this diagnosis. Options for treatment include multiple pin fixation (acute instability) or fusion of the LT interval (static or chronic instability). In patients with additional ulnar positive variation and ulnocarpal impaction, both the LT instability and the ulnocarpal impaction are well managed with an ulnar-shortening osteotomy. Ligament reconstructions have fallen out of favor because of late recurrent instability.

c. Axial Carpal Instability—Secondary to violent trauma causing intercarpal disruption of the proximal and distal rows as well as the intermetacarpal bases in a longitudinal fashion. These injuries have been classified by Garcia-Elias into axial-radial, axial-ulnar, and combined. They are treated with reduction and pinning, as well as prolonged casting.

2. CIND (Carpal Instability Nondissociative)—Ligamentous disruption leading to instability between rows (radiocarpal or midcarpal). These patients present with complaints of subluxations that may or may not be painful, but that give them a feeling of giving way and an unreliable clunking wrist. Generally, patients with CIND midcarpal instability are ligamentously lax, but it also occurs after trauma. Cineradiographic examination will show a sudden shift of the proximal carpal row with active radial or ulnar deviation (catch-up clunk). Nonoperative management with immobilization is tried first; if this fails the most reliable option for treatment is a fusion across the midcarpal joint. Ligament reconstruction does not yield lasting results in most series. Of all the wrist instabilities, midcarpal instability is the most amenable to treatment with splints. Ulnar translation is a radiocarpal CIND that occurs after global rupture of the extrinsic carpal ligaments. Immediate open repair, reduction and pinning is indicated, because late repairs yield poor results. Radiographic diagnosis of ulnar translation is made when >50% of the lunate width is ulnarly translated off the lunate fossa of the radius (Fig. 6-26). The more common CIND radiocarpal instability results from malunion of the distal radius, and treatment is directed at correcting the malunion.

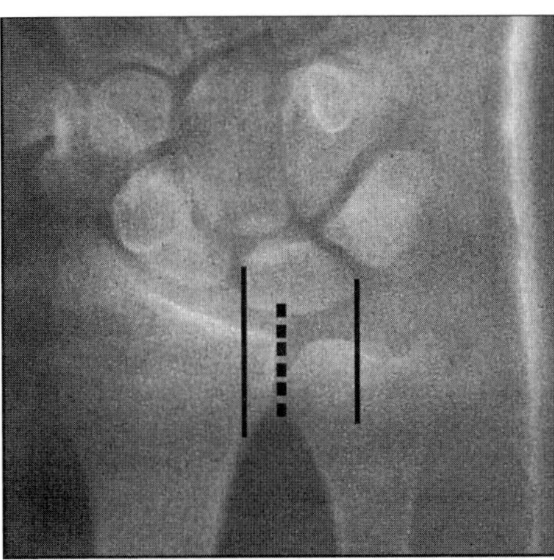

FIGURE 6-26 ■ Ulnar translation. The lunate width *(solid lines)* is normally 50% or more in contact with the radius. A line from the sigmoid notch *(dotted line)* shows more than 50% of the lunate lying ulnar to the radius; therefore ulnar translation instability is present.

3. CIC (Carpal Instability Combined)—Ligamentous disruption both within and between rows.

a. Classic example is the perilunate dislocation. The arc of this injury can course through bone (i.e., transscaphoid or transradial styloid perilunar injury), which is known as the greater arc. When the disruption courses though ligaments around the lunate, this is known as the lesser arc. It can involve a combination of both the greater and lesser arcs. Radiographs will demonstrate breaks in Gilula's arcs as well as signs of instability in the involved intervals, as previously described. Mayfield described four stages of perilunar instability proceeding from radial to ulnar around the lunate involving the following joints: (1) SL, (2) SL and CL, (3) SL and CL and LT, (4) lunate dislocates from the radiocarpal joint, usually in a volar direction. This injury is treated by open reduction pin fixation and a prolonged period of casting (8–12 weeks). The efficacy of direct repair of the disrupted volar ligaments has not been definitively shown to be beneficial. **Poor outcome correlates most closely with a persistently elevated SL gap**.

b. Scaphocapitate Syndrome—This is an uncommon variant of the perilunate dissociation wherein the arc of injury proceeds through the neck of the capitate and the proximal fragment rotates

90–180 degrees. This obviously could lead to a midcarpal arthritis problem if not recognized and dealt with. If recognized early, treat with open reduction and fixation of the capitate fragment. If recognized late, options include excision of the fragment with or without interposition grafts, ORIF if the cartilage is still good, or a midcarpal fusion may be necessary.

C. Limited Arthrodesis—Most reliable way to correct instability if the patient is willing to sacrifice motion. Fusion across a joint is associated with the following percentage loss of motion: radiocarpal, 55–60%; midcarpal, 20–35%; between two bones in the same row, 10–20%.

D. Other Common Causes of Wrist Pain

1. Scaphoid Fracture

   a. The major blood supply is from the radial artery, branches of which enter at the dorsal ridge and supply the proximal 80% of the bone. There is another group of vessels, which are branches of the superficial palmar branch of the radial artery, that enter the bone in the distal tubercle and supply the distal 30%. Because of the arrangement of the vascular supply, fractures of the proximal fifth of the scaphoid are associated with an AVN rate of 100%; those of the proximal third are associated with an AVN rate of 33%.

   b. Incidence of Fracture Location Within the Bone—Waist, 65%; proximal third, 25%; distal third, 10%

   c. Treatment—A bone scan has a specificity of 98% and a sensitivity of 100% and is therefore the best test to diagnose an occult scaphoid fracture. It should be positive within 24 hours of injury. The vast majority of stable scaphoid fractures are well treated by casting. It is important to start immobilization early because nonunion rates are significantly increased when immobilization is delayed beyond 4 weeks from fracture. The type of cast is controversial, and literature support can be found for nearly anything; therefore this remains surgeon's preference. However Gellman and coworkers demonstrated that time to union and rates of delayed union and nonunion are diminished with a long arm-thumb-spica cast. There is evidence that pulsed electromagnetic fields are helpful with delayed unions. Unstable scaphoid fractures have a higher incidence of nonunion and malunion (which can be problematic) and are best treated by early ORIF. Criteria for instability include displacement greater than 1 mm, capitolunate angle greater than 15 degrees, an SL angle >60 degrees, and proximal pole fractures. Vertical oblique fractures and comminuted fractures are inherently unstable and are best treated with ORIF or percutaneous fixation. Results of percutaneous screw fixation of reducible unstable fractures are superior to those from closed treatment.

2. Scaphoid Nonunion—Can lead to advanced collapse and progressive arthritis. Two types of bone grafts are generally used to treat this problem: the inlay (Russe) graft, which has a union rate of 92% and is used in nonunions not associated with adjacent carpal collapse and excessive flexion deformity (humpback scaphoid); and the interposition (Fisk) graft, which is an opening-wedge graft designed to restore scaphoid length and angulation. This will usually correct the adjacent carpal instability. Union rates are reported as between 72% and 95%. The most reliable sign of a vascular proximal pole is punctuate bleeding at the time of surgery. If bleeding is obvious, the union rate is 92%; if bleeding is questionable, the union rate is 71%; if there is no bleeding, the union rate is 0%. MRI is unreliable in predicting the presence of punctuate bleeding at surgery. After successful surgery, the progression of arthritis is slower but still occurs in 40–50% of patients. It is therefore desirable to attempt to obtain union. If initial surgery fails, repeat bone grafting is 50–80% successful. Vascularized bone grafts harvested from the distal radius are now popular in management of these difficult cases, and they may offer improved results. Vascularized grafts are more successful than nonvascular grafts when treating nonunion in the face of AVN. However, published series are limited at this time. A distal radius vascularized bone pedicle graft based on the 1–2 intercompartmental supraretinacular artery (1–2 intercompartmental supra-retinacular artery [ICSRA]) has shown accelerated healing in many cases.

3. Scapholunate Advanced Collapse (SLAC Wrist)—Progressive arthritis due to SL interval disruption with flexion deformity of the scaphoid and DISI of the proximal carpal row. As a consequence of the instability, concentric joint surfaces are malaligned, leading to force concentration and arthritis. Watson has classified SLAC into three stages (Fig. 6-27). Stage I: arthritis between the scaphoid and radial styloid; stage II: arthritis between the scaphoid and the entire scaphoid facet of the radius (in scaphoid nonunion advanced collapse [SNAC], the proximal pole of the scaphoid and corresponding surface of the radius are spared from arthritis because they

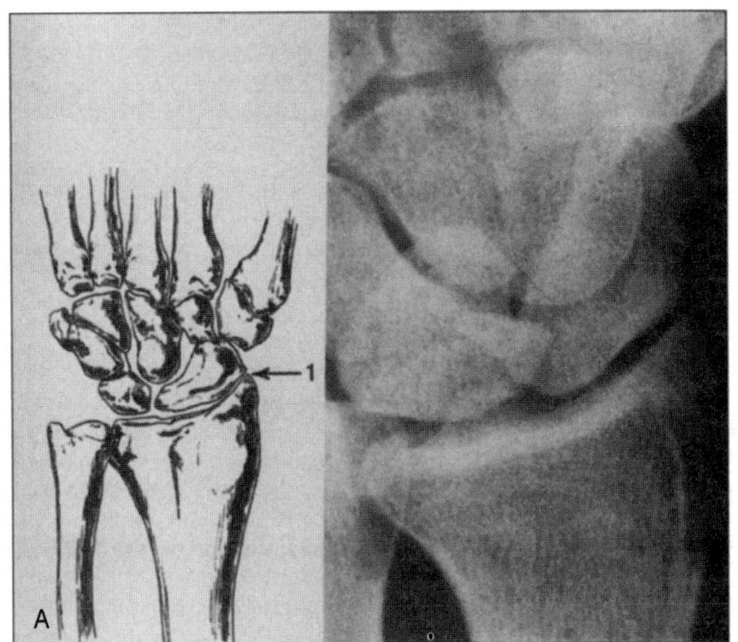

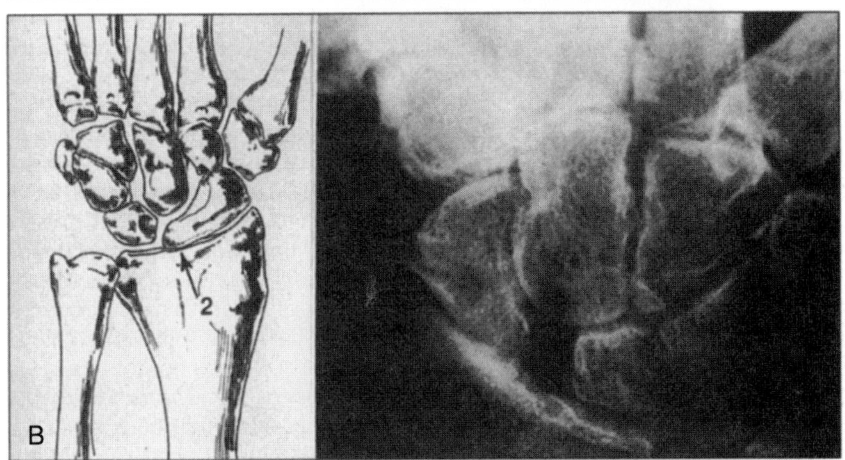

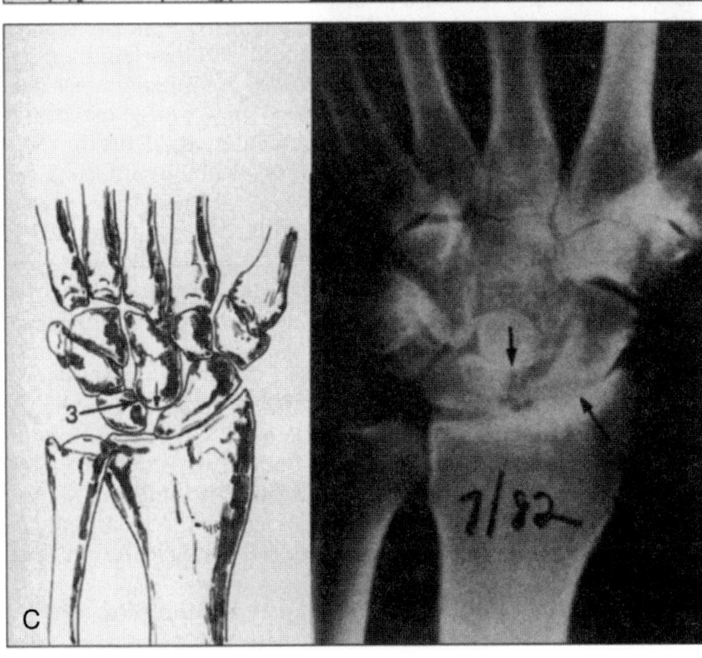

FIGURE 6-27 ■ Scapholunate advanced collapse. *A,* Early degenerative changes noted at the tip of the radial styloid and distal-radial aspect of the scaphoid *(arrow)* (stage I). *B,* Degenerative process has progressed to articular surface between distal radius and scaphoid *(arrow)*; radiograph *(right)* shows scapholunate dissociation, joint cartilage loss, and osteophyte formations (stage II). *C,* Progression of degeneration from the radioscaphoid (arrow pointing up in radiograph, *right*) to the capitolunate articulation (*arrow pointing down in radiograph, right*) with preservation of the radiolunate joint (stage III). (From Watson, H.K., and Ballet, F.L.: The SLAC wrist: Scapholunate advanced collapse pattern of degenerative arthritis. J. Hand Surg. [Am.] 9:358–365, 1984.)

are not loaded); stage III: stages I and II plus arthritis between the capitate and lunate. Options for treatment are based on stage. Stage I: radial styloidectomy and scaphoid stabilization (e.g., STT fusion); stage II: scaphoid excision and four-corner fusion, proximal row carpectomy, wrist fusion; stage III: scaphoid excision and four-corner fusion, wrist fusion. *Results of treatment:* wrist fusion: best pain relief and good grip strength, no motion; proximal row carpectomy and scaphoid excision four-corner fusion: essentially equivalent in several long-term studies. Concepts for treatment of SNAC are similar to those for SLAC. However, unlike SLAC, in SNAC when the wrist is in fixed DISI and the scaphocapitate joint is not arthritic, excision of the distal half of the scaphoid consistently relieves pain, improves both motion and grip strength.

4. Hamate Hook Fracture—Presents with history of blunt trauma to the palm, usually sports associated with a club (golf club, tennis racket); they also often have paresthesias involving the ring and small fingers. A CT scan is the best test to confirm the diagnosis. It is treated with excision of fracture fragment. ORIF can be done but has little benefit. When evaluating be aware of the bipartite hamate (os hamuli proprius); smooth cortical surfaces are the clue.
5. STT Arthritis—Second most common degenerative condition in the wrist. It is well treated with an STT fusion after a trial of nonoperative management to include splints, NSAIDs, and steroid injections.
6. AVN of the Scaphoid (Preiser's Disease)—A rare condition. The diagnosis is based on radiographic evidence of sclerosis and fragmentation of the proximal pole of the scaphoid without evidence of fracture. The average age of onset is 40 years. It is treated with immobilization, which is effective in 20% of cases. Operative treatment includes drilling, revascularization, allograft replacement, vascularized bone grafts, a salvage procedure such as proximal row carpectomy, or scaphoid excision and four-corner fusion.
7. AVN of the Capitate—Also rare with only sporadic case reports. It is treated with immobilization. If this fails, excision of the necrotic portion and tendon interposition arthroplasty has had good early results.
8. Kienbock's Disease (AVN of the Lunate)—The etiology remains controversial but involves both biomechanical and anatomic factors that create a lunate that is susceptible to repetitive microtrauma. The principle biomechanical factor is negative ulnar variation. Anatomic factors include the shape of the lunate bone and the type of vascular supply. Lunates with a proximal ulnar apex (type I) tend to coexist with ulnarnegative variation, whereas lunates that are square (type II) or rectangular (type III) are seen in ulnar-neutral or ulnar-positive variation, receptively. Patterns of blood supply of the lunate and their incidence: Y (60%), I (30%), X (10%). The radiographic stages are described in Table 6-14.

   Treatment—Initial treatment of stage 1 is immobilization and anti-inflammatory drugs; 50% of patients treated in this manner have continued daily symptoms. Failing a trial of nonoperative management or initial presentation of a more advanced stage, the condition is generally treated operatively. Revascularization procedures have encouraging early results; however, long-term follow-up is lacking and the results do not appear to be better than less technical alternatives. The recommended treatment for stage 1–3A is a joint leveling procedure. Radial shortenings and ulnar lengthenings have similar results, but the nonunion rate for ulnar lengthenings is higher. Patients who are initially ulnar neutral can be treated with a wedge osteotomy of the radius or an intercarpal fusion (STT, SC). Stage 3B requires dealing with the intercarpal collapse pattern (DISI). This is usually done with a limited intercarpal fusion (STT) or proximal row carpectomy. Stage 4 is treated with wrist fusion, limited intercarpal fusion, or proximal row carpectomy in an attempt to obliterate or remove the arthritic portions of the joint. Effects of various procedures on radiolunate loads (percentage decrease): STT fusion (3%), scaphocapitate fusion (12%), capitohamate fusion (0%), ulnar lengthening or radial shortening of 4 mm (45%), capitate shortening and capitohamate arthrodesis (66%, but radioscaphoid load increases by 26%).
9. Triangular fibrocartilage complex (TFCC) Anatomy—Dorsal radioulnar ligament, volar radioulnar ligament, articular disk, meniscus

Table 6-14. RADIOGRAPHIC STAGES OF KIENBOCK'S DISEASE

STAGE	CHARACTERISTICS
1	No visible changes in the lunate, changes seen on MRI
2	Sclerosis of the lunate
3A	Sclerosis and fragmentation of the lunate
3B	Stage 3A with fixed rotation of the scaphoid
4	Degenerative arthritis of the adjacent intercarpal joints

homologue, ulnar collateral ligament, ECU subsheath, origins of the ulnolunate and LT ligaments. The periphery is well vascularized, whereas the radial central portion is relatively avascular (Fig. 6-28).

10. Classification of TFCC abnormalities—Treatment of class 1 lesions (Table 6-15): All traumatic lesions of the TFCC are initially managed with immobilization and anti-inflammatory medication, if seen acutely, and are not associated with instability patterns, subluxations, or displaced fractures on radiograph. Failing this, persistent symptoms usually require operative treatment. Arthroscopic resection of the torn portion is possible for type 1A lesions, and type 1B lesions are amenable to repair. Type 1C is usually managed with an arthroscopically assisted limited open repair. Type 1D can be managed with partial excision or direct repair with ulnar shortening.

Treatment of class 2 lesions (Table 6-16): These abnormalities represent a pathologic progression of disease associated with ulnar-positive variation and impaction between the ulnar head and proximal pole of the lunate. Nonoperative treatment is tried first with immobilization, NSAIDs, and avoidance of aggravating activities (steroid injections are also worthwhile). Surgical treatment involves decompression of the ulnocarpal

Table 6-15. CLASS 1: TRAUMATIC TFCC INJURIES

CLASS	CHARACTERISTICS	TREATMENT
1A	Central perforation or tear	Resection of unstable flap back to a stable rim
1B	Ulnar avulsion with or without ulnar styloid fracture	Repair of the rim to its origin at the ulnar styloid
1C	Distal avulsion (origins of UL and UT ligaments)	Advancement of the distal volar rim to the triquetrum (bone anchor)
1D	Radial avulsion (involving the dorsal and/or volar radioulnar ligaments)	Direct repair to the radius to preserve the TFCC contribution to DRUJ stability

TFCC, triangular fibrocartilage complex; UL, ulnolunate; UT, ulnotriquetral; DRUJ, distal radioulnar joint.

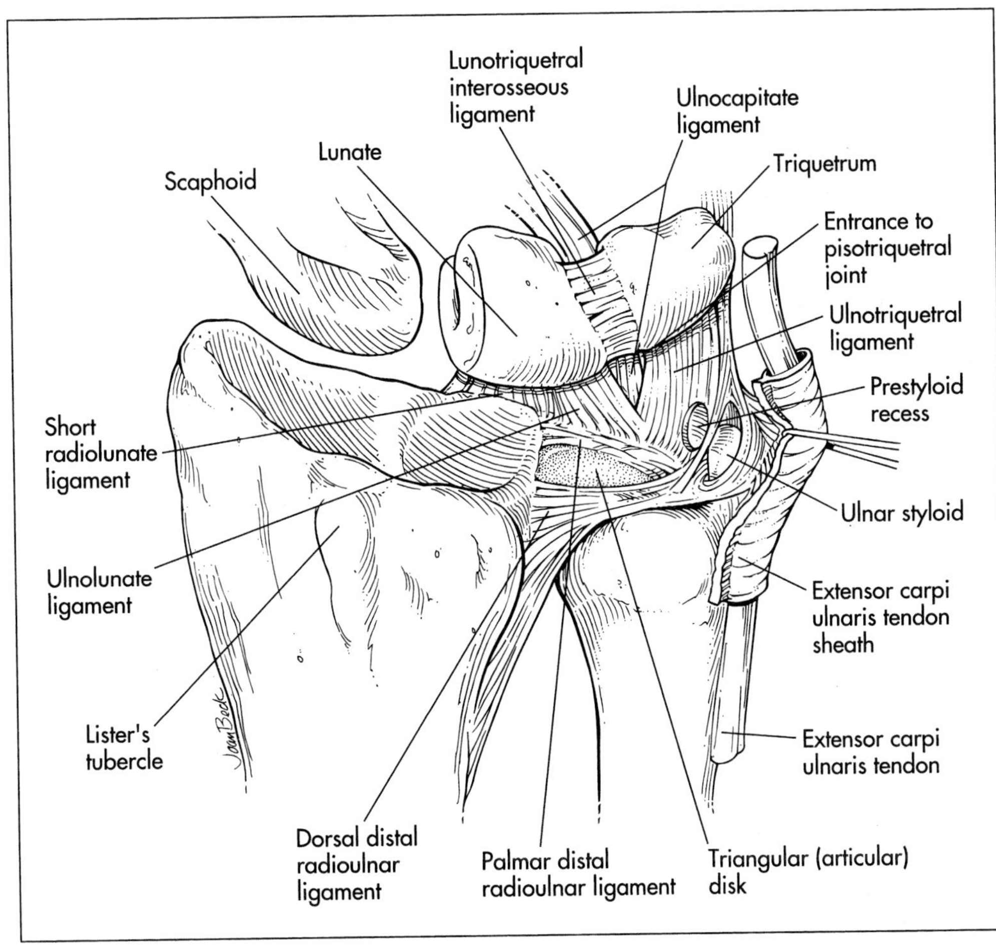

FIGURE 6-28 ■ Anatomy of the triangular fibrocartilage complex (TFCC). (From Cooney, W.P., Linscheid, R.L., and Dobyns, J.H.: The Wrist: Diagnosis and Operative Treatment. St. Louis, C.V. Mosby, 1998.)

Table 6-16. CLASS 2: DEGENERATIVE TFCC TEARS (ULNOCARPAL IMPACTION SYNDROME)

CLASS	CHARACTERISTICS
2A	TFCC wear (thinning)
2B	2A + lunate and/or ulnar chondromalacia
2C	TFCC perforation + lunate and/or ulnar chondromalacia
2D	2C + LT ligament disruption
2E	2D + ulnocarpal and DRUJ arthritis

TFCC, triangular fibrocartilage complex; LT, lunotriquetral; DRUJ, distal radioulnar joint.

articulation. This has been traditionally done with a diaphyseal ulnar shortening. This approach has the additional advantage of tightening the ulnocarpal ligaments and is recommended when concomitant LT instability is present. Other options not requiring osteotomy include the wafer (class 2A–C) or arthroscopic wafer (class 2C) resections of the ulnar head. Positive ulnar variance greater than 2 mm is a contraindication to wafer resection, and it is best managed with diaphyseal shortening. Class 2E lesions are managed with limited ulnar head resections as described by Bowers or Watson or a Suave-Kapandji procedure (arthrodesis of DRUJ and creation of a proximal pseudarthrosis at the level of the ulnar neck). Darrach's resection of the distal ulna is considered a salvage procedure because of problems with impingement and instability of the residual ulnar stump.

11. Ulnar Styloid Impaction Syndrome—Seen in patients with excessively long ulnar styloids. Impaction occurs between the styloid tip and the triquetrum. Excessive ulnar styloid length is determined by subtracting the ulnar variance from the ulnar styloid length and dividing this by the width of the ulnar head (ulnar styloid process index >0.22 is elevated). This pathologic entity is treated with avoidance of aggravating activities, NSAIDs, and cortisone injections. Failing this, excellent results have been reported with partial ulnar styloidectomy.
12. Tendinitis
    a. De Quervain's Tenosynovitis—A stenosing tenosynovial inflammation of the first dorsal compartment of the wrist. It is most common in women 30–50 years old. The provocative examination maneuver is the Finkelstein test (wrist ulnar deviation with the thumb held in patient's clenched fist). It is initially managed with splints, activity modification, NSAIDs, and steroid injections. Surgical treatment involves release of the first dorsal compartment on its dorsal side. Surgical pitfalls include injury to the sensory branch of the radial nerve or failure to recognize and decompress the EPB lying in a separate compartment.
    b. Flexor Carpi Radialis Tendinitis—Occurs where the flexor carpi radialis tendon passes under the ridge on the trapezium. It is usually well managed with a brief period of immobilization and NSAIDs or a steroid injection. Surgical decompression is rarely necessary but effective in recalcitrant cases.
    c. Intersection Syndrome—An inflammation of a potential space between the thumb outriggers (APL, EPB) and the radial wrist extensors. An inflamed bursa in this region has been found in some patients. It tends to occur after repetitive wrist dorsiflexion activities in the work place. Examination often reveals crepitus over the area with resisted wrist dorsiflexion and thumb extension. It is treated with a wrist splint and a steroid injection. Recalcitrant cases are managed by surgical débridement of the area. Some have suggested that this condition is really a tenosynovitis of the second dorsal compartment and that release of this compartment is an important part of the procedure.
    d. Snapping ECU—The sixth dorsal compartment is unique because it has a subsheath that is critical to the stability of the ECU. When these fibers, which also contribute to the TFCC, are attenuated, the ECU can subluxate in an ulnar and volar direction. This snapping of the ECU can lead to tendinitis. Treatment involves the usual trial of nonoperative means and includes a splint that restricts forearm pronation and supination. Failing this, reconstruction of the ECU subsheath utilizing a extensor retinaculum flap is indicated.
13. Ganglions, Ganglion Cysts—Account for 60–70% of soft-tissue tumors of the hand. These synovial cysts appear predominantly on the dorsum of the wrist (70%). In this location the origin is almost always from the SL ligament. They also are seen on the volar wrist (20%), deriving their origin from the radiocarpal or STT joints. They are also seen on the volar aspect of a digit at the metacarpal phalangeal flexion crease (volar retinacular ganglion cyst). The cyst fluid is a gelatinous (apple jelly-like) material with a high concentration of hyaluronic acid. Recurrence rates after aspiration are between 15% and 20%. When they are properly excised with a swath of joint capsule surrounding the stalk of the cyst, *recurrence*

rates are less than 10% for dorsal cysts, and as high as 20% for volar cysts.

VIII. Arthritis

A. Radiographic Differentiation Osteoarthritis/RA

B. Osteoarthritis (OA)—Common locations in upper extremities include the trapeziometacarpal joint of the thumb, DIP joint (Heberden's nodes), carpus (STT, pisotriquetral joint), and less commonly, the PIP joint (Bouchard's nodes). Primary OA tends to occur in females >40 years old, and there is a questionable genetic predisposition.

1. Mucous Cyst—A ganglion-type cyst emanating from an arthritic DIPJ. Nail deformity is common. Rupture is dangerous because there is a direct communication with the joint that could lead to septic arthritis. Spontaneous resolution occurs in 20–60% of patients. Surgical treatment is indicated in an impending rupture. Surgical treatment includes excision of the cyst and underlying osteophytes. Skin coverage can be an issue and local rotational flap may be needed.
2. DIP Joint OA—Patients complain of pain, deformity, and appearance. Treatment is fusion of the joint. Most reliable technique regarding fusion rates is with a screw. Nonunion after fusion occurs in 10%. Index and middle fingers are fused in extension. The ring and small fingers are fused in some degree of flexion, although some women may prefer full extension for cosmetic reasons.
3. PIP Joint OA—Same complaints as DIP joint OA. Treatment is fusion, especially for the index finger, to preserve pinch strength. Silicone replacement arthroplasty can be considered for the other digits. Surface replacement prosthesis are available, and provide improved lateral stability and ROM as compared with silicone prosthesis. Results are similar with volar or dorsal approach to PIP arthroplasty. Recommended position for small-joint arthrodesis is described in Table 6-17. PIP fusion rates are best with screws; however, plates, K-wires, and tension band techniques are also acceptable.
4. Thumb Basilar Arthritis (CMC Joint)
   a. Anatomy—This joint is a biconcave saddle joint. Important ligaments include the anterior oblique (holds the Bennett's fracture fragment), intermetacarpal ligament, posterior oblique ligament, and dorsoradial capsule (this is the ligament that disrupts in a dorsal CMC joint dislocation from trauma). Joint reactive force is 13 × applied pinch force. The anterior oblique (beak) ligament is the primary restraint to subluxation.
   b. Classification (Eaton et al., 1984)
      I Pre-arthritis (slight joint space widening)
      II Slight narrowing CMC joint
      III Marked narrowing CMC joint (STT not involved)
      IV Pantrapezial arthritis
   c. Physical Findings—Include swelling, painful CMC grind test, and crepitus. Metacarpal adduction and web space contractures develop late.
   d. Treatment—Nonoperative measures include NSAIDs, splints, and steroid injections. If a trial of nonoperative treatment fails, operative options include arthrodesis (stages II, III) of the CMC joint, which may be a good choice for patients who are heavy laborers. The advantages include good pain relief, stability, and length preservation. Disadvantages include decreased ROM, nonunion rate of 12%, and the STT joint not treated. Options for treatment in stages II and III include metacarpal extension osteotomy and trapezial resection and ligament suspension. Extension osteotomy has gained popularity, 93% are improved at an average 7-year follow-up. Trapezial resection and suspension arthroplasty (stages II, III, IV) has emerged as the favored approach in most patients. Reconstruction of the anterior oblique ligament function has prevented excessive shortening of the thumb ray, which was a problem with the simple anchovy procedure. A wide variety of techniques exist, all with similar clinical results, producing 80–90% good or excellent results. Though shortening of the ray with pinch has been documented, this does not correlate with deterioration of the clinical result. If the MCPJ hyperextends beyond 30 degrees, this must be addressed as well with volar capsulodesis, EPB tendon transfer, or

Table 6-17. POSITION FOR SMALL JOINT ARTHRODESIS

JOINT	POSITION
Distal interphalangeal	10–20 degrees of flexion
Proximal interphalangeal	30–45 degrees of flexion, cascading from index to small finger in 5-degree increments
Thumb metacarpophalangeal	15 degrees of flexion 10 degrees of pronation
Thumb carpal-metacarpal	30–40 degrees of palmar abduction 30–35 degrees of radial abduction 15 degrees of pronation

sesamoid fusion; otherwise a swan neck deformity will develop over time. Silicone replacement arthroplasty is ill advised, because of prosthesis fracture, subluxation, and silicone synovitis.

5. Erosive OA—Is seen in middle-aged women (F/M ratio = 10 : 1). The arthritis is confined to the IP joints. Radiographs demonstrate cartilage destruction, osteophytes, and subchondral erosions (gull wing deformity). The disease is self-limited, and patients are relatively asymptomatic; after 10 years of intermittently acute disease, bony ankylosis can occur late in 10–15% of patients. Occasionally fusions can be used to correct deformity.
6. Pulmonary Hypertrophic Osteoarthropathy—Periosteal new bone formation in association with clubbing of the fingers. Patients complain of diffuse pain with morning joint stiffness. Up to 12% of patients with bronchogenic carcinoma have it.

C. Inflammatory Arthritis

1. Arthritis Mutilans—Seen in patients with RA or psoriatic arthritis. Digits develop gross instability with bone loss (pencil-in-cup deformity, wind chime fingers). It is treated by restoring length and stability with interposition bone graft and fusion.
2. Rheumatoid Arthritis
   a. Rheumatoid Nodules—Seen in 20–25% of patients with RA. *They constitute the most common extra-articular manifestation of the disease* and are associated with aggressive disease. They are usually found over the olecranon, ulnar border of forearm, and over IP joints dorsally. Symptoms include esthetic compromise, pain, and ulcerations. Treatment involves corticosteroids or surgical excision. Both are associated with a high recurrence rate and incidence of breakdown or ulceration.
   b. Caput Ulnae Syndrome—Synovitis in the DRUJ leads to capsular and ligamentous stretching and bone and cartilage damage. As the ECU subsheath stretches, the ECU will subluxate into a volar and ulnar position. This leads to supination of the carpus away from the ulnar head, further stretching dorsal restraints. This developing instability allows the ulna to subluxate in a dorsal direction. When this occurs, it adds to increased pressures in the overlying extensor compartments, which are already elevated by synovitis. This increased pressure causes ischemic necrosis and rupture of the extensor tendons (Vaughn-Jackson syndrome). It is critical to differentiate this from extensor lag caused by PIN palsy secondary to elbow synovitis. A positive tenodesis test (MPJ extension with passive wrist flexion) confirms integrity of the extensor tendons and suggests PIN palsy as the cause of extensor lag. Tendons can also rupture via attrition over sharp bone. If this problem is recognized before the ulna subluxates, synovectomy can dramatically slow the disease process. Darrach's resection of ulnar head remains the gold standard for treating this problem. The distal ulnar stump is stabilized with volar capsule. The ECU is relocated dorsally with a retinacular flap. The Suave-Kapandji ulnar pseudarthrosis has the advantage of preserving the TFCC and ulnar buttress and is therefore a good option in younger patients before the carpus has slid in an ulnar direction. Silicone ulnar head replacement is out.
   c. Sudden Loss of Ability to Extend the Digits—Differential diagnosis includes tendon rupture (loss of passive tenodesis), subluxation of extensors into ulnar valleys (inspection), subluxation of MCPJs (radiographs), PIN compressive neuropathy at the elbow secondary to synovitis (can still extend the wrist actively and tenodesis effect intact). Can have multiple causes, which makes the diagnosis challenging.
   d. Tendon Rupture—EDM is the most common, followed by EDC to ring and small finger, followed by the EPL. MPJs are passively correctable but cannot be actively maintained, have no tenodesis effect, and the tendon defect is usually palpable. It is treated with dorsal tenosynovectomy, Darrach's procedure and primary repair (rarely possible), tendon transfer (Table 6-18), or intercalated tendon graft.
   e. Attritional Rupture of the FPL (Mannerfelt-Norman syndrome)—*Most common flexor tendon rupture in RA*. It requires

Table 6-18. COMMONLY USED EXTENSOR TENDON TRANSFERS

RUPTURED TENDON	TRANSFER
EPL	EIP to EPL
EDM	Just leave it and deal with tenosynovitis and caput ulnae
EDM and EDC5	EIP to EDC5
EDM, EDC5, EDC4	EDC4 side to side to EDC3, EIP to EDM
Multiple	Motor choices are EIP, FDS (ring), wrist extensor or flexor

EPL, extensor pollicis longus; EIP, extensor indicis proprius; EDM, extensor digiti minimi; EDC, extensor digitorum communis; FDS, flexor digitorum superficialis.

exploration, because a spike of bone in the carpal tunnel can go on to rupture the index flexors. It is treated with interposition graft or an FDS tendon transfer.

f. Radiocarpal Destruction—Synovitis causes capsular distension and previously mentioned changes in the DRUJ lead to supination, radial rotation, and ulnar and volar translocation of the carpus. SL disruption can lead to rotatory subluxation of the scaphoid and carpal collapse. When this is seen before significant destruction has occurred, synovectomy is the treatment of choice. Transfer of the ECRL to ECU can redistribute forces to diminish radial rotation and volar subluxation (Clayton's procedure). Of patients so treated, 50–60% have arrest of the destruction at the wrist. A radiolunate fusion is a good intermediate choice, particularly after a previous Darrach's resection of the ulna. It centralizes the lunate and diminishes further ulnar and volar subluxation. Wrist arthrodesis remains the gold standard for advanced disease. Bilateral fusions are not contraindicated. Total wrist arthroplasty is an option in low-demand patients with adequate bone stock, minimal deformity, and intact extensors. Silicone replacement arthroplasty had a reoperation rate of 41% at postoperative 5.8 years in one study. The biaxial prosthesis (metal and plastic) had a 24% failure rate at 6.5 years in one study. Newer designs show improved results in 4- to 10-year follow-up.

g. Etiology of MPJ Ulnar Drift
   (1) Joint synovitis leads to stretching of the radial hood sagittal fibers, which are weaker than their ulnar counterparts.
   (2) The extrinsic extensors drift into the ulnar valleys.
   (3) The lax collateral ligaments from joint synovitis permit ulnar deviation.
   (4) Synovitis damage in the joint further destabilizes it.
   (5) The ulnar intrinsics contract and become an ulnar and volar deforming force.
   (6) Radial deviation of the wrist alters the vector of pull on the extrinsic extensors toward the ulnar direction.
   (7) Flexor sheath synovitis distends the flexor retinaculum, allowing the flexors to shift in an ulnar direction.
   (8) Descent of the ring and small finger metacarpals, from altered pull of the ECU, contributes to the ulnovolar deforming forces, transmitting it through the juncturae tendons and the intervolar plate ligaments.

h. Treatment of MPJ Disease—Early: synovectomy, extensor tendon centralization, ulnar intrinsic release with or without crossed intrinsic transfer. Late: arthroplasty. Long-term results from MCP arthroplasty: overall patient satisfaction 70%, total arc of motion 40 degrees, implant breakage rate variable (10–20%), recurrent ulnar drift (6–10 degrees), infection and particulate synovitis are rare. It is critically important that wrist deformity is addressed at the same time. Persistent radial deviation of the wrist dooms MCP reconstruction to failure.

i. PIP Swan Neck Deformities—Caused by multiple factors that lead to an imbalance of forces and can include terminal tendon rupture and DIP mallet, synovitis attenuation volar plate, FDS rupture, intrinsic tightness from MPJ disease (Table 6-19).

j. PIP Boutonnière Deformity—Synovitis leads to attenuation of central slip, volar subluxation of lateral bands, tightness of transverse retinacular ligament, and volar plate contracture (Table 6-20). Best treated with PIP arthrodesis. Central slip repair or reconstruction has a high recurrence rate.

k. Rheumatoid Thumb Deformity
   Treatment thumb deformity—Type 1: stage 1 (MCP and IP passively correctable): synovectomy and extensor hood reconstruction. Stage 2 (MCP fixed and IP passively correctable): MCPJ fusion or arthroplasty. Stage 3 (fixed MCP and IP): IP fusion MCP arthroplasty or IP and MCP fusion if carpometacarpal (CMC) is normal.

Table 6-19. TREATMENT OF RHEUMATOID SWAN NECK DEFORMITY

TYPE	DESCRIPTION	TREATMENT
I	PIP supple in all MCPJ positions	Proximal Fowler's tenotomy, sublimis tenodesis, SORL reconstruction
II	PIP flexion limited with MCPJ hyperextension	Intrinsic release and/or reconstruction MCPJ
III	PIP flexion limited in all MCPJ positions	Closed manipulation with or without pinning
IV	Rigid deformity with ankylosis on radiograph	Arthrodesis

PIP, proximal interphalangeal; SORL, spiral oblique retinacular ligament; MCPJ, metacarpophalangeal joint.

Table 6-20. TREATMENT OF RHEUMATOID BOUTONNIÈRE DEFORMITY

STAGE	DESCRIPTION	TREATMENT
Stage I	Synovitis and mild deformity	Synovectomy, splints and lateral band, or distal Fowler's tenotomy
Stage II	Moderate deformity (30–40 degrees flexion), but passive extension is possible	Synovectomy, combined with central slip reconstruction, lateral band reconstruction, or distal Fowler's tenotomy
Stage III	Fixed flexion contracture	Arthoplasty or fusion
IVC		Preganglionic: nonrepairable, pseudomeningocele, denervation

Type 2: determine stage of involvement at CMC and MCP and treat based on recommendations for types 1 and 3.

Type 3: stage 1 (CMC pain, minimal deformity): splinting/medical management or CMC arthroplasty. Stage 2 (passively correctable, CMC and MCP): CMC arthroplasty, MCP fusion or tenodesis. Stage 3 (CMC dislocation, fixed MCP, and adducted thumb): CMC arthroplasty, MCP fusion, first web release.

Type 4: stage 1 (passively correctable deformities): synovectomy, UCL reconstruction, adductor fascia release. Stage 2 (fixed deformity): MP arthroplasty (with UCL reconstruction) or fusion.

Type 5: MP stabilized in flexion by volar capsulodesis or fusion.

TYPE	DESCRIPTION	DISEASE LOCATION
Type 1	Boutonnière	MPJ (dorsal capsule)
Type 2	Type 1 with CMC joint subluxation	MCPJ and CMC
Type 3	Swan neck	CMC (adducted MC)
Type 4	Gamekeeper	MCPJ (UCL)
Type 5	Swan neck with disease at the MPJ, CMC OK	MCPJ (volar plate)

3. Gout—90% of cases occur in men, primary is idiopathic, secondary is associated with diseases with high metabolic turnover, such as psoriasis, hemolytic anemia, leukemia, hyperparathyroidism, drugs. *Monosodium urate crystals* are seen.

   Eighty percent of patients with elevated uric acid levels never have a gout attack. *The diagnosis can only be made by joint aspiration and inspection for crystals.* Radiographic findings include soft-tissue densities (tophi), intra-articular erosions at the joint margins, extra-articular erosions (punched-out appearance with overhanging lip). Treat acute attacks with IM injection of adrenocorticotropic hormone (ACTH) (40 U), indomethacin, or cochicine. Cyclosporin A, used in transplant surgery, impairs renal urate clearance and can precipitate a gout attack.
4. Calcium Pyrophosphate Deposition (CPPD) Disease (Pseudogout)—*Calcium pyrophosphate dihydrate crystals.* Associated diseases include hemochromatosis, hyperparathyroidism, gout, RA, hypophosphatemia, systemic lupus erythematosus, ochronosis, Wilson's disease (copper deposition), hemophilia. Chondrocalcinosis is present in 7% of patients. Long-term dialysis can cause a pyrophosphate-like arthropathy. Can cause pseudorheumatoid acute wrist inflammation mimicking sepsis. Radiographs show calcification of fibrocartilage structures such as the TFCC. It is treated with ACTH injection, splints for comfort. Recurrent cases managed with colchicine (0.6 mg po bid). Surgery is rarely necessary.
5. Systemic Lupus Erythematosus (SLE)—90% of these patients have arthritis in a rheumatoid-like pattern. Other characteristics include marked joint laxity, deformity, Raynaud's phenomenon, facial butterfly rash, positive ANA, high titer of anti-DNA antibodies. Treatment is primarily medical (corticosteroids). Splinting is usually not successful, and soft-tissue reconstructions tend to stretch out. Fusions are the most reliable procedures in these patients; however, success has been reported with MCP arthroplasties.
6. Scleroderma (Systemic Sclerosis)—Hand manifestations include Raynaud's phenomenon in 90% of these patients, PIP flexion contractures, skin ulcers, septic arthritis, and calcific deposits. CREST (calcinosis, Raynaud's, esophageal problems, sclerodactyly, telangiectasia) is a form of the disease. Surgical involvement usually deals with refractory Raynaud's with periadventitial digital sympathectomy. Arthrodesis is helpful for PIP flexion deformities with dorsal skin ulcers over fixed flexed joints. Symptomatic calcific deposits (calcinosis circumscripta) can be treated by débridement. Refractory finger tip ulcers are best treated with conservative tip amputation.
7. Psoriatic Arthritis (Seronegative Spondyloarthropathy)—Skin manifestations precede joint involvement by several years. RA and ANA tests are usually negative, human

leukocyte antigen studies are often positive. Clinical manifestations include onychodystrophy, distal phalanx acrolysis, PIP fusions, MCP erosions, and wrist fusions. The arthritis can be isolated to DIP joint and is differentiated from degenerative joint disease (DJD) by centripetal erosions, which actually cause joint space widening, advancing to pencil-in-cup deformity, in which there is a whittling of the middle phalanx and widening of the base of the distal phalanx. Treatment is primarily medical, with methotrexate usually yielding excellent relief. Surgery is indicated when destroyed, unstable, or stiff joints cause significant functional problems. They may benefit from either resection arthroplasty or fusion.

8. Juvenile Rheumatoid Arthritis—There are three clinical types: (1) systemic or Still's disease, (2) polyarticular, and (3) pauciarticular. Laboratory studies are not diagnostic. Hand involvement is most common in the polyarticular variant. Unlike the adult variety, deformities are wrist ulnar deviation and flexion with MCP stiffness in an extended position. Nonoperative treatment is favored so as to avoid damaging open growth plates. Splinting can aid autofusions in progress to fuse in a functional position. Tenosynovectomy can provide pain relief but usually does not improve motion. Corrective osteotomies are usually deferred until skeletal maturity.

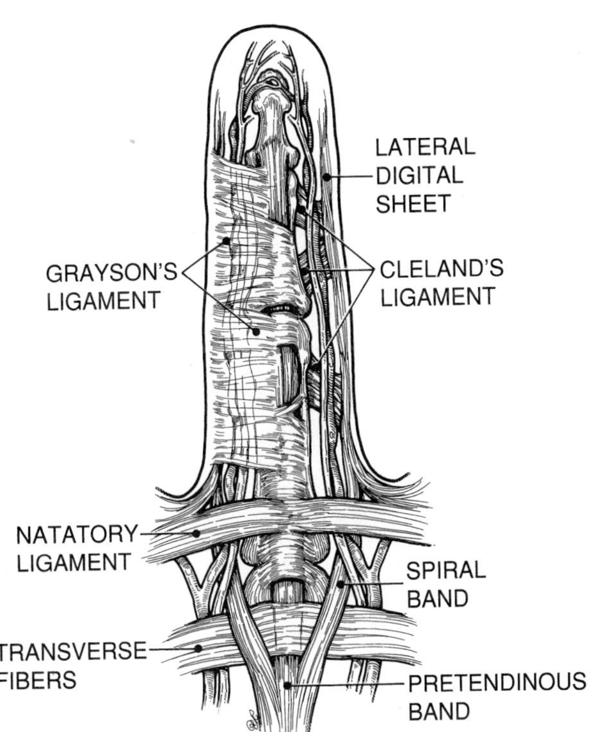

FIGURE 6-29 ■ Parts of the normal digital fascia that become diseased. Grayson's ligament, shown on the left, is an almost continuous sheet of thin fascia in the same plane as the natatory ligament. Cleland's ligaments, shown on the right, do not become diseased. The lateral digital sheet receives fibers from the natatory ligament and the spiral band. The spiral bands pass on either side of the metacarpophalangeal joint, deep to the neurovascular bundles, to reach the side of the finger. (From McFarlane, R.M.: Patterns of the diseased fascia in the fingers in Dupuytren's contracture. Plast. Reconstr. Surg. 54:31–44, 1974.)

IX. Dupuytren's Disease—Divided into three stages: (1) proliferative stage: large myofibroblasts, minimal extracellular matrix, with a lot of cellular gap junctions, very vascular; (2) involutional stage: dense myofibroblast network, ratio of type III to type I collagen increased; (3) residual stage: myofibroblasts disappear and a smaller population of fibrocytes become the predominant cell line. The offending cell is the myofibroblast, characterized by cytoplasmic monofilament bundles composed of cytoskeletal proteins. The cell of origin remains obscure. Other cells that contribute to contraction include the "mobile fibroblasts." Involved fascial components include the peritendinous bands, spiral bands, natatory ligaments, Grayson's ligaments, Cleland's ligaments, and lateral digital sheath (Fig. 6-29). Named cords include the central cord, spiral cord, lateral cord, retrovascular cord, abductor digiti minimi cord, and first web space intercommissural cord (Fig. 6-30). The *spiral cord* is composed of the peritendinous aponeurosis, spiral band, lateral digital sheath, and Grayson's ligament. *The only part of the web coalescence not involved in the spiral cord is the natatory ligament.* The spiral cord always puts the neurovascular bundle at risk. As IP contracture increases, the neurovascular bundle is pushed volarly, proximally, and toward the midline. The incidence is higher in northern Europeans and persons of Celtic origin. Disease onset is rare before the age of 40. The male/female ratio has been reported to be from 2:1 to 10:1. There is a high incidence of Dupuytren's in the HIV-positive population (increased activity oxygen free radicals). It is inherited as an autosomal dominant trait with variable penetrance (accounting for the fact that only 10% of patients have a positive family history). Dupuytren's diathesis is associated with aggressive early onset of the disease involving hands, feet, (lederhosen disease) and the penis (Peyronie's disease). Disease associations include alcoholism, diabetes, epilepsy, and chronic pulmonary disease. Occupational hand trauma does not bring on the disease, but it can possibly exacerbate it by microtrauma to early nodules. Nonoperative treatments are proven to be ineffective. Corticosteroid injections in nodules not associated with a cord can slow down the progression of the disease (Ketchum) Indications for surgery include MCP flexion contracture of >30 degrees and/or PIP flexion contractures greater than 30 degrees. The current trend is to move away from early surgery for PIP flexion contractures. Regional palmar fasciotomy of involved rays through various skin incisions is the currently favored surgical intervention.

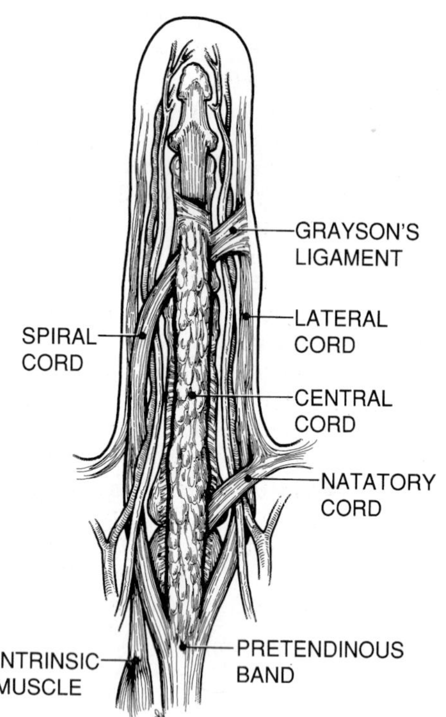

FIGURE 6-30 ■ The change in the normal fascia bands to diseased cords. (From Green, D.H., Hotchkiss, R.M., Pederson, W.C., and Lampert, R., eds.: Green's Operative Hand Surgery, 4th ed. New York, Churchill Livingstone, 1998. Courtesy of Dr. R.M. McFarlane.)

Segmental aponeurectomies have been shown to be as effective as regional fasciotomies in two studies. Total palmar fasciotomy is no longer favored because it does not completely prevent recurrence and has a high complication rate. The open palm technique of McCash may be the procedure of choice in older patients who are at high risk for stiffness. Leaving the wounds open reduces edema, hematoma, and pain and allows for early motion. The open palm technique is associated with the lowest rate of complications. Dermofasciectomy is generally reserved for those patients who have a strong diathesis or a recurrence. Skin grafting of residual defects remains controversial. If possible it is best to wait until the disease reaches the involutional stage because recurrence rates are lower. *The best predictor of central neurovascular bundle displacement is the presence of a PIP joint flexion contracture (77% positive predictive value);* second is the presence of an interdigital soft-tissue mass (71% positive predictive value). Meticulous hemostasis is essential because hematoma is the most common complication of Dupuytren's surgery. Active motion is generally started 5–7 days postoperatively. A night-time extension splint is worn for 6 months. Continuous passive motion has not been shown to be helpful. Long-term recurrence rates are around 50%. Flare reactions are more common in women. Concomitant CTR increases incidence of postoperative flare reaction.

X. Nerve Injury/Paralysis/Tendon Transfers— Classification (Seddon, 1943): type 1 (neuropraxia): nerve contusion involving conduction block without wallerian degeneration. There is a variable order of recovery and the prognosis is excellent. On physical exam Tinel's sign is negative. Type 2 (axonotmesis): conduction block with wallerian degeneration. Axons and myelin sheaths degenerate but endoneural tubes remain intact. Sequential order of neurologic return at a rate dependent on the magnitude of injury is usual. Type 3 (neurotmesis): conduction block with all layers of the nerve disrupted and wallerian degeneration. No recovery without operative repair can be expected. There is an orderly sequence of return at a rate of 1 mm/day in adults and 3–5 mm/day in children after successful repair. Classification (Sunderland, 1951): first degree: same as neuropraxia. Second degree: same as axonotmesis. Third degree: *most variable degree of ultimate recovery,* axonal injury associated with endoneurial scarring. Fourth degree: nerve is in continuity, but at the level of injury there is complete scarring across the nerve, preventing regeneration. Tinel's sign is present at the level of injury, but it does not move distally with time. Fifth degree: same as neurotmesis. After transection of a peripheral nerve, the distal segment undergoes wallerian degeneration (axoplasm and myelin are degraded and removed by phagocytosis). Existing Schwann's cells that produce myelin proliferate and line up on the basement membrane. This distal tube receives sprouting axons. The nerve cell body swells and enlarges, and the rate of structural protein production increases. There are multiple sprouts from each proximal axon, which connect into the distal stump and migrate at a rate of 1 mm/day. **Age is the single most important factor influencing the success of nerve recovery, with a noticeable change after the age of 30.** The level of injury is the second most important factor. Distal repairs have a better prognosis than proximal ones. The nature of the injury, with sharp lacerations doing better than crush avulsion injuries, is also noteworthy. Delayed repairs yield a loss of 1% of neural function for each week beyond the third week from injury (time limit: 18 months for repair). Specificity of regenerating axons depends on deletion of erroneously migrating motor axons after initial random regeneration along both motor and sensory pathways. Nerve growth factors are thought to affect the rate of nerve regeneration but not specificity. EMG tests the innervation of muscle. Signs of denervation are fibrillations, and these can be seen as early as 2–4 weeks postinjury. Technique of nerve repair—epineural: epineurium repaired in a tension free fashion. Fascicular: repairs the perineural sheaths. This has not been demonstrated to improve functional results clinically or experimentally. Group fascicular (three indications): median nerve in the distal third of the forearm, ulnar nerve in the distal third of the forearm, and the sciatic nerve in the thigh. If the gap is >2.5 cm, nerve grafting is usually necessary.

Fibrin glue provides for better histologic result, but functional results are statistically the same as with suture anastomosis. Schwann's cells in the nerve graft survive and are eventually replaced by Schwann's cells migrating from either end of the graft.

A. Brachial Plexus Palsy—Any one patient can have any and all degrees of injury at any level along the plexus. Knowledge of brachial plexus anatomy is critical to understanding the physical exam and diagnosis of brachial plexus lesions (Fig. 6-31). Absent fascial attachment to the dura causes the lower elements of the plexus C8 and T1 roots to suffer the most severe injury. It is important to assess the energy of the injury via the history because high-energy injuries are associated with more severe damage, such as rupture of plexal segments and root avulsions. The goal is to determine the extent of nerve injury and from this decide whether early surgical intervention is indicated or a period of further observation for recovery is warranted. Important signs of injury severity include Horner's sign on the affected side, which usually shows up 3–4 days after injury and correlates with C8 and/or T1 root avulsions. Severe pain in an anesthetized limb correlates with root avulsion because it represents deafferentation and the presence or absence of rhomboid; serratus anterior function can also help identify level of the injury. A standard and complete motor sensory evaluation is documented to assist with preoperative planning and recovery assessment. Radiographs of the cervical spine, chest clavicle, and scapula are done. Inspiration and expiration chest radiographs can demonstrate a paralyzed diaphragm, indicating a severe upper root injury. Fracture of the transverse processes indicates a high-energy injury with likely root avulsion. Scapulothoracic dissociation is often associated with root avulsion and major vascular injury. CT and MRI are both useful, and they have largely supplanted traditional myelography. MRI demonstrates: T2—highlights the fat content of the cervical spinal cord and nerve roots (empty sleeves); T1—highlights the water content that is present in a pseudomeningocele. Findings consistent with significant injury include pseudomeningocele, empty root sleeves, and cord shift away from midline. Sensory and motor evoked potentials are more useful than standard EMG and NCV. They should be done 3–6 weeks postinjury to allow wallerian degeneration to occur. Stimulation is done over Erb's point, and recordings are taken

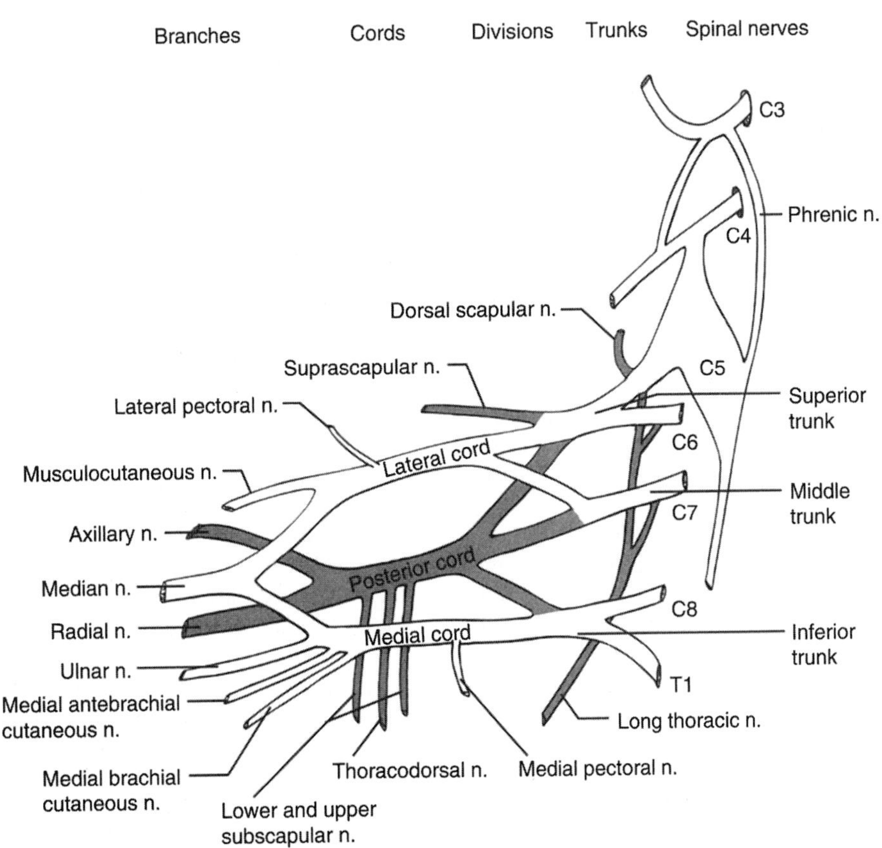

FIGURE 6-31 ■ Brachial plexus anatomy. (From Brushart, T.M., and Wilgis, E.F.: Brachial plexus and shoulder girdle injuries. In B.D. Browner and J.B. Jupiter, eds.: Skeletal Trauma, 2nd ed. WB Saunders, p. 1696.)

over the cortex with scalp electrodes. Positive readings provide evidence of roots that are in continuity with the spinal cord. Negative readings cannot differentiate among avulsion, rupture, or axonotmesis. Modern series indicate that there is a reverse relationship between time from injury to operation and outcome. Even in cases with total clinical brachial plexopathy, less than 24% of patients have avulsion of all five roots. Therefore there should almost always be something to repair or graft; if not, nerve transfers can be done. Immediate surgical exploration is indicated in penetrating trauma and iatrogenic injuries. One study showed that many patients with gunshot wounds to the plexus improved with time. Therefore it is reasonable to observe these patients for 3 months in the absence of a major vascular injury. Early surgical intervention (3 weeks–3 months postinjury) is indicated in patients with total or near-total plexus involvement or patients with less than this but a high-energy injury. It is clear that recovery in this situation is improved by neurologic repair or reconstruction. The delayed surgical approach (3–6 months postinjury) is reserved for patients with low-energy injuries and/or patients with partial upper level palsy. It is preferable to wait and observe for recovery. If recovery plateaus early, surgery would be warranted. *The best clinical sign of improvement and effective nerve regeneration is an advancing Tinel's sign*. If surgery is going to be done at all, it should be done within the first 6 months after injury, if possible. An isolated C8–T1 injury in an adult is best treated with early tendon transfers. The problem is that the distance between the injury site and the hand intrinsic muscles makes reinnervation unlikely. The surgical priorities of repair are as follows: (1) elbow flexion (musculocutaneous n.), (2) shoulder stabilization (suprascapular n.), (3) brachiothoracic pinch (pectoral nerve), (4) sensation in C6–7 distribution (lateral cord), (5) wrist extension and finger flexion (lateral and posterior cords). Direct repair is infrequently possible without excessive traction; therefore nerve grafts are often used. Donor sites include the sural, medial brachial, and medial antebrachial cutaneous nerves. Vascularized nerve graft includes the ulnar nerve when there is proven avulsion of C8 and T1. The nerve is mobilized on its branches from the superior ulnar collateral artery. Nerve regeneration appears to be quicker, but ultimate recovery is not significantly better than standard graft techniques. Nerve transfer is indicated when there are an insufficient number of proximal axon resources (i.e., multiple root avulsions). In this circumstance it is necessary to turn to extraplexal sources to get axons. Commonly used sources include the spinal accessory nerve (1700 axons), intercostal nerve (1300 axons), motor branches of cervical plexus (3400–4000 axons), contralateral lateral pectoral nerve (400–600 axons). In general, repair and reconstruction does improve the prognosis. Infraclavicular injuries have a better prognosis than supraclavicular; the fewer the avulsed roots the better. Results of nerve transfer thus far have been mixed.

B. Obstetrical Brachial Plexopathy—Associated with a high birth weight (>4000 g), difficult presentation (shoulder dystocia), cephalopelvic disproportion, and forceps delivery. The muscle grading system used to evaluate these patients is as follows: M0—no contraction; M1—contraction without movement; M2—contraction with slight movement; M3—complete movement. Complete recovery is possible if the biceps and deltoid are graded M1 by 2 months. Results, though still good, are incomplete if biceps and deltoid do not contract until 3.5 months. If biceps is not graded M3 by 5 months, results will be highly unsatisfactory. Early surgery is indicated if, at 1 month, the arm is completely flail and Horner's sign is present. If at 1 month the hand shows signs of recovery but the shoulder does not, there is still a chance for spontaneous recovery. If at 3 months biceps function is evident, surgery is not recommended. In cases in which there is no biceps function, an EMG is obtained. Total absence of electrical evidence of reinnervation indicates corresponding root avulsion. In indicated cases, the results of surgical reconstruction are far better than the expectant approach. Unlike adults, reinnervation of the hand intrinsics is possible in infants. The results of nerve grafting are better in infants than they are in adults. Palliative treatment of the sequelae of birth palsies is difficult, and the results are rarely satisfactory.

C. Tendon Transfers—Indicated to replace a paralyzed muscle, replace ruptured or avulsed tendon or muscle, and restore balance to a paralyzed hand (e.g., cerebral palsy). Tendon transfers are generally deferred until tissue equilibrium is achieved, passive mobility is restored, and donors with adequate power and excursion are available. Important definitions and relationships to understand include force that is proportional to the cross-sectional area of the muscle, amplitude (Table 6-21) that is proportional to length of the muscle, work capacity that is equal to force times the length (F × L), and power that is work per unit of time. Other important principles include selecting a motor that is expendable. Synergistic transfers are easier to rehabilitate. Synergistic actions

Table 6-21. AMPLITUDE (THE 3-5-7 RULE)

Wrist flexors or extensors	33 mm
EDC, FPL, EPL	50 mm
FDS/FDP	70 mm

EDC, extensor digitorum communis; FPL, flexor pollicus longus; EPL, extensor pollicus longus; FDS, flexor digitorum superficialis; FDP, flexor digitorum profundus.

are those that occur together in normal function (e.g., finger flexion and wrist extension). The motor will decrease one grade in strength after transfer. A straight line of pull is best. Transfers should have only one function per motor unit. Try to restore sensibility before transfer, if possible. The selection of a transfer is based on a careful assessment of the patient. The key questions are (1) what is missing, (2) what is available for transfer, and (3) what are the options for transfer. This plus a familiarity with classic transfers will usually lead to an acceptable solution. (Table 6-22).

D. Cerebral Palsy—The typical deformities include wrist and finger flexion, thumb-in-palm deformity, forearm pronation, and elbow flexion. Initial management involves physical therapy and night-time static extension splints. Botulinum toxin is temporarily effective when severe spasticity is present. Intrathecal baclofen infusion has been effective in reducing spasticity in double blind studies. Children with motion disorders do not do well with surgery. The best results are in children with spastic contractures and voluntary control, an IQ of 50–70 or higher, and the ability to place the hand on the knee or head within 5 seconds. The better the sensibility, the better patients will do with surgery. In poor surgical candidates, surgery is done for hygiene alone and involves (1) shoulder derotational osteotomy or lengthening of subscapular and/or pectoralis; (2) elbow: when contracture is >60 degrees, biceps/brachialis lengthening capsulotomy; musculocutaneous nerve neurectomy can help for mild contracture <30 degrees; flexor pronator slide is not a good procedure for function because it corrects too many problems, not allowing for independent

Table 6-22. CLASSIC TENDON TRANSFERS

PALSY	LOSS	TRANSFER
Radial	Wrist extension	Pronator teres to ECRB
	Finger extension	FCU to EDC II–V
		FCR to EDC II–V
		FDS III to EPL and EIP, FDS IV to EDC III–V
		Palmaris longus to EPL
Low ulnar	Thumb extension	FDS to radial lateral band
	Hand intrinsics (interosseous and ulnar lumbricals)	ECRL to lateral band
		EDQ EIP to lateral band
		FCR + graft to lateral band
		Metacarpal phalangeal capsulodesis
	Thumb adduction	ECRL + graft to adductor pollicis
		Brachioradialis + graft to adductor pollicis
	Index abduction	EIP to first dorsal interosseous
		Abductor pollicis longus to first dorsal interosseous
		ECRL to first dorsal interosseous
High ulnar	Low problems + FDP	Suture to functioning FDP index and long index and long finger
	Ring and small	
Low median	Opposition	FDS ring to abductor pollicis brevis (FCU pulley)
		EIP to thumb proximal phalanx (routed around the ulna for line of pull)
		Abductor digiti quinti to abductor pollicis brevis
		Palmaris longus to abductor pollicis brevis
High median	Thumb IP flexion	Brachioradialis to flexor pollicis longus
	Index and long finger flexion	Suture to functioning FDP ring and small or ECRL to FDP index and long if additional power needed
Low median and ulnar	Plus opposition transfer	
	Thumb adduction	ECRB + graft to abductor tubercle of thumb
	Thumb abduction	EIP to abductor pollicis brevis
	Index abduction	Abductor pollicis longus to first dorsal interosseous
	Clawed fingers	Brachioradialis + four-tailed free graft to the A2 pulley
	Volar sensibility	Neurovascular island flap from back of hand
High median and ulnar	Thumb adduction	ECRB + graft to abductor tubercle of thumb
	Thumb IP flexion	Brachioradialis to FPL
	Thumb abduction	EIP to abductor pollicis brevis
	Index abduction	Abductor pollicis longus to first dorsal interosseous
	Finger flexion	ECRL to FDP
	Clawed fingers	Tenodesis of all MP joints with free tendon graft from dorsal carpal ligament routed deep to transverse metacarpal ligament to extensor apparatus
	Wrist flexion	ECU to FCU
	Volar sensibility	Neurovascular island flap from back of hand

FCU, flexor carpi ulnaris; EDC, extensor digitorum communis; FDS, flexor digitorum superficialis; EPL, extensor pollicis longus; EIP, extensor indicis proprius; ECRL, extensor carpi radialis longus; EDQ, extensor digiti quinti; FDP, flexor digitorum profundus; ECRB, extensor carpi radialis brevis; ECU, extensor carpi ulnaris.

adjustment; (3) wrist: arthrodesis (SIMPLIFY THE MACHINE); and (4) fingers: superficialis to profundus transfer and FPL lengthening. Surgery for the good candidate is aimed at improving function. Wrist extension is classically achieved with the Green transfer (FCU to ECRB around the ulnar border of the forearm). This should only be done in patients who have active digital extension with the wrist positioned in neutral preoperatively; otherwise, overcorrection may impair digital release. Other available motors include the brachioradialis. Overcorrection with this transfer is not a frequent problem and it exhibits a multiplier effect with elbow motion. The ECU is another option. This transfer can also diminish hyperulnar deviation, especially when combined with a fractional lengthening of the FCU. It can also be transferred to the EDC if digital extensors are weak. Inadequate release is corrected with a flexor lengthening.

Z-lengthening is probably the most controlled method, with 1 degree of extension achieved for each 0.5 mm of lengthening. Tendon transfers to the extensors are indicated only when there are no significant joint contractures and when there is a muscle available for transfer that is only active in the release phase. The other alternative is to transfer the FDS through the interosseous membrane. Favored muscles include FCU, ECU, and ECRB. Thumb-in-palm deformity is treated surgically with release or lengthening of the adductor pollicis, first dorsal interosseous, flexor pollicis brevis, and flexor pollicis longus. Web space deepening plasty and augmentation of thumb extension and abduction with transfer of brachioradialis, palmaris longus, or flexor digitorum sublimis is also done. When the MCP joint is unstable in hyperextension, this is managed with a volar capsulodesis or an arthrodesis. For spastic thumb-in-palm deformity with interphalangeal hyperextension, the EPL is redirected along the axis of the first dorsal compartment.

XI. Congenital Hand Disorders

Limb Embryology—The limb bud appears during the fourth week of gestation. At 33 days the hand is a paddle without individual digits. Digital separation begins at 47 days (7 weeks) and is complete by 54 days (8 weeks) (Fig. 6-32). At 7 weeks the condensation that will give rise to each of the bones

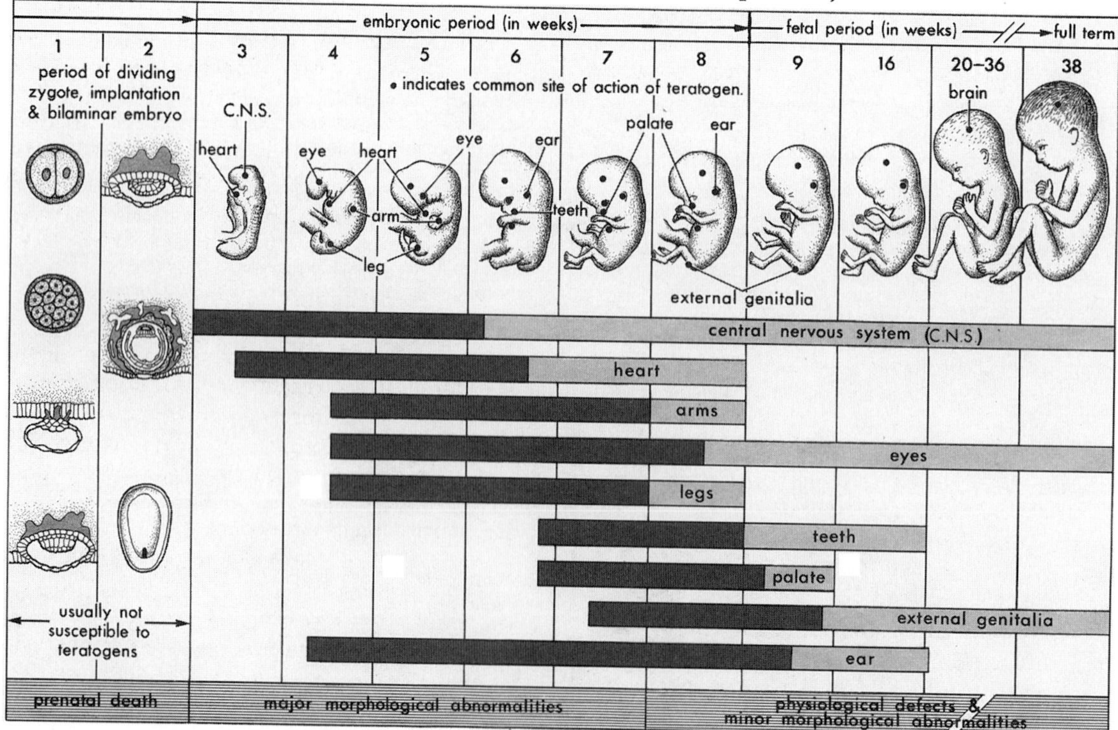

FIGURE 6-32 ■ Hand development begins in the fourth week and is complete at the end of the eighth week. The arms, legs, heart, and central nervous system are all in critical phases of development during this time. Thus there is an association with deformity in these systems in many hand deformities. (From Moore, K.L.: The Developing Human, 2nd ed. WB Saunders, Philadelphia, 1977.)

of the hand is evident. (See Chapter 11, Anatomy, for ossification order of carpal and digital bones.) Consultation with a geneticist is important in the early management to assist in diagnosing disorders outside the musculoskeletal system that are associated with 80% of the heritable limb deficiencies.

A. Failure of Part Formation
   1. Transverse absence relates to all congenital amputations, including: true transverse absence, constriction ring syndrome, and symbrachydactyly. The absence of nubbins differentiates symbrachydactyly from constriction ring syndrome, which does not have nubbins. These deformities are generally not associated with syndromes and occur most commonly at the proximal forearm level. Surgical management of transverse absence includes any or all of the following: free phalangeal transfer, ulnar post reconstruction, and free toe to hand transfer. Free phalangeal transfer is a good choice when: (1) there is suitable soft-tissue envelope (symbrachydactyly), (2) there is adequate proximal bony support, and (3) the child is <15 months old, because survival of the growth plate diminishes with age. Intact periosteum and collateral ligament repair improve survival and function. Ulnar post reconstruction is a good choice when there is not an adequate soft-tissue envelope. This procedure involves distraction manoplasty followed by interposition corticocancellous graft or on-top plasty with an adjacent metacarpal. The goal is to provide for opposable posts for rudimentary pinch. Toe to hand transfer should be carefully considered in all cases. Although survival is possible, the vestigial nature of the structures used to motor the transferred toe make functional results usually poor. The exception to this is in amputation due to constriction ring syndrome, wherein functional results are much better because there are suitable proximal parts to connect to the transferred toe. The Krukenberg reconstruction, radial-ulnar division for prehension, is reserved for blind patients who perform poorly with a prosthesis because of the absence of visual control. Candidates for prosthetic devices are fit with a passive device at 6 to 9 months, and they are advanced to a body-powered device at 15 to 24 months.
   2. Longitudinal Absence
      a. Radial Club Hand—Both extremities affected in 50–72% of cases. Associated anomalies include Holt-Oram syndrome, TAR (thrombocytopenia-absent radii), Fanconi's anemia, and VATER syndrome. Classification: stage I, deficient distal radial epiphysis; stage II, complete but short = hypoplasia; stage III, present proximally = partial aplasia; stage IV, completely absent = total aplasia (most common). The humerus is often short in these children. The ulna is curved and thick and only 60% of normal length. Carpal bone fusion and absence is also seen. Treatment begins with early passive motion therapy. Elbow stiffness is a contraindication to surgical intervention. Centralization involves any or all of the following and is done at 6–12 months of age: resection of varying amounts of carpus, shortening of the ECU, and, when necessary, angular osteotomy of the ulna. It is important to preserve the distal ulnar physis. In children with particularly resistant stiffness, a two-stage centralization using a distraction external fixator in the first stage is indicated. In those with absent thumbs, thumb reconstruction is performed at about 18 months.
      b. Ulnar Club Hand—Less common than radial club hand. It is not associated with cardiac or hematologic problems, but is associated with other musculoskeletal anomalies. Most commonly associated anomalies include proximal femoral focal deficiency, fibula deficiency, phocomelia, and scoliosis. The wrist is stable, and the elbow is the problem. Ulnar digits are often absent and, if present, are syndactylized. Classification: stage I, hypoplasia of the ulna; stage II, partial aplasia of the ulna; stage III, total aplasia of the ulna; stage IV, radiohumeral synostosis. Ulnar club hand is treated with syndactyly release and digital rotation osteotomies done early (12–18 months of age). In type IV, an osteotomy of the radius may be necessary to obtain elbow motion. This is generally reserved for those children who have bilateral deformity and those with severe elbow flexion contractures and/or fixed hyperpronation deformity ("hand on flank"). Type II may be associated with a radial head dislocation, which may require radial head resection and creation of a one-bone forearm. A fibrocartilaginous band connecting the carpus to the ulna is present in types II and IV. There is considerable controversy over the benefit of resecting this abnormal structure.
      c. Cleft Hand—The true cleft hand is often bilateral and familial, involves the feet, and has associated absent metacarpals, differentiating it from symbrachydactyly. The severity of this anomaly varies widely from a cleft between middle and ring fingers to oligodactylous (absent) radial digits and syndactylous ulnar digits. Cleft closure and thumb web construction are the top priorities. Syndactyly, when present, should be

released early because it is between digits of different lengths and growth potential. Thumb reconstruction may require anything from web space deepening, to tendon transfers, to rotational osteotomies, to toe to hand transfer. Web deepening should not precede cleft closure because it may compromise flaps for the cleft closure. Transverse bones should be removed because they widen the cleft with growth.

B. Failure of Part Differentiation
   1. Radioulnar Synostosis—Bilateral in 60% of cases. Examination reveals fixed pronation deformity exceeding 50 degrees in 50% of cases. The radius is heavy and bowed, whereas the ulna is straight and narrow. When this disorder is unilateral and minor, it is best not to intervene. If pronation deformity is significant, a rotational osteotomy is done through the synostosis at age 5, setting the forearm at 10–20 degrees of pronation. If it is bilateral, the dominant side is set at 30–45 degrees of pronation, and the nondominant side is set at 20–35 degrees of supination.
   2. Symphalangism (Congenital Digital Stiffness)—Hereditary symphalangism is autosomal dominant and associated with correctable hearing loss. It is more common in the ulnar digits. Nonhereditary symphalangism is seen with syndactyly, Apert's syndrome, and Poland's syndrome. Indications for surgery in infancy do not exist. Appearance and function can sometimes be improved by angular osteotomies in adolescence.
   3. Camptodactyly (Congenital Digital Flexion Deformity)—Usually occurs at the PIP joint in the small finger. There are two types. Type I is seen in infancy and affects the sexes equally; it responds to splinting and stretching. Type II is seen in adolescent girls. This is rarely a functional problem, though the deformity gets worse during the adolescent growth spurt. It is due to abnormal lumbrical insertion or an abnormal FDS origin and/or insertion. If full PIP extension can be achieved actively with the MCP held in flexion and there are no profound secondary radiographic changes, the digit can be explored and the abnormal tendon can be transferred to the radial lateral band. Type III multiple digits are involved with more severe contracture and is usually associated with a syndrome. If associated with arthrogryposis, the anatomic abnormalities are more complex. Skin grafts, tendon lengthening, and capsulotomy can yield limited improvement. In general, nonoperative treatment is favored for all three types. **Kirner's deformity** is a specific deformity involving an apex dorsal and ulnar curvature of the distal phalanx. Epiphyseal arrest or osteochondrosis has been implicated as an etiologic factor. Operative treatment while the epiphysis is open is generally avoided; however, there is one report of successful results with hemiepiphysiodesis. If a functional problem exists after skeletal maturity, corrective osteotomies can improve the angular deviation.
   4. Clinodactyly (Congenital Curvature of the Digit in the Radioulnar Plane)—There are three types: type I, minor angulation—normal length (very common); type II, minor angulation, short phalanx—present in 25% of children with Down's syndrome and 3% of others; type III, marked angulation—delta phalanx. The delta phalanx has a C-shaped epiphysis and longitudinally bracketed diaphysis. When the involved digit is too long, especially when the delta phalanx is an extra bone, early excision is done. When the delta phalanx replaces a normal digit of a consequently short finger, opening-wedge osteotomy is done.
   5. Flexed Thumb—The two main causes are congenital trigger thumb and congenital clasped thumb.
      a. Congenital Trigger Thumb—Involves flexion only at the IP joint. If it does not resolve spontaneously, it will respond to A1 pulley release. This is usually deferred until the child is 6–12 months old.
      b. Congenital Clasped Thumb—Exhibits deficient active thumb extension and slight limitation of passive extension. The types are differentiated based on passive mobility. Supple clasped thumbs are a result of a weak or absent EPL and EPB. The rigid variety is associated with hypoplastic extensors, MCPJ contractures, ulnar collateral ligament deficiency, thenar muscle hypoplasia, and inadequate first web space skin. This condition is initially treated with splinting for 3–6 months. If the child does not experience active extension or if significant flexion contractures exist, surgery is indicated. The supple variety is treated with a tendon transfer to the EPL. Complex cases may require any or all of the following: capsular release MPJ/CMC, muscular release of adductor pollicis (ADP)/flexor pollicis brevis/first dorsal interosseous, FPL Z-lengthening, extensor tendon transfer, opposition transfer, first web space deepening plasty.
   6. Arthrogryposis (Congenital Curved Joints)—Results from a defect in the motor unit as a whole at some point between the anterior horn cell and the muscle itself. It may be either neurogenic (90%) or myopathic (10%). The resultant immobility in fetal life produces the characteristic joint contractures, which tend to be symmetric. Classification: type I, single localized deformity (e.g., forearm pronation,

complex clasped thumb); type II, full expression (absence of shoulder musculature, thin tubular limbs, elbows extended, wrists flexed and ulnarly deviated, fingers fixed in intrinsic plus, thumb adducted, no flexion creases); type III, same as type II plus polydactyly and involvement of systems other than neuromuscular. In type I cases, correction of isolated deformity is usually achieved surgically. Type II cases are treated with therapy, splints, and serial casts to diminish contractures. Tendon transfers to replace essential motors are deferred until passive joint mobility is restored. The main goals in these children are one elbow that extends, one elbow that flexes, and wrist extension. Occasional arthrodesis of PIP joints is required to improve digital posture.

7. Syndactyly—**The most common congenital hand anomaly**. Syndactyly is classified based on the absence (simple) or presence (complex) of bony connections and whether the joining extends to the tip of the finger (complete) or stops somewhere short of that (incomplete). Acrosyndactyly refers to fusion between the more distal portions of the digit with proximal fenestration as is seen in constriction ring syndrome. When syndactyly presents alone, it is autosomal dominant with reduced penetrance and variable expression yielding a positive family history in 10–40% of cases. Syndactyly ray involvement is remembered with the mnemonic 5-15-50-30, which stands for thumb-index (5%), index-middle (15%), middle-ring (50%), ring-small (30%). Generally, syndactylized digits are released at around 1 year of age. The exceptions to this rule are in acrosyndactyly, in which distal releases should be accomplished in the neonatal period, and in syndactyly between rays of unequal length, which should not be delayed beyond 6 months. Both sides of the same digit are never separated on the same day so as to protect the circulation. The new web is constructed with a local skin flap. Full-thickness skin grafts are always required to obtain sufficient coverage. **Poland's syndrome** is a rare, nongenetic disorder characterized by four things: (1) unilateral short fingers, (2) *simple complete syndactyly*, (3) hand hypoplasia, and (4) ipsilateral absence of the sternocostal head of the pectoralis major. **Apert's syndrome** includes the following anomalies: acrocephaly, hypertelorism, and bilateral complex syndactyly with symphalangism. In this condition the index, middle, and ring fingers often share a common nail. Simple syndactyly between small and ring fingers is present. There is usually a deficient thumb web with a shortened and radially deviated thumb and a delta proximal phalanx.

Table 6-23. PREAXIAL POLYDACTYLY THUMB CLASSIFICATION

TYPE	DESCRIPTION	FREQUENCY
I	Bifid distal phalanx	2%
II	Duplicated distal phalanx	15%
III	Bifid proximal phalanx	6%
IV	**Duplicated proximal phalanx**	**43% (most common)**
V	Bifid metacarpal	10%
VI	Duplicated metacarpal	4%
VII	Triphalangia	20%

The general approach is to release the border digits before age 1, with construction of two digits out of the central three 6 months later.

C. Duplication

1. Preaxial Polydactyly (Thumb Duplication)—Usually unilateral and sporadic and not associated with syndromes except in type VII. Type VII associations include Holt-Oram syndrome, Fanconi's anemia, Blackfan-Diamond anemia, hypoplastic anemia, imperforate anus, cleft palate, and tibia defects. Wassel has classified this condition based on the complete or incomplete duplication of each phalanx (Table 6-23).

   The goal of surgical correction is to construct a thumb that is at least 80% of the size of the contralateral normal thumb. A type 1 combination is known as the Bilhaut-Celoquet procedure. It involves removing the central composite tissue segments from each thumb and combining the two into one. Though this seems the logical thing to do, there are significant problems with this approach. These problems include stiffness residua (from tendon scarring and nonlevel joints), size or angular deformity (from physeal arrest), and nail deformity (from germinal matrix scarring). Generally, this procedure is avoided unless there is no other way to obtain a thumb of sufficient size. The type II combination involves preserving the skeleton and nail of one of the thumbs and augmenting this with soft tissues from the other thumb. This allows for obtaining good size-match and tendon and ligament balance. This, if possible, is generally the favored approach. In Wassel types IV and VI, the ulnar thumb is retained so that integrity of the all-important ulnar collateral ligament is maintained. It is important to trim the metacarpal head on the side of skeletal excision to avoid an unsightly prominence. Division of anomalous tendon insertions, radial collateral ligament reconstruction, and reattachment of the intrinsics are also done. The type III combination (segmental digital transfer or "on-top plasty") is sometimes done for types V, VI, and VII when there is a clearly superior proximal segment on one digit and a clearly superior distal segment on the other digit. This involves a transfer of the superior distal segment to the superior proximal segment on a neurovascular pedicle with retained tendons.

2. Postaxial Polydactyly (Small Finger Duplication)—There are two types: type A, well-formed digit, and type B, a rudimentary skin tag. This disorder is 10 times more common in African Americans compared with whites. Associated anomalies are rare in African Americans because the condition is inherited as an autosomal dominant trait. In whites, however, a thorough genetic and physical work-up is needed. Virtually every body system and 17 chromosome abnormalities have been associated with postaxial polydactyly in whites. Vestigial digits are either tied off in the nursery or amputated before 1 year of age. The type A digit is managed with a type 2 combination with preservation of the radial digit and appropriate augmentation of soft-tissue structures from the ulnar digit.
3. Central Polydactyly—Most commonly associated with syndactyly. Early surgery is indicated to prevent angular deformity with growth. Impaired motion may result from interposed digit or symphalangism of adjacent digits. Tendons, nerves, and vessels may be shared to the point that only one finger from three skeletons may be obtainable. Angular deviation may require ligament reconstruction, osteotomy, or both.

D. Overgrowth—Macrodactyly is a nonhereditary, congenital digital enlargement. Ninety percent of cases are unilateral, 70% involve more than one digit. The adult analog is lipofibromatous hamartoma of the median nerve. Affected digits correspond with anatomic neural innervation, with median nerve being the most common. Angular deviation, joint stiffness, and involved nerve compression syndromes also occur. Classification: static—present at birth and growth is linear with other digits; progressive—not always evident at birth, but growth compared with normal digits is exponential. The severely affected single digit is best amputated. When the thumb or multiple digits are involved, the following procedures may offer improvement: epiphyseal ablation, angular and/or shortening osteotomies, longitudinal narrowing osteotomies, nerve stripping and defatting. All are associated with the following risks: increased stiffness and impaired neurovascular status.

Table 6-24. BLAUTH'S CLASSIFICATION OF THUMB HYPOPLASIA

Type I	Minor hypoplasia, all structures present, just a small thumb
Type II	Adduction contracture, MCP joint ulnar collateral ligament instability, thenar hypoplasia, normal skeleton with respect to articulations
Type IIIA	Extensive intrinsic and extrinsic musculotendinous deficiencies, intact CMC joint
Type IIIB	Extensive intrinsic and extrinsic musculotendinous deficiencies, basal metacarpal aplasia, CMC joint not intact
Type IV	Total or subtotal aplasia of the metacarpal, rudimentary phalanges, thumb attached to hand by skin bridge (pouce flottant)
Type V	Complete absence of the thumb

MCP, metacarpophalangeal; CMC, carpometacarpal.

E. Undergrowth—Thumb hypoplasia has been classified by Blauth (Table 6-24).

Type I requires no treatment. Types IIIB–V are best treated with pollicization. The critical structure is the CMC joint. Absence of the CMC joint requires thumb amputation and pollicization. Types II and IIIA are treated with reconstruction, addressing the following issues: stabilization of the MCPJ ulnar collateral ligament, web deepening plasty, opponens transfer if opposition is insufficient (Huber's transfer has the following advantages: amplitude and direction of pull are equal to replaced motors, tension is automatically set, thenar eminence will have a more normal appearance), extrinsic flexor and extensor exploration with correction of any anomalies to include tendon graft, if needed.

F. Constriction Ring Syndrome—Occurs sporadically with no evidence of hereditary predisposition. It manifests in four ways: (1) simple constriction rings, (2) rings with distal deformity with or without lymphedema, (3) acrosyndactyly, and (4) amputations. Early (neonatal period) surgery is indicated when edema may jeopardize circulation. Release is accomplished with multiple circumferential Z-plasties. Acrosyndactyly is managed by early release, preferably in the neonatal period.

G. Congenital Dislocation of the Radial Head—Clues suggestive of congenital dislocation rather than post-traumatic include bilateral involvement, other congenital anomalies, familial occurrence, irreducible by closed means. Some helpful radiographic clues include hypoplastic capitellum, short ulna with long radius, and a convex radial head. Sixty percent of the time this occurs with malformation syndromes or connective tissue disorders. In 40% of cases the defect is isolated. The inheritance pattern can be dominant or recessive. The only accepted surgical indications are pain, limited motion, or cosmetic dissatisfaction. In these instances radial head excision is indicated once the child reaches skeletal maturity.

H. Madelung's Deformity—Results from a disruption of the volar ulnar epiphysis of the distal radius. As the child grows, the distal radius exhibits excessive radial inclination and radiopalmar tilt. Symptoms arise from ulnocarpal impaction, restricted forearm rotation, and median nerve irritation and usually do not present until the child is an adolescent. If the deformity is not painful, no treatment is necessary. Corrective osteotomies of the radius with or without distal ulna recession are the preferred operative approach. Severe deformities may benefit from a distraction external fixator so as not to compromise circulation or nerve function with a single-stage correction.

XII. Hand Tumors (See also Chapter 8, Orthopaedic Pathology)

A. Benign Tumors

1. Localized Nodular Tenosynovitis—(xanthoma, localized pigmented villonodular synovitis, giant cell tumor of tendon sheath)—Age range 10–75. This is a firm, lobulated, nontender mass usually located on the volar surface of the fingers. Joint involvement occurs in 20% of cases, with bone erosions 10% of the time. Marginal excision is the treatment of choice. The recurrence rate is 10%. Pathology: gross; solid, tan, lobulated mass; micro: collagen stroma, giant cells, polyhedral histiocytes, hemosiderin.
2. Neurolemmoma—Most common solitary peripheral nerve tumor. It has a Schwann's cell origin. The age range is 20–70. These tumors are not associated with sensory/motor deficit. They are eccentric in the nerve and encapsulated. They can therefore be shelled out of the nerve without disrupting axons as opposed to neurofibroma. The treatment is marginal excision.
3. Glomus Tumor—A tumor of perivascular temperature regulating bodies; 75% occur in the hand; 50% of these are subungual, and 50% occur with erosions in the distal phalanx. Nail ridging is a common finding. The symptom complex involves the following triad: pain, cold intolerance, and exquisite tenderness to touch. MRI is helpful in making the diagnosis. Treatment is marginal excision.
4. Epidermal Inclusion Cyst—A common, painless, slow-growing mass emanating from a penetrating injury that drives keratinizing epithelium into subcutaneous tissues. It is treated with marginal excision and has a low recurrence rate.
5. Ganglion—**Most common hand mass**. Presentation may occur in a variety of areas, such as the dorsum of the wrist, volar wrist, DIP joint (mucous cyst), and digital flexor retinaculum. These lesions are firm, well circumscribed, often fixed to deep tissue but not to the overlying skin, and translucent. Surgical excision requires adequate exposure to delineate the joint of origin so that the stalk and a portion of the adjacent capsule can be excised. *Volar wrist cysts have a higher recurrence rate than dorsal cysts after surgical excision*. Nonoperative management such as aspiration has a higher recurrence rate than surgery but most often is tried before surgery because the risk is extremely low. Arthroscopic ganglionectomy is being studied as to its efficacy in several centers.
6. Calcinosis—May be secondary to degeneration. Symptoms include pain and erythema. Treatment includes rest, heat, and anti-inflammatory medication or injection. Surgical excision of large deposits is indicated in refractory cases. Calcinosis circumscripta can be seen in SLE, RA, and scleroderma, and it may be associated with Raynaud's phenomenon.
7. Dejerine-Sottas Disease—Localized swelling of a peripheral nerve due to hypertrophic interstitial neuropathy. Usually seen in the median nerve, and it may require carpal tunnel release. The lesion cannot be shelled out of the nerve without sacrificing axons.
8. Turret Exostosis—Traumatic subperiosteal hemorrhage that leads to extraperiosteal new bone formation. These lesions can be symptomatic if they form under the nail or under the extensor expansion on a digit. They are treated with excision after the bone matures so as to minimize recurrence.
9. CMC Boss—This represents a degenerative osteophyte located at the index and long finger CMC joint. Symptomatic lesions are best treated with excision and CMC fusion.
10. Enchondroma—The age range is 10–60. It is a benign cartilage tumor causing a radiolucent lobulated mass in the diaphyseal and/or metaphyseal portions of the bone. It is usually seen in the metacarpal, proximal, and middle phalanges and is rare in the distal phalanx. It causes symmetric fusiform expansion of the bone with endosteal scalloping and calcifications within the mass. It is most often incidentally noted in association with a pathologic fracture or other hand trauma. If noted with a pathologic fracture through the tumor, the fracture is managed in the standard fashion. Once the fracture is healed, the treatment is curettage and bone grafting of

the lesion if it is symptomatic or associated with more than one pathologic fracture.

11. Osteoid Osteoma—The age range is 10–30. Location is more common in the phalanx but it also occurs in the carpus. Classically, the pain is worse with alcohol and better with aspirin, except in fingertips, where aspirin does not seem to help. The diagnosis is often difficult, but plain films, bone scans, tomograms, and MRI are all helpful in localizing the nidus. Treatment involves excision of the nidus.
12. Giant Cell Tumor of Bone—These lesions are not entirely benign and can occasionally be very aggressive. The age range is in the third decade of life. Symptoms can include pain, but it is also noted incidentally when investigating other hand trauma. It is typically located in tubular bones (epiphyseal region); the third most common location is the distal radius. It is multicentric 18% of the time; cortical thinning and breakthrough can be seen on radiographs. Curettage alone has a high recurrence rate of 20–80%. Intercalary resection or amputation may be needed, especially when cortical breakthrough is visible. If there is no breakthrough, curettage and packing with polymethacrylate can be successful. If intercalary resection is done, the distal radius can be effectively reconstructed with a free fibula graft (either vascularized or nonvascularized).
13. Pigmented Subungual Lesions—Should go through usual blood break-down color changes and grow distally with the nail. If not, biopsy is indicated because there is a risk of subungual melanoma.
14. Melanoma—Lesions <1 mm thick are treated with local resection with a 1-cm margin. Lesions that are thicker should undergo sentinel node biopsy, even if nodes are negative clinically. If the biopsy is positive, radical node dissection is done. If the nodes are positive clinically, node dissection is done.

B. Malignancies—Rare in the hand. The most common primary malignancy is squamous cell carcinoma. The most common bony malignancy is chondrosarcoma. The most common metastasis to the hand is lung CA, and the most common location is distal phalanx. The most common primary sarcoma is epithelioid sarcoma.

XIII. Nails

A. Structure—The ventral germinal matrix produces the largest amount of nail keratin. The sterile matrix lies under the nail. The lunula is the junction of the sterile and germinal matrix. The hyponychium lies between distal nail and tip skin and is a barrier to microorganisms. The eponychium is the distal margin of the nail fold, whereas the perionychium is the lateral margin.

B. Nail Bed Injury—The best results are from early accurate repair. Though there are conflicting reports in the literature; a subungual hematoma involving >50% of the surface area of the nail is often associated with a significant nail bed injury. Removal of nail and repair of the nail bed with a 6-0 absorbable suture is indicated in this circumstance. Distal phalanx fractures with step-off of the dorsal cortex are associated with nail deformity. They should be reduced. The nail plate or synthetic substitute should be replaced after nail bed repair to preserve the eponychial fold and to diminish postoperative pain. If the nail bed is avulsed, the avulsed segment can be replaced, if available, as a free nail bed graft. Other options include a reversed dermal graft, nail matrix graft from the toe, or a split-thickness matrix graft from injured finger or a toe. As a secondary reconstructive effort, a vascularized wrap-around flap can be considered in selected patients.

C. Split Nail Deformity—Reconstruction requires excision of scarred nail bed and dorsal roof. Small defects can be closed primarily. Larger defects require full- or split-thickness toenail bed graft or a reverse dermal graft.

D. Hook Nail Deformity—Caused by loss of bony support or aggressive tip closure that brings the nail bed over the tip of the finger. The nail plate will follow the bed over the edge like a lemming over the cliff. It is treated by replacing the sterile matrix to the dorsum of the finger and tip closure with a local flap. The antenna procedure is a method in which the sterile matrix is suspended on K wires and volar soft-tissue loss is replaced with a cross-finger flap. In recalcitrant cases, a vascularized composite flap from the toe can be considered.

XIV. Elbow

A. Anatomy—The articular geometry of the ulnohumeral joint provides significant stability to the elbow, particularly when the joint is in extension. Primary ligament stability comes from the anterior band of the medial collateral ligament. The ulnar lateral collateral ligament provides stability to the radiocapitellar joint. When this ligament is incompetent, posterolateral rotatory instability can develop. The functional range of motion of the elbow is 30–130 degrees with 50 degrees of pronation and 50 degrees of supination.

B. Distal Biceps Tendon Rupture—Rare condition, but is generally seen in young, active males. When identified, the tendon should be repaired because there is a significant loss of power forearm supination and elbow flexion. Traditionally, the two-incision approach has been used (Boyd and Anderson); however, a single anterior approach utilizing suture anchors is gaining in popularity. Early reports are inconclusive but would suggest that there may be a diminished incidence of radioulnar synostosis with a single incision. Results with both techniques are not significantly different.

C. Epicondylitis
   1. Lateral (Tennis Elbow)—A common inflammation of the origin of the ECRB tendon. Typically, an insufficient healing response occurs, leaving the origin vulnerable to secondary injury. In that light it can be a difficult problem to treat, requiring patience. Tenderness over the lateral epicondyle and pain reproduced with resisted wrist extension that is worse when the elbow is also in extension are the clinical clues. Nonoperative measures include rest, NSAIDs, a counterforce brace (strap), and corticosteroid injections. It is usually a good idea to engage in a prolonged course of nonoperative treatment (9–12 months) because the vast majority of patients will get better. Recalcitrant cases are managed with release of the ECRB origin from the lateral epicondyle and débridement of "granulation tissue." It is important to remember that in 5% of these cases there will be a coexistent radial tunnel syndrome that should also be released to be complete.
   2. Medial (Golfer's Elbow)—This disorder is less common. It is also best treated with a long trial of nonoperative treatment. Refractory cases often respond to débridement of the medial epicondyle and reattachment of the flexor-pronator group. It is important to rule out cubital tunnel syndrome preoperatively so that an opportunity to transpose the ulnar nerve is not missed.

D. Rheumatoid Elbow—Principally, these patients are managed medically and with cortisone injections. When these measures lose their efficacy or joint destruction yields mechanical problems, surgical measures can be considered.
   1. Synovectomy—Radial head excision done through a lateral approach is effective in properly selected patients. Patients with stability and remaining articular cartilage and uncontrollable painful synovitis will do the best after synovectomy. Arthoscopic synovectomy with a limited exposure for radial head excision has also been done with similar success.
   2. Interposition Arthroplasty—Yields results that are less predictable than with total elbow arthroplasty. It remains a reasonable choice for young, active patients, with 75–80% good results having been reported. It involves resection and contouring the articular surfaces, which are then covered with fascia. Many use a distraction external fixator to allow for early motion in a controlled fashion to diminish instability and encourage a useful arc of motion.
   3. Total Elbow Arthroplasty—Has emerged as a reliable procedure for advanced stages of RA of the elbow. The principal indications are pain, loss of motion, and instability. The semiconstrained design is associated with the best results and implant survival rates. It is also used in properly selected post-traumatic arthritis cases, with good results.

E. Stiff Elbow—Principally managed with physical therapy to include the use of a dynamic splint. Contractures that are primarily intrinsic (secondary to intra-articular arthritis) are best managed with either total elbow arthroplasty or distraction interposition arthroplasty, depending on the patient's activity level and age. Intrinsic contractures that involve only the olecranon and the olecranon fossa can be well treated with osteophyte excision and clearing the olecranon fossa with a Cloward drill. Contractures that are primarily extrinsic (secondary to capsular contractures) are well managed with extrinsic capsular release. A technique called the "column procedure" has been described, which allows for a safe anterior and posterior capsular release through a single lateral approach, with reliable good results reported.

Selected Bibliography

ANATOMY AND PATHOPHYSIOLOGY

Smith, R.J.: Intrinsic muscles of the fingers: Function, dysfunction and surgical reconstruction. AAOS Instructional Course Lectures, vol. 24. St. Louis, C.V. Mosby, 1975, pp. 200–220.

COMPRESSIVE NEUROPATHY

Agee, J.M., McCarroll, H.R., Tortosa, R., et al.: Endoscopic release of the carpal tunnel: A randomized prospective multicenter study. J. Hand Surg. [Am.] 17:987–995, 1992.

Buch-Jaeger, N., and Foucher, G.: Correlation of clinical signs with nerve conduction tests in the diagnosis of carpal tunnel syndrome. J. Hand Surg. [Br.] 19:720–724, 1994.

Dellon, A.L.: Review of results for ulnar nerve entrapment at the elbow. J. Hand Surg. [Am.] 14:688–670, 1989.

Gelberman, R.H., Pfeffer, G.B., Galbraith, R.T., et al.: Results of treatment of severe carpal tunnel syndrome without internal neurolysis of the median nerve. J. Bone Joint Surg. [Am.] 69:896–903, 1987.

Gundberg, A.B.: Carpal tunnel decompression in spite of normal electromyography. J. Hand Surg. 8:348–349, 1983.

Hartz, C.R., Linschied, R.L., Gramse, R.R., et al.: The pronator teres syndrome: Compressive neuropathy of the median nerve. J. Bone Joint Surg. [Am.] 63:885–890, 1981.

Learmonth, J.R.: A technique for transplanting the ulnar nerve. Surg. Gynecol. Obstet. 75:92–93, 1942.

Leffert, R.D.: Anterior submuscular transposition of the ulnar nerve. J. Hand Surg. 7:147–155, 1982.

Lubahn, J.D., Cermak, M.B.: Uncommon nerve compression syndromes of the upper extremity. J. Am. Acad. Orthop. Surg. 6:378–386, 1998.

Posner, M.A.: Compression ulnar neuropathies at the elbow: II. Treatment. J. Am. Acad. Orthop. Surg. 6:289–297, 1998.

Posner, M.A.: Compression ulnar neuropathy at the elbow I. Etiology and diagnosis. J. Am. Acad. Orthop. Surg. 6:282–288.

Ritts, G.D.: Radial tunnel syndrome: A 10 yr surgical experience. Clin. Orthop. 219:201–205, 1987.

Spinner, M.: The anterior interosseous nerve syndrome. J. Bone Joint Surg. [Am.] 52:84–94, 1970.

Szabo, R.M, Steinberg, D.R.: Nerve entrapment syndromes in the wrist. J. Am. Acad. Orthop. Surg. 115–123, 1994.

Wood, V.E.: Thoracic outlet syndrome. Orthop. Clin. North Am. 19:131–146, 1988.

TENDON INJURIES

Bishop, A.T., Topper, S.M., and Bettinger, P.C.: Flexor mechanism reconstruction and rehabilitation. In Peimer, C.A., ed.: Surgery of the Hand and Upper Extremity. New York, McGraw Hill, 1996, pp. 1133–1162.

Gelberman, R.H., Vande Berg, J.S., Lundborg, G.N., et al.: Flexor tendon healing and restoration of the gliding surface. J. Bone Joint Surg. [Am.] 65:70–80, 1983.

LaSalle, W.E., and Strickland, J.W.: An evaluation of the two stage flexor tendon reconstruction technique. J. Hand Surg. 8:263–267, 1983.

Leddy, J.P., and Packer, J.W.: Avulsion of the profundus tendon insertion in athletes. J. Hand Surg. 2:66–69, 1977.

Lister, G.D., Kleinert, H.E., Kutz, J.E., et al.: Primary flexor tendon repair followed by immediate controlled mobilization. J. Hand Surg. 2:441–451, 1977.

Manske, P.R.: Nutrient pathways of flexor tendons in primates. J. Hand Surg. 7:436–444, 1982.

Manske, P.R., Gelberman, R.H., Vande Berg, J.S., et al.: Intrinsic flexor tendon repair. J. Bone Joint Surg. [Am.] 66:385–396, 1984.

Newport, M.L.: Extensor tendon injuries in the hand. J. Am. Acad. Orthop. Surg. 5:59–66, 1997.

Parkes, A.: The lumbrical plus finger. J. Bone Joint Surg. [Br.] 53:236–239, 1971.

Stern, P.J., and Kastrup, J.J.: Complications and prognosis of treatment of mallet finger. J. Hand Surg. [Am.] 13A:329–334, 1988.

Strickland, J.W., and Glogovac, S.V.: Digital function following flexor tendon repair in zone II: A comparison of immobilization and controlled passive motion techniques. J. Hand Surg. 5:537–543, 1980.

Strickland, J.W.: Flexor tendon injuries. I. Foundations of treatment. J. Am. Acad. Orthop. Surg. 3:44–54, 1995.

Strickland, J.W.: Flexor tendon injuries. II. Flexor tendon injuries: Operative technique. J. Am. Acad. Orthop. Surg. 3:55–62, 1995.

Verdan, C.: Syndrome of quadrigia. Surg. Clin. North Am. 40:425–426, 1966.

Wehbe, M.A., and Schneider, L.H.: Mallet fractures. J. Bone Joint Surg. [Am.] 66:658–669, 1984.

HAND INFECTIONS

Abrams, R.A., Botte, M.J.: Hand infections: Treatment recommendations for specific types. J. Am. Acad. Orthop. Surg. 4:219–230, 1996.

Chuinard, R.G., and D'Ambrosia, R.D.: Human bite infections of the hand. J. Bone Joint Surg. [Am.] 59:416–418, 1977.

Glickel, S.Z.: Hand infections in patients with acquired immunodeficiency syndrome. J. Hand Surg. [Am.] 13:770–775, 1988.

Gunther, S.F., Elliott, R.C., Brand, R.L., et al.: Experience with atypical mycobacterial infection in the deep structures of the hand. J. Hand Surg. 2:90–96, 1977.

Hitchcock, T.F., and Amadio, P.C.: Fungal infections. Hand Clin. 5:599–611, 1989.

Louis, D.S., and Silva, J., Jr.: Herpetic whitlow: Herpetic infections of the digits. J. Hand Surg. 4:90–94, 1979.

Neviaser, R.J.: Closed tendon sheath irrigation for pyogenic flexor tenosynovitis. J. Hand Surg. 3:462–466, 1978.

Schecter, W., Meyer, A., Schecter, G., et al.: Necrotizing fasciitis of the upper extremity. J. Hand Surg. 7:15–19, 1982.

VASCULAR OCCLUSION/DISEASE

Flatt, A.E.: Digital artery sympathectomy. J. Hand Surg. 5:550–556, 1980.

Jones, N.F.: Acute and chronic ischemia of the hand: Pathophysiology, treatment, and prognosis. J. Hand Surg. [Am.] 16:1074–1083, 1991.

Koman, L.A., and Urbaniak, J.R.: Ulnar artery insufficiency—a guide to treatment. J. Hand Surg. 6:16–24, 1981.

Lankford, L.L.: Reflex sympathetic dystrophy. In Omer, G., and Spinner, M., eds.: Management of Peripheral Nerve Problems. Philadelphia, W.B. Saunders, 1986.

Phillips, C.S., and Murphy, M.S.: Vascular problems of the upper extremity: A primer for the orthopedic surgeon. J. Am. Acad. Orthop. Surg. 6:401–408, 2002.

Tsuge, K.: Treatment of established Volkmann's contracture. J. Bone Joint Surg. [Am.] 57:925–929, 1975.

REPLANTATION

Boulas, H.J.: Amputations of the fingers and hand: Indications for replantation. J. Am. Acad. Orthop. Surg. 6:100–105, 1998.

Fassler, R.R.: Fingertip injuries: Evaluation and treatment. J. Am. Acad. Orthop. Surg. 4:84–92, 1996.

Gupta, A., Wolff, T.W.: Management of the mangled hand and forearm. J. Am. Acad. Orthop. Surg. 3:226–236, 1995.

Nissenbaum, M.: Class IIA ring avulsion injuries: An absolute indication for microvascular repair. J. Hand Surg. [Am.] 9:810–815, 1984.

Russell, R.C., O'Brien, B., Morrison, W.A., et al.: The late functional results of upper limb revascularization and replantation. J. Hand Surg. [Am.] 9:623–633, 1984.

Schlenker, J.D., Kleinert, H.E., and Tsai, T.: Methods and results of replantation following traumatic amputation of the thumb in sixty-four patients. J. Hand Surg. 5:63–70, 1980.

Tamai, S.: Twenty years' experience of limb replantation—review of 293 upper extremity replants. J. Hand Surg. 7:549–555, 1982.

Urbaniak, J.R., Evans, J.P., and Bright, D.S.: Microvascular management of ring avulsion injuries. J. Hand Surg. 6:25–30, 1981.

Urbaniak, J.R., Roth, J.H., Nunley, J.A., et al.: The results of replantation after amputation of a single finger. J. Bone Joint Surg. [Am.] 67:611–619, 1985.

MICROSURGERY

Godina, M.: Early microsurgical reconstruction of complex trauma of the extremities. Plast. Reconstr. Surg. 78:285–292, 1986.

Hans, C.S., Wood, M.B., Bishop, A.T., et al.: Vascularized bone transfer. J. Bone Joint Surg. [Am.] 74:1441–1449, 1992.

Lister, G., et al.: Emergency free flaps to the upper extremity. J. Hand Surg. [Am.] 13:22–28, 1988.

Lister, G.D., Kallisman, M., and Tsai, T.: Reconstruction of the hand with free microvascular toe to hand transfer: Experience with 54 toe transfers. Plast. Reconstr. Surg. 71:372–384, 1983.

Manktelow, R.T., Zuker, R.M., and McKee, N.H.: Functioning free muscle transplantation. J. Hand Surg. [Am.] 9:32–39, 1984.

Matev, I.B.: Thumb reconstruction through metacarpal bone lengthening. J. Hand Surg. 5:482–487, 1980.

Morrison, W.A., O'Brien B., and MacLeod, A.M.: Thumb reconstruction with a free neurovascular wrap-around flap from the big toe. J. Hand Surg. 5:575–583, 1980.

Scheker, L.R., Kleinert, H.E., and Hanel, D.P.: Lateral arm composite tissue transfer to ipsilateral hand defects. J. Hand Surg. [Am.] 12:665–672, 1987.

Stern, P.J., and Lister, G.D.: Pollicization after traumatic amputation of the thumb. Clin. Orthop. 155:85–94, 1981.

Wood, M.B., and Irons, G.B.: Upper extremity free skin flaps transfer: Results and utility compared with conventional distant pedicle skin flaps. Ann. Plast. Surg. 11:523–526, 1983.

WRIST PAIN/INSTABILITY

Bednar, J.M., Osterman, A.L.: Carpal instability. J. Am. Acad. Orthop. Surg. 1:10–17, 1993.

Bowers, W.H: Distal radioulnar joint arthroplasty: the hemi-resection interposition technique. J Hand Surg. 10A:169–178, 1985.

Chidgey, L.K.: The distal radioulnar joint: Problems and solutions. J. Am. Acad. Orthop. Surg. 3:95–109, 1995.

Chun, S., and Palmer, A.K.: The ulnar impaction syndrome: Follow-up of ulnar shortening osteotomy. J. Hand Surg. [Am.] 18:46–53, 1993.

Cooney, W.P.: Evaluation of chronic wrist pain by arthrography, arthroscopy and arthrotomy. J. Hand Surg. 18:815–822, 1993.

Fernandez, D.L.: A technique for anterior wedge-shaped grafts for scaphoid nonunions with carpal instability. J. Hand Surg. [Am.] 9:733–737, 1984.

Gelberman, R.H., et al.: The vascularity of the lunate bone and Kienbock's disease. J. Hand Surg. 5:272–278, 1980.

Gelberman, R.H., Wolock, B.S., and Siegel, D.B.: Current concepts review: Fractures and non-unions of the carpal scaphoid. J. Bone Joint Surg. [Am.] 71:1560–1565, 1989.

Gellman, H., Caputo, R.J., Carter, V., Aboulafia, A., et al.: J. Bone Joint Surg. [Am.] 71(3):354, 1989.

Green, D.P.: The effect of avascular necrosis on Russe bone grafting for scaphoid nonunion. J. Hand Surg. [Am.] 10:597, 1985.

Green, D.P., and O'Brien, E.T.: Classification and management of carpal dislocations. Clin. Orthop. 149:55–72, 1980.

Herbert, T.J., and Fischer, W.E.: Management of the fractured scaphoid using a new bone screw. J. Bone Joint Surg. [Br.] 66:114–123, 1984.

Horii, E., Garcia-Elias, M., Bishop, A.T., et al.: Effect of force transmission across the carpus in procedures used to treat Kienbock's disease. J. Hand Surg. [Am.] 15:393–400, 1990.

Jebson, P.J., Adams, B.D.: Wrist arthrodesis: Review of current techniques. J. Am. Acad. Orthop. Surg. 9:53–60, 2001.

Joseph, R.B., Linschied, R.L., Dobyns, J.H., et al.: Chronic sprains of the carpometacarpal joints. J. Hand Surg. 6:172–180, 1981.

Lavernia, C.J., Cohen, M.S., and Taleisnik, J.: Treatment of scapholunate dissociation by ligamentous repair and capsulodesis. J. Hand Surg. [Am.] 17:354–359, 1992.

Linschied, R.L., Dobyns, J.H., Beabout, J.W., et al.: Traumatic instability of the wrist: Diagnosis, classification and pathomechanics. J. Bone Joint Surg. [Am.] 54:1612–1632, 1972.

Mayfield, J.K., Johnson, R.P., and Kilcoyne, R.K.: Carpal dislocations: Pathomechanics and progressive perilunar instability. J. Hand Surg. 5:226–241, 1980.

Palmer, A.K.: Triangular fibrocartilage complex lesions: A classification. J. Hand Surg. [Am.] 14:594–606, 1989.

Regan, D.S., Linschied, R.L., and Dobyns, J.H.: Lunotriquetral sprains. J. Hand Surg. [Am.] 9:502–514, 1984.

Ruby, L.K., Stinson, J., and Belsky, M.R.: The natural history of scaphoid nonunion. J. Bone Joint Surg. [Am.] 67:428–432, 1985.

Shin, A.Y., Battaglia, M.J., Bishop, A.T.: Lunotriquetral instability: Diagnosis and treatment. J. Am. Acad. Orthop. Surg. 8:170–179, 2000.

Taleisnik, J.: Post-traumatic carpal instability. Clin. Orthop. 149:73–82, 1980.

Topper, S.M., Wood, M.B., and Cooney, W.P.: Athletic injuries of the wrist. In Cooney, W.P., Linschied, R.L., and Dobyns, J.H., eds.: The Wrist: Diagnosis and Operative Treatment. St. Louis, Mosby–Year Book, 1998, pp. 1030–1074.

Topper, S.M., Wood, M.B., and Ruby, L.K.: Ulnar styloid impaction syndrome. J. Hand Surg. [Am.] 22:699–704, 1997.

Trousdale, R.T., Amadio, P.C., Cooney, W.P., et al.: Radio-ulnar dissociation. J. Bone Joint Surg. [Am.] 74:1486–1497, 1992.

Trumble, T., Glisson, R.R., Seaber, A.V., et al.: A biomechanical comparison of methods for treating Kienbock's disease. J. Hand Surg. [Am.] 11:88–93, 1986.

Viegas, S.F., Patterson, R.M., Peterson, P.D., et al.: Ulnar sided perilunate instability: An anatomic and biomechanical study. J. Hand Surg. [Am.] 15:268–278, 1990.

Walsh, J.J., Berger, R.A., Cooney, W.P.: Current status of scapholunate interosseous ligament injuries. J. Am. Acad. Orthop. Surg. 10:32–42, 2002.

Watson, H.K., and Ballet, F.L.: The SLAC wrist: Scapholunate advanced collapse pattern of degenerative arthritis. J. Hand Surg. [Am.] 9:358–365, 1984.

Watson, H.K., and Hempton, R.F.: Limited wrist arthrodesis: 1. The triscaphoid joint. J. Hand Surg. 5:320–327, 1980.

Weiss, A.P., Weiland, A.J., Moore, J.R., et al.: Radial shortening for Kienbock disease. J. Bone Joint Surg. [Am.] 73:384–391, 1991.

ARTHRITIS

Bamberger, H.B., Stern, P.J., Kiefhaber, T.R., et al.: Trapeziometacarpal joint arthrodesis: A functional evaluation. J. Hand Surg. [Am.] 17:605–611, 1992.

Brown, F.E., and Brown, M.L.: Long-term results after tenosynovectomy to treat the rheumatoid hand. J. Hand Surg. [Am.] 13:704–708, 1988.

Burton, R.I., and Pellegrini, V.D., Jr.: Surgical management of basal joint arthritis of the thumb. Part II: Ligament reconstruction with tendon interposition arthroplasty. J. Hand Surg. [Am.] 11:324–332, 1986.

Carroll, R.E., and Hill, N.A.: Arthrodesis of the carpometacarpal joint of the thumb. J. Bone Joint Surg. [Br.] 55:292–294, 1973.

Cobb, T.K., and Bechenbaugh, R.D.: Biaxial total-wrist arthroplasty. J. Hand Surg. [Am.] 21:1011, 1996.

Eaton, R.G., Lane, L.B., Litter, J.W., et al.: Ligament reconstruction for the painful thumb carpometacarpal joint: A long-term assessment. J. Hand Surg. [Am.] 9:692–699, 1984.

Imbriglia, J.E., Broudy, A.S., Hagberg, W.C., et al.: Proximal row carpectomy: Clinical evaluation. J. Hand Surg. [Am.] 15:426–430, 1990.

Kirschenbaum, D., Schneider, L.H., Adams, D.C., et al.: Arthroplasty of the metacarpophalangeal joints with use of silicone rubber implants in patients who have rheumatoid arthritis. J. Bone Joint Surg. [Am.] 75:3–12, 1993.

Mannerfelt, L., and Norman, O.: Attritional ruptures of the flexor tendons in RA caused by bony spurs in the carpal tunnel. J. Bone Joint Surg. [Br.] 51:270, 1969.

Millender, L.H., and Nalebuff, E.A.: Arthrodesis of the rheumatoid wrist. J. Bone Joint Surg. [Am.] 55:1026–1034, 1973.

Nalebuff, E.A., and Garrett, J.: Opera-glass hand in rheumatoid arthritis. J. Hand Surg. 1:210–220, 1976.

DUPUYTREN'S DISEASE

Benson, L.S., Williams, C.S., Kahle, M.: Dupuytrens contracture. J. Am. Acad. Orthop. Surg. 6:24–35, 1998.

Hill, N.A.: Current concepts review: Dupuytren's contracture. J. Bone Joint Surg. [Am.] 67:1439–1443, 1985.

Ketchum, L. D.: The injection of nodules of Dupuytren's disease with triamcinone acetonide. J Hand Surg. 25A(6):1157–62, 2003.

McFarlane, R.M.: The current status of Dupuytren's disease. J. Hand Surg. 8:703–709, 1983.

Schneider, L.H., Hankin, F.M., and Eisenberg, T.: Surgery of Dupuytren's disease: A review of the open palm method. J. Hand Surg. [Am.] 11:23–27, 1986.

Seyfer, A., and Hueston, J.: Dupuytren's contracture. Hand Clin. 7:617–776, 1991.

Strickland, J.W., and Bassett, R.L.: The isolated digital cord in Dupuytren's contracture: Anatomy and clinical significance. J. Hand Surg. [Am.] 10:118–124, 1985.

NERVE INJURY, TENDON TRANSFERS, PARALYSIS

Aziz, W., Singer, R.M., and Wolff, T.W.: Transfer of the trapezius for flail shoulder after brachial plexus injury. J. Bone Joint Surg. [Br.] 72:701–704, 1990.

Brand, P.: Biomechanics of tendon transfers. Hand Clin. 4:137–154, 1988.

Dellon, A.L., Curtis, R.M., and Edgerton, M.T.: Reeducation of sensation in the hand after nerve inury and repair. Plast. Reconstr. Surg. 53:297–305, 1974.

Eversmann, W.W.: Tendon transfers for combined nerve injuries. Hand Clin. 4:187–199, 1988.

Freehafer, A.A.: Tendon transfers in patients with cervical spinal cord injury. J. Hand Surg. [Am.] 16:804–809, 1991.

Gaul, J.S., Jr.: Intrinsic motor recovery: A long term study of ulnar nerve injury. J. Hand Surg. 7:502–508, 1982.

Gellman, H., Nichols, D.: Reflex sympathetic dystrophy in the upper extremity. J. Am. Acad. Orthop. Surg. 5:13–322, 1997.

Gilbert, A., and Razaboni, R.: Indications and results of brachial plexus surgery in obstetrical palsy. Orthop. Clin. North Am. 19:91, 1988.

Hentz, V.R., Brown, M., and Keoshian, L.A.: Upper limb reconstruction in quadriplegia: Functional assessment and proposed treatment modifications. J. Hand Surg. 8:119–131, 1983.

House, J.H., and Shannon, M.A.: Restoration of strong grasp and lateral pinch in tetraplegia: A comparison of two methods of thumb control in each patient. J. Hand Surg. [Am.] 10:22–29, 1985.

Inglis, A.E., and Cooper, W.: Release of the flexor-pronator origin for flexion deformities of the hand and wrist in spastic paralysis. J. Bone Joint Surg. [Am.] 48:847–857, 1966.

Keenan, M.E., Korchek, J.I., Botte, M.J., et al.: Results of transfer of the flexor digitorum superficialis tendons to the flexor digitorum profundus in adults with acquired spasticity of the hand. J. Bone Joint Surg. [Am.] 69:1127–1132, 1987.

Kline, D.G.: Civilian gunshot wounds to the brachial plexus. J. Neurosurg. 70:166–174, 1989.

Lee, S.K., Wolfe, S.W.: Peripheral nerve injury and repair. J. Am. Acad. Orthop. Surg. 8:243–252, 2000.

Leffert, R.D.: Clinical diagnosis, testing, and electromyographic study in brachial plexus traction injuries. Orthop. Clin. North Am. 237:24–31, 1988.

Millesi, H., Meissl, G., and Berger, A.: Further experience with interfascicular grafting of the median ulnar and radial nerves. J. Bone Joint Surg. [Am.] 58:209–218, 1976.

Riordan, D.C.: Tendon transfers in hand surgery. J. Hand Surg. 8:748-753, 1983.
Seddon, H.: Three types of nerve injury. Brain 66:237-288, 1943.
Sedel, L.: The results of surgical repair of brachial plexus injuries. J. Bone Joint Surg. [Br.] 64:54-66, 1982.
Skoff, H., and Woodbury, D.F.: Current concepts review: Management of the upper extremity in cerebral palsy. J. Bone Joint Surg. [Am.] 67:500-503, 1985.
Smith, R.J.: Tendon Transfers of the Hand and Forearm. Boston, Little, Brown, 1987.
Stern, P.J., and Caudle, R.J.: Tendon transfers for elbow flexion. Hand Clin. 4:297-307, 1988.
Stewart, J.D.: Electrodiagnostic techniques. Hand Clin. 2:677, 1986.
Sunderland, S.: A classification of peripheral nerve injuries producing loss of function. Brain 74:491-516, 1951.
Szabo, R.M., and Gelberman, R.H.: Operative treatment of cerebral palsy. Hand Clin. 1:525-543, 1985.
Terzis, J., Faibisoff, B., and Williams, H.B.: The nerve gap: Suture under tension vs. graft. Plast. Reconstr. Surg. 56:166-170, 1975.

CONGENITAL HAND DISORDERS

Blauth, W.: The hypoplastic thumb. Arch. Orthop. Unfallchir. 62(3): 225-246, 1967.
Buck-Gramcko, D.: Congenital malformations. J. Hand Surg. [Am.] 15:150-152, 1990 (editorial).
Buck-Gramcko, D.: Pollicization of the index finger. J. Bone Joint Surg. [Am.] 53:1605-1617, 1971.
Buck-Gramcko, D.: Radialization as a new treatment for radial club hand. J. Hand Surg. [Am.] 10:964-968, 1985.
Cleary, J.E., and Omer, G.E.: Congenital proximal radioulnar synostosis. J. Bone Joint Surg. [Am.] 67:539-545, 1985.
Eaton, C.J., and Lister, G.D.: Syndactyly. Hand Clin. 6:555-575, 1990.
Eaton, C.J., and Lister, G.D.: Toe transfer for congenital hand defects. Microsurgery 12:186-195, 1991.
Gallant, G.G., Bora, W.: Congenital deformities of the upper extremity. J. Am. Acad. Orthop. Surg. 4:162-171, 1996.
Gilbert, A.: Toe transfers for congenital hand defects. J. Hand Surg. 7:118-124, 1982.
Kleinman, W.B.: Management of thumb hypoplasia. Hand Clin. 6:617-641, 1990.
Lamb, D.W.: Radial club hand. J. Bone Joint Surg. [Am.] 59:1-13, 1977.
Light, T.R., and Manske, P.R.: Congenital malformations and deformities of the hand. AAOS Instr. Course Lect. 38:31-71, 1989.
Manske, P.R.: Thumb reconstruction. Hand Clin. 8:1-196, 1992.
Marks, T.W., and Bayne, L.G.: Polydactyly of the thumb: Abnormal anatomy and treatment. J. Hand Surg. 3:107-116, 1978.
Miller, J.K., Wenner, S.M., and Kruger, L.M.: Ulnar deficiency. J. Hand Surg. [Am.] 11:822-829, 1986.
Siegert, J.J., Cooney, W.P., and Dobyns, J.H.: Management of simple camptodactyly. J. Hand Surg. [Br.] 15:181-189, 1990.
Swanson, A.B.: A classification for congenital limb malformation. J. Hand Surg. 8:693-702, 1983.
Tada, K., and Yonenobu, K.: Duplication of the thumb: A retrospective review of 237 cases. J. Bone Joint Surg. [Am.] 65:584-598, 1983.
Tsuge, K.: Treatment of macrodactyly. J. Hand Surg. [Am.] 10:968-969, 1985.
Upton, J., and Tan, C.: Correction of constriction rings. J. Hand Surg. [Am.] 16:947-953, 1991.
Weckesser, E.C.: Congenital clasped thumb. J. Bone Joint Surg. [Am.] 37:1417-1428, 1968.

HAND TUMORS

Amadio, P.C., and Lombardi, R.M.: Metastatic tumors of the hand. J. Hand Surg. [Am.] 12:311, 1987.
Angelides, A.B., and Wallace, P.F.: The dorsal ganglion of the wrist: Its pathogenesis, gross and microscopic anatomy, and surgical treatment. J. Hand Surg. 1:228-235, 1976.
Carroll, R.E., and Berman, A.T.: Glomus tumors of the hand. J. Bone Joint Surg. [Am.] 54:691-703, 1972.
Creighton, J., Peimer, C., Mindell, E., et al.: Primary malignant tumors of the upper extremity: Retrospective analysis of one hundred twenty-six cases. J. Hand Surg. [Am.] 10:808-814, 1985.
Doyle, L.K., Ruby, L.K., Nalebuff, E.A., et al.: Osteoid osteoma of the hand. J. Hand Surg. [Am.] 10:408-410, 1985.
Fleegler, E.J., and Zeinowicz, R.J.: Tumors of the perionychium. Hand Clin. 1:128, 1990.
Frassica, F.J., Amadio, P.C., Wold, L.E., et al.: Primary malignant bone tumors of the hand. J. Hand Surg. [Am.] 14:1022, 1989.
Kuur, E., Hansen, S.L., and Lindequist, S.: Treatment of solitary enchondromas in fingers. J. Hand Surg. [Br.] 14:109-112, 1989.
Moore, J.R., Weiland, A.J., and Curtis, R.M.: Localized nodular tenosynovitis: Experience with 115 cases. J. Hand Surg. [Am.] 9:412-417, 1984.
Rock, M., Pritchard, D., and Unni, K.: Metastases from histologically benign giant cell tumor of bone. J. Bone Joint Surg. [Am.] 64:269-274, 1984.
Steinberg, B., Gelberman, R.H., Mankin, H., et al.: Epithelioid sarcoma in the upper extremity. J. Bone Joint Surg. [Am.] 74:28-35, 1992.
Strickland, J.W., and Steichen, J.B.: Nerve tumors of the hand and forearm. J. Hand Surg. 2:285-291, 1977.

NAILS

Ashbell, T.S., Kleinert, H.K., Putcha, S., et al.: The deformed fingernail, a frequent result of failure to repair nail bed injuries. J. Trauma 7:177-190, 1967.
Louis, D.S., Palmer, A.K., and Burney, R.E.: Open treatment of digital tip injuries. J.A.M.A. 244:697-698, 1980.
Schenck, R., and Cheema, T.A.: Hypothenar skin grafts for fingertip reconstruction. J. Hand Surg. [Am.] 9:750-753, 1984.
Shephard, G.H.: Treatment of nail bed avulsions with split thickness nail bed grafts. J. Hand Surg. 8:49-54, 1983.
Shibata, M., Seki, T., Yoshizu, T., et al.: Microsurgical toenail transfer to the hand. J. Plast. Reconstr. Surg. 88:102-109, 1991.
Zook, E.G., Guy, R.J., and Russell, R.C.: A study of nail bed injuries: Causes, treatment, and prognosis. J. Hand Surg. [Am.] 9:247-252, 1984.
Zook, E.G., Van Beek, A.L., Russell, R.C., et al.: Anatomy and physiology of the perionychium: A review of the literature and anatomic study. J. Hand Surg. 5:528-536, 1980.

ELBOW

Boyd, H.B., and Anderson, M.D.: A method for reinsertion of the distal biceps brachii tendon. J. Bone Joint Surg. [Am.] 43:1041, 1961.
Ferlic, D.C., Patchett, C.E., and Clayton, M.L.: Elbow synovectomy in rheumatoid arthritis: Long term results. Clin. Orthop. 220:119-125, 1987.
Mansat, P., and Morrey, B.F.: The column procedure: A limited lateral approach for extrinsic contracture of the elbow. J. Bone Joint Surg. [Am.] 80:1603-1615, 1998.
Morrey, B.F., Askew, L.J., An, K.N., et al.: A biomechanical study of normal elbow motion. J. Bone Joint Surg. [Am.] 63:872, 1981.
Nirschl, R.P., and Pettrone, F.A.: Tennis elbow. J. Bone Joint Surg. [Am.] 61:832-839, 1979.
O'Driscoll, S.W., Bell, D.F., and Morrey, B.F.: Posterolateral rotatory instability of the elbow. J. Bone Joint Surg. [Am.] 73:440, 1991.

Acknowledgments

I would like to acknowledge the following surgeons for their previous contributions to the development of this chapter: Mark D. Miller, MD, James F. Bruce, MD, and Steve Topper, MD.

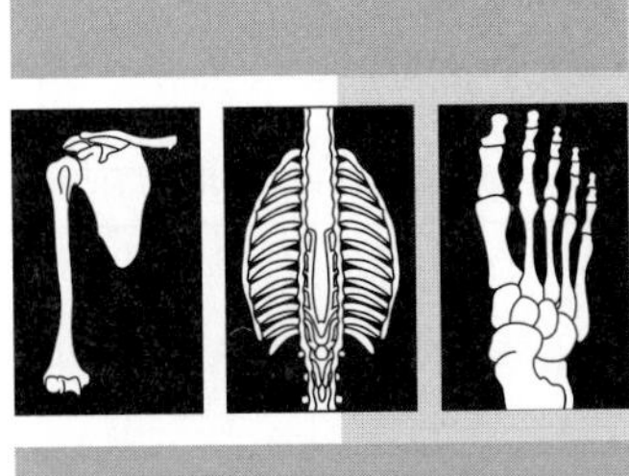

7 Spine

WILLIAM C. LAUERMAN
BRIAN R. MCCALL

I. Introduction

A. Anatomy—See Chapter 11, Anatomy.

B. History and Physical Examination (Table 7-1)—A complete history is critical to fully assess complaints, including evaluation of localized pain (tumor, infection), mechanical pain (instability, discogenic disease), radicular pain (herniated nucleus pulposus [HNP], stenosis), night pain (tumor), and systemic symptoms, such as fever or unexplained weight loss (infection, tumor). The physical examination must be complete to evaluate both the spine and the neurologic function of the extremities. Localized hip and shoulder pathology may simulate spine disease and must also be evaluated. The examination must include the following:

EXAMINATION	FEATURES
Inspection	Overall alignment in sagittal and coronal planes (sciatic scoliosis)
Gait	Wide-based (myelopathy), forward-leaning (stenosis), antalgic
Palpation	Localized posterior swelling (trauma), acute gibbus deformity, tenderness
Range of motion	Flexion/extension, lateral bend, full versus limited
Neurologic assessment	Motor, sensory, reflexes, long tract signs (Tables 7-2, 7-4)
Special tests	Straight-leg raise, Spurling's test, Waddell's signs of inorganic pathology

C. Objective Tests—Plain radiographs (wait 4-6 weeks), add flexion/extension for suspected instability. Magnetic resonance imaging (MRI) (HNP, stenosis, soft tissue, tumor, infection) is excellent for further imaging. Computed tomographic (CT) scans with fine cuts ± myelographic dye (bony anatomy) is particularly helpful after previous surgery. Bone scan, helpful in evaluating metastatic disease, may be negative with multiple myeloma. Laboratory evaluation: C-reactive protein and erythrocyte sedimentation rate for infection, metabolic screen, serum/urine protein electrophoresis for myeloma, complete blood count (often high normal white blood cell [WBC] count with infection, anemia with myeloma).

D. Back Pain—Ubiquitous complaint, second only to upper respiratory infection as cause of office visits, with 60-80% lifetime prevalence. Standard work-up, beginning with history (most important) and progressing to physical examination (see Table 7-1). Radiographic and laboratory studies rarely help in acute case. Some important considerations in the evaluation of back pain include the following:

1. Age—Children may be affected by congenital or, more commonly, developmental disorders, infection, or primary tumors. Young adults are more likely to suffer from disc disease, spondylolisthesis, or acute fractures. In older adults spinal stenosis, metastatic disease, and osteopenic compression fractures are more common.
2. Radicular Signs and Symptoms—Often associated with disc herniation or spinal stenosis. Intraspinal pathologic conditions or other entities associated with cord or root impingement may be responsible. Herpes zoster is a rare cause of lumbar radiculopathy with pain preceding the skin eruption.
3. Systemic Symptoms—Careful history-taking can lead to the diagnosis of metabolic disease, ankylosing spondylitis (young adult, men > women), tumor, or infection (confirmed with laboratory studies). Associated signs and symptoms may be essential to the diagnosis (e.g., ophthalmologic symptoms with spondyloarthropathies; other joint involvement with rheumatoid arthritis [RA] or osteoarthritis). Metastatic tumor should be considered in patients with a history of cancer, pain at rest,

Table 7-1. DIFFERENTIAL DIAGNOSIS OF DISORDERS IN THE L-SPINE

EVALUATION	BACK STRAIN	HNP	SPINAL STENOSIS	SPONDYLOLISTHESIS/ INSTABILITY	TUMOR	SPONDYLO-ARTHROPATHY	METABOLIC	INFECTION
Predominant pain (leg versus back)	Back	Leg	Leg	Back	Back	Back	Back	Back
Constitutional symptoms				+	+		+	
Tension sign		+						
Neurologic examination		+	+ After stress					
Plain x-ray studies			+	+	±	+	+	±
Lateral motion x-ray studies				+				
CT scan		+	+		+			+
Myelogram		+	+					
Bone scan					+	+	+	+
ESR					+	+		+
Ca/P/alk phos					+			

HNP, herniated nucleus pulposus; ESR, erythrocyte sedimentation rate; CT, computed tomography; Ca/P/alk phos, calcium alkaline phosphatase.
From Weinstein, J.N., and Wiesel, S.W.: The Lumbar Spine. Philadelphia, WB Saunders, 1990, p. 360.

systemic symptoms, and in those older than age 50. Many patients with fibromyalgia have chronic back pain, often refractory to localized treatment. Fibromyalgia is more common in women, and is associated with sleep disturbance, irritable bowel syndrome, and dysmenorrhea. Excessive generalized tenderness, on both sides of the midline, is the hallmark physical finding.

4. Referred Pain—"Back pain" can often be viscerogenic, vascular, or related to other skeletal areas (especially with hip arthritis). Careful history-taking and physical examination are essential. Common areas of referred back pain include peptic ulcer disease, cholecystitis, nephrolithiasis, pancreatitis, pelvic inflammatory disease, and abdominal aortic aneurysm.
5. Psychogenic—Psychological disturbances play an important role in some patients with chronic low back disorders. Evidence of secondary gain (especially compensation or litigation) and inappropriate (Waddell's) signs, symptoms, and maneuvers can help identify these patients. Nevertheless, one must be wary of real pathologic conditions, even in such patients.
6. History of Back Pain—Perhaps the most important risk factor for future pain, especially with frequent disabling episodes and short intervals between episodes. Compensation work situations, smoking, and age over 30 are also associated with development of persistent disabling lower back pain. The incidence of disabling pain actually declines after age 60.

II. Cervical Spine

A. Cervical Spondylosis—Chronic disc degeneration and associated facet arthropathy. Resultant syndromes include discogenic neck pain (axial pain), radiculopathy (root compromise), myelopathy (cord compression), and combinations. Cervical spondylosis typically begins at age 40–50, is seen in men > women, and most commonly occurs at the C5–C6 > C6–C7 levels. Risk factors include frequent lifting, cigarette smoking, and a history of excessive driving.

1. Pathoanatomy—Involves the disc and four other articulations (Fig. 7-1): two facet joints and two uncovertebral joints (of Luschka). The cervical cord becomes compromised when the diameter of the canal (normally about 17 mm) is reduced to less than 13 mm (measurable on plain lateral radiograph). With neck extension, the cord is pinched between the degenerative disc and spondylotic bar anteriorly and the hypertrophic facets and infolded ligamentum flavum posteriorly. With neck flexion the canal dimension increases slightly to relieve pressure on the cord. Progressive collapse of the cervical discs results in loss of

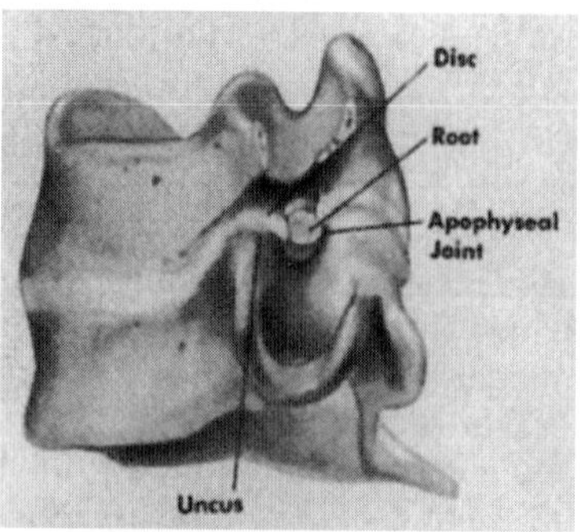

FIGURE 7-1 ■ Cervical root impingement. (From Rothman, R.H., and Simeon, F.A.: The Spine, 2nd ed. Philadelphia, WB Saunders, 1982, p. 452.)

normal lordosis of the cervical spine and chronic anterior cord compression across the kyphotic spine/anterior chondro-osseous spurs. Spondylotic changes in the foramina, primarily from chondro-osseous spurs of the joints of Luschka, may restrict motion and may lead to nerve root compression. Soft-disc herniation is usually posterolateral, between the posterior edge of the uncinate process and the lateral edge of the posterior longitudinal ligament, resulting in acute radiculopathy. Anterior herniation may cause dysphagia (rare). Myelopathy may be seen with large central herniation or spondylotic bars with a congenitally narrow canal. Ossification of the posterior longitudinal ligament, resulting in cervical stenosis and myelopathy, is common in Asians but may also be seen in non-Asians.

2. Signs and Symptoms—Degenerative discogenic neck pain may present with the insidious onset of neck pain without neurologic signs or symptoms, exacerbated by excess vertebral motion. Occipital headache is common. Radiculopathy can involve one or multiple roots, and symptoms include neck, shoulder, and arm pain, paresthesias, and numbness. Findings may overlap because of intraneural intersegmental connections of sensory nerve roots. Mechanical stress such as excessive vertebral motion, in particular, rotation and lateral bend with a vertical compressive force (Spurling's test), may exacerbate these symptoms. The lower nerve root at a given level is usually affected (see Table 7-2). Myelopathy may be characterized by weakness (upper > lower extremity), decreased manual dexterity, ataxic broad-based shuffling gait, sensory changes, spasticity and, rarely, urinary retention. The most worrisome complaint is lower-extremity weakness (corticospinal tracts). Patients may complain of urinary urgency or frequency. "Myelopathy hand" and the "finger escape sign" (small finger spontaneously abducts because of weak intrinsics) suggest cervical myelopathy. Upper motor neuron findings such as hyperreflexia, Hoffmann's sign, inverted radial reflex (ipsilateral finger flexion when eliciting the brachioradialis reflex), clonus, or Babinski's sign may be present. Additionally, the upper extremities may have radicular (lower motor neuron) signs along with evidence of myelopathy distally. Funicular pain, characterized by central burning and stinging ± Lhermitte's phenomenon (radiating lightning-like sensations down the back with neck flexion) may also be present with myelopathy.

3. Diagnosis—Largely based on history and physical examination. Plain radiographs, including oblique views, should be assessed for changes in uncovertebral and facet joints, alignment, osteophytes (bars), and disc space narrowing, and to measure the sagittal canal diameter. However, radiographic changes of the degenerated cervical spine may not correlate with symptoms: 70% of patients, by the age of 70, will have degenerative changes on x-ray film. CT-myelography or MRI demonstrates neural compressive pathology well, although false-positive MRI scans are common: 25% of asymptomatic patients over age 40 will have findings of either HNP or foraminal stenosis on cervical MRI. Therefore correlation with history and physical examination is critical. MRI is also useful for detecting intrinsic changes in the spinal cord (myelomalacia—area of bright signal in the cord on T2) as well as disc degeneration. Discography is controversial and is rarely used for cervical spine disorders. Electrodiagnostic studies have a high false-negative rate but may be helpful in select cases for differentiating peripheral nerve compression from more central compression and diseases, such as amyotrophic lateral sclerosis.

4. Treatment—Nonsteroidal anti-inflammatory drugs (NSAIDs), moist heat, cervical isometric exercises, use of a collar, traction, and pain clinic modalities are helpful in most cases of discogenic neck pain and radiculopathy. Indications for surgery include myelopathy with motor/gait impairment or radiculopathy with persistent disabling pain and weakness. Surgery for discogenic neck pain is less rewarding. Anterior Smith-Robinson discectomy and

Table 7-2. FINDINGS IN NERVE ROOT COMPRESSION

LEVEL	ROOT	MUSCLES AFFECTED	SENSORY LOSS	REFLEX
C3–C4	C4	Scapular	Lateral neck, shoulder	None
C4–C5	C5	Deltoid, biceps	Lateral arm	Biceps
C5–C6[a]	C6	Wrist extensors, biceps, triceps (supination)	Radial forearm	Brachioradialis
C6–C7	C7	Triceps, wrist flexors (pronation)	Middle finger	Triceps
C7–C8	C8	Finger flexors, interossei	Ulnar hand	None
C8–T1	T1	Interossei	Ulnar forearm	None

[a]Most common.

fusion is preferred technique. Posterior foraminotomy is useful for single-level radiculopathy. For multilevel spondylosis and myelopathy, more extensive decompression is necessary. The anterior approach involves excision of osteophytes and corpectomy with a strut graft fusion plus or minus instrumentation. Anterior plating may increase fusion rate in multilevel discectomies with fusion and will protect a strut graft in multilevel corpectomies, although plating may actually contribute to nonunion following strut grafting. Adjunctive posterior plating may be employed in cases involving prior laminectomy or following multilevel corpectomy and strut grafting. Posterior approaches include canal-expansive laminoplasty (commonly used for ossification of the posterior longitudinal ligament), which can help decrease the incidence of instability associated with multilevel laminectomy. Overall alignment should be lordotic for this approach to be successful. Laminoplasty has been found to limit range of motion postoperatively and has a significant rate of axial neck pain as well. Multilevel laminectomy may fail owing to failure to adequately relieve anterior compression or secondary to progressive kyphosis, which may require anterior decompression and fusion with a strut graft for salvage. Successful anterior decompression and fusion results in 70–90% improvement in pain and neurologic function. Complications of the anterior approach include neurologic injury (<1%), pseudarthrosis of 12% for single-level fusions, 30% for multilevel fusions (treated with posterior wiring or plating or repeat anterior fusion with plating if symptomatic), upper airway obstruction after multilevel corpectomy, or injury to other neck structures, including the recurrent laryngeal nerve (increased with right-side approach). Complications of laminectomy include subluxation if facets are sacrificed, leading to a swan neck deformity, muscle ischemia, and direct spinal cord injury with quadriparesis. Radicular symptoms may be alleviated after decompression, but gait changes may not.

B. Cervical Stenosis—May be congenital or acquired (traumatic, degenerative). Absolute (anteroposterior canal diameter <10 mm) or relative (10–13 mm diameter) stenosis predisposes the patient to the development of radiculopathy, myelopathy, or both from relatively minor soft- or hard-disc pathology or trauma. Pavlov's (Torg's) ratio (canal/vertebral body width) should be 1.0. A ratio <0.80 or a sagittal diameter of <13 mm is considered a significant risk factor for later neurologic involvement. Minor trauma such as hyperextension may lead to a central cord syndrome, even without overt skeletal injury. In relative stenosis, radicular symptoms usually predominate. CT-myelography and MRI are helpful. Evaluation may include somatosensory evoked potentials, which help identify cord compromise in absolute stenosis. Surgery may serve a prophylactic function but is usually reserved for patients who develop myelopathy or radiculopathy. Surgical approaches are similar to those previously described.

C. Rheumatoid Spondylitis—Cervical spine involvement is common in RA (up to 90%) and is more common with long-standing disease and multiple joint involvement. Neck pain, decreased range of motion, crepitation, and occipital headaches are the most common complaints. Neurologic impairment in patients with RA usually occurs gradually (weakness, decreased sensation, hyperreflexia) and is often overlooked or attributed to other joint disease. Surgery may not reverse significant neurologic deterioration, especially if a tight spinal canal is present, but it can stabilize it. Therefore it is essential to look for subtle signs of early neurologic involvement and to assess the space available for the cord (SAC). Indications for surgical stabilization include instability, pain, neurologic deficit due to neural compression, impending neurologic deficit (based on objective studies), or some combination. Patients with RA should have flexion/extension films before elective surgery.

1. Atlantoaxial Subluxation—Most common, 50–80% of cases. Usually a result of pannus formation at the synovial joints between the dens and the ring of C1, resulting in destruction of the transverse ligament, the dens, or both. Anterior subluxation of C1 on C2 is most common, but posterior and lateral subluxation can also occur. Findings on examination may include limitation of motion, upper motor neuron signs, and weakness. Plain radiographs that include patient-controlled flexion and extension views are evaluated to determine the anterior atlantodens interval (ADI) as well as the SAC, which is the posterior ADI. Instability is present with motion of >3.5 mm on flexion and extension views, although radiographic instability in RA is common and is not necessarily an indication for surgery. A 7-mm difference may imply disruption of the alar ligaments. A difference of >9–10 mm or **SAC of <14 mm** is associated with an increased risk of neurologic injury and usually requires surgical treatment. Myelopathy, progressive neurologic impairment and progressive instability are also indications for surgical stabilization, usually a posterior C1–C2 fusion. Transarticular screw fixation (Magerl's) across C1–C2 eliminates the need for halo immobilization associated with wiring, but preoperative CT must be assessed to evaluate the position of the vertebral aa. Atlantoaxial subluxation that is not reducible may require removal of the posterior arch of C1 for cord

decompression followed by occiput-C2 fusion. Anterior cord compression because of pannus often resolves following posterior fusion (PSF); odontoidectomy should be reserved as a secondary procedure and is only rarely necessary. Neurologic impairment with RA has been classified by Ranawat.

GRADE	CHARACTERISTICS
I	Subjective paresthesias, pain
II	Subjective weakness; upper motor neuron findings
III	Objective weakness; upper motor neuron findings (A = ambulatory; B = nonambulatory)

Surgery is less successful in Ranawat IIIB patients, but should still be considered. Complications include pseudarthrosis (10–20%) and adjacent segment involvement on long-term follow-up. Extension of the fusion to the occiput lessens the nonunion rate. An SAC of <14 mm is a relative indication for prophylactic fusion, even in the absence of myelopathy.

2. Cranial Settling (Basilar Invagination)—Second most common (40%). Cranial migration of the dens from erosion and bone loss between the occiput and C1–C2. Often seen in combination with fixed atlantoaxial subluxation. Measurement techniques are shown in Figure 7-2. Landmarks may be difficult to identify, with Ranawat's line probably the most easily reproducible. Progressive cranial migration (>5 mm) or neurologic compromise may require operative intervention (occiput-C2 fusion). Somatosensory evoked potentials may be helpful in evaluation. When brain stem compromise is significant with functional impairment, transoral or anterior retropharyngeal odontoid resection may be required.

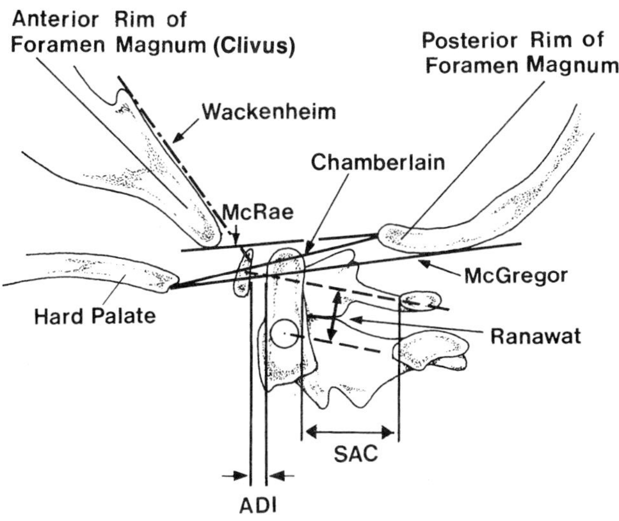

FIGURE 7-2 ■ Common measurements in C1–C2 disorders.

If there is any suggestion of cranial settling in cases of atlanto-axial interval (AAI), occipitocervical fusion is the conservative approach.

3. Subaxial subluxation—Occurs in 20% of cases. Commonly seen in combination with upper C-spine instability. Because the joints of Luschka and facet joints are affected by RA, subluxation may occur at multiple levels. Lower cervical spine involvement is more common in males, with steroid use, with seropositive RA, in patients with rheumatoid nodules, and in those with severe RA. Subaxial subluxation of >4 mm or >20% of the body is indicative of cord compression. A cervical height index (cervical body height/width) of <2.00 approaches 100% sensitivity and specificity in predicting neurologic compromise. Posterior fusion and wiring is sometimes required for subluxation >4 mm with intractable pain and neurologic compromise.

D. Cervical Spine and Cord Injuries

1. Introduction—Spinal cord injuries occur most commonly in young males involved in motor vehicle accidents, falls, and diving accidents. Gunshot wounds are an increasing cause. Findings may be subtle; the significant morbidity and mortality rates associated with missed injuries have led to current emphasis on cervical spine protection after polytrauma. Missed cervical spine injuries are most common in the presence of decreased level of consciousness, alcohol/drug intoxication, head injury, and in patients with multiple injuries. Facial injuries, hypotension, and localized tenderness or spasm should be investigated. Careful neurologic examination to document the lowest remaining functional level and to assess for the possibility of sacral sparing, or sparing of posterior column function indicating an incomplete spinal cord injury, is essential. Neurologic level by American Spine Association standards is defined as the most caudal level with normal motor and sensory function bilaterally. Spinal cord injury presenting within 8 hours without contraindications should be given a bolus dose of methylprednisolone (30 mg/kg) initially and then a drip (5.4 mg/kg) each hour for 23 hours, if started within 3 hours, or for 47 hours otherwise. Relative contraindications include pregnancy, age younger than 13 years, concomitant infection, penetrating spinal wounds, and uncontrolled diabetes. GI prophylaxis should be given. Spinal shock usually involves a 24- to 72-hour period of paralysis, hypotonia, and areflexia. At its conclusion, the progressive onset of spasticity, hyperreflexia, and clonus develops over days to weeks. The return of the bulbocavernosus reflex (anal sphincter contraction in response to squeezing the glans

penis or tugging on the Foley catheter) signifies the end of spinal shock, and for **complete** injuries further neurologic improvement is minimal. Injuries below the thoracolumbar level (conus or cauda equina) may permanently interrupt the bulbocavernosus reflex. Neurogenic shock (secondary to loss of sympathetic tone) can be differentiated from hypovolemic shock based on the presence of relative bradycardia in neurogenic shock, in contrast to the presence of tachycardia and hypotension with hypovolemic shock. Swan-Ganz monitoring is helpful in this setting because neurogenic and hypovolemic shock often occur concurrently. Hypovolemic shock is treated with fluid resuscitation, whereas selective vasopressors are effective in neurogenic shock.

2. Prognosis—The Frankel classification is useful when considering functional recovery from spinal cord injury.

FRANKEL GRADE	FUNCTION
A	Complete paralysis
B	Sensory function only below injury level
C	Incomplete motor function (grade 1–2/5) below injury level
D	Fair to good (useful) motor function (grade 3–4/5) below injury level
E	Normal function (grade 5/5)

3. Radiographic Evaluation—Includes complete cervical spine series (C1–T1; multiple-level injuries are common [10–20%]), oblique views (facet subluxation, dislocations, fractures); tomograms (dens fractures and facet joint injuries) may be helpful. On the lateral, 85% of C-spine fractures are detected. CT scanning is useful for evaluating C1 fractures and assessing bone in the canal but may miss an axial plane fracture (type II odontoid). Fine-cut CT scanning is employed to assess poorly visualized (on plain film) areas of the C-spine in the initial trauma work-up. Myelography may be used in patients with an otherwise unexplained neurologic deficit. MRI has advantages for demonstrating posterior ligamentous disruption, disc herniation, canal compromise, and the status of the spinal cord.
4. Cord Injuries—May be complete (no function below a given level) or incomplete (with some sparing of distal function). Most cord injury is due to contusion or compression, not transection. With complete injuries, an improvement of one nerve root level can be expected in 80% of the patients, and approximately 20% recover two functioning root levels. Several categories of incomplete lesions exist. These syndromes are classified based on the area of the spinal cord that has been the most severely damaged. Central cord syndrome is the most common and is often seen in patients with pre-existing cervical spondylosis who sustain a hyperextension injury. The cord is anteriorly compressed by osteophytes and posteriorly by the infolded ligamentum flavum. The cord is injured in the central gray matter, which results in proportionately greater loss of motor function to the upper extremities than to the lower extremities, with variable sensory sparing. The second most common cord injury is anterior cord syndrome, in which the damage is primarily in the anterior two-thirds of the cord, sparing the posterior columns (proprioception and vibratory sensation). These patients demonstrate greater motor loss in the legs than in the arms. CT scan may demonstrate bony fragments compressing the anterior cord. The anterior cord syndrome has the worst prognosis. The Brown-Séquard syndrome damages half of the cord, causing ipsilateral motor loss, position/proprioception loss, and contralateral pain, and temperature loss (usually two levels below the insult). This injury, usually the result of penetrating trauma, carries the best prognosis. Single-root lesions can occur at the level of the fracture, most commonly C5 or C6, leading to deltoid or biceps weakness; they are usually unilateral. A summary of the syndromes is presented in Table 7-3.
5. Specific Cervical Spine Injuries—See Chapter 10, Adult Trauma, for classification and treatment of cervical spine injuries.

Table 7-3. SPINAL CORD INJURY SYNDROMES

SYNDROME	PATHOLOGY	CHARACTERISTICS	PROGNOSIS
Central	Age >50, extension injuries	Affects upper > lower extremities, motor and sensory loss	Fair
Anterior	Flexion-compression (vertebral A)	Incomplete motor and some sensory loss	Poor
Brown-Séquard	Penetrating trauma	Loss of ipsilateral motor function, contralateral pain and temperature sensation	Best
Root	Foramina compression/herniated nucleus pulposus	Based on level—weakness	Good
Complete	Burst/canal compression	No function below injury level	Poor

6. Treatment—Discussed in Chapter 10, Adult Trauma. It basically includes immobilization (collar for undisplaced, stable fractures; skeletal traction, halo vest, or surgery for unstable fractures) and immediate application of skeletal traction to realign the spine in the presence of a displaced fracture with or without neurologic injury. Skeletal traction requires the placement of Gardner-Wells tongs (pins parallel to the external auditory meatus) and the addition of 5–10 pounds initially, with 5–7 pounds per cervical level with sequential radiographs between the additions of weight. If necessary, anterior decompression for incomplete injuries with persistent cord compression (can lead to improvement of one to three levels, even with complete injuries) and stabilization may be indicated. Late decompression for up to 1 year may be effective in improving root return. Laminectomies are contraindicated except in the rare case of posterior compression from a fractured lamina. Gunshot wounds are treated nonoperatively except with esophageal or colonic perforation.
7. Complications—Numerous; include neurologic injury, nonunion, and malunion. Autonomic dysreflexia can follow cervical and upper thoracic spinal cord injuries. It is commonly related to bladder overdistention or fecal impaction and manifests with pounding headache (from severe hypertension), anxiety, profuse head and neck sweating, nasal obstruction, and blurred vision. Urinary catheterization or rectal disimpaction and supportive treatment usually relieve symptoms. Instability in the cervical spine can occur late and is associated with >3.5 mm of subluxation and >11 degrees of difference in angulation between adjacent motion segments.

E. Sports-Related Cervical Spine Injuries
1. Burner (Stinger) Syndrome—Common injury associated with stretching the upper brachial plexus by bending the neck away from the depressed shoulder or neck extension toward the painful shoulder in the setting of foraminal stenosis (root irritation). Athlete will complain of burning dysesthesia with weakness in the involved extremity. Fracture or acute HNP should be ruled out. The athlete with a neck injury should be further evaluated for cervical pain, tenderness, or persisting neurologic symptoms.
2. Transient Quadriplegia—Most commonly seen after axial load injury (spearing), but may also be seen after forced hyperextension or hyperflexion. Presents with bilateral burning paresthesia and weakness or paralysis. High association with cervical stenosis (Torg's ratio <0.8) as well as instability, HNP, and congenital fusions. No definitive association with future permanent neurologic injury. Patients with concurrent pathologic conditions, including instability, HNP, degenerative changes, or symptoms that lasted more than 36 hours, should be prohibited from contact sports.

F. Other Cervical Spine Problems—Ankylosing spondylitis and neuromyopathic conditions can cause severe flexion deformities of the cervical spine. Patients with ankylosing spondylitis must be carefully evaluated for occult fracture because of the problem of pseudarthrosis and progressive kyphotic deformity. Severe chin-on-chest deformity in ankylosing spondylitis, with the inability to look straight ahead, occasionally represents a major functional limitation and is often associated with severe hip flexion contractures as well as a flexion deformity of the lumbar spine. Treatment usually begins by addressing the hip and lumbar disorder but may ultimately require cervicothoracic laminectomy, osteotomy, and fusion for correction of the neck deformity. This procedure is performed under local anesthesia with brief general anesthesia, and immobilization postoperatively is carried out in a halo cast. Traction, surgical release of contracted sternocleidomastoid muscles, and posterior fusion are sometimes required for severe neuromyopathic conditions.

III. Thoracic/Lumbar Spine

A. HNP
1. Introduction—Disc degeneration with aging includes loss of water content, annular tears, and myxomatous changes, resulting in herniation of nuclear material. Changes in proteoglycan metabolism, secondary immunologic factors, and structural factors also play a role. Discs can protrude (bulging nucleus, intact annulus), extrude (through the annulus but confined by the posterior longitudinal ligament), or be sequestrated (disc material free in canal). HNP is usually a disease of young and middle-age adults; the disc nucleus desiccates and is less likely to herniate in older patients.
2. Thoracic Disc Disease—Relatively uncommon (1% of all HNPs), it usually involves the middle to lower thoracic levels, with T11–T12 being the most common and 75% occurring between T8–T12. Thoracic HNP can be divided into central, posterolateral, and lateral herniations. It usually presents with the onset of back or chest pain that may progress to radicular symptoms (band-like chest or abdominal discomfort, numbness, paresthesias, leg pain) and/or myelopathy (sensory changes, paraparesis, bowel/bladder/sexual dysfunction). Physical findings may be difficult to elicit but may include localized tenderness, sensory pinprick level, upper motor neuron signs with leg hyperreflexia, weakness, and abnormal rectal examination (with normal UE findings). Radiographs may show

disc narrowing and calcification or osteophytic lipping. Underlying Scheuermann's disease may predispose patients to develop HNP. Myelo-CT or MRI should demonstrate thoracic HNP. MRI is useful for ruling out cord disorder, but there is a high false-positive rate, requiring close clinical correlation. Immobilization, analgesics, and nerve blocks are sometimes helpful for radiculopathy. Surgery, usually through an anterior transthoracic approach or costotransversectomy (including anterior discectomy and hemicorpectomy as needed), is recommended in the presence of myelopathy or persistent unremitting pain with documented pathologic conditions. Thoracoscopic discectomy can also be employed. Posterior approach to a thoracic HNP is contraindicated because of the high rate of neurologic injury.

3. Lumbar Disc Disease—Major cause of increased morbidity and causes major financial impact in the United States. Most often involves the L4–L5 disc (the "backache disc"), followed closely by L5–S1. Most herniations are posterolateral (where the posterior longitudinal ligament is the weakest) and may present with back pain and nerve root pain/sciatica involving the lower nerve root at that level. Central prolapse is often associated with back pain only; however, acute insults may precipitate a cauda equina compression syndrome (Fig. 7-3). This syndrome is a surgical emergency that most commonly presents with bilateral buttock and lower-extremity pain, as well as bowel or bladder dysfunction (usually urinary retention), saddle anesthesia, and varying degrees of loss of lower-extremity motor or sensory function. Digital rectal examination and evaluation of perianal sensation are important for the immediate diagnosis. Immediate myelography (or MRI) and surgery (if the test results are positive) are indicated to arrest progression of neurologic loss although the prognosis is guarded for recovery in most cases.

   a. History and Physical Examination—An acute injury or precipitating event should be sought, and the location of symptoms (especially pain radiating to the extremity), character of pain, postural changes (neurogenic claudication), effect of increased intrathecal pressure, and a complete review of symptoms (including psychiatric history) should be elicited.

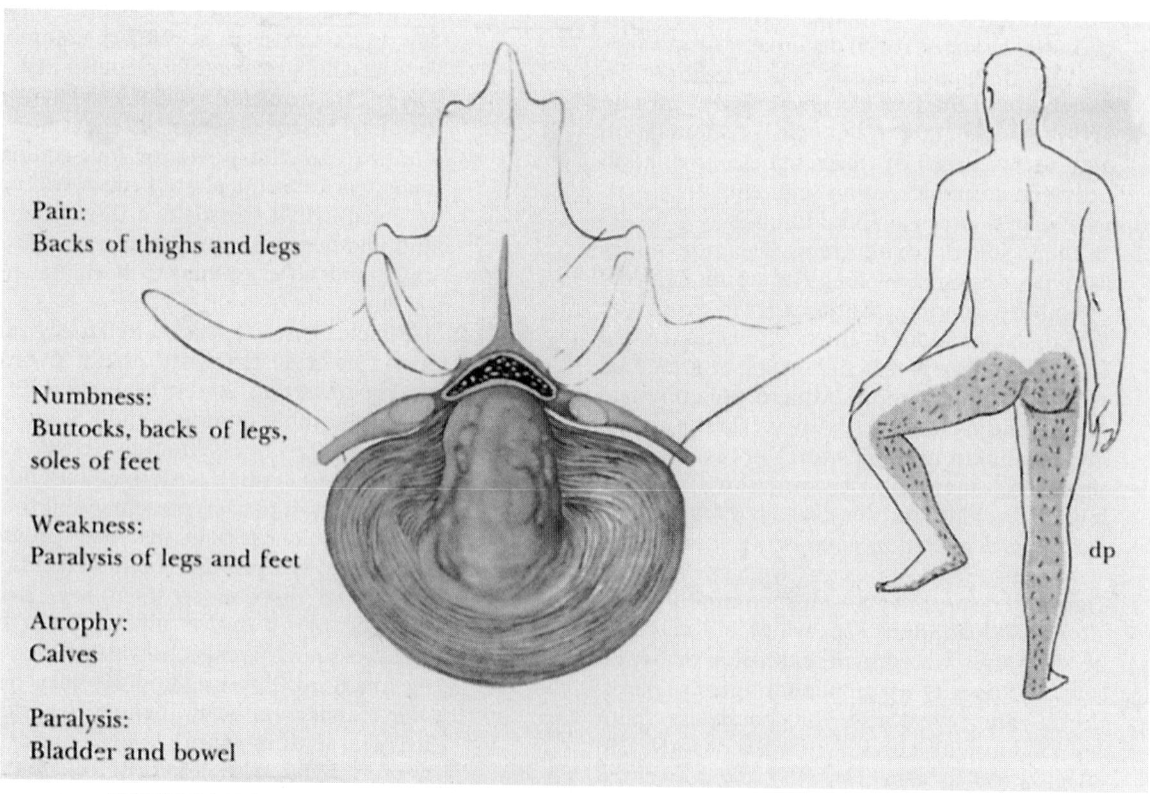

FIGURE 7-3 ■ Cauda equina syndrome. (From DePalma, A.F., and Rothman, R.H.: The Intervertebral Disc. Philadelphia, WB Saunders, 1970, p. 194.)

Occupational risks, such as jobs requiring prolonged sitting and repetitive lifting, are also important factors. Intradiscal pressure is lowest when lying supine and highest when sitting and flexed forward with weights in hands. Referred pain in mesodermal tissues of the same embryologic origin, often to the buttocks or posterior thighs, must be differentiated from true radicular pain due to nerve root impingement, with symptoms that typically reach distal to the knee. Psychosocial evaluation, pain drawings, and psychologic testing are helpful in some cases. The finding of an "inverted V" triad of hysteria, hypochondriasis, and depression on the Minnesota Multiphasic Personality Inventory has been identified as a significant adverse risk factor in lumbar disc surgery. Physical examination should include observation (change in posture, gait), palpation of the posterior spine (spasm, localized tenderness), measurement of range of motion (ROM) (decreased flexion), hip examination, vascular evaluation (distal pulses), abdominal and rectal examination, and neurologic evaluation. Tension signs such as straight-leg raising or the bowstring sign (L4–L5 or L5–S1) and the femoral nerve stretch test (L2–L3 or L3–L4) are important findings that suggest HNP and are essential when considering a patient for discectomy. A positive contralateral straight-leg raising test (pain in the affected buttock/leg when raising the opposite leg) is most specific for HNP. Specific findings by level are presented in Table 7-4. A large central disc herniation at one level may impinge on more than one nerve root. Inappropriate signs and symptoms (Waddell's) are also important to note. Inappropriate symptoms include pain at the tip of the "tailbone," pain plus numbness, or giving way of the whole leg. Nonorganic physical signs include tenderness with light touch in nonanatomic areas, simulation (light axial loading), distraction testing, pain with pelvic rotation, negative sitting (and positive supine) straight-leg raising test, regional nonanatomic disturbances (such as a stocking-glove distribution), and overreaction.

b. Diagnostic Tests—Plain radiographs are indicated before proceeding with special tests to rule out other disorders, such as isthmic defects. However, most plain radiographic findings are nonspecific, and plain radiography can usually be deferred for 6 weeks. Myelography, CT, or MRI is effective **when used as a confirmatory study**. CT is noninvasive and helpful for demonstrating bony stenosis and identifying lateral pathologic conditions. Combined with myelography (invasive), imaging of neural compression may be improved. MRI is superior for identifying cord disorders, neural tumors, and disc disorders. It is noninvasive, involves no ionizing radiation, and gives a "myelogram" effect on the T2 images. Multiplanar views allow imaging of central, foraminal, and extraforaminal stenosis. In addition, MRI demonstrates the state of hydration of the discs and visualizes the marrow of the vertebral bodies, thus representing an excellent modality to screen for tumor or infection. False-positive MRI is common (35% of those <40 years old; 93% of those >60 years old) and therefore require correlation with the history and physical examination. MRI is the imaging modality of choice for most back disorders. Electromyography (EMG) and nerve conduction velocity (NCV) testing (which demonstrate fibrillations 3 weeks after nerve root pressure) are not usually helpful and rarely provide more information than a good physical examination. Thermography does not have proven efficacy in the evaluation of disc disease or any other disorder of the spine.

c. Treatment—Activity modification, NSAIDs, moist heat, and progressive ambulation are successful in returning most patients to

Table 7-4. FINDINGS IN LUMBAR DISC DISEASE

LEVEL	NERVE ROOT	SENSORY LOSS	MOTOR LOSS	REFLEX LOSS
L1–L3	L2, L3	Anterior thigh	Hip flexors	None
L3–L4	L4	Medial calf	Quadriceps, tibialis anterior	Knee jerk
L4–L5	L5	Lateral calf, dorsal foot	EDL, EHL	None
L5–S1	S1	Posterior calf, plantar foot	Gastrocnemius/soleus	Ankle jerk
S2–S4	S2, S3, S4	Perianal	Bowel/bladder	Cremasteric

EDL, extensor digitorum longus; EHL, extensor hallicus longus.

their normal function. More than half of patients who seek treatment for low back pain recover in 1 week, and 90% recover within 1–3 months. Half of patients with sciatica recover in 1 month. This treatment is followed by back rehabilitation and fitness programs. Aerobic conditioning and education are the most important factors in avoiding missed work days due to disc disease and in returning patients to work. Instruction should include avoiding rotation and flexion due to increased disc pressure associated with these activities. If patients fail to improve within 6 weeks of conservative care, further evaluation is indicated. Those patients with predominantly low back pain may require bone scan, MRI, and medical work-up to rule out spinal tumors or infection. If these study results are normal, back rehabilitation is continued. In patients who have predominantly leg pain (sciatica) who fail conservative therapy, a trial of lumbar epidural steroids may be helpful, although it has not been proved effective in controlled studies. Additional studies (CT [± myelogram] or MRI) are undertaken in patients who after 6–12 weeks continue to be symptomatic with pain, neurologic deficit, and positive nerve tension signs. These studies are, as a rule, preoperative tests and should be done to confirm clinical suspicions. Patients with positive study results, neurologic findings, tension signs, and predominantly sciatic symptoms without mitigating psychosocial factors are the best candidates for surgical discectomy. Standard partial laminotomy and discectomy are most commonly performed. Operative positioning requires the abdomen to be free to decrease pressure on the inferior vena cava, and consequently, on the epidural veins. With proper indications, 95% of patients have initially good or excellent results, although as many as 15–20% of patients have significant backache on long-term follow-up.

Percutaneous discectomy currently has limited indications in the treatment of lumbar disc disease, with no long-term follow-up studies proving its efficacy. It is contraindicated in the presence of a sequestered fragment or spinal stenosis. Endoscopic discectomy does allow direct visualization and can address sequestered fragments and lateral recess stenosis. Intradiscal enzyme therapy has fallen out of favor because of its questionable efficacy and serious complications (anaphylaxis and transverse myelitis). Indications for all these minimally invasive treatments for disc herniations are similar to those for open surgery (leg pain, tension signs, neurologic deficits, positive study results).

d. Complications—Fortunately rare but can be devastating.

4. Vascular Injury—May occur during attempts at disc removal if curettes are allowed to penetrate the anterior longitudinal ligament. Intraoperative pulsatile bleeding due to deep penetration is treated with rapid wound closure, intravenous (IV) fluids and blood, repositioning the patient, and a transabdominal approach to find and stop the source of bleeding. Mortality may exceed 50%. Late sequelae of vascular injuries may include delayed hemorrhage, pseudoaneurysm, or arteriovenous fistula formation.
5. Nerve Root Injury—More common with anomalous nerve roots. Dural tears (1% incidence) should be repaired primarily when they occur to avoid the development of a pseudomeningocele or spinal fluid fistula. Adequate exposure, as well as hemostasis, lighting, magnification, and careful surgical technique, is important for diminishing the incidence of the "battered root syndrome."
6. Failed Back Syndrome—Often the result of poor patient selection, but other causes include recurrent herniation (usually acute recurrence of signs/symptoms following a 6- to 12-month pain-free interval), herniation at another level, discitis (3–6 weeks postoperatively, with rapid onset of severe back pain), unrecognized lateral stenosis (may be most common), and vertebral instability. Epidural fibrosis occurs at about 3 months postoperatively, and may be associated with back or leg pain; responds poorly to re-exploration. Scar can best be differentiated from recurrent HNP with a gadolinium-enhanced MRI.
7. Dural Tear—More common during revision surgery and should be repaired immediately if it is recognized. Fibrin adhesive sealant may be a useful adjunct for effecting dural closure. Bed rest and subarachnoid drain placement is advocated if cerebrospinal fluid leak is suspected postoperatively.
8. Wound Infection—(Approximately 1% in open discectomy.) Similar to infection elsewhere. Increased risk in diabetics. Incision and drainage and removal of loose graft may be required.
9. Cauda Equina Syndrome—Secondary to extruded disc, surgical trauma, hematoma. Suspect with postoperative urinary retention. Digital rectal examination is used to diagnose initially. Further imaging may be necessary.

B. Discogenic Back Pain—Patients complain of back pain greater than leg pain and may have a paucity of physical findings, no radiculopathy, and negative tension signs. X-ray may show disc-space narrowing, but this is nondiagnostic. MRI reveals decreased signal intensity in the disc space on T2 (dark disc). Discography is a useful preoperative study to correlate MRI findings with a clinically significant pain generator. The study should be performed at multiple levels to include all abnormal levels on MRI and one or more normal levels. The procedure should elicit pain similar, after injection, to that usually described by the patient (concordant pain) and should involve at least 1 minimally painful, nonconcordant level to be considered positive. Treatment consists of conservative therapy with NSAIDs, therapy, and conditioning. If extended nonoperative treatment has failed, and if the patient has a positive MRI and discogram, interbody fusion can be performed either from an anterior or retroperitoneal approach or through a posterior midline (posterior lumbar interbody fusion) or posterior transforaminal approach. Fusion is performed with structural constructs (femoral ring allografts or interbody fusion cages) in the disc space. Intradiscal electrothermy (IDET) involves percutaneously heating the fibers of the annulus fibrosus to reconfigure the collagen fibers, restoring the mechanical integrity of the disc. This may be effective in early conditions (<50% loss of disc height), but not in more advanced disease; long-term follow-up suggests that symptomatic improvement often lasts less than 1 year.

C. Lumbar Segmental Instability—Present when normal loads produce abnormal spinal motion. The most common symptom is mechanical back pain, although "dynamic" stenosis can occur, leading to radicular symptoms. The most consistent clinical sign is the "instability catch" (sudden, painful catch with extension from a flexed position). Degenerative lumbar disc disease is indicated by disc space narrowing. A combination of annulus damage and disc space narrowing may cause reduction in the disc's ability to resist rotatory forces. Continuing degeneration or facet subluxation may then lead to instability. Radiographically, traction spurs (horizontal and below disc margin), angular changes >10 degrees (20 degrees at L5–S1) on flexion films, and translatory motion >3–4 mm (6 mm at L5–S1) with flexion-extension views are all characteristic of lumbar instability but are difficult to quantify and may not correlate with clinical symptoms. Iatrogenic instability can occur after removal of a total of one or more facet joints during surgery. Surgical treatment options do not have clearly defined indications but posterolateral fusion is the standard treatment. The use of pedicle screw instrumentation is well established, with fusion rates approaching 90% in nonsmokers for one or two level fusions. Anatomic landmark for pedicle screw insertion in the lumbar spine is the intersection of the transverse process, pars intraarticularis, and lateral aspect of the superior articular facet.

D. Spinal Stenosis
   1. Introduction—Spinal stenosis is narrowing of the spinal canal or neural foramina, producing nerve root compression, root ischemia, and a variable syndrome of back and leg pain. Central stenosis produces compression of the thecal sac, whereas lateral stenosis involves compression of individual nerve roots either in the subarticular (lateral) recess (by the medial overgrowth of the superior articular facet at a given facet joint) or in the intervertebral foramen. Stenosis usually does not become symptomatic until patients reach late middle age; it affects men somewhat more often than women.
   2. Central Stenosis
      a. Introduction—Can be congenital (idiopathic or developmental in achondroplastic dwarfs) or acquired. Acquired stenosis, the most common type, is usually degenerative owing to enlargement of osteoarthritic facets with medial encroachment, but it can be secondary to degenerative spondylolisthesis, post-traumatic, postsurgical, or due to various disease processes (e.g., Paget's, fluorosis). Pre-existing "trefoil" canal shapes, a congenitally narrow canal, or medially placed facets may limit the ability to tolerate minor acquired encroachment. Central stenosis represents compression of the thecal sac, with absolute stenosis defined as a cross-sectional area of <100 mm^2 or <10 mm of anteroposterior diameter as seen on CT cross-section. Soft-tissue structures, including hypertrophied ligamentum flavum, facet capsule, and bulging disc may contribute as much as 40% to thecal sac compression. Central stenosis is more common in men, because their spinal canal is smaller at the L3–L5 levels than that of women, and afflicts an older population than does lateral recess stenosis.
      b. Symptoms—Include insidious pain and paresthesias with ambulation or prolonged standing, relieved sitting, or with flexion of the spine. Patients commonly complain of lower-extremity pain, most commonly in the buttock and thigh, numbness, or "giving way." A history of radiating leg pain in a true dermatomal distribution, although typical in patients with HNP, is relatively uncommon in those with spinal stenosis. Neurogenic claudication, which occurs in about 50% of patients with stenosis, usually can be differentiated from vascular claudication by history. Physical examination is also important. Stenosis patients will typically have pain

with extension, have normal extremity perfusion and pulses, and have few neurologic findings. Abnormal neurological examinations are found in fewer than 50%. Standing treadmill tests can be a sensitive provocative evaluation of neurogenic claudication.

ACTIVITY	VASCULAR CLAUDICATION	NEUROGENIC CLAUDICATION
Walking	Distal-proximal pain, calf pain	Proximal-distal thigh pain
Uphill walking	Symptoms develop sooner	Symptoms develop later
Rest	Relief with sitting or bending	
Bicycling	Symptoms develop	Symptoms do not develop
Lying flat	Relief	May exacerbate symptoms

c. Imaging—Further work-up may include plain radiographs on which disc degeneration, interspace narrowing, medially placed facets, and flattening of the lordotic curve are commonly seen; subluxation and degenerative changes of the facet joints may be seen. Plain CT, postmyelo-CT, and MRI are standard imaging modalities. Careful inspection of these studies is necessary to assess lateral nerve root entrapment by medial hypertrophy of the superior facet, the tip of the superior facet, soft-tissue thickening, osteophyte formation off the posterior vertebral body (uncinate spur), or a combination of these problems. Central stenosis is a diminution in the area of the thecal sac and is produced by thickening of the ligamentum flavum and/or posterior protrusion of the disc, in combination with enlarged facet joints. Simply looking for the "bony" measurements results in underestimating the degree of stenosis; soft-tissue contribution to thecal sac narrowing must be considered. Bone scan or MRI may help to rule out malignancy. EMG/NCV testing may be used, but sensitivity is variable and depends on the examiner. NCV testing is sometimes helpful in differentiating radiculopathy from peripheral neuropathy.

d. Treatment—Rest, Williams' flexion exercises, NSAIDs, and weight reduction are important in management of patients with stenosis. Lumbar epidural steroids may be helpful for short-term relief but have shown variable results in controlled studies. Transforaminal nerve block can be quite effective when the involved roots can be identified, and should be considered in most cases before moving to surgery. Surgery is indicated in patients with positive study results and persistent, unacceptably impaired quality of life. Adequate decompression of the identified disorder typically includes laminectomy and partial medial facetectomy, which can usually be done without destabilizing the spine, thus avoiding fusion. Fusion is indicated in patients with surgical instability (removal of one facet or more), pars defects (including postsurgical) with disc disease, symptomatic radiographic instability, degenerative or isthmic spondylolisthesis, and degenerative scoliosis.

3. Lateral Stenosis—Impingement of nerve roots lateral to the thecal sac as they pass through the lateral recess and into the neural foramen. Often associated with facet joint arthropathy (superior articular process enlargement) and disc disease (Fig. 7-4). The three-joint complex (disc and both facets) must be considered when evaluating lateral stenosis. Nerve root compression can occur at more than one level and must be completely decompressed to relieve symptoms. Compression can be subarticular (lateral recess stenosis), which consists of compression between the medial aspect of a hypertrophic superior articular facet and the posterior aspect of the vertebral body and disc. Hypertrophy of the ligamentum flavum and/or ventral facet joint capsule and vertebral body osteophyte/disc exacerbates the stenosis. Foraminal stenosis can be produced by intraforaminal disc protrusion, impingement of the tip of the superior facet, uncinate spurring, or a combination. Subarticular stenosis, which is more common, affects the traversing (lower) nerve root (L5 root at L4-5), whereas foraminal stenosis affects the exiting (upper) root (L4) at a motion segment. Lateral stenosis is most frequently seen in combination with central

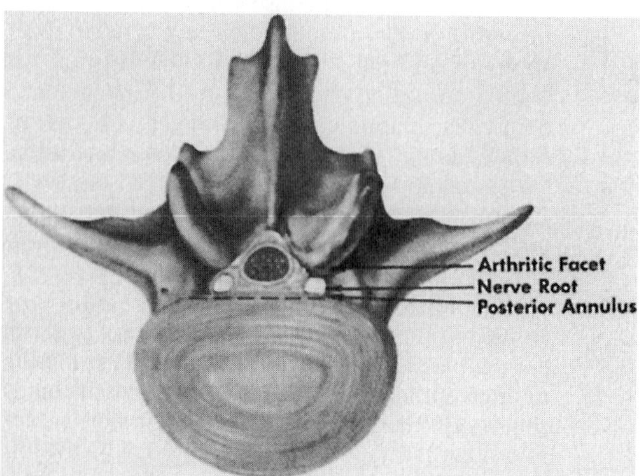

FIGURE 7-4 ■ Lateral stenosis. Note nerve root entrapment laterally on the right by arthritic facet and bulging posterior annulus. (From Rothman, R.H., and Simeon, F.A.: The Spine, 2nd ed. Philadelphia, WB Saunders, 1982, p. 194.)

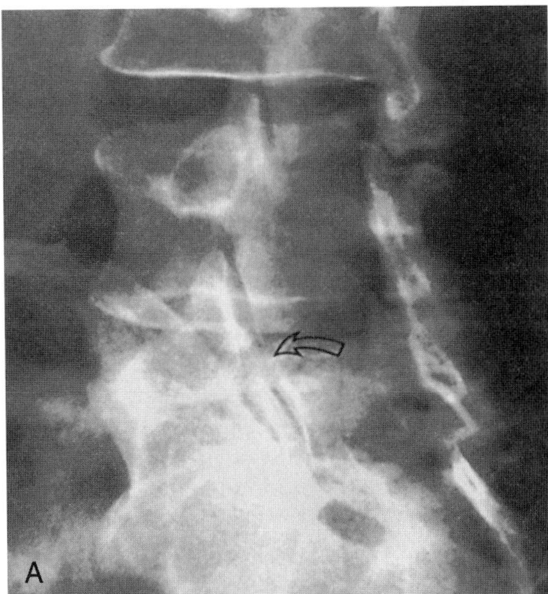

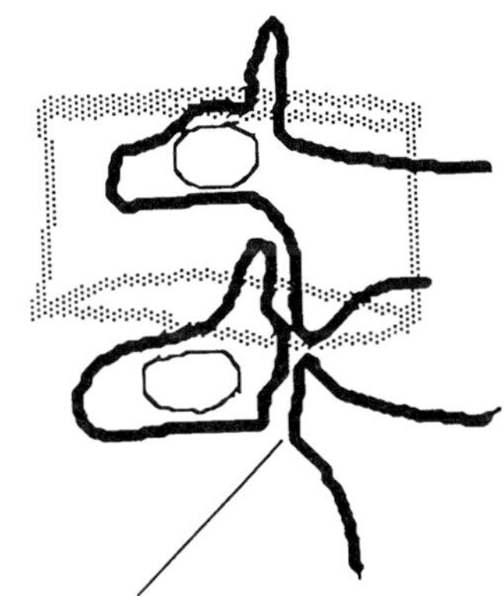

FIGURE 7-5 ■ Spondylolysis. Note disruption of "collar on Scottie dog." (From Helms, C.A.: Fundamentals of Skeletal Radiology. Philadelphia, WB Saunders, 1989, p. 101.)

stenosis but can appear as an isolated entity usually involving middle-age or even young adults with symptoms of radicular pain unrelieved by rest and without tension signs. Lower lumbar areas are most commonly involved because the foramina decrease in size as the nerve root size increases. Pain may be the result of intraneural edema and demyelination. Substance P may be released as a response to spinal nerve root irritation. After failure of nonoperative treatment, decompression of the hypertrophied lamina and ligamentum flavum and partial facetectomy are usually successful. Fusion may be necessary if instability is present or created.

4. Extraforaminal Lateral Root Compression ("Far Out Syndrome" [Wiltse's])—Involves L5 root impingement between the sacral ala and the L5 transverse process. It is usually seen in degenerative scoliosis, isthmic spondylolisthesis, or extraforaminal herniated discs. It must be specifically sought on special radiographs (25-degree caudocephalic [Ferguson's] view), CT, or MRI.

E. Spondylolysis and Spondylolisthesis

1. Spondylolysis—Defect in the pars interarticularis. It is one of the most common causes of low back pain in children and adolescents. The defect in the pars is thought to be a fatigue fracture from repetitive hyperextension stresses (most common in gymnasts, football linemen), to which there may be a hereditary predisposition. Plain lateral radiographs demonstrate 80% of lesions, with another 15% visible on oblique radiographs, which show a defect in the "neck of the Scottie dog" as described by Lachapelle (Fig. 7-5). CT, bone scan, and more recently, single-photon emission computed tomography (SPECT) scanning may be helpful in identifying subtle defects; increased uptake is more compatible with acute lesions that have the potential to heal. Bracing or casting (a single-thigh pantaloon spica) has been advocated for acute lesions, but treatment is usually aimed at symptomatic relief rather than fracture healing and includes activity restriction, flexion exercises, and bracing. Nonunion is common and may have normal scans.
2. Spondylolisthesis—Forward slippage of one vertebra on another. Can be classified into six types (Newman, Wiltse, McNab) (Table 7-5; Figs. 7-6, 7-7). Severity of slip in spondylolisthesis

Table 7-5. TYPES OF SPONDYLOLISTHESIS

CLASS	TYPE	AGE	PATHOLOGY/OTHER
I	Dysplastic	Child	Congenital dysplasia of S1 superior facet
II	Isthmic[a]	5–50	Predisposition leading to elongation/fracture of pars (L5–S1)
III	Degenerative	Older	Facet arthrosis leading to subluxation (L4–L5)
IV	Traumatic	Young	Acute fracture/other than pars
V	Pathologic	Any	Incompetence of bony elements
VI	Postsurgical	Adult	Excessive resection of neural arches/facets

[a]Most common.

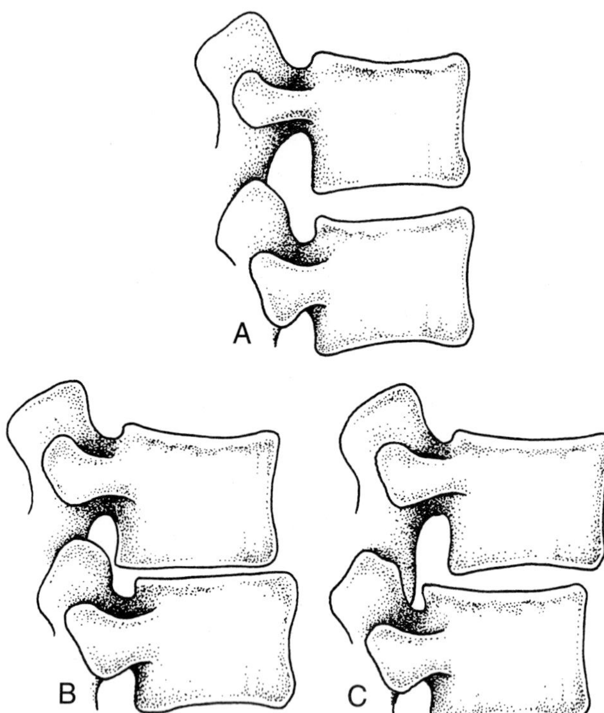

FIGURE 7-6 ■ Degenerative spondylolisthesis. *A,* Normal. *B,* Retrolisthesis—disc narrowing is greater than posterior joint degeneration. *C,* Anterolisthesis—posterior joints are more degenerated than the disc. (From Weinstein, J.N., and Wiesel, S.W.: The Lumbar Spine. Philadelphia, WB Saunders, 1990, p. 84.)

is based on the amount or degree (as compared with S1 width): I, 0–25%; II, 25–50%; III, 50–75%; IV, >75%; V, >100% (spondyloptosis). Other measurements, including the sacral inclination (normally >30 degrees) and the slip angle (normally <0 degrees, signifying lordosis at the L5–S1 disc), are also useful for quantifying lumbopelvic deformity, which affects cosmesis as well as prognosis (Fig. 7-8).

3. Childhood Spondylolisthesis—Usually at L5–S1, is typically type II, and usually presents with back pain (instability), hamstring tightness, deformity, or alteration in gait ("pelvic waddle"). Although the onset of symptoms may occur at any time in life, screening studies identify the occurrence of the slippage as being most common at 4–6 years. Spondylolisthesis is most common in whites, boys, and youngsters involved in hyperextension activities, and it is remarkably common in Eskimos (>50%). It is thought to result from shear stress at the pars interarticularis associated with repetitive hyperextension. Severe slips are rare and are often associated with radicular findings (L5), cauda equina dysfunction, kyphosis of the lumbosacral junction, and "heart-shaped" buttocks. Spina bifida occulta, thoracic hyperkyphosis, and Scheuermann's disease are associated with spondylolisthesis.

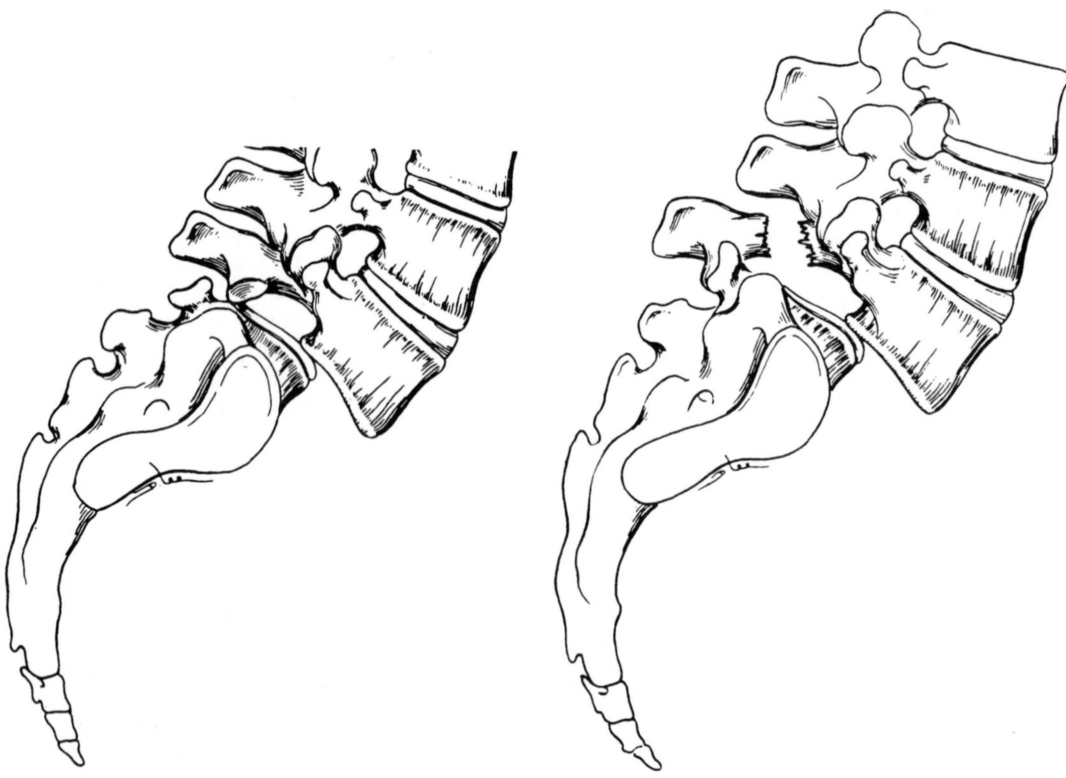

FIGURE 7-7 ■ Spondylolisthesis. (From Rothman, R.H., and Simeon, F.A.: The Spine, 2nd ed. Philadelphia, WB Saunders, 1982, p. 264.)

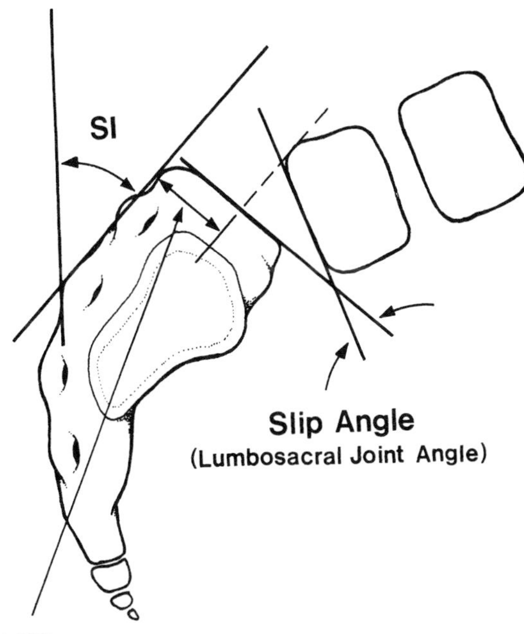

FIGURE 7-8 ■ Measurements used for evaluation of spondylolisthesis. (Modified from Wiltse, L.L., and Winter, R.B.: Terminology and measurement of spondylolisthesis. J. Bone Joint Surg. [Am.] 65:768–772, 1983.)

a. Low-Grade Disease (<50% Slip)—Spondylolysis or mild spondylolisthesis may require bone scan or CT for diagnosis and usually responds to nonoperative treatment consisting of activity modification and exercise. Adolescents with a grade I slip may return to normal activities, including contact sports, once they are asymptomatic. Those with asymptomatic grade II spondylolisthesis are restricted from activities such as gymnastics or football. Progression is uncommon, but risk factors include young age at presentation, female gender, a slip angle of >10 degrees (see Fig. 7-9), a high-grade slip, and a dome-shaped or significantly inclined sacrum (>30 degrees beyond vertical). Furthermore, patients with type I or dysplastic spondylolisthesis are at higher risk for slip progression and the development of cauda equina dysfunction because the neural arch is intact. Patients with a greater than 25% slip, or with L4–5 or L3–4 spondylolisthesis, have a higher risk of low back pain than the general population. Surgery for patients with a low-grade slip generally consists of L5–S1 posterolateral fusion in situ and is usually reserved for those with intractable pain who have failed nonoperative treatment or those demonstrating progressive slippage. Wiltse has popularized a paraspinal muscle-splitting approach to the lumbar transverse process and sacral alae that is frequently utilized in this setting. L5 radiculopathy is uncommon in children with low-grade slips and rarely if ever requires decompression. Repair of the pars defect using a lag screw (Buck's) or tension band wiring (Bradford's) with bone grafting has been reported. It may be indicated in young patients with slippage less than 25% and a pars defect at L4 or above.

b. Grades III and IV Spondylolisthesis and Spondyloptosis (Grade V)—Commonly cause neurologic abnormalities. L5–S1 isthmic spondylolisthesis causes an L5 radiculopathy (contrast with S1 radiculopathy in L5–S1 HNP). Prophylactic fusion is recommended in children with slippage of more than 50%. It often requires bilateral posterolateral fusion in situ, usually at L4–S1 (L5 is too far anterior to effect L5–S1 fusion) with or without instrumentation. Nerve root exploration is controversial but is usually limited to children with clear-cut radicular pain or significant weakness. Reduction of spondylolisthesis has been associated with a 20–30% incidence of L5 root injuries (most transient) and should be utilized cautiously. A cosmetically unacceptable deformity and L5–S1 kyphosis so severe that the posterior fusion mass from L4 to the sacrum would be under tension without reversal of the kyphosis are the most commonly cited indications. In situ fusion leaves a patient with a high-grade slip and LS kyphosis with such severe compensatory hyperlordosis above the fusion that long-term problems frequently ensue. Reduction in this setting is gaining widespread acceptance. Close neurologic monitoring should be done during the procedure and for several days afterward to identify postoperative neuropathy. Posterior decompression, fibular interbody fusion, and posterolateral fusion without reduction has been reported with excellent long-term results (Bohlman). The Gill procedure, consisting of removal of the loose elements without fusion, is contraindicated.

4. Degenerative Spondylolisthesis—More common in African Americans, diabetics, and women over age 40; it is most common at the L4–L5 level (see Fig. 7-8). It is reported to be more common in patients with transitional L5 vertebrae and with sagittally oriented facet joints. Degenerative spondylolisthesis frequently results in central and lateral recess stenosis with L5 radiculopathy owing to root compression in the lateral recess between the hypertrophic and subluxated inferior facet of

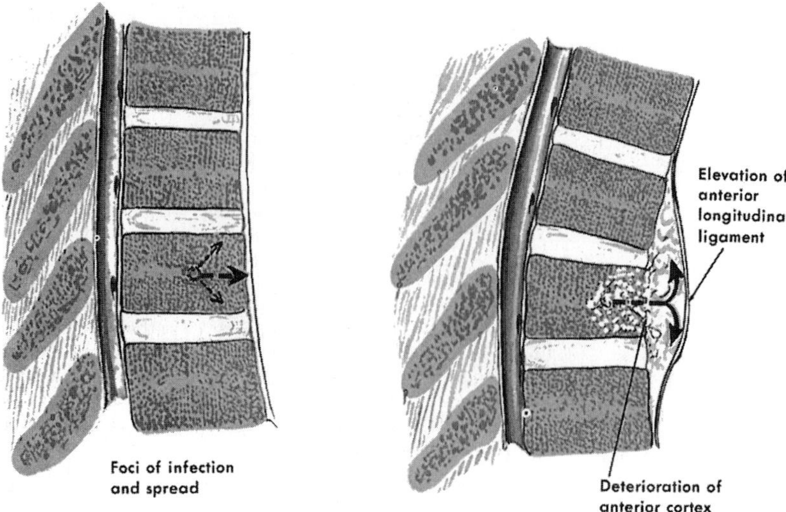

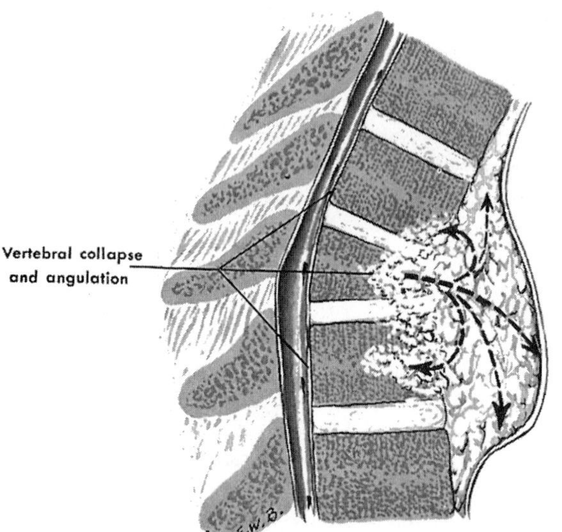

FIGURE 7-9 ■ Pathogenesis of spinal tuberculosis. (From Tachdjian, M.O.: Pediatric Orthopaedics, 2nd ed. Philadelphia, WB Saunders, 1990, p. 1450.)

L4 and the posterosuperior body of L5. The operative treatment of degenerative spondylolisthesis involves decompression of the nerve roots and stabilization by posterolateral fusion. The addition of hardware is controversial and may be indicated for concurrent scoliotic deformity, severe slips, and failed fusions.

5. Adult Isthmic Spondylolisthesis—While often asymptomatic, isthmic spondylolisthesis in an adult may cause back and radicular pain. Nonoperative treatment includes rest, corset, NSAIDs, and flexion exercises. It is essential to assess for other common sources of back pain before assuming that spondylolisthesis is the cause; MRI scanning is a useful tool in this setting. Isthmic L5-S1 spondylolisthesis frequently causes radicular symptoms in the adult, resulting from compression of the exiting L5 root in the L5-S1 foramen; compression may involve hypertrophic fibrous repair tissue at the pars defect, uncinate spur formation off the posterior L5 body, and bulging of the L5-S1 disc. Operative treatment is favored in the presence of radicular symptoms and usually involves thorough foraminal decompression and fusion, with or without pedicular screw fixation. Compromised results in workers' compensation patients have been reported.

F. Thoracolumbar Injuries

1. Introduction—The thoracolumbar spine is the most common site for vertebral column injuries. Although the classification and treatment of

these injuries is included in Chapter 10, Adult Trauma, some points need to be emphasized here. The upper thoracic spine (T1–T10) is stabilized by the ribs and the facet orientation, as well as the sternum, and is less susceptible to trauma. At the thoracolumbar junction, however, there is a fulcrum of increased motion, and this area is more commonly affected by spinal trauma. Two anatomic points also bear noting: (1) the middle T-spine is a vascular "watershed" area, and vascular insult can lead to cord ischemia; and (2) the spinal cord ends and the cauda equina begins at the level of L1–L2, so lesions below the L1 level carry a better prognosis because nerve roots, not cord, are affected.

2. Stable Versus Unstable Injuries—The three-column system (Denis) has been proposed for evaluating spinal injuries and determining which are stable or unstable. The anterior column is composed of the anterior longitudinal ligament and the anterior two-thirds of the annulus and vertebral body. The middle column consists of the posterior third of the body and annulus and the posterior longitudinal ligament. The posterior column comprises the pedicles, facets, spinous processes, and posterior ligaments, including the interspinous and supraspinous ligaments, ligamentum flavum, and facet capsules. Disruption of the middle column (seen as widening of the interpedicular distances on anteroposterior radiographs or a change in height of the posterior cortex of the body on lateral views) suggests an unstable injury that may require operative fixation. In addition, disruption of the posterior ligamentous complex in the face of anterior fracture or dislocation is a strong indication of instability and of the potential need for surgical stabilization. Exceptions may include the upper thoracic spine, which is inherently more stable, and bony Chance's fractures. Nonpathologic compression fractures of three sequential vertebrae lead to an increase in risk of post-traumatic kyphosis.
3. Treatment—May be either operative or nonoperative (bracing or casting) for stable fractures, with a well-aligned spine with less than 20–30 degrees of kyphosis and no neurologic compromise. Operative intervention includes decompression for progressive neurologic deficit (emergency) or for incomplete neurologic deficit. May be accomplished anteriorly via vertebrectomy and stabilization or posteriorly via a transpedicular route. Posterior instrumentation with restoration of height and sagittal alignment may decompress the canal by repositioning the "posterolateral complex." Historically, posterior instrumentation and fusion have extended three levels above and two levels below the injury to stabilize the fracture. Constructs are created either in compression (fracture/dislocations, Chance's fractures, or shear fractures) or in distraction (burst fractures) to reduce and stabilize the injury. Newer, more rigid segmental systems with multiple hooks, wires, and screws or rod-sleeve constructs have supplanted the standard Harrington system and allow restoration of the normal sagittal contour of the spine. Pedicle screw systems are available that purport to limit instrumentation levels to one above and one below the injury. High rates of screw breakage and progressive kyphosis have been reported. The goals of surgery include stabilization of the fracture and preservation or improvement of neural function in all patients, as well as more rapid entry into rehabilitation and a shorter hospital stay for patients with complete injuries. Rehabilitation following spinal cord injury is discussed more fully in Chapter 9, Rehabilitation.
4. Complications—The most common long-term complication of a thoracolumbar fracture, treated with or without surgery, is pain. Unfortunately, the relationship between chronic pain and "stability," deformity, pseudarthrosis, and many other factors is unclear. Various types of post-traumatic deformity are noted, including scoliosis caudal to a complete injury (an age-related phenomenon with 100% occurrence in those <10 years old) and progressive kyphosis (common with unrecognized posterior ligamentous injury). Symptomatic flat back of the lumbar spine results in a forward flexed posture and easy fatigue (occurs with uncontoured distraction instrumentation). Other complications include late progressive neurologic loss and pain due to the development of post-traumatic syringomyelia. Late development of a neuropathic spine with gross bony destruction and bony spicules in the soft tissue has also been described.

G. Other Thoracolumbar Disorders

1. Destructive Spondyloarthropathy—Seen in hemodialysis patients with chronic renal failure. Typically involves three adjacent vertebrae with two intervening discs. Changes include subluxation, degeneration, and narrowing of the disc height. Although the process may resemble infection, it probably represents crystal or amyloid deposition.
2. Facet Syndrome—Inflammation or degeneration of the lumbar facet joints. May cause pain that is characteristically in the low back, with radiation down one or both buttocks and posterior thighs that is worse with extension. Selective injections of local anesthetic can be

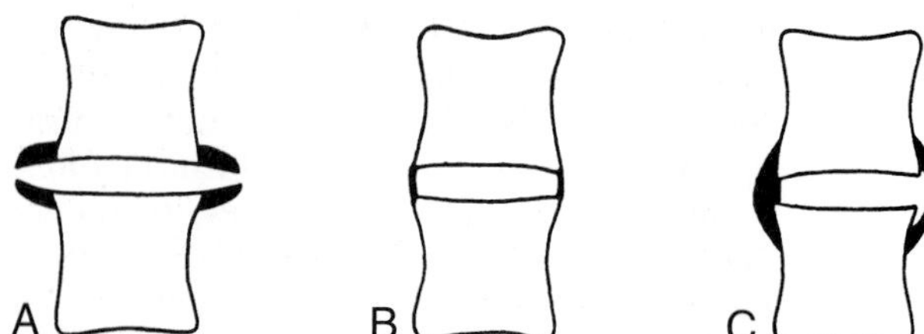

FIGURE 7-10 ■ Differential diagnoses of *(A)* osteophytes (degenerative joint disease), *(B)* marginal syndesmophytes (ankylosing spondylitis), and *(C)* nonmarginal syndesmophytes (DISH). (From Rothman, R.H., and Simeon, F.A.: The Spine, 2nd ed. Philadelphia, WB Saunders, 1982, p. 924.)

helpful in the diagnosis of this condition, but anesthetic/steroid injections into the facet joint as a treatment modality are less effective (<20% with excellent pain relief). The significance of the facet syndrome is debated, and no widely accepted treatment regimen exists. There is no proof that surgery (facet rhizotomy or fusion) is beneficial.

3. Diffuse Idiopathic Skeletal Hyperostosis (DISH)—Forestier's disease. Defined by the presence of nonmarginal syndesmophytes (differentiated from ankylosing spondylitis, which has marginal syndesmophytes [Fig. 7-10]) at three successive levels. DISH can occur anywhere in the spine but is most common in the T-spine and is more often seen on the right side. DISH is associated with chronic lower back pain and is more common in patients with diabetes and gout. The prevalence of DISH has been found to be as high as 28% in autopsy specimens. Although there appears to be no relationship between DISH and spinal pain, DISH is associated with extraspinal ossification at several joints, including an increased risk of heterotopic ossification following total hip surgery.
4. Ankylosing Spondylitis—HLA-B27-positive patients are usually young men who present with insidious onset of back and hip pain during the third or fourth decade of life. Sacroiliac joint obliteration and marginal syndesmophytes allow radiographic differentiation from DISH. Ankylosing spondylitis may result in fixed cervical, thoracic, or lumbar hyperkyphosis. It occasionally causes marked functional limitation, primarily due to the inability of affected patients to face forward. Extension osteotomy and fusion of the lumbar spine with compression instrumentation can successfully balance the head over the sacrum. Assessment for hip flexion contractures or cervicothoracic kyphosis is mandatory. The cervical spine may be corrected by a C7–T1 osteotomy and fusion under local anesthesia. Complications of osteotomies include nonunion, loss of correction, and neurologic and aortic injury. It has multiple medical associations, most notably pulmonary fibrosis, and aortic regurgitation.
5. Adult Scoliosis—Usually defined as scoliosis in patients over age 20, it is more symptomatic than its childhood counterpart (discussed in Chapter 2, Pediatric Orthopaedics). Cause is usually idiopathic but can also be neuromuscular, degenerative (secondary to degenerative disc disease or osteoporosis), post-traumatic, or postsurgical. Curves are usually thoracic (secondary to unrecognized adolescent scoliosis) or lumbar/thoracolumbar (most common in adults). Although the association between pain and scoliosis is controversial, back pain is the most common presenting complaint and appears to be related to curve severity and location (lumbar curves more painful). Pain usually begins in the convexity of the curve and later moves to the concavity, reflecting a more refractory condition. Radicular pain and stenosis can occur and may require surgical decompression. Other complaints include cosmetic deformity, cardiopulmonary problems (thoracic curves >60–65 degrees may alter pulmonary function tests; curves >90 degrees may affect mortality), and neurologic symptoms (secondary to stenosis). There is no demonstrated association between curve progression and pregnancy. Progression is unlikely in curves <30 degrees. Right thoracic curves >50 degrees are at highest risk for progression (usually 1 degree/year), followed by right lumbar curves. Myelography with CT or MRI is useful for the evaluation of nerve root compression in stenosis. MRI, facet injections, and/or discography may be utilized to evaluate symptoms in the lumbar spine. Nonoperative treatment includes NSAIDs, weight reduction, therapy, muscle strengthening, facet joint injections, and orthotics (used with activity). The uncertain correlation between adult scoliosis and back pain makes conservative management, including a thorough evaluation for other common causes of back pain, essential. Surgery is usually reserved for symptomatic curves >50–60 degrees in young adults and up to 90 degrees and beyond in older patients, for progressive curves, for patients with cardiopulmonary compromise (worsening pulmonary function tests in severe curves), and for patients with refractory spinal stenosis. Operative risk is high (up to 25% complication rate in older patients), and complications include pseudarthrosis (15% with posterior fusion only, highest risk in lumbar spine), urinary tract infection, instrumentation problems, infection (up to 5%), and neurologic deficits. Additionally, long

convalescence is usually required. Combined anterior release and fusion and posterior fusion and instrumentation may be beneficial for large (>70 degrees), more rigid curves (as determined on side-bending films) or curves in the lumbar spine. Preservation of normal sagittal alignment with fusion is critical. Fusion to the sacrum is associated with more complications (pseudarthrosis, instrumentation failure, loss of normal lordosis, and pain) and should be avoided when possible. Achieving a successful result, including fusion to the sacrum, is enhanced by combined anterior and posterior fusion.The ideal implant for instrumentation in these cases has not been found; commonly used instrumentation for sacral fixation includes Galveston's fixation and sacral pedicle or alar screw constructs. Clinical and experimental evidence exists demonstrating the benefit of structural interbody grafting (femoral ring allograft or mesh cage), at L5-S1 and L4-5, to decrease the stress on the sacropelvic fixation.

6. Postlaminectomy Deformity—Progressive deformity (usually kyphosis) resulting from a prior wide laminectomy. Laminectomy in children is followed by a high risk (90%) of deformity. Fusion plus internal fixation may be considered prophylactic for young patients who require extensive decompression. Fusion utilizing pedicular screw fixation is best for reconstruction in the adult lumbar spine.

H. Kyphosis

1. Introduction—Kyphosis in adults may be idiopathic (old Scheuermann's), post-traumatic, secondary to trauma or ankylosing spondylitis, or a result of metabolic bone disease. Progressive kyphosis secondary to multiple osteoporotic compression fractures is usually treated with exercises, bracing, and medical management of the underlying bone disease. Surgical attempts at correction and stabilization are marked by high complication rate.An underlying malignancy as a cause of the osteopenia should be considered; evaluation with MRI is sensitive for determining the presence of tumor.Vertebroplasty and kyphoplasty, percutaneous techniques designed to relieve pain (both) and correct deformity (kyphoplasty) have been proposed for acute and subacute compression fractures. Precise indications for these techniques, such as number of levels and timing, have not been defined, and long-term outcome data regarding their efficacy are lacking.
2. Nontraumatic Adult Kyphosis—Severe idiopathic or congenital kyphosis may be a source of back pain in the adult, particularly when present in the thoracolumbar or lumbar spine.When the symptoms fail to respond to nonoperative management (see the preceding discussion on adult scoliosis), posterior instrumentation and fusion of the entire kyphotic segment, using a compression implant, may be indicated. Anterior fusion in conjunction is performed for curves not correcting to 55 degrees or less on hyperextension lateral radiographs.
3. Post-traumatic Kyphosis—May be seen following fractures of the thoracolumbar spine treated nonoperatively, particularly when the posterior ligamentous complex has been disrupted; fractures treated by laminectomy without fusion; and fractures for which fusion has been performed unsuccessfully. Progressive kyphosis may produce pain at the fracture site, with radiating leg pain and/or neurologic dysfunction if there is associated neural compression. Operative options include posterior fusion with compression instrumentation for milder deformities; combined anterior and posterior osteotomies, instrumentation, and fusion for more severe deformities; and anterior spinal cord or cauda equina decompression combined with posterior instrumentation and fusion for cases involving neurologic dysfunction. Some all-posterior approaches such as pedicle subtraction osteotomy address anterior pathology and can achieve 30 degrees of correction per level.

IV. Sacrum and Coccyx

A. Sacroiliac Joint Pain—Elicited with the patient lying on the affected side without support (Gaenslen's test); direct compression; or flexion, abduction, and external rotation (FABER test) of the involved extremity. Local injections may have a diagnostic and therapeutic role. Orthotic management (trochanteric cinch) can be helpful. Fusion is not indicated unless an infection is present.

B. Idiopathic Coccygodynia—Pain and point tenderness over the coccyx. More common in women, may occur after pregnancy, minor trauma, or idiopathically. Occasionally associated with a fracture, four types have been identified based on morphology of the coccyx. Symptoms may last 1-2 years, but are almost always self-limited. Treatment should be conservative and may include a sitting donut, NSAIDs, stretching exercises, and local injection. Surgery is associated with a high failure rate and significant risk of complications.

C. Sacral Insufficiency Fracture—Occurs in older patients with osteopenia, often without a history of trauma. Complaints include low back and groin pain. Diagnosed with technetium bone scan (H-shaped uptake pattern is diagnostic) or CT scan. Treatment is nonoperative with rest, analgesics, and ambulatory aids until symptoms resolve.

V. Spine Tumors and Infections

A. Introduction—The spine is a frequent site of metastasis, and certain tumors with a predilection for the spine have unique manifestations in vertebrae. Tumors of the vertebral body include histiocytosis X, giant cell tumor, chordoma, osteosarcoma, hemangioma, metastatic disease, and marrow cell tumors. Tumors of the posterior elements include aneurysmal bone cysts, osteoblastoma, and osteoid osteoma. Radiographic changes include absent pedicle, cortical erosion or expansion, and vertebral collapse. Bone scans can be helpful in cases of protracted back pain or night pain. MRI is the diagnostic test of choice. Malignant tumors have decreased T1 and increased T2 intensity, the sensitivity of which is increased with use of gadolinium. Malignant tumors occur more commonly in lower (lumbar > thoracic > cervical) spinal levels and in the vertebral body. Complete surgical excision is difficult and usually consists of tumor debulking and stabilization. Adjuvant therapy is essential. For more details on these tumors, refer to Chapter 8, Orthopaedic Pathology.

B. Metastasis—Most common tumors of the spine, spreading to the vertebral body first and later to the pedicles. Red flags for possible spinal metastasis include a history of cancer, recent unexplained weight loss, night pain, and age >50 years. Most tumors are osteolytic and are not demonstrated on plain films until >30% destruction of the vertebral body has occurred. Breast, lung, and prostate metastases are most common, the latter being blastic. CT-guided needle biopsy is often possible, and surgery for diagnosis can be avoided. Poor prognosis is associated with neurologic dysfunction, proximal lesions, long duration of symptoms, and rapid growth of the metastasis. Radiation therapy and chemotherapy are the mainstays of treatment unless the tumor is destabilizing and progressive or causes spinal cord or cauda equina dysfunction. Radiosensitivity varies among primary tumor types: prostate and lymphoid tumors are quite radiosensitive; breast cancer is 70% sensitive, 30% are resistant; gastrointestinal and renal cell tumors are quite radioresistant. Surgical indications include progressive neurologic dysfunction unresponsive to radiation therapy, persistent pain despite radiation therapy, need for a diagnostic biopsy, and pathologic instability. In cases of neurologic deficit and/or spinal instability, anterior decompression and stabilization (preserving intact posterior structures) have a role and may result in recovery of neurologic function. Posterior stabilization or a circumferential approach is indicated in cases with multiple levels of destruction, involvement of both anterior and posterior columns, or translational instability. Life expectancy should play an important role as to whether surgical treatment is performed. Methylmethacrylate may be useful as an anterior strut but should only be utilized as an adjunct because of the high complication rate. Iliac crest graft is favored if life expectancy is >6 months. Anterior internal fixation may be indicated to maximize immediate stability and rehabilitation.

C. Primary Tumors

1. Osteoid Osteoma and Osteoblastoma—Common in the spine. May present with painful scoliosis in a child. Pain is typically relieved by aspirin. Bone scan can help localize the level, and thin-cut CT scans can direct surgical excision. Scoliosis (the lesion is typically at the apex of the convexity) resolves with early resection (within 18 months) in a child <11 years of age. If no scoliosis exists, NSAIDs are the mainstay of treatment. If they do not alleviate the pain, resection may be required. Osteoblastomas typically occur in the posterior elements in older patients, with neurologic involvement in more than half. This presentation typically requires resection and posterior fusion.
2. Aneurysmal Bone Cyst—May represent degeneration of other, more aggressive tumors. These cysts typically occur during the second decade of life. They occur in the posterior elements but may also involve the anterior elements. Treatment is excision and/or radiation therapy.
3. Hemangioma—Typically seen in asymptomatic patients. Symptomatic patients over age 40 may seek treatment after small spinal fractures. Classically has "jailhouse striations" on plain films and "spikes of bone" demonstrated on CT. Vertebrae are typically normally sized and not expanded (as in Paget's disease). Treatment is observation or radiation therapy in cases of persistent pain after pathologic fracture. Anterior resection and fusion are reserved for refractory cases or pathologic collapse and neural compression, but massive bleeding may be encountered.
4. Eosinophilic Granuloma—Usually seen in children younger than 10 years. Seen more often in the thoracic spine; may present with progressive back pain. Classically causes vertebral flattening (vertebra plana—Calvé's disease), which is seen on lateral radiographs. Biopsy may be required for diagnosis unless the radiographic picture is classic or histiocytosis has already been diagnosed. Chemotherapy is useful for the systemic form. Bracing may be indicated in children to prevent progressive kyphosis. Low-dose radiation therapy may be indicated in the presence of neurologic deficits; otherwise, symptoms are usually self-limited. At least 50% reconstitution of vertebral height may be expected.
5. Giant Cell Tumor—Most commonly seen in the fourth and fifth decades of life. Destroys the vertebral body in an expansile fashion. Surgical excision and bone grafting comprise the usual recommended treatment. High recurrence rate

is reported. Radiation therapy should be avoided because of the possibility of malignant degeneration of the tumor.

6. Plasmacytoma/Multiple Myeloma—Also common in the spine, causing osteopenic, lytic lesions. Pain, pathologic fractures, and diffuse osteoporosis are common. Increased calcium and decreased hematocrit levels are common, as well as abnormal protein studies. Treatment is radiation therapy (3000–4000 cGy ± chemotherapy). Surgery is reserved for instability and in patients with refractory neurologic symptoms.
7. Chordoma—Classically a slow-growing lytic lesion in the midline of the anterior sacrum or the base of the skull. May occur in other vertebrae (cervical most common). These tumors may present with intra-abdominal complaints and a presacral mass. Radiation therapy and surgery are favored. Surgical excision can include up to half of the sacral roots (i.e., all roots on one side) and still maintain bowel and bladder function. Recurrence rate is high, but aggressive attempts at surgical excision are indicated. Although a complete cure is rare, patients typically survive 10–15 years after diagnosis.
8. Osteochondroma—Arises in the posterior elements. It is seen commonly in the cervical spine. Treatment is excision, which may be necessary to rule out sarcomatous changes.
9. Neurofibroma—Can present with enlarged intervertebral foramina seen on oblique radiographs.
10. Malignant Primary Skeletal Lesions—Osteosarcoma, Ewing's sarcoma, and chondrosarcoma are uncommon in the spine. When they do occur they are associated with a poor prognosis. Chemotherapy and irradiation are the mainstays of treatment, but aggressive surgical excision may have a role. Lesions may actually be metastases, which are treated palliatively.
11. Lymphoma—Can present with "ivory" vertebrae. Usually associated with a systemic disease, lymphoma is treated after histologic diagnosis by irradiation and/or chemotherapy.

D. Spinal Infections

1. Disc Space Infection—Bloodborne infection can primarily invade the disc space in children. *Staphylococcus aureus* is the most common offender, but gram-negative organisms are common in older patients. Children (mean age 7, although all age groups are affected) commonly present with inability to walk, stand, or sit; back pain/tenderness; and restricted range of motion. Laboratory studies may be normal except for an elevated erythrocyte sedimentation rate, C-reactive protein, and WBC count (often high normal or mildly elevated). Radiographic findings include disc space narrowing and endplate erosion, but these findings do not occur until 10 days to 3 weeks following onset, and their absence is unreliable. MRI scan is the diagnostic test of choice, although bone scan is also useful in the diagnosis. Treatment includes bed rest, immobilization, and antibiotics.
2. Pyogenic Vertebral Osteomyelitis—Seen with increasing frequency but still associated with a significant (6–12 week) delay in diagnosis. Older debilitated patients and IV drug addicts are at increased risk. A history of pneumonia, urinary tract infection, skin infection, or immunologic compromise (transplant patients, RA, diabetes [DM]) is common. The organism is usually hematogenous in origin (*S. aureus*, 50–75% of cases). A history of unremitting spinal pain at any level is characteristic, and tenderness, spasm, and loss of motion are seen. Forty percent of neurologic deficits are seen in older patients, in patients with infections at more cephalad levels of the spine, in patients with debilitating systemic illnesses such as diabetes or RA, and in patients with delayed diagnoses. Plain radiographic findings include osteopenia, paraspinous soft-tissue swelling (loss of psoas shadow), erosion of the vertebral endplates, and disc destruction. Disc destruction, seen on plain radiographs or MRI, is **atypical of neoplasms**. Bone scanning is sensitive for a destructive process. MRI is both sensitive for detecting infection and specific in differentiating infection from tumor. Gadolinium enhances sensitivity. Tissue diagnosis via blood cultures or aspirate of the infection is mandatory; when made, 6–12 weeks of intravenous antibiotics is the treatment of choice. Bracing may be used adjunctively. Open biopsy is indicated when a tissue diagnosis has not been made, and an anterior approach or costotransversectomy is used. Anterior débridement and strut grafting are reserved for refractory cases, typically associated with abscess formation, or cases involving neurologic deterioration, extensive bony destruction, or marked deformity. Posterior surgery is usually ineffective for débridement; posterior stabilization is only occasionally required following anterior débridement and strut grafting.
3. Spinal Tuberculosis—The most common extrapulmonary location of tuberculosis is in the spine. Originating in the metaphysis of the vertebral body and spreading under the anterior longitudinal ligament, spinal tuberculosis can cause destruction of several contiguous levels or can result in skip lesions (15%) or abscess formation (50%) (see Fig. 7-10). On early plain x-ray studies, vertebral body destruction anteriorly, with preservation of the disc, distinguishes tuberculosis from pyogenic infection. About two-thirds of patients have abnormal chest radiographs, and 20% have a negative purified protein derivative of tuberculin (PPD) test

or are anergic. Severe kyphosis, sinus formation, and (Pott's) paraplegia are late sequelae. Spinal cord injury may occur secondary to direct pressure from the abscess, bony sequestra (good prognosis), or rarely, meningomyelitis (poor prognosis). Chemotherapy is the mainstay of treatment. Surgical indications are neurologic deficit, spinal instability, progressive kyphosis, or advanced disease with caseation, fibrosis, and avascularity limiting antibiotic penetration. Radical anterior débridement of the infection followed by uninstrumented autogenous strut grafting (Hong Kong procedure) is the accepted surgical treatment. Advantages include less progressive kyphosis, earlier healing, and decrease in sinus formation. Adjuvant chemotherapy beginning 10 days before surgery is recommended.

Selected Bibliography

REVIEWS

GENERAL INFORMATION

Boden, S.D.: The use of radiographic imaging studies in the evaluation of patients who have degenerative disorders of the lumbar spine. J. Bone Joint Surg. [Am.] 78:114–125, 1996.

Boden, S.D., and Wiesel, S.W.: Lumbar spine imaging: Role in clinical decision making. J. Am. Acad. Orthop. Surg. 4:238–248, 1996.

CERVICAL SPONDYLOSIS, STENOSIS

Bohlman, H.H.: Cervical spondylosis and myelopathy. AAOS Instr. Course Lect. 44:81–98, 1995.

Law, M.D., Bernhardt, M., and White, A.A.: Evaluation and management of cervical spondylotic myelopathy. AAOS Instr. Course Lect. 44:99–110, 1995.

Levine, M.J., Albert, T.J., and Smith, M.D.: Cervical radiculopathy: Diagnosis and nonoperative management. J. Am. Acad. Orthop. Surg. 4:305–316, 1996.

RHEUMATOID SPONDYLITIS

Monsey, R.D.: Rheumatoid arthritis of the cervical spine. J. Am. Acad. Orthop. Surg. 5:240–248, 1997.

CERVICAL SPINE INJURY

Botte, M.J., Byrne, T.P., Abrams, R.A., et al.: Halo skeletal fixation: Techniques of application and prevention of complications. J. Am. Acad. Orthop. Surg. 4:44–53, 1996.

Slucky, A.V., and Eismont, F.J.: Treatment of acute injury of the cervical spine. AAOS Instr. Course Lect. 44:67–80, 1995.

DISC DISEASE

Eismont, F.J., and Currier, B.: Current concepts review: Surgical management of lumbar intervertebral-disc disease. J. Bone Joint Surg. [Am.] 71:1266, 1989.

LUMBAR STENOSIS

Spivak, J.M.: Degenerative lumbar spinal stenosis. J. Bone Joint Surg. [Am.] 80:1053–1067, 1998.

SPONDYLOLISTHESIS

Hensinger, R.N.: Current concepts review: Spondylolysis and spondylolisthesis in children and adolescents. J. Bone Joint Surg. [Am.] 71:1098, 1989.

Larsen, J.M., and Capen, D.A.: Pseudarthrosis of the lumbar spine. J. Am. Acad. Orthop. Surg. 5:153–162, 1997.

Lauerman, W.C., and Cain, J.E.: Isthmic spondylolisthesis in the adult. J. Am. Acad. Orthop. Surg. 4:201–208, 1996.

THORACOLUMBAR INJURY

Bohlman, H.H.: Current concepts review: Treatment of fractures and dislocations of the thoracic and lumbar spine. J. Bone Joint Surg. [Am.] 67:165, 1985.

Slucky, A.V., and Potter, H.G.: Use of magnetic resonance imaging in spinal trauma: Indications, techniques, and utility. J. Am. Acad. Orthop. Surg. 6(3):134–145, 1998.

DEFORMITY

Bradford, D.S.: Adult scoliosis: Current concepts of treatment. Clin. Orthop. 229:70, 1988.

Tribus, C.B.: Scheuermann's kyphosis in adolescents and adults: Diagnosis and management. J. Am. Acad. Orthop. Surg. 6:36–43, 1998.

OTHER

Tay, B.K., Deckey, J., Hu, S.S.: Spinal infections. J. Am. Acad. Orthop. Surg. 10:188-197, 2001.

Belanger, T.A., Rowe, D.E.: Diffuse idiopathic skeletal hyperostosi: Musculoskeletal manifestations. J. Am. Acad. Orthop. Surg. 9:258-267, 2001.

Kambin, P., McCullen, G., Parke, W., et al.: Minimally invasive arthroscopic spinal surgery. AAOS Instr. Course Lect. 46:143–161, 1997.

Regan, J.J., Yuan, H., and McCullen, G.: Minimally invasive approaches to the spine. AAOS Instr. Course Lect. 46:127–141, 1997.

RECENT ARTICLES

GENERAL INFORMATION

Sidhu, K.S., and Herkowitz, H.H.: Spinal instrumentation in the management of degenerative disorders of the lumbar spine. Clin. Orthop. 335:39–53, 1997.

BACK PAIN

Jensen, M.E.: MRI of the lumbar spine in people without back pain. N. Engl. J. Med. 331:69, 1994.

CERVICAL SPONDYLOSIS, STENOSIS

Bernhardt, M., Hynes, R.A., Blume, H.W., et al.: Cervical spondylotic myelopathy. J. Bone Joint Surg. [Am.] 75:119, 1993.

Bohlman, H.H., Emery, S.E., Goodfellow, D.B., et al.: Robinson anterior cervical diskectomy and arthrodesis for cervical radiculopathy. J. Bone Joint Surg. [Am.] 75:1298–1307, 1993.

Emery, S.E., Bohlman, H.H., Bolesta, M.J., et al.: Anterior cervical decompression and arthrodesis for the treatment of cervical spondylotic myelopathy: Two to seven year follow-up. J. Bone Joint Surg. [Am.] 80:941–951, 1998.

Ghanayem, A.J., Leventhal, M., and Bohlman, H.H.: Osteoarthrosis of the atlanto-axial joints: Long-term follow-up after treatment with arthrodesis. J. Bone Joint Surg. [Am.] 78:1300–1308, 1996.

Iwasaki, M., and Ebara, S.: Expansive laminoplasty for cervical radiculomyelopathy due to soft disc herniation. Spine 21:32–38, 1996.

Johnson, M.J., and Lucas, G.L.: Value of cervical spine radiographs as a screening tool. Clin. Orthop. 340:102–108, 1997.

McAfee, P.C., Hohlman, H.H., Ducker, T.B., et al.: One-stage anterior cervical decompression and posterior stabilization: A study of one hundred patients with minimum two years of follow-up. J. Bone Joint Surg. [Am.] 77:1791, 1995.

Zdeblick, T.A., Hughes, S.S., Riew, K.D., et al.: Failed anterior cervical discectomy and arthrodesis: Analysis and treatment of thirty-five patients. J. Bone Joint Surg. [Am.] 79:523–532, 1997.

RHEUMATOID SPONDYLITIS

Boden, S.D., Dodge, L.D., Bohlman, H.H., et al.: Rheumatoid arthritis of the cervical spine: A long-term analysis with predictors of paralysis and recovery. J. Bone Joint Surg. [Am.] 75:1282, 1993.

CERVICAL SPINE INJURY

Anderson, P.A., and Bohlman, H.H.: Anterior decompression and arthrodesis of the cervical spine: Long-term motor improvement. Part II—Improvement in complete traumatic quadriplegia. J. Bone Joint Surg. [Am.] 74:683-692, 1992.

Bohlman, H.H., and Anderson, P.A.: Anterior decompression and arthrodesis of the cervical spine: Long term motor improvement. Part I—Improvement in incomplete traumatic quadriparesis. J. Bone Joint Surg. [Am.] 74:671-682, 1992.

McAfee, P.C., Bohlman H.H., Ducker, T.B., et al.: One-stage anterior cervical decompression and posterior stabilization. J. Bone Joint Surg. [Am.] 77:1791, 1995.

Torg, J.S., Naranja, R.J., Pavlov, H., et al.: The relationship of developmental narrowing of the cervical spinal canal to reversible and irreversible injury of the cervical spinal cord in football players: An epidemiological study. J. Bone Joint Surg. [Am.] 78:1308-1314, 1996.

DISC DISEASE

Atlas, S.J., Deyo, R.A., Keller, R.B., et al.: The Maine lumbar spine study: Part II. Spine 21:1777-1786, 1996.

Brown, C.W., Deffner, P.A., et al.: The natural history of thoracic disc herniations. Spine 17:S97-S102, 1992.

Komori, H., and Shinomiya, K.: The natural history of HNP with radiculopathy. Spine 21:225-229, 1996.

Stillerman, C.B., Chen, T.C., et al.: Experience in the surgical management of 82 symptomatic thoracic disc herniations and review of the literature. J Neurosurg. 88:623-633, 1998.

LUMBAR STENOSIS

Grob, D., Humke, T., and Dvorak, J.: Degenerative lumbar spinal stenosis: Decompression with and without arthrodesis. J. Bone Joint Surg. [Am.] 77:1036-1041, 1995.

Katz, J.N., and Lipson, S.J.: Seven to ten year outcome of decompressive surgery for degenerative lumbar spinal stenosis. Spine 21:92-98, 1996.

Riew, K.D., Yin, Y., et al.: The effect of nerve-root injection on the need for operative treatment of lumbar radicular pain. A prospective, randomized, controlled, double-blind study. J. Bone Joint Surg. [Am.] 82:1589-1596, 2000.

Stewart, G., and Sachs, B.L.: Patient outcomes after reoperation on the lumbar spine. J. Bone Joint Surg. [Am.] 78:706-711, 1996.

SPONDYLOLISTHESIS

Carpenter, C.T., and Dietz, J.W.: Repair of a pseudarthrosis of the lumbar spine: A functional outcome study. J. Bone Joint Surg. [Am.] 78:712-720, 1996.

Carragee, E.J.: Single-level posterolateral arthrodesis, with or without posterior decompression, for the treatment of isthmic spondylolisthesis in adults: A prospective, randomized study. J. Bone Joint Surg. [Am.] 79:1175-1180, 1997.

Fischgrund, J.S., Mackay, M., Herkowitz, H.N., et al.: Degenerative lumbar spondylolisthesis with spinal stenosis: A prospective, randomized study comparing decompressive laminectomy and arthrodesis with and without spinal instrumentation. Spine 22:2807-2812, 1997.

Goel, V.K., and Gilbertson, L.G.: Basic science of spinal instrumentation. Clin. Orthop. 335:10-31, 1997.

Herkowitz, H.N., and Kurz, L.T.: Degenerative lumbar spondylolisthesis with spinal stenosis: A prospective study comparing decompression with decompression and intertransverse process arthrodesis. J. Bone Joint Surg. [Am.] 73:802-808, 1991.

Jinkins, J.R., Rauch, A.: Magnetic resonance imaging of entrapment of lumbar nerve roots in spondylolitic spondylolisthesis. J. Bone Joint Surg. 76:1643-1648, 1994.

Thomsen, K., and Christensen, F.B.: The effect of pedicle screw instrumentation on functional outcome and fusion rates in posterolateral lumbar spinal fusion: A prospective, randomized clinical study. Spine 22:2813-2822, 1997.

Zdeblick, T.: A prospective randomized study of lumbar fusion. Spine 18:983-991, 1993.

THORACOLUMBAR INJURY

Delamarter, R.B., Sherman, J., and Carr, J.B.: Pathophysiology of spinal cord injury: Recovery after immediate and delayed decompression. J. Bone Joint Surg. [Am.] 77:1042, 1995.

Kaneda, K., and Taneichi, H.: Anterior decompression and stabilization with the Kaneda device for thoracolumbar burst fractures associated with neurological deficits. J. Bone Joint Surg. [Am.] 79:69-83, 1997.

DEFORMITY

Barr, J.D., Barr, M.S., et al.: Percutaneous vertebroplasty for pain relief and spinal stabilization. Spine 25:923-928, 2000.

Dickson, J.H., and Mirkovic, S.: Results of operative treatment of idiopathic scoliosis in adults. J. Bone Joint Surg. [Am.] 77:513-523, 1995.

Lieberman, I.H., Dudeney, S., et al.: Initial outcome and efficacy of "kyphoplasty" in the treatment of painful osteoporotic compression fractures. Spine 26:1631-1638, 2001.

Weinstein, S.L., Dolan, L.A., et al.: Health and function of patients with untreated idiopathic scoliosis. A 50-year natural history study. J.A.M.A. 289:559-567, 2003.

INFECTIONS, TUMORS

Bauer, H.C.: Posterior decompression and stabilization for spinal metastases: Analysis of sixty-seven consecutive patients. J. Bone Joint Surg. [Am.] 79:514-522, 1997.

Carragee, E.J.: Pyogenic vertebral osteomyelitis. J. Bone Joint Surg. [Am.] 79:874-880, 1997.

COMPLICATIONS

Klein, J.D., and Hey, L.A.: Perioperative nutrition and postoperative complications in patients undergoing spinal surgery. Spine 21:2676-2682, 1996.

McDonnell, M.F., and Glassman, S.D.: Perioperative complications of anterior procedures on the spine. J. Bone Joint Surg. [Am.] 78:839-847, 1996.

Wang, J.C., Bohlman, H.H., et al.: Dural tears secondary to operations on the lumbar spine: Management and results after a two-year minimum follow-up of eighty-eight patients. J. Bone Joint Surg. 80:1728-1732, 1998.

CLASSIC ARTICLES

GENERAL INFORMATION

Boden, S.D., Davis, D.O., Dina, T.S., et al.: Abnormal magnetic resonance scans of the lumbar spine in asymptomatic subjects. J. Bone Joint Surg. [Am.] 72:403, 1990.

Boden, S.D., McCown, P.R., Davis, D.O., et al.: Abnormal MRI scans of cervical spine in asymptomatic subjects: A prospective investigation. J. Bone Joint Surg. [Am.] 72:1178-1184, 1990.

Garfin, S.R., Bottle, M.J., Walters, R.L., et al.: Complications in the use of the halo fixation device. J. Bone Joint Surg. [Am.] 68:320, 1986.

Macnab, I.: The blood supply of the lumbar spine and its application to the technique of intertransverse lumbar fusion. J. Bone Joint Surg. [Br.] 53:628, 1971.

White, A.A., III, Johnson, R.M., Panjabi, M.M., et al.: Biomechanical analysis of clinical stability in the cervical spine. Clin. Orthop. 109:85-96, 1975.

BACK PAIN

Deyo, R.H., Diehl, A.K., and Rosenthal, M.: How many days of bed rest for acute low back pain? A randomized clinical trial. N. Engl. J. Med. 315:1064-1070, 1986.

Frymoyer, J.W.: Back pain and sciatica. N. Engl. J. Med. 318:291-300, 1988.

Frymoyer, J.W., Pope, M.H., Clements, J.H., et al.: Risk factors in low back pain: An epidemiological survey. J. Bone Joint Surg. [Am.] 65:213-218, 1983.

Nachemson, A.: Work for all: For those with low back pain as well. Clin. Orthop. 179:77-85, 1983.

CERVICAL SPONDYLOSIS, STENOSIS

Emery, S.E. Cervical spondylotic myelopathy: Diagnosis and treatment. J. Am. Acad. Orthop. Surg. 9:376–388, 2001.

Fielding, J.W., Hensinger, R.N., and Hawkins, R.J.: Os odontoideum. J. Bone Joint Surg. [Am.] 62:376, 1980.

Gore, D.R., and Sepic, S.B.: Anterior cervical fusion for degenerated or protruded discs: A review of one hundred forty-six patients. Spine 9:667–671, 1984.

Gore, D.R., Sepic, S.B., Gardner, G.M., et al.: Neck pain: A long-term follow-up of 205 patients. Spine 12:1–5, 1987.

Herkowitz, H.N., Kurz, L.T., and Overholt, D.P.: Surgical management of cervical soft disk herniation: A comparison between anterior and posterior approach. Spine 15:1026–1030, 1990.

Hirabayashi, K., and Satomi, K.: Operative procedure and results of expansive open-door laminoplasty. Spine 13:870–876, 1988.

Smith, G.W., and Robinson, R.A.: The treatment of certain cervical spine disorders by anterior removal of the intervertebral disk and interbody fusion. J. Bone Joint Surg. [Am.] 40:607–623, 1958.

Zdeblick, T.A., and Bohlman, H.H.: Cervical kyphosis and myelopathy: Treatment by anterior corpectomy and strut-grating. J. Bone Joint Surg. [Am.] 71:170, 1989.

RHEUMATOID SPONDYLITIS

Brooks, A.L., and Jenkins, E.B.: Atlanto-axial arthrodesis by the wedge compression method. J. Bone Joint Surg. [Am.] 60:279, 1978.

Clark, C.R., Goetz, D.D., and Menezes, A.H.: Arthrodesis of the cervical spine in rheumatoid arthritis. J. Bone Joint Surg. [Am.] 71:381–392, 1989.

Pellicci, P.M., Ranawat, C.S., Tsairis, P., et al.: A prospective study of the progression of rheumatoid arthritis of the cervical spine. J. Bone Joint Surg. [Am.] 63:342, 1981.

Rana, N.A.: Natural history of atlanto-axial subluxation in rheumatoid arthritis. Spine 14:1054–1056, 1989.

Ranawat, C.S., O'Leary, P., Pellicci, P., et al.: Cervical spine fusion in rheumatoid arthritis. J. Bone Joint Surg. [Am.] 61:1003, 1979.

CERVICAL SPINE INJURY

Allen, B.L., Jr., Ferguson, R.L., Lehmann, T.R., et al.: A mechanistic classification of closed, indirect fractures and dislocation of the lower cervical spine. Spine 7:1–27, 1982.

Anderson, L.D., and D'Alozono, R.T.: Fractures of the odontoid process of the axis. J. Bone Joint Surg. [Am.] 56:1663, 1974.

Bohlman, H.H.: Acute fractures and dislocations of the cervical spine: An analysis of 300 hospitalized patients and review of the literature. J. Bone Joint Surg. [Am.] 61:1119–1142, 1979.

Clark, C.R., and White, A.A., III: Fractures of the dens: A multicenter study. J. Bone Joint Surg. [Am.] 67:1340–1348, 1985.

Fielding, J.W., and Hawkins, R.J.: Atlanto-axial rotatory fixation: Fixed rotatory subluxation of the atlanto-axial joint. J. Bone Joint Surg. [Am.] 59:37, 1977.

Gallie, W.E.: Fractures and dislocations of the cervical spine. Am. J. Surg. 46:495, 1939.

Johnson, R.M., Hart, D.L., Simmons, E.F., et al.: Cervical orthoses: A study comparing their effectiveness in restricting cervical motion in normal subjects. J. Bone Joint Surg. [Am.] 59:332, 1977.

Kang, J.E., Figgie, M.P., and Bohlman, H.H.: Sagittal measurements of the cervical spine in subaxial fractures and dislocations: An analysis of two hundred eighty-eight patients with and without neurologic deficits. J. Bone Joint Surg. [Am.] 76:1617–1628, 1994.

Levine, A.M., and Edwards, C.C.: The management of traumatic spondylolisthesis of the axis. J. Bone Joint Surg. [Am.] 67:217–226, 1985.

Torg, S., Pavlov, H., Genuario, S.E., et al.: Neurapraxia on the cervical spinal cord with transient quadriplegia. J. Bone Joint Surg. [Am.] 68:1354–1370, 1986.

DISC DISEASE

Albrand, O.W., and Corkill, G.: Thoracic disc herniation: Treatment and prognosis. Spine 4:41–46, 1979.

Bell, G.R., and Rothman, R.H.: The conservative treatment of sciatica. Spine 9:54–56, 1984.

Bohlman, H.H., and Zdeblick, T.A.: Anterior excision of herniated thoracic discs. J. Bone Joint Surg. [Am.] 70:1038, 1988.

Hanley, E.N., and Shapiro, D.E.: The development of low back pain after excision of a lumbar disk. J. Bone Joint Surg. [Am.] 71:719–721, 1989.

Kostuik, J.P., Harrington, I., Alexander, D., et al.: Cauda equina syndrome and lumbar disc herniation. J. Bone Joint Surg. [Am.] 68:386, 1986.

Waddell, G., Kummell, E.G., Lotto, W.M., et al.: Failed lumbar disk surgery and repeat surgery following industrial injuries. J. Bone Joint Surg. [Am.] 61:201–207, 1979.

Weber, H.: Lumbar disc herniation: A controlled, prospective study with ten years of observation. Spine 8:131, 1983.

LUMBAR STENOSIS

Kirkaldy-Willis, W.H.: The relationship of structural pathology to the nerve root. Spine 9:49–52, 1984.

Kirkaldy-Willis, W.H., Wedge, J.H., Yong-Hing, K., et al.: Pathology and pathogenesis of lumbar spondylosis and stenosis. Spine 4:319, 1978.

Spengler, D.M.: Current concepts review: Degenerative stenosis of the lumbar spine. J. Bone Joint Surg. [Am.] 69:305, 1987.

SPONDYLOLISTHESIS

Boxall, D., Bradford, D.S., Winter, R.B., et al.: Management of severe spondylolisthesis in children and adolescents. J. Bone Joint Surg. [Am.] 61:479, 1979.

Bradford, D.S.: Closed reduction of spondylolisthesis and experience in 22 patients. Spine 13:580, 1988.

Bradford, D.S., and Boachie-Adjei, O.: Treatment of severe spondylolisthesis by anterior and posterior reduction and stabilization: A long-term follow-up study. J. Bone Joint Surg. [Am.] 72:1060, 1990.

Frederickson, B.W., Baker, D., McHolick, W.J., et al.: The natural history of spondylolysis and spondylolisthesis. J. Bone Joint Surg. [Am.] 66:699–707, 1984.

Gill, G.G., Manning, J.G., and White, H.L.: Surgical treatment of spondylolisthesis without spine fusion. J. Bone Joint Surg. [Am.] 37:493, 1955.

Harris, I.E., and Weinstein, S.D.: Long-term follow-up of patients with grade III and IV spondylolisthesis: Treatment with and without posterior fusion. J. Bone Joint Surg. [Am.] 69:960–969, 1987.

Osterman, K., Lindholm, T.S., and Laurent, L.E.: Late results of removal of the loose posterior element (Gill's operation) in the treatment of lytic lumbar spondylolisthesis. Clin. Orthop. 117:121, 1976.

Peek, R.D., Wiltse, L.L., Reynolds, J.B., et al.: In situ arthrodesis without decompression for grade III or IV isthmic spondylolisthesis in adults who have severe sciatica. J. Bone Joint Surg. [Am.] 71:62, 1989.

Saraste, H.: The etiology of spondylolysis: A retrospective radiographic study. Acta Orthop. Scand. 56:253, 1985.

Wiltse, L.L., and Winter, R.B.: Terminology and measurement of spondylolisthesis. J. Bone Joint Surg. [Am.] 65:768–772, 1983.

Wiltse, L.L., Guyer, R.D., Spencer, C.W., et al.: Alar transverse process impingement of the L5 spinal nerve: The far-out syndrome. Spine 9:31, 1984.

THORACOLUMBAR INJURY

Bohlman, H.H., and Eismont, F.J.: Surgical techniques of anterior decompression and fusion for spinal cord injuries. Clin. Orthop. 154:57, 1981.

Bracken, M.B., Shepard, M.J., Collins, W.F., et al.: A randomized, controlled trial of methylprednisolone or naloxone in the treatment of acute spinal cord injury. N. Engl. J. Med. 322:1405, 1990.

Cain, J.E., DeJung, J.T., Divenberg, A.S., et al.: Pathomechanical analysis of thoracolumbar burst fracture reduction: A calf spine model. Spine 18:1640–1647, 1993.

Cammissa, F.P., Jr., Eismont, F.J., and Green, B.A.: Dural laceration occurring with burst fractures and associated laminar fractures. J. Bone Joint Surg. [Am.] 71:1044–1052, 1989.

Denis, F.: The three-column spine and its significance in the classification of acute thoracolumbar spinal injuries. Spine 8:817–831, 1983.

Ferguson, R.L., and Allen, B.L., Jr.: A mechanistic classification of thoracolumbar spine fractures. Clin. Orthop. 189:77, 1984.

Holdsworth, F.W.: Fractures, dislocations, and fracture-dislocations of the spine. J. Bone Joint Surg. [Am.] 52:1534, 1970.

Kaneda, K., Abumi, K., and Fujiya, M.: Burst fractures with neurologic deficits of the thoracolumbar-lumbar spine: Results of anterior decompression and stabilization with anterior instrumentation. Spine 9:788, 1984.

McAfee, P.C., Bohlman, H.H., and Yuan, H.A.: Anterior decompression of traumatic thoracolumbar fractures with incomplete neurologic deficit using a retroperitoneal approach. J. Bone Joint Surg. [Am.] 67:89–104, 1985.

Mumfred, J., Weinstein, J.N., Spratt, K.F., et al.: Thoracolumbar burst fractures: The clinical efficacy and outcome of nonoperative management. Spine 18:955–970, 1993.

DEFORMITY

Allen, B.L., Jr., and Ferguson, R.L.: The Galveston technique of pelvic fixation with L-rod instrumentation of the spine. Spine 9:388, 1984.

Bradford, D.S., Moe, J.H., Montalvo, F.J., et al.: Scheuermann's kyphosis and roundback deformity: Results of Milwaukee brace treatment. J. Bone Joint Surg. [Am.] 56:740, 1974.

Jackson, R.P., Simmons, E.H., and Stripinis, D.: Incidence and severity of back pain in adult idiopathic scoliosis. Spine 8:749, 1983.

Lauerman, W.C., Bradford, D.S., Ogilvie, J.W., et al.: Results of lumbar pseudarthrosis repair. J. Spinal Disord. 5:128–136, 1992.

Lauerman, W.C., Bradford, D.S., Transfeld, E.E., et al.: Management of pseudarthrosis after arthrodesis of the spine for idiopathic scoliosis. J. Bone Joint Surg. [Am.] 73:222–236, 1991.

Luque, E.R.: Segmental spinal instrumentation of the lumbar spine. Clin. Orthop. 203:126–134, 1986.

Murray, P.M., Weinstein, S.L., and Spratt, K.F.: The natural history and long term follow-up of Scheuermann's kyphosis. J. Bone Joint Surg. [Am.] 75:236–248, 1993.

Sponseller, P.D., Cohen, M.S., Nachemson, A.L., et al.: Results of surgical treatment of adults with idiopathic scoliosis. J. Bone Joint Surg. [Am.] 69:667–675, 1987.

Swank, S., Lonstein, J.E., Moe, J.H., et al.: Surgical treatment of adult scoliosis: A review of two hundred and twenty-two cases. J. Bone Joint Surg. [Am.] 63:268, 1981.

Weinstein, S.L., and Ponseti, I.V.: Curve progression in idiopathic scoliosis. J. Bone Joint Surg. [Am.] 65:447–455, 1983.

Winter, R.B., Lonstein, J.E., and Denis, F.: Pain patterns in adult scoliosis. Orthop. Clin. North Am. 19:339, 1988.

SACRUM

Denis, F., Davis, S., and Comfort, T.: Sacral fractures: An important problem retrospective analysis of 236 cases. Clin. Orthop. 227:67–81, 1988.

Newhouse, K.E., El-Khoury, G.Y., and Buckwalter, J.A.: Occult sacral fractures in osteopenic patients. J. Bone Joint Surg. [Am.] 75:1472–1477, 1992.

Postacchini, F., and Massobrio, M.: Idiopathic coccygodynia: Analysis of fifty-one operative cases and a radiographic study of the normal coccyx. J. Bone Joint Surg. [Am.] 65:1116–1124, 1983.

INFECTIONS, TUMORS

Allen, A.R., and Stevenson, A.W.: A ten-year follow-up of combined drug therapy and early fusion in bone tuberculosis. J. Bone Joint Surg. [Am.] 49:1001, 1967.

Batson, O.B.: The function of the vertebral veins and their role in the spread of metastases. Ann. Surg. 112:138–149, 1940.

Bohlman, H.H., Sachs, B.L., Carter, J.R., et al.: Primary neoplasms of the cervical spine: Diagnosis and treatment of twenty-three patients. J. Bone Joint Surg. [Am.] 68:483, 1986.

Eismont, F.J., Bohlman, H.H., Soni, P.L., et al.: Pyogenic and fungal vertebral osteomyelitis with paralysis. J. Bone Joint Surg. [Am.] 65:19–29, 1983.

Emery, S.E., Chan, D.P.K., and Woodward, H.R.: Treatment of hematogenous pyogenic vertebral osteomyelitis with anterior debridement and primary bone grafting. Spine 14:284, 1989.

Hodgson, A.R., Stock, F.E., Fang, H.S.Y., et al.: Anterior spinal fusion: The operative approach and pathological findings in 412 patients with Pott's disease of the spine. Br. J. Surg. 48:172, 1960.

Kostulk, J.P., Errica, T.J., Gleason, T.F., et al.: Spinal stabilization of vertebral column tumors. Spine 13:250, 1988.

McAfee, P.C., and Bohlman, H.H.: One-stage anterior cervical decompression and posterior stabilization with circumferential arthrodesis: A study of twenty-four patients who had a traumatic or neoplastic lesion. J. Bone Joint Surg. [Am.] 71:78, 1989.

Siegal, T., Tiqva, P., and Siegal, T.: Vertebral body resection for epidural compression by malignant tumors: Results of forty-seven consecutive operative procedures. J. Bone Joint Surg. [Am.] 67:375–382, 1985.

Weinstein, J.N., and MacLain, R.F.: Primary tumors of the spine. Spine 12:843–851, 1987.

COMPLICATIONS

Deyo, R.A., Cherkin, D.C., Loeser, J.D., et al.: Morbidity and mortality in association with operation on the lumbar spine. J. Bone Joint Surg. [Am.] 74:536, 1992.

Eismont, F.J., Wiesel, S.W., and Rothman, R.H.: The treatment of dural tears associated with spinal surgery. J. Bone Joint Surg. [Am.] 63:1132, 1981.

Farey, I.D., McAfee, P.C., Davis, R.F., et al.: Pseudarthrosis of the cervical spine after anterior arthrodesis: Treatment by posterior nerve-root decompression, stabilization and arthrodesis. J. Bone Joint Surg. [Am.] 72:1171, 1990.

Flynn, J.C., and Price, C.T.: Sexual complications of anterior fusion of the lumbar spine. Spine 9:489, 1984.

Kurz, L.T., Garfin, S.F., and Both, R.E.: Harvesting autologous iliac bone grafts: A review of complications and techniques. Spine 14:1324–1331, 1989.

Simpson, J.M., Silveri, C.P., Balderston, M.D., et al.: The results of operation on the lumbar spine in patients who have diabetes mellitus. J. Bone Joint Surg. [Am.] 75:1823–1829, 1993.

OTHER

Detwiler, K.N., Loftus, C.M., Godersky, J.C., et al.: Management of cervical spine injuries in patients with ankylosing spondylitis. J. Neurosurg. 72:210, 1990.

Graham, B., and Can Peteghem, P.K.: Fractures of the spine in ankylosing spondylitis: Diagnosis, treatment, and complications. Spine 14:803–807, 1989.

Simmons, E.H.: Kyphotic deformity of the spine in ankylosing spondylitis. Clin. Orthop. 128:65–77, 1977.

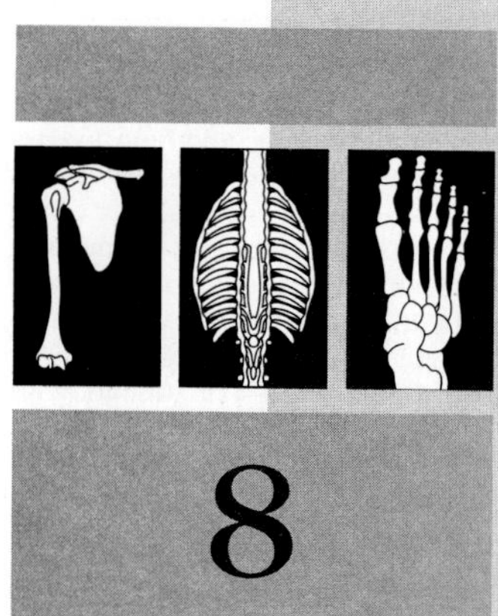

8

Orthopaedic Pathology

FRANK J. FRASSICA
DEBORAH A. FRASSICA
EDWARD F. McCARTHY

I. Introduction

A. Nomenclature—Primary bone lesions can be classified into three types: malignant bone tumors (sarcomas), benign bone tumors, and lesions that simulate bone tumors (reactive and miscellaneous conditions). Common lesions that are not of mesenchymal origin include metastatic bone disease, myeloma, and lymphoma. A common classification system for bone tumors is shown in Table 8-1. Sarcomas are malignant neoplasms of connective tissue (mesenchymal) origin. Sarcomas generally exhibit rapid growth in a centripetal fashion and invade adjacent normal tissues. Each year in the United States there are about 2800 new bone sarcomas. High-grade malignant bone tumors tend to destroy the overlying cortex and spread into the soft tissues. Low-grade tumors are generally contained within the cortex or a surrounding periosteal rim. Sarcomas metastasize primarily via the hematogenous route, with the lungs being the most common site. Benign bone tumors may be small and have a limited growth potential or may be large and destructive. Tumor simulators and reactive conditions are processes that occur in bone but are not true neoplasms (e.g., osteomyelitis, aneurysmal bone cyst, bone island).

B. Staging—Staging systems may be useful for developing evaluation strategies, planning treatment, and predicting prognosis. For musculoskeletal lesions the staging system of the Musculoskeletal Tumor Society (also called the Enneking system) is the most popular and useful. There are two systems: one for malignant lesions and one for benign lesions. For malignant lesions, the system is based on knowing the histologic grade of the lesion (low or high), the anatomic features (intracompartmental or extracompartmental), and the absence (M_0) or presence (M_1) of metastases.

1. Grade—Most malignant lesions are high-grade (G_2) (potential for distant metastases is >20%). Low-grade malignant (G_1) lesions are less common, with less than 10% chance of distant metastases. Grading of tumors requires a morphologic range, and most grading systems are based on three grades: grade 1, well differentiated; grade 2, moderately differentiated; grades 3 poorly differentiated. Grading can be difficult and is based on nuclear anaplasia (degree of loss of structural differentiation), pleomorphism (variations in size and shape), and nuclear hyperchromasia (increased nuclear staining). Commonly graded lesions are shown in Table 8-2. The grade of the tumor most strongly correlates with the potential for metastasis: Grade 1 (low grade), <10%; Grade 2 (intermediate grade), 10–30%; and Grade 3 (high grade), >30%.
2. Tumor Site—The plain radiographs and special studies, such as computed tomography (CT) and magnetic resonance imaging (MRI) scans, are inspected to determine whether the tumor is situated within the bone compartment (intracompartmental, or T_1) or has left the confines of the bone (extracompartmental, or T_2).
3. Metastases—For most lesions a chest radiograph and CT scan of the chest are performed to search for pulmonary lesions. A technetium bone scan is used to exclude the presence of other bone lesions.
4. The staging system can be synthesized into six distinct stages (Table 8-3).

C. Evaluation

1. Clinical Presentation—Most patients with bone tumors present with musculoskeletal pain. The pain is similar whether the bone destruction is secondary to a primary mesenchymal tumor (e.g., osteosarcoma, chondrosarcoma) or because of metastatic bone disease, myeloma, or lymphoma. The pain is typically deep seated and dull and may resemble a toothache.

Table 8-1. CLASSIFICATION OF PRIMARY TUMORS OF BONE*

HISTOLOGY TYPE	BENIGN	MALIGNANT
Hematopoietic		Myeloma
		Lymphoma
Chondrogenic	Osteochondroma	Primary chondrosarcoma
	Chondroma	Secondary chondrosarcoma
	Chondroblastoma	Dedifferentiated chondrosarcoma
	Chondromyxoid fibroma	Mesenchymal chondrosarcoma
		Clear cell chondrosarcoma
Osteogenic	Osteoid osteoma	Osteosarcoma
	osteoblastoma	Parosteal osteosarcoma
		Periosteal osteosarcoma
Unknown origin	Giant cell tumor	Ewing's tumor
	(Fibrous) histiocytoma	Malignant giant cell tumor
		Adamantinoma
Fibrogenic	Fibroma	Fibrosarcoma
	Desmoplastic fibroma	Malignant fibrous histiocytoma
Notochordal		Chordoma
Vascular	Hemangioma	Hemangioendothelioma
		Hemangiopericytoma
Lipogenic	Lipoma	
Neurogenic	Neurilemoma	

*Classification is based on that advocated by Lichtenstein, L.: Classification of primary tumors of bone. Cancer 4:335–341, 1951.

Initially, the pain may be intermittent and related to activity, a work injury, or a sporting injury. The pain usually progresses in intensity and becomes constant. Many patients experience pain at night. As the pain progresses, it is not relieved by nonsteroidal anti-inflammatory

Table 8-2. TYPICAL LOW-GRADE AND HIGH-GRADE BONE AND SOFT-TISSUE TUMORS

LOW-GRADE	HIGH-GRADE
Bone	
Parosteal osteosarcoma	Intramedullary (classic) osteosarcoma
Primary chondrosarcoma	
Secondary chondrosarcoma	Postradiation sarcoma
Hemangioendothelioma	Paget's sarcoma
Chordoma	Fibrosarcoma
Adamantinoma	Malignant fibrous histiocytoma
Soft Tissue	
Myxoid liposarcoma	Malignant fibrous histiocytoma
Lipoma-like liposarcoma	Pleomorphic liposarcoma
Angiomatoid malignant fibrous histiocytoma	Synovial sarcoma
	Rhabdomyosarcoma
	Alveolar cell sarcoma

Table 8-3. STAGING SYSTEM OF THE MUSCULOSKELETAL TUMOR SOCIETY (ENNEKING SYSTEM)

STAGE	GTM	DESCRIPTION
I-A	$G_1T_1M_0$	Low grade Intracompartmental No metastases
I-B	$G_1T_2M_0$	Low grade Extracompartmental No metastases
II-A	$G_2T_1M_0$	High grade Intracompartmental No metastases
II-B	$G_2T_2M_0$	High grade Extracompartmental No metastases
III-A	$G_{1/2}T_1M_1$	Any grade Intracompartmental With metastases
III-B	$G_{1/2}T_2M_1$	Any grade Extracompartmental With metastases

Grade system (G): low grade (G_1) and high grade (G_2). High-grade lesions are intermediate in grade between low-grade, well-differentiated tumors and high-grade, undifferentiated tumors.

Tumor size (T): Determined using specialized procedures, including radiography, tomography, nuclear studies, CT, and MRI. Compartments are used to describe the tumor site. Usually compartments are easily defined based on fascial borders in the extremities. Of note, the skin and subcutaneous tissues are classified as a compartment, and the periosseous potential space between cortical bone and muscle is often considered as a compartment as well.

T_0 lesions are confined within the capsule and within its compartment of origin. T_1 tumors have extracapsular extension into the reactive zone around it, but both the tumor and the reactive zone are confined within the compartment of origin. T_2 lesions extend beyond the anatomic compartment of origin by direct extension or otherwise (e.g., trauma, surgical seeding). Tumors that involve major neurovascular bundles are almost always classified as T_2 lesions.

Metastases (M): Regional and distal metastases both have an ominous prognosis; therefore the distinction is simply between no metastases (M_0) or the presence of metastases (M_1).

drugs (NSAIDs) or weaker narcotics (such as acetaminophen [Tylenol] with codeine). Most patients with a high-grade sarcoma will present with a 1–3 month history of pain. In contrast, with low-grade tumors such as chondrosarcoma, adamantinoma, and chordoma, there may be a long history of mild to moderate pain (6–24 months).

2. Physical Examination—Patients with suspected bone tumors should be examined carefully. The affected site is inspected for soft-tissue masses, overlying skin changes, adenopathy, and general musculoskeletal condition. When metastatic disease is suspected, the thyroid gland, abdomen, prostate, and breasts should be examined as appropriate.
3. Radiography—Plain radiographs in two planes are the first radiographic examinations to be performed. When the clinician suspects malignancy and the radiographs are normal, selected studies may follow. Technetium bone scans are an excellent modality to search for occult malignancies. In patients with myeloma for whom scan results may be negative, a skeletal

survey is more sensitive. MRI is an excellent modality for screening the spine for occult metastases, myeloma, or lymphoma. A chest radiograph should be obtained in all age groups when the clinician suspects a malignant lesion. The radiographs must be carefully inspected to formulate a working diagnosis. The working diagnosis then guides the clinician during further evaluation and treatment. Formulation of the differential diagnosis is based on several clinical and radiographic parameters.

a. Age of the Patient—Knowledge of common diseases in defined age groups is the first step. Certain diseases are uncommon in particular age groups (Table 8-4).
b. Number of Bone Lesions—Is the process monostotic or polyostotic? If there are multiple destructive lesions in middle-age to older patients (ages 40–80), the most likely diagnosis is metastatic bone disease, multiple myeloma, or lymphoma. In young patients (ages 15–40), multiple lytic and oval lesions are most likely a vascular tumor (hemangioendothelioma). In children below age 5, multiple destructive lesions may represent metastatic neuroblastoma or Wilms' tumor. Histiocytosis X may also lead to multiple lesions in the young patient. Fibrous dysplasia and Paget's disease may present with multiple lesions in all age groups.
c. Anatomic Location within Bone—Certain lesions have a predilection for occurring within a certain bone or a particular location. Adamantinoma is a malignant tumor that most commonly occurs in the tibia in young patients. Chondroblastoma most commonly occurs within the epiphysis of long bones. Giant cell tumor typically begins in the metaphysis and extends through the epiphysis to lie just below the cartilage. Ewing's tumor, in many cases, involves the diaphysis. Osteogenic sarcoma most commonly occurs in the metaphysis of the distal femur and proximal tibia but occurs within the diaphysis in about 7% of patients with long-bone lesions.
d. Effect of the Lesion on Bone—High-grade malignant lesions generally spread rapidly through the medullary cavity. Cortical bone destruction occurs early, and the process spreads into the adjacent soft tissues. Low-grade malignant lesions tend to spread slowly, but they can also destroy the cortical bone and produce a soft-tissue mass.
e. Response of the Bone to the Lesion—With high-grade lesions, there is often little ability of the host bone to contain the process; the result is rapid destruction of cortical bone and the presence of a soft-tissue mass. In contrast with low-grade lesions, the host bone can often contain the lesion with a thickened cortex or rim of periosteal bone. With benign or low-grade lesions, there is often a thick periosteal response about the lesion.
f. Matrix Characteristics—If the lesion produces a matrix, it is helpful to determine whether the matrix is cartilage calcification or mineralization of osteoid. Cartilage calcification often appears stippled or may show arcs or rings; osteoid mineralization is often cloud-like.

4. Laboratory Studies—They are often nonspecific. There are a set of routine studies that should be obtained for all patients when there is not an obvious diagnosis (Table 8-5). The studies can be grouped into those for younger patients (up to age 40) and those for older patients (40–80 years).
5. Biopsy—It is generally performed after complete evaluation of the patient. It is of great benefit to both pathologist and surgeon to have a narrow working diagnosis, as it allows accurate interpretation of the frozen section analysis and

Table 8-4. AGE DISTRIBUTION OF VARIOUS BONE LESIONS

AGE	MALIGNANT	BENIGN
Birth to 5 Years	Leukemia Metastatic neuroblastoma Metastatic rhabdomyosarcoma	Osteomyelitis Osteofibrous dysplasia
10–25 Years	Osteosarcoma Ewing's tumor Leukemia	Eosinophilic granuloma Osteomyelitis Enchondroma Fibrous dysplasia
40–80 Years	Metastatic bone disease Myeloma Lymphoma Paget's sarcoma Postradiation sarcoma	Hyperparathyroidism Paget's disease Mastocytosis

Table 8-5. LABORATORY EVALUATIONS FOR YOUNG AND MIDDLE-AGED PATIENTS

Age 5–40 Years
Complete blood count with differential Peripheral blood smear Erythrocyte sedimentation rate
Age 40–80 Years
Complete blood count with differential Erythrocyte sedimentation rate Chemistry group: calcium and phosphate Serum or urine protein electrophoresis Urinalysis

allows definitive treatment of some lesions based on the frozen section. There are several surgical principles, which the clinician must follow.

a. The orientation and location of the biopsy tract is critically important. If the lesion proves to be malignant, the entire biopsy tract must be removed with the underlying lesion. Transverse incisions should be avoided (Fig. 8-1).
b. The surgeon must maintain meticulous hemostasis to prevent hematoma formation and subcutaneous hemorrhage. When possible, biopsies are done through muscles so the muscle layer can be closed tightly. Tourniquets are utilized to obtain tissue in a bloodless field and then are released so bleeding points can be controlled. Avitene, Gelfoam, and Thrombostat sprays are used as necessary. If hemostasis cannot be achieved, a small drain should be brought out of the corner of the wound to prevent hematoma formation. A compression dressing is routinely used on the extremities.
c. A frozen section analysis is done on all biopsy samples to ensure that adequate diagnostic tissue is obtained. Before biopsy, the surgeon should review the radiographs with the pathologist to plan the biopsy site. When possible, the soft-tissue component should be sampled rather than the bony component.
d. It is an important tenet to remember that all biopsy samples should be submitted for bacteriologic analysis if the frozen section does not reveal a neoplasm. Antibiotics should not be delivered until the cultures are obtained.
e. Needle biopsy is an excellent method for achieving a tissue diagnosis and providing minimal tissue disruption. However, open biopsy remains the most reliable technique for avoiding incorrect diagnoses. When the nature of the lesion is obvious based on the radiographic features and adequate tissue can be obtained with needle biopsy, the needle biopsy technique is safe to use. The pathologist must be experienced and comfortable with the small sample of tissue.

6. Surgical Procedures—The goal of treatment of malignant bone tumors is to remove the lesion with minimal risk of local recurrence. Limb salvage is performed when two essential criteria are met: (1) local control of the lesion must be at least equal to that of amputation surgery; and (2) the limb that has been saved must be functional. A wide surgical margin (a cuff of normal tissue around the tumor) is the surgical goal. Surgical procedures are graded according to the system of the Musculoskeletal Tumor Society (Fig. 8-2).
   a. Intralesional—The plane of dissection goes directly through the tumor. When dealing with malignant mesenchymal tumors, an

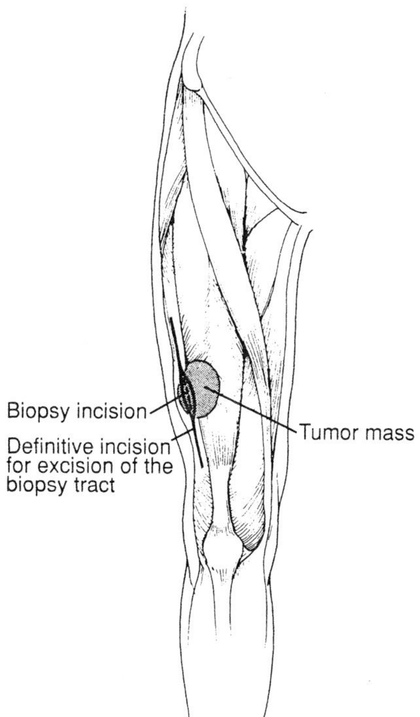

FIGURE 8-1 ■ Lesion in the lateral aspect of the quadriceps mechanism. A short longitudinal incision is made over the lesion. Before incising the skin a second incision line should be drawn to demonstrate how the biopsy tract can be removed at the time of the definitive surgery. (From Sim, F.H., Frassica, F.J., and Frassica, D.A.: Soft tissue tumors: diagnosis, evaluation and management. AAOS 2:209, 1994. Copyright 1994 American Academy of Orthopaedic Surgeons. Reprinted with permission.)

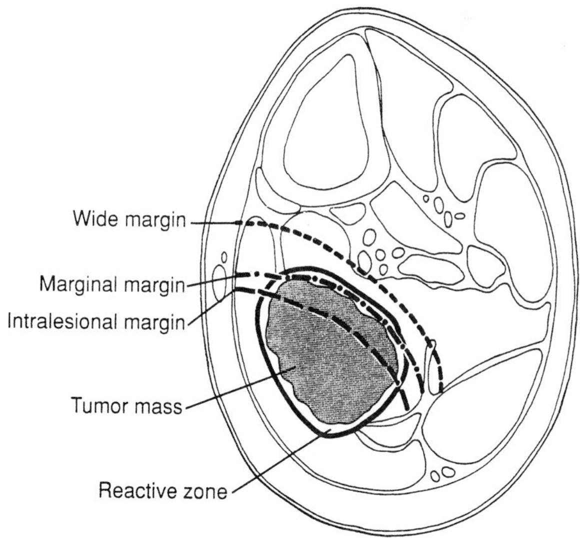

FIGURE 8-2 ■ Types of surgical margin. An intralesional line of resection enters the substance of the tumor. A marginal line of resection travels through the reactive zone of the tumor. A wide surgical margin removes the tumor with a cuff of normal tissue. (From Sim, F.H., Frassica, F.J., and Frassica, D.A.: Soft tissue tumors: diagnosis, evaluation and management. AAOS 2:209, 1994. Copyright 1994 American Academy of Orthopaedic Surgeons. Reprinted with permission.)

intralesional margin results in 100% local recurrence.

b. Marginal—A marginal line of resection goes through the reactive zone of the tumor; the reactive zone contains inflammatory cells, edema, fibrous tissue, and satellites of tumor cells. When resecting malignant mesenchymal tumors, a plane of dissection through the reactive zone will probably result in a local recurrence rate of 25–50%.

c. Wide—A wide surgical resection is accomplished when the entire tumor is removed with a cuff of normal tissue. The local recurrence rate drops below 10% when such a surgical margin is achieved.

d. Radical—A radical margin is achieved when the entire tumor and its compartment (all surrounding muscles, ligaments, and connective tissues) are removed.

7. Adjuvant Therapy

a. Chemotherapy—Multi-agent chemotherapy has a significant impact on both the efficacy of limb salvage and disease-free survival for osteogenic sarcoma and Ewing's tumor. Most protocols utilize preoperative regimens (called neo-adjuvant chemotherapy) for 8–12 weeks. Patients are then restaged and, if appropriate, limb salvage is performed. Patients then undergo maintenance chemotherapy for 6–12 months. Patients with localized disease have up to a 60–70% chance for long-term, disease-free survival with the combination of multi-agent chemotherapy and surgery (osteosarcoma and Ewing's tumor).

b. Radiation Therapy—External beam irradiation is utilized for local control of Ewing's tumor, lymphoma, myeloma, and metastatic bone disease. It is also utilized as an adjunct for the treatment of soft-tissue sarcomas, in which it is used in combination with surgery. The role of surgery in the treatment of Ewing's tumor is evolving. In some centers chemotherapy and surgery are the major forms of treatment, whereas in others traditional chemotherapy and external beam irradiation are preferred.

1. Postirradiation sarcoma is a devastating complication in which a spindle sarcoma occurs within the field of irradiation for a previous malignancy (e.g., Ewing's tumor, breast cancer, Hodgkin's disease). The histology is usually that of an osteosarcoma, fibrosarcoma, or malignant fibrous histiocytoma. Postirradiation sarcomas are probably more frequent in patients who undergo intensive chemotherapy (especially with alkylating agents) and irradiation.

2. Late stress fractures also may occur in weight-bearing bones to which high-dose irradiation has been applied. The subtrochanteric region and the diaphysis of the femur are common sites.

8. Molecular biology: Several bone and soft-tissue neoplasms have been associated with tumor suppressor genes or specific genetic defects. A low level of retinoblastoma (RB) gene has been associated with osteosarcoma. The TB53 gene has been found to also have low levels in both rhabdomyosarcoma and osteosarcoma. Gene translocations have been found in Ewing's sarcoma of bone (11:22) and several soft tissue sarcomas: myxoid liposarcoma (12:16), synovial sarcoma (X:18), and rhabdomyosarcoma (2:13) (Temple).

II. Soft-Tissue Tumors

A. Introduction—Soft-tissue tumors are common. Patients may have small lumps or large masses. Soft-tissue tumors can be broadly classified as benign, malignant (sarcomas), or reactive tumor-like conditions (Table 8-6). Lesions are classified according to the direction of differentiation of the lesion—whether the tumor is tending to produce

Table 8-6. CLASSIFICATION OF SOFT-TISSUE TUMORS

TUMORS AND TUMOR-LIKE LESIONS OF FIBROUS TISSUE	FIBROHISTIOCYTIC TUMORS
Benign	*Benign*
Fibroma	Fibrous histiocytoma
Nodular fasciitis	Atypical fibroxanthoma
Proliferative fasciitis	
Fibromatoses	*Intermediate (Dermatofibrosarcoma protuberans)*
Superficial fibromatoses	*Malignant (Malignant fibrous histiocytoma)*
Palmar and plantar fibromatosis	Storiform–pleomorphic
Knuckle pads	Myxoid (myxofibrosarcoma)
Deep fibromatoses (extra-abdominal fibromatoses)	Giant cell (malignant giant cell tumor of soft parts)
Malignant	Inflammatory (malignant xanthogranuloma, xanthosarcoma)
Adult fibrosarcoma	Angiomatoid
Postradiation fibrosarcoma	

Table 8-6. CLASSIFICATION OF SOFT-TISSUE TUMORS—cont'd

TUMORS AND TUMOR-LIKE CONDITIONS OF ADIPOSE TISSUE

Benign

Lipoma (cutaneous, deep, and multiple)
Angiolipoma
Spindle cell and pleomorphic lipoma
Lipoblastoma and lipoblastomatosis
Intramuscular and intermuscular lipoma
Hibernoma

Malignant

Liposarcoma
  Well differentiated (lipoma-like, sclerosing, inflammatory)
  Myxoid
  Round cell (poorly differentiated myxoid)
  Pleomorphic
  Dedifferentiated

TUMORS OF MUSCLE TISSUE

Smooth Muscle

Benign
  Leiomyoma (cutaneous and deep)
  Angiomyoma (vascular leiomyoma)
Malignant (leiomyosarcoma)

Striated Muscle

Benign (adult rhabdomyoma)
Malignant (rhabdomyosarcoma—predominantly embryonal [including botryoid], alveolar, pleomorphic, and mixed)

TUMORS OF LYMPH VESSELS

Benign (Lymphangioma)

Cavernous
Cystic (cystic hygroma)

Malignant

Lymphangiosarcoma
Postmastectomy lymphangiosarcoma

TUMORS AND TUMOR-LIKE LESIONS OF SYNOVIAL TISSUE

Benign

Giant cell tumor of tendon sheath
  Localized (nodular tenosynovitis)
  Diffuse (florid synovitis)

Malignant

Synovial sarcoma (malignant synovioma), predominantly biphasic (fibrous or epithelial) or monophasic (fibrous or epithelial)
Malignant giant cell tumor of tendon sheath

TUMORS AND TUMOR-LIKE LESIONS OF PERIPHERAL NERVES

Benign

Traumatic neuroma
Morton's neuroma
Neurilemoma (benign schwannoma)
Neurofibroma, solitary
Neurofibromatosis (von Recklinghausen's disease)
  Localized
  Plexiform
  Diffuse

Malignant

Malignant schwannoma
Peripheral tumors of primitive neuroectodermal tissues

TUMORS AND TUMOR-LIKE LESIONS OF CARTILAGE AND BONE-FORMING TISSUES

Benign

Panniculitis ossificans
Myositis ossificans
Fibrodysplasia (myositis) ossificans progressiva
Extraskeletal chondroma
Extraskeletal osteoma

Malignant

Extraskeletal chondrosarcoma
  Well differentiated
  Myxoid (choroid sarcoma)
  Mesenchymal
Extraskeletal osteosarcoma

TUMORS AND TUMOR-LIKE LESIONS OF PLURIPOTENTIAL MESENCHYME

Benign mesenchymoma
Malignant mesenchymoma

TUMORS AND TUMOR-LIKE CONDITIONS OF BLOOD VESSELS

Benign

Hemangioma
Deep hemangioma (intramuscular, synovial, perineural)
Glomus tumor

Intermediate (Hemangioendothelioma)

Malignant

Hemangiosarcoma
Malignant hemangiopericytoma

TUMORS AND TUMOR-LIKE CONDITIONS OF DISPUTED OR UNCERTAIN HISTOGENESIS

Benign

Tumoral calcinosis
Myxoma (cutaneous and intramuscular)

Malignant

Alveolar soft-part sarcoma
Epithelioid sarcoma
Clear cell sarcoma of tendons and aponeuroses
Extraskeletal Ewing's sarcoma

UNCLASSIFIED SOFT TISSUE TUMORS AND TUMOR-LIKE LESIONS

Adapted from Enzinger, F.M., and Weiss, S.W.: Soft Tissue Tumors. St. Louis, CV Mosby, 1983.

collagen (fibrous lesion), fat, or cartilage. The evaluation of patients with soft-tissue tumors must be systematic to avoid errors. Unplanned removal of a soft-tissue sarcoma is the most common error made by surgeons. Delay in diagnosis may also occur if the clinician does not recognize that the lesion is malignant. Patients who have a new soft-tissue mass or a soft-tissue mass that is growing or causing pain should undergo MRI. The MRI should be carefully reviewed with a radiologist to characterize the nature of the mass. If one can determine that the lesion is a benign process such as a lipoma, ganglion cyst, muscle tear, then the lesion is classified as a determinate lesion and one can plan treatment without doing a biopsy. In contrast, if one cannot determine the exact nature of a lesion, the lesion is classified as indeterminate, and either a needle or open biopsy is necessary to determine the exact diagnosis. Then treatment can be planned.

1. Benign Soft-Tissue Tumors—They may occur in all age groups. The lesions vary in their biologic behavior, from tumors that are asymptomatic and self-limited (Enneking stage 1—inactive) to growing and symptomatic (Enneking stage 2—active). Occasionally, benign lesions grow rapidly and invade adjacent tissues (Enneking stage 3—aggressive).
2. Malignant Soft-Tissue Tumors (Sarcomas)—Sarcomas are rare tumors of mesenchymal origin. In the United States each year there are approximately 7000 new cases of soft-tissue sarcomas. Patients often experience an enlarging painless or painful soft-tissue mass. Most sarcomas are large (>5 cm), deep, and firm in character. In some instances they are small and may be present for a long time prior to recognition. Lesions that may be initially small include synovial sarcoma, epithelioid sarcoma, and clear cell sarcoma. Initial radiographic evaluation begins with plain radiographs in two planes. MRI scans are the best imaging modality to define the anatomy and to help characterize the lesion. When a mass is judged to be indeterminate, an open incisional or needle biopsy is performed. Radiation therapy is an important adjunct to surgery in the treatment of soft-tissue sarcomas. The ionizing irradiation can be delivered preoperatively, perioperatively with brachytherapy after loading tubes, or postoperatively. Treatment regimens are often designed to use combinations of the three types of preoperative, postoperative, and external beam irradiation. Poor prognostic factors include: high grade, size greater than 5 cm, and location below the deep fascia.

B. Tumors of Fibrous Tissue—Fibrous tumors are common, and there is a wide range, from small self-limited benign conditions to aggressive, invasive benign tumors. The malignant fibrous tumors are fibrosarcoma and malignant fibrous histiocytoma.

1. Calcifying Aponeurotic Fibroma—This entity presents as a slowly growing, painless mass in the hands and feet in children and young adults, ages 3–30 (Enzinger). Radiographs may reveal a faint mass with stippling. Histologic examination shows a fibrous tumor with centrally located areas of calcification and cartilage formation. Local excision often results in recurrence (in up to 50% of cases); however, the condition appears to resolve with maturity.
2. Fibromatosis
   a. Palmar (Dupuytren's) and Plantar (Lederhosen) Fibromatosis—These disorders consist of firm nodules of fibroblasts and collagen that develop in the palmar and plantar fascia. The nodules and fascia hypertrophy, producing contractures.
   b. Extra-abdominal Desmoid Tumor—It is the most locally invasive of all benign soft-tissue tumors. It commonly occurs in adolescents and young adults. On palpation the tumor has a distinctive "rock-hard" character. Multiple lesions may be present in the same extremity (10–25%). Histologically, the tumor consists of well-differentiated fibroblasts and abundant collagen. The lesion infiltrates adjacent tissues. Surgical treatment is aimed at resecting the tumor with a wide margin. Local recurrence is common. Radiotherapy has been used as an adjunct to prevent recurrence and progression. The behavior of the tumor is capricious in that recurrent nodules may remain dormant for years or grow rapidly for some time and then stop growing.
3. Nodular Fasciitis—It is a common reactive lesion that presents as a painful, rapidly enlarging mass in a young person (age 15–35 years). Half of the cases occur in the upper extremity. Histologically, short, irregular bundles and fascicles, a dense reticulum network, and only small amounts of mature collagen characterize the lesion. Mitotic figures are common, but atypical mitoses are never seen. Treatment consists of excision with a marginal line of resection.
4. Malignant Fibrous Soft-Tissue Tumors—Malignant fibrous histiocytoma and fibrosarcoma are the two malignant fibrous lesions. They have a similar clinical and radiographic presentation and are treated in a similar manner. Patients are generally between the ages of 30 and 80 years. The most common presentation is an enlarging, rather painless mass. When the mass reaches a substantial size (>10 cm), the patient often experiences symptoms. Plain radiographs are usually normal, except in advanced cases where there may be bone erosion or destruction. MRI often shows a deep-seated inhomogeneous mass. Histologically, the two

lesions may be similar, but there are distinctive features. In malignant fibrous histiocytoma the spindle and histiocytic cells are arranged in a storiform (cartwheel) pattern. There are short fascicles of cells and fibrous tissue that appear to radiate about a common center around slit-like vessels (Enzinger). Chronic inflammatory cells may also be present. With fibrosarcoma, there is a fasciculated growth pattern with fusiform or spindle-shaped cells, scanty cytoplasm, and indistinct borders, and the cells are separated by interwoven collagen fibers (Enzinger). In some cases the tissue is organized into a herringbone pattern, which consists of intersecting fascicles in which the nuclei in one fascicle are viewed transversely, whereas in an adjacent fascicle they are viewed longitudinally. Treatment is wide local excision. Radiation therapy is employed in many cases when the size of the tumor exceeds 5 cm. A common scenario is to deliver radiation preoperatively (5000–5500 cGy), followed by resection of the lesion. A final radiation boost (2000 cGy) is then given postoperatively or perioperatively with brachytherapy after loading tubes if the margins are very close or positive.

5. Dermatofibrosarcoma Protuberans—This is a rare, nodular, cutaneous tumor that occurs in early to midadult life (Enzinger). The lesion is low grade. It has a tendency to recur locally, but it only rarely metastasizes, often after repeated local recurrences (Enzinger). In 40% of the cases it occurs on the upper or lower extremities (Enzinger). The tumor grows slowly but progressively. The central portion of the nodules shows uniform fibroblasts arranged in a storiform pattern around an inconspicuous vasculature. Wide resection is the best form of treatment.

C. Tumors of Fatty Tissue—There is a wide spectrum of benign and malignant tumors of fat origin. Each has a particular biologic behavior, which guides evaluation and treatment.

1. Lipomas—Lipomas are common benign tumors of mature fat. They may occur in a subcutaneous, intramuscular, or intermuscular location. Patients often describe a long history of a mass and sometimes a mass that was only recently discovered. Most are not painful. Plain radiographs may show a radiolucent lesion in the soft tissues if the lipoma is deep within the muscle or between the muscle and bone. CT or MRI shows a well-demarcated lesion with the same signal characteristics as mature fat on all sequences. If the patient experiences no symptoms, and the radiographic features are diagnostic of lipoma, no treatment is necessary. If the mass is growing or causing symptoms, excision with a marginal line of resection or an intralesional margin is all that is necessary. Local recurrence is uncommon. There are several variants of which the surgeon must be aware.
   a. Spindle Cell Lipoma—This lesion commonly occurs in male patients (age 45–65 years). The tumor presents as a solitary, painless, growing, firm nodule. Histologically, there is a mixture of mature fat cells and spindle cells. There is a mucoid matrix with a varying number of birefringent collagen fibers (Enzinger). Treatment is excision with a marginal margin.
   b. Pleomorphic Lipoma—This lesion is common in middle-aged patients and presents as a slowly growing mass. Histologically, there are lipocytes, spindle cells, and scattered bizarre giant cells. The lesion may be confused with different types of liposarcoma. Treatment is excision with a marginal margin.
   c. Angiolipoma—This lesion is the only lipoma that is very painful when palpated. Patients usually present with small nodules in the upper extremity that are intensely painful. MRI may show a small fatty nodule or completely normal results. Histologically, the lesion consists of mature fat cells (as in a typical lipoma) and nests of small arborizing vessels.

2. Liposarcoma—Liposarcomas are sarcomas in which the direction of differentiation is toward fatty tissue. They are a heterogeneous group of tumors, having in common the presence of lipoblasts (signet ring–type cells) in the tissue. Liposarcomas virtually never occur in the subcutaneous tissues. Liposarcomas are classified into the following types:

   Well-differentiated liposarcoma (low grade)
      Lipoma-like
      Sclerosing
      Inflammatory
   Myxoid liposarcoma (intermediate grade)
   Dedifferentiated (high grade)
   Round-cell liposarcoma (high grade)
   Pleomorphic liposarcoma (high grade)

   Liposarcomas metastasize according to the grade of the lesion: well-differentiated liposarcomas have a very low rate of metastasis (<10%); intermediate grade, 10–30%; and high grade, >50%.

D. Tumors of Neural Tissue—The two benign neural tumors are neurilemoma and neurofibroma. Their malignant counterpart is neurofibrosarcoma.

1. Neurilemoma (Benign Schwannoma)—This lesion is a benign nerve-sheath tumor. It occurs in the young to middle-aged adult (20–50 years) and is usually asymptomatic except for the presence of the mass. The tumor grows slowly and may wax and wane in size (cystic change). MRI studies may demonstrate an eccentric mass arising from a

peripheral nerve or only show an indeterminate soft tissue mass (low on T1-weighted images and high on T2). Histologically, the lesion is composed of Antoni's A and B areas.

a. Antoni's A—Compact spindle cells, usually having twisted nuclei, indistinct cytoplasm, and occasionally clear, intranuclear vacuoles. When the lesion is highly differentiated, there may be nuclear palisading, whorling of cells, and Verocay's bodies.
b. Antoni's B—Less orderly and cellular, the cells are arranged haphazardly in the loosely textured matrix (with microcystic change, inflammatory cells, and delicate collagen fibers); large, irregularly spaced vessels.
c. When the lesion is predominantly cellular (Antoni's A), the tumor may be confused with a sarcoma. Treatment consists in removing the eccentric mass while leaving the nerve intact.

2. Neurofibroma—It may be solitary or multiple (neurofibromatosis). Most are superficial, grow slowly, and are painless. When they involve a major nerve, they may expand it in a fusiform fashion. Histologically, there are interlacing bundles of elongated cells with wavy, dark-staining nuclei. The cells are associated with wire-like strands of collagen (Enzinger). Small to moderate amounts of mucoid material separate the cells and collagen. Treatment consists of excision with a marginal margin. Neurofibromatosis (von Recklinghausen's disease) is an autosomal dominant trait, with both a peripheral and central form of the disease. In addition to neurofibromas, patients have café-au-lait spots and variable skeletal abnormalities (nonossifying fibromas, scoliosis, and long-bone bowing). Malignant change occurs in 5-30% of patients. The presence of pain and an enlarging soft tissue may herald the presence of conversion to a sarcoma.
3. Neurofibrosarcoma—This is a rare tumor that arises de novo or in the setting of neurofibromatosis. Neurofibrosarcomas are high-grade sarcomas and are treated in a fashion similar to other high-grade sarcomas.

E. Tumors of Muscle Tissue—They are uncommon tumors ranging from benign leiomyoma and rhabdomyoma to the malignant entities of leiomyosarcoma and rhabdomyosarcoma. The benign entities seldom occur on the extremities.

1. Leiomyosarcoma—It may present as a small nodule or a large extremity mass. The lesions may or may not be associated with blood vessels. They may be either low- or high-grade and are treated as other low- and high-grade sarcomas.
2. Rhabdomyosarcoma—This highly malignant tumor is most common in young patients (<20 years of age). The tumor is the most common sarcoma in young patients and may grow rapidly. Histologically, the lesion is composed of spindle cells in parallel bundles, multinucleated giant cells, and racquet-shaped cells. The histologic hallmark is the appearance of cross striations within the tumor cells (rhabdomyoblasts). Rhabdomyoblasts may be difficult to find. Rhabdomyosarcomas are sensitive to multiagent chemotherapy. Wide surgical resection is performed after induction chemotherapy. External beam irradiation plays a prominent role in this tumor.

F. Vascular Tumors—Hemangiomas and glomus tumors are the two principal benign entities, and hemangiopericytoma and angiosarcoma are the less common malignant entities.

1. Hemangioma—This soft-tissue tumor is commonly seen in children and adults. The lesion may occur in a cutaneous, subcutaneous, or intramuscular location. Patients with large tumors complain of symptoms of vascular engorgement (aching, heaviness, swelling). MRI scans demonstrate a heterogeneous lesion with numerous small blood vessels and fatty infiltration. The clinician should examine the patient in both the supine and standing positions. Hemangiomas in the lower extremity will often fill with blood after several minutes. Plain radiographs may reveal small phleboliths. Nonoperative treatment is chosen if local measures adequately control discomfort: NSAIDs, vascular stockings, and activity modification. Many patients can be treated by sclerosing the hemangioma with a sclerosing agent, such as alcohol. This therapy is performed by interventional radiologists. Wide surgical resection is used for resistant cases, but the local recurrence rate is high.
2. Hemangiopericytoma—This rare tumor of the pericytes of blood vessels appears in benign and malignant forms. Within the malignant group, there is a morphologic range from intermediate- to high-grade malignancy. Patients present with a slowly enlarging painless mass. Hemangiopericytoma are malignant and are treated similar to other sarcomas with wide resection and radiation therapy in selected cases.
3. Angiosarcoma—In this rare tumor the tumor cells resemble the endothelium of blood vessels. Angiosarcomas are highly malignant lesions that are very infiltrative with a high local failure rate. Amputation surgery is frequently necessary to achieve local control. Pulmonary metastases are common.

G. Synovial Disorders—These entities include benign conditions, such as ganglia, and synovial proliferative disorders, such as pigmented villonodular synovitis and synovial chondromatosis.

1. Ganglia—It presents as an out pouching of the synovial lining of an adjacent joint. The most common locations include the wrist, foot, and knee. The cyst is filled with gelatinous, mucoid material. Histologically, the cyst wall is made up of paucicellular connective tissue without a true epithelial lining. With MRI scanning,

one finds a homogeneously low signal on T1-weighted images and a very bright signal on T2-weighted images. A contrast agent such as gadolinium is very useful to differentiate cyst from solid neoplasms because the cyst will not enhance (except a small rim at the periphery) and active neoplasms usually will.

2. Pigmented Villonodular Synovitis—This reactive condition (not a true neoplasm) is characterized by an exuberant proliferation of synovial villi and nodules. The process may occur locally within a joint or diffusely. The knee is most commonly affected, followed by the hip and shoulder. Patients present with pain and swelling in the affected joint. Recurrent, atraumatic hemarthroses are the hallmark of this disorder. Arthrocentesis demonstrates a bloody effusion. Cystic erosions may occur on both sides of the joint. Histologically, there are highly vascular villi lined with plump, hyperplastic synovial cells, hemosiderin-stained multinucleated giant cells, and chronic inflammatory cells. Treatment is aimed at complete synovectomy. Knee synovectomy can be accomplished by arthroscopy for resection of all the intra-articular disease, followed by open posterior synovectomy to remove the posterior extra-articular extension. Local recurrence is common (30–50%) despite complete synovectomy. External beam irradiation (3500–4000 cGy) can reduce the rate of local recurrence to 10–20%.
3. Giant Cell Tumor of Tendon Sheath—This benign nodular tumor occurs along the tendon sheaths of the hands and feet. Histologically, the lesion is moderately cellular (sheets of rounded or polygonal cells). There are hypocellular-collagenized zones (Enzinger). Multinucleated giant cells are common, as are xanthoma cells. Treatment consists in resection with a marginal margin. Local recurrence is common and usually treated with repeat excision.
4. Synovial Chondromatosis—This synovial proliferative disorder occurs within joints or bursae, ranging in appearance from metaplasia of the synovial tissue to firm nodules of cartilage. The lesion typically affects young adults who present with pain, stiffness, and swelling. Radiographs may demonstrate fine, stippled calcification. Treatment consists in removing the loose bodies and synovectomy.
5. Synovial Sarcoma—This highly malignant tumor occurs proximal to joints but rarely arises from an intra-articular location. The tumor may be present for years or present as a rapidly enlarging mass. Synovial sarcoma is the most common sarcoma in the foot. Radiographs may show mineralization within the lesion (in up to 25% of cases). The spotty mineralization may even resemble the peripheral mineralization seen in heterotopic ossification. Histologically, the tumor is biphasic, with an epithelial component and a spindle cell component. The epithelial component may show epithelial cells that form glands or nests, or they may line cyst-like spaces. Regional lymph nodes may be involved. All synovial sarcomas are high-grade lesions. Wide surgical resection with adjuvant radiotherapy is the most common method of treatment. Metastases develop in 30–60%. Larger tumors (>5–10 cm) are more prone to distant spread.

H. Other Rare Sarcomas
1. Epithelioid Sarcoma—This rare nodular tumor commonly occurs in upper extremities of young adults. It may also occur about the buttock/thigh, knee, or foot. Epithelioid sarcoma is the most common sarcoma in the hand. The lesion may ulcerate and mimic a granuloma or rheumatoid nodule. Lymph node metastases are common. Histologically, the cells range from ovoid to polygonal, with deeply eosinophilic cytoplasm (Enzinger). Cellular pleomorphism is minimal. The lesions are often misdiagnosed as benign processes. Wide-margin surgical resection is necessary to prevent local recurrence.
2. Clear Cell Sarcoma—This tumor presents as a slowly growing mass associated with tendons or aponeuroses. The lesion most commonly occurs about the foot and ankle but may also involve the knee, thigh, or hand. Microscopically, it is characterized by compact nests or fascicles of rounded or fusiform cells with clear cytoplasm (Enzinger). Multinucleated giant cells are common. Wide surgical resection with adjuvant irradiation is the treatment of choice.
3. Alveolar Cell Sarcoma—It presents as a slowly growing, painless mass in young adults (ages 15–35 years). It most commonly occurs in the anterior thigh. Microscopically, it appears as dense fibrous trabeculae dividing the tumor into an organoid or nest-like arrangement (Enzinger). Cells are large and rounded and contain one or more vesicular nuclei with small nucleoli. Vascular invasion is prominent. Treatment is wide-margin surgical resection with adjuvant irradiation in selected cases.

I. Post-Traumatic Conditions
1. Hematoma—Hematoma may occur after trauma to the extremity. The lesion organizes and resolves with time. Sarcomas may spontaneously hemorrhage into the body of the tumor or following minor trauma and masquerade as a benign process. Clinicians should follow patients with hematomas at 6-week intervals until the mass resolves. MRI scanning is often not able to distinguish a simple hematoma from a sarcoma with spontaneous hemorrhage.
2. Myositis Ossificans (Heterotopic Ossification)—It occurs after single or repetitive episodes of trauma. Occasionally, patients cannot recall the traumatic episode. The most common locations are over the diaphyseal segment of long bones (in the midaspect of the muscle bellies).

As maturation progresses, radiographs show peripheral mineralization with a central lucent area. In most cases the lesion is not attached to the underlying bone, but in some cases it may become fixed to the periosteal surface. Histologically, there is a zonal pattern with mature, trabecular bone at the periphery and immature tissue in the center. When the diagnosis is apparent, nonoperative treatment is all that is necessary.

III. Bone Tumors

A. Introduction—All bone lesions can be subdivided into three groups: benign bone neoplasms, malignant bone neoplasms, and non-neoplastic lesions (also called tumor-like conditions, tumor simulators, and reactive conditions). Lesions can be further subclassified into processes that begin in the bone (intramedullary lesions) and processes that clearly begin outside the intramedullary cavity (surface lesions).

B. Bone-Producing Lesions—There are only three lesions in which the tumor cells produce osteoid: osteoid osteoma, osteoblastoma, and osteosarcoma.

1. Osteoid Osteoma (Fig. 8-3)—This self-limited benign bone lesion produces pain in young patients (ages 5–30 years, although all age groups may be affected). Patients present with pain that increases with time. Most patients have pain at night, which may be strikingly relieved by salicylates. The pain may be referred to an adjacent joint, and when the lesion is intracapsular, it may simulate arthritis. The tumor may produce painful scoliosis, growth disturbances, and flexion contractures. Common locations include the proximal femur, tibial diaphysis, and spine (Fig. 8-4). The radiographs usually show intensely reactive bone and a radiolucent nidus. It may be possible to detect the lesion with special studies only, such as tomograms, CTs, or MRI scans, because of the intense sclerosis. The nidus is by definition always <1.5 cm, although the area of reactive bone sclerosis may be quite long. Technetium bone scan results are always positive and show intense focal uptake. Microscopically, there is a distinct demarcation between the nidus and the reactive bone. The nidus consists of an interlacing network of osteoid trabeculae with variable mineralization. The trabecular organization is haphazard, and the greatest degree of mineralization is in the center of the lesion. Treatment consists of complete removal of the nidus by curettage with hand and power instruments. Patients may also be treated nonoperatively with NSAIDs. About 50% of patients treated with NSAIDs will have their lesions burn out with no further medical or surgical treatment necessary. A new treatment that is gaining popularity is percutaneous radio frequency ablation of the osteoid osteoma. Under CT guidance, a radio frequency probe is placed into the lesion, and the nidus is heated up to 80°C. About 90% of selected patients can be successfully treated with radio frequency ablation.
2. Osteoblastoma (Fig. 8-5)—This rare bone-producing tumor can attain a large size and is not self-limited as is osteoid osteoma. Patients present with pain, and when the lesion involves the spine, neurologic symptoms may be present. Common locations include the spine, proximal humerus, and hip. Radiographically, there is bone destruction with or without the characteristic reactive bone formation in osteoid osteoma. The bone destruction occasionally has a moth-eaten or permeative character simulating a malignancy. Histologically, the lesions show regularly shaped nuclei containing little chromatin but abundant cytoplasm (Dahlin). The tissue is loosely arranged with numerous blood vessels. The lesion does not permeate the normal trabecular bone but, rather, merges with them. Treatment consists of curettage.
3. Osteosarcoma—Spindle cell neoplasms that produce osteoid are arbitrarily classified as osteosarcoma. There are many types of osteosarcoma (Table 8-7 and Fig. 8-6). The lesions that must be recognized (to have a reasonable grasp on the entity osteosarcoma) include high-grade intramedullary osteosarcoma (ordinary or classic osteosarcoma), parosteal osteosarcoma, periosteal osteosarcoma, telangiectatic osteosarcoma, osteosarcoma occurring with Paget's disease, and osteosarcoma following irradiation.
   a. High-Grade Intramedullary Osteosarcoma (Fig. 8-7)—Also called ordinary or classic osteosarcoma, it is the most common type of osteosarcoma and most commonly occurs about the knee in children and young adults (Fig. 8-8). Other common sites include the proximal humerus, proximal femur, and pelvis. Patients present primarily with pain. More than 90% of intramedullary osteosarcomas are high grade and penetrate the cortex early to form a soft-tissue mass (stage IIB lesion). About 10–20% of patients have pulmonary metastases at presentation. Plain radiographs demonstrate a lesion in which there is bone destruction and bone formation. Occasionally, the lesion is purely sclerotic or lytic. MRI or CT scans are useful for defining the anatomy of the lesion in regard to intramedullary extension, involvement of neurovascular structures, and muscle invasion. Histologically, two criteria are utilized: (1) the tumor cells produce osteoid, and (2) the stromal cells are frankly malignant. The lesions may be highly heterogeneous in appearance,

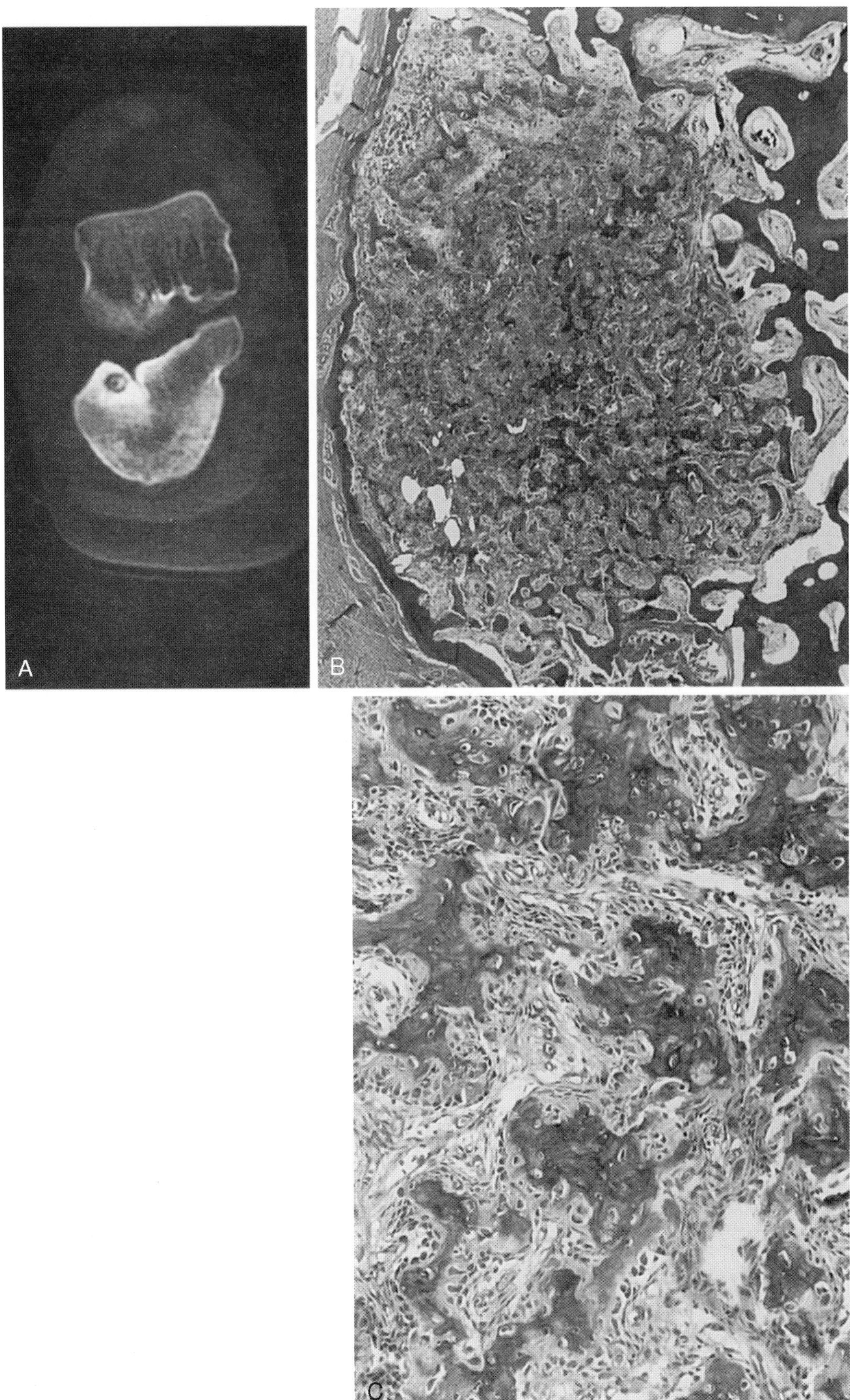

FIGURE 8-3 ■ Osteoid osteoma of the calcaneus. *A,* Radiograph shows a well-circumscribed lytic lesion with dense surrounding bone and a central nidus. *B,* Low-power photomicrograph (×25) shows the nidus. *C,* Higher-power photomicrograph (×160) shows mineralizing new bone with a loose fibrovascular stroma.

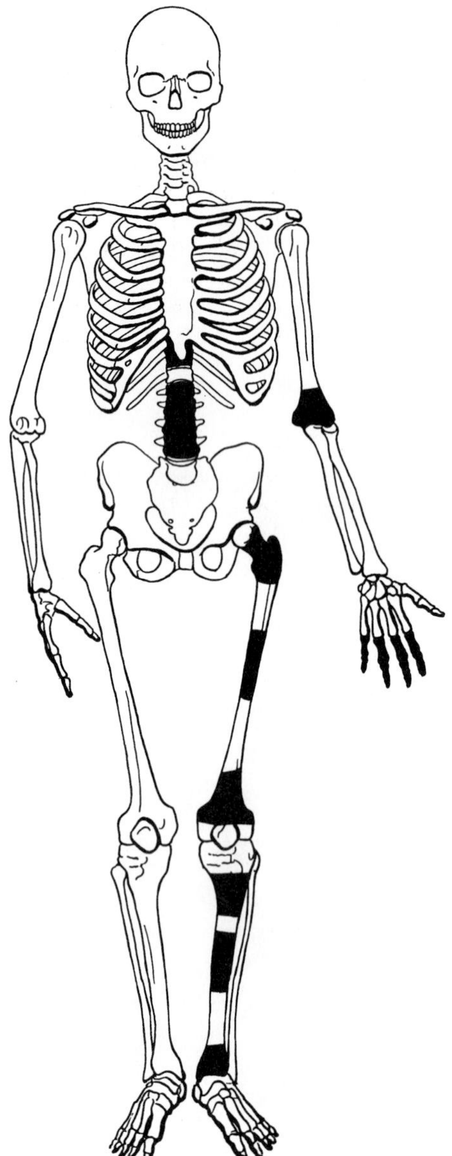

FIGURE 8-4 ■ Skeletal distribution of the most common sites of osteoid osteoma. (From McCarthy, E.F., and Frassica, F.J.: Pathology of Bone and Joint Disorders. Philadelphia, WB Saunders, 1998.)

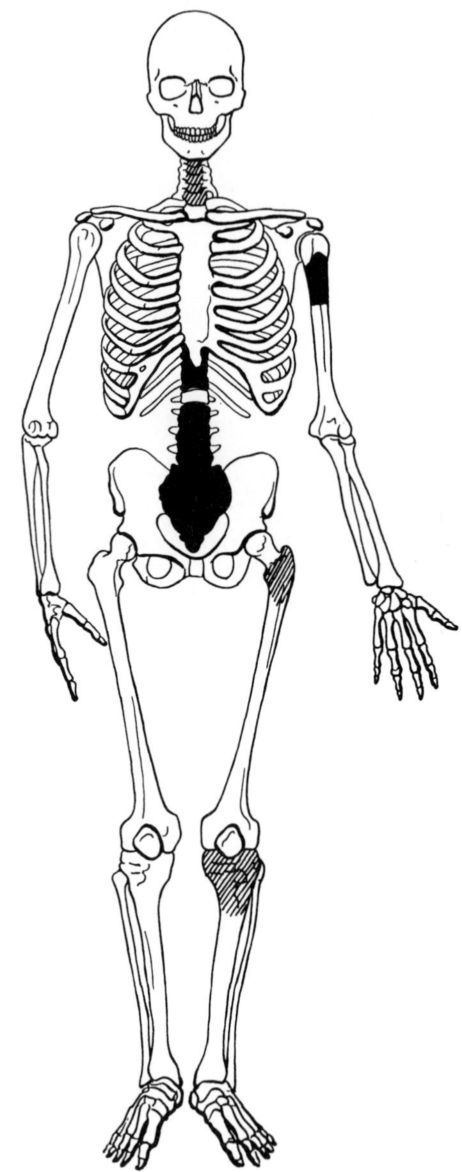

FIGURE 8-5 ■ Skeletal distribution of the most common sites of osteoblastoma. (From McCarthy, E.F., and Frassica, F.J.: Pathology of Bone and Joint Disorders. Philadelphia, WB Saunders, 1998.)

Table 8-7. CLASSIFICATION OF OSTEOSARCOMA

High-grade central osteosarcoma
Low-grade central osteosarcoma
Telangiectatic osteosarcoma
Surface osteosarcomas
Parosteal osteosarcoma
Periosteal osteosarcoma
High-grade surface osteosarcoma
Osteosarcoma of the jaw
Multicentric osteosarcoma
Secondary osteosarcomas
Osteosarcoma in Paget's disease
Postradiation osteosarcoma
Dedifferentiated chondrosarcoma
Osteosarcoma derived from benign precursors

with some lesions being predominantly chondroblastic, osteoblastic, or fibroblastic. Other lesions may contain large numbers of giant cells or predominantly small cells rather than spindle cells. Telangiectatic osteosarcoma is a type in which the lesional tissue can be described as a bag of blood with few cellular elements. The cellular elements present are highly malignant in appearance. The radiographic features of telangiectatic osteosarcoma are those of a destructive, lytic, expansile lesion. Telangiectatic osteosarcomas occur in the same locations as aneurysmal bone cysts, and their radiographic appearances can be confused with each other (Fig. 8-9). Historically, osteosarcoma was treated by amputation; long-term studies show a survival of only 10–20%, with the pulmonary system

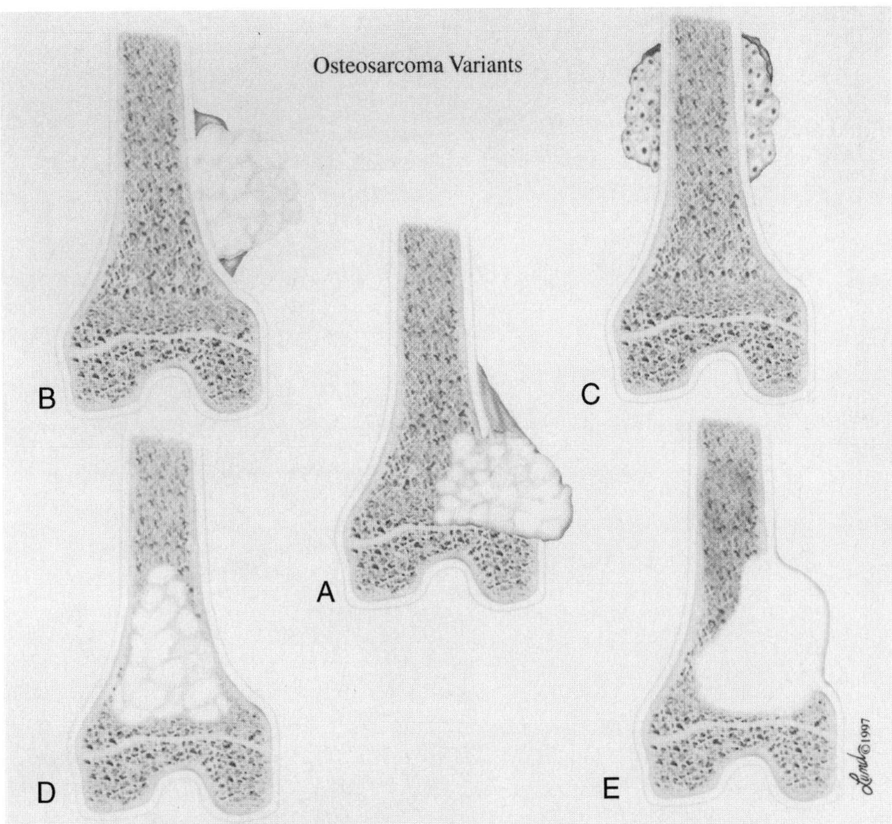

FIGURE 8-6 ■ Artist's depiction of the different types of osteosarcoma of bone. *B* and *C* depict the low-grade variants of osteosarcoma: parosteal osteosarcoma and well-differentiated intramedullary osteosarcoma. Parosteal osteosarcoma arises from the surface of the bone with a broad cortical attachment. The tumor grows in a lobulated fashion. In contrast, well-differentiated intramedullary osteosarcoma stays within the medullary cavity and usually does not break through the cortex. Both of these lesions are heavily mineralized. In contrast, *A* shows a destructive process that has destroyed the distal metaphysis and extended into the soft tissues. The cortical bone destruction and extension into the soft tissues is typical of a high-grade intramedullary osteosarcoma. *C*, which shows a lesion arising from the cortex with a lobular pattern suggestive of cartilage, is a periosteal osteosarcoma. In this surface tumor there is osteoid production by the cells, but there is a predominance of cartilage. *E* shows a very destructive lytic lesion with no bone production. The overlying cortex has been destroyed with extension into the soft tissues. This pattern of bone destruction occurs in telangiectatic osteosarcoma. (From McCarthy, E.F., and Frassica, F.J.: Pathology of Bone and Joint Disorders. Philadelphia, WB Saunders, 1998.)

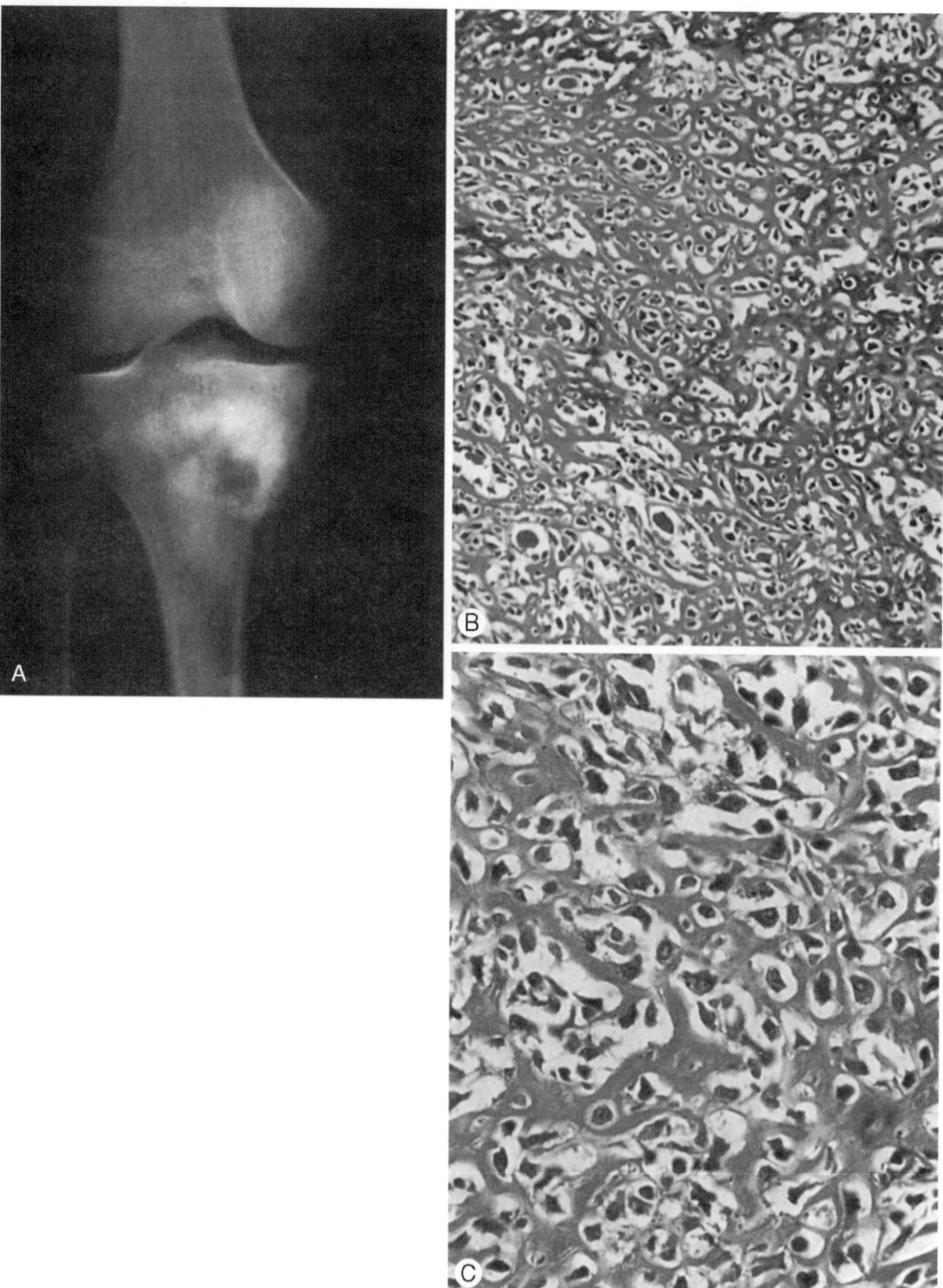

FIGURE 8-7 ■ Conventional osteoblastic osteosarcoma of the proximal tibia. *A,* Radiograph shows a poorly defined osteoblastic lesion in the proximal tibial metaphysis. *B,* Low-power photomicrograph (×160) shows lace-like mineralizing osteoid surrounding atypical osteoblasts. *C,* Higher-power photomicrograph (×400).

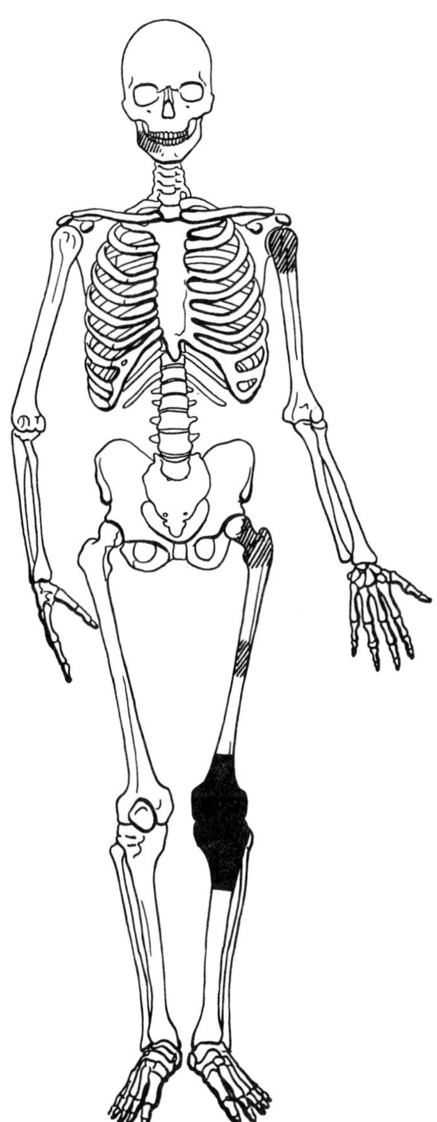

FIGURE 8-8 ■ Conventional osteosarcoma locations. (From McCarthy, E.F., and Frassica, F.J.: Pathology of Bone and Joint Disorders. Philadelphia, WB Saunders, 1998.)

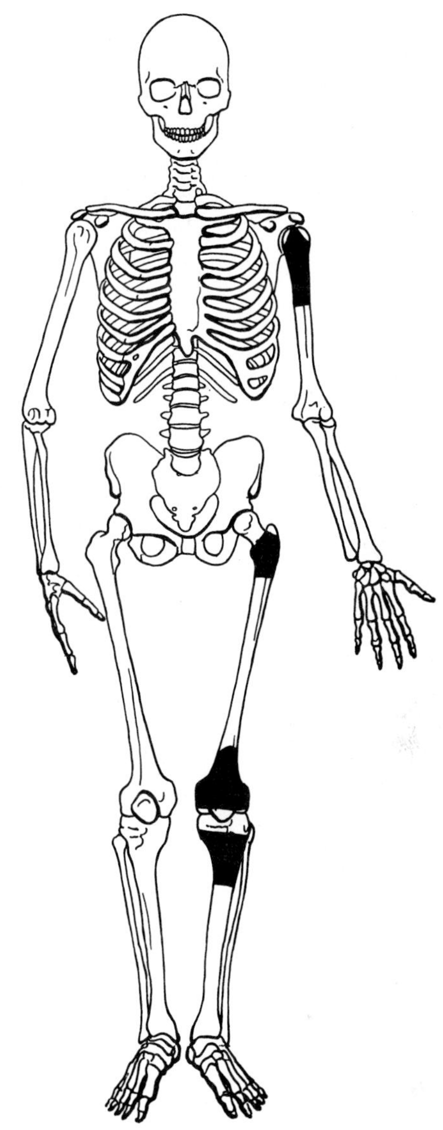

FIGURE 8-9 ■ Telangiectatic osteosarcoma locations. (From McCarthy, E.F., and Frassica, F.J.: Pathology of Bone and Joint Disorders. Philadelphia, WB Saunders, 1998.)

being the most common site of failure. Multi-agent chemotherapy has dramatically improved long-term survival and the potential for limb salvage. It effectively destroys the malignant cells, and in many patients there is total necrosis of the tumor. The chemotherapy kills both the micrometastases that are present in 80–90% of the patients at presentation and sterilizes the reactive zone around the tumor. Preoperative chemotherapy is delivered for 8–12 weeks, followed by resection of the tumor. Staging studies are performed at the end of chemotherapy to ensure that the lesion is resectable. Maintenance chemotherapy is then given for 6–12 months. Long-term survival is approximately 60–70% with these regimens. Prognostic factors that adversely affect survival include: (1) expression of P-glycoprotein, high-serum alkaline phosphatase, high lactic dehydrogenase, vascular invasion, no alteration of DNA ploidy following chemotherapy, and (2) the absence of antishock protein 90 antibodies after chemotherapy.

b. Parosteal Osteosarcoma (Fig. 8-10)—This low-grade osteosarcoma occurs on the surface of the metaphysis of long bones. Patients often complain of a painless mass. The most common sites are the posterior aspect of the distal femur, proximal tibia, and proximal humerus (Fig. 8-11); the lesion is more common in females than in males. The radiographic appearance is characteristic in that it demonstrates a heavily ossified, often lobulated mass arising from

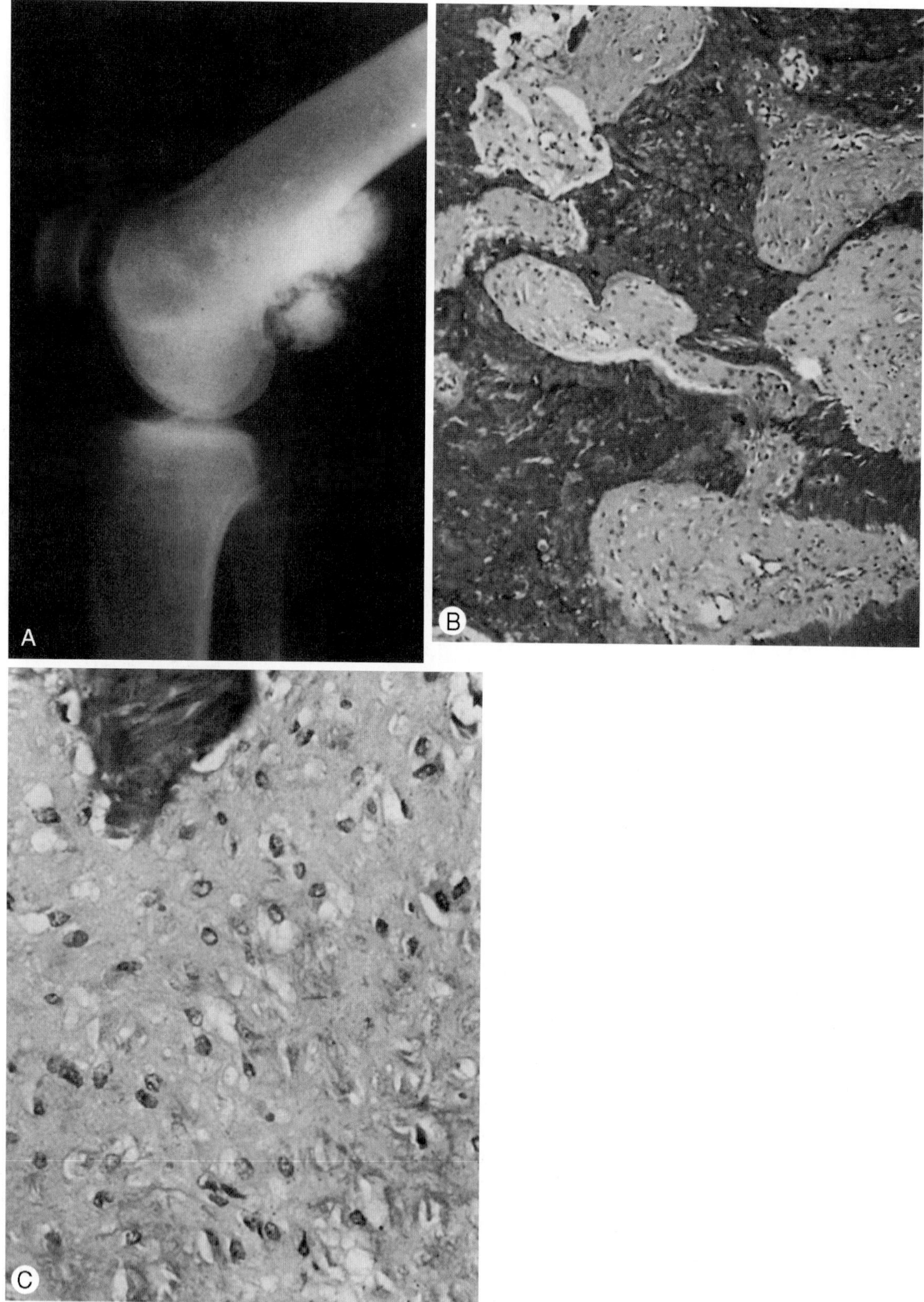

FIGURE 8-10 ■ Parosteal osteosarcoma of the distal femur. *A,* Radiograph shows an exophytic bony mass in the posterior distal femur. *B,* Low-power photomicrograph (×160) shows plates of new bone in a fibrous matrix. *C,* Higher-power photomicrograph (×400) shows a fibrous stroma with atypical cells.

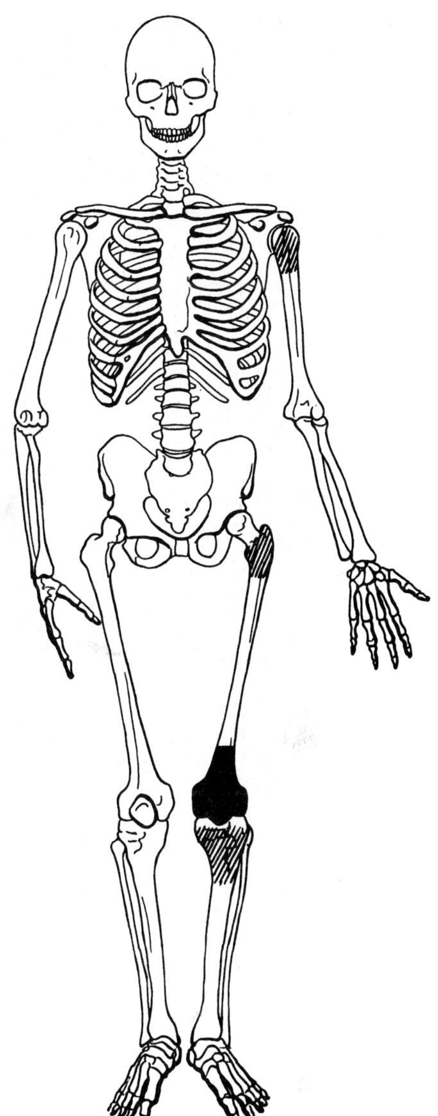

FIGURE 8-11 ■ Skeletal distribution of the most common sites of parosteal osteosarcoma. (From McCarthy, E.F., and Frassica, F.J.: Pathology of Bone and Joint Disorders. Philadelphia, WB Saunders, 1998.)

the cortex. Histologically, the most prominent feature is regularly arranged osseous trabeculae (Dahlin). Between the nearly normal trabeculae are slightly atypical spindle cells. At the periphery of the tumor are spindle cells, which typically invade skeletal muscle. Interestingly, cartilage is frequently present and may be arranged as a cap over the lesion. Treatment of parosteal osteosarcoma is wide-margin surgical resection, which is usually curative. In approximately one-sixth of the lesions that appear radiographically to be parosteal osteosarcoma, there is a high-grade malignancy. In this setting the lesion is called a dedifferentiated parosteal osteosarcoma. For typical low-grade parosteal osteosarcomas, chemotherapy or irradiation is not needed; however, the prognosis is much worse for dedifferentiated parosteal osteosarcomas, and multi-agent chemotherapy is an important component of therapy. When local control has been achieved in parosteal osteosarcoma, the prognosis is excellent, with >95% long-term survival. Invasion into the medullary cavity does not adversely affect long-term survival. Dedifferentiation is a poor prognostic factor.

c. Periosteal Osteosarcoma (Fig. 8-12)—This rare surface form of osteosarcoma occurs most commonly in the diaphysis of long bones (typically the femur or tibia) (Fig. 8-13). The radiographic appearance is fairly constant; a sunburst-type lesion rests on a saucerized cortical depression. Histologically, the lesion is predominantly chondroblastic, and the grade of the lesion is intermediate (grade 2 or 3). Highly anaplastic regions are not found. The prognosis for periosteal osteosarcoma is

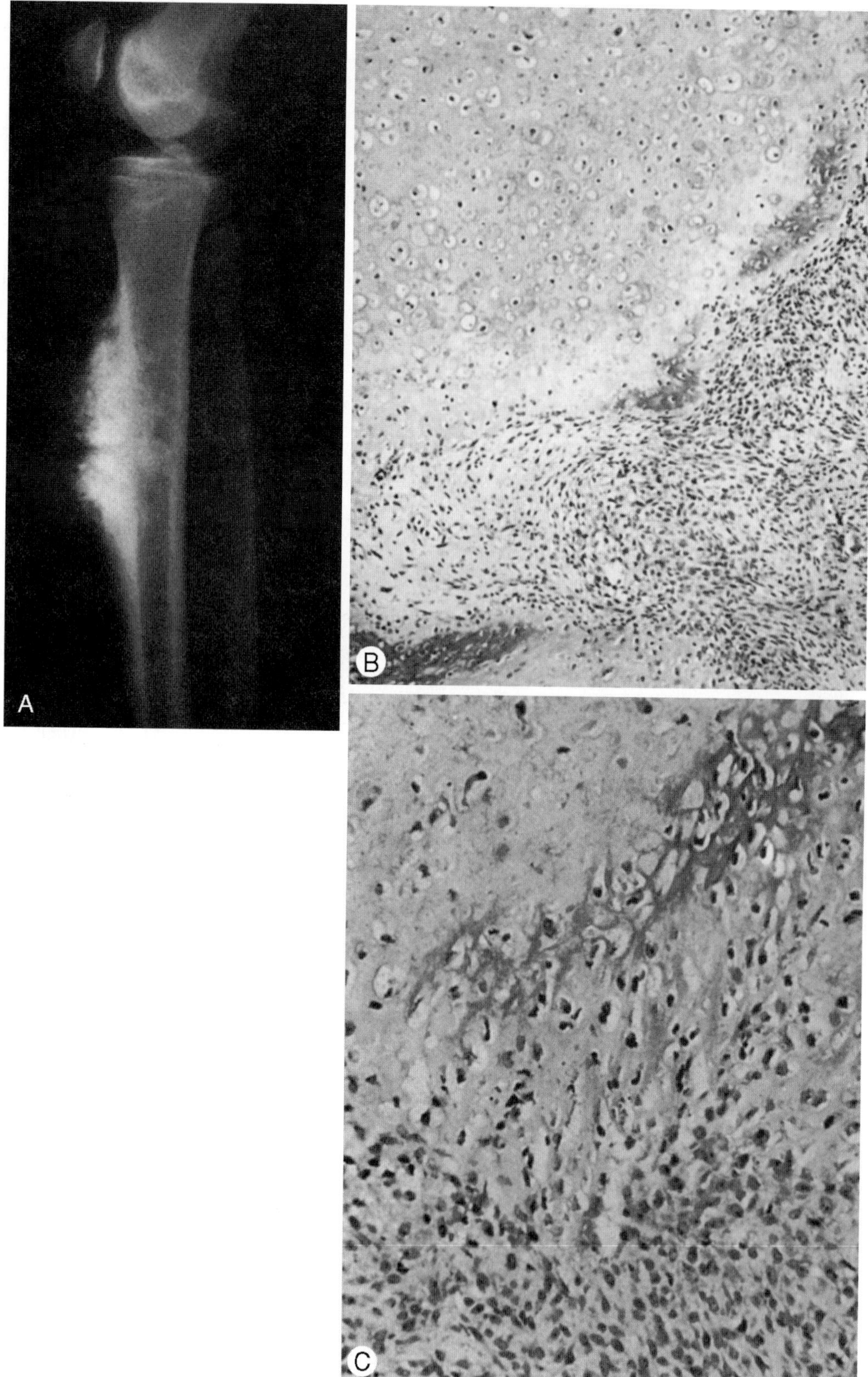

FIGURE 8-12 ■ Periosteal osteosarcoma of the diaphysis of the tibia. *A,* Lateral radiograph showing a surface lesion with bone formation. *B,* Low-power photomicrograph (×160) showing cartilage and bone formation. *C,* Higher-power photomicrograph showing pleomorphism and direct production of osteoid by the tumor cells.

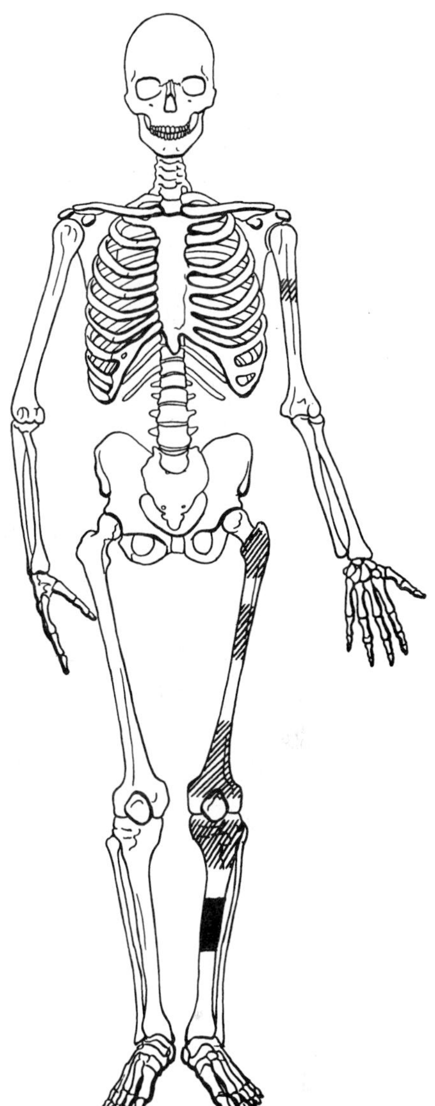

FIGURE 8-13 ■ Skeletal distribution of the most common sites of periosteal osteosarcoma. (From McCarthy, E.F., and Frassica, F.J.: Pathology of Bone and Joint Disorders. Philadelphia, WB Saunders, 1998.)

intermediate between parosteal osteosarcoma (very low-grade) and high-grade intramedullary osteosarcoma. Preoperative chemotherapy, wide-margin surgical resection, and maintenance chemotherapy comprise the preferred treatment. The risk of pulmonary metastases is 20–35%.

C. Chondrogenic Lesions—The principal benign cartilage lesions are chondromas, osteochondroma, chondromyxoid fibroma, and chondroblastoma (Fig. 8-14). The common malignant cartilage tumors are intramedullary chondrosarcoma and dedifferentiated chondrosarcoma. Clear cell chondrosarcoma and mesenchymal chondrosarcoma are rare forms.

1. Chondromas (Fig. 8-15)—These benign cartilage tumors may occur in the medullary cavity or on the surface of the bone (periosteal chondroma). Enchondromas are benign cartilage lesions that are most commonly localized in the metaphysis of long bones, especially the proximal femur and humerus and the distal femur (Fig. 8-16). They are common in the hand, where they usually occur in the diaphysis and metaphysis (Dahlin). Pathologic fractures in the hand are common. Involvement of the epiphysis is rare. Most enchondromas are asymptomatic. Radiographically, in long bones there may be a prominent stippled or mottled calcified appearance. Occasionally, active lesions are purely lytic without evidence of mineralization. Most enchondromas require no treatment other than observation. Histologically, they are composed of small cells that lie in lacunar spaces. The lesion is usually hypocellular, and the cells have a bland appearance (no pleomorphism, anaplasia, or hyperchromasia). In contrast, lesions in the hand may be hypercellular and display worrisome histologic features. When lesions

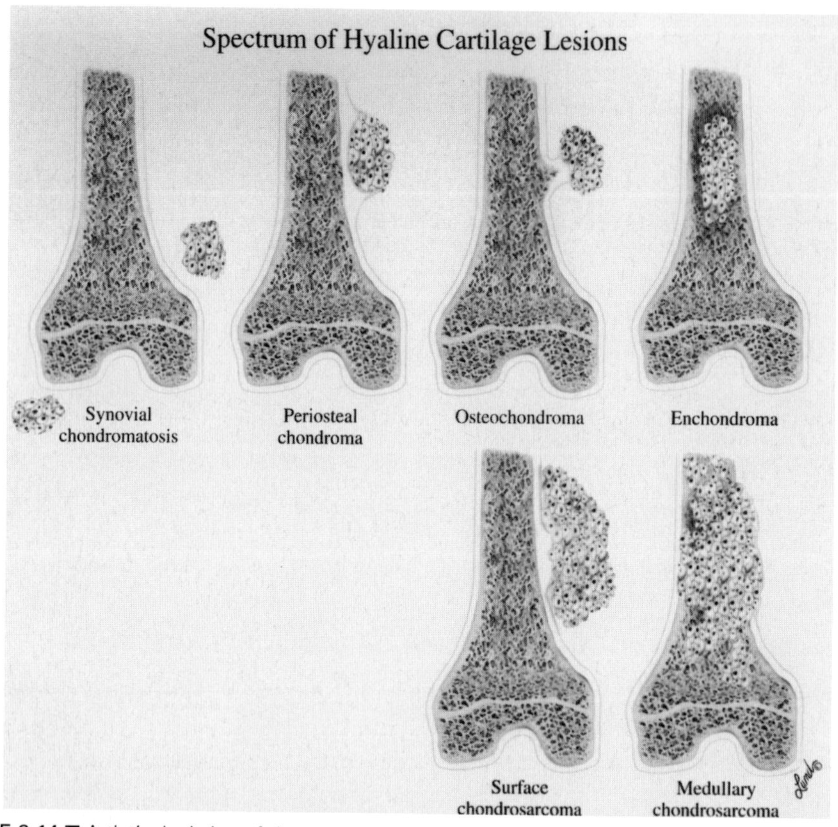

FIGURE 8-14 ■ Artist's depiction of the common types of cartilage tumors. *(Top left)* Lobular pattern of cartilage in synovial chondromatosis. *(Second from left)* Surface tumor of bone composed of mature cartilage that sits in a saucer-shaped depression on the bone's surface. These lesions are called periosteal chondromas. *(Third from left)* Surface tumor in which the cortices are continuous between the surface lesion and the host cortex. On top of the bone sits a thin rim of cartilage (1–3 mm). This lesion is called an osteochondroma and is one of the most common benign cartilage tumors. *(Fourth from left)* Enchondroma. Notice that this benign cartilage tumor sits in the medullary cavity in a quiescent manner. There are no cortical changes, such as erosions, cortical thickening, or cortical bone destruction. In contrast, *(bottom right)* shows destruction of the cortex and extension into the soft tissues. This is a medullary chondrosarcoma with active growth. In this instance the cartilage is growing and destroying the bone rather than being quiescent. (From McCarthy, E.F., and Frassica, F.J.: Pathology of Bone and Joint Disorders. Philadelphia, WB Saunders, 1998.)

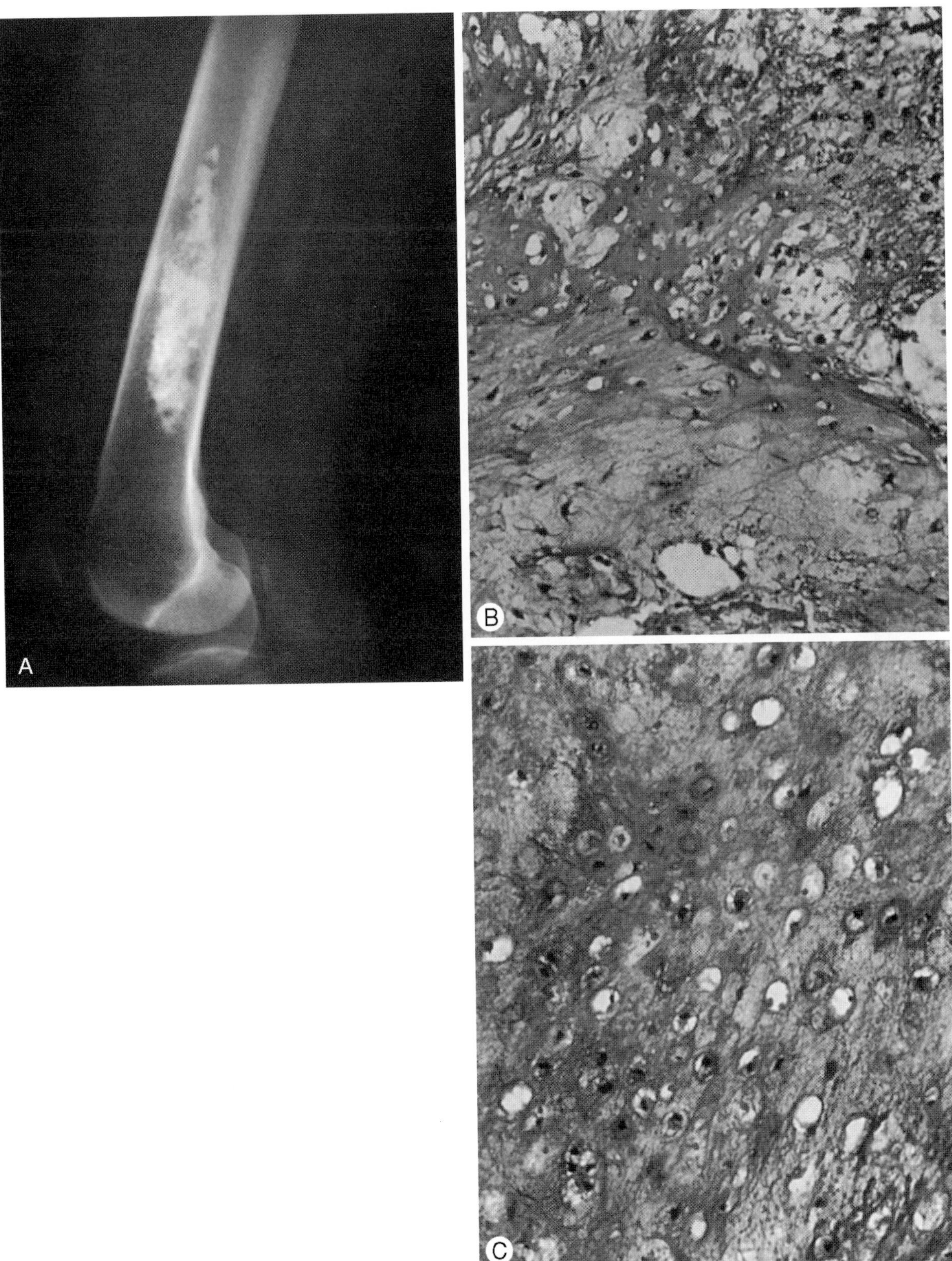

FIGURE 8-15 ■ Enchondroma of the distal femur. *A,* Radiograph shows densely mineralized medullary lesion. *B,* Low-power (×160) photomicrograph shows mineralized hyaline cartilage. *C,* Higher-power (×250) photomicrograph shows bland chondrocytes in lacunae.

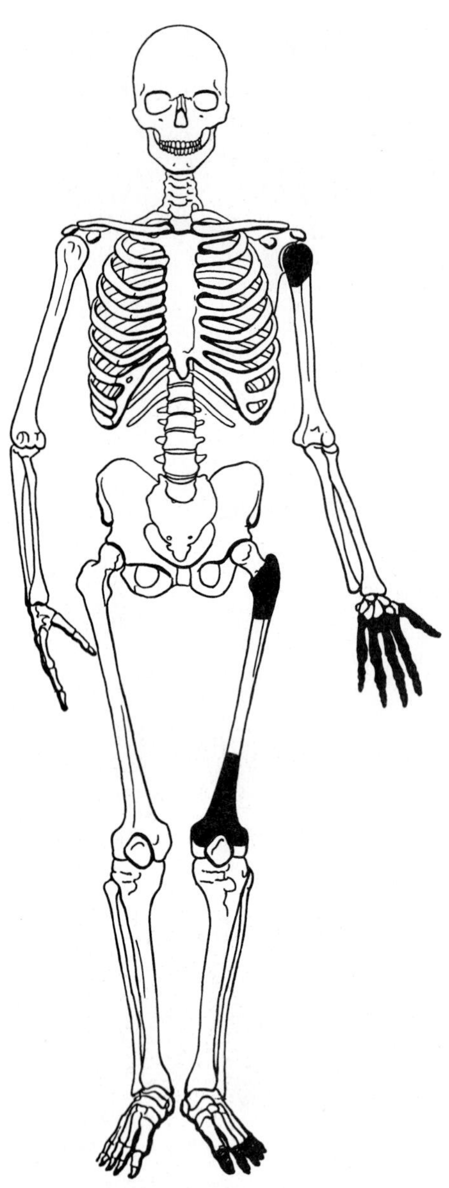

FIGURE 8-16 ■ Skeletal distribution of the most common sites of enchondromas. Note the common location in the phalanges of the hand, the proximal humerus, and distal femur. (From McCarthy, E.F., and Frassica, F.J.: Pathology of Bone and Joint Disorders. Philadelphia, WB Saunders, 1998.)

are not causing pain, serial radiographs are obtained to ensure that the lesions are inactive (not growing). Radiographs are obtained at 3 months and 1 year after presentation. In contrast, periosteal chondromas occur on the surface of long bones (Fig. 8-17). They most commonly occur on the surface of the distal femur, proximal humerus, and proximal femur (Fig. 8-18). Usually, there is a well-demarcated shallow cortical defect and a slight buttress of cortical bone at the edges of the lesion. About a third of periosteal chondromas have a mineralized cartilaginous matrix on the radiograph, whereas two-thirds have no apparent radiographic mineralization. When surgical treatment is necessary, enchondromas are treated by curettage and bone grafting. Periosteal chondromas are usually excised with a marginal margin. Enchondromas may be multiple in the same extremity. When there are many lesions, when the involved bones are dysplastic, and when the lesions tend to unilaterality, the diagnosis of multiple enchondromatosis, or Ollier's disease, is made. If soft-tissue angiomas are also present, the patient has Maffucci's syndrome. Chondrosarcomas virtually never occur in the setting of a previous enchondroma; however, patients with multiple enchondromatosis are at increased risk (Ollier's disease, 30%; Maffucci's syndrome, 100%). Patients with multiple enchondromatosis also have an increased risk of visceral malignancies, such as astrocytomas, and gastrointestinal malignancies.

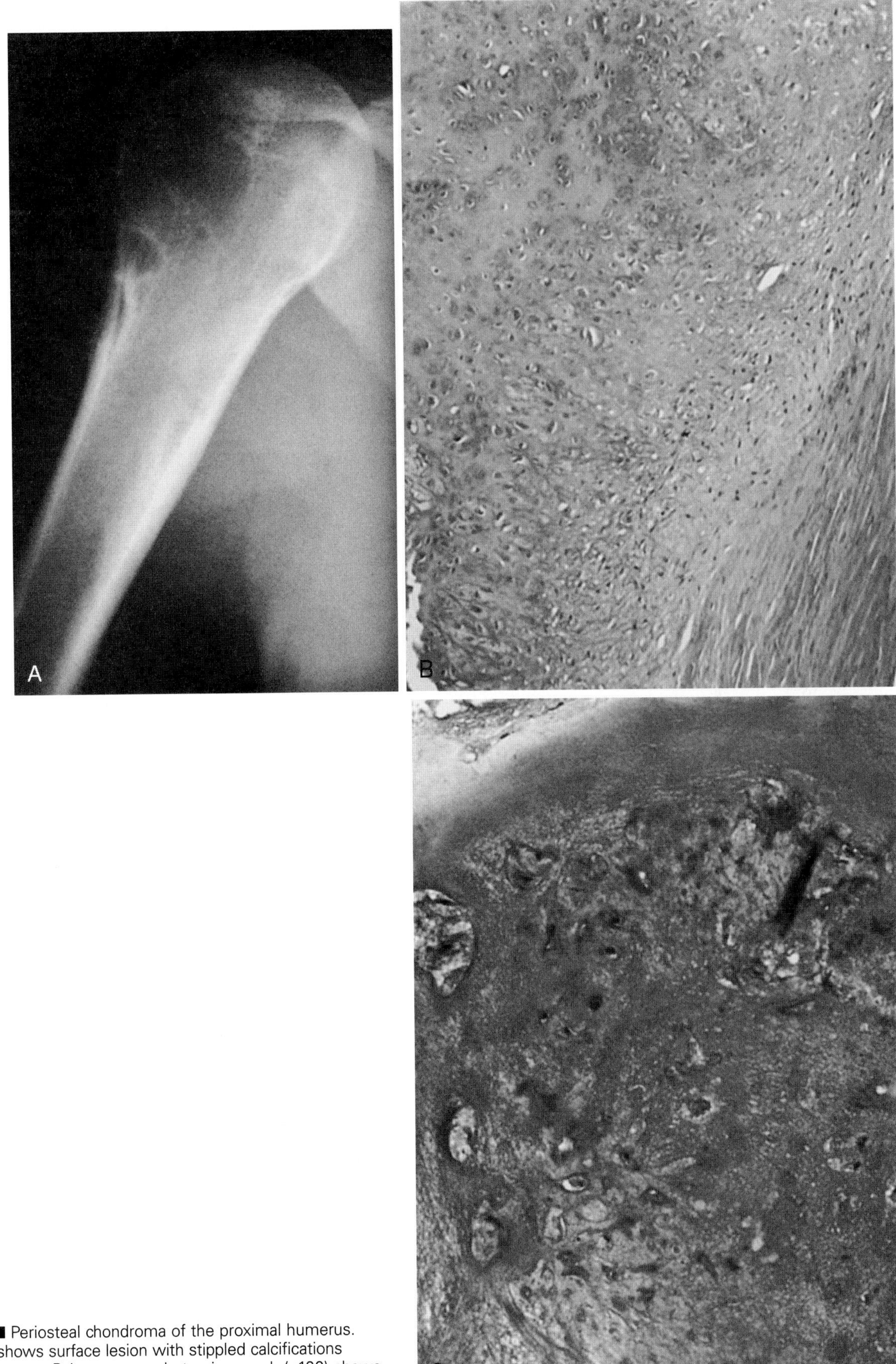

FIGURE 8-17 ■ Periosteal chondroma of the proximal humerus. *A,* Radiograph shows surface lesion with stippled calcifications scalloping the cortex. *B,* Low-power photomicrograph (×100) shows bland hyaline cartilage. *C,* Higher-power photomicrograph (×250).

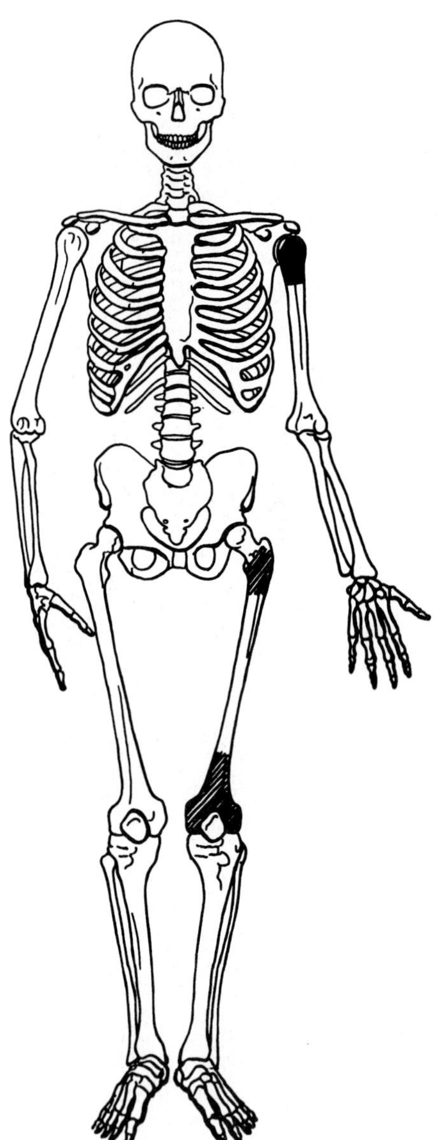

FIGURE 8-18 ■ Periosteal chondroma locations. (From McCarthy, E.F., and Frassica, F.J.: Pathology of Bone and Joint Disorders. Philadelphia, WB Saunders, 1998.)

2. Osteochondroma (Fig. 8-19)—These benign surface lesions probably arise secondary to aberrant cartilage (from the perichondral ring) on the surface of bone (Dahlin). Patients usually present with a painless mass, after trauma, or discovered incidentally when a radiograph is obtained for another reason. They most commonly occur about the knee, proximal femur, and proximal humerus (Fig. 8-20). The characteristic appearance is a surface lesion in which the cortex of the lesion and the underlying cortex are continuous; the medullary cavity of the host bone also flows into (is continuous with) the osteochondroma. The osteochondroma may have a narrow stalk (pedunculated) or a broad base (sessile). These lesions typically occur at the site of tendon insertions, and the affected bone is abnormally wide (Dahlin). Histologically, the underlying cortex is covered by a thin cap of cartilage. Grossly, the cartilage cap is usually only 2–3 mm thick. In a growing child the cap may exceed 1–2 cm. Histologically, the chondrocytes are arranged in linear clusters with an appearance resembling that of the normal physis. When asymptomatic, these lesions are treated with observation only. Patients may experience pain secondary to muscle irritation, mechanical trauma (contusions), or an inflamed bursa over the lesion. In this scenario excision is a logical alternative. Pain in the absence of mechanical factors is a warning sign of malignant change. The development of a sarcoma in an osteochondroma is rare, far less than 1%. Destruction of the subchondral bone, mineralization of a soft-tissue mass, and an

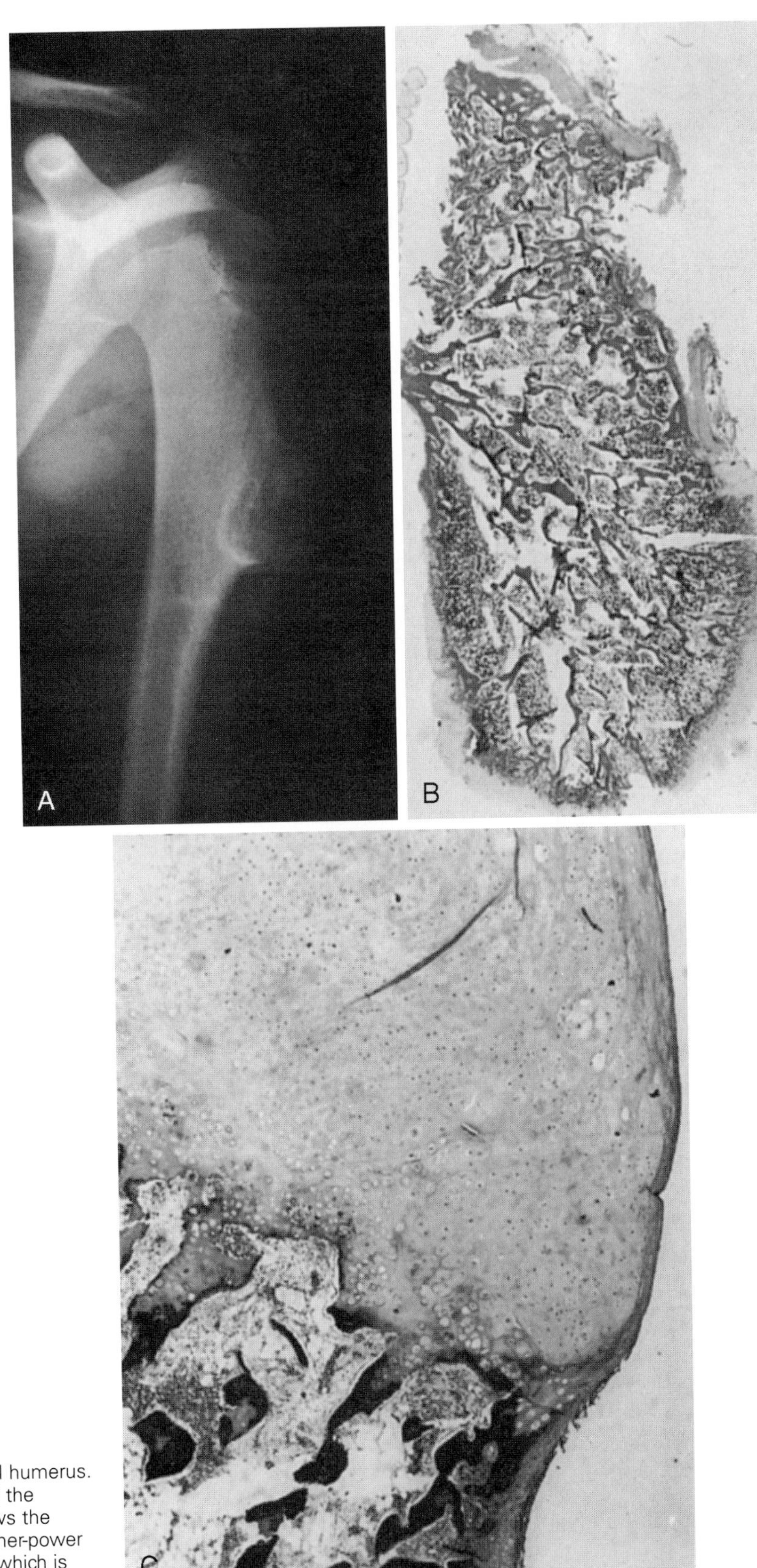

FIGURE 8-19 ■ Osteochondroma of the proximal humerus. *A*, Radiograph shows sessile osteochondroma of the proximal humerus. *B*, Photomicrograph (×6) shows the osteochondroma with a cartilaginous cap. *C*, Higher-power photomicrograph (×25) shows the cartilage cap, which is undergoing endochondral ossification.

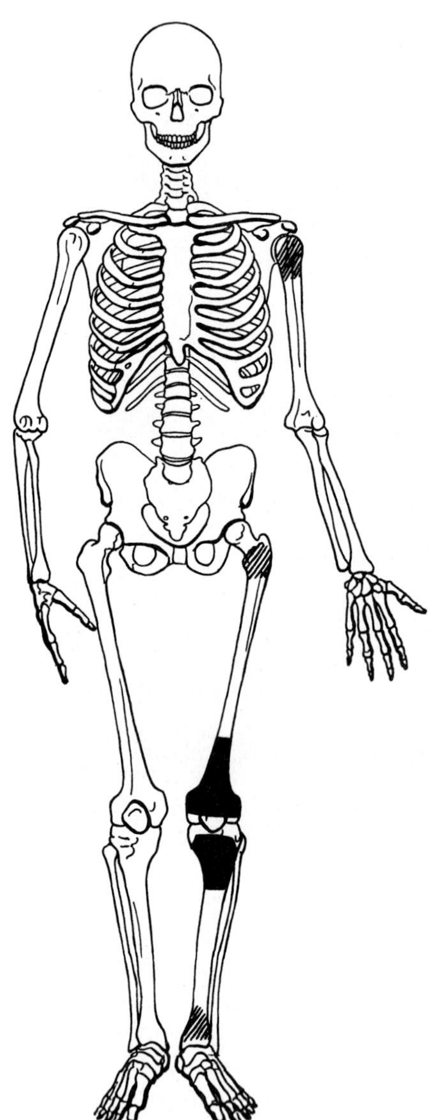

FIGURE 8-20 ■ Skeletal distribution of the most common sites of osteochondromas. (From McCarthy, E.F., and Frassica, F.J.: Pathology of Bone and Joint Disorders. Philadelphia, WB Saunders, 1998.)

inhomogeneous appearance are radiographic changes of malignant transformation. When a malignant change occurs, a low-grade chondrosarcoma is usually present, although a dedifferentiated chondrosarcoma may rarely occur. When a chondrosarcoma develops in an osteochondroma the lesion is termed a "secondary chondrosarcoma." The prognosis is usually excellent; these low-grade tumors seldom metastasize. Multiple exostoses is a common disorder characterized by multiple osteochondromas. The osteochondromas are often sessile in nature and large. This is an autosomal dominant condition with mutations in the EXT1 and EXT2 gene loci. Secondary chondrosarcomas more commonly develop in patients with multiple exostoses (risk is approximately 10%).

3. Chondroblastoma (Fig. 8-21)—These benign cartilage tumors are centered in the epiphysis in young patients (most have open physes). The most common locations are the distal femur, proximal tibia, and proximal humerus (Fig. 8-22). Although the lesion is usually in the epiphysis, it may also occur in an apophysis. Another common location is the triradiate cartilage of the pelvis. Patients usually present with pain referable to the involved joint. Radiographically, there is a central region of bone destruction that is usually sharply demarcated from the normal medullary cavity by a thin rim of sclerotic bone (Dahlin). There may or may not be mineralization within the lesion. Histologically, the basic proliferating cells are thought to be chondroblasts. There are scattered multinucleated giant cells

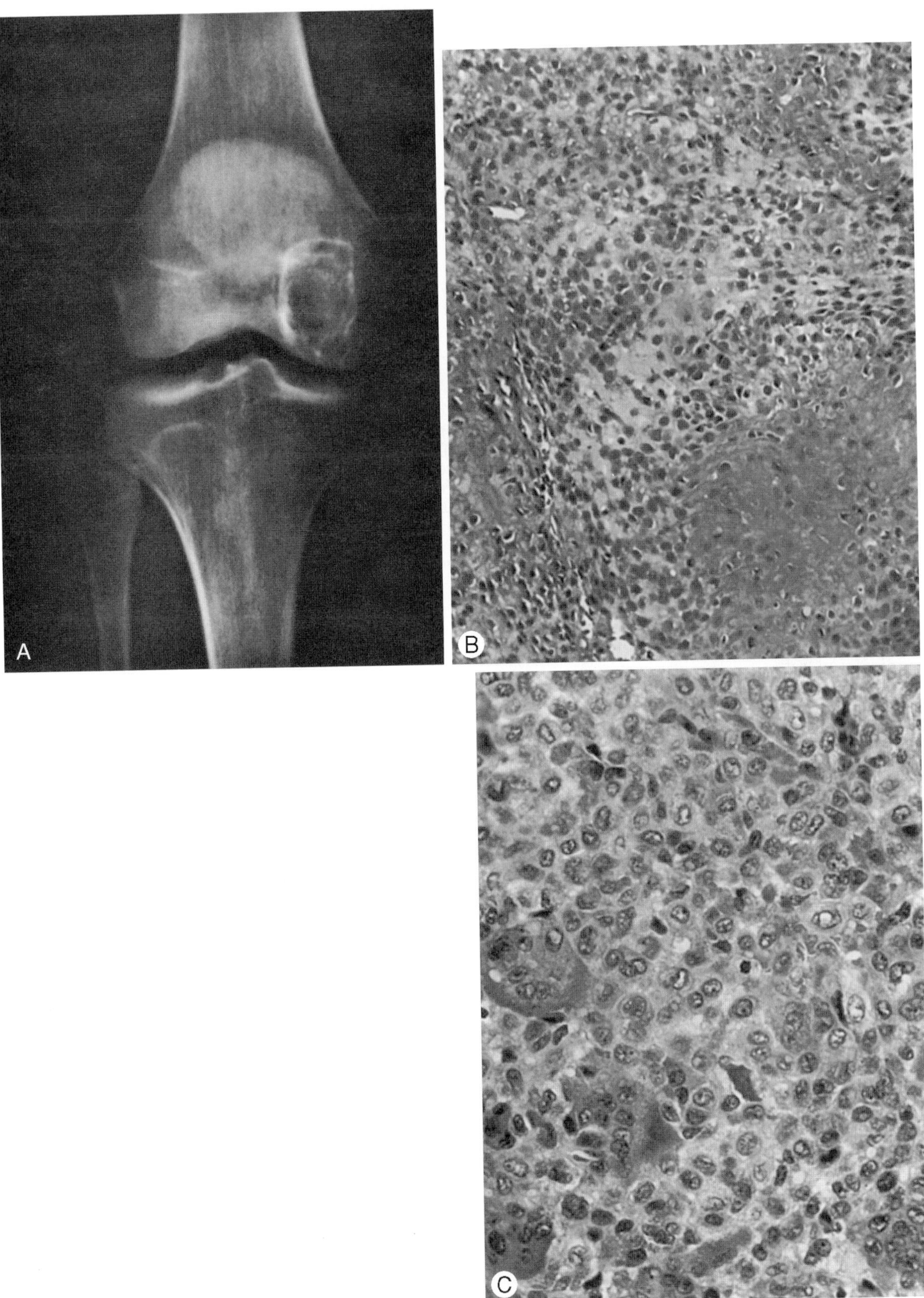

FIGURE 8-21 ■ Chondroblastoma of the distal femur. *A*, Radiograph shows a well-circumscribed lytic lesion with a sclerotic rim in the distal femoral epiphysis. *B*, Low-power photomicrograph (×160) shows cellular stroma in a chondroid matrix. *C*, Higher-power photomicrograph (×400) shows rounded stromal cells with multinucleated giant cells.

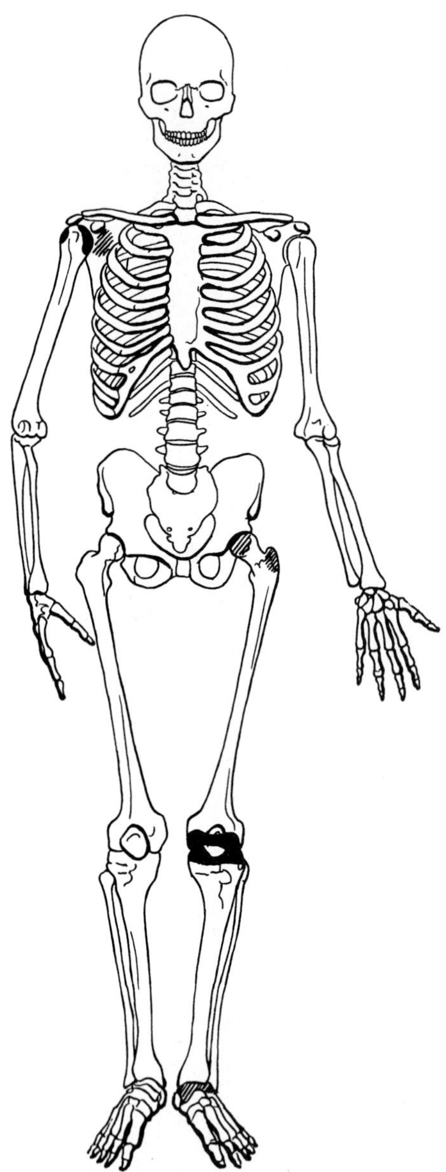

FIGURE 8-22 ■ Skeletal distribution of the most common sites of chondroblastomas. Chondroblastomas begin exclusively in either the epiphysis or apophysis. They commonly occur in the distal femur, proximal tibia, femoral head, greater trochanteric apophysis, and the proximal humeral epiphysis called (Codman's tumor). (From McCarthy, E.F., and Frassica, F.J.: Pathology of Bone and Joint Disorders. Philadelphia, WB Saunders, 1998.)

throughout the lesion and zones of chondroid substance. Mitotic figures may be found. Chondroblastomas are treated by curettage (intralesional margin) and bone grafting. About 2% of benign chondroblastomas metastasize to the lungs. There may be genetic abnormalities in chromosomes 5 and 8 (Temple).

4. Chondromyxoid Fibroma (Fig. 8-23)—These rare, benign cartilage tumors contain variable amounts of chondroid, fibromatoid, and myxoid elements. The lesion is more common in males and tends to involve long bones (especially the tibia). The pelvis and distal femur are other common locations (Fig. 8-24). Patients present with pain of variable duration (months to years). Radiographically, there is a lytic, destructive lesion that is eccentric and sharply demarcated from the adjacent normal bone. Usually, no matrix mineralization is seen radiographically. The tumor grows in lobules, and there is often a condensation of cells at the periphery of the lobules. The chondroid element may vary from small to heavy concentrations. Treatment is resection with a marginal line of resection. There may be a genetic rearrangement on chromosome 6 at position q13 (6q13) (Temple).
5. Intramedullary Chondrosarcoma (Fig. 8-25)—This malignant neoplasm of cartilage cells occurs in adults and the older age groups.

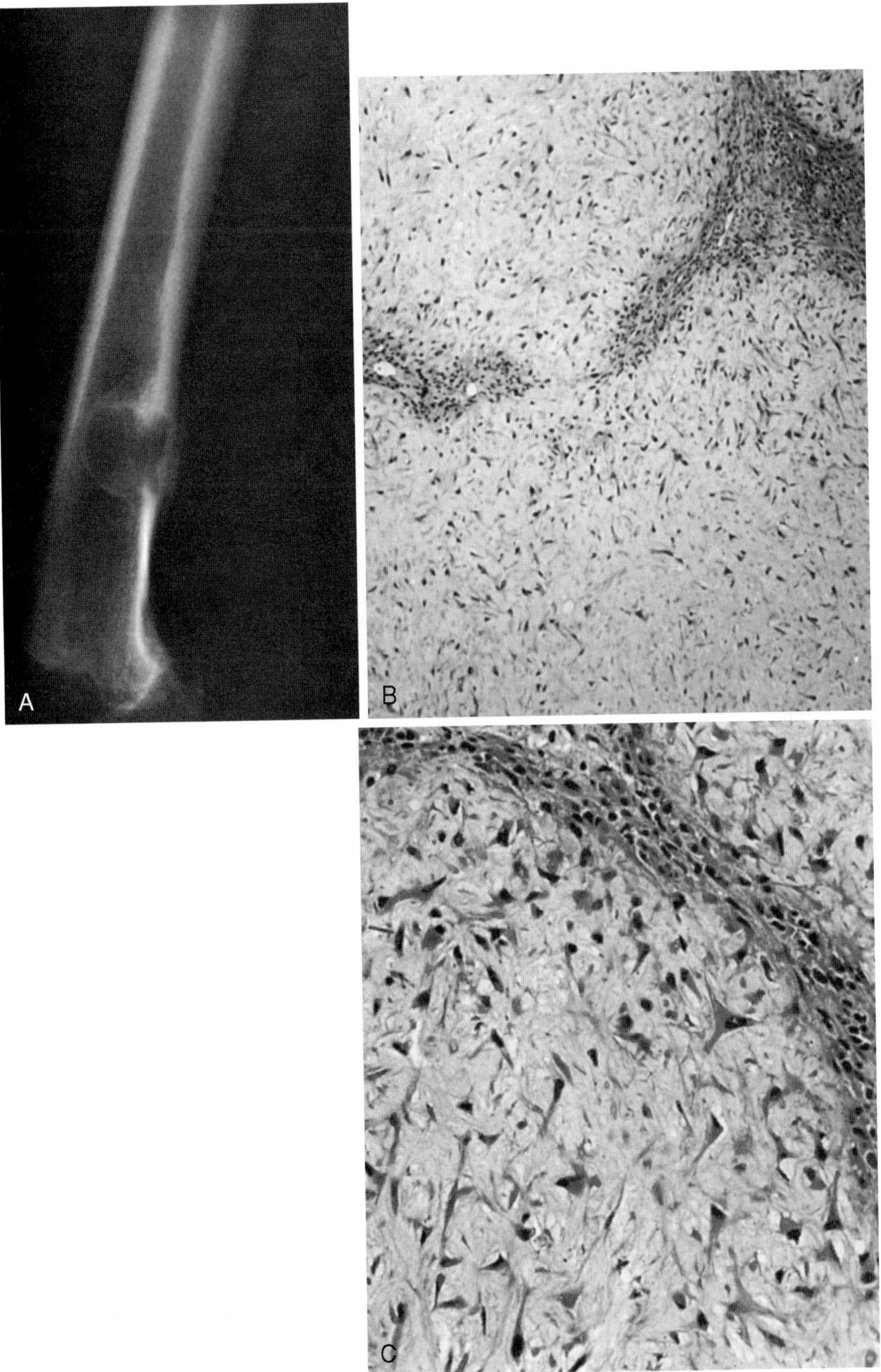

FIGURE 8-23 ■ Chondromyxoid fibroma of the femur. *A,* Radiograph shows well-circumscribed lytic lesion in the distal femur with a rim of sclerotic bone. *B,* Low-power photomicrograph (×100) shows lobules of fibromyxoid tissue. *C,* Higher-power photomicrograph (×250) shows myxoid stroma with stellate cells.

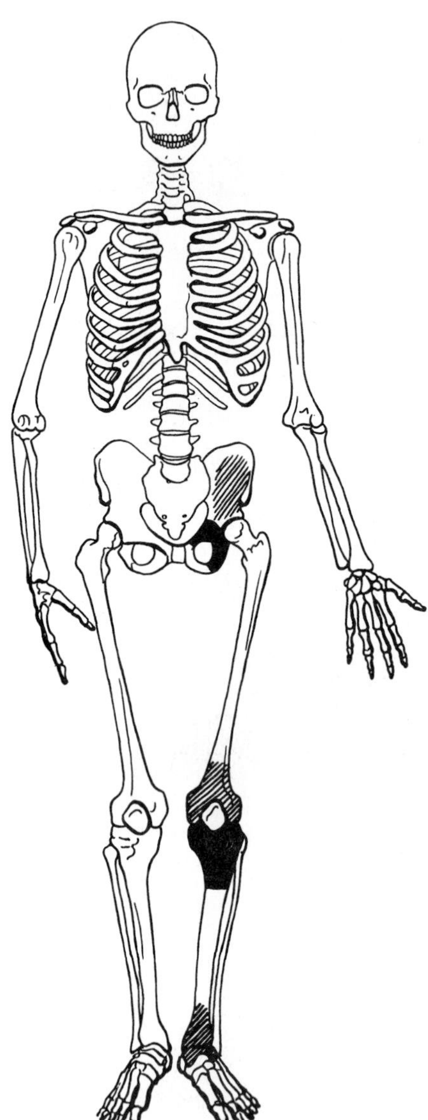

FIGURE 8-24 ■ Skeletal distribution of the most common sites of chondromyxoid fibroma. The tibia and pelvis are common locations. (From McCarthy, E.F., and Frassica, F.J.: Pathology of Bone and Joint Disorders. Philadelphia, WB Saunders, 1998.)

The most common locations include the shoulder and pelvic girdles, knee, and spine. Patients may have pain or a mass. Plain radiographs are usually diagnostic, with bone destruction, thickening of the cortex, and mineralization consistent with cartilage within the lesion (Fig. 8-26). About 85% of patients will have prominent cortical changes. A soft-tissue mass is often present in patients who have had symptoms for a long time. It may be extremely difficult to differentiate malignant cartilage based on histologic features alone. The clinical, radiographic, and histologic features of a particular lesion must be combined to avoid incorrect diagnoses. The criteria for the diagnosis of malignancy include: (1) many cells with plump nuclei, (2) more than an occasional cell with two such nuclei, and (3) especially giant cartilage cells with large single or multiple nuclei with clumps of chromatin (Dahlin). Chondromas of the hand, lesions in patients with Ollier's disease and Maffucci's syndrome, and periosteal chondromas may have atypical histopathologic features; however, their behavior is that of a benign cartilage lesion and, hence they are not malignant lesions. In these lesions there may be hypercellularity and worrisome nuclear features; however, the biologic behavior is innocent. More than 90% of chondrosarcomas are grade 1 or grade 2 lesions. Grade 3 lesions are uncommon and they behave as other highly malignant bone tumors. Treatment consists of wide-margin surgical resection. For typical low-grade (grades 1 and 2) chondrosarcoma there is no role for chemotherapy or irradiation.

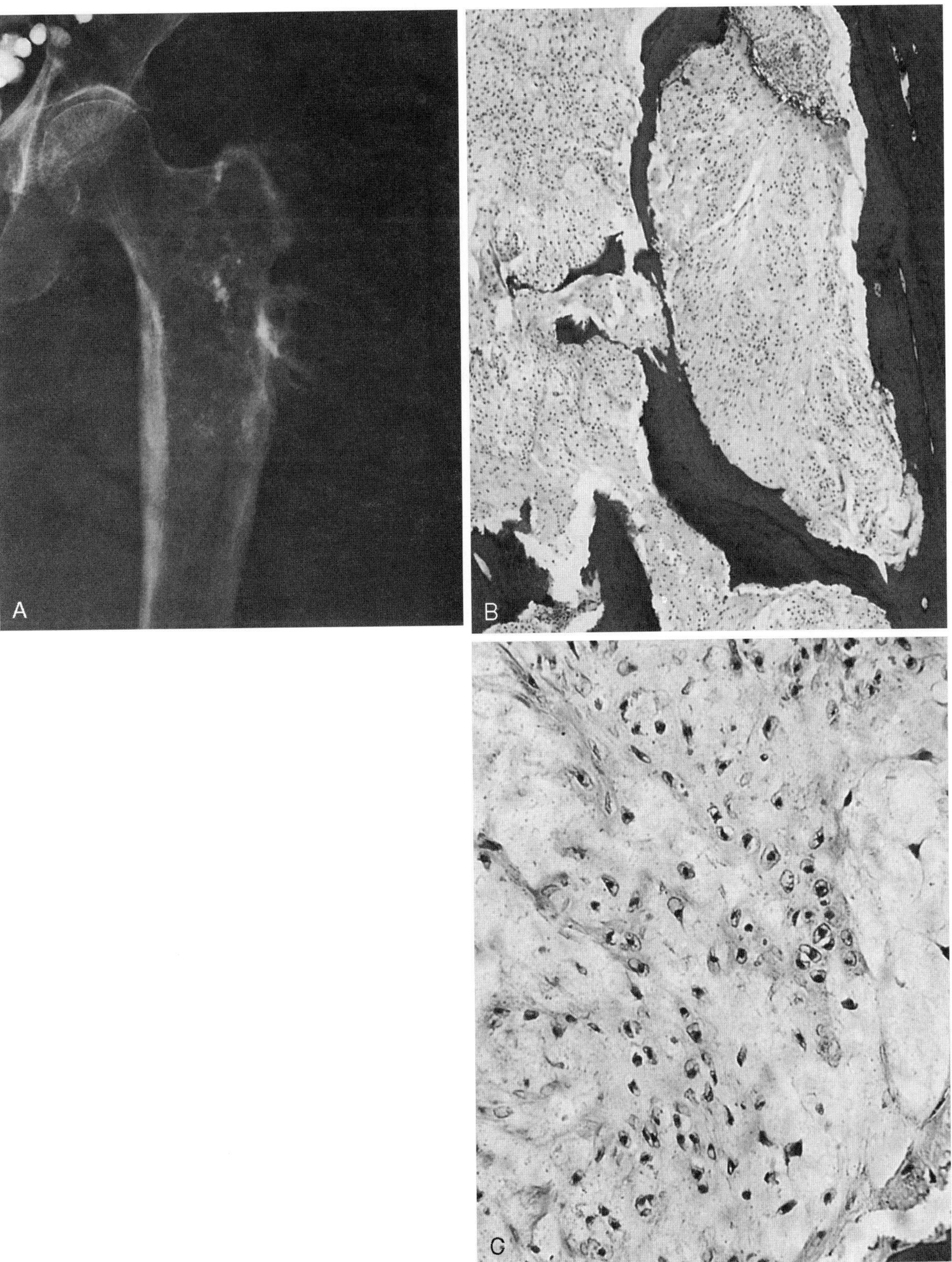

FIGURE 8-25 ■ Central (intramedullary) chondrosarcoma of the proximal femur. *A,* Radiograph shows an expansile lytic lesion in the proximal femur with stippled calcifications. *B,* Low-power photomicrograph (×40) shows cartilage with a permeative growth pattern. *C,* Higher-power photomicrograph (×250) shows cellular cartilage.

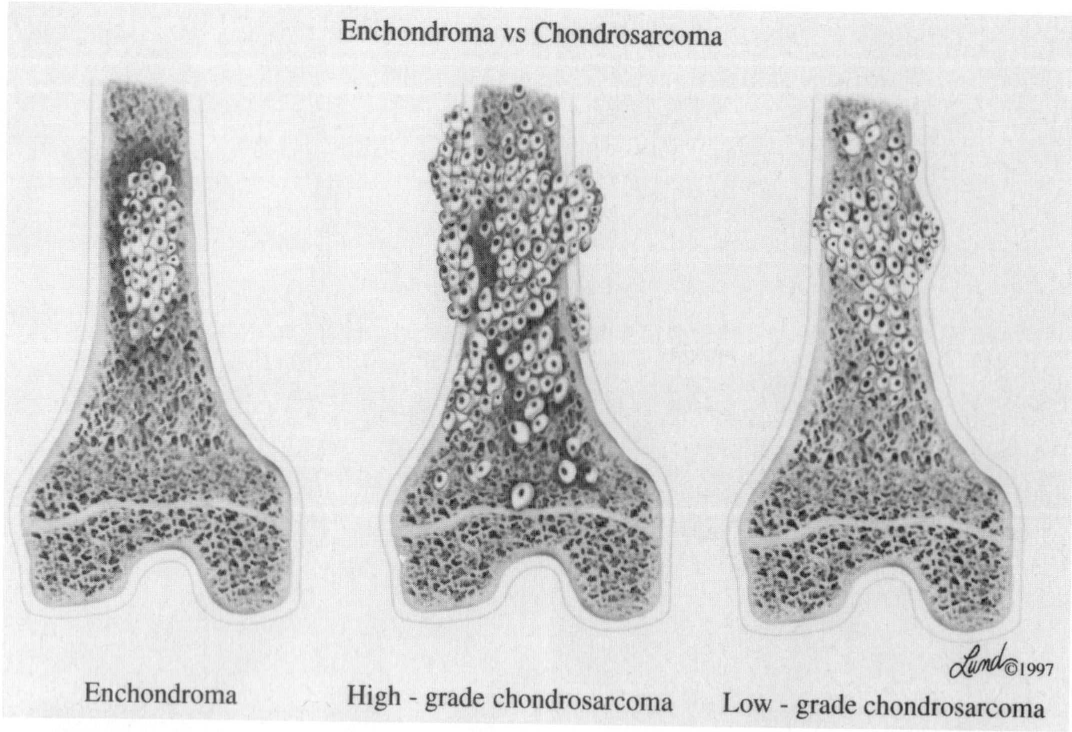

FIGURE 8-26 ■ Artist's depiction of the three types of intramedullary cartilage tumors: enchondroma, high-grade chondrosarcoma, and low-grade chondrosarcoma. Enchondromas are inactive intramedullary hyaline cartilage tumors. Note that the cortices are not involved. There is no cortical erosion, thickening, expansion, or breakthrough. In contrast, the high-grade chondrosarcoma *(middle)* shows destruction of the cortex and extension into the soft tissues. Low-grade chondrosarcoma *(right)*. Note the cortical erosion with expansion of the cortex but no breakthrough. (From McCarthy, E.F., and Frassica, F.J.: Pathology of Bone and Joint Disorders. Philadelphia, WB Saunders, 1998.)

6. Dedifferentiated Chondrosarcoma (Fig. 8-27)—These lesions are the most malignant cartilage tumors. They have a bimorphic histologic and radiographic appearance. Histologically, there is a low-grade cartilage component that is intimately associated with a high-grade spindle cell sarcoma (osteosarcoma, fibrosarcoma, malignant fibrous histiocytoma). The most common locations include the distal and proximal femur and the proximal humerus (Fig. 8-28). Radiographically, in more than 80% of the lesions there is a typical chondrosarcoma with a superimposed highly destructive area. Patients present with a picture similar to that of low-grade chondrosarcoma, including pain and decreased function. The prognosis is poor, and long-term survival is less than 10%. Wide-margin surgical resection and multi-agent chemotherapy are the principal methods of treatment.

D. Fibrous Lesions—Truly fibrous neoplasms of bone are not common and number only three: metaphyseal fibrous defect (fibroma), desmoplastic fibroma, and fibrosarcoma.

1. Metaphyseal Fibrous Defect (Fig. 8-29)—This is a common lesion occurring in young patients. Most of these lesions resolve spontaneously and are probably not true neoplasms. Common names for this lesion include nonossifying fibroma, nonosteogenic fibroma, cortical desmoid, fibromatosis, and xanthoma. The most common locations are the distal femur, distal tibia, and proximal tibia. Most patients are asymptomatic, and the lesion is discovered incidentally. The radiographic appearance is characteristic, with the lytic lesion that is metaphyseal, eccentric, and surrounded by a sclerotic rim. The cortex may be slightly expanded and thinned. Histologically, there is a cellular, fibroblastic connective tissue background with the cells arranged in whorled bundles (Dahlin). There are numerous giant cells, lipophages, and various amounts of hemosiderin pigmentation. Treatment is observation if the radiographic appearance is characteristic and there is not an excessive risk of pathologic fracture. If more than 50–75% of the cortex is involved and the patient is symptomatic, curettage and bone grafting are performed.
2. Desmoplastic Fibroma—This lesion is a rare, low-grade malignant fibrous tumor of bone. Radiographically, the lesion is purely lytic.

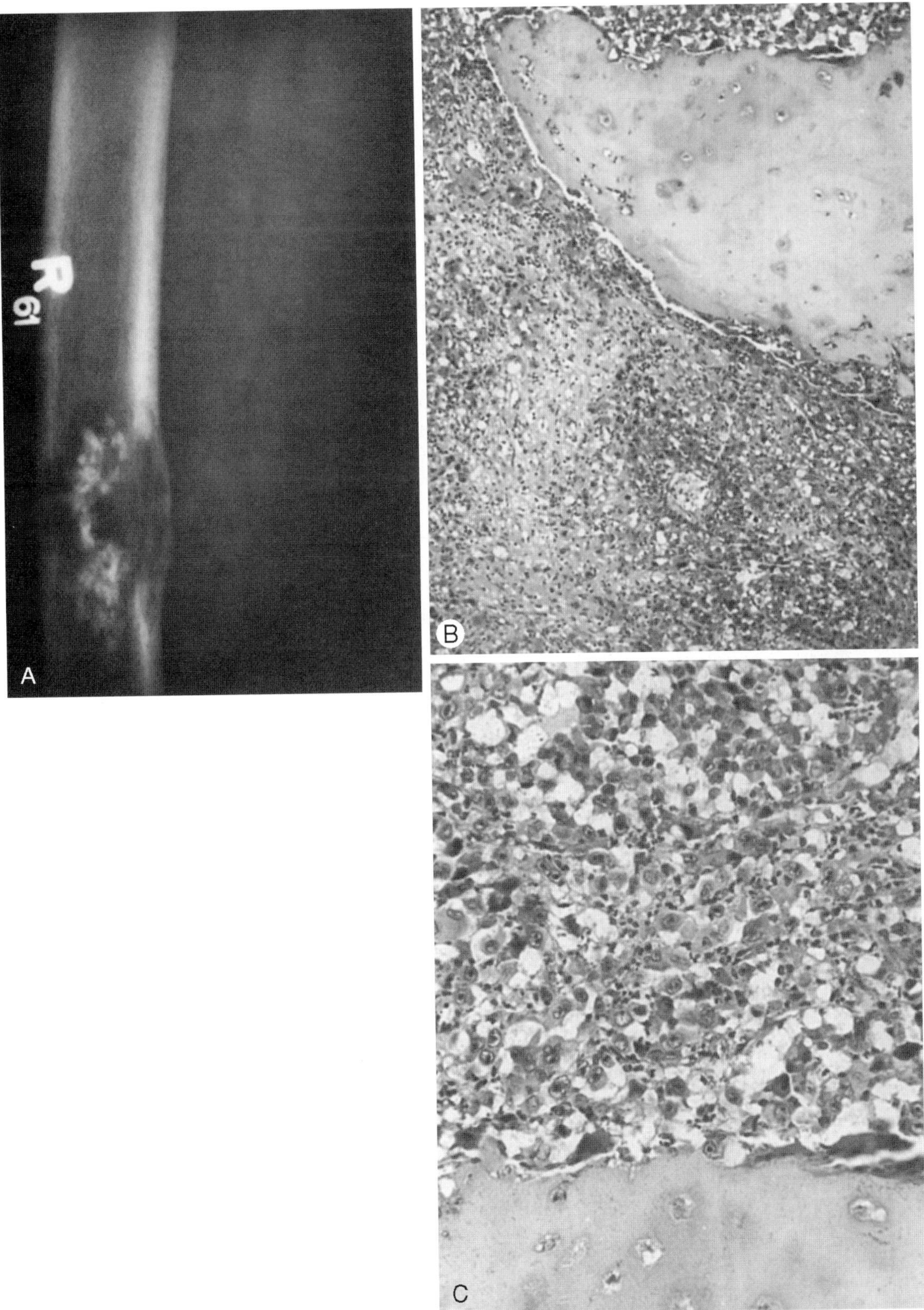

FIGURE 8-27 ■ Dedifferentiated chondrosarcoma of the femur. *A*, Radiograph shows focal dense mineralization surrounded by a poorly defined lytic lesion. *B*, Low-power photomicrograph (×100) shows an island of hyaline cartilage surrounded by a cellular neoplasm. *C*, Higher-power photomicrograph (×250) shows hyaline cartilage adjacent to pleomorphic rounded cells.

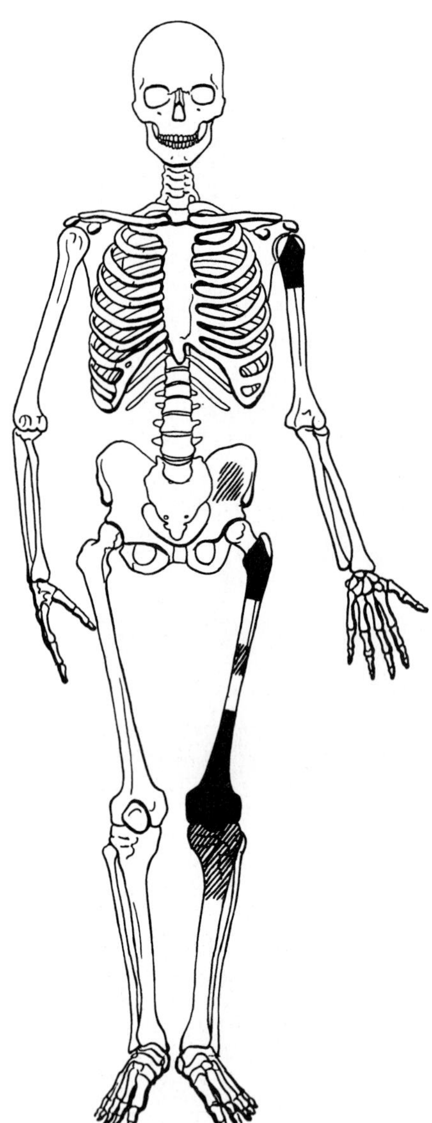

FIGURE 8-28 ■ Skeletal distribution of the most common sites of dedifferentiated chondrosarcoma. The femur and humerus are the most common sites. (From McCarthy, E.F., and Frassica, F.J.: Pathology of Bone and Joint Disorders. Philadelphia, WB Saunders, 1998.)

Because the process is low-grade, there will often be residual or reactive trabeculations (or corrugations) of bone. Histologically, this lesion is composed of abundant collagen and mature fibroblasts with no cellular atypia. Wide surgical resection is the treatment.

3. Fibrosarcoma (Fig. 8-30)—This malignant tumor of bone has a presentation and localization similar to that of osteosarcoma. The tumor affects primarily an older age group but does occur during all decades of life. Patients present with pain and swelling as with any other malignant bone tumor. Radiographically, there is bone destruction that is typically in a permeative pattern. The histologic features are the same as those of soft-tissue fibrosarcoma, with spindle cells, variable collagen production, and a herringbone pattern. Treatment consists in wide-margin surgical resection. Although the prognosis is poor, the role of chemotherapy has not been fully defined; effective regimens for the older patient have not been adequately explored.

E. Histiocytic Lesions

1. Malignant Fibrous Histiocytoma (Fig. 8-31)—These malignant bone tumors have proliferating cells with a histiocytic quality. The nuclei are often indented; the cytoplasm is usually abundant and may be slightly foamy; the nucleoli are often large; and multinucleated giant cells are usually a prominent feature (Dahlin). There may be variable amounts of fibrous tissue found within the lesion, and the fibrogenic areas have a storiform appearance. Chronic inflammatory cells are frequently found. Patients present with pain and swelling.

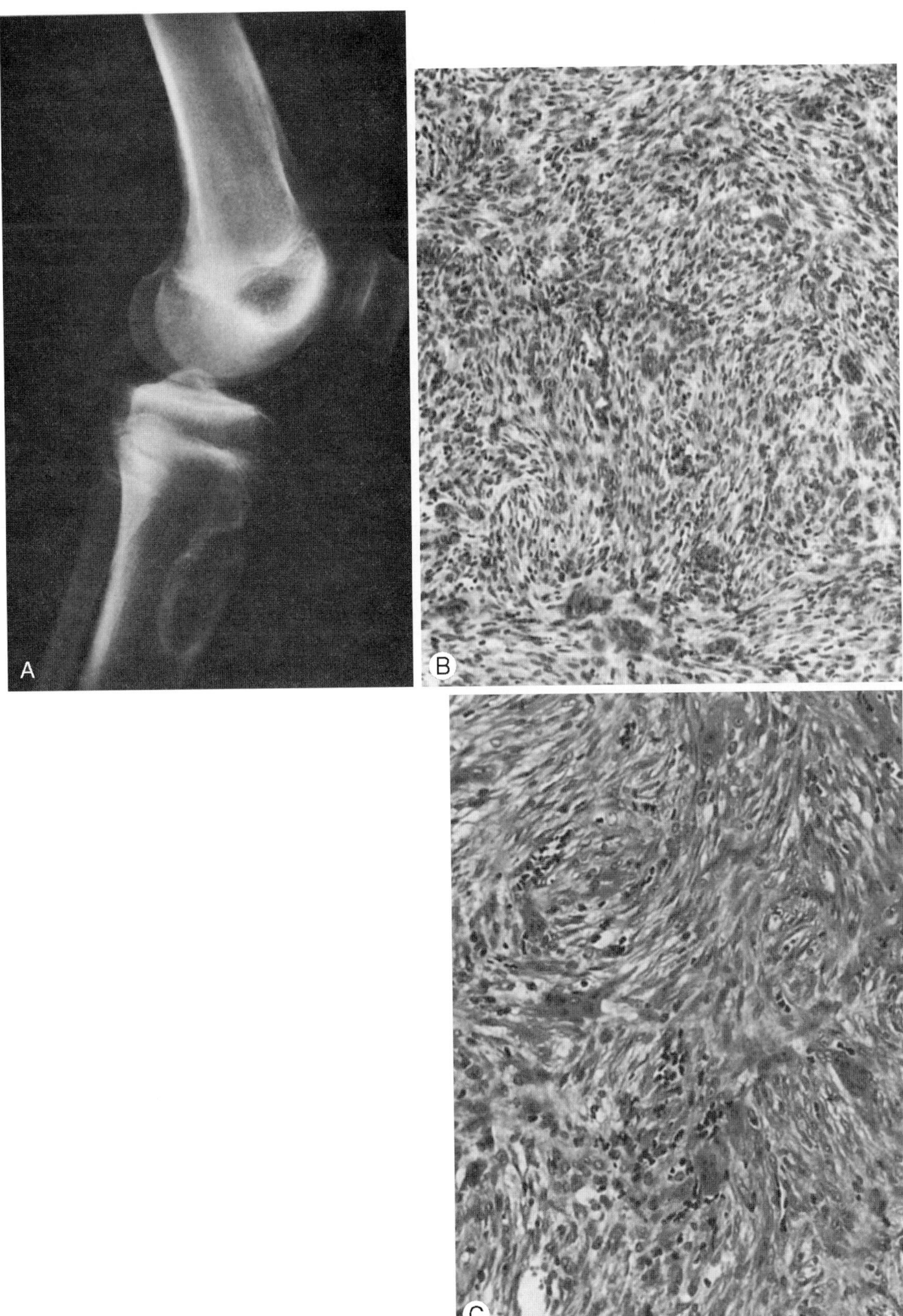

FIGURE 8-29 ■ Nonossifying fibroma of the proximal tibia. *A,* Radiograph shows a scalloped, well-circumscribed lesion with a sclerotic rim in the proximal tibial metaphysis. *B,* Low-power photomicrograph (×160) showing spindle cells in a storiform pattern and occasional multinucleated giant cells. *C,* Higher-power photomicrograph (×250).

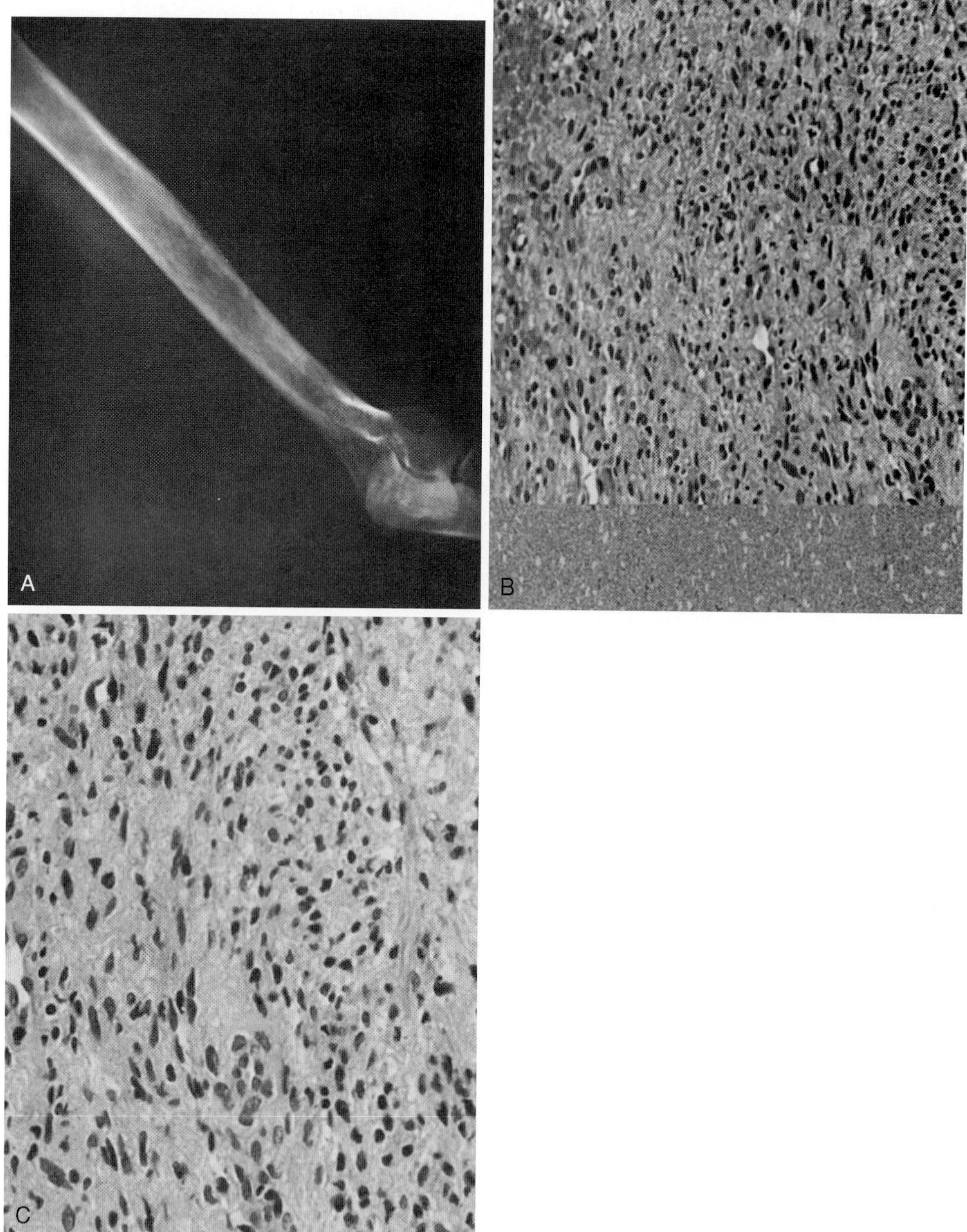

FIGURE 8-30 ■ Fibrosarcoma of the humerus. *A,* Radiograph shows a permeative lesion in the midshaft of the humerus. *B,* Low-power photomicrograph (×250) shows atypical spindle cells. *C,* Higher-power photomicrograph (×400).

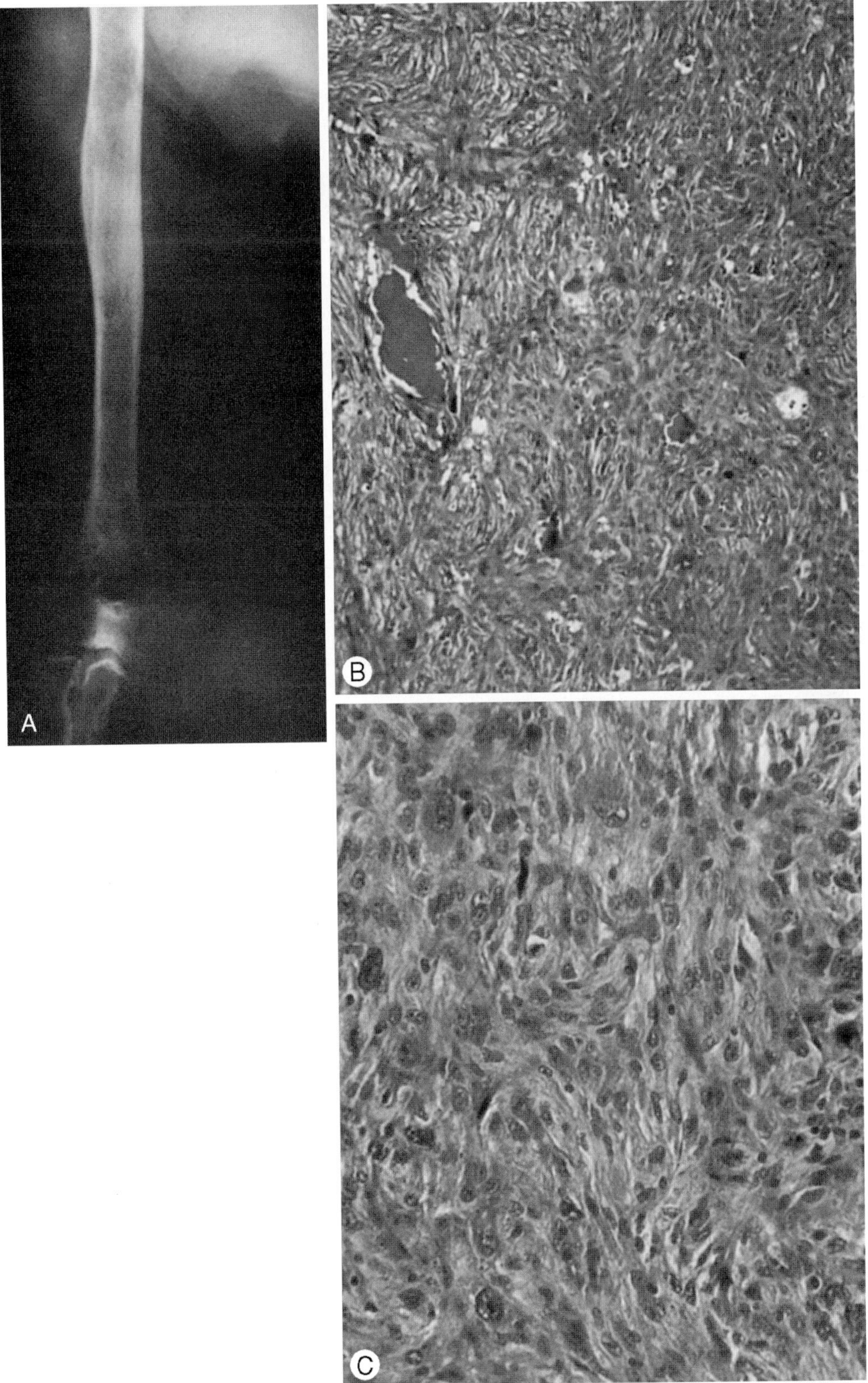

FIGURE 8-31 ■ Malignant fibrous histiocytoma of the humerus. *A,* Radiograph shows poorly defined lytic lesions in the proximal and distal humerus. *B,* Low-power photomicrograph (×200) shows spindle cells arranged in a storiform pattern. *C,* Higher-power photomicrograph (×400) shows a uniform population of pleomorphic cells.

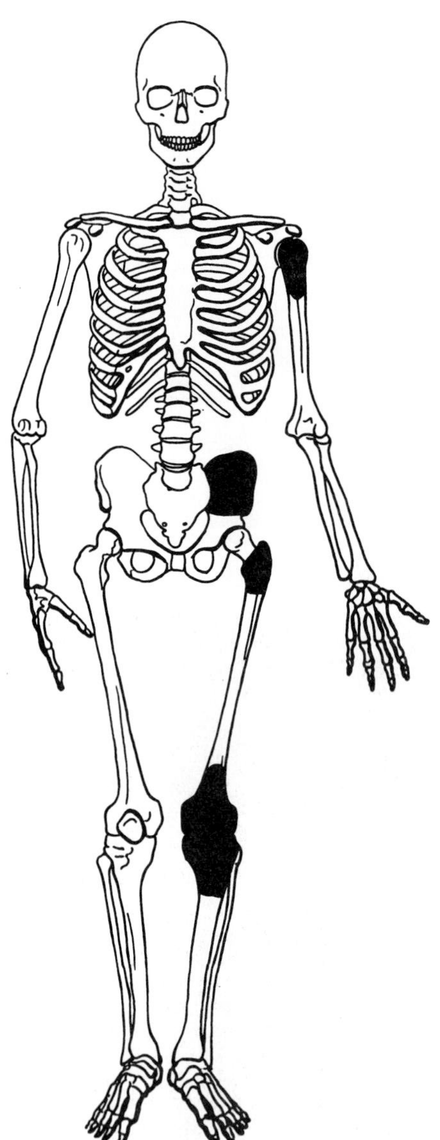

FIGURE 8-32 ■ Skeletal distribution of the most common sites of malignant fibrous histiocytoma. (From McCarthy, E.F., and Frassica, F.J.: Pathology of Bone and Joint Disorders, Philadelphia, WB Saunders, 1998.)

The most common locations include the distal femur, proximal tibia, proximal femur, ilium, and proximal humerus (Fig. 8-32). Radiographs usually demonstrate a destructive lesion with either purely lytic bone destruction or a mixed pattern of bone destruction and formation. Treatment is wide surgical excision. Most patients are candidates for multi-agent chemotherapy, although few studies have shown chemotherapy to be efficacious for this tumor.

F. Notochordal Tissue (Fig. 8-33)—Chordoma is a malignant neoplasm in which the cell of origin derives from primitive notochordal tissue. This lesion occurs predominantly at the ends of the vertebral column (spheno-occipital region and sacrum) (Fig. 8-34). About 10% of chordomas occur in the vertebral bodies (cervical, thoracic, and lumbar regions). Patients present with an insidious onset of pain. Lesions in the sacrum may present as pelvic pain, low back pain, hip pain, or with primarily gastrointestinal symptomatology (obstipation, constipation, loss of rectal tone). In the vertebral bodies there may be a wide variation in neurologic symptoms because of nerve compression. Patients with a long-standing history of undiagnosed pelvic or low back pain should undergo a rectal examination; more than half of sacral chordomas are palpable with digital examination. Plain radiographs often do not reveal the true extent of sacrococcygeal chordomas. The sacrum is difficult to evaluate on plain radiographs because of overlying bowel gas and fecal material. In addition, the anteroposterior pelvic view reveals bone destruction only at the sacral cortical margins and neural foramina; these areas are not typically involved early. CT scans show midline bone destruction and

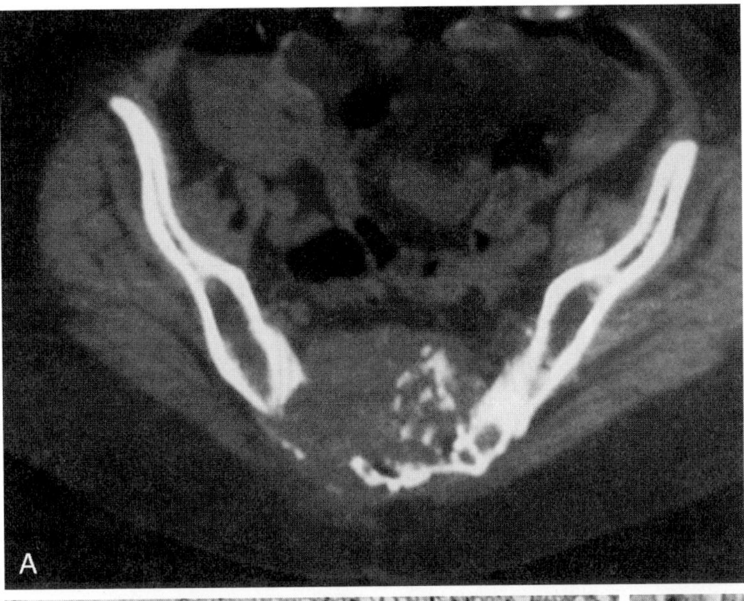

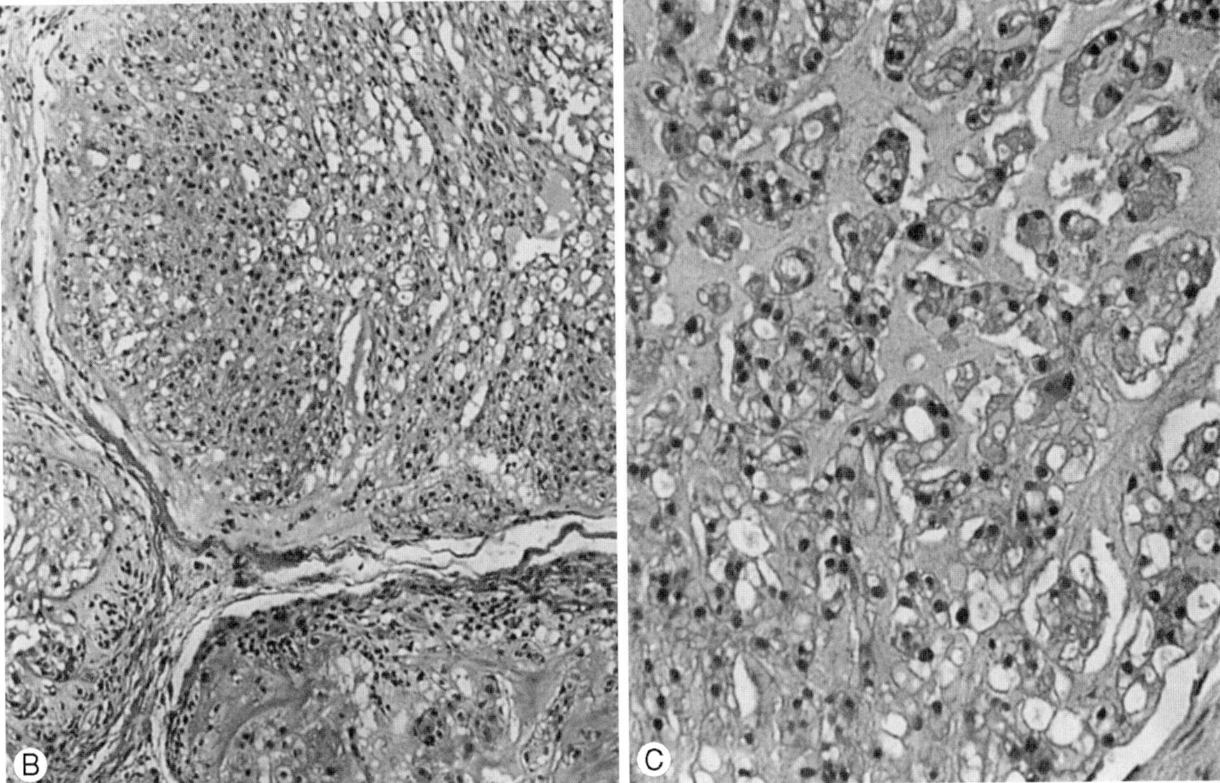

FIGURE 8-33 ■ Chordoma of the sacrum. *A,* CT scan shows a destructive lesion in the sacrum. *B,* Low-power photomicrograph (×100) shows a lobular arrangement of tissue. *C,* Higher-power photomicrograph (×250) shows nests of physaliferous cells.

a soft-tissue mass. The sacrum is often expanded, and the soft-tissue mass may show irregular mineralization. In the vertebral bodies one often sees areas of both bone formation and bone destruction. The tumor grows in distinct lobules. The chordoma cells sometimes have a vacuolated appearance and are called physaliferous cells. The chordoma cells are often in strands in a mass of mucus. Treatment is resection with a wide surgical margin. Radiation therapy may be added if a wide margin is not achieved. Chordomas metastasize in 30–50% of cases, and they often take the patient's life because of local extension.

G. Vascular Tumors—Vascular tumors of bone represent a heterogeneous group of disorders.

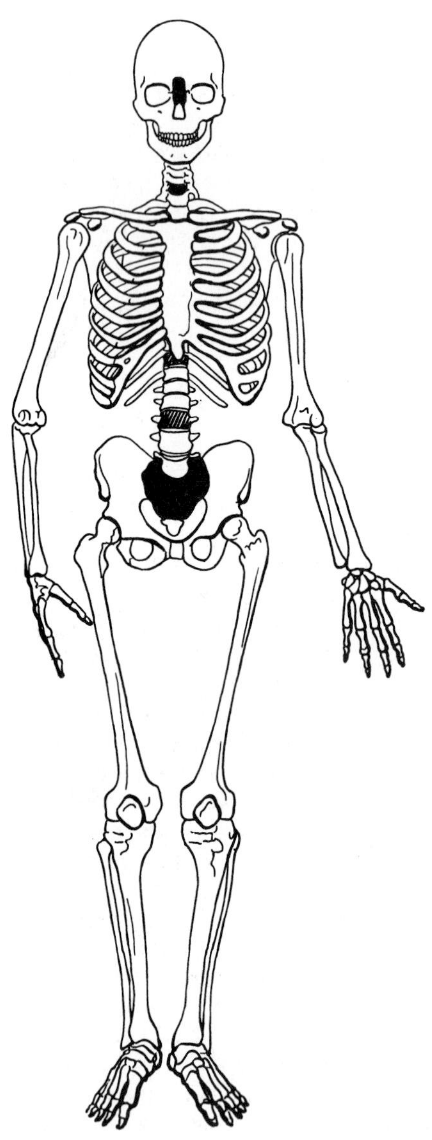

FIGURE 8-34 ■ Skeletal distribution of the most common sites of chordoma. Chordomas occur exclusively in the spine, with 50% being sacrococcygeal, 40% in the spheno-occipital region, and 10% in the vertebra. (From McCarthy, E.F., and Frassica, F.J.: Pathology of Bone and Joint Disorders. Philadelphia, WB Saunders, 1998.)

Benign conditions include hemangioma, lymphangioma, and perhaps vanishing bone disease (Gorham's disease or massive osteolysis). Malignant entities include hemangioendothelioma (hemangiosarcoma) and hemangiopericytoma.

1. Hemangiomas (Fig. 8-35)—These tumors most commonly occur in vertebral bodies. Patients may present with pain or pathologic fracture. Vertebral hemangiomas have a characteristic appearance, with lytic destruction and vertical striations or a coarsened honeycomb appearance (Dahlin). Occasionally, patients have more than one bone involved. Histologically, there are numerous blood channels. Most lesions are cavernous in nature, although some may be a mixture of capillary and cavernous blood spaces.
2. Hemangioendothelioma— Malignant vascular tumors of bone are rare. Patients may be in any age group and present with pain. Multifocal involvement of the bones of the same extremity is common. Radiographs show a predominantly lytic lesion with no reactive bone formation. The low-grade lesions often have residual trabecular bone. Histologically, the tumor cells form vascular spaces. The lesions range from very well-differentiated (easily recognizable vascular spaces) to very undifferentiated tumors (difficult to recognize the vasoformative quality of the tumor). Low-grade multifocal lesions may be treated with radiation alone.

H. Hematopoietic Tumors—Lymphoma and myeloma are the two malignant hematopoietic tumors.

1. Lymphoma (Fig. 8-36)—Lymphoma of bone is common and occurs in three scenarios: (1) as a solitary focus (primary lymphoma of bone), (2) in association with other osseous sites and

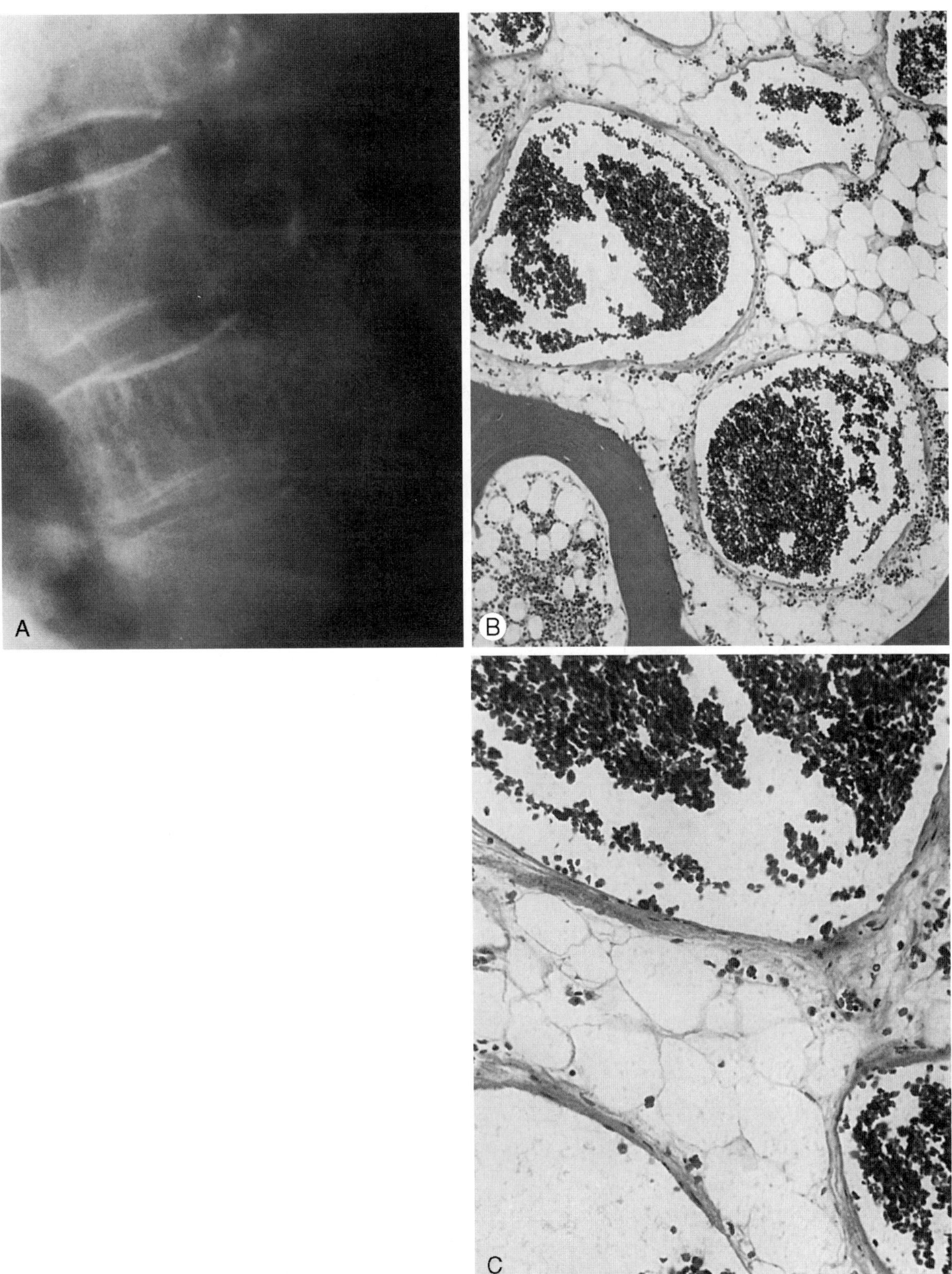

FIGURE 8-35 ■ *A,* Hemangioma of the vertebra. *B,* Low-power photomicrograph shows dilated vascular spaces in the marrow (×50). *C,* Higher-power photomicrograph (×100) shows endothelial-lined spaces.

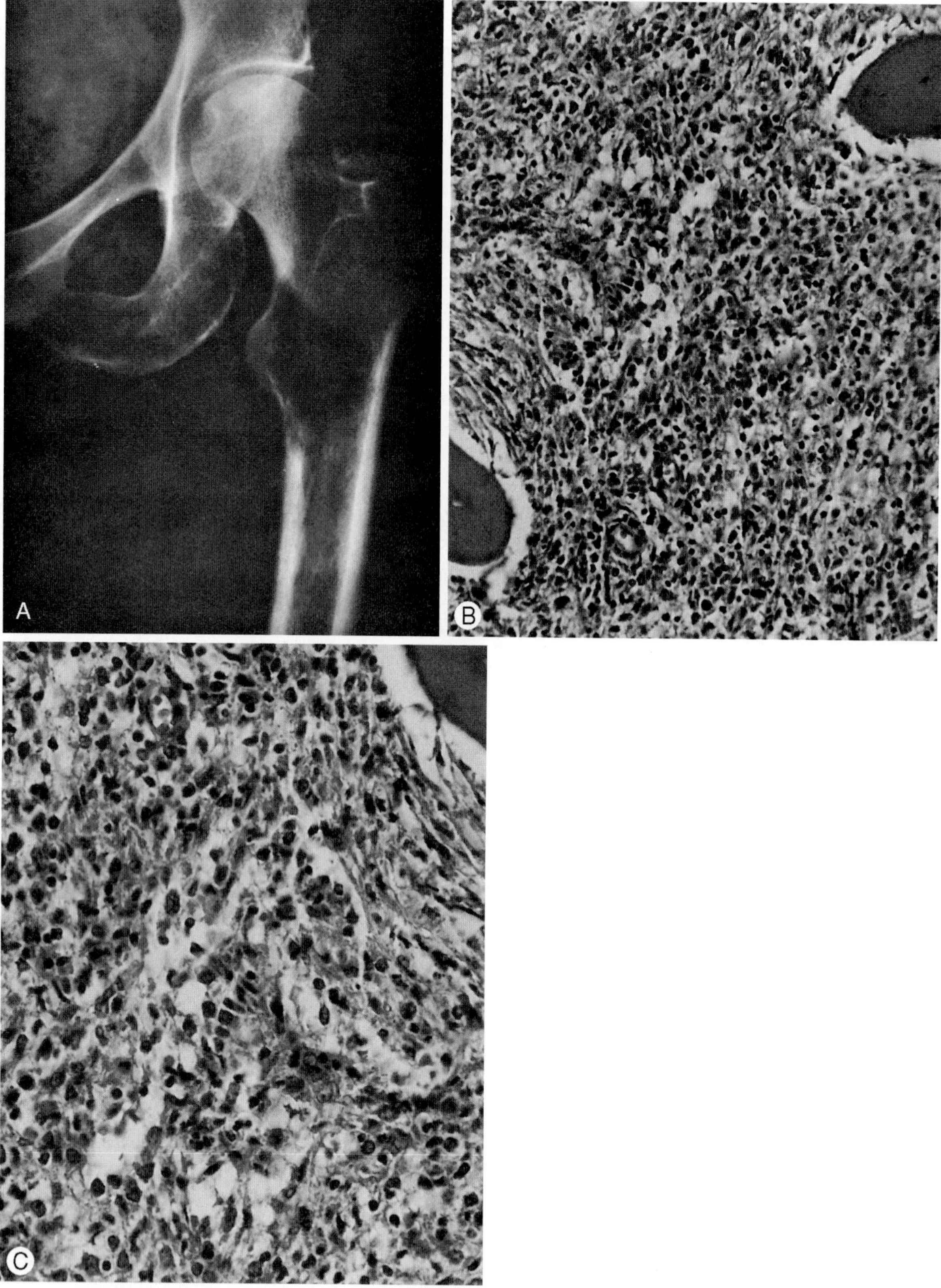

FIGURE 8-36 ■ Lymphoma of bone. *A,* Radiograph shows a poorly circumscribed lytic lesion in the proximal femur and the ischium. *B,* Low-power photomicrograph (×200) shows marrow replacement by a uniform population of lymphoid cells. *C,* Higher-power photomicrograph (×400).

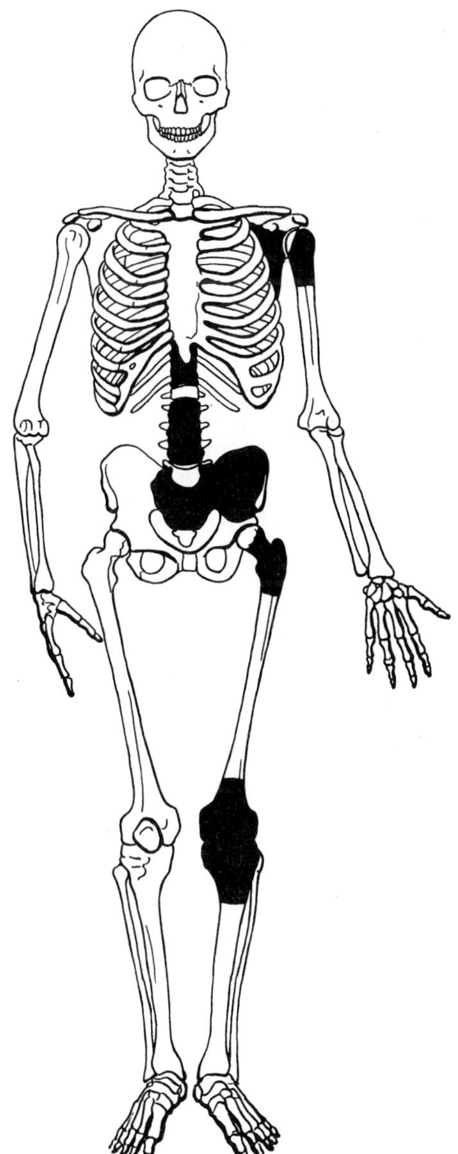

FIGURE 8-37 ■ Skeletal distribution of the most common sites of lymphoma of bone. The knee, pelvis, and vertebra are common sites. (From McCarthy, E.F., and Frassica, F.J.: Pathology of Bone and Joint Disorders. Philadelphia, WB Saunders, 1998.)

nonosseous sites (nodal disease and soft-tissue masses), and (3) as metastatic foci (Dahlin). Malignant lymphoma affects individuals at all decades of life. Patients generally present with pain. Large soft-tissue masses may be present. The most common locations include the distal femur, proximal tibia, pelvis, proximal femur, vertebra, and shoulder girdle (Fig. 8-37). The radiographs often show a lesion that involves a large portion of the bone (long lesion). Bone destruction is common and often has a mottled appearance. Reactive bone formation admixed with bone destruction is common. The cortex may be thickened. A mixed cell infiltrate is usually present. Most lymphomas are large cell B lymphomas. Treatment centers on multi-agent chemotherapy and irradiation. Surgery is generally only used to stabilize fractures.

2. Myeloma—Plasma cell dyscrasias represent a wide range of conditions, from benign monoclonal gammopathy (Kyle's disease) to multiple myeloma. There are three plasma cell dyscrasias with which the orthopaedist must be familiar: multiple myeloma, solitary myeloma, and osteosclerotic myeloma.
   a. Multiple Myeloma (Fig. 8-38)—This plasma cell disorder commonly occurs in patients between 50 and 80 years of age. Patients usually present with bone pain, most commonly in the spine and ribs, or a pathologic fracture. Fatigue is a common complaint secondary to the associated anemia. Symptoms may be related to complications, such as renal insufficiency, hypercalcemia, and the deposition of amyloid. Serum creatinine levels are elevated in about 50% of patients. Hypercalcemia is present in about a third of patients. The classic radiographic appearance is punched-out lytic lesions. The involved bone may show expansion and a "ballooned" appearance. Osteopenia may be the only finding. Histologically, the classic appearance is sheets of plasma cells. Well-differentiated plasma cells have an eccentric nucleus and a peripherally clumped chromatic "clock face" (Fig. 8-39). There is a perinuclear clear zone (halo) that represents the Golgi apparatus. In contrast, undifferentiated tumors lack some or all of these features, and the cells are anaplastic. The treatment of myeloma is multi-agent chemotherapy; surgical stabilization with irradiation is used for impending and complete fractures. Prognosis is related to the stage of disease, with an overall median survival of 18–24 months.
   b. Solitary Myeloma—It is important to differentiate solitary myeloma from multiple myeloma because of the more favorable prognosis in patients with the former. Diagnostic criteria include (1) solitary lesion on skeletal survey, (2) histologic confirmation of plasmacytoma, and (3) bone marrow plasmacytosis of 10% or less. Patients with serum protein abnormalities and Bence-Jones proteinuria of less than 1 g/24 h at presentation are not excluded if they meet the aforementioned criteria. The radiographic and histologic features are the same as for multiple myeloma. Treatment is external-beam irradiation to the lesion (4500 cGy); when necessary, prophylactic internal fixation is performed.

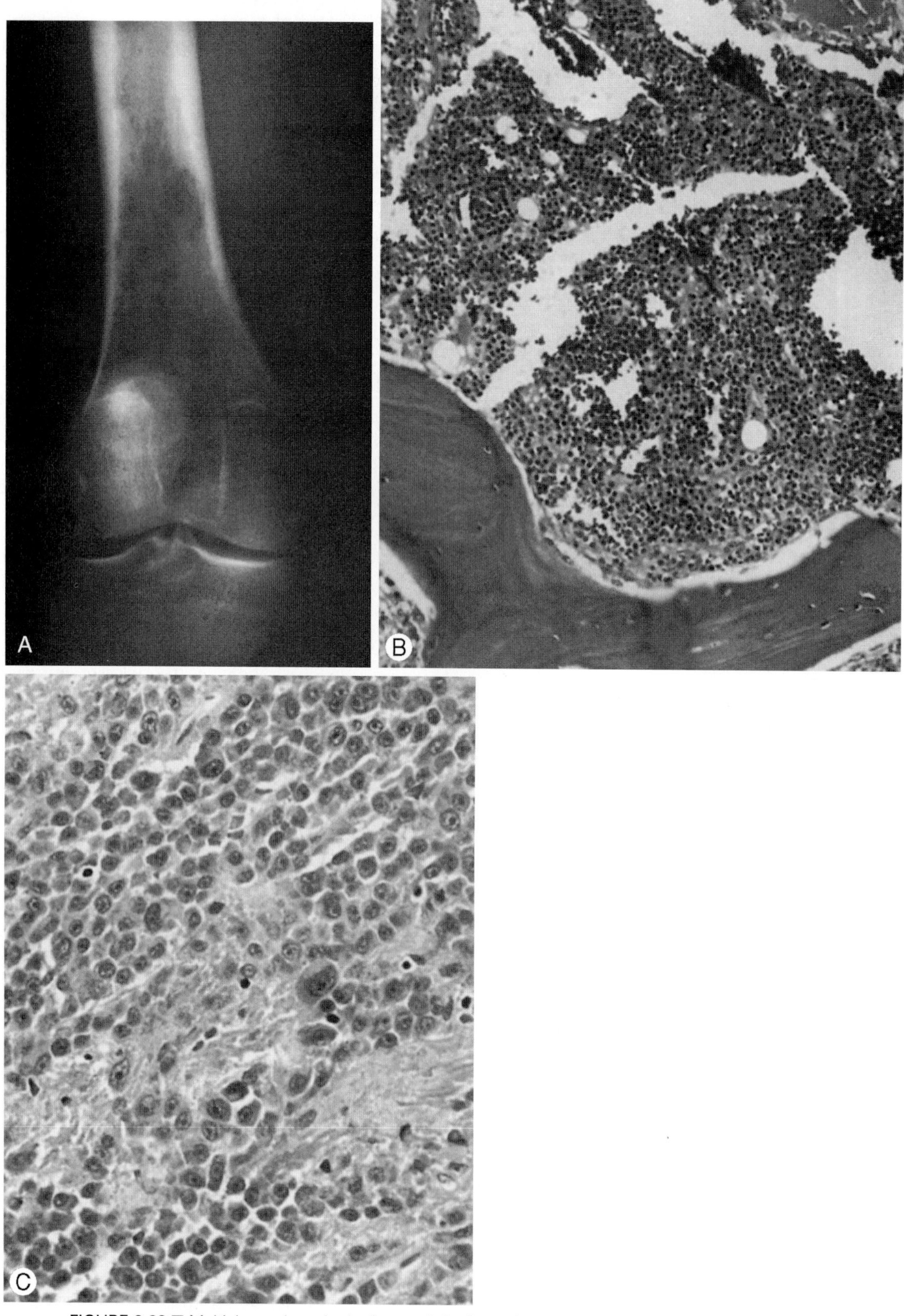

FIGURE 8-38 ■ Multiple myeloma in the femur. *A,* Radiograph shows a poorly circumscribed lytic lesion in the distal femur. *B,* Radiograph shows marrow replacement by a uniform population of cells. *C,* Higher-power photomicrograph (×400) shows sheets of atypical plasma cells.

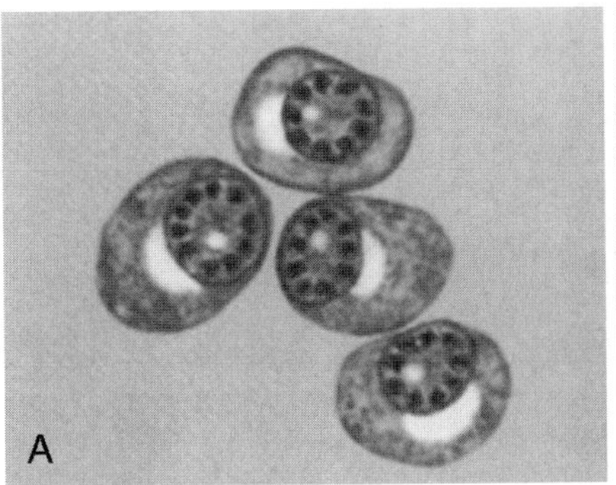

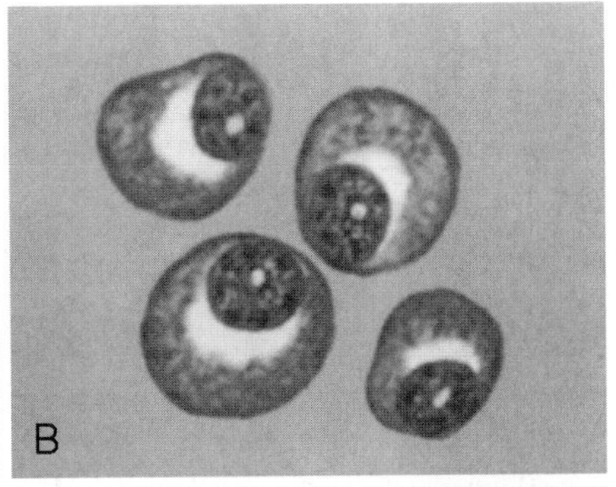

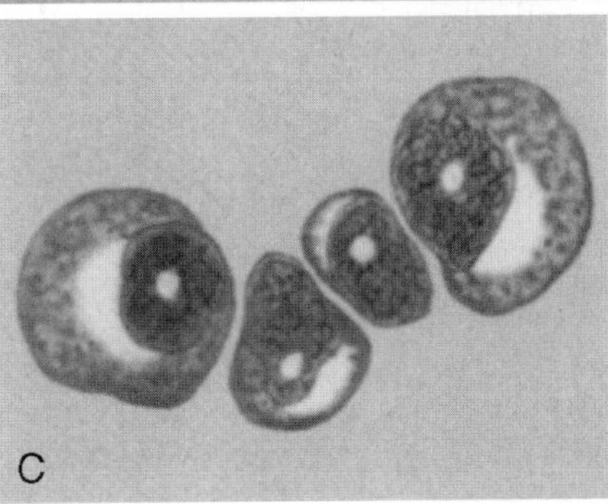

FIGURE 8-39 ■ Myeloma cells. *A,* Plasma cells from a well-differentiated case of myeloma that resemble plasma cells seen in benign inflammatory cases. *B,* Plasma cells of intermediate maturity. *C,* Plasma cells that are immature and less well-differentiated. (From Frassica, F.J., Frassica, D.A., and Sim, F.H.: Myeloma of bone. In Stauffer, R.N., ed.: Advances in Operative Orthopaedics, vol. 2. St. Louis, Mosby–Year Book, 1994, p. 362.)

c. Osteosclerotic Myeloma—This form is a rare variant in which bone lesions are associated with a chronic inflammatory demyelinating polyneuropathy. Generally, the diagnosis of osteosclerotic myeloma is not made until the polyneuropathy is recognized and evaluated. Sensory symptoms (tingling, pins and needles, coldness) are noted first, followed by motor weakness. Both the sensory and motor changes begin distally, are symmetric, and proceed proximally. Severe weakness is common, but bone pain is not characteristic. Radiographic studies may show a spectrum from purely sclerotic to a mixed pattern of lysis and sclerosis. The lesions usually involve the spine, pelvic bones, and ribs; the extremities are generally spared. Patients may have abnormalities outside the nervous system and have a constellation of findings termed the POEMS syndrome (polyneuropathy, organomegaly, endocrinopathy, M protein, and skin changes). Treatment is a combination of chemotherapy, radiotherapy, and plasmapharesis. The neurologic changes may not improve with treatment.

I. Tumors of Unknown Origin—The three principal tumors of unknown origin are giant cell tumor, Ewing's tumor, and adamantinoma.

1. Giant Cell Tumor (Fig. 8-40)—This distinctive neoplasm has poorly differentiated cells (Dahlin). The lesion is a benign but aggressive process. Further confusion results from the fact that this benign tumor may rarely (<2% of the time) metastasize to the lungs (benign metastasizing giant cell tumor). Unlike most bone tumors, which occur more commonly in males, giant cell tumor is more common in females. The lesion is uncommon in children with open physes. The lesion is most common in the epiphysis of long bones, and about 50% of lesions occur about the knee; the vertebra and sacrum are involved in about 10% of cases (Fig. 8-41). Multicentricity occurs in fewer than 1% of patients. Patients present with pain that is usually referable to the joint involved. Radiographs show a purely lytic destructive lesion in the metaphysis that extends into the epiphysis and often borders the subchondral bone. Early in the symptomatic phase, the radiographs may appear normal; a small lytic focus is difficult to detect. The basic proliferating cell has a round-to-oval or even spindle-shaped nucleus (Dahlin). The giant cells appear to have the same nuclei as the proliferating mononuclear cells. Mitotic figures may be numerous. Giant cell tumors may undergo a number of secondary degenerative changes, such as aneurysmal bone cyst formation, necrosis, fibrous repair, foam cell formation, and reactive new bone (Fig. 8-42). Treatment is aimed at removing the lesion with preservation of the involved joint. Extensive exteriorization (removal of a large cortical window over the lesion), curettage with hand and power instruments, and chemical cauterization with phenol are performed. The large resulting defect is usually

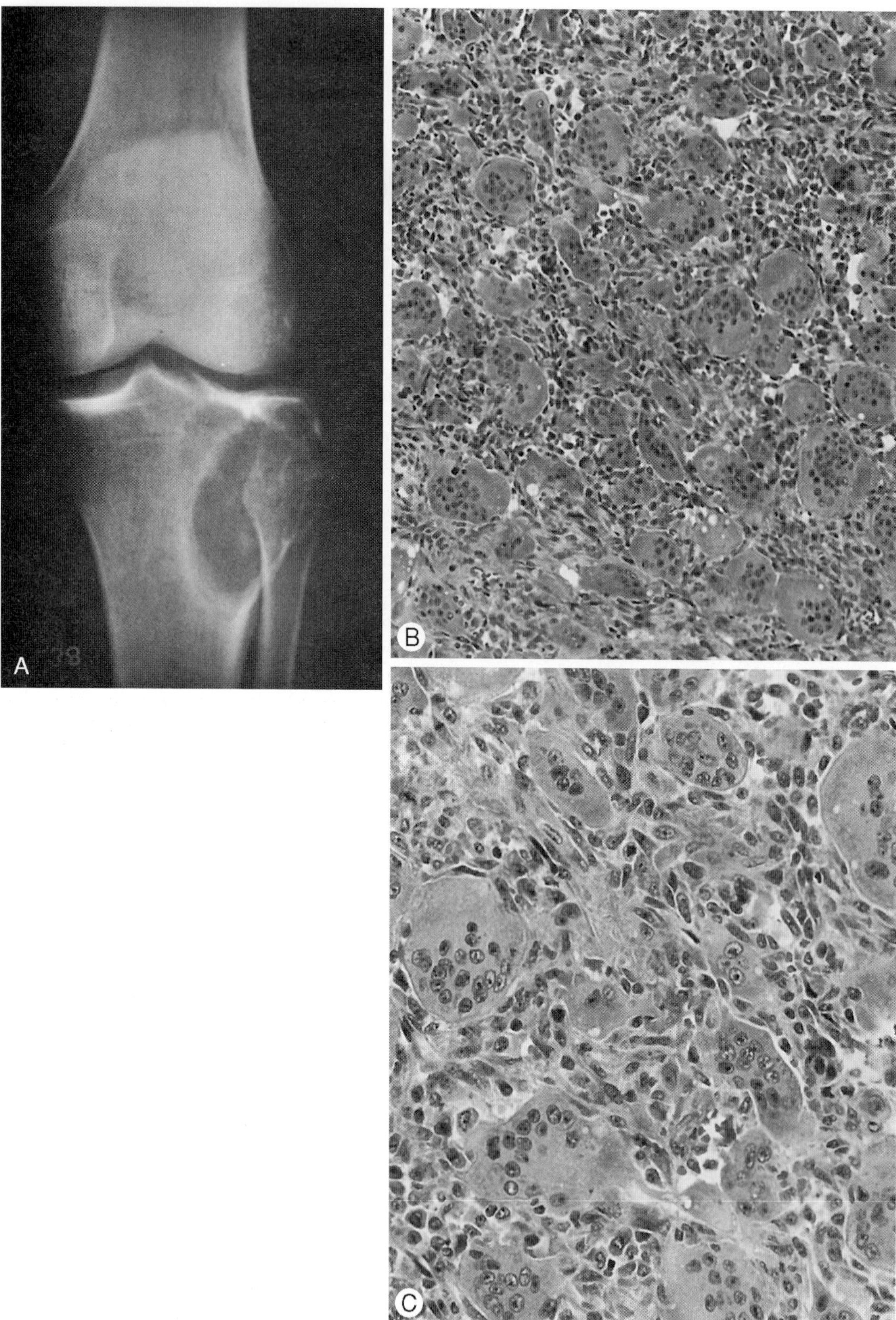

FIGURE 8-40 ■ Giant cell tumor of the proximal tibia. *A,* Radiograph shows a well-circumscribed lytic lesion in the proximal tibia involving both the epiphysis and the metaphysis. *B,* Low-power photomicrograph (×160) shows sheets of multinucleated giant cells. *C,* Higher-power photomicrograph (×300).

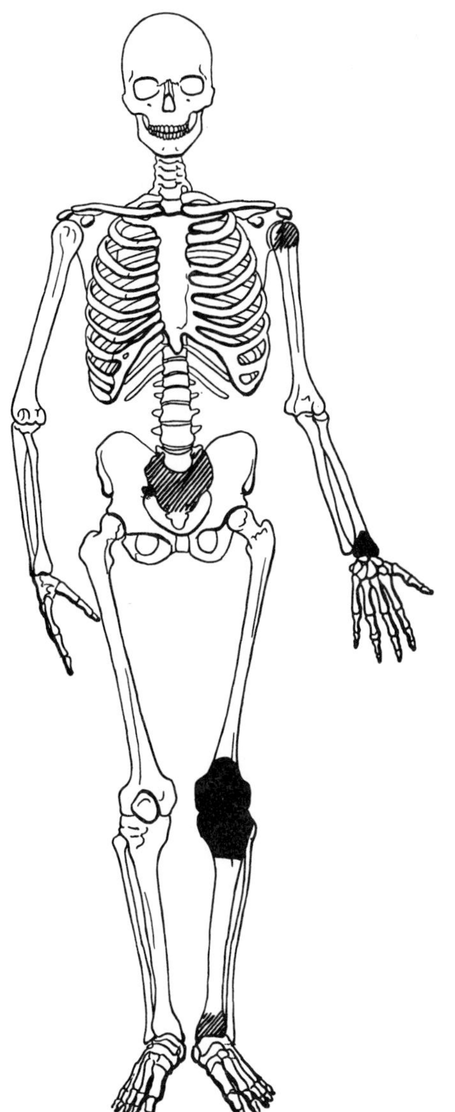

FIGURE 8-41 ■ Skeletal distribution of the most common sites of giant cell tumor of bone. The knee, distal radius, and proximal humerus are the most common sites. (From McCarthy, E.F., and Frassica, F.J.: Pathology of Bone and Joint Disorders. Philadelphia, WB Saunders, 1998.)

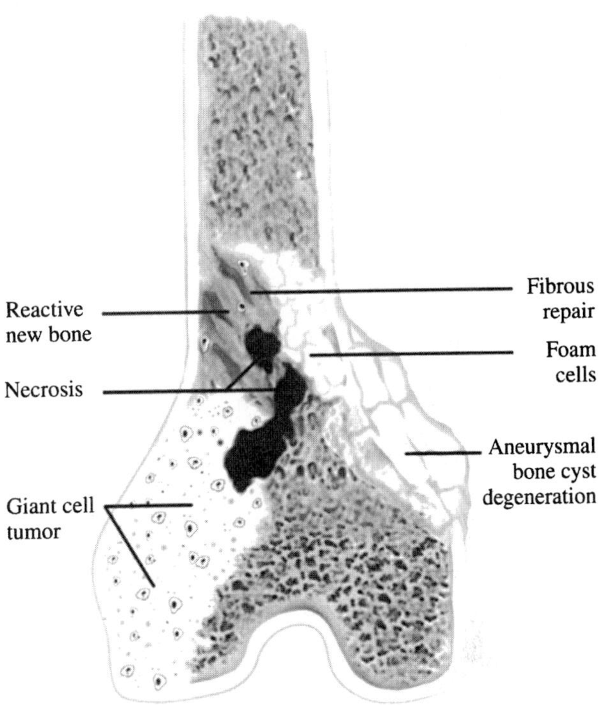

FIGURE 8-42 ■ Artist's depiction of the secondary changes seen in giant cell tumor of bone. Giant cell tumor of bone may undergo many secondary changes, including aneurysmal bone cyst formation in which the tumor causes marked expansion of the bone with ballooning out of the cortex. Necrosis and cyst formation are also common. Fibrous repair, reactive new bone, and foam cells may often be found. (From McCarthy, E.F., and Frassica, F.J.: Pathology of Bone and Joint Disorders. Philadelphia, WB Saunders, 1998.)

reconstructed with subchondral bone grafts and methyl methacrylate. Local control using this treatment regimen has a success rate of 85–90%.

Malignancy may occur in two forms in giant cell tumor: primary malignant giant cell tumor and secondary malignant giant cell tumor. Secondary malignant giant cell tumor occurs following radiation to a giant cell tumor or after multiple local recurrences. The most common scenario is that a patient has a large, aggressive giant cell tumor that is inoperable. The patient then receives irradiation, and a sarcoma (osteosarcoma, fibrosarcoma, or malignant fibrous histiocytoma) develops in the irradiated field 3–50 years following the irradiation (called the latency period). A small number of patients may have the development of a high-grade sarcoma following multiple local recurrences.

2. Ewing's Tumor (Fig. 8-43)—This distinctive, small, round-cell sarcoma occurs most commonly in children and young adults; most children are older than 5 years. When a small blue cell tumor is found in a child younger than 5 years, metastatic neuroblastoma and leukemia should be excluded. In patients older than 30 years of age, metastatic carcinomas must be excluded. Patients generally present with pain, and fever may be present. Laboratory tests may show an elevated erythrocyte sedimentation rate, leukocytosis, anemia, and an elevated white blood cell count. The most common locations include the pelvis, distal femur, proximal tibia, femoral diaphysis, and proximal humerus (Fig. 8-44). Radiographs often show a large destructive lesion that involves the metaphysis and diaphysis; the

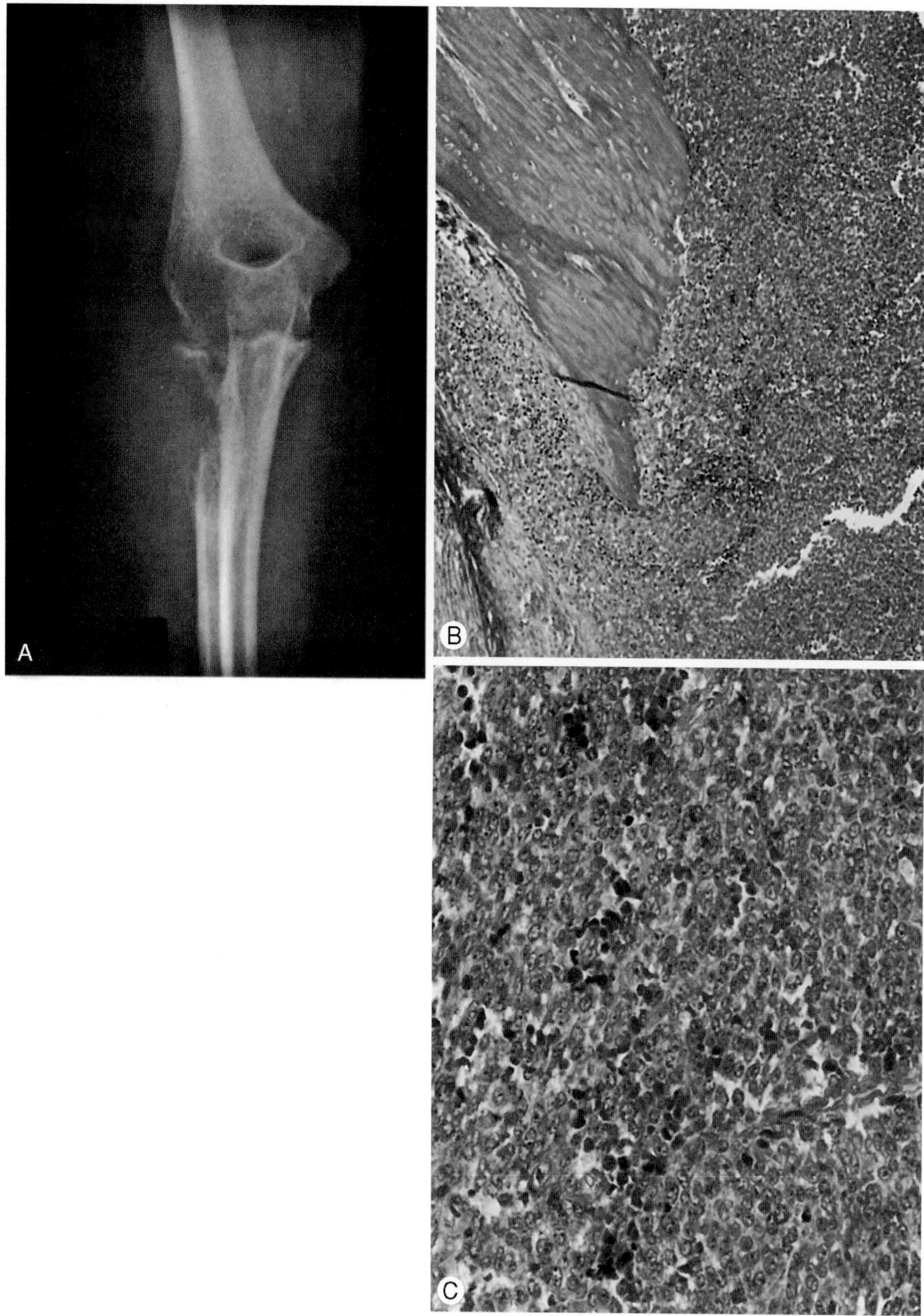

FIGURE 8-43 ■ Ewing's sarcoma of the proximal radius. *A,* Radiograph shows a destructive expansile lesion in the proximal radius. *B,* Low-power photomicrograph (×100) shows bone surrounded by a highly cellular neoplasm. *C,* Higher-power photomicrograph (×400) shows sheets of round cells.

lesion may be purely lytic or have variable amounts of reactive new bone formation. The periosteum may be lifted off in multiple layers, giving a characteristic but uncommon onion skin appearance. There is often a large soft-tissue component. Treatment involves a multimodality approach with (1) multi-agent chemotherapy, (2) irradiation, and (3) surgical resection. Traditionally, most lesions have been treated with chemotherapy and irradiation, but the role of surgery is becoming more prominent. Long-term survival with multimodality treatment may be as high as 60–70%. There is a consistent chromosomal translocation (11:22) with the formation of a fusion protein (EWS-FLI 1) (Temple). Poor prognostic factors include: (1) spine and pelvic tumors, (2) tumors greater than 100 cm^3, (3) poor response to chemotherapy (less than 90% necrosis), and (4) elevated lactic dehydrogenase levels (Temple).

3. Adamantinoma (Fig. 8-45)—This rare tumor of long bones contains epithelial-like islands of cells. The tibia is the most common site, although rarely, other long bones are involved (fibula, femur, ulna, radius) (Fig. 8-46). Most patients are young adults and present with pain of months' to years' duration. The typical radiographic appearance is that of multiple, sharply circumscribed, lucent defects of different sizes, with sclerotic bone interspersed between the zones and extending above and below the lucent zones (Dahlin). Typically, one of the lesions in the midshaft is the largest and is associated with cortical bone destruction. Histologically, the cells have an epithelial

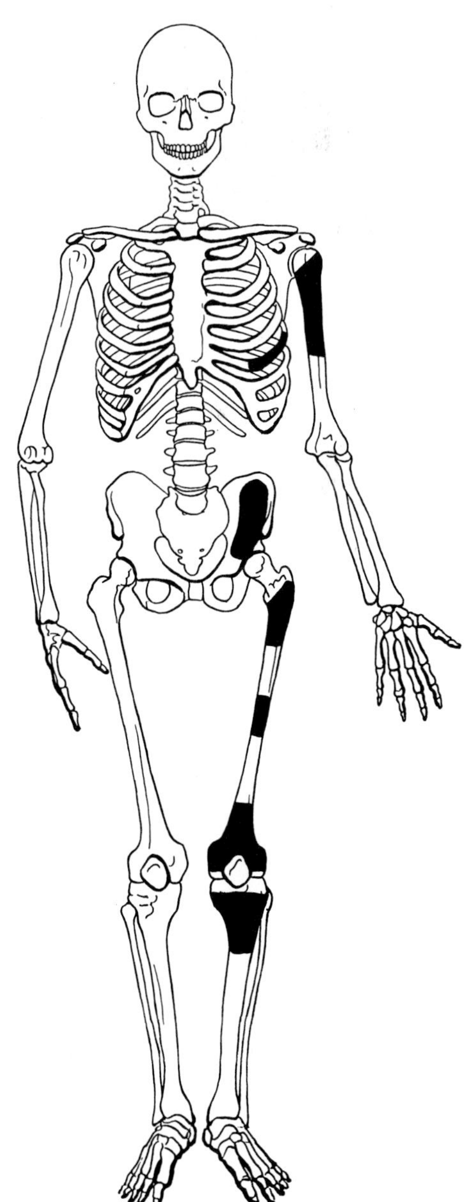

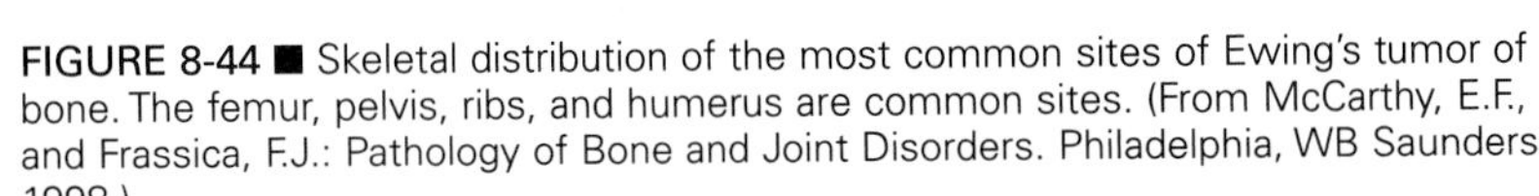

FIGURE 8-44 ■ Skeletal distribution of the most common sites of Ewing's tumor of bone. The femur, pelvis, ribs, and humerus are common sites. (From McCarthy, E.F., and Frassica, F.J.: Pathology of Bone and Joint Disorders. Philadelphia, WB Saunders, 1998.)

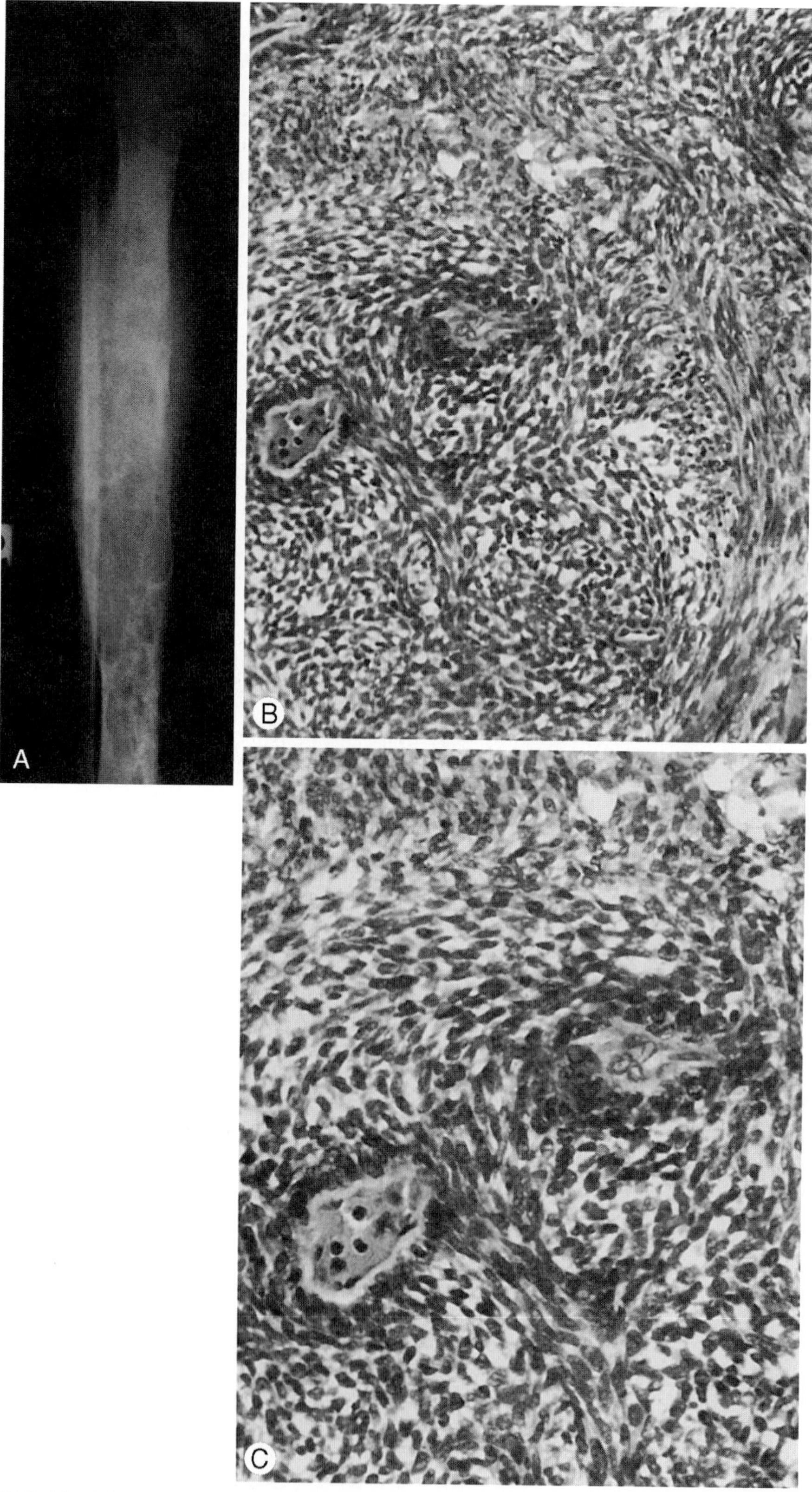

FIGURE 8-45 ■ Adamantinoma of the tibia. *A,* Radiograph shows a bubbly symmetric lytic lesion in the tibial diaphysis. *B,* Low-power photomicrograph (×250) shows biphasic differentiation with spindle cells and epithelioid cells. *C,* Higher-power photomicrograph (×400).

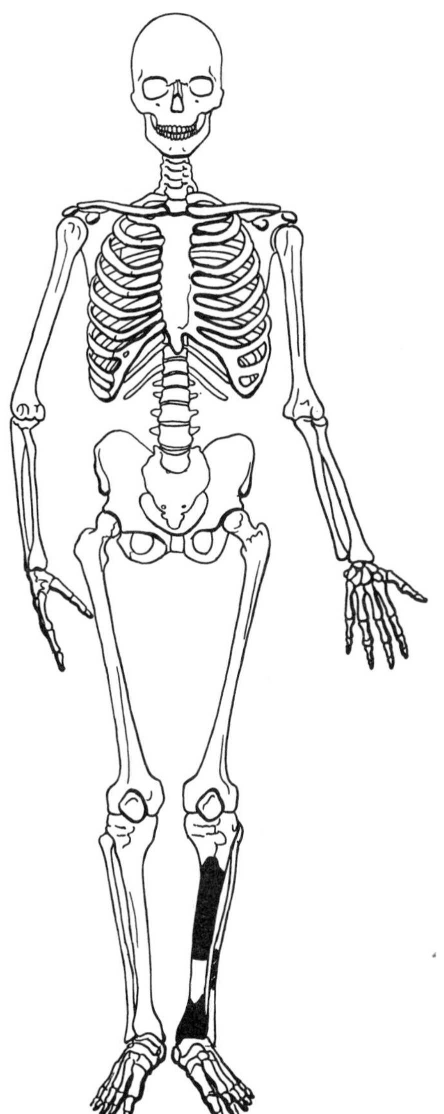

FIGURE 8-46 ■ Skeletal distribution of the most common sites of adamantinoma. This peculiar tumor most commonly affects the tibia. (From McCarthy, E.F., and Frassica, F.J.: Pathology of Bone and Joint Disorders, Philadelphia, WB Saunders, 1998.)

Table 8-8. TUMOR-LIKE CONDITIONS (TUMOR SIMULATORS)

Young Patient
Eosinophilic granuloma
Osteomyelitis
Avulsion fractures
Aneurysmal bone cyst
Fibrous dysplasia
Osteofibrous dysplasia
Heterotopic ossification
Unicameral bone cyst
Giant cell reparative granuloma
Exuberant callus
Adult
Synovial chondromatosis
Pigmented villonodular synovitis
Stress fracture
Heterotopic ossification
Ganglion cyst
Older Adult
Metastatic bone disease
Mastocytosis
Hyperparathyroidism
Paget's disease
Bone infarcts
Bone islands
Ganglion cyst
Cyst secondary to joint disease
Epidermoid cyst

quality and are arranged in a palisading or glandular pattern; the epithelial cells occur in a fibrous stroma. Treatment of this low-grade malignant lesion is wide-margin surgical resection. The lesion may metastasize either early or after multiple failed attempts at local control.

J. Tumor-like Conditions—There are many lesions that simulate primary bone tumors and must be considered in the differential diagnosis (Table 8-8). These lesions range from metastases to reactive conditions.

1. Aneurysmal Bone Cyst (Fig. 8-47)—This non-neoplastic reactive condition may be aggressive in its ability to destroy normal bone and extend into the soft tissues. The lesion may arise primarily in bone or be found in association with other tumors, such as giant cell tumor, chondroblastoma, chondromyxoid fibroma, and fibrous dysplasia. It may also occur within a malignant tumor. Three-fourths of patients with an aneurysmal bone cyst are <20 years of age. Patients experience pain and swelling, which may have been present for months or years. The characteristic radiographic finding is an eccentric, lytic, expansile area of bone destruction in the metaphysis; in classic cases there is a thin rim of periosteal new bone surrounding the lesion. The plain radiograph may demonstrate the periosteal bone if it is mineralized, and the MRI scan usually shows the periosteal layer going all around the lesion. The essential histologic features are cavernous blood-filled spaces without an endothelial lining (Dahlin). There are thin strands of bone present in the fibrous tissue of the septae. Benign giant cells may be numerous. Treatment is careful curettage and bone grafting. Local recurrence is common in children with open physes.
2. Unicameral Bone Cyst (Fig. 8-48)—This lesion occurs most commonly in the proximal humerus and is characterized by cystic, symmetric expansion with thinning of the involved cortices; other common sites are the proximal femur and distal tibia. The cause is unknown, but it probably results from some disturbance of the physis. Patients generally present with pain, usually after a fracture due

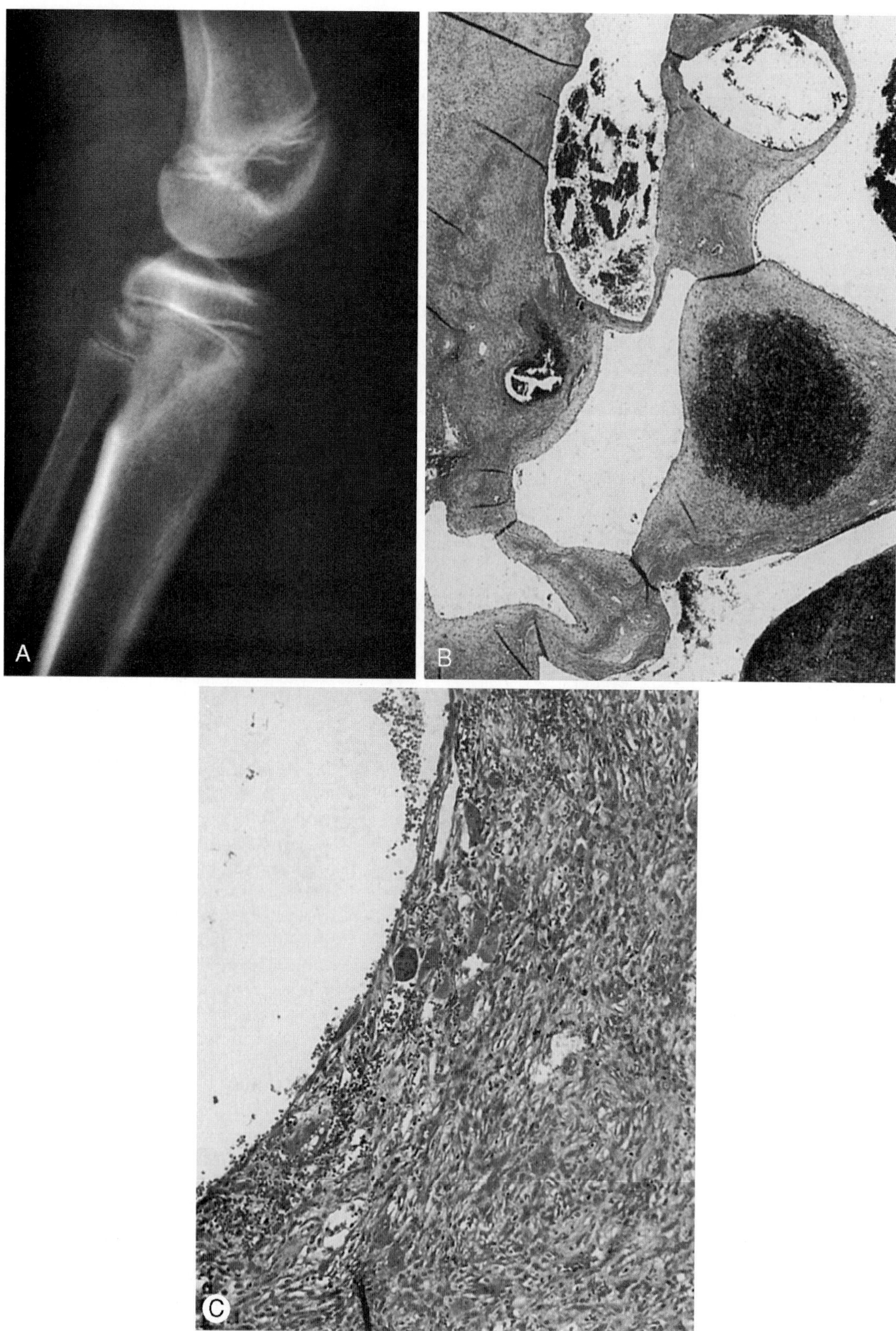

FIGURE 8-47 ■ Aneurysmal bone cyst of the proximal tibia. *A,* Radiograph shows a well-defined lytic lesion in the posterior tibial metaphysis. *B,* Low-power photomicrograph (×25) shows blood-filled lakes. *C,* Higher-power photomicrograph (×50) shows the wall of the cyst with fibroblasts and occasional multinucleated giant cells.

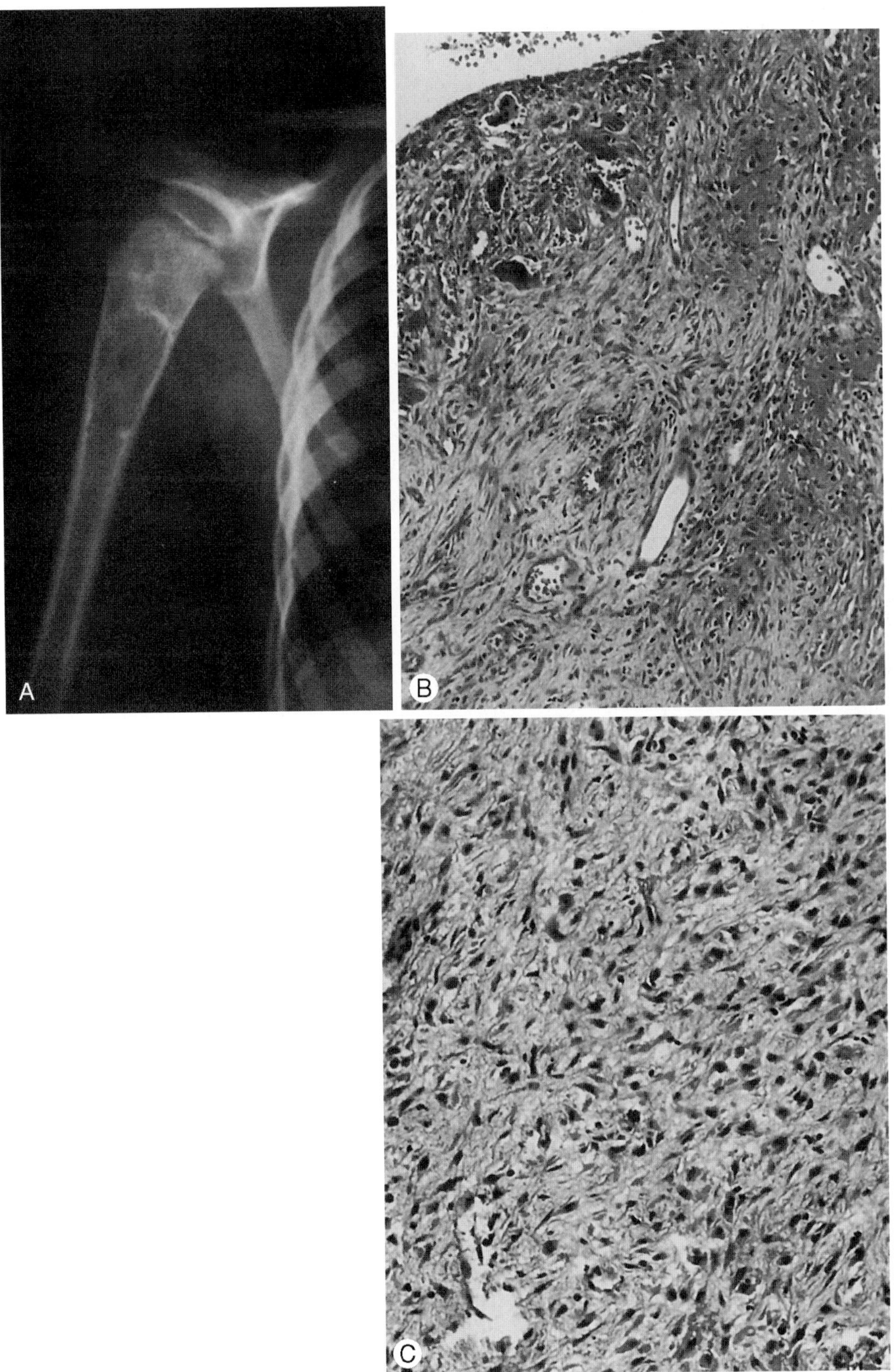

FIGURE 8-48 ■ Unicameral bone cyst of the humerus. *A,* Radiograph shows a symmetric, midline, well-circumscribed lytic lesion in the humeral metaphysis. *B,* Low-power photomicrograph (×160) shows the fibrous tissue membrane with reactive bone and occasional multinucleated giant cells. *C,* High-power field.

to minor trauma (e.g., sporting event, throwing a baseball, wrestling). The radiographic picture is characteristic, with a central lytic area and symmetric thinning of the cortices. The bone is often expanded; however, the width of the bone generally is no greater than the width of the physis. The lesion often appears trabeculated. When the cyst abuts the physeal plate, the process is called *active*; when there is normal bone intervening, the cyst is termed *latent*. Histologically, the cyst has a thin fibrous lining; the lining of the cyst contains fibrous tissue, giant cells, hemosiderin pigment, and a few chronic inflammatory cells (Dahlin). Treatment of unicameral bone cyst begins with aspiration to confirm the diagnosis, followed by methyl prednisolone acetate injection. Curettage and bone grafting are reserved for recalcitrant lesions, especially in the proximal femur where pathologic fractures can lead to severe hip disability.

3. Histiocytosis X (Fig. 8-49)—This disease of the reticuloendothelial system may manifest in a range from eosinophilic granuloma (usually in a single bone and self-limited) to Letterer-Siwe disease (which is a fulminant fatal form). Eosinophilic granuloma of bone is the most common manifestation where only a single bone or occasionally multiple bones are involved. Patients present with pain and swelling. The radiographs often show a highly destructive lesion with a well-defined margination. The cortex may be destroyed with periosteal reaction, and there may be a soft-tissue mass simulating a malignant bone tumor. There may be expansion of the involved bone. Any bone may be involved. Histologically, the proliferating Langerhans' cell with an indented or grooved nucleus is the characteristic cell. The cytoplasm is eosinophilic, and the nuclear membrane has a crisp border. Mitotic figures may be common. Eosinophilic granuloma is a self-limited process, and several forms of treatment have been successful, including low-dose irradiation (600–800 cGy), curettage and bone grafting, and observation. When the articular surface is in jeopardy or an impending fracture is a possibility, curettage and bone grafting are a logical choice. Low-dose irradiation is effective for most lesions and is associated with low morbidity. Hand-Schuller-Christian disease is characterized by both bone lesions and visceral involvement; the classic triad, which occurs in fewer than a fourth of patients, includes (1) exophthalmus; (2) diabetes insipidus; and (3) lytic skull lesions. Letterer-Siwe disease occurs in young children and is usually fatal.

   In time the term *Histiocytosis X* will be replaced with *Langerhans' cell histiocytosis*. The proliferating cell is the Langerhans' cell (from the dendritic system in the skin). Langerhans' cell granulomatosis has three principal forms: solitary (analogous to eosinophilic granuloma of bone), multiple (no visceral involvement), and multiple sites with visceral involvement (analogous to Hand-Schuller-Christian disease and Letterer-Siwe disease).

4. Fibrous Dysplasia (Fig. 8-50)—This developmental abnormality of bone is characterized by monostotic or polyostotic involvement. Yellow or brown patches of skin may accompany the bone lesions (Dahlin). When, in addition to the skin abnormalities, there are endocrine abnormalities (especially precocious puberty) with multiple bone lesions, the condition is called McCune-Albright syndrome. Virtually any bone may be involved, with the proximal femur being the most common. Radiographs may show a variable appearance with a highly lytic or ground-glass appearance; there is often a well-defined rim of sclerotic bone around the lesion. The major histologic feature is proliferation of fibroblasts, which produce a dense, collagenous matrix (Dahlin). There are often trabeculae of osteoid and bone within the fibrous stroma. Cartilage may be present in variable amounts. The bone fragments are present in a disorganized fashion and have been likened to "alphabet soup" and "Chinese letters." Treatment of fibrous dysplasia is symptomatic. Internal fixation and bone grafting are used in areas of high stress where nonoperative treatment would not be effective; most patients do not need surgical treatment.
5. Osteofibrous Dysplasia—This rare variant of fibrous dysplasia primarily involves the tibia and is usually confined to the cortices. Bowing is very common, and children may develop pathologic fractures. The lesion typically presents in children younger than age 10. This diagnosis can be made radiographically. In general a biopsy is not necessary. When performed, the biopsy shows fibrous tissue stroma and a background of bone trabeculae with osteoblastic rimming. Nonoperative treatment is preferred until the child reaches maturity.
6. Paget's Disease—This condition is characterized by abnormal bone remodeling. The disease is most commonly diagnosed during the fifth decade of life. The process may be monostotic or polyostotic. Patients usually present with pain. Radiographs demonstrate coarsened trabeculae and remodeled cortices; the coarsened trabeculae give the bone a blastic appearance. Histologically, the characteristic features are irregular broad trabeculae, reversal or cement lines, osteoclastic activity, and fibrous vascular tissue between the trabeculae (Dahlin). Medical treatment of Paget's disease is aimed at retarding the activity of the osteoclasts; agents used include diphosphonates, calcitonin, and methotrexate. The older

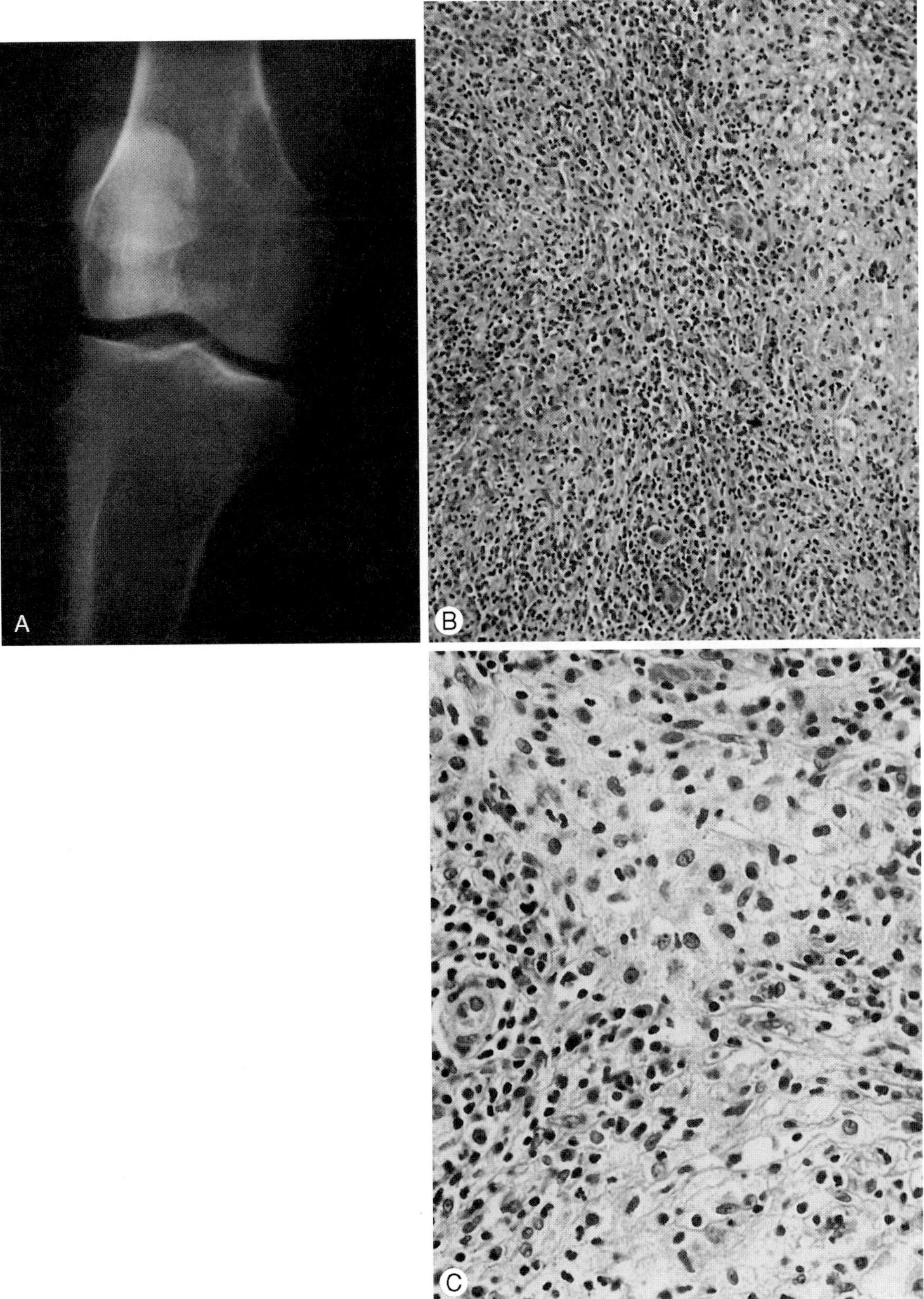

FIGURE 8-49 ■ Eosinophilic granuloma of the distal femur. *A,* Radiograph shows a well-circumscribed lesion with a sclerotic rim in the femoral metaphysis. *B,* Low-power photomicrograph (×160) shows a heterogeneous population of inflammatory cells with an aggregation of histiocytes. *C,* Higher-power photomicrograph (×400) shows nests of Langerhans' histiocytes.

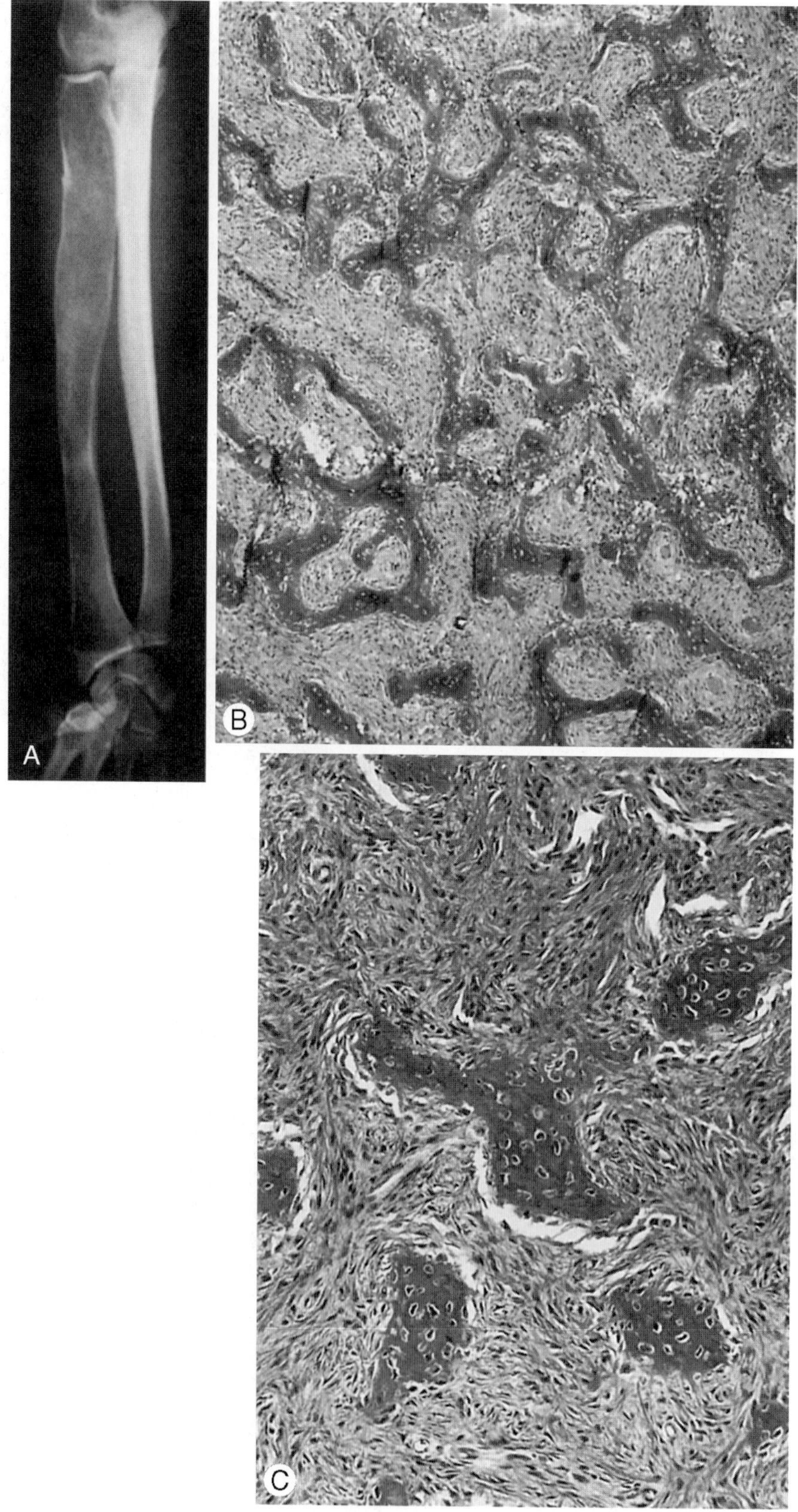

FIGURE 8-50 ■ Fibrous dysplasia of the radius. *A,* Radiograph shows a long, symmetric, ground-glass lytic lesion of the radius. *B,* Low-power photomicrograph (×50) shows seams of osteoid in a fibrous background. *C,* Higher-power photomicrograph (×160) shows osteoid surrounded by bland fibrous tissue.

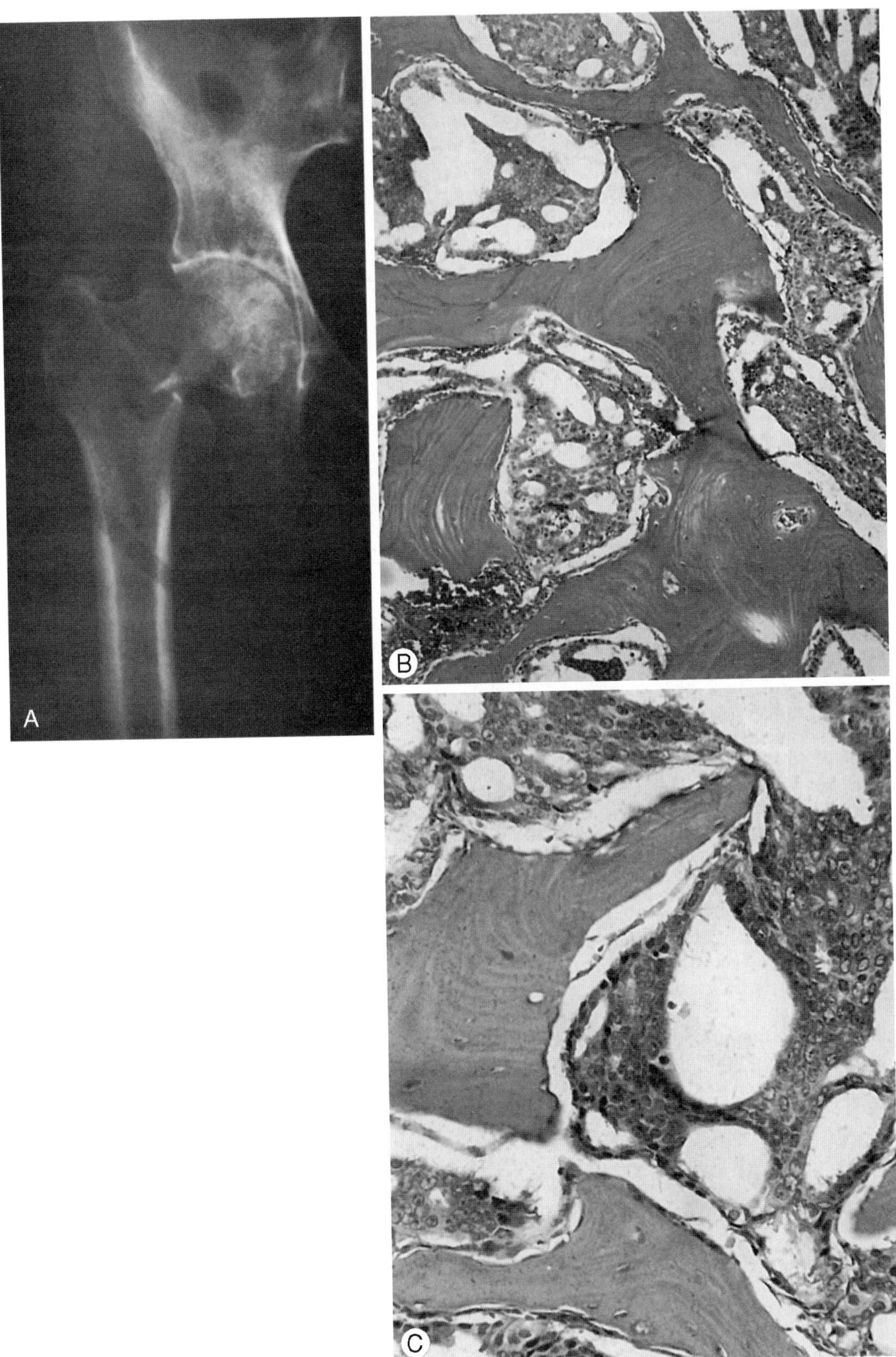

FIGURE 8-51 ■ Metastatic carcinoma. *A*, Radiograph shows a lytic lesion in the femoral neck and the ilium. *B*, Low-power photomicrograph (×100) shows the glandular arrangement of cells in the marrow space. *C*, Higher-power photomicrograph (×400).

diphosphonates (e.g., Didronel) stopped both osteoclastic activity and new bone formation; Didronel may cause osteomalacia and cannot be used for more than 6 months. Pamidronate, which can be used only intravenously, does not inhibit bone formation and has become one of the most useful agents in the diphosphonate class of medications. Patients may present with degenerative joint disease, fracture, or neurologic encroachment; joint degeneration is common in the hip and knee. Prior to replacement, arthroplasty patients should be treated to decrease bleeding at the time of surgery. Fewer than 1% of patients with Paget's disease develop malignant degeneration with the formation of a sarcoma within a focus of Paget's disease; the symptoms of a Paget's sarcoma are the abrupt onset of pain and swelling. The radiographs usually demonstrate cortical bone destruction and the presence of a soft-tissue mass. Paget's sarcomas are deadly tumors with a poor prognosis (long-term survival is <20%).

7. Metastatic Bone Disease (Fig. 8-51)—This tumor is the most common entity that destroys the skeleton in older patients. When a destructive bone lesion is found in a patient over age 40, metastases must be considered first; the five carcinomas that are most likely to metastasize to bone are breast, lung, prostate, kidney, and thyroid. The most common locations are the pelvis, vertebral bodies, ribs, and proximal limb girdles. The pathogenesis of skeletal metastases is probably related to Batson's vertebral vein plexus. The venous flow from the breast, lung, prostate, kidney, and thyroid drains into the vertebral vein plexus (Fig. 8-52). The plexus has intimate connections to the vertebral bodies, pelvis, skull, and proximal limb girdles. The radiographs most commonly demonstrate a destructive lesion that may be purely lytic, a mixed pattern of bone destruction and formation, or a purely sclerotic lesion. The histologic hallmark is epithelial cells in a fibrous stroma; the epithelial cells are often arranged in a glandular pattern. Interestingly, the bone destruction is caused not by the tumor cells themselves but rather by activation of osteoclasts (Fig. 8-53). To combat the osteoclastic bone destruction, many patients are now treated with antiresorptive agents (diphosphates) such as intravenous Pamidronate. Treatment of metastatic bone disease is aimed at controlling pain and maintaining the independence of the patient. Prophylactic internal fixation is performed when impending fracture is present. There are many criteria for fixation. Conditions that put the patient most at risk are the following:
   a. More than 50% destruction of the diaphyseal cortices
   b. Permeative destruction of the subtrochanteric femoral region
   c. More than 50–75% destruction of the metaphysis
   d. Persistent pain following irradiation

   Patients older than age 40 with a single destructive bone lesion, without a known primary tumor, must still be considered to have metastatic disease. Simon outlined a diagnostic strategy that identifies the primary lesion in up to 80–90% of patients (Table 8-9).

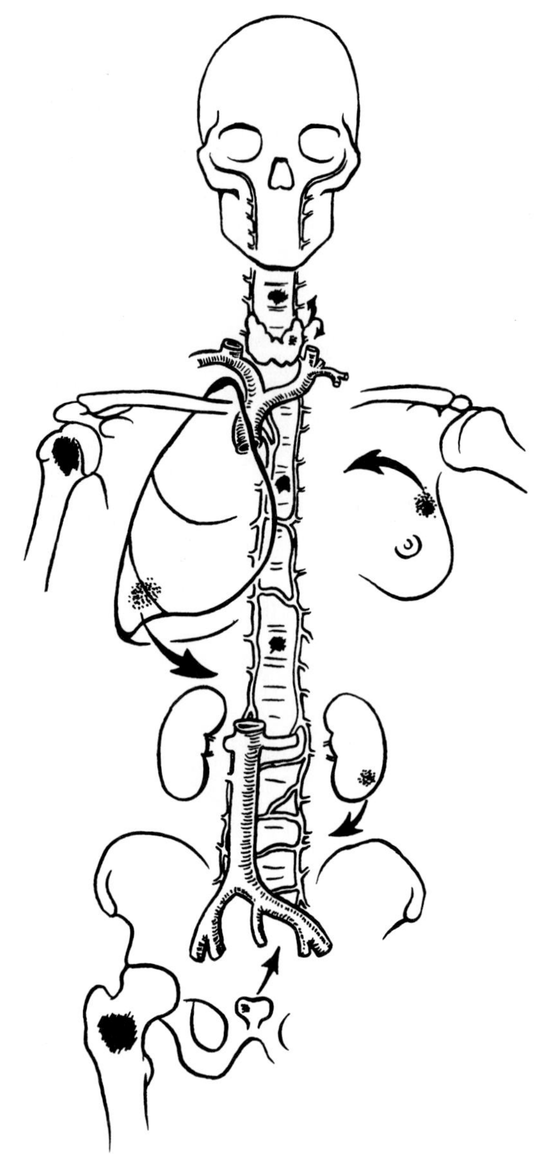

FIGURE 8-52 ■ Artist's depiction of Batson's venous plexus. This plexus is longitudinal and valveless and extends from the sacrum to the skull. The breast, lung, kidney, prostate, and thyroid glands all connect to this system. Tumor cells can enter this system and spread to the vertebra, ribs, pelvis, and proximal limb girdle. (From McCarthy, E.F., and Frassica, F.J.: Pathology of Bone and Joint Disorders. Philadelphia, WB Saunders, 1998.)

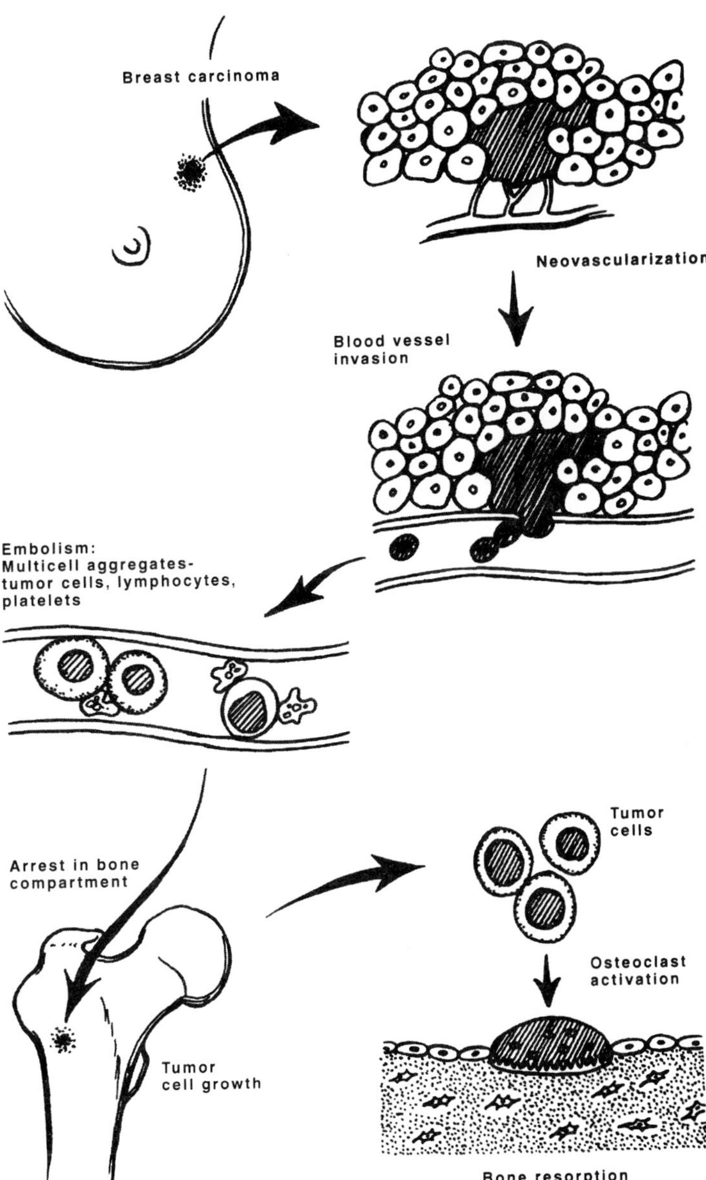

FIGURE 8-53 ■ The mechanism of bone metastases is complex. Metastatic cells spread into the venous system by vascular invasion and lodge in the medullary cavity. These tumor cells activate osteoclasts, which resorb the host bone. (From McCarthy, E.F., and Frassica, F.J.: Pathology of Bone and Joint Disorders. Philadelphia, WB Saunders, 1998.)

8. Osteomyelitis—Bone infections often simulate primary tumors. Occult infections may occur in all age groups. Patients may present with fever, chills, and bone pain; most commonly, though, patients present with bone pain without systemic symptoms. The radiographs may be nonspecific. Bone destruction and bone formation are usually the characteristic findings of chronic infections; acute infections often produce cortical bone destruction and periosteal elevation. Serpiginous tracts and irregular areas of bone destruction suggest infection rather than neoplasm. Histologically, the lesion is usually apparent with (1) edema of the granulation tissue, (2) numerous new blood vessels, and (3) a mixed cell population of inflammatory cells, plasma cells,

Table 8-9. EVALUATION OF THE OLDER PATIENT WITH A SINGLE BONE LESION AND SUSPECTED METASTASES OF UNKNOWN ORIGIN

Plain radiographs in two planes of the affected limb
Technetium bone scan to detect multiple lesions
Radiographic studies to search for occult neoplasms
- Chest radiograph and CT of the chest (to search for occult lung cancer)
- CT of the abdomen or ultrasonography of the abdomen (to detect renal cell cancer *or lymphoma*)
- Skeletal survey (if myeloma is suspected)
- Screening laboratory studies
- Complete blood count with differential
- Erythrocyte sedimentation rate
- Chemistry group: liver function test, calcium, phosphorus, alkaline phosphatase
- Serum or urine immunoelectrophoresis

polymorphonuclear leukocytes, eosinophils, lymphocytes, and histiocytes. Occasionally, a chronic infection is complicated by a squamous cell carcinoma. One should always biopsy material that has been sent for culture and culture material that has been sent for biopsy. The treatment of osteomyelitis is removal of all dead tissue and appropriate antibiotic therapy.

Selected Bibliography

TEXTBOOKS

McCarthy, E.F., and Frassica, F.J.: Pathology of Bone and Joint Disorders. Philadelphia, WB Saunders, 1998.

Mirra, J.M.: Bone Tumors: Clinical, Radiologic, and Pathologic Correlations. Philadelphia, Lea and Febiger, 1989.

Sim, F.H.: Diagnosis and Management of Metastatic Bone Disease: A Multidisciplinary Approach. Raven Press, New York, 1988.

Simon, M.A., and Springfield, D.: Surgery for Bone and Soft Tissue Tumors. Lippincott-Raven, Philadelphia, 1998.

Unni, K.K.: Dahlin's Bone Tumors: General Aspects and Data on 11,087 Cases. Lippincott-Raven, Philadelphia, 1996.

Wold, L.E., McLeod, R.A., Sim, F.H., et al.: Atlas of Orthopaedic Pathology. Philadelphia, WB Saunders, 1990.

REVIEWS

American Joint Committee on Cancer. Soft tissues. In Beahrs, O.H., and Myers, M., eds.: Manual for Staging of Cancer, 3rd ed. Philadelphia, JB Lippincott, 1988.

Enneking, W.F.: Clinical Musculoskeletal Pathology, 3rd ed. Gainesville, University of Florida Press, 1990.

Frassica, F.J., Chang, B.W., Ma, L.D., et al.: Soft tissue sarcomas: General features, evaluation, imaging, biopsy, and treatment. Curr. Orthop. 11:105–113, 1997.

Frassica, F.J., Gitelis, S.G., and Sim, F.H.: Metastatic Bone Disease: General Principles, Pathogenesis, Pathophysiology and Biopsy. Instr. Course Lect. 41:293–300, 1992.

Mindell, E.R.: Chordoma. J. Bone Joint Surg. [Am.] 63:501–505, 1981.

Orthopaedic Knowledge Update Home Study Syllabus I, II, III. Chicago, American Academy of Orthopaedic Surgeons, 1984, 1987, 1990.

Sim, F.H., Frassica, F.J., and Frassica, D.A.: Soft tissue tumors: Evaluation, diagnosis, and management. J. Am. Acad. Orthop. Surg. 2(4):202–211, 1994.

Simon, M.A.: Current concepts review: Biopsy of musculoskeletal tumors. J. Bone Joint Surg. [Am.] 64:1253, 1982.

RECENT ARTICLES

Bell, R.S., O'Sullivan, B., Liu, F.F., et al.: The surgical margin in soft tissue sarcoma. J. Bone Joint Surg. [Am.] 71:370, 1989.

Berrey, B.H., Jr., Lord, C.F., Gebhardt, M.C., et al.: Fractures of allografts: Frequency, treatment, and end results. J. Bone Joint Surg. [Am.] 72:825, 1990.

Choong, P.F.M., Pritchard, D.J., Rock, M.G., et al.: Survival after pulmonary metastectomy in soft tissue sarcoma: Prognostic factors in 214 patients. Acta Orthop. Scand. 66:561–568, 1995.

Frassica, F.J., Frassica, D.A., Pritchard, D.J., et al.: Ewing sarcoma of the pelvis: Clinicopathological features and treatment. J. Bone Joint Surg. [Am.] 75:1457–1465, 1993.

Frassica, F.J., Waltrip, R.L., Sponseller, P.D., et al.: Clinicopathologic features and treatment of osteoid osteoma and osteoblastoma in children and adolescents. Orthop. Clin. North Am. 27:559–574, 1996.

O'Connor, M.I., and Sim, F.H.: Salvage of the limb in the treatment of malignant pelvic tumors. J. Bone Joint Surg. [Am.] 71:481, 1989.

Rougraff, B.T., Kneisl, J.S., and Simon, M.A.: Skeletal metastases of unknown origin: A prospective study of a diagnostic strategy. J. Bone Joint Surg. [Am.] 75:1276, 1993.

Rosenthal, D.I., Hornicek, F.J., Wolfe, M.W., et al.: Percutaneous radiofrequency coagulation of osteiod osteoma compared with operative treatment. J. Bone Joint Surg. 80:815–821, 1998.

Peabody, T., Monson, D., Montag, A., et al.: A comparison of the prognoses for deep and subcutaneous sarcomas of the extremities. J. Bone Joint Surg. [Am.] 76:1167, 1994.

Rock, M.G., Sim, F.H., Unni, K.K., et al.: Secondary malignant giant cell tumor of bone: Clinicopathologic assessment of nineteen patients. J. Bone Joint Surg. [Am.] 68:1073, 1986.

Simon, M.A., and Bierman, J.S.: Biopsy of bone and soft tissue lesions. J. Bone Joint Surg. [Am.] 75:616, 1993.

Temple, H.T., Clohisy, D.R. Musculoskeletal oncology. Chapter 17 in Orthopaedic Knowledge Update. American Academy of Orthopaedic Surgeons, Rosemont, IL, 2002.

Yaw, K.M., and Wurtz, D.: Resection and reconstruction for bone tumor in the proximal tibia. Orthop. Clin. North Am. 22:133–148, 1991.

Yazawa, Y., Frassica, F.J., Chao, E.Y.S., et al.: Metastatic bone disease: A study of the surgical treatment of 166 pathological humeral and femoral shaft fractures. Clin. Orthop. Rel. Res. 251:213, 1990.

CLASSIC ARTICLES

Bell, R.S., O'Sullivan, B., Liu, F.F., et al.: The surgical margin in soft tissue sarcoma. J. Bone Joint Surg. [Am.] 71:370, 1989.

Berrey, B.H., Jr., Lord, C.F., Gebhardt, M.C., et al.: Fractures of allografts: Frequency, treatment, and end results. J. Bone Joint Surg. [Am.] 72:825, 1990.

Eilber, F.R., Eckhardt, J., and Morton, D.L.: Advances in the treatment of sarcomas of the extremity: Current status of limb salvage. Cancer 54:2695–2701, 1984.

Enneking, W.F., Spanier, S.S., and Goodman, M.A.: A system for the surgical staging of musculoskeletal sarcoma. Clin. Orthop. 153:106–120, 1980.

Enneking, W.F., Spanier, S.S., and Malawer, M.M.: The effect of the anatomic setting on the results of surgical procedures for soft parts sarcoma of the thigh. Cancer 47:1005–1022, 1981.

Heare, T.C., Enneking, W.F., and Heare, M.J.: Staging techniques and biopsy of bone tumors. Orthop. Clin. North Am. 20:273, 1989.

Madewell, J.E., Ragsdale, B.D., and Sweet, D.E.: Radiologic and pathologic analysis of solitary bone lesions. Part I. Internal margins. Radiol. Clin. North Am. 19:715–748, 1981.

Mankin, H.J., Doppelt, S.H., Sullivan, T.R., et al.: Osteoarticular and intercalary allograft transplantation in the management of malignant tumors of bone. Cancer 50:613–630, 1982.

Mankin, H.J., Lange, T.A., and Spanier, S.S.: The hazards of biopsy in patients with malignant primary bone and soft tissue tumors. J. Bone Joint Surg. [Am.] 64:1121–1127, 1982.

Medsger, T.A., Jr.: Twenty-fifth rheumatism review: Paget's disease. Arthritis Rheum. 26:281–283, 1983.

Merkow, R.L., and Lane, J.M.: Current concepts of Paget's disease of bone. Orthop. Clin. North Am. 15:747–764, 1984.

Miller, M.D., Yaw, K.M., and Foley, H.T.: Malpractice maladies in the management of musculoskeletal malignancies. Contemp. Orthop. 23:577–584, 1991.

Pritchard, D.J., Lunke, R.J., Taylor, W.F., et al.: Chondrosarcoma: A clinicopathologic and statistical analysis. Cancer 45:149–157, 1980.

Ragsdale, B.D., Madewell, J.E., and Sweet, D.E.: Radiologic and pathologic analysis of solitary bone lesions. Part II. Periosteal reactions. Radiol. Clin. North Am. 19:749–783, 1981.

Sim, F.H., Beauchamp, C.P., and Chao, E.Y.S.: Reconstruction of musculoskeletal defects about the knee for tumor. Clin. Orthop. 221:188–201, 1987.

Simon, M.A.: Biopsy of musculoskeletal tumors. J. Bone Joint Surg. [Am.] 64:1253–1257, 1982.

Simon, M.A.: Current concepts review: Limb salvage for osteosarcoma. J. Bone Joint Surg. [Am.] 70:307–310, 1988.

Simon, M.A., and Nachman, J.: The clinical utility of pre-operative therapy for sarcomas. J. Bone Joint Surg. [Am.] 68:1458–1463, 1986.

Springfield, D.S., Schmidt, R., Graham-Pole, J., et al.: Surgical treatment for osteosarcoma. J. Bone Joint Surg. [Am.] 70:1124–1130, 1988.

Sweet, D.E., Madewell, J.E., and Ragsdale, B.D.: Radiologic and pathologic analysis of solitary bone lesions. Part III. Matrix patterns. Radiol. Clin. North Am. 19:785–814, 1981.

Wuisman, P., and Enneking, W.F.: Prognosis for patients who have osteosarcoma with skip metastasis. J. Bone Joint Surg. [Am.] 72:60, 1990.

Zimmer, W.D., Berquist, T.H., McLeod, R.A., et al.: Bone tumors: Magnetic resonance imaging versus computed tomography. Radiology 155:709–718, 1985.

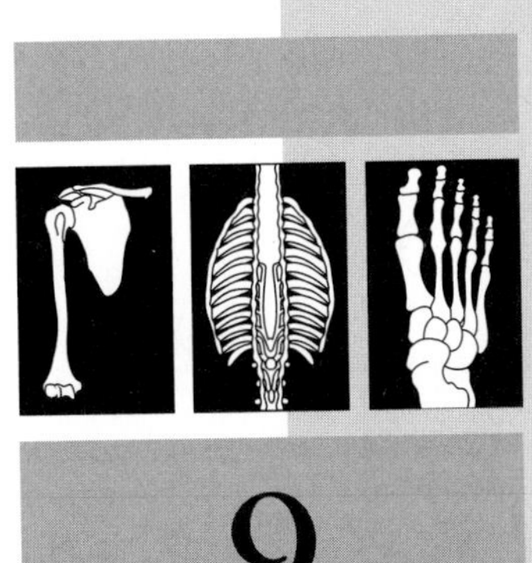

9

Rehabilitation: Gait, Amputations, Prosthetics, Orthotics

FRANK A. GOTTSCHALK

I. Gait

A. Walking—The process of moving from one location to another. Walking is a cyclic, energy-efficient activity. It requires that one foot be in contact with the ground at all times **(single-limb support)**, with a period when both limbs are in contact with the ground **(double-limb support)** (Fig. 9-1). The **step** is the distance between **initial swing and initial contact** of the same limb. **Stride** is initial contact to initial contact of the same limb (Fig. 9-2). **Velocity** is a function of cadence (steps per unit time) and stride length. Running involves a period when neither limb is in contact with the ground. Prerequisites for normal gait include stance-phase stability, swing-phase ground clearance, pre-position of the foot before initial contact (heel strike), and energy-efficient step length and speed. **Stance phase occupies 60%** of the cycle from initial contact, progression through loading response, midstance, terminal stance, and preswing. **Swing phase is 40% of the cycle** and starts at initial swing (toe off), proceeds with limb acceleration to midswing, when the limb decelerates at terminal swing before the next cycle (Figs. 9-3 and 9-4). During initial swing, the **hip and knee flex**, and the ankle starts dorsiflexion.

B. Gait Dynamics—Multiple phases of gait contribute to an energy-efficient process by lessening excursion of the center of body mass. The head, neck, trunk, and arms represent 70% of body weight. **The center of gravity** of this mass is located just **anterior to T10, which is 33 cm above the hip joints** in an individual of average height (184 cm). The resultant gait pattern resembles a sinusoidal curve.

C. Determinants of Gait (Motion Patterns)
In mechanical terms there are six independent degrees of freedom.

1. Pelvic Rotation—The pelvis rotates about a vertical axis, **horizontal rotation**, alternately to the left and right of the line of progression, lessening the center-of-mass deviation in the horizontal plane and reducing impact at initial floor contact.
2. Pelvic List—The non-weight-bearing, **contralateral side drops 5 degrees**, reducing superior deviation.
3. Knee Flexion at Loading—The stance-phase limb is flexed 15 degrees to dampen the impact of initial loading.
4. Foot and Ankle Motion—Through the subtalar joint, damping of the loading response occurs, leading to stability during midstance and efficiency of propulsion at push-off.
5. Knee Motion—Works together with the foot and ankle to decrease necessary limb motion. The knee flexes at initial contact and extends at midstance.
6. **Lateral pelvic displacement** relates to transfer of body weight onto limb —The motion is 5 cm over the weight-bearing limb, narrowing the base of support and increasing stance-phase stability.

D. Muscle Action—Agonist and antagonist muscle groups work in concert during the gait cycle to effectively advance the limb through space. The hip flexors advance the limb forward during swing phase and are opposed during terminal swing before initial contact by the decelerating action of the hip extensors. **Most muscle activity is eccentric, which is muscle lengthening while contracting,** and allows an antagonist muscle to dampen the activity of an agonist and act as a "shock absorber" (Fig. 9-5). **Isocentric** contraction is muscle length remaining constant during contraction (Table 9-1). Some muscle activity can be concentric, in which the muscle shortens to move a joint through space.

E. Pathologic Gait—Abnormal gait patterns are caused by multiple factors.

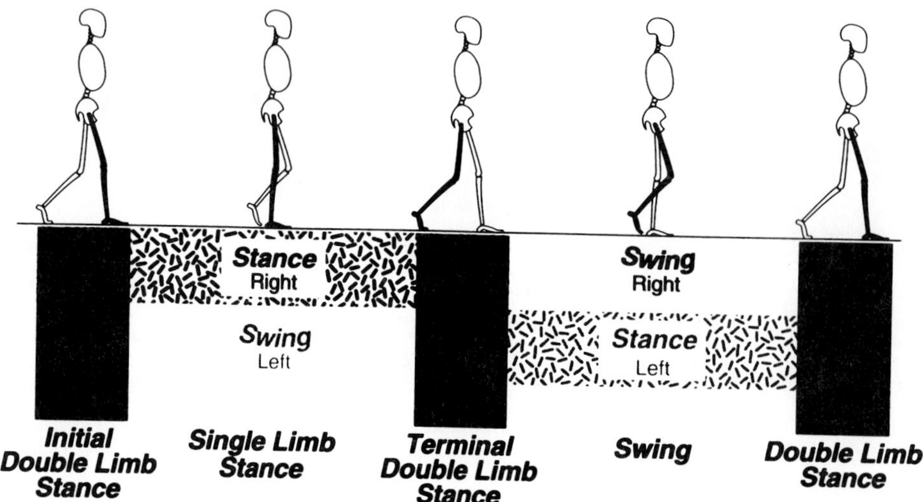

FIGURE 9-1 ■ Subdivisions of stance and their relationship to bilateral floor contact pattern. (Reprinted from Perry, J.: Gait Analysis, Normal and Pathological Function, 1992, with permission from SLACK, Inc.)

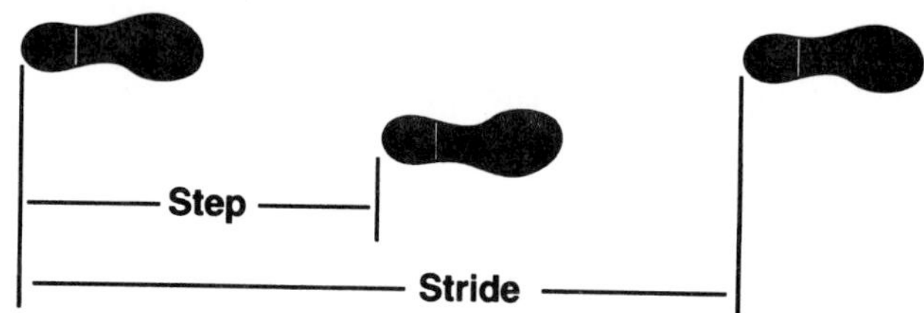

FIGURE 9-2 ■ Step versus stride. (Reprinted from Perry, J.: Gait Analysis: Normal and Pathological Function, 1992, with permission from SLACK, Inc.)

1. Muscle weakness or paralysis decreases the ability to normally move a joint through space. A walking pattern develops based on the specific muscle or muscle group involved and the ability of the individual to achieve a substitution pattern to replace that muscle's action (Table 9-2).
2. Neurologic conditions may alter gait by producing muscle weakness, loss of balance, reduced coordination between agonist and antagonist muscle groups (i.e., spasticity), and joint contracture. Hip scissoring is associated with overactive adductors, and knee flexion contracture may be caused by hamstring spasticity. **Equinus deformity** of the foot and ankle may result in steppage gait and back setting of the knee.
3. Pain in a limb creates an **antalgic gait** pattern in which the individual shortens stance phase to lessen the time that the painful limb is loaded. Contralateral swing phase is more rapid.
4. Joint abnormalities alter gait by changing the range of motion of that joint or by producing pain. Arthritis of hip and knee may have joint contractures and reduced range of motion. **Anterior cruciate deficient knee has quadriceps avoidance gait**, which is a lower than normal net quadriceps moment during midstance.
5. Hemiplegia—Prolongation of stance and double limb support is characteristic. Associated problems are **ankle equinus**, limitation of knee flexion, and increased **hip flexion**.

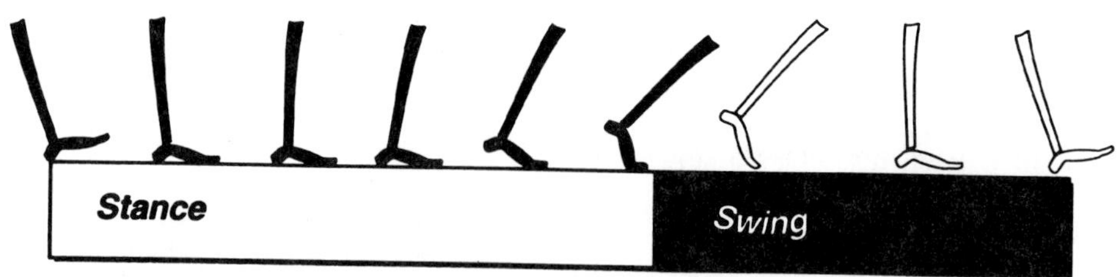

FIGURE 9-3 ■ Divisions of the gait cycle. Clear and shaded bars represent duration of each phase. (Reprinted from Perry, J.: Gait Analysis: Normal and Pathological Function, 1992, with permission from SLACK, Inc.)

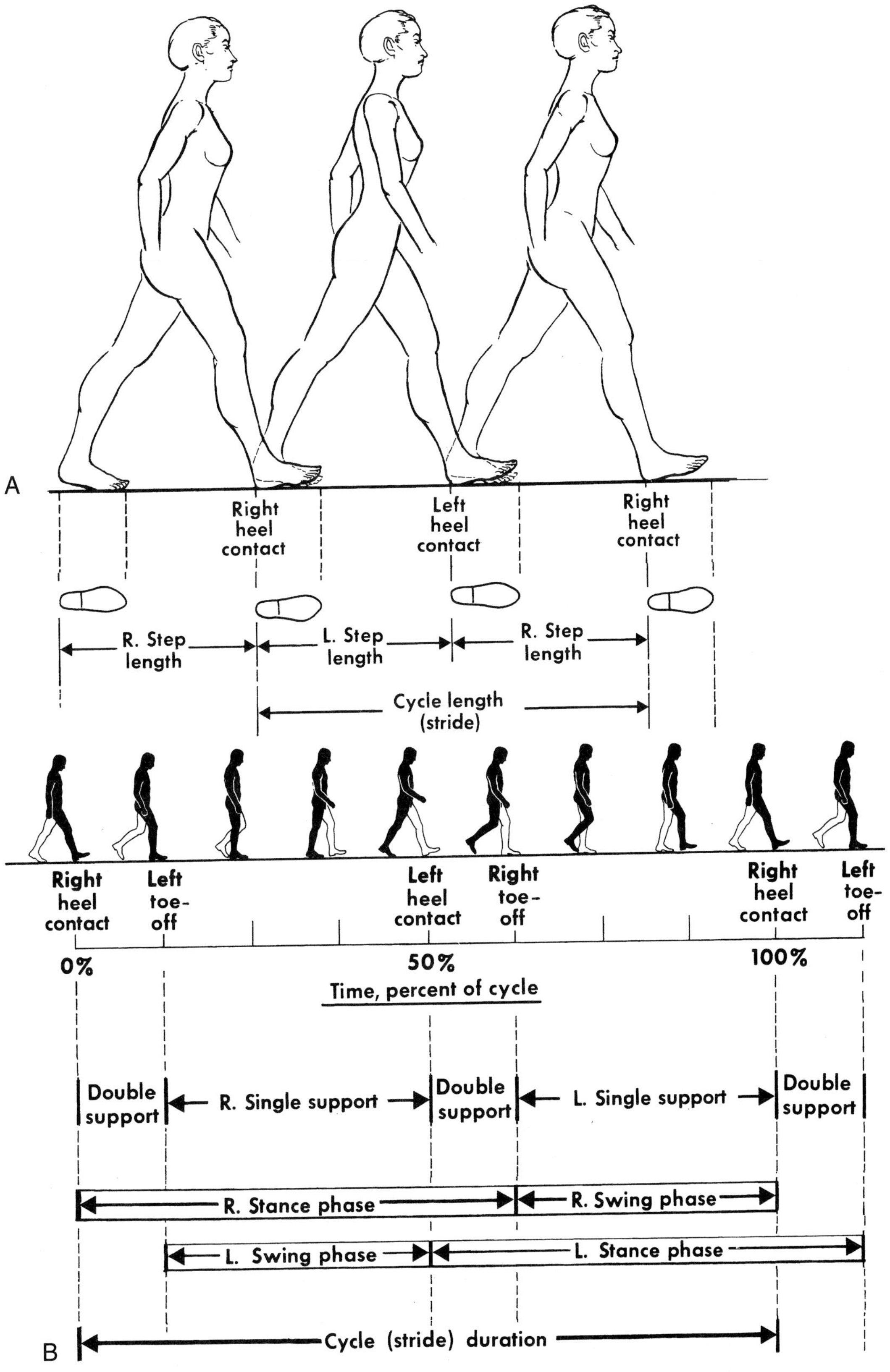

Time Dimensions of Walking Cycle

FIGURE 9-4 ■ Distance and time dimensions of walking cycle. *A,* Distance (length). *B,* Time. (From Inman, V.T., Ralston, H., and Todd, F.: Human Walking. Baltimore, Williams & Wilkins, 1982, p.26.)

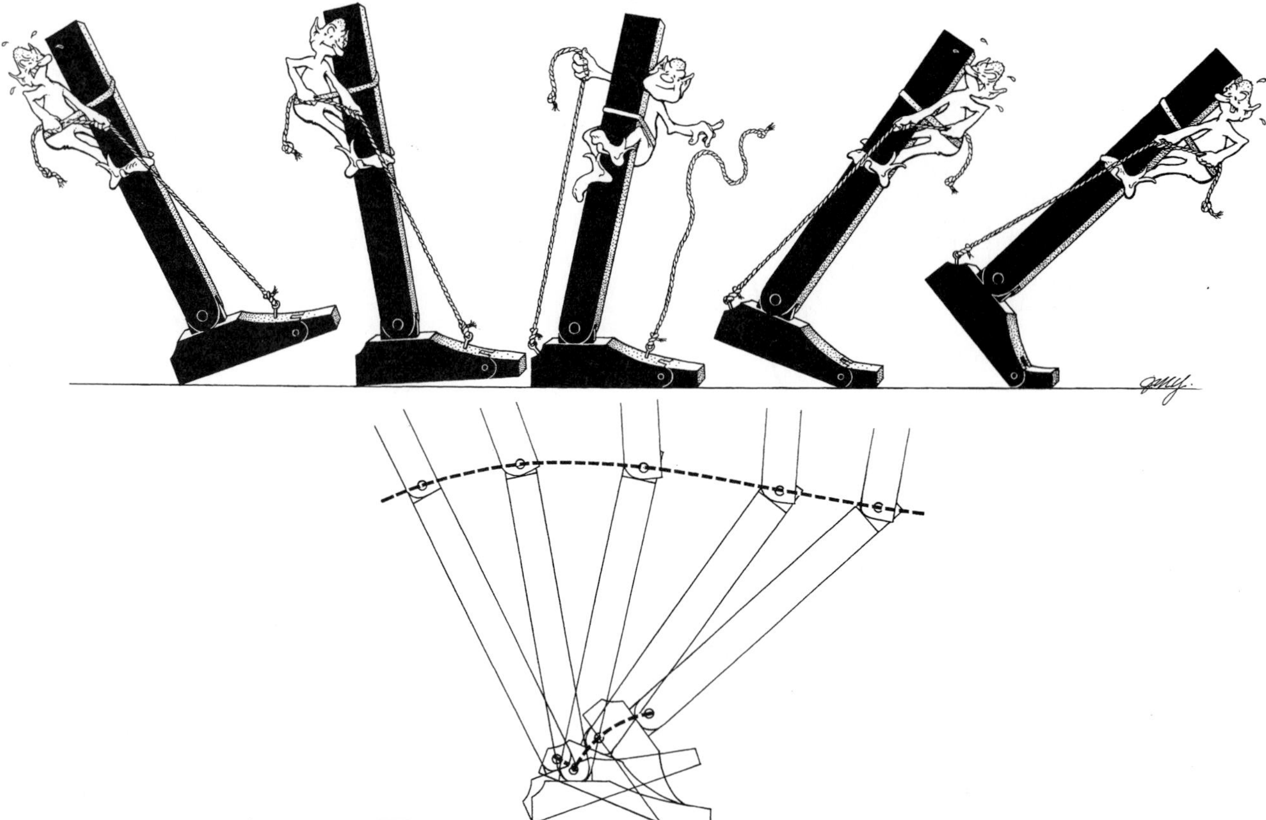

FIGURE 9-5 ■ Effect of ankle motion, controlled by muscle action, on pathway of knee. The smooth and flattened pathway of the knee during stance phase is achieved by forces acting from the leg on the foot. Foot slap is restrained during initial lowering of the foot; afterward, the plantar flexors raise the heel. (From Inman, V.T., Ralston, H., and Todd, F.: Human Walking. Baltimore, Williams & Wilkins, 1982, p. 11.)

Table 9-1. MUSCLE ACTION AND FUNCTION

MUSCLE	ACTION	FUNCTION
Gluteus medius	Eccentric	Controls pelvic tilt at midstance
Gluteus maximus	Concentric	Powers hip extension
Iliopsoas	Concentric	Powers hip flexion
Hip adductors	Eccentric	Control lateral sway (late stance)
Hip abductors	Eccentric	Control pelvic tilt (midstance)
Quadriceps	Eccentric	Stabilizes knee at heel strike
Hamstrings	Eccentric	Control rate of knee extension (stance)
Tibialis anterior	Concentric	Dorsiflexes ankle at swing
	Eccentric[a]	Slows plantar flexion rate (heel strike)
Gastrocnemius/soleus	Eccentric	Slows dorsiflexion rate (stance)

[a]Predominant role.

Surgical correction of equinus is 1 year after onset. Gait impairment may be excessive plantar flexion, weakness, and balance problems.

6. Crutches and Canes—Crutches increase stability by providing two additional loading points. **Canes** help shift the center of gravity to the affected side when the cane is used in the opposite hand. This **decreases the joint reaction** forces of the lower limb and reduces pain.
   Forces across the knee may be **4–7 times body weight**, and **70%** of load across knee occurs through the **medial compartment**.

II. Amputations—Amputation of all or part of a limb is done for peripheral vascular disease, trauma, tumor, infection, or congenital anomaly. It is often an alternative to limb salvage and should be considered a reconstructive procedure. Because of the psychologic implications and the alteration of body self-image, a multidisciplinary-team approach should be taken to return the patient to maximum level of independent function. The process should be considered the first step in the rehabilitation of the patient rather than a failure of treatment.

Table 9-2. GAIT ABNORMALITIES CAUSED BY MUSCLE WEAKNESS

MUSCLE	PHASE	DIRECTION	TYPE OF GAIT	TREATMENT
Gluteus medius	Stance	Lateral	Abductor lurch	Cane
Gluteus maximus	Stance	Backward	Lurch (hip hyperextension)	
Quadriceps	Stance	Forward	Lurch/back knee gait	AFO
	Swing	Forward	Abnormal hip rotation	
Gastrocnemius/soleus	Stance	Forward	Flat foot (calcaneal) gait	±AFO
	Swing	Forward	Delayed heel rise	
Tibialis anterior	Stance	Forward	Foot drop/slap	AFO
	Swing	Forward	Steppage gait	

AFO, ankle-foot orthosis.

A. Metabolic Cost of Amputee Gait—The metabolic cost of walking is increased with proximal-level amputations, being inversely proportional to the length of the residual limb and the number of functional joints preserved. With more-proximal amputation, patients have a decreased self-selected, maximum walking speed. **Oxygen consumption is increased** with more-proximal-level amputation; thus the transfemoral amputee with peripheral vascular disease uses close to maximum energy expenditure during normal self-selected–velocity walking (Table 9-3).

B. Load Transfer—The soft-tissue envelope acts as an interface between the bone of the residual limb and the prosthetic socket. Ideally, it is composed of a mobile, securely attached muscle mass covering the bone end and full-thickness skin that tolerates the direct pressures and pistoning within the prosthetic socket. It is rare for the prosthetic socket to achieve a perfect intimate fit. A nonadherent soft-tissue envelope allows some degree of mobility, or "pistoning," of the bone within the soft-tissue envelope, thus eliminating the shear forces that produce tissue breakdown and ulceration. Load transfer (i.e., weight-bearing) occurs by either direct or indirect means. Direct load transfer (i.e., end– weight-bearing) is accomplished with knee disarticulation or ankle disarticulation (Syme's amputation). Intimacy of the prosthetic socket is necessary only for suspension. When the amputation is performed through a long bone (i.e., transfemoral or transtibial), the end of the stump does not take all the weight and the load is transferred indirectly by the total contact method. This process requires an intimate prosthetic socket fit and **7–10 degrees of flexion of the knee for transtibial** amputation **and 5–10 degrees of adduction and flexion of the femur** for transfemoral amputation (Fig. 9-6).

Table 9-3. ENERGY EXPENDITURE FOR AMPUTATION

AMPUTATION LEVEL	% ENERGY ABOVE BASELINE	SPEED (m/min)	O_2 COST (mL/kg/m)
Long transtibial	10	70	0.17
Average transtibial	25	60	0.20
Short transtibial	40	50	0.20
Bilateral transtibial	41	50	0.20
Transfemoral	65	40	0.28
Wheelchair	0–8	70	0.16

C. Amputation Wound Healing—Depends on several factors, which include vascular inflow, nutrition, and an adequate immune status. Patients with malnutrition or immune deficiency have a high rate of wound failure or infection. **A serum albumin level below 3.5 g/dl** indicates a malnourished patient. **An absolute lymphocyte count below 1500/mm³** is a sign of immune deficiency. If possible, amputation surgery should be delayed in patients with stable gangrene until these values can be improved by nutritional support, usually in the form of oral hyperalimentation. In severely affected patients, nasogastric or percutaneous gastric feeding tubes are sometimes essential. When infection or severe ischemic pain requires urgent surgery, open amputation at the most distal, viable level, followed by open wound management, can be accomplished until wound healing can be optimized. Oxygenated blood is a prerequisite for wound healing and **a hemoglobin concentration of more than 10 g/dl** is necessary. Amputation wounds generally heal by collateral flow, so arteriography is rarely useful for predicting wound healing. Doppler ultrasonography has been used as the measure of vascular inflow to predict wound healing in the ischemic limb. An absolute Doppler pressure of 70 mm Hg was originally described as the minimum inflow to support wound healing. The ischemic index is the ratio of the Doppler pressure at the level being tested to the brachial systolic pressure. It is generally accepted that patients require **an ischemic index of 0.5 or greater** at the surgical level to support wound healing. The ischemic index at

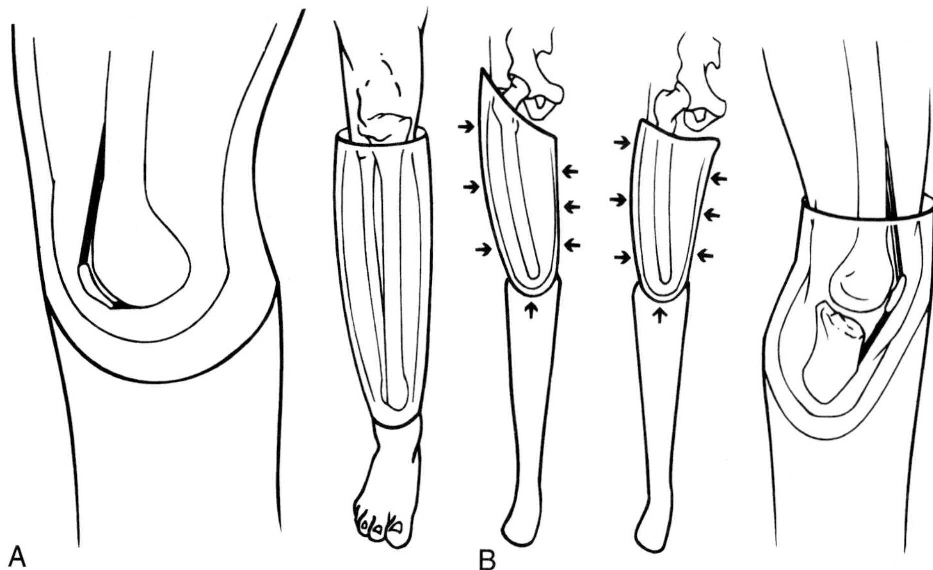

FIGURE 9-6 ■ *A,* Direct load transfer is accomplished in the *(left)* through-knee and *(right)* Syme's ankle disarticulation amputations. *B,* Indirect load transfer is accomplished in above-knee amputations with either *(left)* a standard quadrilateral socket or *(center)* an adducted narrow medial-lateral socket. The below-knee amputation *(right)* transfers weight indirectly with the knee flexed approximately 10 degrees. (From Pinzur, M.: New concepts in lower limb amputation and prosthetic management. Instr. Course Lect. 39:361, 1990.)

the ankle (i.e., the ankle-brachial index) has evolved as the gold standard for assessing adequate inflow to the ischemic limb.

Standard Doppler ultrasonography measures arterial pressure. In the normal limb the **area under the Doppler waveform** tracing is a measure of flow. These values are falsely elevated and nonpredictive in at least 15% of patients with diabetes and peripheral vascular disease, because of the **noncompressibility and noncompliance of calcified peripheral arteries**. The **toe pressures ischemic index(0.5)** are more accurate in these patients. Transcutaneous partial pressure of oxygen ($TcpO_2$) is the present gold standard measure of vascular inflow. It records the oxygen-delivering capacity of the vascular system to the level of contemplated surgery. Values **greater than 40 mm Hg** correlate with acceptable wound-healing rates without the false-positive values seen in noncompliant peripheral vascular diseased vessels. **Pressures less than 20 mm Hg** are predictive for poor healing potential.

D. Pediatric Amputation—Pediatric amputations are usually the result of congenital limb deficiencies, trauma, or tumors. Congenital amputations are a result of **failure of formation**. The present classification system is based on the original work of a 1975 Conference of the International Society for Prosthetics and Orthotics (ISPO) and a subsequent International Organization for Standardization (ISO) standard. Deficiencies are either longitudinal or transverse, with the potential for intercalary deficits. Amputation is rarely indicated in congenital upper limb deficiency; even rudimentary appendages can be functionally useful. In the lower limb, amputation of an unstable segment may allow direct load transfer and enhanced walking (e.g., Syme's amputation for fibular hemimelia). In the growing child, disarticulations should be performed only when possible to maintain maximal residual limb length and to prevent terminal bony overgrowth. Such **overgrowth occurs most commonly in the humerus**, fibula, tibia, and femur, in that order; it is most common in diaphyseal amputations. Numerous surgical procedures have been described to resolve this problem, but **the best method is surgical revision** of the residual limb with adequate resection of bone or autogenous osteochondral stump capping (Fig. 9-7).

E. Trauma—The absolute indication for amputation after trauma is an ischemic limb with a vascular injury that cannot be repaired. Severe open tibia fractures that are managed by limb salvage are often associated with high mortality and morbidity due to infection, increased energy expenditure for ambulation, and decreased potential to return to work. Grade IIIB and IIIC open fractures of the tibia and fibula treated by limb salvage generally have poor functional outcomes and multiple complications and surgeries. Early amputation in the appropriate patient may prevent emotional, marital, financial, and addictive problems. Most grade IIIB and IIIC tibia fractures occur in young

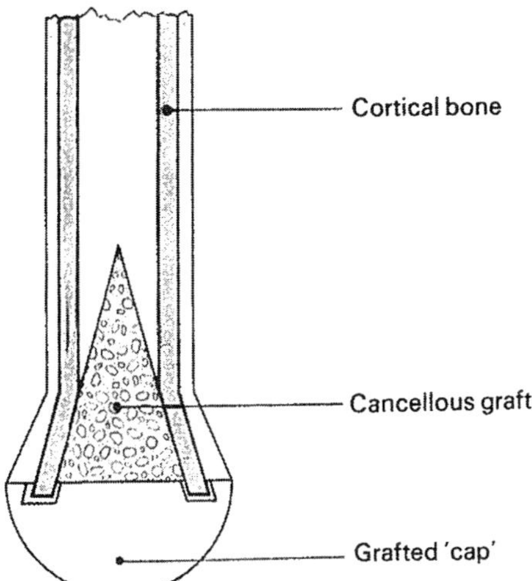

FIGURE 9-7 ■ Diagram of the stump-capping procedure. The bone end has been split longitudinally. (From Bernd, L., Blasius, K., Lukoschek, M., et al.: The autologous stump plasty: treatment for bony overgrowth in juvenile amputees. J. Bone Joint Surg. 73-B:203–206, 1991.)

males who are laborers and who may be more likely to return to gainful employment after amputation and prosthetic fitting. Guidelines for immediate or early amputation of mangled limbs differ between upper and lower limbs. When a salvaged upper limb remains sensate and has prehensile function, it will often function better than an amputation with prosthetic replacement. Maintaining as much length as possible is key to subsequent prosthetic use. Sensation is not as crucial in the lower limb, where current prostheses more closely approximate normal function. The salvaged lower extremity with an insensate plantar weight-bearing surface **(loss of tibialis posterior nerve),** with associated major functional muscle and bone loss, is unlikely to provide a durable limb for stable walking and is a potential source of early or late sepsis. Lack of plantar sensation may be because of a neurapraxia that can resolve. In the absence of other major factors amputation should not be done. The grading scales for evaluating mangled extremities are not absolute predictors but provide reasonable guidelines for determining whether salvage is appropriate.

F. Peripheral Vascular Disease—For patients to learn to walk with a prosthesis and care for their stump and prosthesis, they must possess certain **cognitive capacities:** (1) memory, (2) attention, (3) concentration, and (4) organization. Patients with cognitive deficits or psychiatric disorders have a low likelihood of becoming successful prosthesis users. A majority of patients are diabetic with inherent immune deficiency. The most important risk factors for amputation in diabetic patients are the presence of peripheral neuropathy and development of deformity and infection. Most others are malnourished patients with peripheral vascular disease of sufficient magnitude to require amputation and have disease in their coronary and cerebral arteries. Appropriate consultation with physical therapy, social work, and psychology departments is important to determine rehabilitation potential. Medical consultation will help determine cardiopulmonary reserve. The vascular surgeon should determine whether vascular reconstruction is feasible or appropriate. The **biologic amputation level** is the most distal functional amputation level with a high probability of supporting wound healing. This level is determined by the presence of adequate viable local tissue to construct a residual limb capable of supporting weight-bearing, an adequate vascular inflow, and serum albumin and total lymphocyte count sufficient to aid surgical wound healing. Amputation-level selection is determined by combining the biologic amputation level with the rehabilitation potential to determine the amputation level that maximizes ultimate functional independence.

G. Musculoskeletal Tumors—Advances in chemotherapy and allograft or prosthetic reconstruction have made limb salvage a viable option in extremity sarcomas. The primary goal of tumor surgery is to remove the tumor with adequate surgical margins. If adequate margins can be achieved with limb salvage, the decision can then be based on expected functional outcome. There is still controversy in the literature when limb salvage is compared with amputation regarding energy expenditure to ambulate, quality-of-life measures, and function with activities of daily living. Expected functional outcome should include the psychosocial and body-image values associated with limb salvage. These concerns should be balanced with the apparent improved task performance and **reduced concern for late mechanical injury** associated with amputation and prosthetic limb fitting.

H. Technical Considerations—Skin flaps should be full thickness and avoid dissection between tissue planes. Periosteal stripping should be sufficient to allow for bone transection; this minimizes regenerative bone overgrowth. Wounds should not be sutured under tension.

Muscles are best secured directly to bone at resting tension **(myodesis)** rather than to antagonist muscle **(myoplasty)**. Stable residual limb muscle mass can improve function by reducing atrophy and providing a stable soft-tissue envelope over the end of the bone. All transected nerves form neuromas. The nerve end should come to lie deep in a soft-tissue envelope, away from potential pressure areas. Crushing the nerve may contribute to postoperative phantom or limb pain.

Rigid dressings postoperatively help reduce swelling, decrease pain, and protect the stump from trauma. Early postoperative fitting is done between 5 and 21 days in selected patients.

I. Complications
1. **Pain—Phantom limb sensation**, the feeling that all or part of the amputated limb is present, occurs in almost all adults who have undergone amputation. It usually decreases with time. **Phantom pain** is a burning, painful sensation in the amputated part. It is diminished by prosthetic use, physical therapy, compression, and transcutaneous nerve stimulation. A common cause of residual pain is complex regional pain syndrome (reflex sympathetic dystrophy) or causalgia. Amputation should **not** be performed for this condition.

   Localized stump pain is often related to bony or soft-tissue problems. Referred pain to the limb occurs in a frequent number of cases.
2. **Edema**—Postoperative edema occurs after amputation. It may impede wound healing and place significant tension on the tissues. Rigid dressings and soft compression help reduce the problem. Swelling occurring after stump maturation is usually caused by poor socket fit, medical problems, or trauma. Persistence of chronic swelling may lead to **verrucous hyperplasia**, which is a wart-like overgrowth of skin with pigmentation and serous discharge. It should be treated by a total-contact cast, which is changed regularly to accommodate the reduced edema.
3. **Joint Contractures**—Usually noted as **hip and knee flexion contractures**, which can be produced at the time of surgery by anchoring the respective muscles with the joints in a flexed position. These can be avoided by ensuring correct positioning of the amputated limb.
4. **Wound Failure**—Occurs most often in diabetic and vascular patients. If not amenable to local care, **wedge excision** of soft tissue and bone with closure without tension is preferred treatment.

J. Upper-Limb Amputations (Fig. 9-8)—Wrist disarticulation has two advantages over transradial amputation.
1. Preservation of more forearm rotation because of preservation of the distal radioulnar joint;
2. Improved prosthetic suspension because of the flare of the distal radius.

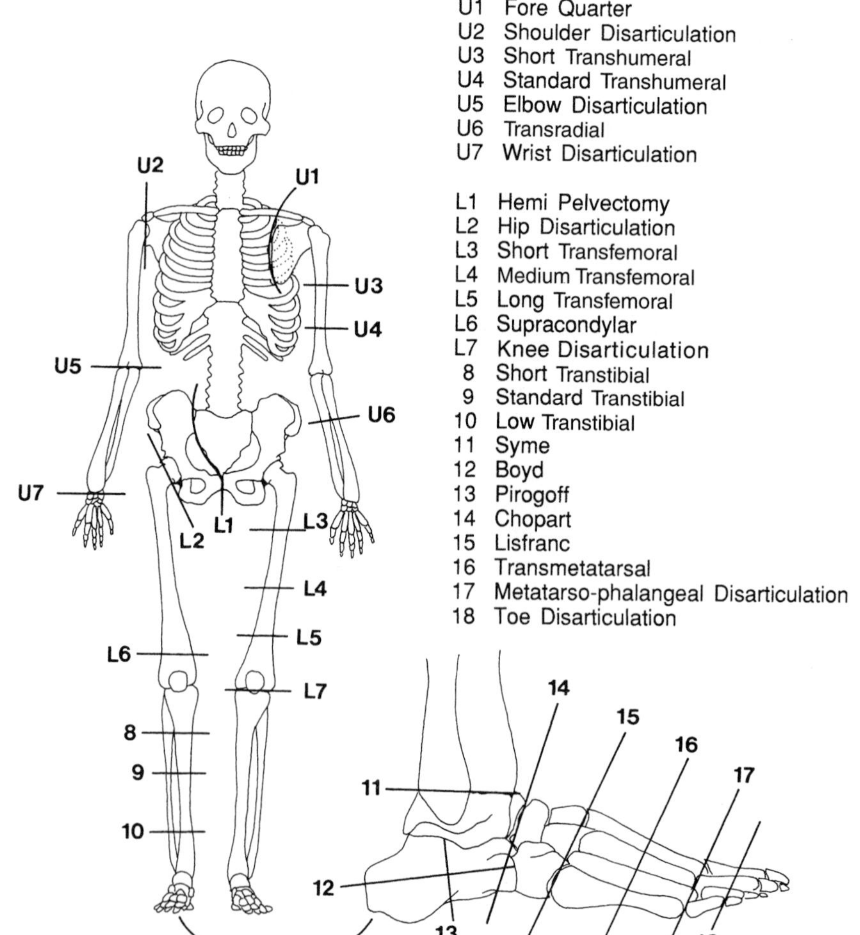

FIGURE 9-8 ■ Composite illustration of common amputation levels.

Wrist disarticulation provides challenges to the prosthetist that may outweigh its benefits. Cosmetically, the prosthetic limb is longer than the contralateral limb; and if myoelectric components are used, the motor and battery cannot be hidden within the prosthetic shank. High levels of function can be obtained at this level of amputation. Forearm rotation and strength are directly related to the length of the **transradial** (below-elbow) residual limb. The optimal length is the junction of the middle and distal thirds of the forearm, where the soft-tissue envelope can be repaired by myodesis and the components of a myoelectric prosthesis can be hidden within the prosthetic shank. Because function at this level is accomplished prosthetically only by opening and closing the terminal device, elbow joint retention is essential. The length and shape of elbow disarticulation provide improved suspension and lever-arm capacity. To improve suspension and reduce the need for shoulder harnessing, a 45–60-degree distal humeral osteotomy is performed. Patients with **complete brachial plexus** injury and a nonfunctioning hand and forearm may be **best treated** by a **transradial amputation** or elbow disarticulation, which can be fitted with a prosthesis. When not due to Raynaud's or Buerger's diseases, gangrene of the upper limb represents end-stage disease, especially in the diabetic patient. These patients experience a high mortality rate and do not survive beyond 24 months. Localized amputations are unlikely to heal. When surgery becomes necessary, amputation should be performed at the **trans-radial** level to achieve wound healing during the final months of the patient's life.

K. Lower-Limb Amputations (see Fig. 9-8)—Ischemic patients generally ambulate with a propulsive gait pattern, so they suffer little disability from toe amputation. Traumatic amputees lose some late-stance-phase stability with toe amputation. The great toe should be amputated distal to the insertion of the flexor hallucis brevis. **Isolated second-toe amputation** should be performed just distal to the proximal phalanx metaphyseal flare, leaving it to act as a buttress and prevent late hallux valgus. Single outer (first or fifth) ray resections function well in standard shoes. Resection of more than one ray leaves a narrow forefoot that is difficult to fit in shoes and often results in a late equinus deformity. Central ray resections are complicated by prolonged wound healing and rarely outperform midfoot amputation.
   1. Transmetatarsal and Lisfranc Tarsal-Metatarsal Amputation—There is little functional difference between these two. The long plantar flap acts as a myocutaneous flap and is preferred to fish-mouth dorsal-plantar flaps. Transmetatarsal amputation should be through the proximal metaphyses to prevent late plantar pressure ulcers under the residual bone ends. Percutaneous tendo Achilles lengthening should be performed with the Lisfranc amputation to prevent the late development of equinus or equinovarus. Late varus can be corrected with transfer of the tibialis anterior tendon to the neck of the talus. Some authors have reported reasonable functional outcomes with hindfoot amputation (i.e., Chopart's or Boyd's), but most experts recommend avoiding these levels if possible in diabetic and vascular patients. Although children have been reported to function reasonably well, adults retain an **inadequate lever arm** and are prone to experience **fixed equinus** of the heel if tendo Achilles lengthening and tibialis anterior tendon transfer are not performed.
   2. Ankle Disarticulation (Syme's Amputation)—Allows direct load transfer and is rarely complicated by late residual limb ulcers or tissue breakdown. It provides a stable gait pattern that rarely requires prosthetic gait training after surgery. Surgery should be performed in one stage, even in ischemic limbs with insensate heel pads. A **patent tibialis posterior artery** is necessary to ensure healing. The malleoli and metaphyseal flares should be removed from the tibia and fibula, but the remaining tibial articular surface should be retained to provide a resilient residual limb. The heel pad should be secured to the tibia either anteriorly through drill holes or posteriorly by securing the tendo Achilles.
   3. Transtibial (Below-Knee) Amputation—Should be performed with a long posterior myocutaneous flap as the preferred method of creating a soft-tissue envelope. Optimal bone length is at least 12–15 cm below the knee joint or longer, if adequate gastrocnemius or soleus can be used to construct a durable soft-tissue envelope. Posterior muscle should be secured to the beveled anterior tibia by myodesis. Rigid dressings are preferred during the early postoperative period, and early prosthetic fitting may be started 5–21 days after surgery, if the residual limb is capable of transferring load and the patient has satisfactory physical reserve.
   4. Knee Disarticulation (Through-Knee Amputation)—Current technique uses a long posterior flap with gastrocnemius muscle as end padding. Alternative is to use sagittal skin flaps and cover the end of the femur with gastrocnemius to act as a soft-tissue envelope end pad. The **patella tendon** is sutured to the **cruciate ligaments** in the notch, leaving the patella on the anterior femur. This level is generally used in the nonwalker who can support wound healing at the transtibial or distal level. Knee disarticulation is muscle-balanced,

provides an excellent weight-bearing platform for sitting, and provides a lever arm for transfer. When performed in a potential walker, it provides **a direct load transfer** (end-bearing) residual limb.

5. Transfemoral (Above-Knee) Amputation—Increases energy cost for walking. Peripheral vascular disease trans-femoral amputees are unlikely to become good walkers, so salvaging the limb at the knee disarticulation, or transtibial level, is critical to maintaining functional walking independence. With greater length, the lever arm, suspension, and limb advancement are optimized. The optimal transfemoral bone length is 12 cm above the knee joint to accommodate the prosthetic knee. Adductor myodesis is important for maintaining femoral adduction during the stance phase to allow optimal prosthetic function (Fig. 9-9). The major deforming force is into abduction and flexion. Adductor myodesis at normal muscle tension eliminates the problem of **adductor roll** in the groin. Sectioning of **adductor magnus** results in a loss of **70% of adductor pull** (Fig. 9-10). Rigid dressings are difficult to apply and maintain at this level. Elastic compression dressings are used and may be suspended about the opposite iliac crest. Hip disarticulation is infrequently performed, and only an occasional few of these amputees become meaningful prosthetic users because of the high energy requirements for walking. Post-trauma or tumor patients occasionally use the prosthesis for limited activity. These patients sit in their prosthesis and must use their torso to achieve momentum to "throw" the limb forward to advance it.

III. Prosthetics

A. Upper Limb—The shoulder provides the center of radius of the functional sphere of the upper limb. The elbow acts as the caliper to position the hand at a workable distance from that center to perform tasks. Multiple-joint–segment tasks are usually done simultaneously, whereas upper-limb prostheses perform these same tasks sequentially; thus joint- and residual-limb-length salvage is directly correlated with functional outcome. Motion at the retained joints is essential to maximize that function. Residual limb length is important for prosthetic socket suspension and providing the lever arm necessary to "drive" the prosthesis through space. Limb salvage is more critical for the upper limb, where sensation is critical to function. An insensate prosthesis provides less function than a partially sensate, partially functional salvaged limb. After amputation, prosthetic fitting should be done as soon as possible, even before complete wound healing has occurred. Outcomes of prosthetic limb use vary from **70% to 85%** when **prosthetic fitting occurs within 30 days** of amputation, for **transradial amputation**, in contrast with <30% when started late. **Myoelectric prostheses** provide good cosmesis and are used for **sedentary work**. They can be used in any position, including overhead activity, and are most successful in the midlength **transradial** amputee, where only the terminal device needs to be activated. Body-powered prostheses are used for heavy labor. The **terminal device** is activated by **shoulder flexion and abduction. Elbow flexion and extension are controlled by shoulder extension and depression.** Optimal mechanical efficiency of figure-eight harnesses requires the harness

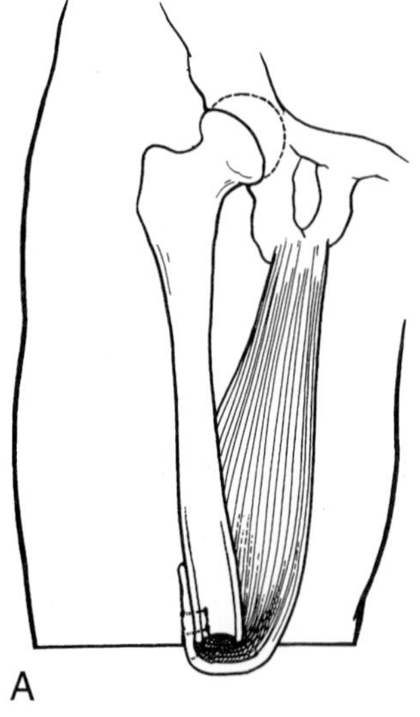

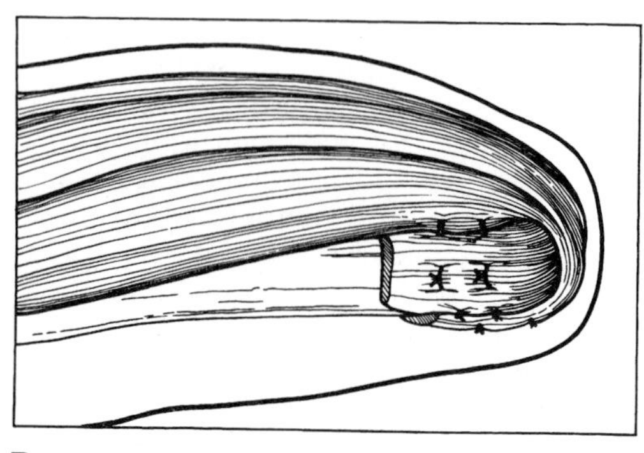

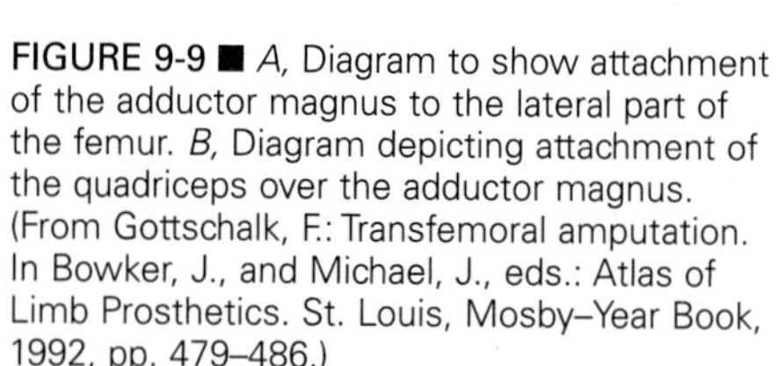

FIGURE 9-9 ■ *A,* Diagram to show attachment of the adductor magnus to the lateral part of the femur. *B,* Diagram depicting attachment of the quadriceps over the adductor magnus. (From Gottschalk, F.: Transfemoral amputation. In Bowker, J., and Michael, J., eds.: Atlas of Limb Prosthetics. St. Louis, Mosby–Year Book, 1992, pp. 479–486.)

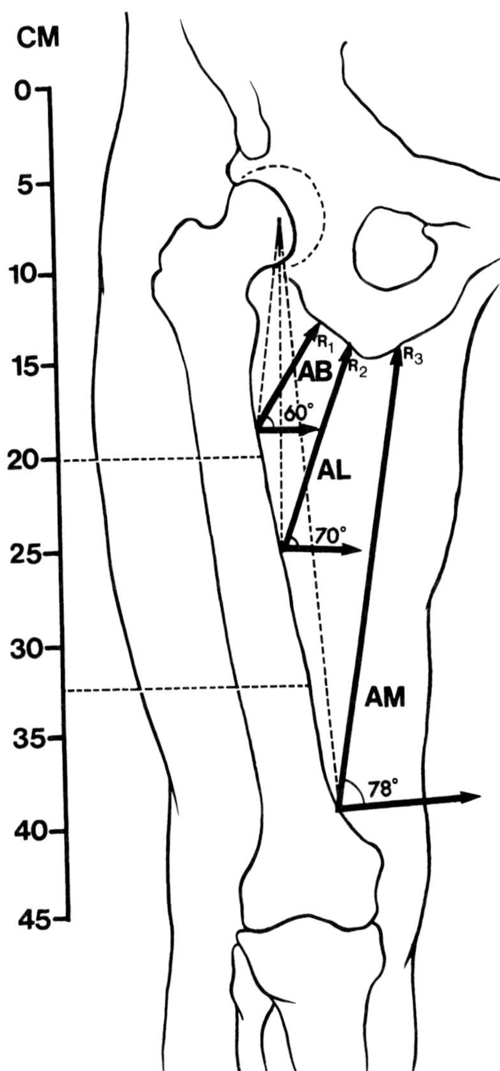

FIGURE 9-10 ■ Diagram of moment arms of the three adductor muscles. Loss of the distal attachment of adductor magnus (AM) will result in a loss of 70% of the adductor pull. *AB*, adductor brevis;*AL*, adductor longus.(From Gottschalk, F.A., Kourosh, S., Stills, M., et al.: Does socket configuration influence the position of the femur in above-knee amputation? J. Prosthet. Orthot. 2:94–102, 1989.)

ring to be at the spinous process of C7 and slightly to the **nonamputated side**.

When the residual forearm is so short as to preclude an adequate lever arm for driving the prosthesis through space, **supracondylar suspension (Munster socket) and step-up hinges** can be used to augment function. Elbow disarticulation and transhumeral (above-elbow) amputations require two motions to develop prehension, making both levels significantly less efficient and the prosthesis heavier than that for amputation at the **transradial** level. The **best function** with the least weight at the lowest cost is provided by **hybrid prosthetic systems** combining myoelectric, traditional body-powered, and body-driven switch components. These levels provide minimal function because the patient must sequentially control two joints and a terminal device. When the lever-arm capacity of the humerus is lost in proximal transhumeral or shoulder disarticulation amputations, limited function can be achieved with a manual universal shoulder joint positioned by the opposite hand, combined with lightweight hybrid prosthetic components.

B. Lower Limb
   1. Prosthetic Feet—Several designs are available and are classified into five classes. The single-axis foot is based on an ankle hinge that provides dorsiflexion and plantar flexion. The disadvantages of the single-axis foot include poor durability and cosmesis. The SACH (solid ankle, cushioned heel) foot has been the standard for decades and was appropriate for general use in low-demand patients. It may lead to **overload problems** on the nonamputated foot, and its use is being discontinued. **Articulated dynamic response** feet allow inversion/eversion and rotation of the foot and are useful for activities on uneven surfaces. They may absorb loads and **decrease shear forces** to the residual limb.
   2. Most **dynamic-response feet** have a **flexible keel** and are the new standard for general use (Fig. 9-11). Correct **dynamic prosthetic foot selection requires** information about the patient's height, **weight, activity level**, access for maintenance, cosmesis, and funding. Dynamic response feet may be grouped into articulated and nonarticulated feet, which have short or long keels.

      The **keel deforms under load,** becoming a spring and allowing dorsiflexion, thereby decreasing the loading on the sound side and providing a spring-like response for push off. Posterior projection of the keel provides a response at heel strike for smooth transition through stance phase. A sagittal split allows for

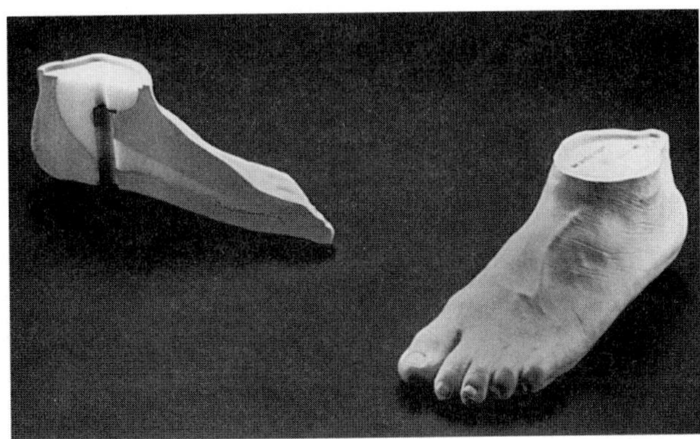

FIGURE 9-11 ■ Cosmetic appearance of a dynamic-response foot (Seattle foot) and cross-section to show internal configuration. (Courtesy of MIND, Seattle, WA.)

moderate inversion or eversion. **Shortened keels** are not as responsive and are indicated for the moderate-activity ambulator, whereas **long keels** are for very high-demand activities. Separate prosthetic feet for running and lower-demand activities may be indicated. The dynamic-response feet, including the Seattle foot, Carbon Copy II/III, and the Flex Foot, allow amputees to undertake most normal activities (Fig. 9-12).

3. Prosthetic Shanks—The structural link between prosthetic components. Two varieties exist—endoskeletal, with a soft exterior and load-bearing tubing inside, and exoskeletal, with a hard, load-bearing exterior shell. **Rotator units** are sometimes added for patients involved in twisting activities (e.g., golf).
4. Prosthetic Knees—Used in transfemoral and knee disarticulation prostheses and chosen based on patient needs. Prosthetic knees provide controlled knee motion in the prosthesis. **Alignment stability** (the position of the prosthetic knee in relation to the patient's line of weight-bearing) is important in design and fitting of prosthetic knees. Placing the **knee center of rotation posterior** to the weight line allows control in the stance phase but makes flexion difficult. Alternatively, with the knee center of rotation anterior to the weight line, flexion is made easier but at the expense of control. Only the **polycentric knee** takes advantage of both options by having a variable center of rotation. Six basic types of knees are available.
   a. **Polycentric** (Four-Bar Linkage) Knee—has a **moving instant center of rotation** that provides for different stability characteristics during the gait cycle and may allow increased flexion for sitting. It is recommended for patients with transfemoral amputations, patients with knee disarticulations, and bilateral amputees (Fig. 9-13).
   b. **Stance-Phase Control** (Weight-Activated, or Safety) Knee—Functions like a constant-friction knee during the swing phase but "freezes" by application of a high-friction housing when weight is applied to the limb. Its use is **primarily reserved for older** patients, high-level amputees, or use on uneven terrain.
   c. **Fluid-Control** (Hydraulic and Pneumatic) **Knee**—Allows adjustment of cadence response by changing resistance to knee flexion via a piston mechanism. The design prevents excessive flexion and is extended earlier in the gait cycle, allowing a more fluid gait.

      The knee is best used in active patients who prefer greater utility and variability at the expense of more weight.
   d. Constant-Friction Knee—A hinge that is designed to dampen knee swing via a screw or rubber pad that applies friction to the knee bolt. It is a general utility knee and may be used on uneven terrain. It is the most common knee used in childhood prosthetics. Its major disadvantages are that it allows only single-speed walking and

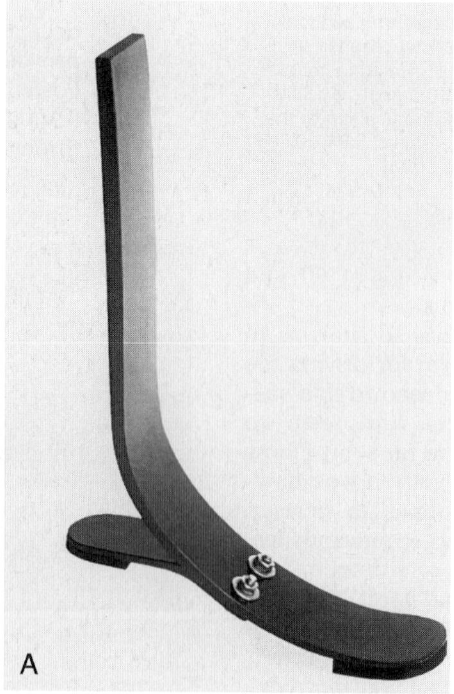

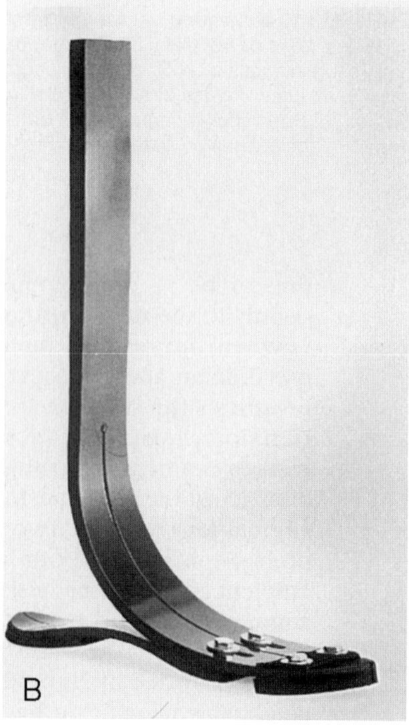

FIGURE 9-12 ■ *A*, Flex Foot with carbon-fiber leaf and posterior projection of keel for heel strike. *B*, Flex Foot with split toe configuration and spring leaf design. (Courtesy of Flex Foot, Inc., Aliso Viejo, CA.)

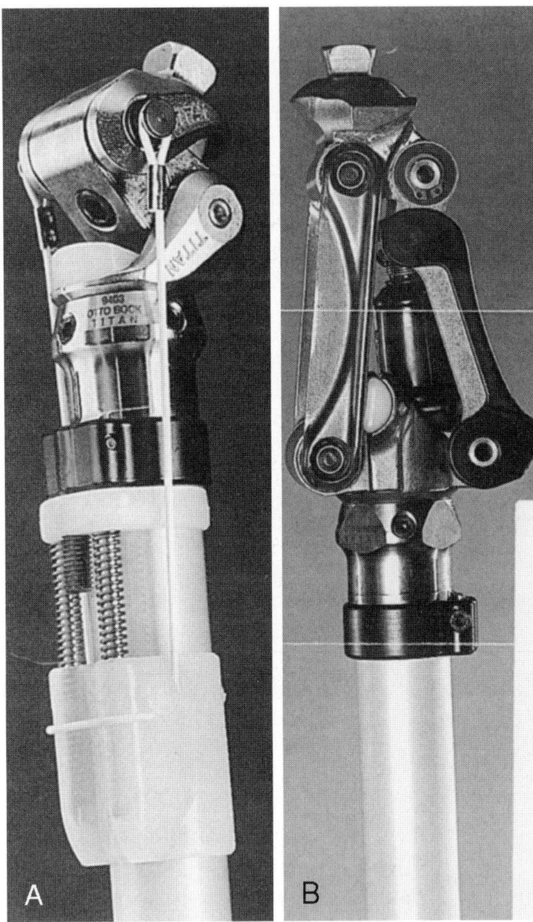

FIGURE 9-13 ■ *A*, Stance-phase control unit for transfemoral prosthesis. *B*, Modular endoskeletal four-bar knee with hydraulic swing-phase control unit. (Courtesy of Otto Bock Orthopaedic Industries, Minneapolis.)

relies solely on alignment for stance-phase stability and is therefore not recommended for older, weaker patients.

e. Variable-Friction (Cadence Control) Knee—Allows resistance to knee flexion to increase as the knee extends by employing a number of staggered friction pads. This knee allows walking at different speeds but is not durable and is not available in endoskeletal systems.

f. Manual Locking Knee—Consists of a constant-friction knee hinge with a positive lock in extension that can be unlocked to allow function similar to that of a constant-friction knee. The knee is often left locked in extension for more stability. The knee has limited indications and is used primarily in weak, unstable patients, those patients just learning to use prostheses, and blind amputees.

g. Summary—Information on the various types of prosthetic knees is summarized in Table 9-4.

5. Suspension Systems—Suspension is provided in modern lower-extremity prosthetics primarily through socket design and **suspension sleeves**. The use of straps and belts is usually for supplementation. Sockets are prosthetic components designed to provide comfortable functional control and even- pressure distribution on the amputated stump. Sockets can be hard (rigid or unlined) or soft (lined with a resilient material and/or flexible shell). In general, suction and socket contour are the primary suspension modalities used. The suction socket provides an airtight seal via a pressure differential between the socket and atmosphere. Total-contact support of the residual limb surface prevents edema formation.

   a. Transtibial Suspension—**Gel liner suspension** systems with a locking pin are the preferred method of suspension. Liners are made from silicone, urethane, or thermoplastic elastomer. The sleeve rolls onto the stump, and the locking pin is then locked into the socket (Fig. 9-14). The liners provide suspension through **suction and friction** and act as the socket interface. Prosthetic socks worn over the liner accommodate volume fluctuation. This suspension allows unrestricted knee flexion and minimal pistoning.

   Prosthetic sleeves use friction and negative pressure for suspension. The sleeves fit

Table 9-4. CHARACTERISTICS OF VARIOUS PROSTHETIC KNEES

KNEE	ACTION	ADVANTAGES	DISADVANTAGES
Constant friction	Limits flexion	Durable, long res istance	Decreased stability
Variable friction	Varies with flexion	Variable cadence	Durability poor
Stance control	Friction brake	Stability during stance	Durability poor, difficult on stairs
Polycentric	Instant center moves	Stable, increased flexion	Durability poor, heavy
Manual locking	Unlock to sit	Maximum stability	Abnormal gait
Fluid control	Deceleration in swing	Variable cadence	Weight, cost

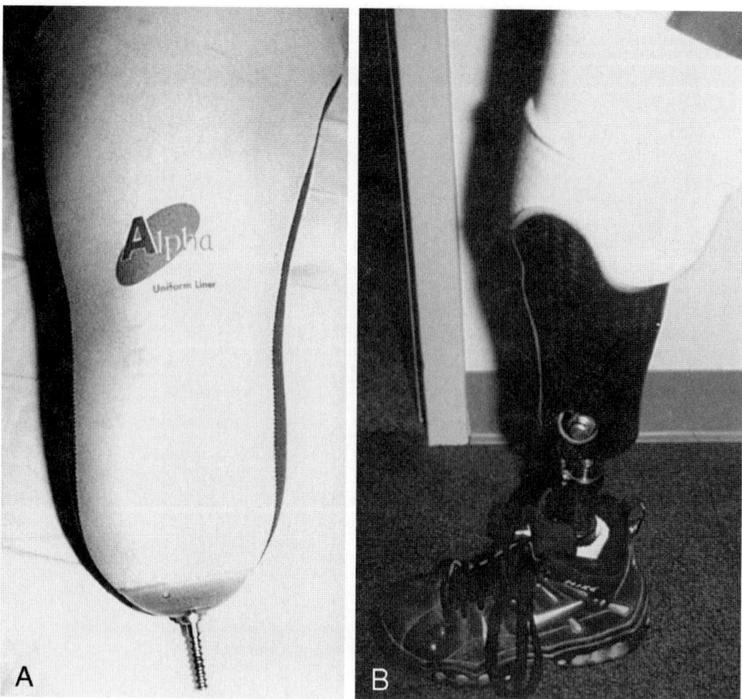

FIGURE 9-14 ■ *A*, Gel liner suspension with locking pin. *B*, Trans-tibial prosthesis with liner locked in place.

snugly to the upper third of the tibial prosthesis and are made from neoprene, latex, silicone, or thermoplastic elastomers.

Supracondylar suspension is recommended when the residual limb is less than 5 cm long. The socket is designed to increase the surface area for pressure distribution by raising the medial and lateral socket brim. A wedge may be used in the soft liner.

Supracondylar-suprapatellar suspension encloses the patella in the socket and has a bar proximal to the patella. This design also provides medial-lateral stability, and no additional cuffs or straps are required. Corset-type prostheses can lead to verrucous hyperplasia and thigh atrophy but reduce socket loads, control the direction of swing, and provide some additional weight support.

b. Transfemoral Suspension—Vacuum (suction) suspension is frequently used. It relies on **surface tension, negative pressure,** and **muscle contraction**. A one-way expulsion valve helps maintain negative pressure, and no belts or straps are required. **Stable body weight** is required for this intimate fit. Roll-on silicone or **thermoplastic liners** may be used with or without locking pins. The **total-elastic suspension** belt, made of neoprene, fastens around the waist and spreads over a larger surface area (Fig. 9-15). It is an excellent auxiliary suspension. **Silesian belts** are used to prevent **socket rotation** in limbs with redundant tissue. Such belts also prevent the socket from slipping off when suction sockets are fitted to short transfemoral stumps and the patient sits.

c. Transfemoral Sockets—Quadrilateral sockets wherein the posterior brim provides a shelf for the ischial tuberosity have been the classic. The design made it difficult to keep the femur in adduction. **Ischial containment** (narrow medial-lateral) sockets distribute the proximal and medial concentration of forces more evenly as well as enhance socket rotational control (Fig. 9-16). The ischium and ramus are contained within the socket of these more anatomic, comfortable, and functional designs. Socket design for transfemoral prosthesis allows **for 10 degrees of adduction** of the femur (to stretch the gluteus medius, allowing adequate strength for midstance stability) **and 5 degrees of flexion** (to stretch the gluteus maximus and allow for greater hip extension).

d. Transtibial Sockets—Patella tendon bearing loads all areas of the residual limb that are **weight tolerant** (i.e., patella tendon, medial tibial flare, anterior compartment, gastrocnemius, and fibular shaft). The anterior wedge shape of the socket helps control rotation of the socket on the limb.

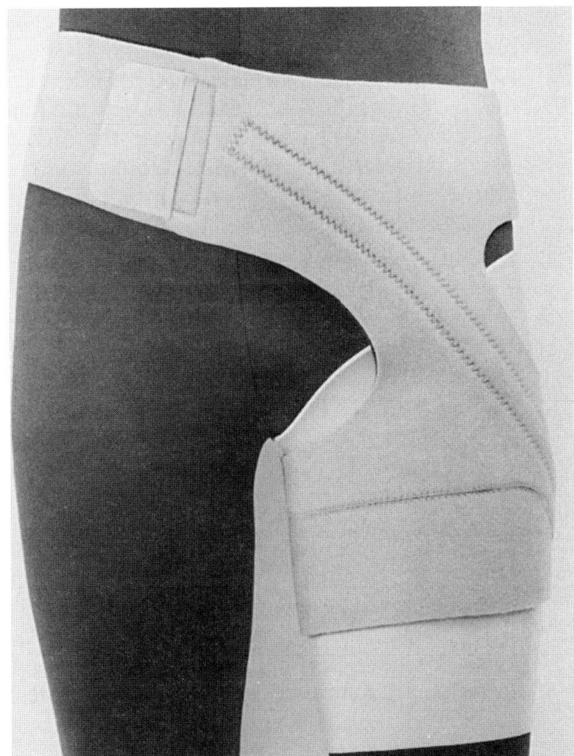

FIGURE 9-15 ■ Total-elastic suspension belt for suspending a trans-femoral socket. (Courtesy of Syncor Manufacturers, Green Bay, WI.)

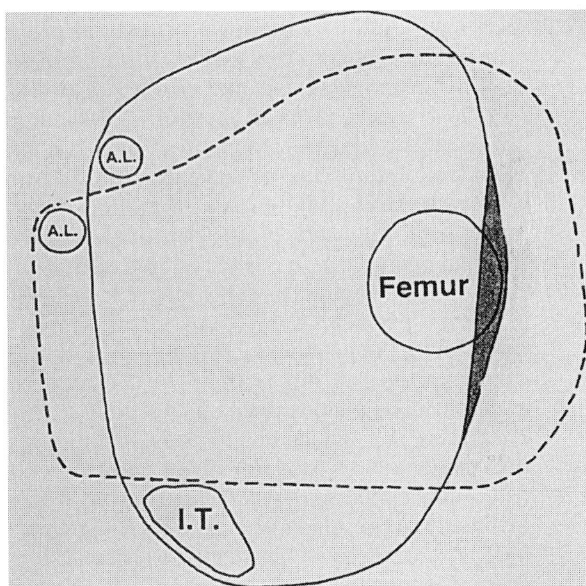

FIGURE 9-16 ■ Comparison of transfemoral sockets. Note inclusion of the ischial tuberosity and narrow medial-lateral design of newer contoured adducted trochanteric-controlled alignment method (CAT-CAM) socket shown in solid line. *AL*, adductor longus; *IT*, ischial tuberosity. (From Sabolich, J.: Contoured adducted trochanteric controlled alignment method. Clin. Prosthet. Orthop. 9:13–17, 1985.)

Weight-intolerant areas include tibial crest and tubercle, distal fibula and fibular head, peroneal nerve, and hamstring tendons. The patellar tendon-bearing supracondylar/suprapatellar socket has proximal extensions over the distal femoral condyles and over the patella.

Total–surface-bearing is different from total contact, in which different areas have different loads. With total–surface-bearing, pressure is distributed more equally across the entire surface of the transtibial residual limb, and the interface liner material in the socket is important. Urethane liners cope with multidirectional forces by easy material distortion and recovery to original shape. Another liner is made of mineral oil gel with reinforcing fabric. These liners provide good shock-absorbing abilities and reduce skin problems.

6. Common Prosthetic Problems
   a. Transtibial—Pistoning during **swing phase** of gait is usually caused by an **ineffective suspension system**. Pistoning in the **stance phase** is due to poor **socket fit** or volume changes in the stump (may require a change in stump sock thickness). Alignment problems are common and are listed in Table 9-5. Pressure-related pain or redness should be corrected with relief of the prosthesis in the affected area. Other problems may be related to the foot—**too soft a foot results in excessive knee extension,** whereas **too hard a foot causes knee flexion and lateral rotation of the toes.**
   b. Transfemoral—Excessive prosthetic length and weak hip abductors or flexors can lead to circumduction, vaulting, and lateral trunk bending. Hip flexion contractures and insufficient anterior socket support can lead to excessive lumbar lordosis (compensatory). Inadequate prosthetic

Table 9-5. PROSTHETIC FOOT GAIT ABNORMALITIES

FOOT POSITION	GAIT ABNORMALITY
Inset	Varus strain, pain (proximedial, distolateral), circumduction
Outset	Valgus strain, pain (proxilateral, distomedial), broad-based gait
Forward placement	Increased knee extension (patellar pain) but stable
Posterior placement	Increased knee flexion/instability
Dorsiflexed foot	Increased patellar pressure
Plantar-flexed foot	Drop off, patellar pressure

knee flexion can lead to terminal knee snap. Medial whip (heel in, heel out) can be caused by a varus knee, excessive external rotation of the knee axis, or muscle weakness. Lateral whip (heel out, heel in) is caused by the opposite (valgus knee, internal rotation at knee, and weakness). Table 9-6 summarizes common transfemoral prosthetic gait problems.

c. Stair Climbing—In general, amputees climb stairs by leading with their normal limb and descend by leading with their prosthetic limb ("the good goes up and the bad comes down").

IV. Orthoses

A. Introduction—The primary function of an orthosis is control of motion of certain body segments. Orthoses are used to protect long bones or unstable joints, support flexible deformities, and occasionally substitute for a functional task. They may be static, dynamic, or a combination of these. **With few exceptions, orthoses are not indicated for correction of fixed deformities or for spastic deformities that cannot be easily controlled manually.** Orthoses are named according to the joints they control and the method used to obtain/maintain that control (e.g., a short-leg, below-the-knee brace is an ankle-foot orthosis (AFO).

B. Shoes—Specific shoes can be used by themselves or in conjunction with foot orthoses. Extra-depth shoes with a high toe box to dissipate local pressures over bony prominences are recommended for diabetic patients. The plantar surface of an insensate foot is protected by use of a pressure-dissipating material. A paralytic or flexible foot deformity can be controlled with more rigid orthoses. SACH heels absorb the shock of initial loading and lessen the transmission of force to the midfoot as the foot passes through the stance phase. A rocker sole can lessen the bending forces on an arthritic or stiff midfoot during midstance as the foot changes from accepting the weight-bearing load to pushing off. It is useful in treating metatarsalgia, hallux rigidus, and other forefoot problems. For the rocker sole to be effective, it must be rigid.

C. **Medial heel outflare** is used to treat severe flat foot of most causes. A foot orthosis is also necessary. Most foot orthoses are used to:

1. Align and support the foot
2. Prevent, correct, or accommodate foot deformities
3. Improve foot function

Three main types of foot orthoses are used: rigid, semirigid, and soft. Rigid foot orthoses limit joint motion and stabilize flexible deformities. **Soft orthoses** have best shock-absorbing ability and are used to accommodate fixed deformities of the feet, especially neuropathic, dysvascular, and ulcerative disorders.

D. AFO—This most commonly prescribed lower-limb orthosis is used to control the ankle joint. It may be fabricated with metal bars attached to the shoe or thermoplastic elastomer. The orthosis may be rigid, preventing ankle motion, or it can allow free or spring-assisted motion in either plane.

After hindfoot fusions, the primary orthotic goals are absorption of the ground reaction forces, protection of the fusion sites, and protection of the midfoot. The thermoplastic foot section achieves medial-lateral control with high trimlines. When subtalar motion is present, an **articulating AFO** permits motion by a mechanical ankle joint design. Primary factors in **orthotic joint selection** include range of motion, durability, adjustability, and **biomechanical implication** on knee joint. A posterior leaf spring AFO provides stance-phase stability for ankle instability in **stance phase.**

E. Knee-Ankle-Foot Orthosis (KAFO)—This orthosis extends from the upper thigh to the foot. It is generally used to control an unstable or paralyzed knee joint. It provides mediolateral stability with prescribed amounts of flexion or extension control. A subset of KAFOs are designated KOs. Knee orthoses can be made of elastic for treatment of patellar pathology or of metal and plastic in the case of anterior cruciate ligament instability.

F. Hip-Knee-Ankle-Foot Orthosis (HKAFO)—This orthosis provides hip and pelvic stability but is rarely used for the adult paraplegic because of the cumbersome nature of the orthosis and the magnitude of effort in achieving minimal gains. Experimentally, it is being used in conjunction with

Table 9-6. PROSTHETIC GAIT ABNORMALITIES

GAIT ABNORMALITY	PROSTHETIC PROBLEM
Lateral trunk bending	Short prosthesis, weak abductors, poor fit
Abducted gait	Poor socket fit medially
Circumducted gait	Prosthetic too long, excess knee friction
Vaulted gait	Prosthetic too long, poor suspension
Foot rotation at heel strike	Heel too stiff, loose socket
Short stance phase	Painful stump, knee too loose
Knee instability	Knee too anterior, foot too stiff
Medial/lateral whip	Excessive knee rotation, tight socket
Terminal snap	Quadriceps weakness, insecure patient
Foot slap, knee hyperextension	Heel too soft
Knee flexion	Heel too hard
Excessive lordosis	Hip flexion contracture, socket problems

implanted electrodes and computerized functional stimulation of paraplegics. In children with upper-level lumbar myelomeningocele, the reciprocating gait orthoses are modified HKAFOs that can be used for standing and simulated walking.

G. Elbow Orthoses—Hinged-elbow orthoses provide minimal stability in the treatment of ligament instabilities. Dynamic spring-loaded orthoses have been successfully used in the treatment of flexion or extension contracture.

H. Wrist and Hand Orthoses (WHO)—The most common use of wrist and hand orthoses today is for postoperative care after injury or reconstructive surgery. These devices are static or dynamic. The opponens splint is successful in pre-positioning the thumb but impairs tactile sensation. Wrist-driven hand orthoses are used in lower cervical quadriplegics. They may be body-powered by tenodesis action or motor-driven. Weight and cumbersomeness are the major limiting factors.

I. Fracture Braces—Fracture bracing remains a valuable treatment option for isolated fractures of the tibia and fibula. Prefabricated fracture orthoses can be used in simple foot and ankle fractures, ankle sprains, and simple hand injuries.

J. Pediatric Orthoses—Many dynamic orthoses are used in children to control motion without total immobilization. The Pavlik harness has become the mainstay for early treatment of developmental dislocation of the hip. Several dynamic orthoses have been used for containment in Perthes' disease.

K. Spine
   1. Cervical Spine—Numerous orthoses are used to immobilize the cervical spine. Effective immobilization ranges from the various types of collars, to posted orthoses that gain purchase about the shoulders and under the chin, to the halo vest, which achieves the most stability by the nature of its fixation into the skull.
   2. Thoracolumbar—Orthoses used for stabilizing mechanical back pain rely on increasing body cavity pressure. Three-point orthoses achieve their control by the length of their lever arm and the subsequent limitation of motion.

V. Surgery for Stroke and Closed Head Injury—The orthopaedic surgeon can play a role in the early management of adult-acquired spasticity secondary to stroke or closed brain injury when the spasticity interferes with the rehabilitation program. Interventional modalities may include orthotic prescription, serial casting, or motor point nerve blocks with short-acting (bupivacaine HCl) or long-acting (phenol 3–4% in glycerol or Botox) agents. Splinting a joint (e.g., the ankle) at neutral is not sufficient to prevent the development of a contracture (e.g., an equinus contracture). When functional joint ranging is insufficient to control deformity, intervention is often indicated. Local anesthetic injections of the posterior tibial nerve or sciatic nerve before casting relieves pain and allows for maximum correction of the deformity. Open nerve blocks may be warranted to avoid injecting mixed nerves with large sensory contributions. Surgical intervention in adult-acquired spasticity is delayed until the patient **achieves maximum spontaneous motor recovery (6 months for stroke and 12–18 months for traumatic brain injury)**. When patients reach a plateau in functional progress, or when their deformity impedes further progress, intervention may be considered. Invasive procedures in this population should be an adjunct to a standard functional rehabilitation program, not an alternative. When surgery is considered as a method of improving function, patients should be **screened for** (1) cognitive deficits, (2) motivation, and (3) body-image awareness. Patients should not be confused and must have adequate short-term memory and the capacity for new learning. In addition to specific cognitive strengths, motivation is necessary for patients to utilize functional gains and participate in their rehabilitation program. Body-image awareness is essential for surgical intervention to become meaningful and potentially beneficial. Patients who lack the awareness of a limb or its position in space should undergo therapy directed toward improving these deficits before embarking on surgical intervention.

A. Lower Limb—**Balance** is the **best predictor** of a patient's ability to ambulate after acquired brain injury. The mainstay of treatment for the dynamic ankle equinus component of this gait deviation is to achieve ankle stability in neutral position during initial floor contact (i.e., initial contact and stance) as well as floor clearance during swing phase. An adjustable AFO with **ankle dorsiflexion and a plantar flexion stop** at neutral is often used during the recovery period, followed by a rigid AFO once the patient has plateaued in recovery. When the dynamic equinus overpowers the holding power of the orthosis and patients "walk out" of their brace, motor-balancing surgery is indicated. The **equinus deformity is treated** by percutaneous tendo Achilles lengthening. The dynamic varus-producing force in adults is the result of out-of-phase tibialis anterior muscle activity during the stance phase. This dynamic varus deformity is corrected by either **split or complete lateral transfer** of the tibialis anterior muscle.

B. Upper Limb—There is a paucity of literature dealing with acquired spasticity in the upper limb. Invasive intervention can be considered for functional and nonfunctional goals. Surgical release of static contracture is generally performed to assist nursing care or hygiene when the fixed contracture and/or spastic component results in skin maceration or breakdown. A functional use of static contracture release is to improve upper-extremity "tracking" (i.e., arm swing) during walking. Most upper-extremity surgery performed in this patient population has the goal of increasing prehensile hand function. The goal may be simply to improve placement, enabling use of the hand as a "paperweight," or to achieve improved fine motor control. In patients with prehensile potential, surgery may allow the "one-handed" patient to be "two-handed" by increasing involved hand function from no function to assistive, or from assistive to independent. When the goal of surgery is to improve function, patients must first be screened for cognitive capacity, motivation, and body-image awareness. Patients must have the cognitive skills and learning capability to participate in their therapy after surgery and to functionally make use of their newly acquired skills at the completion of their rehabilitation program. If they are not motivated, they will not participate in the prolonged effort necessary to achieve meaningful functional improvement. Patients with poor stereognosis or neglect (i.e., poor body-image awareness) find that their involved hand "drifts" in space and is not "available" for use if they have not been carefully trained in visual-compensation techniques. Once it has been determined that the patient has the potential to make functional upper-extremity gains with surgery, he or she is graded on the basis of hand placement, proprioception and sensibility, and voluntary motor control. Dynamic electromyography is used when delineation of phasic motor activity is essential. Muscle unit lengthening, by fractional musculotendinous or step-cut methods, of the agonist deforming muscle units is combined with motor-balancing tendon transfers of the antagonists to achieve muscle balance and improved prehensile hand function.

VI. Spinal Cord Injury—The functional level in a patient with spinal cord injury is determined by the **most distal intact functional dermatome** (sensory level) and **the most distal motor level** where most of the muscles at that level function at least at a "fair" motor grade.

A. Mobility—Spinal cord injury level determines mobility. C4 and higher levels require high back and head support. At C5, mouth-driven accessories can control a motorized wheelchair. Various body-powered or motor-driven orthoses can assist functional prehension, such as a ratchet wrist hand orthosis. C6 levels can operate manual wheelchairs and use a flexor hinge wrist and hand orthosis. Transfers are dependent at C4, assisted at C5, and independent at C6 (Table 9-7).

B. Activities of Daily Living—Patients at the C6 level can groom and dress themselves. Patients at the C7 level can cut meat. Bowel and bladder function can be controlled via rectal stimulation and intermittent catheterization.

C. Psychosocial Factors—Men may be impotent but can often achieve a reflex erection.

D. Autonomic Dysreflexia—This potentially catastrophic hypertensive event can occur with injuries above T5. It is usually caused by an **obstructed urinary catheter** or fecal impaction.

E. Surgery—Spinal fusion is frequently used to expedite rehabilitation and prevent the late development of pain or deformity at the fracture level. Anterior and/or posterior fusion with internal fixation should be performed soon after injury so as to facilitate early rehabilitation. Spasticity and contracture can produce problems in hygiene or the development of pressure ulcers. Percutaneous, or open, motor nerve blocks with phenol can be used to treat these deformities. When the deformity is a static contracture, muscle release or disarticulation may improve sitting or transfer potential. Tendon transfers can be used in the upper limb to eliminate the need for an orthosis or allow the patient to achieve function with an orthosis.

Table 9-7. SPINAL CORD INJURY TREATMENT BY FUNCTIONAL LEVEL

FUNCTIONAL LEVEL	WORKING	NOT WORKING	TREATMENT/MOBILITY
Above C4	—	Diaphragm, upper-extremity muscles	Respirator-dependent
C4	Diaphragm/trapezius	Upper-extremity muscles	Wheelchair chin/puff
C5	**Elbow flexors**	**Below elbow**	**Electric wheelchair, rachet**
C6	Wrist extensors	Elbow extensors	Wheelchair, flexor hinge
C7	**Elbow extensor**	**Grasp**	**Wheelchair, independent**
C8	Finger flexors to middle finger		
T1	Intrinsic muscles	Abdominals/lower-extremity muscles	Wheelchair, independent
T2–T12	Upper-extremity muscles, abdominals	Lower-extremity muscles	Wheelchair, HKAFO (nonfunctional ambulation)
L1	Upper-extremity muscles, abdominals, quadriceps	Lower-extremity muscles	KAFO; minimal ambulation
L2	Iliopsoas	Knee/ankle	KAFO, household ambulation
L3	**Quadriceps**	**Ankle**	**AFO, community ambulation**
L4	Tibialis anterior	Toe, plantar flexors	AFO, community ambulation
L5	Ext. hallucis longus, ext. digitorum longus	Plantar flexors	AFO, independent
S1	Gastrocnemius/soleus	Bowel/bladder	±Metatarsal bar

HKAFO, hip-knee-ankle-foot orthosis; KAFO, knee-ankle-foot orthosis; AFO, ankle-foot orthosis.

VII. Postpolio Syndrome—Polio is a viral disease affecting the anterior horn cells of the spinal cord. Postpolio syndrome is not a reactivation of the polio virus. It is an aging phenomenon whereby more nerve cells become inactive. These patients use a high proportion of their capacity for normal activities of daily living. With aging and the drop-off of muscle units, they no longer have the reserves to perform their daily activities. Treatment comprises prescribed limited exercise combined with periods of rest, so muscles are maintained but not overtaxed. Standard polio surgeries, combining contracture release, arthrodesis, and tendon transfer, are indicated when deformity overcomes functional capacity. The use of lightweight orthoses is important in helping patients to remain functionally independent. The syndrome occurs after middle age.

Selected Bibliography

GAIT

Inman, V.T., Ralston, H., and Todd, F.: Human Walking. Baltimore, Williams & Wilkins, 1981.
Perry, J.: Gait Analysis: Normal and Pathological Function. New York, Slack (McGraw Hill), 1992.
Ounpuu, S.: The biomechanics of running: A kinematic and kinetic analysis. Instr. Course Lect. 39:305, 1990.

AMPUTATIONS AND PROSTHETICS

Bowker, J., and Michael, J., eds.: Atlas of Limb Prosthetics. St. Louis, Mosby-Year Book, 1992.
Pinzur, M., Gold, J., Schwartz, D., et al.: Energy demands for walking in dysvascular amputees as related to the level of amputation. Orthopaedics 15:1033, 1992.
Waters, R.L., Perry, J., Antonelli, D., et al.: Energy cost of walking of amputees: The influence of level of amputation. J. Bone Joint Surg. [Am.] 58:42, 1976.
Wyss, C., Harrington, R., Burgess, E., and Matsen, F.: Transcutaneous oxygen tension as a predictor of success after an amputation. J. Bone Joint Surg. [Am.] 70:203, 1988.
Gottschalk, F. (ed.): Symposium on amputation. Clin. Orthop. 361:2-115, 1999.
Day, H.: The Proposed International Terminology for the Classification of Congenital Limb Deficiencies—The Recommendations of a Working Group of ISPO. London, Spastics International Medical Publications, Heinemann Medical Books, Philadelphia, J.B. Lippincott, 1975.
Bernd, L., Blasius, K., Lukoschek, M., et al.: The autologous stump plasty: Treatment for bony overgrowth in juvenile amputees. J. Bone Joint Surg. [Br.] 73:203-206, 1991.
Gottschalk, F.: Traumatic amputations. In Bucholz, R.W., and Heckman, J.D., eds.: Fractures in Adults. Philadelphia, Lippincott Williams & Wilkins, 2001, pp. 391-414.
Gottschalk, F., and Fisher, D.: Complications of amputation. In Conenwett, J.L., Gloviczki, P., Johnston, K.W., et al., eds.: Rutherford Vascular Surgery. Philadelphia, WB Saunders, 2000, pp. 2213-2248.
Lagaard, S., McElfresh, E., and Premer, R.: Gangrene of the upper extremity in diabetic patients. J. Bone Joint Surg. [Am.] 71:257, 1989.
Gottschalk, F., Kourosh, S., Stills, M., et al.: Does socket configuration influence the position of the femur in above-knee amputation? J. Prosthet. Orthot. 2:94-102, 1989.

ORTHOTICS

Goldberg, B., and Hsu, J., eds.: Atlas of Orthoses and Assistive Devices, AAOS, 3rd ed. St. Louis, Mosby-Year Book, 1997.

STROKE AND CLOSED HEAD INJURY

Braun, R.: Stroke and brain injury. In Green, D., ed.: Operative Hand Surgery, pp. 227-254. New York, Churchill Livingstone, 1988.
Pinzur, M., Sherman, R., Dimonte-Levine, P., et al.: Adult-onset hemiplegia: Changes in gait after muscle-balancing procedures to correct the equinus deformity. J. Bone Joint Surg. [Am.] 68:1249-1257, 1986.

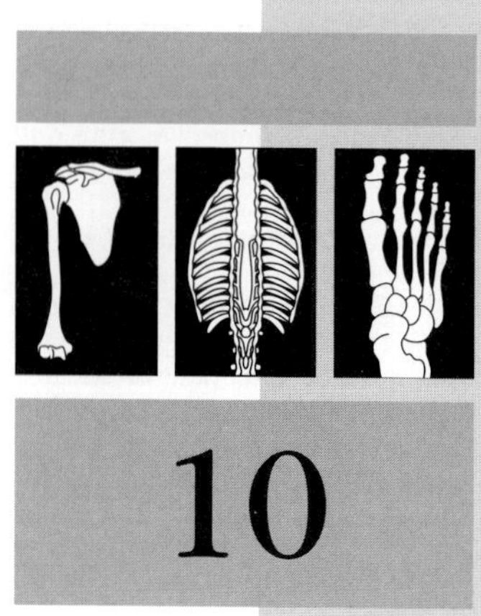

10

Trauma

C. MICHAEL LECROY
BRIAN MULLIS
DAVID B. CARMACK
TODD A. MILBRANDT
D. GREG ANDERSON

SECTION 1

Trauma Treatments

I. **Introduction**—Care of the injured patient is the foundation of orthopaedic surgery. Orthopaedic trauma surgery has developed into a strong subspecialty in recent years, focusing on the care of the multiply injured patient. Additionally, specific expertise in the management of pelvic/acetabular fractures, spinal column injuries, periarticular fractures, and limb reconstruction/salvage are the domain of the orthopaedic trauma surgeon. Nevertheless, a sound grounding in fracture care is essential for the general orthopaedic surgeon and orthopaedic residents. This chapter presents a detailed review and update of current principles in the care of injuries.

A. Advanced Trauma Life Support (ATLS)—ATLS provides our current guidelines for the evaluation and resuscitation of injured patients. An orthopaedic surgeon was the impetus for the creation of ATLS by the American College of Surgeons (ACS). He and his family were in a plane crash. Some died and his other injured family members were cared for by the local trauma system, which was grossly inadequate by current medical standards. His ordeal made him aware of the absence of a nationally recognized trauma care program, hence the creation of ATLS by the ACS.

1. ATLS evaluation is divided into primary and secondary surveys. The primary survey identifies any immediate life-threatening injuries (e.g., shock, airway obstruction, pneumothorax, pericardial tamponade). Attention is directed to (in order of importance) airway, breathing, circulation, disability (neurologic status), and environment (e.g., exposure). Initial mandatory radiographic evaluation includes lateral C-spine, anteroposterior (AP) chest, and AP pelvis views. Hemorrhagic shock is the most common form (systolic blood pressure [SBP] < 90 mm Hg) (Table 10-1), followed by neurogenic and cardiogenic shock. Immediate attention to life-threatening injuries are addressed—*compromised airway*—endotracheal intubation, cricothryoidotomy; *pneumothorax*—needle thoracostomy, tube thoracostomy; *pericardial tamponade*—needle pericardiocentesis; *active hemorrhage*—direct pressure, tourniquet; *hypotension*—injection of 2 liters of lactated Ringer's solution, blood. The secondary survey consists of a more thorough assessment, identifying limb-threatening injuries. Evaluation of occult sources of hemorrhage includes chest,

Table 10-1. CLASSIFICATION OF HEMORRHAGIC SHOCK

CLASS	BLOOD VOLUME LOSS (%)	TREATMENT
I	Up to 15	Fluid replacement
II	15 to 30	Fluid replacement
III	30 to 40	Fluid replacement and blood replacement
IV	>40 (emergently life threatening)	Fluid replacement and blood replacement

From Brinker M.R., ed.: Review of Orthopaedic Trauma. Philadelphia, WB Saunders, 2001, p. 2.

Table 10-2. DPL VS. ULTRASOUND VS. CT IN BLUNT ABDOMINAL TRAUMA

	DPL	ULTRASOUND	CT SCAN
Indication	Document bleeding if ↓ BP	Document fluid if ↓ BP	Document organ injury if BP normal
Advantages	Early diagnosis and sensitive; 98% accurate	Early diagnosis; noninvasive and repeatable; 86–97% accurate	Most specific for injury; 92–98% accurate
Disadvantages	Invasive; misses injury to the diaphragm or retroperitoneum	Operator dependent; bowel gas and subcutaneous air distortion; misses diaphragm, bowel, and some pancreatic injuries	Cost and time; misses diaphragm, bowel, and some pancreatic injuries

From American College of Surgeons, Committee on Trauma: *Advanced trauma life support: student manual*, ed 6, Chicago, 1997, American College of Surgeons.
DPL, Diagnostic peritoneal lavage; *BP*, blood pressure.

abdomen, pelvis, and extremities. Diagnostic peritoneal lavage, computed tomographic (CT) scan, and focused abdominal ultrasound examination (FAST) are used to evaluate abdominal hemorrhage (Table 10-2).

2. Pertinent trauma scoring systems include the injury severity score (ISS), Glasgow Coma Scale (GCS), and Mangled Extremity Severity Score (MESS). Head injures are common causes of early death and are evaluated by the GCS (Table 10-3). A GCS score of <8 is significant for major head injury. The ISS grades the patient's level of injury. ISS is the sum of the squares for the highest Abbreviated Injury Score (AIS) grades in the three most severely injured ISS body regions (Table 10-4). ISS >18 reflects multiply injured trauma patients and can indicate the need to transfer to a trauma center. The mangled extremity severity score has been used as an indicator of limb salvageability. A total score of >7 has been shown retrospectively to be positive predictor for limb amputation, although this has been challenged recently by results from the Lower Extremity Assessment Project (LEAP) study (Table 10-5). Limb salvage criteria remain a controversial area. The only absolute criteria for limb amputation are warm ischemia time >6 hours, a nonreconstructable defect, and if further limb salvage attempts would threaten the patient's life.

Table 10-3. GLASGOW COMA SCALE*

RESPONSE TO ASSESSMENT	SCORE
Eye Opening	
Spontaneous	4
To speech	3
To pain	2
None	1
Best Motor Response	
Obeys commands	6
Localizes pain	5
Normal withdrawal (flexion)	4
Abnormal withdrawal (flexion)—decorticate	3
Extension—decerebrate	2
None (flaccid)	1
Verbal Response	
Oriented	5
Confused conversation	4
Inappropriate words	3
Incomprehensible sounds	2
None	1

From Brinker M.R. ed.: Review of Orthopaedic Trauma. Philadelphia, WB Saunders, 2001, p. 2.

*To calculate a Glasgow Coma Scale score, add the score for Eye Opening with the scores for Best Motor Response and Verbal Response. The best possible score is 15, and the worst possible score is 3.

B. Soft Tissue Trauma—Early evaluation and recognition of nerve, vessel, and muscular injuries will directly affect the overall outcome.

1. Soft tissue injury with closed fractures has been classified by Tscherne (Table 10-6).
2. Vascular trauma, specifically, arterial disruption (leading to distal ischemia) needs to be identified as soon as possible. Initial evaluation includes the documentation of distal pulses (radial, ulnar, dorsalis pedis, and posterior tibial). A palpable pulse rules out an immediate limb-threatening condition. Arterial disruption is commonly associated with penetrating trauma, dislocations (specifically knee), and blunt trauma. Objective signs of arterial damage are described by Frykman as hard and soft signs. Examples of hard signs include pulselessness, massive bleeding at injury, rapidly expanding hematoma, palpable thrill, or audible bruit over a hematoma. Soft signs include a history of arterial bleeding at the scene, proximity of a wound to the artery in question, nonpulsatile hematoma over an artery, and neurologic deficit originating in a nerve adjacent to a named artery. Either one hard sign or two or more soft signs are significant for an arterial lesion that requires further vascular work up. Noninvasive evaluation includes calculating the ankle brachial index (ABI). An ABI of 0.9 or

Table 10-4. ABBREVIATED INJURY SCORE

ABBREVIATED INJURY SCORE EXAMPLES	SCORE
Head	
Crush of head or brain	6
Brain stem contusion	5
Epidural hematoma (small)	4
Face	
Optic nerve laceration	2
External carotid laceration (major)	3
Le Fort III fracture	3
Neck	
Crushed larynx	5
Pharynx hematoma	3
Thyroid gland contusion	1
Thorax	
Open chest wound	4
Aorta, intimal tear	4
Esophageal contusion	2
Myocardial contusion	3
Pulmonary contusion (bilateral)	4
Two or three rib fractures	2
Abdomen and Pelvic Contents	
Bladder perforation	4
Colon transection	4
Liver laceration >20% blood loss	3
Retroperitoneal hematoma	3
Splenic laceration—major	4
Spine	
Incomplete brachial plexus	2
Complete spinal cord C4 or below	5
Herniated disc with radiculopathy	3
Vertebral body compress >20%	3
Upper Extremity	
Amputation	3
Elbow crush	3
Shoulder dislocation	2
Open forearm fracture	3
Lower Extremity	
Amputation	
Below knee	3
Above knee	4
Hip dislocation	2
Knee dislocation	2
Femoral shaft fracture	3
Open pelvic fracture	3
External	
Hypothermia 31–30°C	3
Electrical injury with myonecrosis	3
Second-degree to third-degree burns—20–29% body surface area	3

From Browner, B.D., et al., eds.: Skeletal Trauma, 3rd ed. Philadelphia, WB Saunders, 2003, p.135.

Table 10-5. MESS (MANGLED EXTREMITY SEVERITY SCORE) VARIABLES

COMPONENT	POINTS
Skeletal and Soft Tissue Injury	
Low energy (stab; simple fracture; "civilian gunshot wound")	1
Medium energy (open or multiplex fractures, dislocation)	2
High energy (close-range shotgun or "military" gunshot wound, crush injury)	3
Very high energy (same as above plus gross contamination, soft tissue avulsion	4
Limb Ischemia (Score is Doubled for Ischemia >6 hr)	
Pulse reduced or absent but perfusion normal	1
Pulseless; paresthesias, diminished capillary refill	2
Cool, paralyzed, insensate numb	3
Shock	
Systolic blood pressure always >90 mm Hg	0
Hypotensive transiently	1
Persistent hypotension	2
Age (yr)	
<30	0
30–50	1
>50	2

From Johansen, K., et al. J. Trauma 30:568, 1990.

Table 10-6. CLASSIFICATION OF CLOSED FRACTURES WITH SOFT TISSUE DAMAGE

FRACTURE TYPE	DESCRIPTION
Type 0	Minimal soft tissue damage. Indirect violence. Simple fracture patterns. Example: Torsion fracture of the tibia in skiers.
Type I	Superficial abrasion or contusion caused by pressure from within. Mild to moderately severe fracture configuration. Example: Pronation fracture-dislocation of the ankle joint with soft tissue lesion over the medial malleolus.
Type II	Deep, contaminated abrasion associated with localized skin or muscle contusion. Impending compartment syndrome. Severe fracture configuration. Example: Segmental "bumper" fracture of the tibia.
Type III	Extensive skin contusion or crush. Underlying muscle damage may be severe. Subcutaneous avulsion. Decompensated compartment syndrome. Associated major vascular injury. Severe or comminuted fracture configuration.

From Tscherne, H.; Oestern, H. J.: Die Klassifizierung des Weichteilschadens bei offenen und geschlossenen Frakturen. Unfallheilkunde 85:111–115, 1982. Copyright Springer-Verlag.

greater reflects no arterial injury. An ABI of less than 0.9 has a strong positive predictive value of requiring an arterial repair. Definitive evaluation of a suspected arterial injury requires an angiogram. Arterial damage requiring repair is a surgical emergency and needs to be accomplished within 6 hours of injury. Surgical fasciotomies distal to the arterial repair are required because of the high incidence of reperfusion associated-compartment syndrome. In general the forearm and leg do not require both vessels (ulnar artery/radial artery, anterior tibial artery /posterior tibial artery) for limb viability or function. Arterial repair and skeletal stability should be coordinated, providing a stable platform for the arterial repair.

3. Compartment syndrome occurs when the end-capillary perfusion pressure is less than intracompartmental pressure. Pain out of proportion to the apparent injury and pain with passive stretch are the most reliable indicators in the alert patient. In the obtunded patient with a clinical suspicion of compartment syndrome, documented intracompartmental pressures are mandatory. Pressure measurements of greater than 30 mm Hg, or within 30 mm Hg of diastolic blood pressure (DBP), require surgical fasciotomy (controversy exists as to which absolute numerical value is consistent with a clinical compartment syndrome), which is a surgical emergency. Treatment of compartment syndrome after a delayed diagnosis is controversial; it depends on the presence of infection, open wounds, and need for débridement/fasciotomy.
4. Nerve injury/deficit is associated with both penetrating and blunt trauma. Nerve injuries are commonly described as neuropraxia (nerve stretch), axonotemesis (partial destruction of axon, epineurium intact), and neurotmesis (complete disruption of nerve). Early recognition of neurologic deficit, related to peripheral nerve injury, is essential for preoperative planning. Certain fracture patterns and dislocations are commonly associated with nerve deficits—anterior glenohumeral dislocation (axillary nerve), humeral shaft fracture (radial nerve), radial head fracture/Monteggia fracture (posterior interosseus nerve), supracondylar pediatric humerus fracture (anterior interosseus nerve), hip dislocation (sciatic nerve), and knee dislocation (peroneal nerve and tibial nerve).
5. Bites—Those resulting in evenomation (from snakes, insects, etc.) can cause extensive soft tissue destruction and may lead to compartment syndrome and myonecrosis. Venoms include hemotoxins, cytotoxins, and neurotoxins. Systemic symptoms can be severe. Signs include swelling, ecchymosis, and bullae formation.
   a. Treatment includes potential direct débridement/suction, possible tourniquet, and hospitalization. Monitoring, antibiotics, and administration of antivenin are appropriate. Antivenin can result in serum sickness, which can require systemic corticosteroids. Fasciotomies are sometimes needed for resultant compartment syndrome.
6. Cold Injuries—Freezing injuries are the most common cause of bilateral upper and lower extremity amputations. Injury may be direct (freezing of tissues with ice crystals in the extracellular space) or indirect (vascular damage).
   a. Treatment—Based on restoring core body temperature, rapid rewarming of the extremity, débridement, and physical therapy. Sometimes anticoagulation and sympathectomy are required. Psychosocial factors often are important.
7. Heat Injuries—Burns require close management. Treatment is based on burn depth.
   a. Epidermis—Edema, erythema: symptomatic care
   b. Dermis—Blisters, blanching: topical antibiotic, splint, range-of-motion (ROM) exercises
   c. Subcutaneous—Waxy, dry: excision, split-thickness skin grafting
   d. Deep—Exposed tissue: amputation, flap, reconstruction
      (1) Burns can also result in compartment syndrome and sometimes require escharotomy/fasciotomy. Contractures are common and often require plasties or releases. Infection is also common.
8. Electrical Injuries—Ignition (burns at site of direct contact), conductant (tunnels along neurovascular structures; primary cause of bilateral high upper-extremity amputations), and arc (high-voltage current jumps across flexor surfaces of joints, leading to late contractures). Alternating current is more dangerous than direct current. Current density zones resulting from electrical burns are charred (unrecognizable tissue), gray-white (tissue necrosis), and red (thrombosis).
   a. Treatment—Initial débridement of all necrotic muscle and tissue fasciotomy, second-look débridement (at 2 to 3 days), and finally, definitive flap coverage or amputation. Acute amputation may be required.
9. Chemical Burns—Follow exposure to noxious agents. Severity is based on concentration, duration of contact, penetrability, amount, and mechanism of injury. The mainstay of treatment is copious irrigation. Hydrofluoric acid burns can be successfully treated with calcium gluconate. White phosphorus burns are treated with a 1% copper sulfate solution.
10. High-Pressure Injection Injuries—Occur from accidental injection from paint or grease guns. They usually involve the hand (paint gun injuries are more common and severe because they lead to soft tissue necrosis; grease gun injuries

cause fibrosis). A seemingly innocuous entry wound may cover an area of extensive soft tissue destruction. Treatment includes intravenous (IV) antibiotics and thorough irrigation and débridement (I&D).

C. Joint Injuries
   1. Dislocations—Document direction of joint dislocation with radiographs in AP and lateral planes. Document neurovascular status of limb before any reduction maneuver. In general all dislocated joints should undergo a closed reduction attempt. If required, a general anesthetic and open reduction is accomplished. Repeat neurovascular exam is documented postreduction. If the reduction is unstable, splinting, bridging external fixation, or skeletal traction is used.
   2. Penetrations—"Open Joints" indicate contamination within the true joint space. Historically, diagnosis has relied on looking for saline extravasation after a saline injection into the joint. Recent studies show that this technique has an unacceptably high false-negative rate. Therefore a strong clinical suggestion of contamination should guide the decision for an I&D.

D. Fracture Management—Fractures are described as "open" or "closed," and most fractures are further classified into types by their anatomic location.
   1. Open fractures are most commonly described by the Gustillo and Anderson classification. A strong suspicion of open fracture is required in the initial evaluation, if there are any adjacent wounds, until proved otherwise. Grading of the fracture type is predicated on the amount of energy absorbed by the soft tissue envelope and bone (Table 10-7).
      a. Treatment—Initially all open fractures should have local sterile irrigation, be covered with a betadine-soaked sterile dressing, and splinted. An IV (gram-positive coverage) cephalosporin should be administered (1 gm). If there is a higher level of contamination, IV (gram-negative coverage) aminoglycoside is added (1 mg/kg). For gross contamination (barn yard and clostridium infections), high-dose IV penicillin is added (4 million units). Intravenous therapy is traditionally continued for 24 hours after the last I&D. A tetanus booster should be given for contaminated wounds. Formal radical débridement and irrigation should be accomplished within 6 hours (nationally recognized standard). Débridement principles include wound extension (visualizing entire zone of injury), removing all devitalized bone, and removing all devitalized tissue, followed by copious sterile irrigation. Wound cultures have not been found to be helpful. Antibiotic bead pouches have been shown to decrease infection rates in the initial débridement. Skeletal stabilization (external fixation or internal fixation) should be accomplished after débridement, providing a platform for soft tissue recovery. Highly contaminated wounds or severely damaged soft tissues should be returned to the operating room every 48 hours, until the wound is clean and only viable soft tissues remain. Exposed bone requires soft tissue coverage (rotational flap or free flap), which should be accomplished as soon as possible (traditionally within 5 days). Reported infection rates in open fractures (with appropriate initial care) range from 5–30%. If bone grafting is required, a staged approach is common (planned bone grafting at 6–8 weeks).
   2. Radiographic Evaluation—Injury radiographs include AP and lateral views of the affected area. In general both joints proximal and distal to the fracture should be imaged in the AP and lateral planes to rule out fracture extension. Traction radiographs are very helpful for preoperative planning. Often, a CT scan is essential in preoperative planning (intra-articular fractures, pelvic/acetabular fractures, and spine fractures). Acute nondisplaced fractures can be diagnosed with magnetic resonance imaging (MRI) (femoral neck, scaphoid). Bone scans can be used to diagnose stress fractures that are 24 hours old. Special radiographic views are listed in Table 10-8.

Table 10-7. CLASSIFICATION OF OPEN FRACTURES

FRACTURE TYPE	DESCRIPTION
Type I	Skin opening of 1 cm or less, quite clean. Most likely from inside to outside. Minimal muscle contusion. Simple transverse or short oblique fractures.
Type II	Laceration more than 1-cm long, with extensive soft tissue damage, flaps, or avulsion. Minimal to moderate crushing component. Simple transverse or short oblique fractures with minimal comminution.
Type III	Extensive soft tissue damage including muscles, skin, and neurovascular structures. Often a high-velocity injury with severe crushing component.
Type IIIA	Extensive soft tissue laceration, adequate bone coverage. Segmental fractures, gunshot injuries.
Type IIIB	Extensive soft tissue injury with periosteal stripping and bone exposure. Usually associated with massive contamination.
Type IIIC	Vascular injury requiring repair.

From Gustilo, R.B., et al. I. Trauma 24:742, 1984.

Table 10-8. SPECIAL RADIOGRAPHIC VIEWS FOR SPECIFIC INJURIES

INJURY/LOCATION	EPONYM/DESCRIPTION	TECHNIQUE
Hand and Wrist		
Hand injuries		AP, lat., & obl., digit: dental film
4th & 5th MC	Reverse obl.	Hand placed 45 degrees tilted
MC head	Brewerton	30 degrees pronated from full supination
Gamekeeper's thumb		Street view (with anesthesia)
	Robert	AP hypersupinated (dorsum on cassette)
1st MC-trapezium	Burnam	Robert with 15-degree cephalic tilt
Hamate hook/CT	CT view	Tangential through carpal tunnel
Dorsal carpal chip	Dorsal tangential	Tangential of dorsal carpus
Wrist—unlar var.	Zero rotation	AP, shoulder and elbow at 90 degrees
Carpal instability	Motion	Cineradiography
Radial wrist	Pronation oblique	AP with 45 degrees' pronation
Ulnar wrist	Bura	Sup. obl,; AP with 35 degrees' supination
Scaphoid	Series	PA/lat./obl. fist, PA in ulnar deviation
Forearm and Elbow		
Forearm	Tuberosity	AP elbow with 20-degree tilt to olecranon
Radial head		45-degree lateral of elbow, magnification
Elbow		Check fat pad, ant. humeral line, radius-capitellum
Elbow contracture	AP/lateral	AP humerus, AP forearm
Shoulder		
Shoulder	Trauma	True AP (scapula—45 degrees obl.), scapular lat. (Y)
Shoulder	Axillary lateral	Through axilla with arm abducted
Tuberosities	AP ER/IR	AP with arm in full extension & internal rotation
Impingement	Caudal tilt	AP with 30-degree caudal tilt
Impingement	Supraspinatus outlet	Scapula lat. with 10-degree caudal tilt
Hill Sachs	Stryker Notch	Supine, hand on head, 10-degree cephalic tilt
Bankart	West Point	Prone axillary lat. with 25-degree lat. & post. tilt
Bankart	Garth	Apical obl. with 45-degree caudal & AP tilt
AC injury	Stress	AP both AC (large cassette) with 10 pounds **hanging** weight
AC injury	Alexander	Scapular lat. with shoulders forward
AC arthritis	Zanca	10-degree cephalic tilt of AC
SC injury	Hobbs	PA, patient leans over cassette
SC injury	Serendipity	40-degree cephalic tilt center on manubrium
Clavicle		AP 30-degree cephalic tilt
Spine		
C-spine	Series	AP/lat./obls., open-mouth odontoid
C7	Swimmer's view	Lat. through maximally abducted arm
Instability	Flex/Ext	AP with flexion & extension
L-spine	Series	AP, lat., obliques (foramina), L5/S1 spot lat.
Pelvis and Hip		
Pelvic injury	Inlet	45–50 degrees caudad (assess AP displacement)
Pelvic injury	Outlet	45 degrees cephalad (assess SI superior displacement)
Pelvic injury-Judet	Iliac obl.	Oblique on ilium (**post. column, ant. wall**)
Pelvic injury-Judet	Obturator obl.	Oblique on obturator foramen (**ant. column, post. wall**)
Pelvic injury	Push-pull	Outlet view with stress (assess stability)
SI Injury		Judet views centered on SI joints
Hip	Surgical lat.	Lat. from opposite side with that hip flexed
Femoral neck		AP with 15 degrees' internal rotation
Knee		
Knee AP & lat.		AP with 5 degrees' flexion, lat. with 30 degrees' flexion
Osteochondroid Fx	Notch	Prone 45 degrees from vertical
Knee DJD	Rosenberg	Weight-bearing PA with 45 degrees' flexion
Patella	Merchant	45 degrees' flexion, cassette perpendicular to tibia
Tibial plateau		AP with 10-degree caudal tilt
Foot and Ankle		
Ankle	Mortise	AP with 15 degrees' internal rotation
Ankle	Stress	AP with lat. stress, lat. with drawer
Foot	Weight bearing	AP % lat. weight bearing
Midfoot		Include obliques
Talus	Canale	AP with 75-degree cephalic tilt, pronate 15 degree
Talar Neck		AP with 15-degrees' pronation
Subtalar	Broden	45-degree rotation lat. with varying tilts
Calcaneus	Harris	AP standing, 45-degree tilt
Sesamoid		Tangentials with dorsiflexed toes

3. Stabilization
   a. Initial stabilization with a splint should immobilize both joints proximal and distal to the fracture. Pelvic ring injuries (anterior-posterior compression [APC]) benefit from a "pelvic binder," or early pelvic external fixation, to reduce macromotion and promote hemostasis. Skeletal traction can be needed for femur fractures, acetabular fractures, cervical injuries, and pelvic fractures (vertical shear).
   b. Internal and External Fixation—Preoperative planning will determine intraoperative equipment requirements. A well-planned surgical tactic will provide skeletal stabilization (staged with external fixation versus early primary internal fixation), and decrease infection rates and soft tissue complications.
4. Perioperative Fracture Considerations
   a. Thromboprophylaxis—Deep venous thrombosis (DVT) prevalence is significant in the fracture population. All fracture patients need some form of DVT prophylaxis while in hospital (mechanical or chemoprophylaxis). Certain fracture types are associated with a high incidence of DVT—Pelvic ring injuries, acetabular fractures, hip fractures, femur fractures. Duration and type of thromboprophylaxis postoperatively remains controversial. Fatal pulmonary embolism can result from a DVT. Suspected DVT (limb swelling, calf tenderness [Homan sign]) is commonly diagnosed with duplexultrasonography. Some centers use IV contrast venography, magnetic resonance venography, and a D-Dimer blood analysis as well. The gold standard for DVT detection remains IV contrast venography. A confirmed DVT in a fracture patient is treated with anticoagulation (low-molecular-weight heparin versus coumadin) for 3 months, generally, or an inferior vena cava (IVC) filter.
   b. Fat Embolism Syndrome—Typically occurs after pelvic or femur fractures, with clinical symptoms 24–72 hours after inciting event. Symptoms include hypoxia, confusion, tachycardia, and petechiae. Treatment consists of supportive care (oxygen, IV hydration) and monitoring.
   c. Acute Respiratory Distress Syndrome (ARDS)—Early lone-bone fracture fixation has been shown to decrease the incidence of ARDS in polytrauma patients. Reaming of long bone fractures is associated with increased intravascular fat presence, but is not associated with an increased incidence of ARDS (controversial in pulmonary contusion patients).
   d. Postoperative Weight-Bearing Status—In the elderly hip fracture population, it has been shown that compliance with weight-bearing restrictions is not realistic. These patients either bear weight as they can tolerate it or do not bear weight, which should be determined by surgeon intraoperatively.
5. Fracture Developments
   a. Delayed Union—Failure of expected healing progression (depending on particular fracture). Need to rule out infection.
      (1) Interventions—Ultrasound therapy, electrical stimulation, bone grafting (autograft, injection of marrow elements, allograft, demineralized bone matrix [DBM], bone morphogenic proteins [BMPs]), and revision fixation
   b. Nonunion—Failure or halting of healing progression (failure of healing progression on three successive monthly radiographs, displacement, hardware loosening/failure. Need to rule out infection.
      (1) Types—Hypertrophic, oligotrophic, atrophic, infected, and synovial pseudarthrosis (Fig. 10-1).
      (2) Interventions—Hardware revision (provide stable construct), bone grafting (autograft, injection of marrow elements, allograft [DBM], BMPs). Current studies suggest equal efficacy of BMPs when compared with autograft, although autograft remains the gold standard when bone grafting nonunions.
   c. Segmental Bone Loss—Diaphyseal defects can be reconstructed with distraction ontogenesis (bone transport), direct bone grafting (iliac crest bone grafting [ICBG]), vascularized fibular grafts, allografts, and prosthetic cages with autograft. Selection of grafting techniques depends of surgeon experience, size/length of defect, and presence of infection.
   d. Heterotopic Ossification (HO)—Associated with closed head injury, acetabular surgery involving abductor stripping, and periarticular elbow surgery, as well as many other injuries. Prophylaxes include postoperative low-dose indomethacin (Indocin) (25 mg po tid × 6 weeks) or postoperative local radiation (800 rads). HO develops postoperatively within 3–6 months. Activity of HO is studied with bone scan. When HO matures and bone scan activity decreases, patient is a candidate for HO resection.
   e. Osteomyelitis—Acute or chronic osteomyelitis presents a significant problem in fracture healing.
      (1) Acute osteomyelitis can be treated with repeated aggressive I&D and maintenance of the hardware to maintain skeletal stabilization. Deep cultures will guide antimicrobial therapy (typically 6-week course of antibiotic). It is

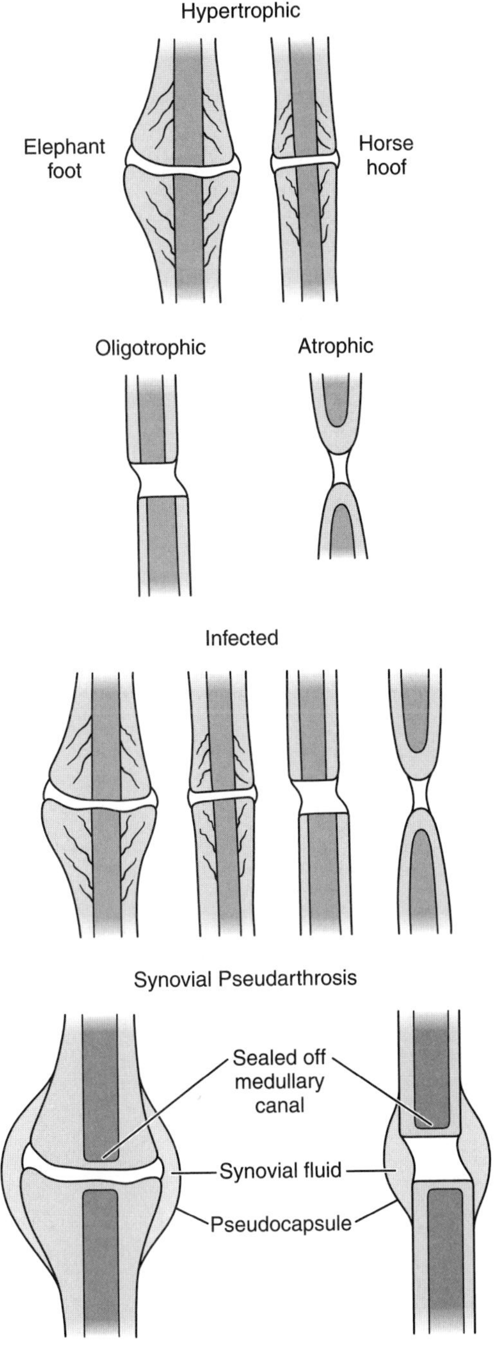

FIGURE 10-1 ■ Classification of nonunions. (From Browner, B.D., et al., eds.: Skeletal Trauma, 3rd ed. Philadelphia, WB Saunders, 2003, p. 532.)

possible to eradicate infection with an aggressive approach.

(2) Chronic osteomyelitis is much more difficult to treat. If nonunion exits, all hardware needs to be removed and devitalized/infected bone needs to be aggressively débrided. Temporary stabilization with external fixation and antibiotic rods/spacers can be used. The decision to place new internal fixation, after a planned interval, in an infected area depends on the desired objective (complete blood count [CBC], erythrocyte sedimentation rate [ESR], C-reactive protein [CRP], frozen specimen evaluation) and subjective findings. Commonly, evaluation of infected bone includes—plain x-ray studies, nuclear medicine studies, MRI, and intraoperative examination. The only way to completely eradicate chronic osteomyelitis is resection of infected bone. Bony healing is possible in the presence of infection, but this needs to be identified and treated appropriately (e.g., hardware removal after union, antibiotics, etc.).

f. Gunshot Wounds (GSWs)—Soft tissue and bony destruction is based on the velocity of the missile (kinetic energy = $\frac{1}{2} mv^2$). Low-velocity GSWs (<2000 ft/sec—most handguns) cause less soft tissue destruction, and treatment usually consists of local entry/exit wound débridement. Treatment of fractures resulting from low-velocity GSWs is similar to closed fracture treatment. High-velocity GSWs (>2000 ft/sec—military/hunting rifles) can cause massive soft tissue destruction and require aggressive radical débridement of devitalized tissue. Timing of fixation of high-velocity GSWs depends on wound conditions. Partially jacketed, unjacketed, and hollow-point bullets cause greater soft tissue destruction. Shotgun wounds, especially at short range, often result in type III wounds (Gustilo and Anderson classification) because of extensive soft tissue injury. The wadding has a high potential for contamination of wounds and must be sought at the time of débridement. Intra-articular missiles should be removed because of the potential for lead intoxication and the certainty of continued articular damage. Nerve injuries associated with GSWs are often temporary (neuropraxia) and are caused by the blast effect of missiles traversing the tissue. Arteriograms should be used liberally if there is any question of an arterial injury.

SECTION 2

Upper and Lower Extremity Injuries and Pelvic Injuries

I. Shoulder

A. **Sternoclavicular Injury**
   1. Evaluation/Classification
      a. Anterior Dislocation
      b. Posterior Dislocation
      c. Spontaneous Atraumatic Subluxation
   2. Treatment
      a. Anterior Dislocation—Closed reduction with bump between shoulders
      b. Posterior Dislocation—Closed reduction with towel clip in operating room with thoracic surgery backup or open reduction and ligamentous reconstruction
      c. Spontaneous Atraumatic Subluxation—Nonoperative
   3. Complications
      a. Bump (Cosmetic)
      b. Degenerative Joint Disease (DJD)
      c. Mediastinal Impingement with Posterior Dislocation

B. **Clavicle Fracture**
   1. Evaluation/Classification
      a. Medial third (5%)
      b. Middle third (85%)
      c. Distal third (10%)
      d. Neer—(Fig. 10-2)
         (1) Nondisplaced interligamentous (coracoclavicular [CC]-acromioclavicular [AC]). Fracture medial to CC ligaments. Conoid torn, trapezoid attached to distal fragment
         (2) Fracture extends to AC joint
         (3) Periosteal sleeve fracture with ligaments attached to periosteum
         (4) Comminuted fracture with ligaments attached to an inferior fragment
   2. Treatment
      a. Figure of eight brace or sling for medial third, middle third, and distal third types I, IV, and V.
      b. Open reduction and internal fixation (ORIF) for distal third type II (IIA and IIB).
      c. Closed treatment, late excision arthroplasty if required for distal third type III.
   3. Complications
      a. Skin Compromise
      b. Vascular Injury
      c. Pneumothorax
      d. Nerve Injury (Rare)
      e. Nonunion (1-5%)

C. **Acromioclavicular Joint (AC) Injury**
   1. Evaluation/Classification
      a. Rockwood—(Fig. 10-3)
         (1) AC sprain
         (2) AC ligament disruption, intact CC ligament
         (3) AC and CC tear (25-100% subluxation)
         (4) Clavicle through trapezius posteriorly
         (5) Detachment of deltoid and trapezius muscles (100-300% subluxation)
         (6) Inferior dislocation of clavicle
   2. Treatment
      a. 7-10 days rest/immobilization
      b. Sling for 2 weeks, rehabilitation, late excision arthroplasty if required
      c. Conservative versus repair (controversial)
      d. Reduce and repair
   3. Complications
      a. Joint stiffness
      b. Deformity
      c. CC ligament and soft tissue calcification
      d. AC DJD

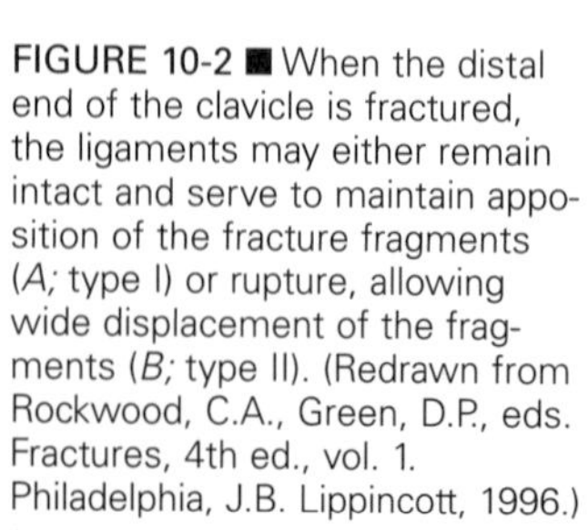

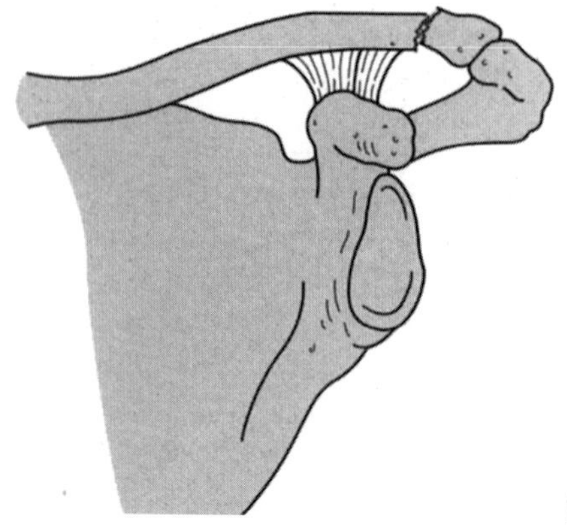

A

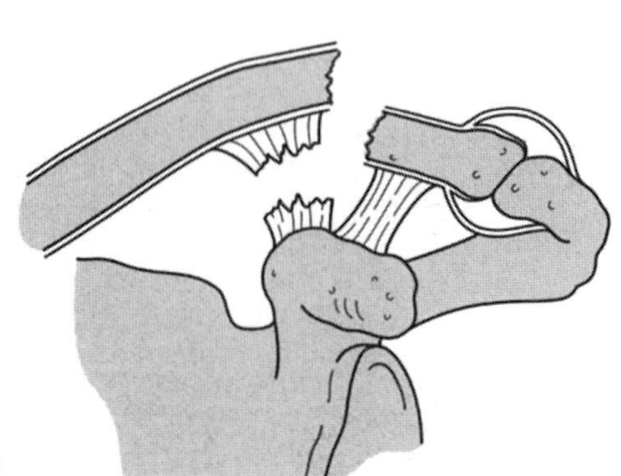

B

FIGURE 10-2 ■ When the distal end of the clavicle is fractured, the ligaments may either remain intact and serve to maintain apposition of the fracture fragments (*A;* type I) or rupture, allowing wide displacement of the fragments (*B;* type II). (Redrawn from Rockwood, C.A., Green, D.P., eds. Fractures, 4th ed., vol. 1. Philadelphia, J.B. Lippincott, 1996.)

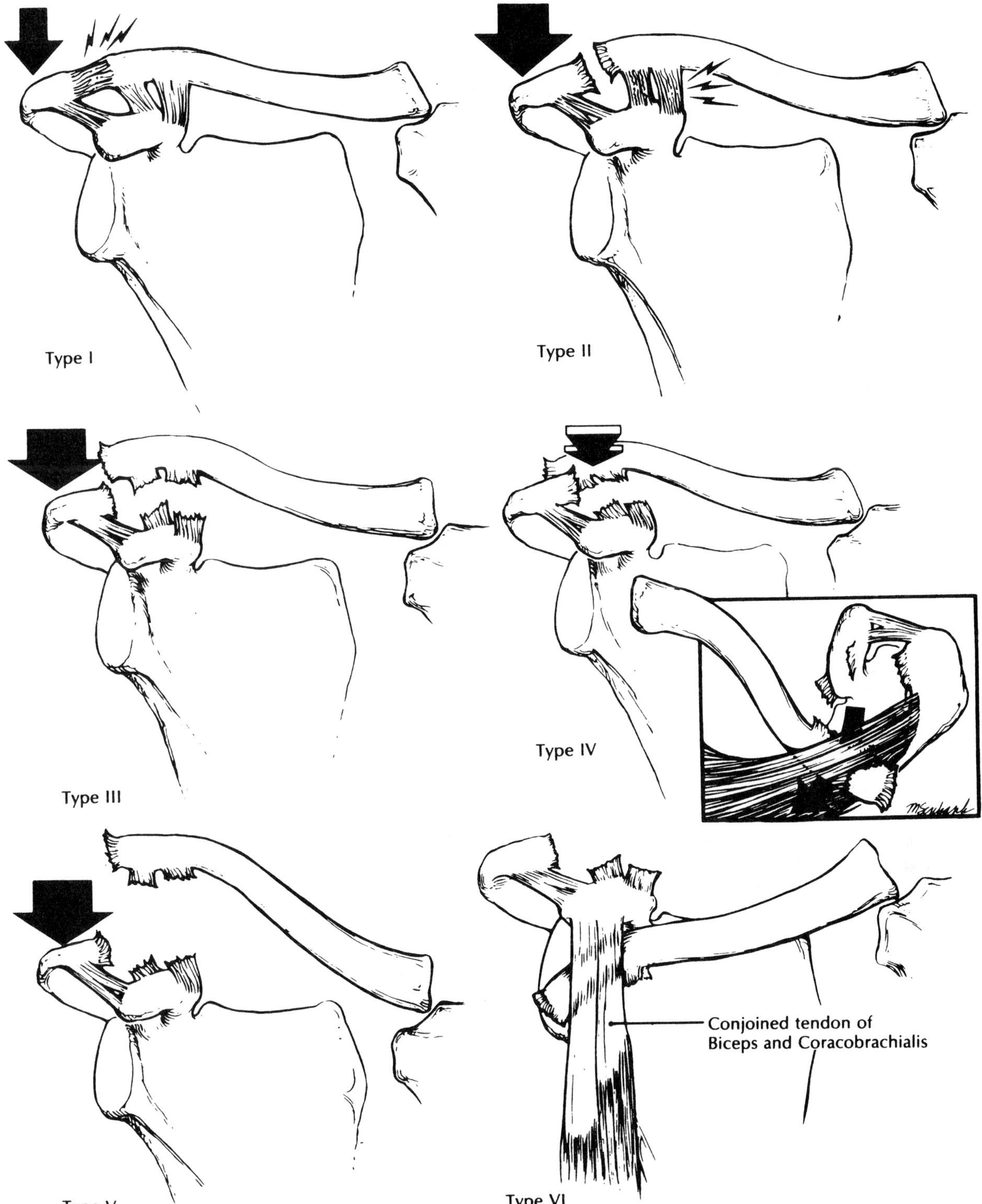

FIGURE 10-3 ■ Classification of acromioclavicular injuries. (From Neer, C.S., and Rockwood, C.A.: Fractures and dislocations of the shoulder. In Rockwood, C.A., and Green, D.P., eds.: Fractures in Adults, 2nd ed. Philadelphia, JB Lippincott, 1984, p. 871. reprinted by permission.)

e. Associated fractures
f. Distal clavicle osteolysis

D. **Scapular Fracture**
1. Evaluation/Classification
a. Zdravkovic and Damholt
(1) Body
(2) Apophyseal fractures, including the coracoid and acromion
(3) Fractures of the superolateral angle, including the neck and glenoid
2. Treatment
a. Most treated conservatively
b. ORIF of large displaced fragments
c. ORIF of large unstable fractures (glenoid with displaced clavicle fracture) or >40 degrees angulation of neck
3. Complications
a. Associated Injuries (Common with Type II)—Clavicle and rib fractures, pneumothorax, vascular and plexus injuries, closed head injury (CHI), pulmonary contusion

E. **Glenoid Fracture**
1. Evaluation/Classification
a. Ideberg
(1) Anterior avulsion fracture
(2) Transverse/oblique fracture—Inferior glenoid free
(3) Upper third glenoid and coracoid
(4) Horizontal glenoid fracture through body
(5) Combination of (2) and (4)
2. Treatment
a. Conservative management
b. ORIF if >25% of glenoid fossa involved with humeral subluxation and intra-articular step-off >5 mm
3. Complications
a. Traumatic DJD

F. **Scapulothoracic Dissociation**
1. Evaluation/Classification
a. Seen on scapular lateral or chest radiograph
2. Treatment
a. Closed reduction and immobilization for 3–6 weeks
3. Complications
a. Vascular and plexus injuries
b. Associated clavicular fracture

G. **Lateral Dissociation** (Closed Forequarter Amputation)
1. Evaluation/Classification
a. Complete neurovascular exam is critical
2. Treatment
a. Arteriography and immediate vascular repair
b. ORIF of clavicle, AC, and SC joints if partial or complete plexus injury exists
3. Complications
a. Poor prognosis
b. High incidence of neurovascular injury

H. **Proximal Humerus Fracture**
1. Evaluation/Classification
a. Neer—Four parts consist of greater tuberosity, lesser tuberosity, head, and shaft (Fig. 10-4)

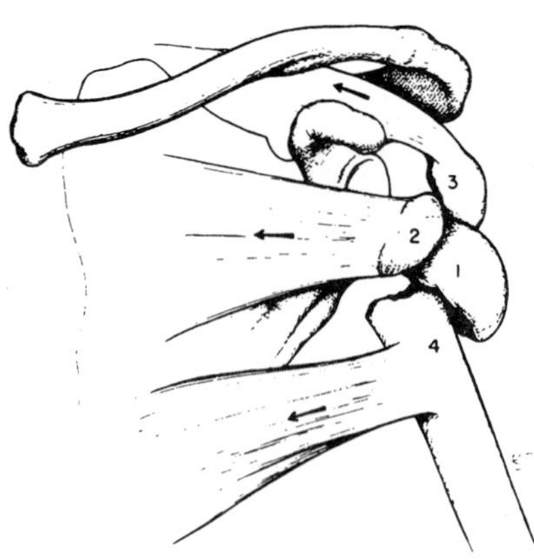

FIGURE 10-4 ■ Proximal humeral fracture. Four parts: *1,* head; *2,* lesser tuberosity; *3,* greater tuberosity; *4,* humeral shaft. (From Neer, C.S., and Rockwood, C.A.: Fractures and dislocations of the shoulder. In Rockwood, C.A., and Green, D.P., eds.: Fractures in Adults, 2nd ed. Philadelphia, JB Lippincott, 1984, p. 696.)

b. Displaced if parts >1 cm apart or 45 degrees angulated
c. Classification based on displacement of fragments
2. Treatment
a. One-Part Fractures—Sling, early ROM (1–2 weeks), and isometric exercises (most common)
b. Two-Part Fractures—Surgical neck fracture; if stable, closed reduction then early ROM; if unstable, closed reduction/percutaneous pinning (CRPP) versus ORIF; ORIF for greater or lesser tuberosity fractures
c. Three-Part Fractures—ORIF for a young patient, total shoulder arthroplasty (TSA) for an elderly patient
d. Four-Part Fractures—ORIF for a young patient, TSA for an elderly patient, nonoperative treatment if valgus is impacted in elderly patient
3. Complications
a. Missed dislocation
b. Adhesive capsulitis (moist heat, gentle ROM)
c. Malunion (reconstruction or TSA required)
d. Avascular necrosis (AVN) (TSA required)
e. Nonunion (surgical neck, tuberosity fractures—require ORIF)
f. Disrupted rotator cuff
g. High rate of AVN with ORIF in four-part

I. **Anterior Shoulder Dislocation** (Fig. 10-5)
1. Evaluation/Classification
a. Axillary lateral critical in diagnosis
2. Treatment
a. Closed reduction, 4 weeks' immobilization in a young patient, 2 weeks in an elderly patient
3. Complications
a. In <20 year old (yo), 85% recurrence rate
b. High incidence of rotator cuff tear in >40 yo

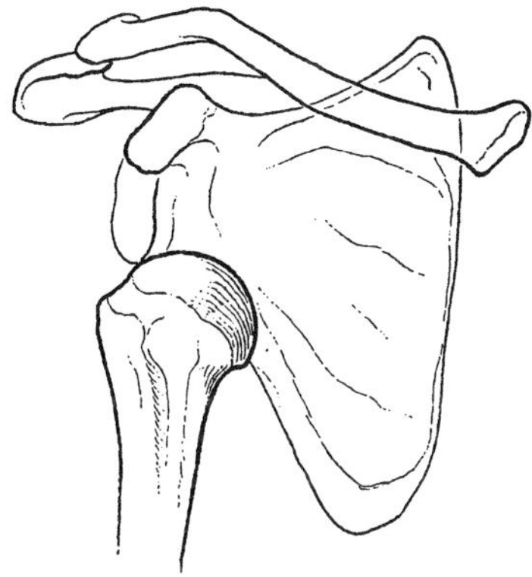

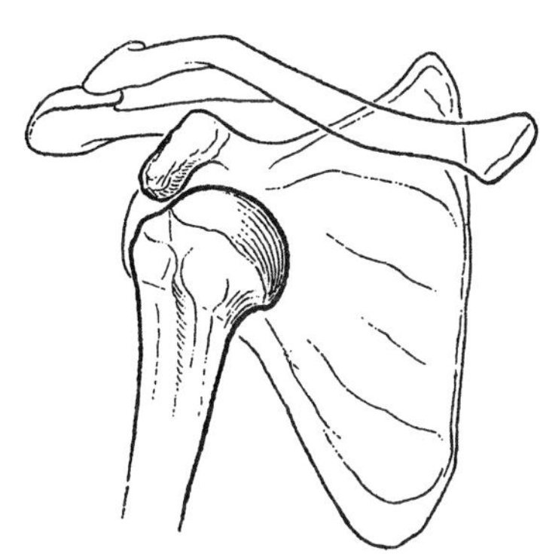

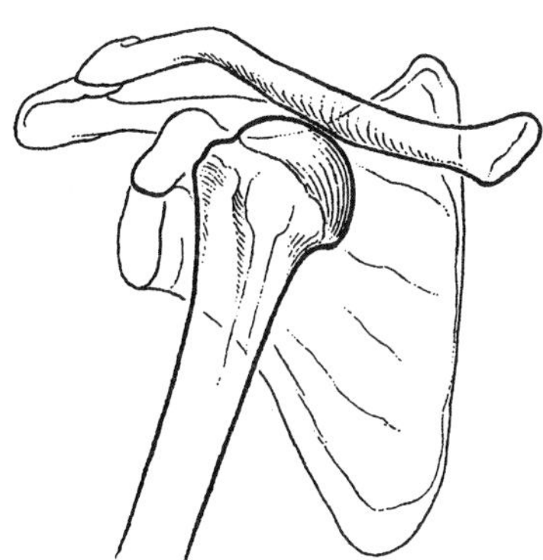

FIGURE 10-5 ■ Anterior shoulder dislocation. *Top*, Subglenoid. *Middle*, Subcoracoid. *Bottom*, Subclavicular. (From Connolly, J.F., ed.: DePalma's The Management of Fractures and Dislocations, an Atlas, 3rd ed. Philadelphia, WB Saunders, 1981, p. 617.)

J. **Posterior Shoulder Dislocation** (Fig. 10-6)
  1. Evaluation/Classification
    a. Seizure or electrical shock
  2. Treatment
    a. Closed reduction and immobilization for 4 weeks
  3. Complications
    a. Lesser tuberosity fracture common

K. **Inferior Shoulder Dislocation—Luxatio erecta** (Fig. 10-7)
  1. Evaluation/Classification
    a. Abducted arm and inability to lower it
  2. Treatment
    a. Reduction and immobilization
  3. Complications
    a. Neurovascular injury and compressive neuropathy or thrombosis of axillary artery (60%)
    b. Rotator cuff tear

II. Humerus

A. **Shaft Fracture**
  1. Evaluation/Classification
    a. Descriptive—Location and fracture pattern
  2. Treatment
    a. Functional brace if <20 degrees anterior angulation, <30 degrees valgus/varus angulation, or <3 cm shortening
    b. ORIF if open fracture, floating elbow, polytrauma, CHI, pathologic
  3. Complications
    a. Radial Nerve Palsy in 5–10% of Cases—Observe unless follows reduction or open fracture
    b. Exploration of Holstein-Lewis fracture (long spiral oblique in distal third) is controversial

B. **Supracondylar Fractures** (Fig. 10-8)
  1. Evaluation/Classification
    a. Rare in adults
    b. High, low, abduction, and adduction (Fig. 10-9)
  2. Treatment
    a. ORIF
  3. Complications
    a. Neurovascular injury
    b. Compartment syndrome
    c. Nonunion
    d. Malunion
    e. Contracture
    f. Decreased ROM (fibrosis, bony block)

C. **Distal Single-Column (Condyle) Fractures** (Fig. 10-10)
  1. Evaluation/Classification
    a. Milch (lateral > medial)
      (1) Lateral trochlear ridge intact
      (2) Fracture through lateral trochlear ridge
  2. Treatment
    a. Type I, Undisplaced—Immobilize in supination (lateral condyle), pronation (medial condyle)
    b. Type II, Displaced—CRPP
    c. Type III—ORIF
  3. Complications
    a. Cubitus valgus (lateral)
    b. Cubitus varus (medial)
    c. Ulnar nerve neurapraxia
    d. DJD

D. **Distal Bicolumn Fractures** (Fig. 10-11)
  1. Evaluation/Classification

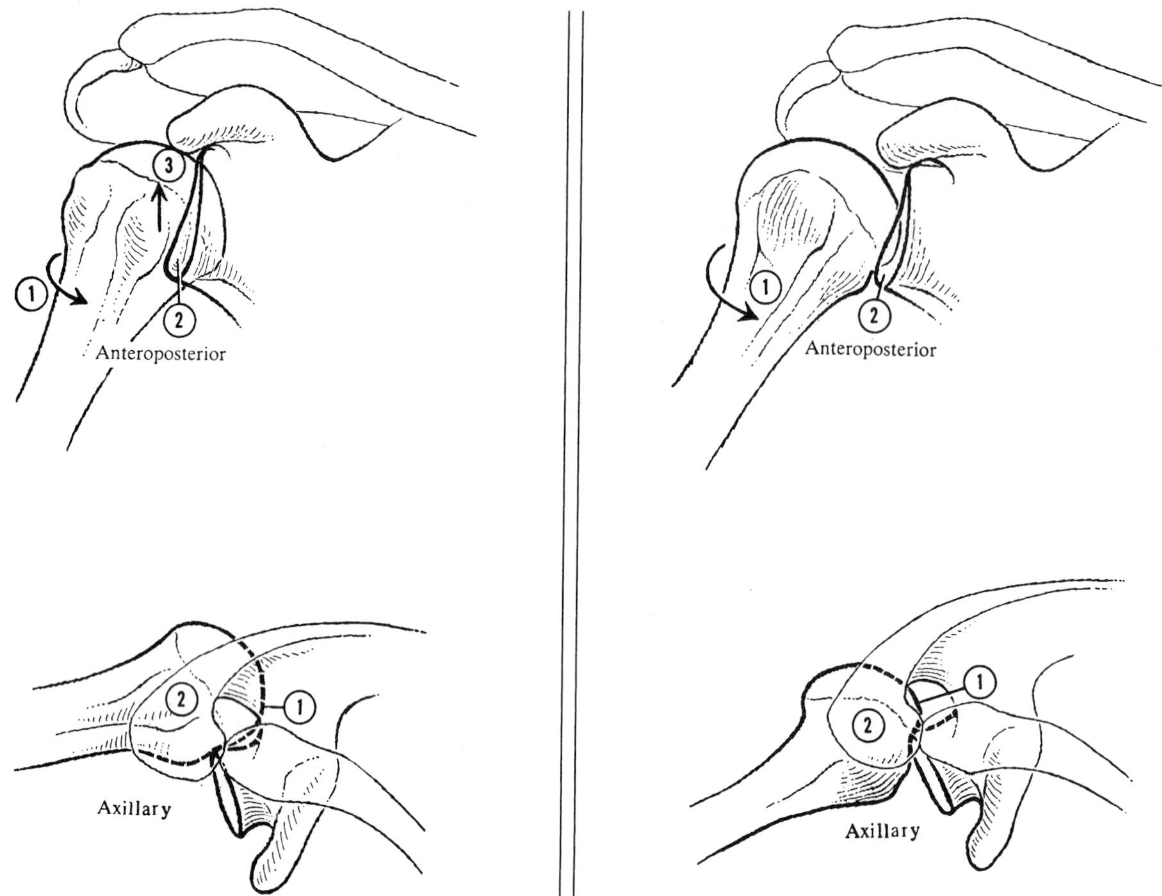

FIGURE 10-6 ■ Posterior shoulder dislocation. *Left*, Subacromial. *Right*, Subcoracoid. (From Connolly, J.F., ed.: DePalma's The Management of Fractures and Dislocations, an Atlas, 3rd ed. Philadelphia, WB Saunders, 1981, p. 633.)

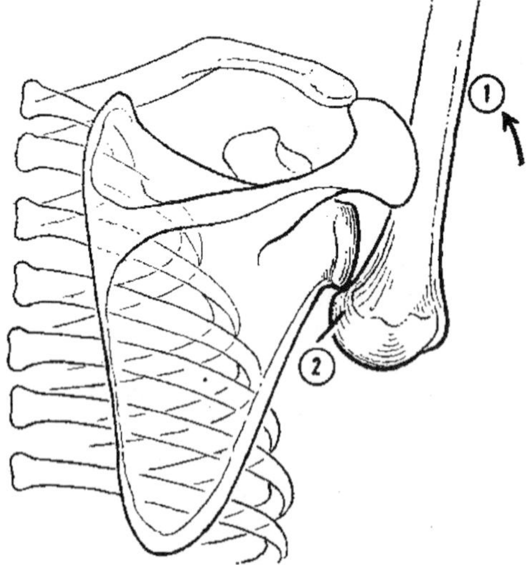

FIGURE 10-7 ■ Luxatio erecta. (From Connolly, J.F., ed.: DePalma's The Management of Fractures and Dislocations, an Atlas, 3rd ed. Philadelphia, WB Saunders, 1981, p. 622.)

a. Jupiter
   (1) High T—Transverse fracture proximal or at upper olecranon fossa
   (2) Low T (Common)—Transverse fracture just proximal to trochlea
   (3) Y—Oblique fracture lines through both columns with distal vertical fracture
   (4) H—Trochlea is free fragment (risk of AVN)
   (5) Medial Lambda—Proximal fracture exits medially
   (6) Lateral Lambda—Proximal fracture exits laterally
   (7) Multiplane—T type with additional fracture in coronal plane

2. Treatment
   a. ORIF—Posterior approach, fix condyles first, then epitrochlear ridge to humeral metaphysis
   b. Mobilize within 3–4 weeks
   c. Arthroplasty for elderly patients

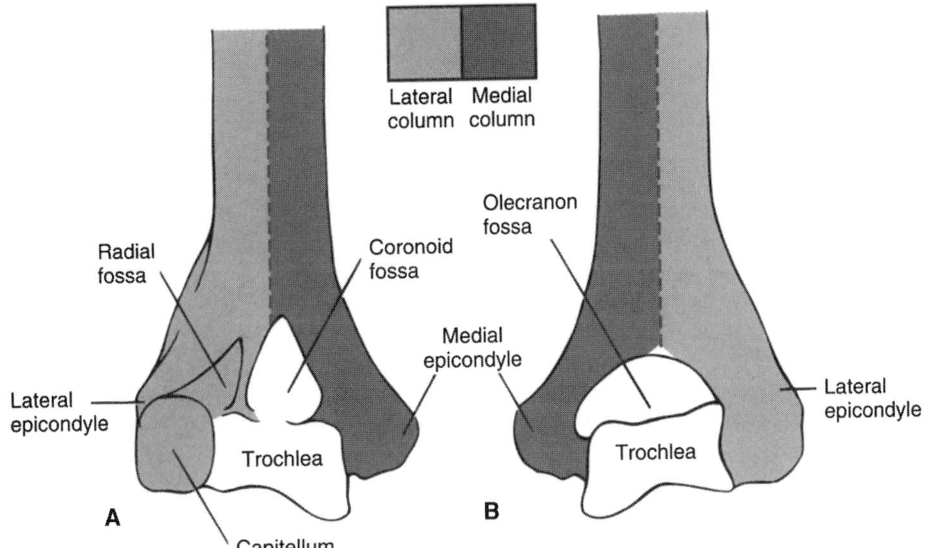

FIGURE 10-8 ■ Anterior *(A)* and posterior *(B)* views of the medial and lateral columns of the distal humerus. (From Browner, B.D., et al. eds.: Skeletal Trauma, 2nd ed. Philadelphia, WB Saunders, 1998, p. 1485.)

3. Complications
   a. Stiffness
   b. Heterotopic ossification
   c. Infection
   d. Ulnar neuropathy (Treat with transposition)

E. **Capitellum Fractures** (Fig. 10-12)
1. Evaluation/Classification
   a. Bryan and Morrey
      Type I—Hahn-Steinthal; complete fracture of capitellum
      Type II—Kocher-Lorenz; sleeve fracture of articular cartilage
      Type III—Comminuted
      Type IV (McKee's modification)—Coronal shear fracture including capitellum and trochlea (Fig. 10-13)
2. Treatment
   a. Splint 2–3 weeks if nondisplaced, ORIF if >2-mm displacement
   b. Splint 2–3 weeks if nondisplaced and excise displaced fragments
   c. Excise if displaced
   d. ORIF
3. Complications
   a. Nonunion with ORIF (1–11%)
   b. Olecranon osteotomy nonunion
   c. Ulnar nerve neuropathy
   d. Heterotopic ossification with ORIF (4%)
   e. AVN of capitellum

III. Elbow

A. **Olecranon Fracture** (Fig. 10-14)
1. Evaluation/Classification
   a. Colton
      (1) Undisplaced (<2 mm)
      (2) Displaced
         (a) Avulsion fracture
         (b) Oblique/transverse fracture
         (c) Comminuted fracture
         (d) Fracture-dislocation
2. Treatment
   a. Splint at 45–90 degrees for 4 weeks
   b. Tension band or fragment excision with triceps reconstruction
   c. Oblique-bicortical screw; transverse-tension band
   d. Plate fixation on dorsal (tension) side
   e. ORIF, no early excision
3. Complications
   a. Decreased ROM
   b. DJD
   c. Nonunion
   d. Ulnar nerve neurapraxia
   e. Instability

B. **Coronoid Fracture**
1. Evaluation/Classification
   a. Regan and Morrey (Fig. 10-15)
      Type I—Tip avulsion
      Type II—Single or comminuted fracture involving ≤50% coronoid
      Type III—Single or comminuted fracture involving ≥50% coronoid
2. Treatment
   a. Type I and II—Early mobilization (consider hinged orthosis)
   b. ORIF
3. Complications
   a. Instability (medial collateral ligament [MCL])
   b. DJD

C. **Radial Head Fracture**
1. Evaluation/Classification
   a. Mason—(Fig. 10-16)
      Type I—Undisplaced
      Type II—Displaced single fracture
      Type III—Comminuted

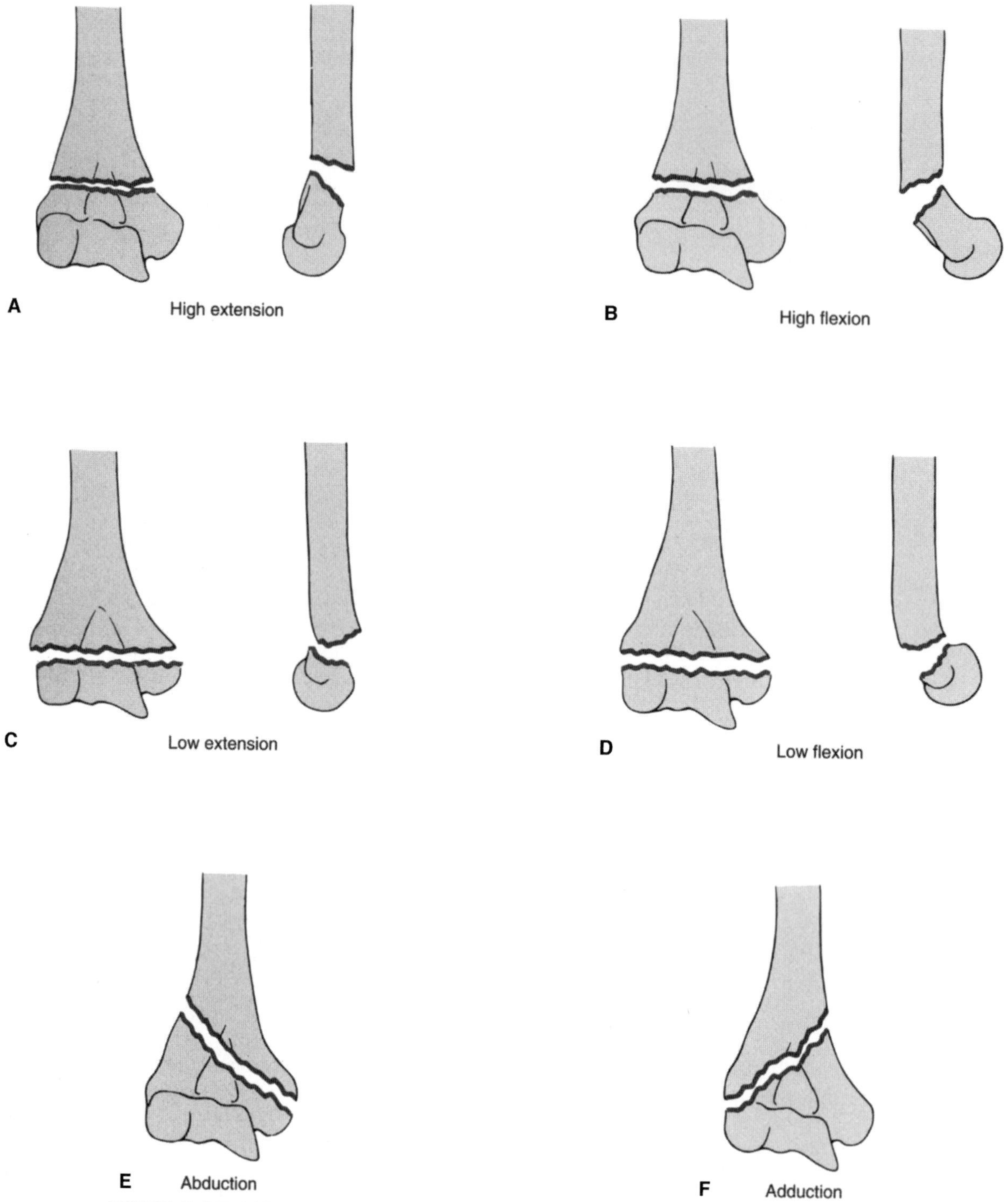

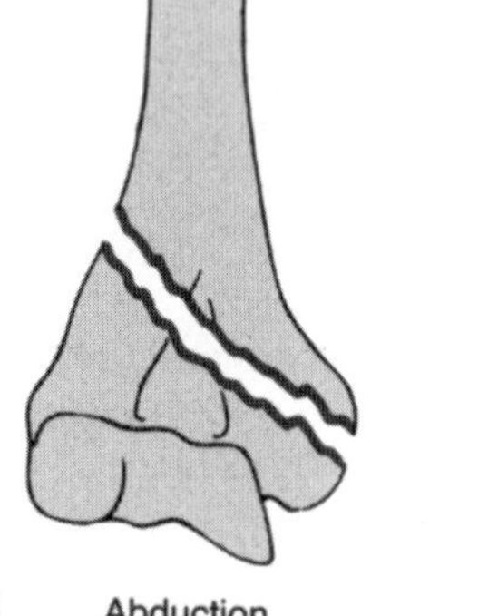

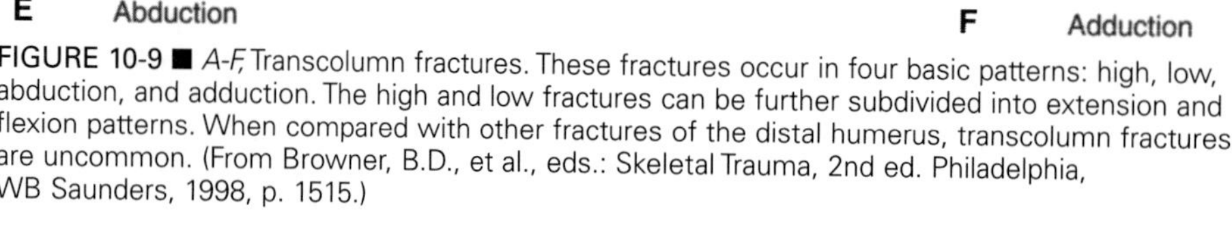

FIGURE 10-9 ■ *A-F,* Transcolumn fractures. These fractures occur in four basic patterns: high, low, abduction, and adduction. The high and low fractures can be further subdivided into extension and flexion patterns. When compared with other fractures of the distal humerus, transcolumn fractures are uncommon. (From Browner, B.D., et al., eds.: Skeletal Trauma, 2nd ed. Philadelphia, WB Saunders, 1998, p. 1515.)

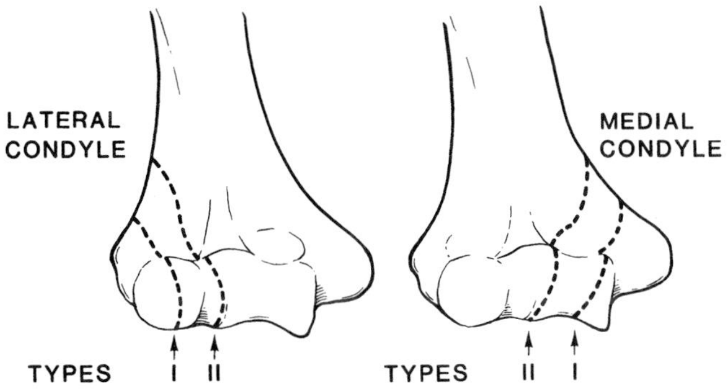

FIGURE 10-10 ■ Humeral condyle fractures. (From Gelman, M.I.: Radiology of Orthopedic Procedures, Problems and Complications, vol. 24, Philadelphia, WB Saunders, 1984, p. 56; reprinted by permission.)

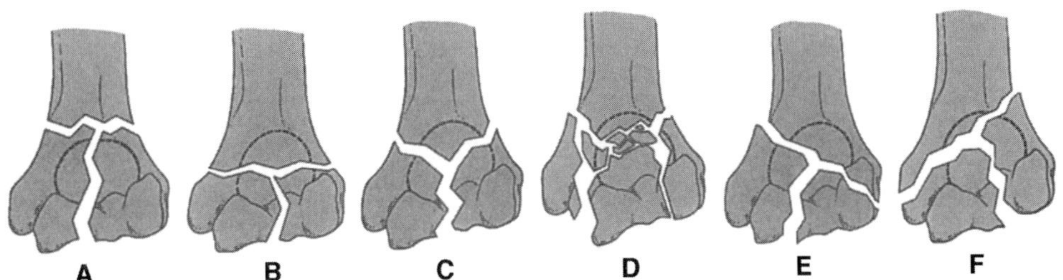

FIGURE 10-11 ■ Bicolumn distal humerus fractures. *A,* High T. *B,* Low T. *C,* Y Pattern. *D,* H Pattern. *E,* Medial lambda. *F,* Lateral lambda. (From Jupiter, J.: Skeletal Trauma, vol. 2, Philadelphia, WB Saunders, 1992, pp. 1159–1163; reprinted by permission.)

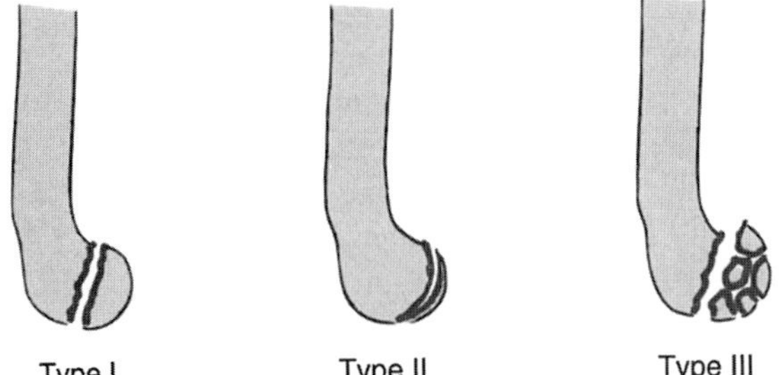

FIGURE 10-12 ■ Fractures of the capitellum can be divided into type I, complete capitellum fracture; type II, the more superficial lesion of Kocher-Lorenz; and type III, comminuted capitellar fracture. (From Browner, B.D., et al., eds.: Skeletal Trauma, 2nd ed. Philadelphia, WB Saunders, 1998, p. 1511.)

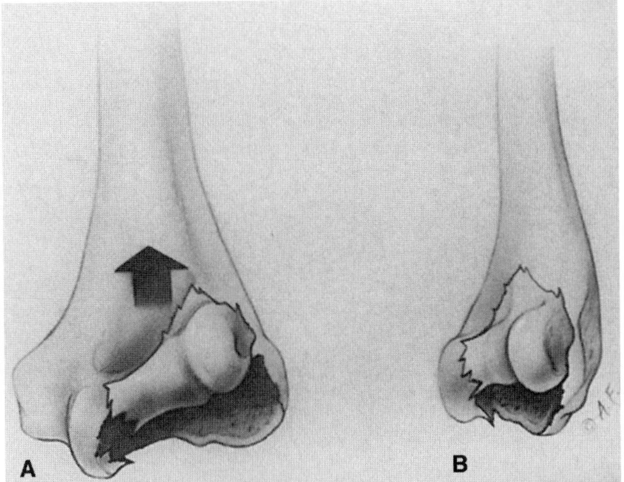

FIGURE 10-13 ■ Coronal shear fracture of the distal humerus. *A,* Diagram showing separation, proximal migration rotation *(arrow)* of the distal fragment, which includes most of the anterior joint surface. *B,* Oblique view. (From Browner, B.D., et al., eds.: Skeletal Trauma, 2nd ed. Philadelphia, WB Saunders, 1998, p. 1512.)

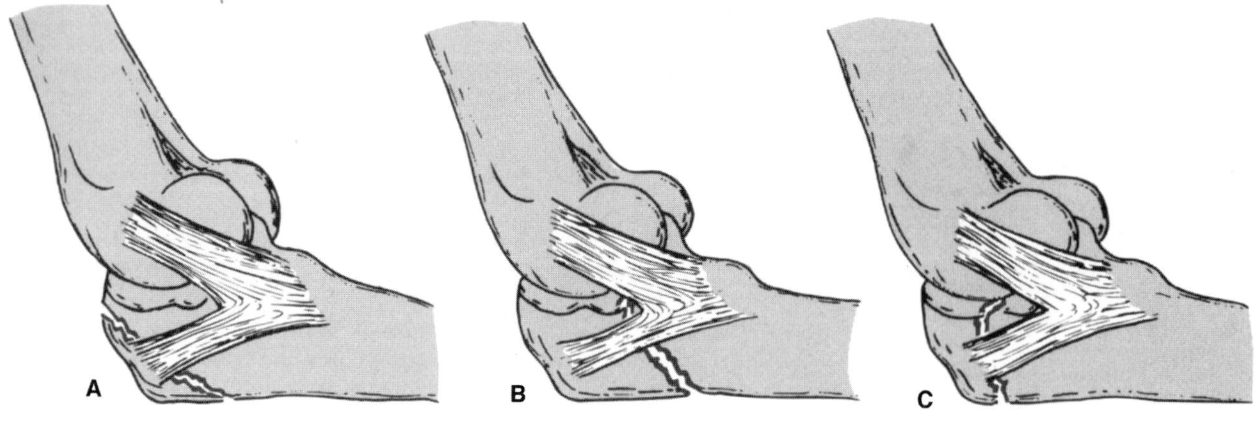

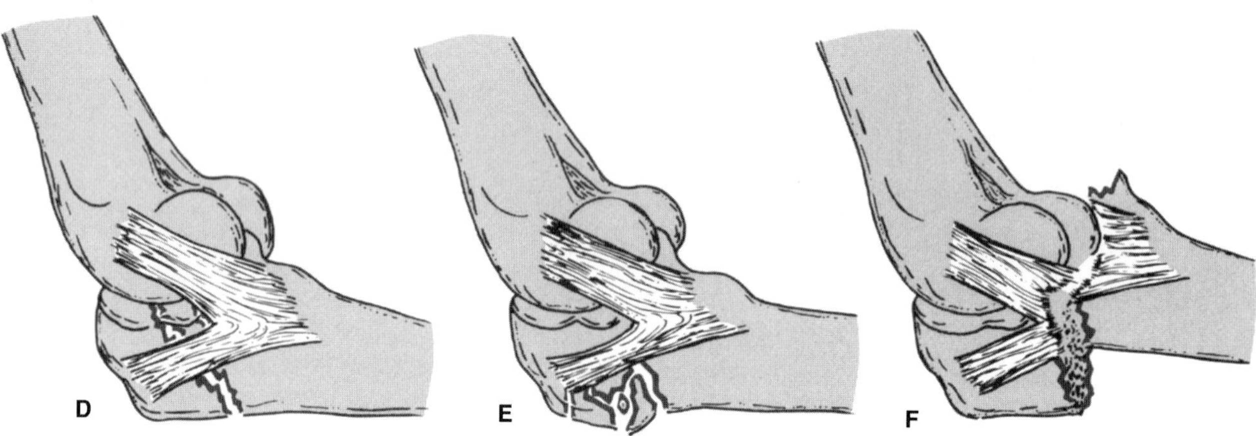

FIGURE 10-14 ■ Colton's classification of olecranon fractures. *A,* Avulsion. *B,* Oblique. *C,* Transverse. *D,* Oblique with comminution. *E,* Comminuted. *F,* Fracture-dislocation. (From Browner, B.D., et al., eds.: Skeletal Trauma, 2nd ed. Philadelphia, WB Saunders, 1998, p. 1469.)

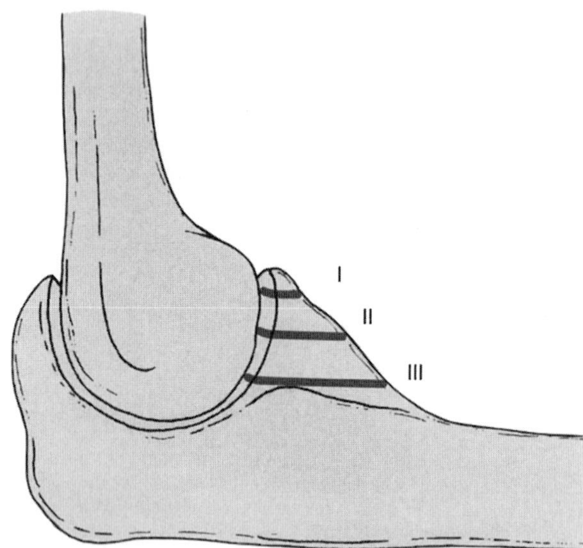

FIGURE 10-15 ■ The coronoid fracture has been classified into three types by Regan and Morrey. (From Browner, B.D., et al., eds.: Skeletal Trauma, 2nd ed. Philadelphia, WB Saunders, 1998, p. 1480.)

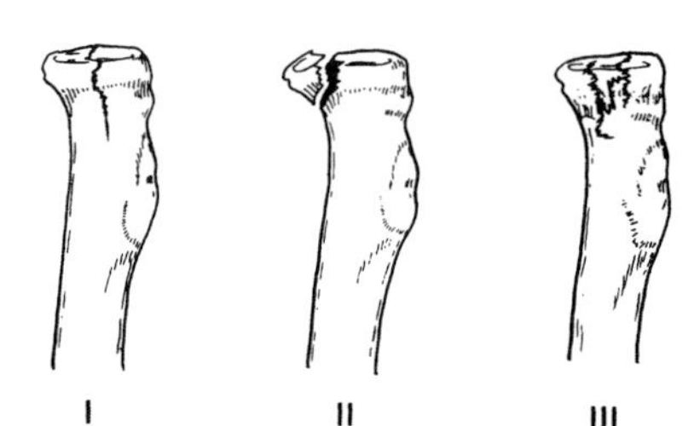

FIGURE 10-16 ■ Classification of radial head fractures. (From Gelman, M.I.: Radiology of Orthopedic Procedures, Problems and Complications, vol. 24, Philadelphia, WB Saunders, 1984, p. 59; reprinted by permission.)

Type IV (Johnson Modification)—Radial head fracture with elbow dislocation

2. Treatment
   a. Nonoperative, early motion ± aspiration
   b. ORIF
   c. For types III and IV—ORIF, MCL repair if unstable, radial head spacer if needed
3. Complications
   a. Decreased ROM
   b. Posterior interosseous nerve (PIN) injury
   c. Intraosseous membrane rupture and distal radioulnar disruption (Essex-Lopresti)
   d. Silastic synovitis

D. **Dislocation** (Fig. 10-17)
1. Evaluation/Classification
   a. Posterolateral (80%), posterior, anterior, medial, lateral, and diversion
2. Treatment
   a. Closed reduction
      (1) Stable—Splint at 90 degrees for 7-10 days
      (2) Unstable—Splint at 90 degrees for 2-3 weeks
3. Complications
   a. Radial head and neck fractures (50-60%),
   b. Epicondyle fractures (10%)
   c. Coronoid fractures (10%)
   d. Median and ulnar nerve injury
   e. Brachial artery injury
   f. Flexion contracture
   g. Heterotopic ossification

IV. Forearm Fractures

A. **Proximal Ulna Fracture and Radial Head Dislocation—Monteggia** (Fig. 10-18)
1. Evaluation/Classification
   a. Bado
      Type I—(60%) Anterior radial head dislocation and apex anterior proximal third ulna fracture
      Type II—(15%) Posterior radial head dislocation and apex posterior proximal third ulna fracture
      Type III—Lateral radial head dislocation and proximal ulnar metaphyseal fracture

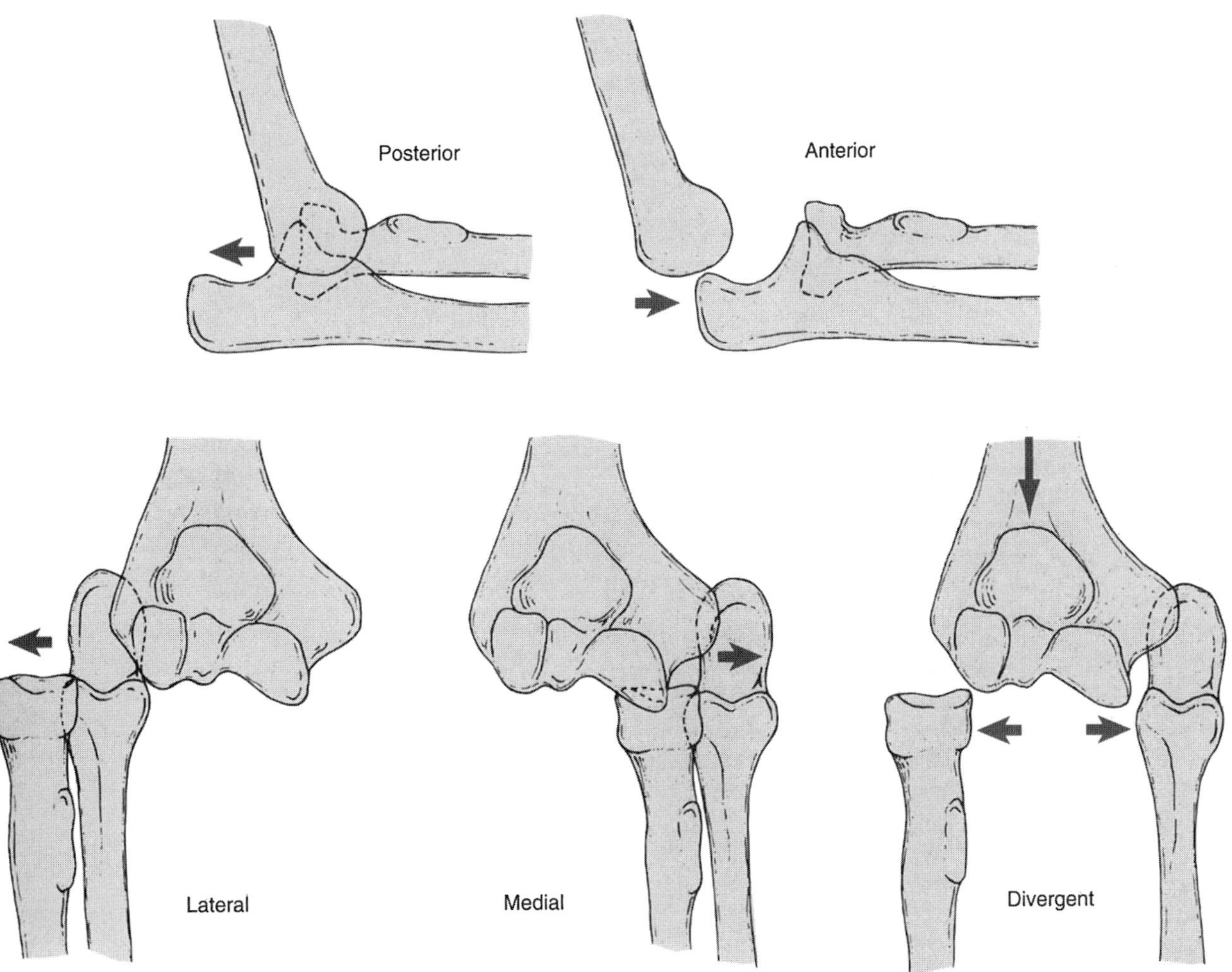

FIGURE 10-17 ■ An elbow dislocation is defined by the direction of the forearm bones. (From Browner, B.D., et al., eds.: Skeletal Trauma, 2nd ed. Philadelphia, WB Saunders, 1998, p. 1475.)

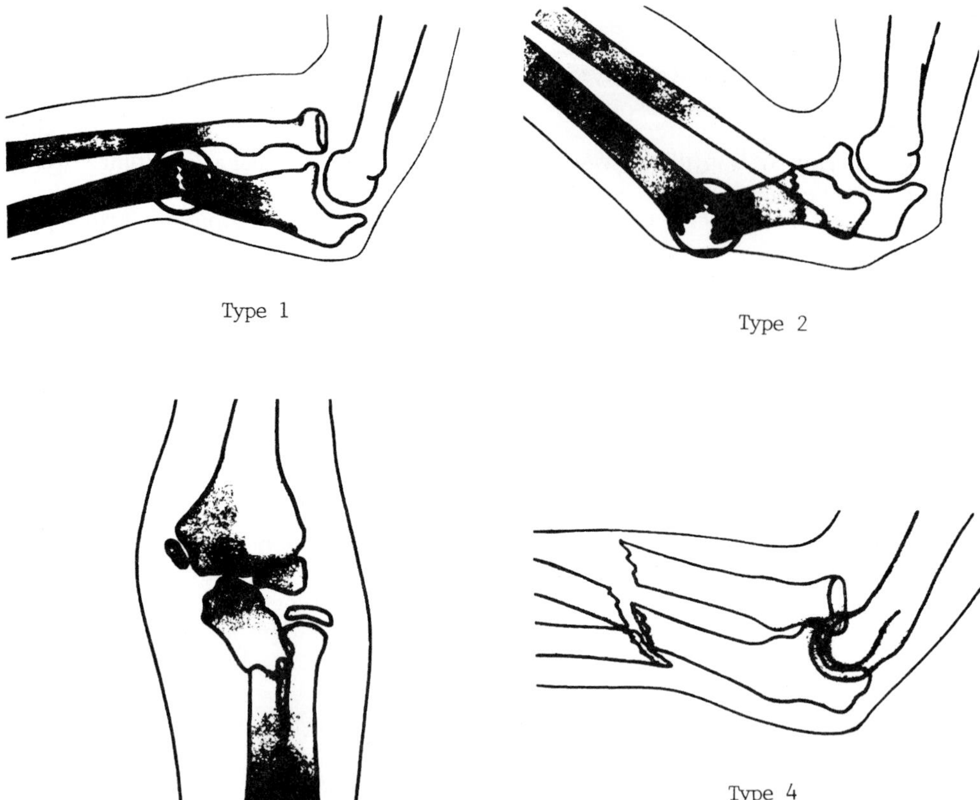

FIGURE 10-18 ■ Classification of Monteggia fractures. (From Reckling, F.W., and Cordell, L.D.: Unstable fracture-dislocations of the forearm. Arch. Surg. 96:1004, 1968; reprinted by permission. Copyright 1968 American Medical Association.)

Type IV—Anterior radial head dislocation with proximal third radius and ulna fractures

2. Treatment

Type I—ORIF, closed reduction head, cast with 110 degrees flexion

Type II—ORIF, closed reduction head, cast with 70 degrees flexion

Type III—ORIF, closed reduction head, cast with 110 degrees flexion

Type IV—ORIF, closed reduction head, cast with 110 degrees flexion

3. Complications
   a. PIN injury (usually resolves spontaneously)
   b. Redislocation/subluxation (inadequate reduction)

B. **Proximal Radius Fractures**
1. Evaluation/Classification
   a. Displaced versus nondisplaced
2. Treatment
   a. Nondisplaced—Long arm cast (LAC) supination, close follow-up
   b. Displaced—Proximal fifth closed, one fifth to two thirds ORIF
3. Complications
   a. Malunion

C. **Radius and Ulna Fractures—"Both Bone"**
1. Evaluation/Classification
   a. Displaced versus nondisplaced
2. Treatment
   a. ORIF
3. Complications
   a. Malunion/nonunion
   b. Vascular injury
   c. PIN injury
   d. Compartment syndrome
   e. Synostosis
   f. Refracture (after plate removal)

D. **Ulna Fractures—"Nightstick"**
1. Evaluation/Classification
   a. Sustained by a direct blow to the ulnar forearm
2. Treatment
   a. Distal two thirds, <50% displaced, <10 degrees angulation—LAC to functional fracture brace with good interosseus mold
   b. Proximal third or >50% displaced or >10 degrees angulation—ORIF

3. Complications
   a. Malunion/nonunion

E. **Distal Third Radius Fractures and Radioulnar Dislocation—Galeazzi or Piedmont**
   1. Evaluation/Classification
      a. Distal radioulnar joint (DRJ) instability indicated by ulnar styloid fracture, widened DRUJ on posteroanterior (PA) view, dislocation on lateral view, ≥5 mm radial shortening
   2. Treatment
      a. ORIF radius with stabilization of DRUJ in supination or CRPP
   3. Complications
      a. Malunion/nonunion
      b. Distal subluxation

V. Wrist

A. **Distal Radius Fracture**—Colles' fracture (dorsal displacement), Smith's fracture (volar displacement)
   1. Evaluation/Classification
      a. Frykman—I-VIII: (even numbers = ulna styloid fracture) I, extra-articular; III, radiocarpal; V, radioulnar; VII, radiocarpal and radioulnar (Fig. 10-19)
      b. Melone—Four parts (shaft, radial styloid, dorsomedial, palmar medial): I, minimal displacement; II, carpus displacement; III, volar spike; IV, volar fragment rotated (Fig. 10-20)
      c. Thomas (not used)
      d. Intra- versus extra-articular
   2. Treatment
      a. Colles' Fracture—Closed reduction and splint, acceptable reduction if <10 degrees change in palmar tilt, <2 mm radial shortening, <5 degrees change in radial angle, <1–2 mm articular step-off; external fixation (ex-fix), percutaneous pin (PCP) fixation (independently or with ex-fix), and ORIF if unacceptable closed reduction
      b. Smith's Fracture—Closed reduction and splint in supination; CRPP or ORIF if needed
   3. Complications
      a. Loss of reduction
      b. Malunion/nonunion
      c. Median nerve neuropathy
      d. Weakness
      e. Tendon adhesion
      f. Instability
      g. Extensor pollicis longus (EPL) rupture
      h. Dorsal intercalated segment instability (DISI) (>15 degrees dorsiflexion [DF])
      i. Ulnar side pain
      j. Complex regional pain syndrome
      k. Volkmann's ischemic contracture

B. **Dorsal Rim (Radius) Fracture**—Dorsal Barton's fracture (Fig. 10-21)
   1. Evaluation/Classification
      a. Two-part dorsal radiocarpal fracture; dislocation is rare

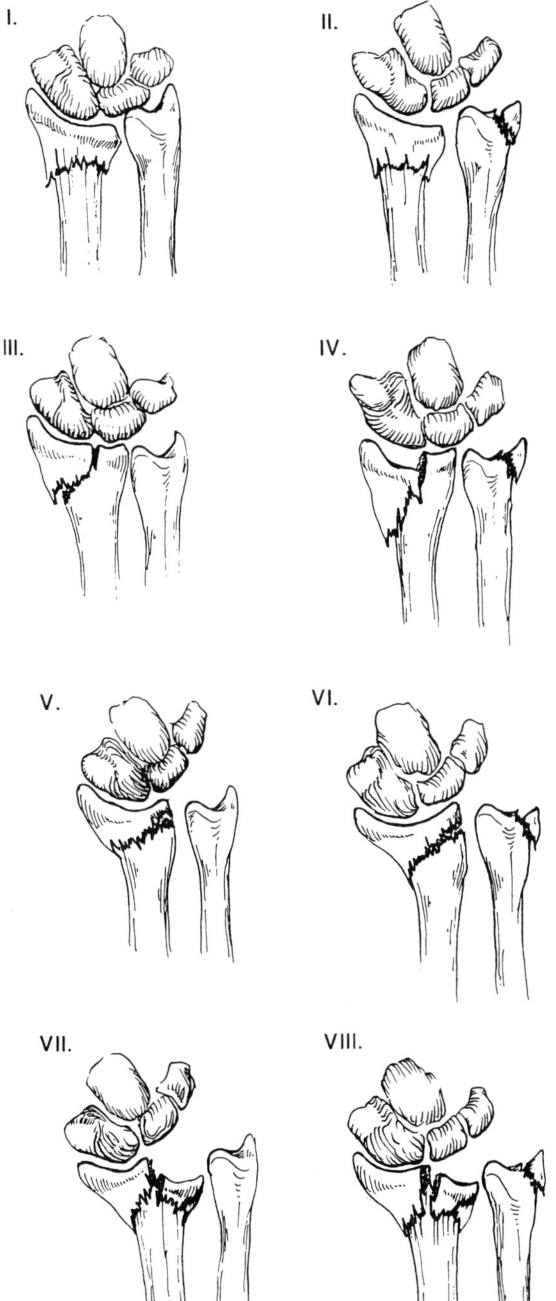

FIGURE 10-19 ■ Frykman's classification of distal radius fractures. Note even numbers with ulnar styloid involvement. (From Kozin, S.H., and Berlet, A.C.: Handbook of Common Orthopaedic Fractures. West Chester, PA, Medical Surveillance, 1989, pp. 17, 19.)

   2. Treatment
      a. Rarely, closed reduction
      b. ORIF with dorsal approach
   3. Complications
      a. Similar to Colles' fracture

C. **Radial Styloid Fracture**—Chauffeur's fracture (Fig. 10-22)
   1. Evaluation/Classification
      a. Usually high-energy trauma in young adult

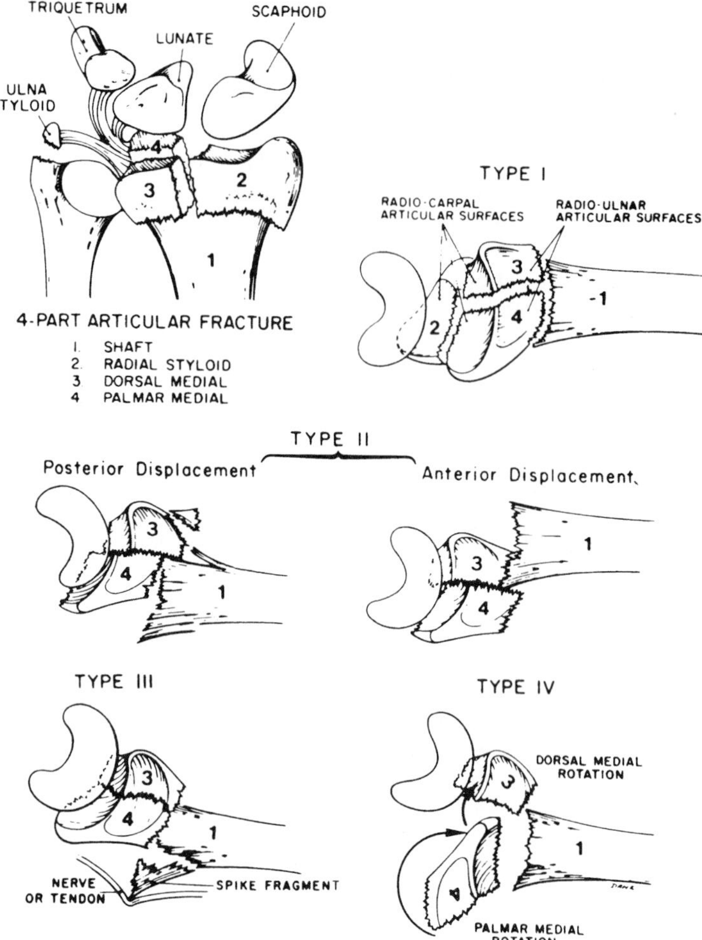

FIGURE 10-20 ■ Melone classification of distal radius fractures. (From Melone, C.P., Jr.: Open treatment for displaced articular fractures of the distal radius. Clin. Orthop. 202:104, 1986; reprinted by permission.)

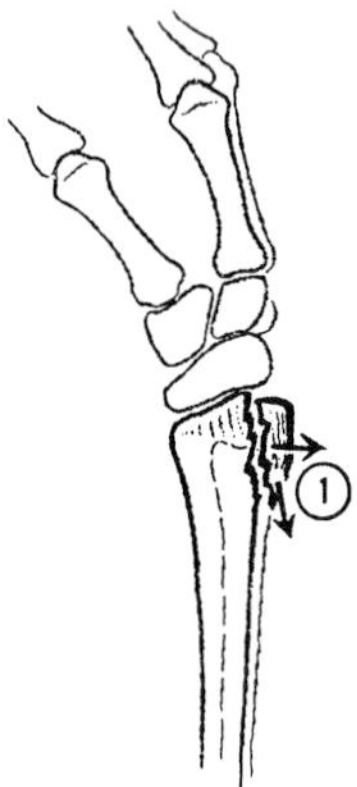

FIGURE 10-21 ■ Dorsal Barton's fracture. (From Connolly, J.F., ed.: Depalma's The Management of Fractures and Dislocations, an Atlas, 3rd ed. Philadelphia, WB Saunders, 1981, p. 1032; reprinted by permission.)

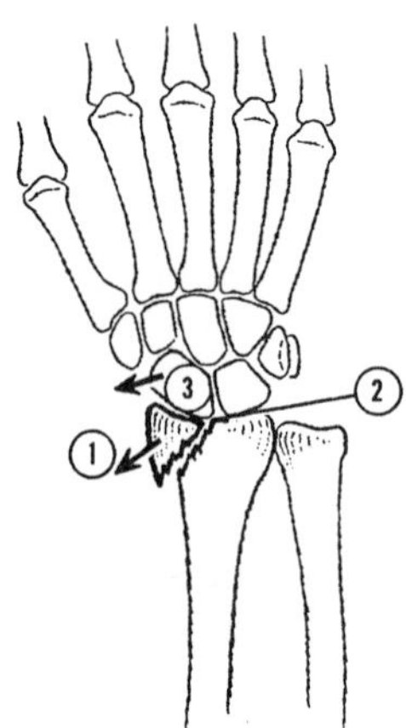

FIGURE 10-22 ■ Radial styloid fractures. (From Connolly, J.F., ed.: Depalma's The Management of Fractures and Dislocations, an Atlas, 3rd ed. Philadelphia, WB Saunders, 1981, p. 1033; reprinted by permission.)

2. Treatment
   a. CRPP or cannulated screw, immobilize in ulnar deviation
3. Complications
   a. Similar to Colles' fracture
   b. Associated perilunate injury (ORIF)

D. **Volar Rim (Radius) Fracture**—Volar Barton's fracture (Fig. 10-23)
1. Evaluation/Classification
   a. Two-part volar radiocarpal fracture-dislocation
2. Treatment
   a. Rarely closed reduction
   b. ORIF with volar approach
3. Complications
   a. Similar to Colles' fracture

E. **Distal Radioulnar Joint (DRUJ) Injury**
1. Evaluation/Classification
   a. Fracture of base of ulnar styloid associated with TFCC tear
2. Treatment
   a. Closed versus ORIF to achieve anatomic reduction of ulnar styloid, immobilize in supination
3. Complications
   a. Osteochondral fracture
   b. Ulnar nerve compression
   c. Instability
   d. Arthrosis
   e. Weak grip
   f. Limited forearm rotation

VI. Carpal

A. **Scaphoid Fracture** (Fig. 10-24)
1. Evaluation/Classification
   a. Based on anatomic location; >1 mm displacement, any angulation, scapholunate (SL) angle >45 degrees, capitolunate (CL) angle >15 degrees
2. Treatment
   a. Nondisplaced distal—Short arm-thumb-spica cast for 8–12 weeks
   b. Nondisplaced proximal and midbody—long arm-thumb-spica cast for 6 weeks, followed by short arm-thumb-spica cast until union
   c. Displaced—ORIF
3. Complications
   a. Nonunion (treat with Russe bone graft)
   b. Instability
   c. Refracture
   d. Nerve injury
   e. DJD
   f. Pain
   g. Missed fracture (bone scan or MRI helpful)

B. **Lunate Fracture**
1. Evaluation/Classification
   a. Osteonecrosis, late; Kienbock's disease
2. Treatment
   a. Ulnar lengthening/radial shortening/resection
3. Complications
   a. Disorganization
   b. Disintegration

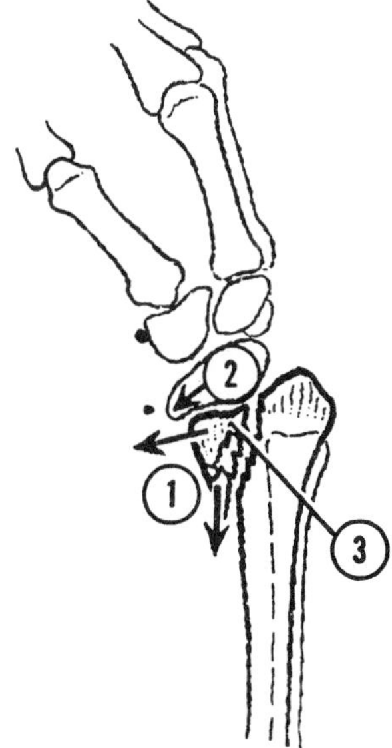

FIGURE 10-23 ■ Volar Barton's fracture. (From Connolly, J.F., ed.: Depalma's The Management of Fractures and Dislocations, an Atlas, 3rd ed. Philadelphia, WB Saunders, 1981, p. 1028; reprinted by permission.)

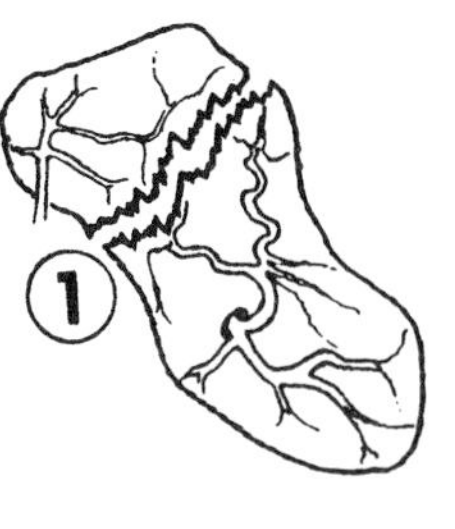

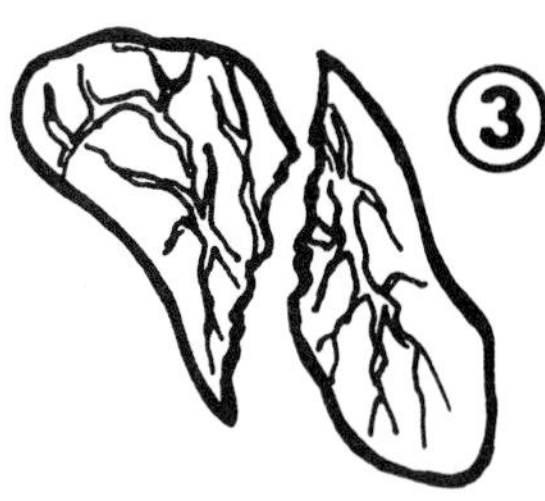

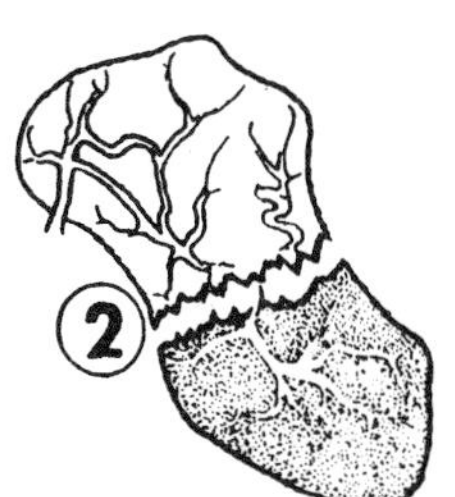

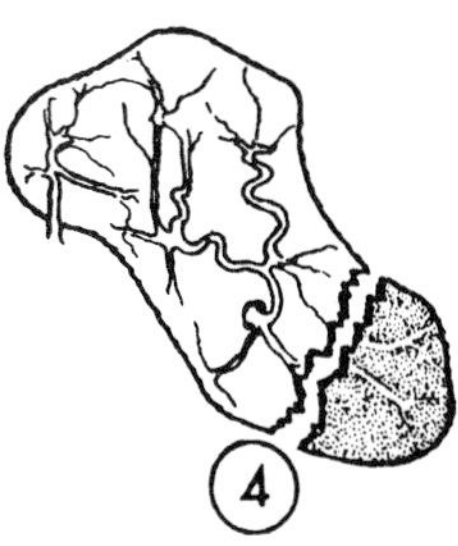

FIGURE 10-24 ■ Classification of scaphoid fractures. *1,* Neck. *2,* Waist. *3,* Body. *4,* Proximal pole. Note progressive risk of avascular necrosis with proximal transverse fractures. (From Weissman, B.N., and Sledge, C.B.: Orthopedic Radiology, Philadelphia, WB Saunders, 1986, p. 1060; reprinted by permission.)

C. **Triquetrum Fracture**
1. Evaluation/Classification
a. Dorsal shear injury (most common and third most common carpal fracture after scaphoid and lunate)
b. Body fracture (rare)
2. Treatment
a. Dorsal shear—Closed treatment for 4-6 weeks, excision of fragment if symptoms continue
b. Body— Closed treatment if nondisplaced, ORIF for displaced fracture
3. Complications
a. Usually asymptomatic

D. **Pisiform Fracture**
1. Evaluation/Classification
a. Uncommon—1-3% of all carpal fractures
2. Treatment
a. Short arm cast (SAC) with 30 degrees of wrist flexion and ulnar deviation for 6 weeks
3. Complications
a. Fifty percent associated with distal radius, hamate, or triquetrum fracture
b. Nonunion (treat with excision)

E. **Trapezium Fracture**
1. Evaluation/Classification
a. Body fracture
b. Trapezial ridge fracture
(1) Base of ridge
(2) Tip of ridge
2. Treatment
a. Body—ORIF for intra-articular displaced fracture
b. Trap ridge I—Attempt closed treatment, early excision for nonunion common
c. Trap ridge II—Closed treatment for 6 weeks (molded abduction of first ray)
3. Complications
a. Body—Associated carpometacarpal (CMC) dislocation or Bennett's fracture
b. Trap ridge I fracture—Chronic pain (requires excision)

F. **Capitate Fracture**
1. Evaluation/Classification
a. Rarely occurs in isolation
2. Treatment
a. ORIF
3. Complications
a. Associated with perilunate dislocations, scaphoid fracture, and CMC fracture/dislocation
b. Osteonecrosis
c. Nonunion (treat by fusion of the capitate of the scaphoid and lunate)

G. **Hamate Fracture**
1. Evaluation/Classification
a. Body Fracture—Uncommon
b. Hook of Hamate Fracture—Common in golf, baseball, racquet sports
2. Treatment
a. Body—Closed treatment for nondisplaced; CRPP or ORIF if displaced or unstable
b. Hook—Closed treatment for 6 weeks if acute; excision or ORIF for chronic nonunion
3. Complications
a. Body—Associated with fourth and fifth CMC fracture/dislocation
b. Hook of Hamate—Ulnar nerve and flexor tendon symptoms or attritional rupture

H. **Perilunate Instability**
1. Evaluation/Classification
a. Mayfield—(Fig. 10-25)
(1) Scapholunate dissociation
(2) Lunocapitate disruption
(3) Lunotriquetral disruption
(4) Lunate dislocation
2. Treatment
a. Early (6-8 weeks)—Open (dorsally), ligament repair and ORIF scaphoid fracture (if present)
b. Late—Triscaphe fusion, proximal row carpectomy, or wrist fusion
3. Complications
a. Rotatory instability of scaphoid

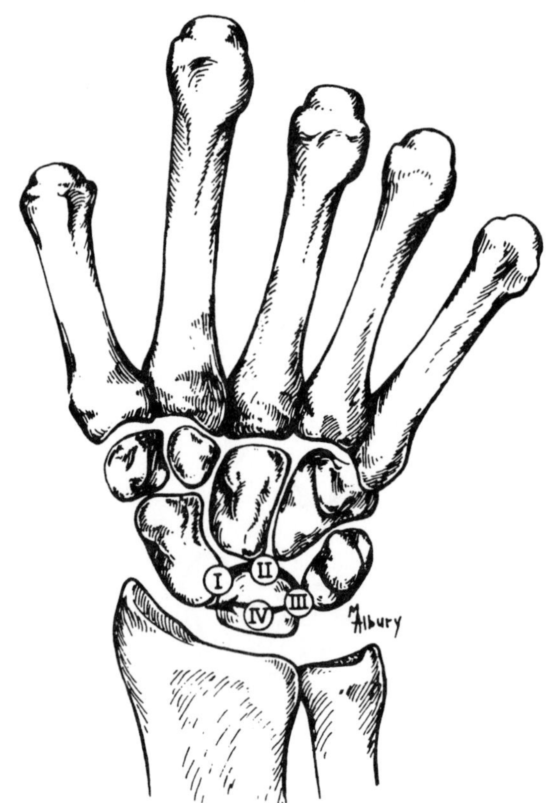

FIGURE 10-25 ■ Perilunar instability—stages. *I*, Scapholunate. *II*, Capitolunate. *III*, Triquetrolunate. *IV*, Dorsal radiocarpal (leading to lunate dislocation). (From Mayfield, J.K.: Mechanism of carpal injuries. Clin. Orthop. 149:50, 1980; reprinted by permission.)

b. Median nerve palsy
c. Late flexor rupture

I. **Rotatory Lunate Dissociation**—Terry Thomas's Sign
1. Evaluation/Classification
a. A 2 mm or larger scapholunate gap versus opposite side
2. Treatment
a. Closed treatment if minor, ORIF if scaphoid fracture is displaced, open repair of ligaments if significant disruption
3. Complications
a. Late DJD

J. **Carpal Instability**
1. Evaluation/Classification
a. DISI—Most common (dorsal SL angle >70 degrees) (Fig. 10-26)
b. Volar intercalated segmental instability (VISI) (volar SL angle <35 degrees)
c. Axial injury
2. Treatment
a. DISI and VISI—CRPP versus ORIF
b. Axial—ORIF
3. Complications
a. DISI and VISI—DJD, stiffness, treatment for chronic instability is controversial
b. Axial—Usually high energy with skin and soft tissue injury, neurovascular injury (ulnar nerve most common), intrinsic muscle injury

VII. Hand

A. Hamatometacarpal Fracture/Dislocation
1. Evaluation/Classification
a. Cain
Type IA—Ligamentous injury
Type IB—Dorsal hamate fracture (most common)
Type II—Comminuted dorsal hamate fracture
Type III—Coronal hamate fracture
2. Treatment
Type IA—Stable, cast; unstable, CRPP
Type IB—Stable, cast; unstable, ORIF
Type II—ORIF, restore dorsal buttress
Type III—ORIF, restore congruent joint surface
3. Complications
a. Delay in diagnosis (CT scan helpful)

B. First CMC Dislocation (Fig. 10-27)
1. Evaluation/Classification
a. True dislocation without fracture is rare
2. Treatment
a. CRPP with traction and pronation
3. Complications
a. Chronic instability

C. First Metacarpophalangeal (MCP) Joint Injury/Dislocation
1. Evaluation/Classification
a. Ulnar Collateral Ligament (UCL) Injury (Most Common)—Gamekeeper's thumb (Fig. 10-28); sprain (does not open

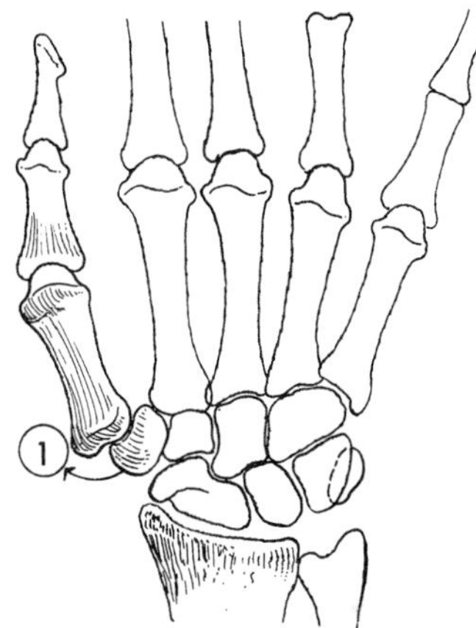

FIGURE 10-27 ■ Subluxation/dislocation of the thumb carpometacarpal joint. (From Connolly, J.F., ed.: Depalma's The Management of Fractures and Dislocations, an Atlas, 3rd ed., Philadelphia, WB Saunders, 1981; p. 1165; reprinted by permission.)

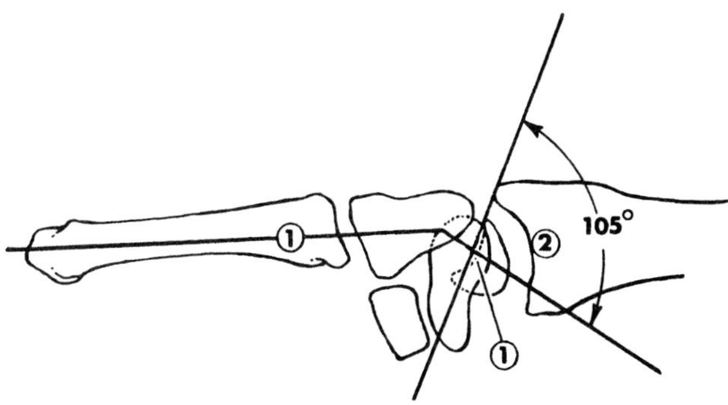

FIGURE 10-26 ■ Dorsal intercalary segmental instability (DISI). Note scapholunate angle >70 degrees, consistent with a DISI pattern. (From Connolly, J.F., ed.: Depalma's The Management of Fractures and Dislocations, an Atlas, 3rd ed. Philadelphia, WB Saunders, 1981, p. 1085; reprinted by permission.)

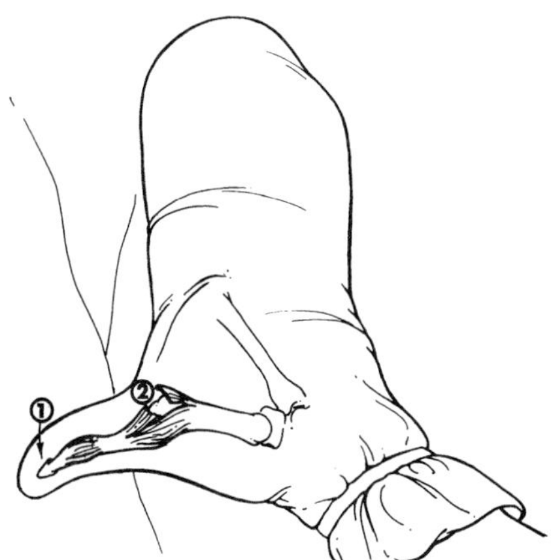

FIGURE 10-28 ■ Gamekeeper's thumb (ulnar collateral ligament injury). (From Connolly, J.F., ed.: Depalma's The Management of Fractures and Dislocations, an Atlas, 3rd ed. Philadelphia, WB Saunders, 1981, p. 1151; reprinted by permission.)

>35–45 degrees with stress) or rupture (interposition of adductor aponeurosis [Stener lesion])
   b. Radial collateral ligament (RCL) injury (rare)
   c. Dorsal Dislocation—Simple or complex (interposition of volar plate) (Fig. 10-29)
2. Treatment
   a. Gamekeeper's Sprain—Thumb-spica cast for 4–6 weeks
   b. Stener Lesion—Open repair
   c. RCL Injury—Splint (late reconstruction if needed)
   d. Simple Dorsal Dislocation—Reduce and immobilize for 3 weeks
   e. Complex Dorsal Dislocation—Open repair
3. Complications
   a. Unrecognized Stener lesion
   b. Chronic pain
   c. Instability

D. **Finger MCP Dislocation**
1. Evaluation/Classification
   a. Collateral ligament injury (uncommon)
   b. Simple dorsal dislocation
   c. Complex dorsal dislocation
   d. Volar dislocation (rare)
2. Treatment
   a. Collateral Ligament—Splint in 50 degrees MCP flexion for 3 weeks, and then buddy tape for 3 weeks; ORIF if an avulsion fracture exists with >2–3 mm displacement or >20% of the articular surface involved
   b. Simple Dorsal—Splint 7–10 days then buddy tape
   c. Complex Dorsal and Volar Dislocations—Open reduction
3. Complications
   a. Loss of motion leads to profound effect on hand function

E. **Proximal Interphalangeal (PIP) Joint Dislocation**
1. Evaluation/Classification
   a. Dorsal Dislocation—Most common (volar plate [VP] disruption)
      (1) Hyperextension—VP avulsion
      (2) Complete dislocation with VP avulsion and bilateral collateral ligament injury
      (3) Fracture/dislocation
   b. Volar (Central Slip)—Boutonnière (Fig. 10-30)
   c. Rotatory
2. Treatment
   a. Dorsal Dislocation and Hyperextension—Closed reduction and buddy tape or extension block splint for 2 weeks
   b. Dorsal Complete Dislocation—Closed reduction and extension block splint in 20 degrees for 3 weeks
   c. Dorsal Fracture/Dislocation—For a stable fracture, extension block splint for 2–3 weeks; for an unstable fracture (involving

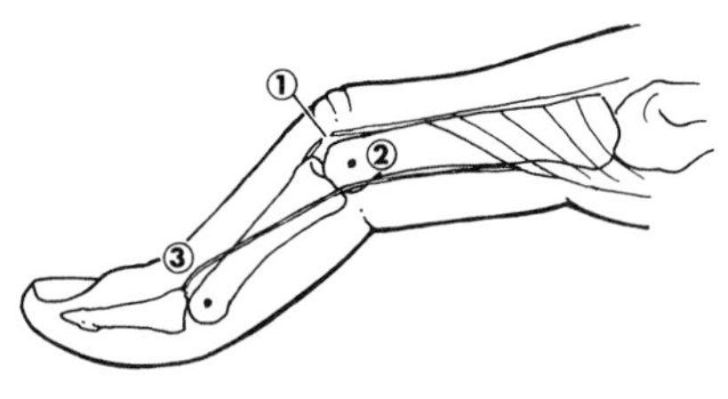

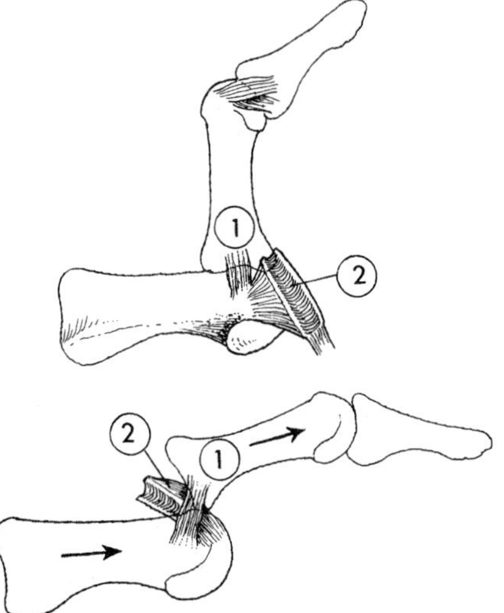

FIGURE 10-29 ■ Thumb metacarpophalangeal (MCP) joint dislocation. *Top,* Simple. *Bottom,* Complex; note interposition of volar plate. (From Connolly, J.F., ed.: Depalma's The Management of Fractures and Dislocations, an Atlas, 3rd ed. Philadelphia, WB Saunders, 1981, p. 1152; reprinted by permission.)

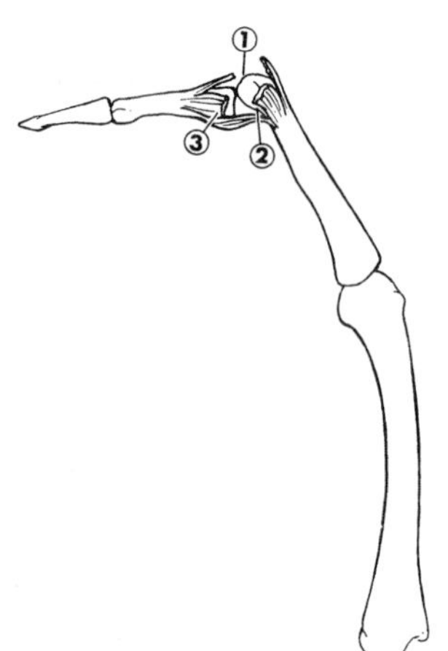

FIGURE 10-30 ■ Boutonnière deformity, an injury to the central slip with volar subluxation of lateral bonds. (From Connolly, J.F., ed.: Depalma's The Management of Fractures and Dislocations, an Atlas, 3rd ed. Philadelphia, WB Saunders, 1981, p. 1149; reprinted by permission.)

>40% articular surface or with subluxation), ORIF; for severe comminution, volar plate arthroplasty
   d. Volar—Attempt closed reduction with flexion and traction, but usually open reduction is needed; extension splint of PIP for 4–6 weeks
   e. Rotatory—ORIF if irreducible or incongruous
3. Complications
   a. Dorsal dislocation—Stiffness, contractures (treat with VP arthroplasty)
   b. Boutonnière late recognition (treat with ORIF or VP arthroplasty)

F. **Distal interphalangeal joint (DIP) dislocation**
1. Evaluation/Classification
   a. Dorsal (most common)
   b. Collateral ligament injury
2. Treatment
   a. Dorsal—Closed reduction and splint for 1–2 weeks; if late diagnosis or irreducible, open reduction
   b. Collateral Ligament—Sprain: buddy tape for 3–6 weeks; tear: open repair
3. Complications
   a. Extensor lag (treatment is 8-week course of splinting, as for Mallet injury

G. **Thumb Metacarpal (MC) Fracture** (Fig. 10-31)
1. Evaluation/Classification
   a. Intra-Articular Volar Ulnar Lip—Bennett's fracture

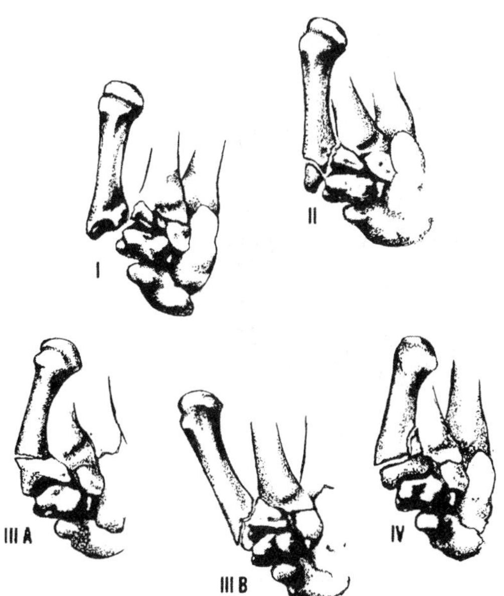

FIGURE 10-31 ■ Classification of first metacarpal base fractures. *I,* Bennett's fracture. *II,* Rolando's fracture. *IIIA,* Transverse extra-articular fracture. *IIIB,* Oblique extra-articular fracture. *IV,* SH II epiphyseal fracture (pediatric). (From Green, D.P., and O'Brien, E.T.: Fractures of the thumb metacarpal. South. Med. J. 65:807, 1972; reprinted by permission.)

   b. Intra-Articular Y or T—Rolando's fracture
   c. Extra-Articular (transverse or oblique)
2. Treatment
   a. Bennett's—CRPP MC to trapezium; ORIF if irreducible
   b. Rolando's—ORIF if large fragment; ex-fix, PCP, and bone graft for comminuted
   c. Extra-Articular—Spica cast for 4 weeks; CRPP if >30 degrees displacement
3. Complications
   a. Bennett's—Displaced by abductor pollicis longus (APL)
   b. Rolando's—DJD

H. **Small MC Base Fractures**—Reverse (or Baby) Bennett
1. Evaluation/Classification
   a. Epibasal
   b. Two-part
   c. Three-part
   d. Comminuted
2. Treatment
   a. Epibasal and Two-Part—CRPP and cast for 6 weeks; ORIF for inadequate articular reduction
   b. Three-Part or Comminuted—CRPP or ORIF
3. Complications
   a. Displaced by extensor carpii ulnaris (ECU)

I. **MC Shaft Fracture**
1. Evaluation/Classification
   a. Transverse
   b. Oblique
   c. Spiral
   d. Comminuted
2. Treatment
   a. Transverse—Closed reduction, immobilize or PCP; accept 10 degrees angulation in second and third metacarpals and 20–30 degrees in fourth and fifth metacarpals; ORIF if irreducible
   b. Oblique and Spiral—CRPP or ORIF
   c. Comminuted—If nondisplaced, splint; if displaced, PCP to adjacent MC or ORIF
3. Complications
   a. Transverse—Compared with the two central metacarpals, the index and long fingers are less tolerant of angulation because of their lesser mobility
   b. Oblique—Shortening common if not treated
   c. Spiral—Digital overlap with flexion if rotation not corrected

J. **MC Neck Fracture**
1. Evaluation/Classification
   a. Fifth—Boxer's Fracture (professional boxer more likely to injure second or third metacarpal)
2. Treatment
   a. Boxer's—Accept up to 40 degrees angulation, Jahss maneuver if needed (flex MCP and apply axial load to reduce neck),

splint in 70 degrees MCP flexion for 2-3 weeks

b. Second or Third Metacarpal—Accept 10-15 degrees angulation; usually requires PCP to adjacent MC or ORIF

3. Complications
   a. Claw deformity with extrinsic tendon imbalance
   b. Prominent MC head in palm (affects grip)
   c. Loss of reduction (no volar buttress)
   d. Nonunion
   e. Contracture of intrinsics

K. **MC Head Fracture**

1. Evaluation/Classification
   a. Vertical
   b. Horizontal
   c. Oblique
   d. Comminuted
2. Treatment
   a. ORIF large fragments, ex-fix if comminuted with early motion
3. Complications
   a. Usually open fracture

L. **Proximal and Middle Phalanx Fracture**

1. Evaluation/Classification
   a. Extra-articular base
   b. Intra-articular base (three types):
      (1) Collateral ligament avulsion
      (2) Compression
      (3) Vertical shear
   c. Diaphyseal
   d. Neck
   e. Condylar
2. Treatment
   a. Extra-Articular—Buddy tape if stable, CRPP or ORIF if unstable
   b. Collateral Ligament—Nondisplaced, buddy tape; displaced or unstable, tension band or ORIF
   c. Compression—ORIF with bone graft if needed
   d. Vertical Shear—CRPP or ORIF
   e. Diaphyseal—Stable and nondisplaced, buddy tape; displaced, closed reduction, SAC with dorsal block; unstable, CRPP or ORIF
   f. Neck—CRPP
   g. Condylar—Nondisplaced, digital splint for 7-10 days; displaced, ORIF
3. Complications
   a. Decreased ROM
   b. Contractures
   c. Malunion/nonunion
   d. Malrotation (may require osteotomy)
   e. Lateral deviation or volar angulation (treat with osteotomy)
   f. Tendon adherence

M. **Distal Phalanx Fracture**

1. Evaluation/Classification
   a. Longitudinal, comminuted, transverse
2. Treatment
   a. Splint for comfort for up to 4 weeks, CRPP if unstable
3. Complications
   a. Nail matrix injury
   b. Subungual hematoma

N. **Extensor Digitorum Longus (EDL) Avulsion**—Mallet finger (Fig. 10-32)

1. Evaluation/Classification
   a. Watson-Jones
      (1) Extensor tendon stretch with 15-30 degrees extensor lag
      (2) Extensor tendon torn with 30-60 degrees extensor lag
      (3) Extensor tendon avulsion flake
      (4) Extensor tendon avulsion fragment—bony mallet
2. Treatment
   a. Extensor Tendon Stretch—Extensor splint for 6 weeks, then 3-4 weeks of night splinting
   b. Extensor Tendon Torn and Avulsion Flake—Extensor splint for 8 weeks, then 3-4 weeks of night splinting; CRPP if patient's occupation precludes splinting
   c. Extensor Tendon Avulsion Fragment—If stable, same as for extensor tendon torn; if unstable (volar displacement, >50% articular surface involved), ORIF
3. Complications
   a. Deformity
   b. Nail bed injury (with ORIF)
   c. Subluxation

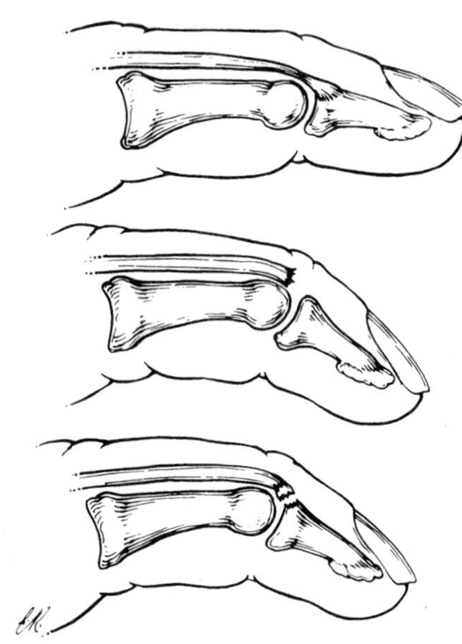

FIGURE 10-32 ■ Mallet finger. *Top to bottom,* Extensor tendon stretch, extensor tendon rupture, bony avulsion. (From Green, D.P., and Rowland, S.A.: Fractures and dislocations in the hand. In Rockwood, C.A., and Green, D.P., eds.: Fractures in Adults, 2nd ed. Philadelphia, JB Lippincott, 1984, p. 319; reprinted by permission.)

O. **Flexor Digitorum Longus (FDL) Avulsion—** Jersey finger (Fig. 10-33)

1. Evaluation/Classification
   a. Leddy
      (1) Tendon retraction to palm-rupturing vincula
      (2) Tendon retracts to PIP held by vinculum
      (3) Large bony fragment catches on A4 pulley at middle phalanx
      (4) (Smith)—Bony avulsion with tendon avulsed from fragment
2. Treatment
   a. Tendon retraction to palm-rupturing vincula—Repair within 7–10 days
   b. Tendon retracts to PIP held by vinculum—Repair within 6 weeks
   c. Large bony fragment catches on A4 pulley at middle phalanx—ORIF
   d. Bony avulsion with tendon avulsed from fragment—Early fixation of bony fragments and tendon
3. Complications
   a. Missed diagnosis can lead to lumbrical plus finger (treat with therapy or fuse DIP late)

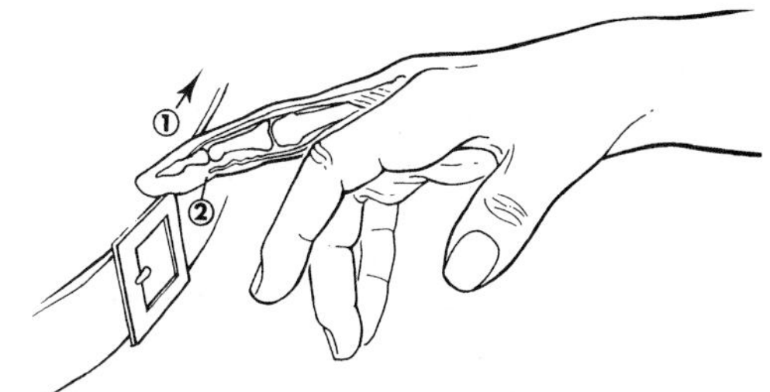

FIGURE 10-33 ■ Avulsion of the flexor digitorum profundus. (From Connolly, J.F., ed.: Depalma's The Management of Fractures and Dislocations, an Atlas, 3rd ed. Philadelphia, WB Saunders, 1981, p. 1149; reprinted by permission.)

VIII. Pelvis

A. **Pelvic Ring Fractures**

1. Evaluation/Classification
   a. Young-Burgess (Fig. 10-34)
      (1) Lateral Compression (LC)
      Type I—Rami + ipsilateral sacral compression
      Type II—Rami + ipsilateral posterior ilium

Pelvic Fracture Classification
(Young & Burgess)

Lateral Compression	AP Compression	Vertical Shear	Combined Mechanism
Type I	Type I	Type I	Anterolateral Force
Type IIA, IIB	Type II	Type II	Anterovertical Force
Type III	Type III	Type III	

FIGURE 10-34 ■ Modified Pennal classification system. (From Orthopaedic Knowledge Update. Chicago, American Academy of Orthopaedic Surgeons.)

Type III—Ipsilateral LC + contralateral APC

(2) Anterior Posterior Compression (APC)
Type I—Symphysis diastasis <2 cm
Type II—Symphysis disrupted + anterior sacroiliac (SI) joint diastasis
Type III—Symphysis disrupted + complete SI dissociation

(3) Vertical Shear (VS)—Malgaigne; Vertical displacement of hemipelvis

(4) Combined Mechanism (CM)

b. Tile
 (1) A—Stable
  (a) Avulsion fractures, iliac wing fractures, transverse sacral fractures
 (2) B—Partially Stable
  (a) Rotationally unstable
  (b) Vertically stable
 (3) C—Unstable
  (a) Rotationally unstable
  (b) Vertically unstable

2. Treatment (Fig. 10-35)—Nonoperative management for stable fractures: Weight-bearing as tolerated (WBAT) (LC type I, APC type I, Tile A, isolated Rami fractures)
 a. Operative Indications
  (1) Symphysis diastasis >2.5 cm
  (2) SI joint displacement >1 cm
  (3) Sacral fracture displacement >1 cm
  (4) Vertical displacement of hemipelvis
  (5) Open fractures
 b. Operative Techniques
  (1) Pubic Symphysis Diastasis
   (a) ORIF (plate fixation) is preferred
    (i) Single plate adequate
    (ii) May perform in conjunction with laparotomy or genitourinary (GU) procedure

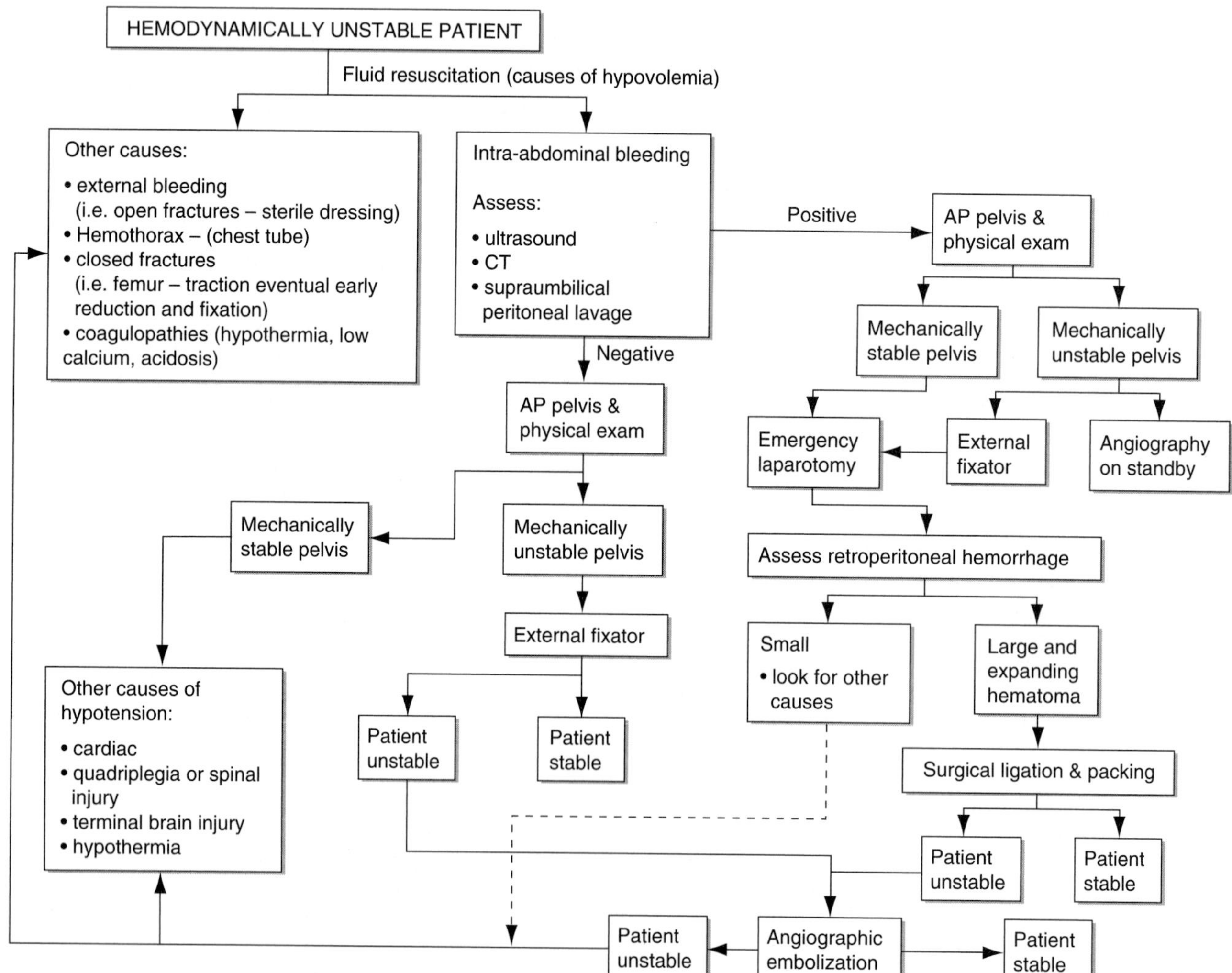

FIGURE 10-35 ■ Protocol for management of pelvic ring disruption in the hemodynamically unstable patient. (Redrawn from Orthopaedic Knowledge Update Trauma 2. Chicago, American Academy of Orthopaedic Surgeons, 2000, p. 233.)

(b) Anterior external fixation
(2) SI Joint Dislocation
(a) Percutaneous iliosacral screw placement
(b) Anterior SI plating
(3) SI Joint Fracture—Dislocation
(a) ORIF posterior plate fixation
(i) Good results in crescent fractures involving posterior ilium
(b) Transiliac sacral bars

3. Complications
a. Life-threatening hemorrhage (worse with APC injuries; venous >arterial)
b. Urogenital injuries—In 20%
c. Malreduction/malunion (75% are painful if residual displacement is >1 cm)
d. Nonunion
e. Leg length discrepancy (>2 cm clinically significant)
f. Neurologic injury—In 8% (iatrogenic injury to L5, S1 nerve roots possible with posterior fixation techniques)
g. DVT or pulmonary embolism (PE)—In 60% and 27%, respectively
h. Infection (increased risk with posterior ORIF; careful evaluation of soft tissue condition necessary)
i. Death (open fractures associated with 30% mortality)

B. **Sacral Fractures**—Occur in 30% of pelvic ring disruptions
1. Evaluation/Classification
a. Denis (Fig. 10-36)
Zone 1—Lateral to foramina
Zone 2—Transforaminal
Zone 3—Medial to foramina
2. Treatment
a. Surgical reduction/fixation indicated for fractures displaced 1 cm
(1) Percutaneous iliosacral screws
(2) Posterior tension band plating
(3) Transiliac sacral bars
b. Open reduction/foraminal decompression indicated if neurologic injuries are present
3. Complications
a. Neurologic Injury—In displaced fractures, 40%. Presence of neurologic injury is most significant factor in outcome
Zone 2—L5 nerve root most common
Zone 3—Central canal involvement with cauda equina syndrome
b. Pain/malunion

C. **Acetabular Fractures**
1. Evaluation/Classification
a. Radiographic Evaluation
(1) AP view of pelvis
(2) Obturator oblique view—Anterior column or posterior wall
(3) Iliac oblique view—Posterior column/anterior wall
(4) Thin-cut CT scan

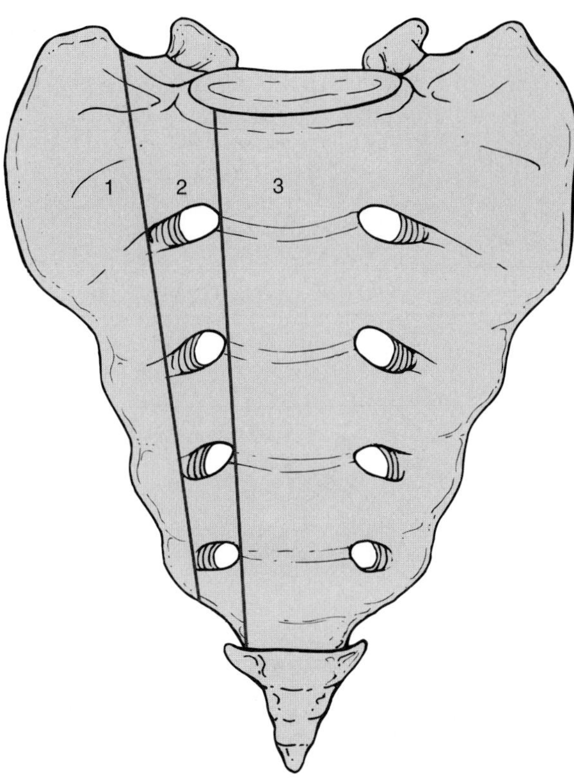

FIGURE 10-36 ■ Denis classification of sacral fractures. (From Browner, B.D., et al., eds.: Skeletal Trauma. Philadelphia, WB Saunders, 1992, p. 820.)

b. Letournel Classification (Fig. 10-37)
(1) Simple Type
(a) Anterior wall
(b) Anterior column
(c) Posterior wall (most common)
(d) Posterior column
(e) Transverse
(2) Associated Types
(a) Posterior column + posterior wall
(b) Transverse + posterior wall (most common)
(c) Anterior with posterior hemitransverse
(d) T-type (involves obturator foramen)
(e) Both columns—"floating acetabulum" (dissociation of articular surface from intact portion of ilium; "Spur sign" obturator oblique x-ray view)

2. Treatment
a. Nonoperative Treatment
(1) Criteria
(a) Nondisplaced or minimally displaced fracture (<2 mm)
(b) Roof arcs >45 degrees
(c) Posterior wall fracture <20%
(d) Secondary congruence in both columns fracture

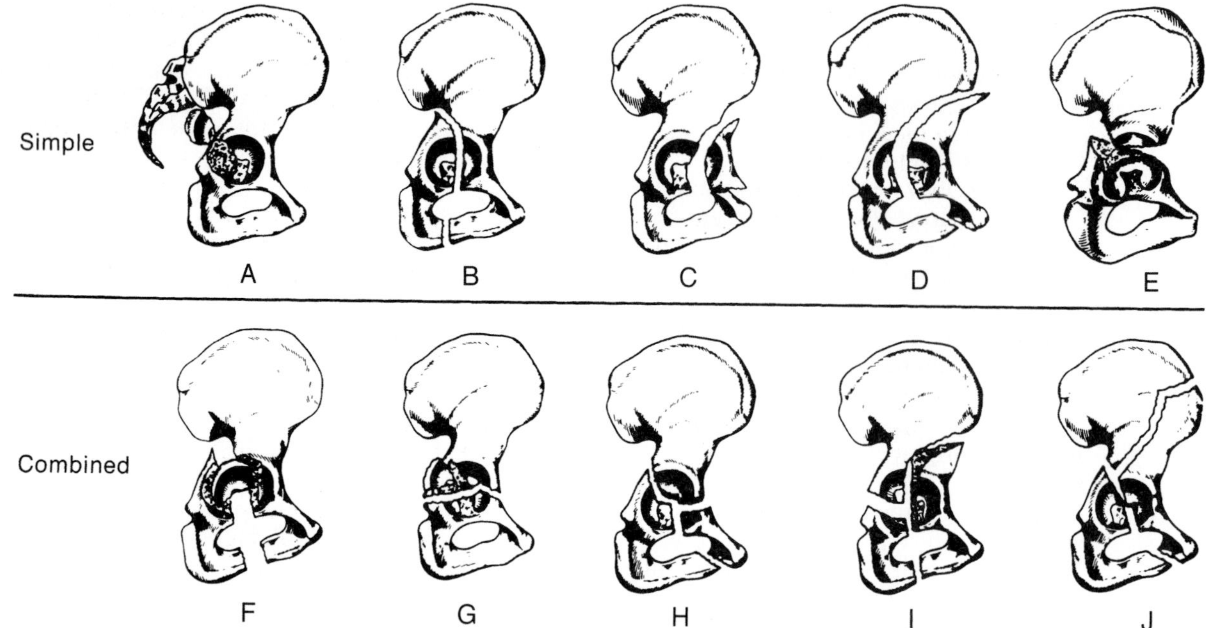

FIGURE 10-37 ■ Letournel classification of acetabular fractures. *A,* Posterior wall. *B,* Posterior column. *C,* Anterior wall. *D,* Anterior column. *E,* Transverse. *F,* Posterior column and posterior wall. *G,* Transverse and posterior wall. *H,* T fracture. *I,* Anterior column and posterior hemitransverse. *J,* Both columns. (From Matta, J.M.: Trauma: Pelvis and acetabulum. In Orthopaedic Knowledge Update II. Chicago, American Academy of Orthopaedic Surgeons, 1987, p. 348.)

(2) Methods
(a) Protected weight-bearing (WB) for 6–8 weeks
(b) Close radiographic follow-up
(3) Relative Contraindications to Surgery
(a) Morbid obesity
(b) Age >60
(c) Open contaminated wound in area
(d) Presence of DVT

b. Operative Treatment
(1) Surgical Indications
(a) Displacement of dome >2 mm
(b) Posterior wall fracture >40%
(c) Marginal impaction
(d) Loose bodies in joint
(e) Irreducible fracture-dislocation
(2) Surgical Approaches
(a) Kocher-Langenbach
(i) Posterior approach
(ii) Posterior wall (PW), posterior column (PC), Transverse, PC + PW, Transverse + PW, T-type fractures
(b) Ilioinguinal
(i) Anterior approach
(ii) Both columns (BC), anterior column (AC), anterior wall (AW) + posterior hemitransverse (PHT) fractures
(c) Extensile
(i) Extended iliofemoral
(ii) Triradiate
(iii) Combined anterior + posterior approaches

3. Complications
a. General Complications
(1) Infection (Increased risk with closed degloving injury of soft tissues—Morel-Lavalle)
(2) Bleeding
(3) Thromboembolic—In 60%
(4) Heterotopic ossification (indomethacin or x-ray (radiation) therapy (XRT) for Kocher-Langenbach extensile approaches)
(5) Neurologic injury
(6) Osteonecrosis (18% posterior fracture patterns)
(7) Post-traumatic DJD (Prevent with anatomic reduction; results of total hip arthroplasty (THA) not as good as for osteoarthritis)
(8) Intra-articular hardware placement (avoid with proper intraoperative fluoroscopy
(9) Abductor muscle weakness

b. Complications of Surgical Approaches
(1) Kocher-Langenbach
(a) Sciatic nerve iatrogenic injury (2–10%)
(b) Damage to femoral head blood supply (medial femoral circumflex artery)
(2) Ilioinguinal
(a) Femoral nerve injury

(b) Lateral femoral cutaneous nerve (LFCN) injury
(c) Thrombosis in femoral vessels
(d) Laceration of corona mortis
(3) Extended iliofemoral
(a) HO (highest incidence)
(b) Possible gluteal muscle necrosis (superior gluteal artery injury)
(4) Combined approaches
(a) Suboptimal simultaneous fracture visualization

D. **Hip Dislocations**
1. Evaluation/Classification
a. Posterior—Most common
(1) Flexion, adduction, internal rotation
b. Anterior
(1) Flexion, abduction, external rotation
2. Treatment
a. Emergent closed reduction (within 6 hours)
b. Open reduction if irreducible
c. Post-reduction CT scan always—Rule out femoral head fracture, intra-articular loose bodies, acetabular fracture
d. Stable hip without associated injuries—protected WB for 2–4 weeks
3. Complications
a. Post-traumatic arthritis—Most common
b. Osteonecrosis—15%
c. Sciatic nerve injury—8–20% (peroneal division)
d. Recurrent dislocation rare

IX. **Femur**
A. **Head Fractures**
1. Evaluation/Classification
a. Associated with hip dislocations
b. In posterior dislocations, 7% incidence
c. CT scan post-reduction to evaluate
d. Pipkin Classification (Fig. 10-38)

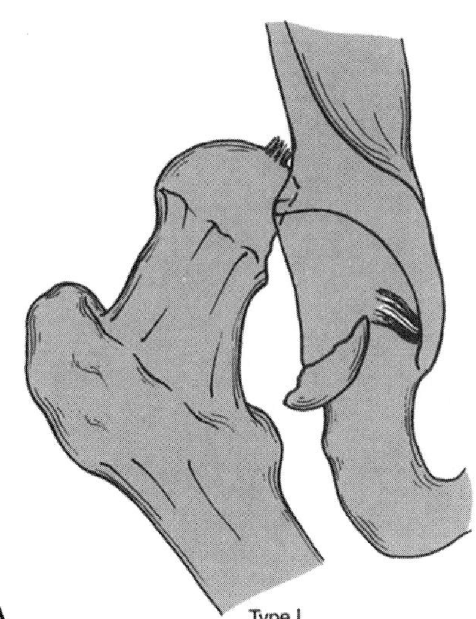

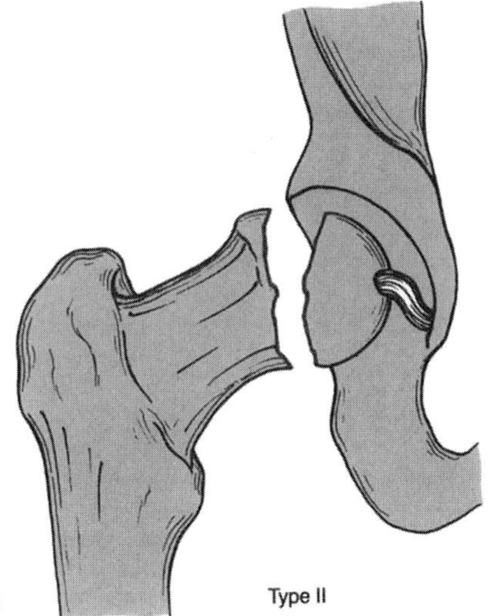

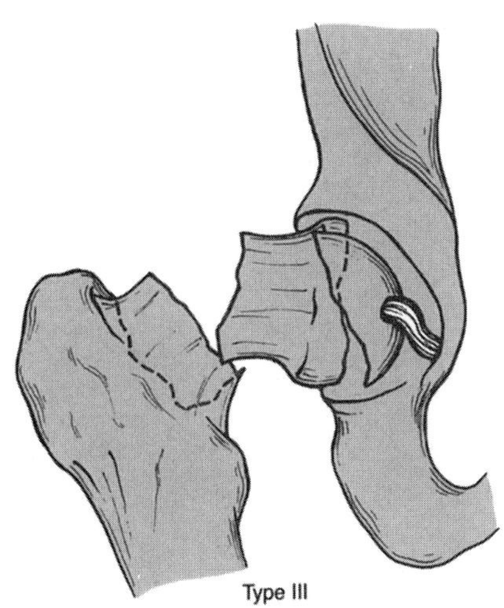

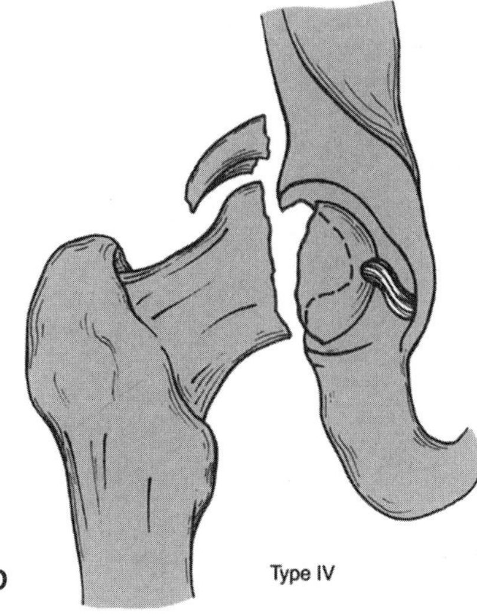

FIGURE 10-38 ■ Pipkin classification of femoral head fractures. (From Browner, B.D., et al., eds.: Skeletal Trauma. Philadelphia, WB Saunders, 1992, p. 1339.)

Type I—Fracture below fovea
Type II—Fracture above fovea
Type III—I or II plus femoral neck fracture
Type IV—I or II plus acetabular fracture

2. Treatment
   a. Reduce hip dislocation
   b. Post-reduction CT scan
   c. Nonoperative Treatment
      (1) Pipkin I, II with anatomic reduction—4–6 weeks touch down weight-bearing (TDWB)
   d. Operative Indications
      (1) >1 mm fracture step-off
      (2) Loose bodies in joint
      (3) Associated neck or acetabular fracture
   e. Pipkin I/II (>1 mm step-off)
      (1) ORIF anterior approach
   f. Pipkin III
      (1) Young patient—ORIF
      (2) Older patient—Endoprosthesis
   g. Pipkin IV
      (1) Treat with acetabular fracture
3. Complications
   a. Same as with hip dislocations, p. 551
   b. High rate of osteonecrosis with Pipkin III

B. **Neck Fractures**
1. Evaluation/Classification
   a. Increasing prevalence
   b. Most common in older patients, women, Caucasians, preexisting medical conditions
   c. MRI to rule out occult fractures
   d. Age of patient most important factor in determining treatment and risk of complications
   e. Garden Classification (Fig. 10-39)
      (1) Nondisplaced
         (a) Incomplete valgus impacted
         (b) Complete fracture
      Displaced
         (c) Displacement of <50%
         (d) Complete displacement
   f. Pauwel's Classification (Fig. 10-40)
      (1) Based on orientation of fracture line
      (2) Increased risk of complications with increased vertical orientation of fracture line
      (3) Pauwel's III—highest risk of osteonecrosis and nonunion
2. Treatment (Fig. 10-41)
   a. Based on physiologic age of patient and degree of displacement

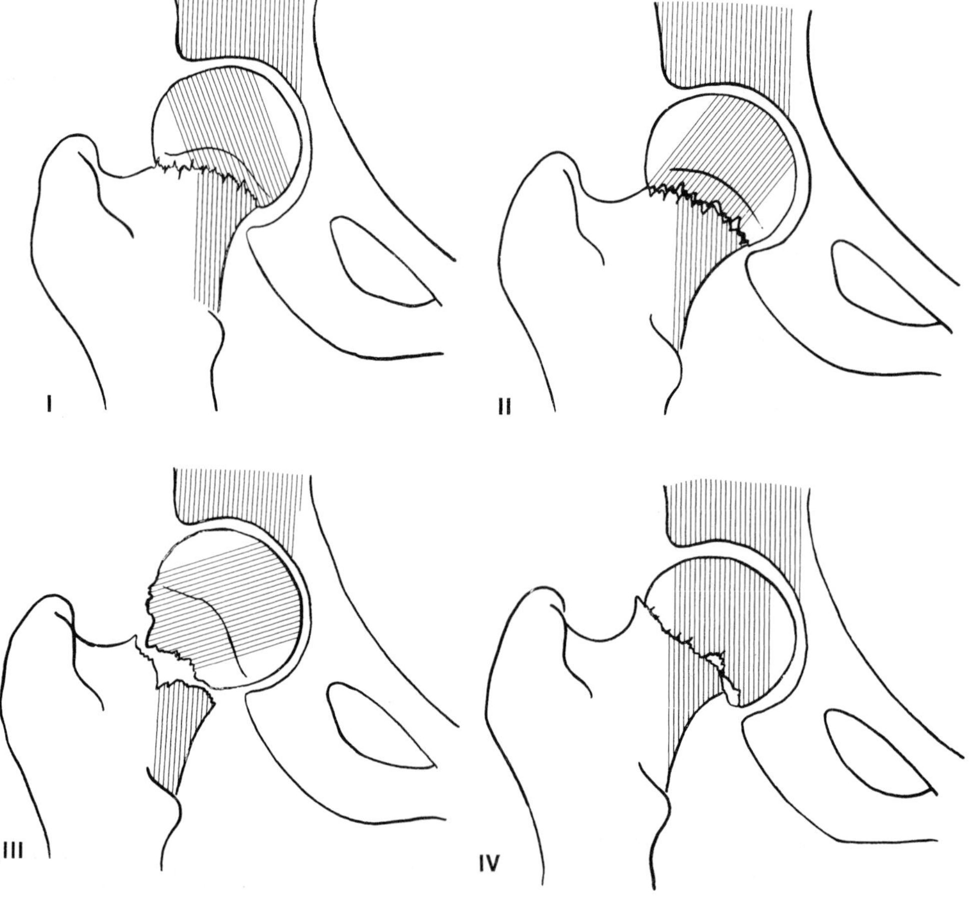

FIGURE 10-39 ■ Garden classification of hip fractures. (From Weissman, B.N., and Sledge, C.B.: Orthopedic Radiology. Philadelphia, WB Saunders, 1986, p. 408.)

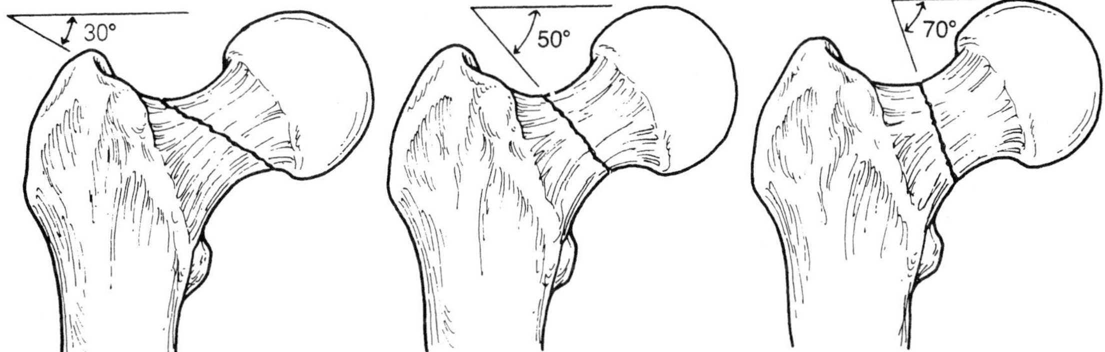

FIGURE 10-40 ■ Pauwel's classification of femoral neck fractures. With progression from type I to type III, there are increasing shear forces placed across the fracture site. (From Evarts, C.M., ed.: Surgery of the Musculoskeletal System, 2nd ed. New York, Churchill Livingstone, 1990, p. 2556.)

b. Fix nondisplaced fractures to prevent displacement
c. Internal Fixation
   (1) Reduction must be anatomic
   (2) Parallel screws (3) at or above lesser trochanter
   (3) Posterior comminution—Add fourth screw
   (4) Basicervical fracture—Sliding hip screw + derotation screw
   (5) Decompression of intracapsular hematoma controversial
d. Prosthetic Replacement
   (1) Hemiarthroplasty
      (a) Debilitated patients
      (b) Metabolic bone disease
      (c) Cemented results > uncemented
      (d) Unipolar versus bipolar controversial
      (e) Posterior approach (increased risk of dislocation) versus anterolateral approach (increased abductor weakness)
   (2) THA
      (a) Older patients with preexisting hip disease (osteoarthritis, rheumatoid arthritis)
e. Young Patient (age <50)
   (1) Displaced fracture is surgical emergency
   (2) Anatomic reduction essential
   (3) Open reduction necessary if anatomic closed reduction not possible

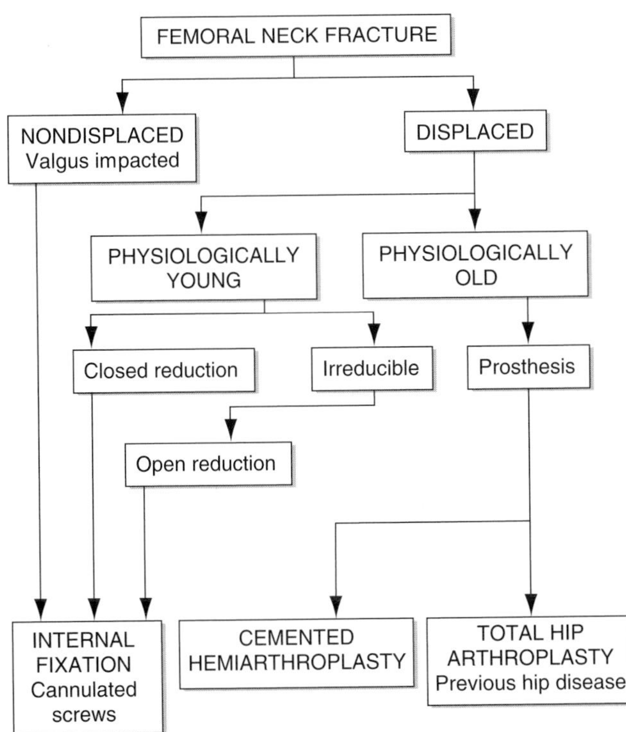

FIGURE 10-41 ■ Treatment algorithm for management of femoral neck fractures. (Redrawn from Orthopaedic Knowledge Update Trauma 2. Chicago, American Academy of Orthopaedic Surgeons, 2000, p. 118.)

(4) Internal fixation with cancellous screws
(5) Increased risk of osteonecrosis and nonunion

f. Older Patient (age >50)
(1) Nondisplaced fracture—Internal fixation
(2) Displaced fracture—Internal fixation versus prosthetic replacement controversial
(3) Decreased perioperative morbidity but increased risk of secondary surgery with internal fixation
(4) Prosthetic replacement in debilitated patient

3. Complications
a. Osteonecrosis—Occurs in 10–45%
(1) Increased risk with increased initial displacement and increased time to reduction
b. Main contribution to femoral head blood supply—Terminal branch of medial femoral circumflex artery (lateral epiphyseal artery) (Fig. 10-42)
c. Nonunion—In 10–30% of displaced fractures
(1) Young patient with no osteonecrosis or <50% head involvement—Valgus intertrochanteric osteotomy

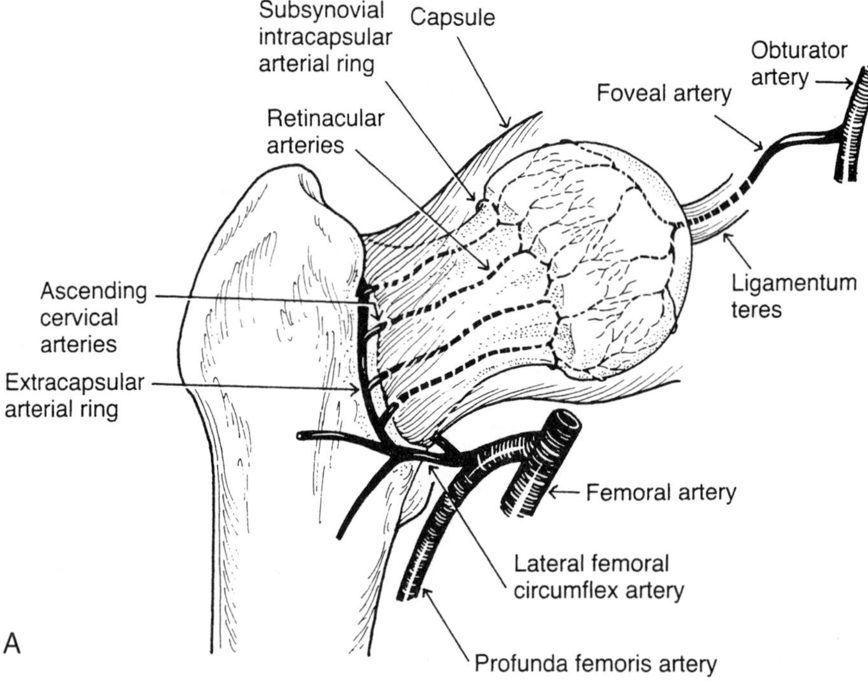

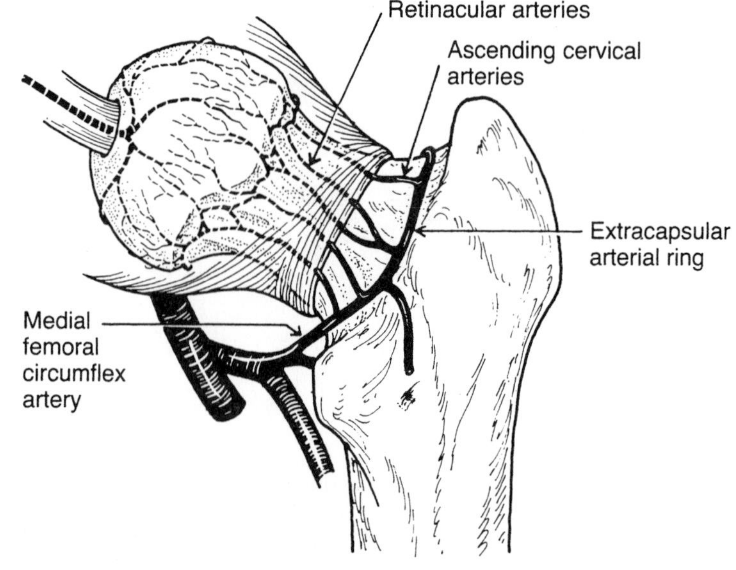

FIGURE 10-42 ■ *A,* Vascular supply of the femoral head and neck, as seen from anterior. Note the location of the retinacular arteries, predisposing them to injury with fracture and displacement of the femoral neck. *B,* Posterior view. Note that the capsule does not extend as far distally on the posterior aspect of the femoral neck as it does anteriorly. (From Evarts, C.M., ed.: Surgery of the Musculoskeletal System, 2nd ed. New York, Churchill Livingstone, 1990, p. 2551.)

(2) Young patient with osteonecrosis and >50% head involvement—Free vascularized fibular graft versus THA
(3) Older patient—Prosthetic replacement

d. Infection
(1) Increased risk in older patients and preoperative delay >48 hours

e. Transfusion Requirement—In 29% of cases
(1) Decreased requirement with internal fixation

f. Mortality—At 1 year in older patients, 30%

C. **Intertrochanteric Fractures**

1. Evaluation/Classification (Fig. 10-43)
a. Risk factors—Osteoporosis, medical comorbidities, positive maternal history (doubles risk)
b. Stable Fractures
(1) Resist medial compressive loads once reduced (two-part fractures)
c. Unstable Fractures
(1) Collapse into varus or shaft displaces medially despite axial reduction (three- and four-part fractures)

2. Treatment
a. Surgical stabilization for all ambulatory patients
b. Early surgery (<48 hours) = decreased 1-year mortality
c. Goal—Neck-shaft axial alignment and correct translation
d. Anatomic reduction of intermediate fragments not necessary
e. Medial displacement osteotomy of no benefit
f. Valgus overreduction in unstable fracture patterns
g. Sliding Hip Compression Screw/Sideplate
(1) Preferred implant
(2) Dynamic interfragmentary compression
(3) "Center/center" position of screw best
(4) Tip-apex distance (TAD) <25 mm—Low risk of cutout (Fig. 10-44)
(5) Medial displacement of shaft in unstable fracture patterns
h. Cephalomedullary Device
(1) Fixed-angle sliding compression screw through intramedullary (IM) nail
(2) Advantages—Implant acts as buttress to prevent excessive fracture collapse and shaft medialization; percutaneous insertion possible
(3) Disadvantage—Potential secondary fracture at tip of nail
i. Reverse Obliquity Fracture
(1) 95-degree fixed-angle device
j. Hemiarthroplasty/THA
(1) Calcar replacement necessary
(2) Most appropriate for treatment failures

3. Complications
a. Implant failure/screw cutout
(1) Occurs in 15% of cases (most common complication)
(2) Decreased risk with proper placement of compression screw

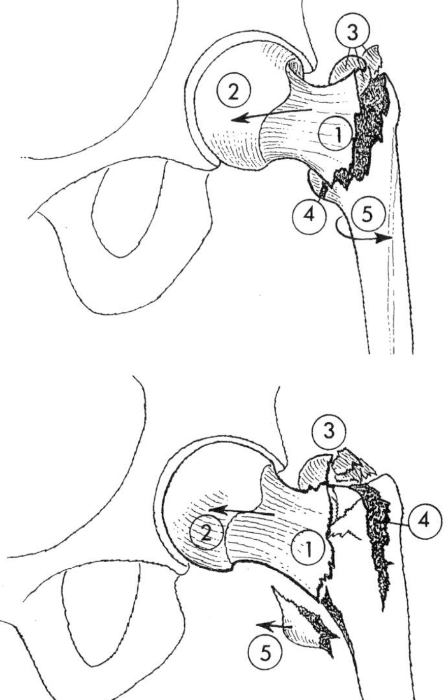

FIGURE 10-43 ■ Intertrochanteric hip fracture classification. *Top,* Stable. *Bottom,* Unstable. (From Connolly, J.F., ed.: Depalma's The Management of Fractures and Dislocations, an Atlas, 3rd ed. Philadelphia, WB Saunders, 1981, p. 1372.)

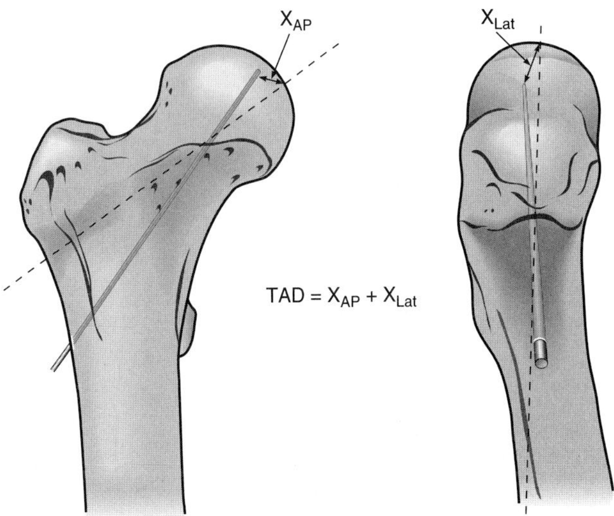

FIGURE 10-44 ■ Tip-apex distance (TAD) should be <25 mm. (Redrawn from Orthopaedic Knowledge Update Trauma 2. Chicago, American Academy of Orthopaedic Surgeons, 2000, p. 127.)

b. Infection
c. Leg length discrepancy (with medial displacement/shortening)
d. Mortality

D. **Subtrochanteric Fractures**

1. Evaluation/Classification
   a. Lesser trochanter to 5 cm distally
   b. Russell-Taylor
      (1) Type I—No piriformis fossa extension
      (2) Type II—with piriformis fossa extension (involves greater trochanter)
      (3) Peritrochanteric fracture—Intertrochanteric extension
2. Treatment
   a. Intramedullary Fixation
      (1) Preserves vascularity
      (2) Load-sharing
      (3) Stronger construct in unstable fracture patterns
      (4) May be contraindicated in Type II fractures
   b. Options
      (1) First-generation IM nail (not recommended)
      (2) Second-generation IM nail
      (3) Cephalomedullary device
   Extramedullary Fixation
      (1) Type II fractures
      (2) Fixed-angle device with long sideplate
      (3) Less strong in unstable fractures
      (4) Bone graft for medial comminution
3. Complications
      (1) Implant failure (Fig. 10-45)
      (2) Strong muscular forces and long lever arms; high compressive forces medially and tensile forces laterally; transition from cancellous to cortical bone
      (3) Nonunion
      (4) Malunion

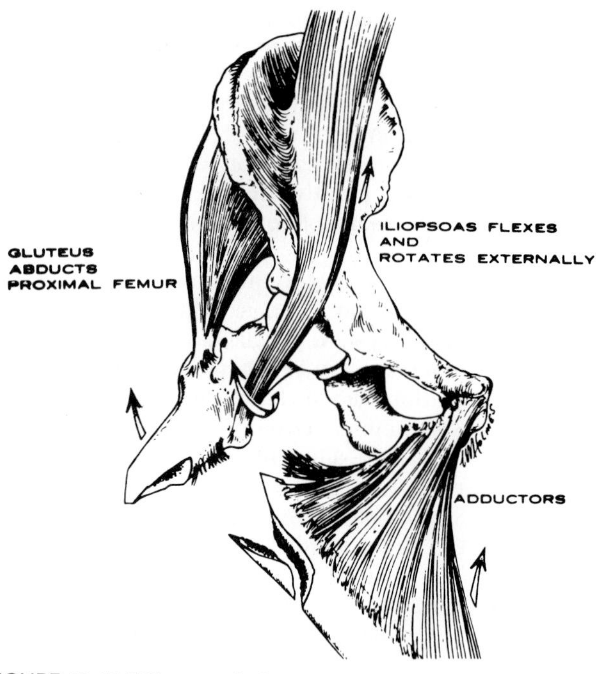

FIGURE 10-45 ■ The muscle forces acting on a type II subtrochanteric fracture. (From Froimson, A.L.: Treatment of comminuted subtrochanteric fractures of the femur. Surg. Gynecol. Obstet. 131:460, 1970.)

      (5) Length or leg rotation
      (6) Infection

E. **Shaft Fractures**

1. Evaluation/Classification
   a. High-energy trauma
   b. Associated injuries common
   c. Winquist and Hanson (Fig. 10-46)—Based on degree of comminution
      (1) Type 0—No comminution
      (2) Type I—<25%, butterfly

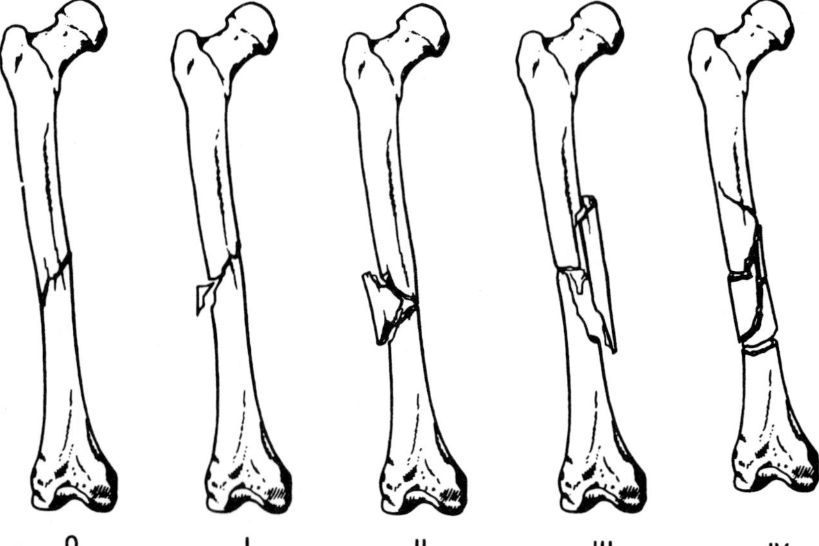

FIGURE 10-46 ■ Winquist and Hanson classification of femoral shaft fractures. (*Note:* type V [not shown] has segmental bone loss.) (From Johnson, K.D.: Femur: Trauma. In Orthopaedic Knowledge Update III, p. 514. Chicago, American Academy of Orthopaedic Surgeons, 1990.)

(3) Type II—25–50%, butterfly
(4) Type III—>50%, comminution
(5) Type IV—Segmental

2. Treatment
a. Little indication for nonoperative treatment
b. Options
(1) External fixation
(a) Indications—Unstable polytrauma patient, severe open fracture, vascular injury
(b) May be safely converted to IM nail within 3 weeks
(c) Disadvantages—Pin tract problems, knee stiffness
(2) Plate Fixation
(a) Usually reserved for special cases (e.g., neck-shaft fractures)
(b) Higher incidence of infection (6%), nonunion (9%), and implant failure (9%)
(3) IM Nailing
(a) Treatment of choice and the gold standard
(b) Union rates are 98–99%
(c) Complications infrequent
c. Factors Associated with IM Nailing
(1) Timing
(a) Early stabilization (<24 hours) associated with decreased pulmonary complications, decreased thromboembolic complications, decreased hospital cost, improved rehabilitation
(b) Consider delaying definitive treatment in presence of severe closed head injury
(2) Locking
(a) Static interlocking recommended; no indication for dynamic locking
(b) Antegrade versus retrograde insertion
(i) Antegrade—Entry point is piriformis fossa; gold standard
(ii) Retrograde—Entry point is intercondylar notch Technically easier; facilitates care of multiply injured patient. Potential complications are knee injury and intra-articular infection
(c) Reaming
(i) Reamed insertion preferred
(ii) Unreamed has theoretic advantage of decreased pulmonary embolization
(iii) Clinical series show no deleterious effect of reaming
(iv) Unreamed—Decreased union rate, increased time to union
(v) Reamer design important—Use sharp reamers, deep flutes, and small shafts and advance slowly
(vi) Consider unreamed nail for bilateral chest injury
(d) Open Fractures
(i) Emergent débridement
(ii) Reamed IM nailing
(iii) Delayed wound closure
(iv) Results comparable to closed fractures
(e) Gunshot Femur Fractures
(i) Low velocity—Reamed IM nailing
(ii) High velocity—Aggressive soft tissue (ST) management; ex-fix versus unreamed nail

3. Complications
a. Infection—Occurs in 1–2% of cases
(1) Treatment—Nail removal after union; reaming of canal
b. Delayed Union
(1) Treatment—Dynamization ± bone grafting
c. Nonunion—Occurs in 1–2% of cases
(1) Treatment—Reamed exchange nailing
d. Pudendal Nerve Injury
(1) Up to 10% with use of perineal post; surgery for penile numbness, impotence
(2) Treatment—Avoid excessive traction
e. HO—Occurs in 25% of cases
(1) Most frequent complication but rarely clinically important
f. Malunion
(1) Most common in distal third of fractures with comminution
(2) Can tolerate up to 15 degrees of malrotation
(3) Nail supine—Increased internal rotation
(4) Nail lateral—Increased external rotation
g. Knee Pain
(1) Increased incidence with retrograde nailing

F. **Ipsilateral Neck-Shaft Fractures**
1. Evaluation/Classification
a. Overall incidence 3%
b. Missed in 30% of cases
c. Usually seen with comminuted fracture midshaft
2. Treatment
a. Neck fracture given priority
b. Anatomic reduction of neck fracture essential
c. Options
(1) Multiple screws for neck + retrograde nail (preferred)
(2) Multiple screws for neck + plate
(3) Antegrade nail with screws anterior to nail
(4) Second-generation nail (not recommended)

G. **Distal Fractures**
1. Evaluation/Classification
a. Young patients—High-energy trauma; significant displacement

b. Older patients—Low energy/osteoporotic bone; less displacement
c. Supracondylar
(1) No intra-articular extension
d. Intercondylar
(1) With intra-articular extension
e. AO/OTA Classification (Fig. 10-47)
(1) 33A—Extra-articular
(2) 33B—Partial articular (unicondylar)
(3) 33C—Complex articular (bicondylar)
2. Treatment
a. Nondisplaced Fractures
(1) Cast brace
(2) Non-weight-bearing (NWB) for 6 weeks
(3) Immediate motion

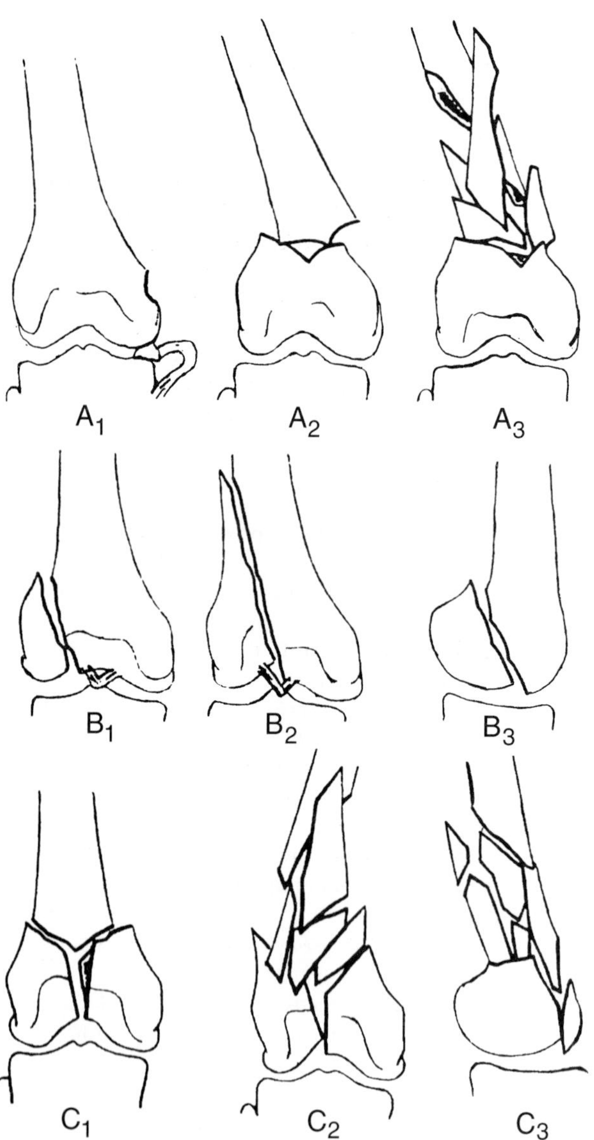

FIGURE 10-47 ■ AO/ASIF classification of supracondylar fractures. *A*, Extra-articular. *B*, Unicondylar. *C*, Bicondylar. (From Johnson, K.D.: Femur: Trauma. In Orthopaedic Knowledge Update III. Chicago, American Academy of Orthopaedic Surgeons, 1990, p. 521.)

b. Displaced Fractures
(1) Principles
(a) Anatomic reduction of joint surface
(b) Stable fixation of articular segment to shaft
(c) Preserve vascularity of fragments
(d) Early motion of knee joint
c. Options
(1) Fixed-Angle Plate Devices
(a) Most stable construct
(b) Union rate—92-96%
(c) Direct reduction lateral approach
(d) Indirect reduction percutaneous techniques complex fractures
(e) May be contraindicated with coronal fractures
(f) Examples—95-degree blade plate, locking compression plate
(2) Nonfixed-Angle Plating
(a) Indicated in severe comminution or coronal plane fractures
(b) Risk—Varus malalignment
(c) If no medial bony support, consider second medial plate + bone graft
(d) Example—Condylar buttress plate
(3) Retrograde IM Nail
(a) Useful in supracondylar fractures
(b) Preferred implant in osteroporotic and periprosthetic fractures
(c) Less axial and rotational stability
3. Complications
a. Vascular Injury
(1) Potential for popliteal artery injury with fracture displacement
b. Nonunion
(1) Union rates better for plate fixation compared with nail fixation
c. Malunion
d. Knee Pain/Stiffness
(1) Increased risk with retrograde nailing

X. Knee

A. Dislocation

1. Evaluation/Classification
a. High-Energy Mechanism
b. Significant Soft Tissue Disruption
c. Beware Underdiagnosis—Up to 50% are reduced
d. Classification (Fig. 10-48)
(1) Anterior (with posterior, most common)
(2) Posterior (with anterior, most common)
(3) Medial
(4) Lateral
(5) Rotatory (posterolateral most common)
2. Treatment
a. Reduce Emergently
b. Revascularize within 6 hours—Reverse saphenous vein graft/fasciotomies
c. Ligament Injury Expected

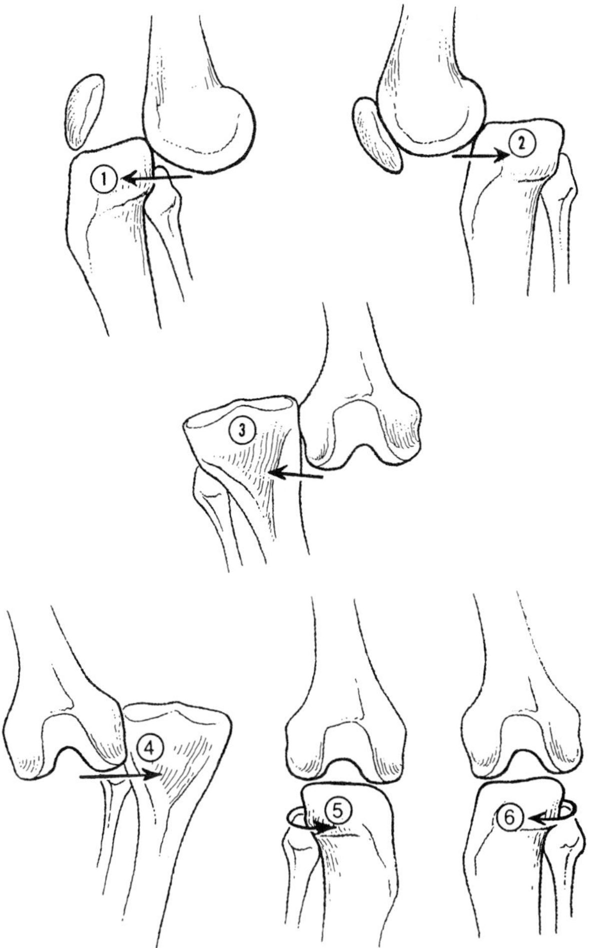

FIGURE 10-48 ■ Dislocations of the knee. *1,* Anterior. *2,* Posterior. *3,* Lateral. *4,* Medial. *5,* Anteromedial. *6,* Anterolateral. (From Connolly, J.F., ed.: Depalma's The Management of Fractures and Dislocations, an Atlas, 3rd ed. Philadelphia, WB Saunders, 1981, p. 1621.)

d. Treatment Options:
   (1) Nonoperative (immobilization)
   (2) Acute repair—Within 3 weeks
   (3) Delayed repair
e. Most important to repair posterior capsule (PCL, posterolateral corner)
f. Treat MCL nonoperatively

3. Complications
   a. Associated vascular injury
      (1) Overall incidence of 30%
      (2) Anterior-posterior dislocations account for 50% of cases
      (3) Ankle-brachial index (ABI) useful—Most sensitive clinical test of arterial injury; normal ABI >0.9
      (4) Treat with surgical exploration/vascular repair if "hard signs" present: Active bleeding, expanding hematoma, absent pulses, bruit, thrill
   b. Neurologic Injury
      (1) Peroneal nerve (23%)
   c. Knee Stiffness
      (1) Most common complication
      (2) Worse with nonoperative management of ligament injury
      (3) Treat with manipulation under anesthesia (MUA) if necessary
   d. Compartment Syndrome
      (1) Associated with long ischemic time/reperfusion
   e. Knee Pain

B. **Patella Fractures**

1. Evaluation/Classification
   a. Mechanism—Direct blow to anterior knee
   b. Distal pole of patella extra-articular (30%)
   c. Inability to actively extend indicative of incompetent extensor mechanism
   d. Classification (Fig. 10-49)
      (1) Transverse—Seen on lateral x-ray view
      (2) Vertical—Seen on sunrise x-ray view
      (3) Comminuted (stellate)
   e. Nondisplaced versus Displaced
      (1) Displacement = 3-mm fragment separation or 2-mm articular step-off

2. Treatment
   a. Nonoperative Treatment
      (1) Nondisplaced fractures
      (2) Minimally displaced fractures with intact extensor mechanism
      (3) Hinged knee brace for 4–6 weeks; WBAT
   b. Operative Treatment
      (1) Displaced fractures
      (2) Preserve patella whenever possible
   c. ORIF
      (1) Anterior tension band wiring
      (2) Kirschner wires or cannulated screws
   d. Partial Patellectomy
      (1) Extra-articular distal pole fractures
      (2) Severely comminuted fractures—Preserve largest pieces and reattach patella ligament anteriorly (Fig. 10-50)

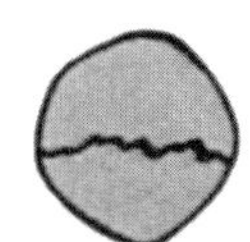

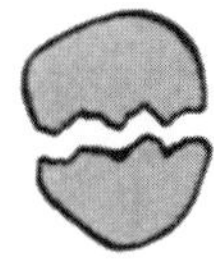

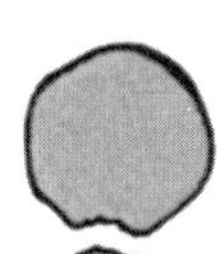

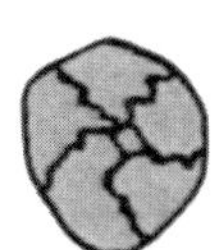

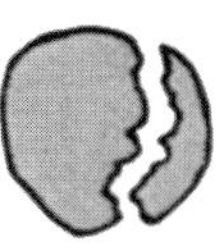

FIGURE 10-49 ■ Types of patellar fractures. (From Weissman, B.N., and Sledge, C.B.: Orthopedic Radiology. Philadelphia, WB Saunders, 1986, p. 553.)

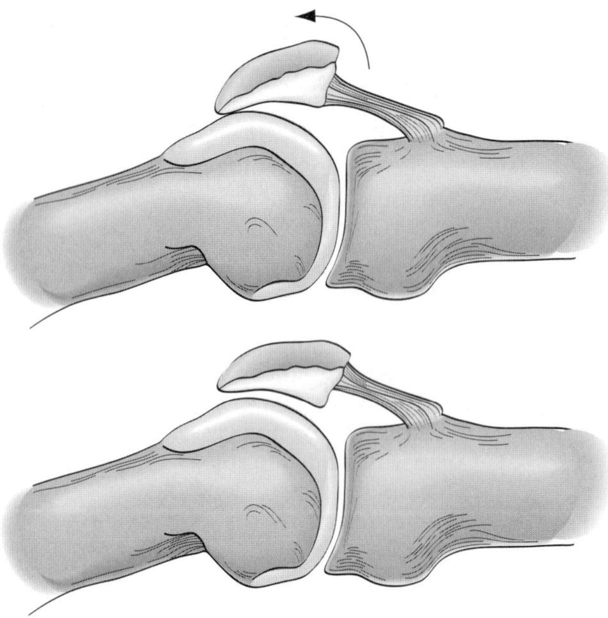

FIGURE 10-50 ■ Anterior reattachment of patellar ligament recommended to prevent tilting of patella superiorly. (Redrawn with permission from Marder, R.A., et al.: Effects of partial patellectomy and reattachment of the patellar tendon on patellofemoral contact areas and pressures. J. Bone Joint Surg. [Am.] 75A:35–45, 1993.)

e. Open Fractures
   (1) Immediate ORIF following wound débridement

3. Complications
   a. Symptomatic hardware—Common
   b. Loss of reduction/fixation—Up to 20%
      (1) Treat with repeat ORIF
   c. Nonunion <5%
   d. Infection
   e. Knee stiffness
      (1) Treatment—Consider MUA

C. **Patellar Dislocations**
1. Evaluation/Classification
   a. Adolescents/young adults
   b. Usually lateral
   c. Injury to medial patellofemoral ligament
2. Treatment
   a. Reduce with knee in full extension
   b. Immobilize with controlled ROM for 6 weeks
3. Complications
   a. High redislocation rate

D. **Patellar Ligament Rupture**
1. Evaluation/Classification
   a. Active adult patients <40 of age
   b. Patellar tendonitis risk factor
   c. Ligament avulsion distal pole
2. Treatment
   a. Direct primary repair indicated
   b. Nonabsorbable sutures
   c. Patellar drill holes or suture anchors
   d. Consider augmentation with cerclage wire or tape
3. Complications
   a. Knee stiffness

E. **Quadriceps Tendon Rupture**
1. Evaluation/Classification
   a. More common than patellar ligament rupture
   b. Older adults (>40) with medical risk factors
   c. Rupture usually intratendinous 2 cm above proximal pole
2. Treatment
   a. Surgical repair indicated for loss of active knee extension
   b. End-to-end primary repair
   c. Worse results with late repair
3. Complications
   a. Knee stiffness

XI. Tibia

A. **Plateau Fractures**
1. Evaluation/Classification
   a. Mechanism—Combination of axial loading and varus/valgus stress
   b. Bimodal distribution
      (1) Males—Peak fourth decade
      (2) Females—Peak seventh decade
   c. CT scan changes classification and/or surgical approach 10–15% of time
   d. MRI to evaluate associated soft tissue injuries (>50%)—MCL >ACL; meniscal tears, 50%
   e. Incidence—Lateral plateau >bicondylar >medial plateau
   f. Schatzker Classification (Fig. 10-51)
      (1) Split fracture
      (2) Split-depressed fracture
      (3) Pure depression fracture
      (4) Medial plateau fracture
      (5) Bicondylar fracture; intact metaphysis
      (6) Bicondylar fracture; metaphyseal-diaphyseal disassociation
   g. AO/OTA Classification (Fig. 10-52)
      (1) 41A—Extra-articular fracture
      (2) 41B—Partial articular fracture (unicondylar)
      (3) 41C—Complete articular fracture (bicondylar)
2. Treatment
   a. Nonoperative Treatment
      (1) <3-mm articular step-off
      (2) Stable knee full extension (<10 degrees varus/valgus instability)
      (3) Cast-brace with early ROM and delayed WB for 4–6 weeks
   b. Operative Treatment
      (1) Articular step-off = 3 mm
      (2) Condylar widening >5 mm
      (3) All medial plateau fractures
      (4) All bicondylar fractures
   c. Plate Fixation
      (1) Direct anatomic reduction
      (2) Rigid fixation

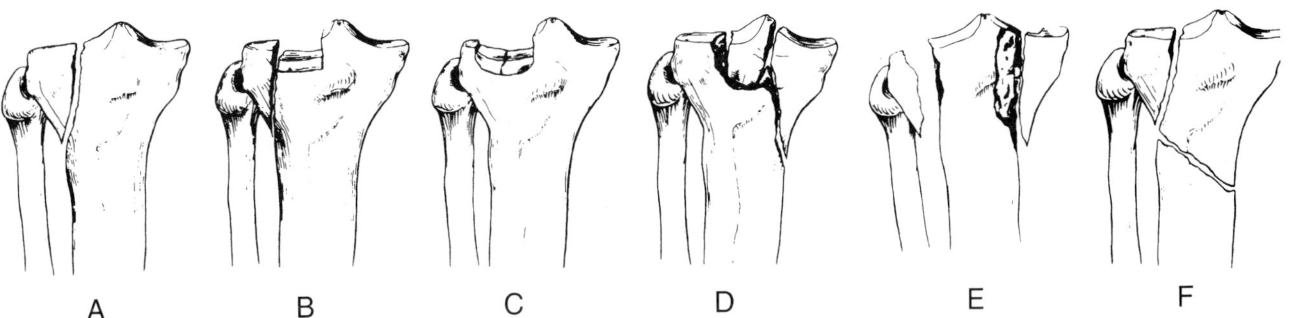

FIGURE 10-51 ■ Diagram of the Schatzker classification of tibial plateau fractures. *A,* type I, cleavage of wedge fracture of the lateral tibial plateau. *B,* type II, lateral split/depression fracture. *C,* type III, pure central depression. *D,* type IV, medial condyle fracture (may involve tibial spine). *E,* type V, bicondylar fracture. *F,* type VI, metaphyseal/diaphyseal disassociation. (From Schatzker, J., McBroom, R., and Bruce, D.: The tibial plateau fracture: the Toronto experience 1968–1975. Clin. Orthop. 138:94–104, 1979.)

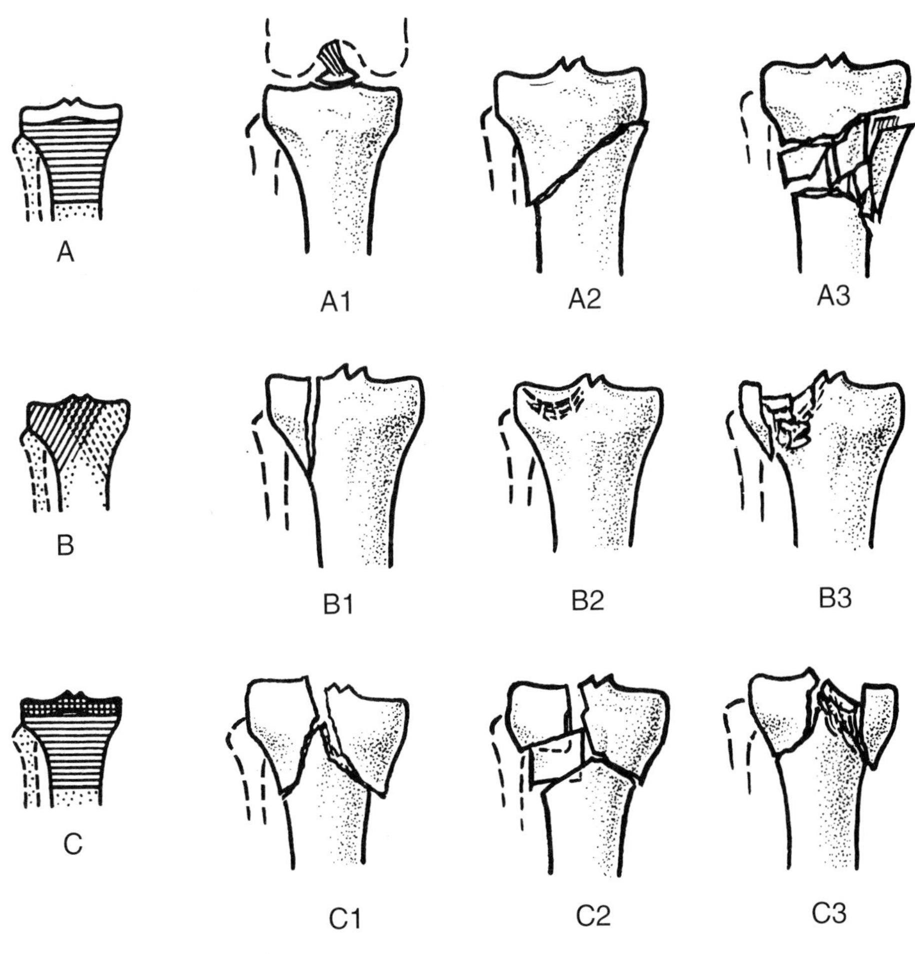

FIGURE 10-52 ■ AO/ASIF universal classification system for tibial plateau fractures (see text). (From Müller, M.E., et al., eds.: The Comprehensive Classification of Fractures of Long Bones. Berlin, Germany, Springer-Verlag, 1990.)

(3) Buttress plate best for unicondylar fractures
(4) Percutaneous plating for bicondylar fractures with fixed-angle implants
(5) Avoid soft tissue complications (no Y incision)
d. External Fixation
(1) Bicondylar fractures
(2) Decreased soft tissue complications
(3) Used with limited open or percutaneous fixation of articular segments
e. Types of External Fixations
(1) Unilateral—Placed medially to prevent varus collapse
(2) Ilizarov—Keep thin wires at least 15 mm from joint
(3) Hybrid Ring—Keep thin wires at least 15 mm from joint
(4) Bridging—Temporary stabilization in significant soft tissue injury
3. Complications
a. Post-Traumatic DJD—May not manifest until 5-7 years after injury
b. Infection—Surgical approach most important factor
c. Malunion—Increased risk with closed treatment
d. Ligamentous Instability—Adversely affects results; prevent with repair of cruciate/collateral ligament injuries
e. Peroneal Nerve Injury
f. Compartment syndrome

B. **Shaft Fractures**
1. Evaluation/Classification
a. Most common long bone fracture
b. Soft tissue injury/management critical determinant of outcome
c. Low Energy—Torsional injury/indirect trauma; fibula fracture at different level; Tscherne O or I soft tissue injury
d. High Energy—Direct trauma; bony comminution; fibula fracture at same level; open fracture or Tscherne II/III
2. Treatment
a. Closed Fractures
(1) Options
(a) Cast immobilization
(b) IM nailing
(c) External fixation
b. Cast Treatment
(1) Low energy fractures
(2) Closed reduction/long leg cast
(3) Early transition to functional brace (4-6 weeks)
(4) Criteria for acceptable alignment
(a) Varus-valgus angulation = 5 degrees
(b) Sagittal plane angulation = 10 degrees
(c) Cortical apposition = 50%
(d) Shortening = 1 cm
(e) Rotational alignment within 10 degrees
c. IM Nailing
(1) Indications
(a) Unacceptable alignment with closed treatment
(b) Significant soft tissue injury
(c) Segmental fracture
(d) Polytrauma/ipsilateral fractures
(e) Morbid obesity
(f) High energy, unstable fractures
(2) IM nailing increased union rate and decreased time to union versus closed treatment for displaced fractures
(3) Static interlocking indicated
(4) Results of reamed superior to results of unreamed
(5) Proximal third fractures—High incidence of valgus and procurvatum malalignment; consider unicortical plating or blocking screws
d. External Fixation
(1) May be indicated in proximal and distal metaphyseal fractures
(2) Diaphyseal fractures—Increased incidence of malalignment compared with IM nailing
(3) Pin tract complications (50%)
e. Open Fractures
(1) Emergent surgical débridement most important step
(2) External fixation versus IM nailing
(a) No difference in infection rates or time to union
(b) IM nailing associated with decreased secondary surgeries, earlier return to WB
(3) Unreamed versus reamed
(a) No apparent adverse effects of reaming
(b) Reaming associated with decreased hardware failure
(4) Limb Salvage—Relative indications for amputation
(a) Warm ischemia >6 hours
(b) Absent plantar sensation
(c) Severe ipsilateral foot trauma
3. Complications
a. Nonunion—Nonhealing past 9 months
(1) Treatment—Dynamization if axially stable; exchange reamed IM nailing if not axially stable. Bone grafting for bone loss
b. Malunion—Increased risk with closed treatment of displaced fractures and with external fixation (compared with IM nailing)
c. Infection—Increased risk with increased severity of soft tissue injury
d. Compartment Syndrome (1-9%)—Pain with passive stretch most sensitive examination finding; compartment pressure within 30 mm Hg diastolic blood pressure

most sensitive indicator; requires emergent fasciotomy
   e. Anterior Knee Pain—Most common complication of tibial nailing (50%); higher with patellar tendon splitting approach
   f. Hardware Failure—Increased risk with unreamed IM nailing
   g. Ankle Stiffness—Most common complication of closed treatment

C. **Femoral and Tibial Shaft Fractures**—"Floating Knee"
   1. Treatment
      a. Antegrade IM nail tibia
      b. Retrograde IM nail femur
   2. Complications
      a. Same as complications described for femoral and tibial shaft fractures

D. **Tibial Plafond Fractures**—Pilon fracture
   1. Evaluation/Classification
      a. High-energy axial loading
         (1) Bone—Comminution/displacement/bone loss
         (2) Soft tissues—Open fractures; Tscherne II/III closed fractures
      b. Fibular fracture associated (75%)
      c. Ruedi and Allgower (Fig. 10-53)
         (1) Minimally/nondisplaced
         (2) Displaced (simple)
         (3) Comminuted
      d. AO/OTA Classification (Fig. 10-54)
         (1) 43A—Extra-articular
         (2) 43B—Partial articular
         (3) 43C—Complete articular
   2. Treatment
      a. No role for nonoperative treatment of displaced fracture
      b. ORIF
         (1) Advantages—Direct anatomic reduction; rigid fixation; early ankle motion
         (2) Disadvantages—High incidence of soft tissue complications (full-thickness flaps, incisions >7 cm apart to prevent)
         (3) Should not be performed acutely
         (4) Staged protocol best—Temporary bridging ex-fix followed by delayed ORIF at 10–14 days
      c. External Fixation
         (1) Decreased risk to soft tissues
         (2) Decreased incidence of wound complications and deep infection compared with ORIF
         (3) Combined with limited or percutaneous internal fixation on delayed basis
         (4) Pin tract problems

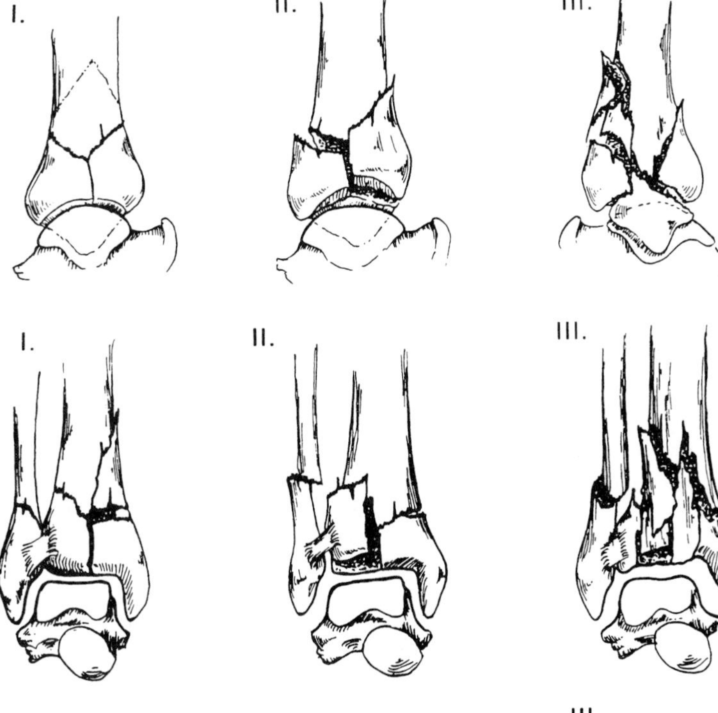

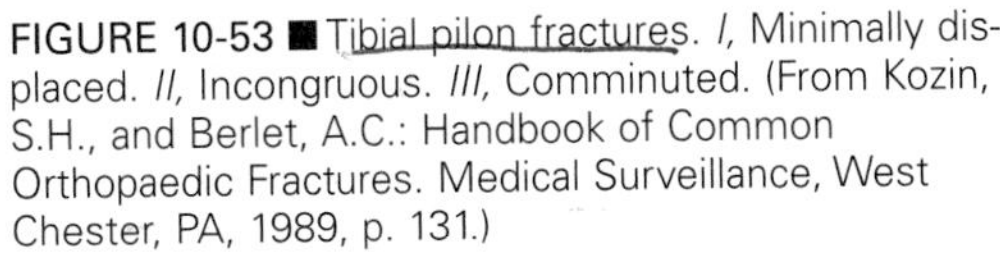

FIGURE 10-53 ■ Tibial pilon fractures. *I*, Minimally displaced. *II*, Incongruous. *III*, Comminuted. (From Kozin, S.H., and Berlet, A.C.: Handbook of Common Orthopaedic Fractures. Medical Surveillance, West Chester, PA, 1989, p. 131.)

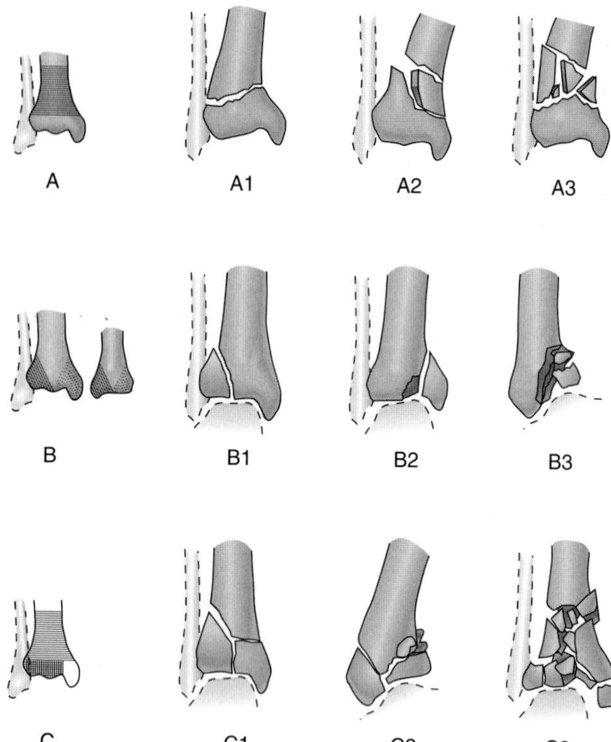

FIGURE 10-54 ■ AO/OTA classification of tibial plafond fractures. (Redrawn with permission from Müller, M.E., et al., eds.: The Comprehensive Classification of Fractures of Long Bones. Berlin, Germany, Springer-Verlag, 1990, p.173.)

3. Complications
    a. Wound slough in 10%
    b. Deep infection in 4–35% of cases
        (1) Increased risk with formal ORIF
    c. Malunion—Varus
    d. Nonunion—Metaphyseal junction
    e. Post-Traumatic Arthrosis—Most common complication

XII. Ankle

A. Fractures

1. Evaluation/Classification
    a. Rotational mechanism
    b. Deep portion of deltoid ligament primary restraint to anterolateral talar displacement
    c. Isolateral malleolar versus bimalleolar versus trimalleolar
    d. AO/OTA Classification (Fig. 10-55)
        (1) Modification of Danis-Weber
        (2) Based on level of fibular fracture
        (3) 44A—Infrasyndesmotic
        (4) 44B—Transyndesmotic
        (5) 44C—Suprasyndesmotic
2. Treatment
    a. Any talar displacement in mortise is indication for anatomic reduction/fixation
    b. 1 mm lateral talar shift = 42% decreased tibiotalar contact area
    c. Medial Malleolar Fracture (Isolated)
        (1) Tip avulsion—Symptomatic treatment
        (2) Nondisplaced or minimally displaced—short leg walking cast (SLWC) versus cast boot
        (3) Displaced—Lag screw fixation
    d. Lateral Malleolar Fracture (Isolated)
        (1) Nonoperative treatment (SLWC versus cast boot) if ankle mortise intact
        (2) Up to 3 mm displacement well tolerated
    e. Bimalleolar Fracture
        (1) ORIF for lateral talar shift (lateral and medial malleoli)
        (2) ORIF superior to closed treatment
        (3) "Functional" bimalleolar—ORIF lateral malleolus; no indication for medial ligament repair
    f. Trimalleolar Fracture
        (1) Fix posterior malleolus >25% or step-off >2 mm
    g. Syndesmosis Disruption
        (1) Suprasyndesmotic fractures
        (2) Measure clear space/overlap 1 cm above joint
        (3) Fixation not required when fibular fracture within 4.5 cm of joint
        (4) Place cortical screw 2 cm above joint; not lag screw
        (5) There is a 30% risk of screw breakage with WB
        (6) Do not remove <3 months
    h. Open Fracture
        (1) Emergent operative débridement
        (2) Immediate ORIF
        (3) Results similar to closed fractures
3. Complications
    a. Wound problems in 4–5% of cases
    b. Deep infection in 1–2% of cases
        (1) Significant increased risk in diabetics (20%)
    c. Post-Traumatic Arthrosis—Rare following anatomic reduction/fixation
    d. Functional Impairment—Common
        (1) Function continues to improve up to 2 years postinjury

B. Achilles Tendon Rupture

1. Evaluation/Classification
    a. Two to four cm above calcaneal insertion
    b. Diagnosis—Thompson calf-squeeze test
    c. Missed diagnosis up to 25%
2. Treatment
    a. Surgical repair associated with:
        (1) Decreased rerupture rate
        (2) Increased plantar flexion strength
    b. Surgical technique—Posteromedial incision, nonabsorbable suture
    c. Percutaneous repair weaker

XIII. Foot

A. Talar Neck Fracture—"Aviator's Astralgus"

GROUPS

Tibia/Fibula, malleolar, infrasyndesmotic lesions (44-A)

1. Isolated (44-A1)

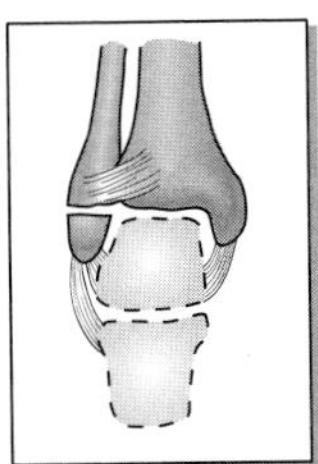

2. With medial malleolar fracture (44-A2)

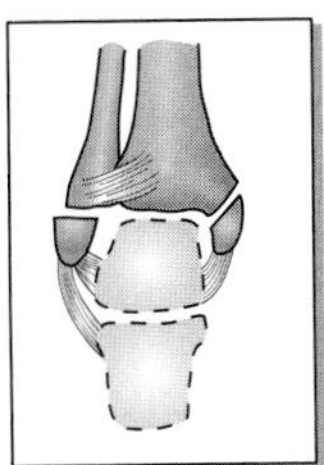

3. With postero-medial fracture (44-A3)

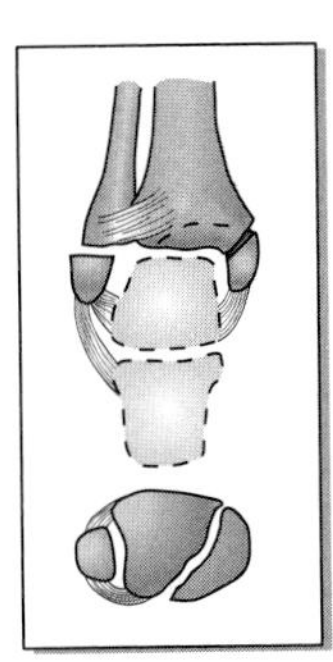

Tibia/Fibula, malleolar, transsyndesmotic fibula fracture (44-A)

1. Isolated (44-B1)

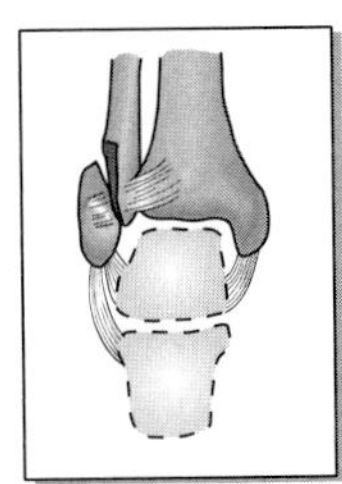

2. With medial lesion (44-B2)

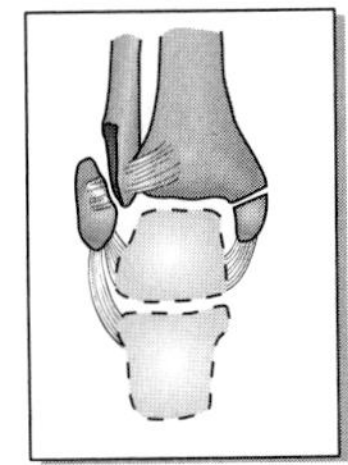

3. With medial lesion and Volkmann (fracture of the postero–leteral rim) (44-A3)

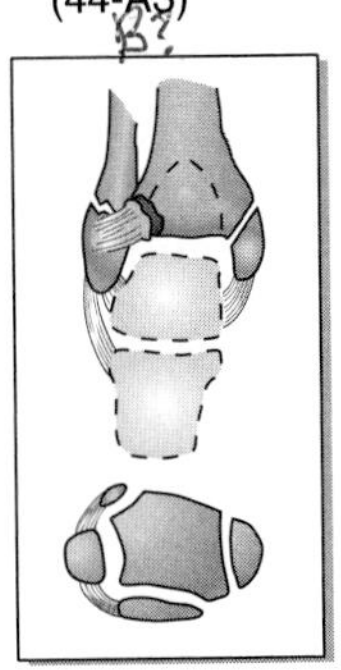

Tibia/Fibula, malleolar, suprasyndesmotic (44-A)

1. Simple diaphyseal fibular fracture (44-C1)

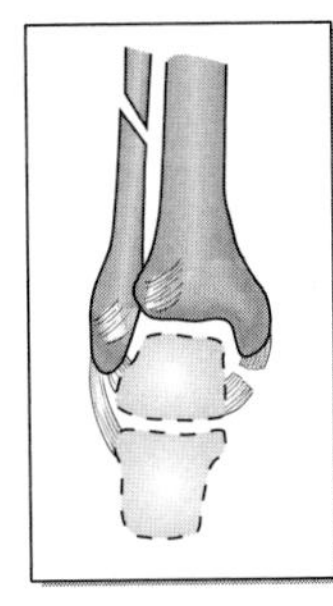

2. Multifragmentary fracture of fibular diaphysis (44-C2)

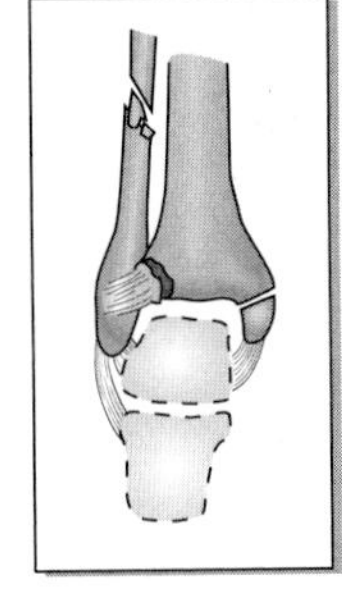

3. Proximal fibula (44-C3)

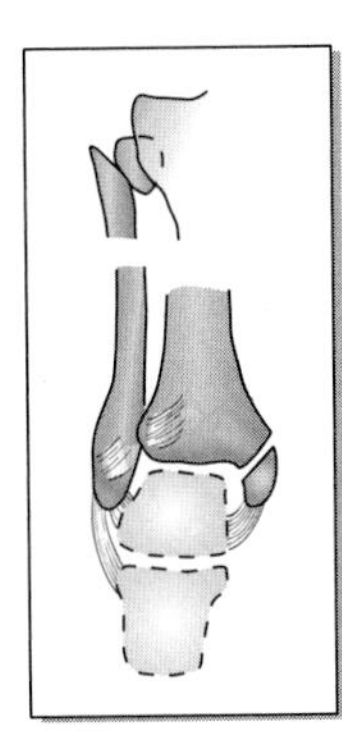

FIGURE 10-55 ■ AO/OTA classification of ankle fractures. (Redrawn from Committee for Coding and Classification: Fracture and dislocation compendium. *J Orthop Trauma* 10(suppl 1):62, 1996.)

1. Evaluation/Classification
   a. Most common fracture of talus (>50%)
   b. Forced dorsiflexion with axial load
   c. Hawkins Classification (Fig. 10-56)
      (1) I—Nondisplaced
      (2) II—Displaced with subtalar dislocation
      (3) III—Displaced with talar body dislocation (subtalar and tibiotalar)
      (4) IV—Displaced with talar body and head dislocation (subtalar, tibiotalar, and talonavicular)
2. Treatment
   a. Displaced fractures require ORIF with anatomic reduction
   b. Dual incisions recommended
   c. Posterior to anterior screws superior

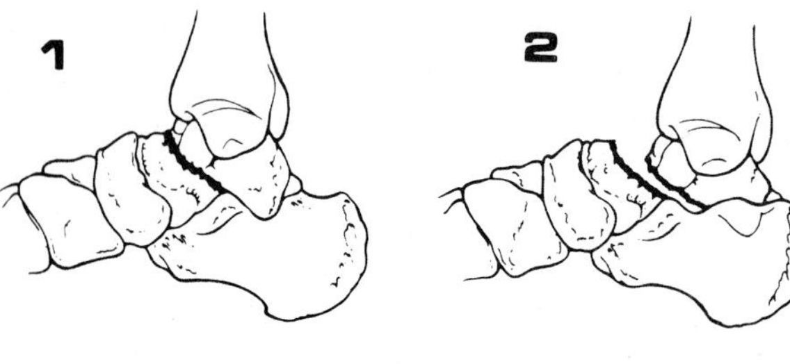

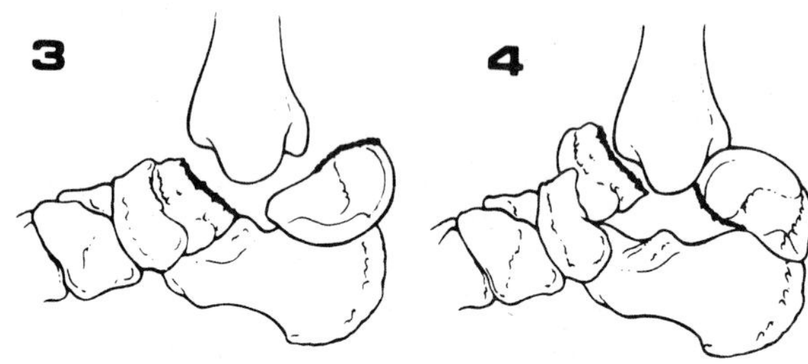

FIGURE 10-56 ■ Hawkins classification of talar neck fractures. (From Sangeorzan, B.J., and Hansen, S.T.: Ankle and foot: trauma. In Orthopaedic Knowledge Update III. Chicago, American Academy of Orthopaedic Surgeons, 1990, p. 616; reprinted by permission.)

d. Postoperative Treatment—NWB for 10–12 weeks

3. Complications
   a. Osteonecrosis—Increased risk with increased initial displacement and nonanatomic reduction
      (1) Hawkins I—<10%
      (2) Hawkins II—20–50%
      (3) Hawkins III—20–100%
      (4) Hawkins IV—100%
      (5) Hawkins Sign—Subchondral lucency on AP x-ray view at 6–8 weeks indicative of intact vascularity
   b. Post-Traumatic Arthritis
      (1) Subtalar—50%
      (2) Tibiotalar—33%
   c. Varus Malunion—25–30%
      (1) Treat with triple arthrodesis

B. **Talar Body and Head Fractures**
1. Evaluation/Classification
   a. Rare
2. Treatment
   a. Anatomic reduction/stable fixation or fragment excision if too small
3. Complications
   a. High rate of complications (osteonecrosis, DJD, pain)

C. **Talar Process Fractures**
1. Evaluation/Classification
   a. Lateral >medial
   b. Often missed; "ankle sprain"
2. Treatment
   a. Nondisplaced—Short leg cast (SLC) for 6 weeks; NWB
   b. Displaced—ORIF (large fragments) versus excision (small fragments)

D. **Subtalar Dislocations**
1. Evaluation/Classification
   a. Medial most common (85%)
2. Treatment
   a. Closed reduction
   b. SLC for 4–6 weeks
3. Complications
   a. Irreducible Medial—Interposed EDB
   b. Irreducible Lateral—Interposed posterior tibial tendon

E. **Calcaneus Fractures**
1. Evaluation/Classification
   a. Axial load
   b. Posterior facet depression + lateral wall blowout
   c. Deformity—Heel shortened, widened, and in varus
   d. Sanders Classification (based on coronal CT image posterior facet)
      (1) Nondisplaced posterior facet
      (2) Single fracture line
      (3) Two-degree fracture line with three posterior facet fragments
      (4) Three fracture lines with four + fragments
2. Treatment
   a. Nonoperative Treatment
      (1) Nondisplaced fractures
      (2) Extra-articular fractures (25%)
      (3) Cast versus cast-boot; early ROM
      (4) Closed reduction cannot restore articular congruity

   Operative Treatment
      (5) Displaced articular fractures
      (6) Goal—Restore calcaneal anatomy (width, height) and reduce articular surfaces
      (7) Extensile lateral approach most common; low profile implants
      (8) No benefit to early surgery
3. Complications
   a. Wound complications in 10–20% of cases (increased risk in smokers, diabetics)
   b. Compartment syndrome occurs in 10%
   c. Heel deformity/malunion
   d. Peroneal impingement
   e. Subtalar arthrosis
   f. Factors Associated with Poor Outcome
      (1) Age >50
      (2) Obesity
      (3) Manual laborer
      (4) Worker's compensation

F. **Navicular Fractures**
1. Evaluation/Classification
   a. Dorsal Lip Avulsion—Most common
   b. Tuberosity Fracture—Posterior tibial tendon avulsion fracture
   c. Body Fracture—Intra-articular
   d. Stress Fracture—Central third

2. Treatment
   a. Dorsal Lip Avulsion—Symptomatic treat (SLC)
   b. Tuberosity Fracture—ORIF if displaced or involves joint
   c. Body Fracture—ORIF
   d. Stress Fracture—SLC NWB for 6 weeks

G. **Cuboid Fractures**—"Nutcracker"
1. Evaluation/Classification
   a. Compression fracture between calcaneus and metatarsal
2. Treatment
   a. ORIF if large fragments and shortening of lateral column
   b. Minimal Impaction—SLC NWB for 6 weeks

H. **Tarsometatarsal Fracture/Dislocation**—Lisfranc
1. Evaluation/Classification
   a. High energy
   b. May be missed
   c. Lisfranc's Ligament—Base of second metatarsal to medial cuneiform
   d. Dorsal Dislocation—Most common (plantar ligaments strongest)
   e. Classification
      (1) Homolateral
      (2) Isolated
      (3) Divergent
2. Treatment
   a. Anatomic reduction necessary
   b. Open treatment indicated if unable to obtain anatomic closed reduction
   c. Screw versus Kirschner-wire fixation (Fig. 10-57)
   d. Postoperative Treatment—Protected WB for 3 months; early ROM midfoot
3. Complications
   a. May be source of significant long-term disability and pain
   b. Altered gait, post-traumatic arthrosis common

I. **Metatarsal Fractures**
1. Evaluation/Classification
   a. Must rule out Lisfranc injury
2. Treatment
   a. Nonoperative Treatment
      (1) Cast/healing shoe
      (2) WB to comfort
   b. Operative Treatment
      (1) Indications—Open fractures, first or fifth metatarsal fractures, multiple metatarsal fractures, displaced articular fractures
      (2) Pinning versus ORIF

J. **Fifth Metatarsal Fractures**—Jones fracture
1. Evaluation/Classification (Fig. 10-58)
   a. Fracture proximal metadiaphyseal junction fifth toe

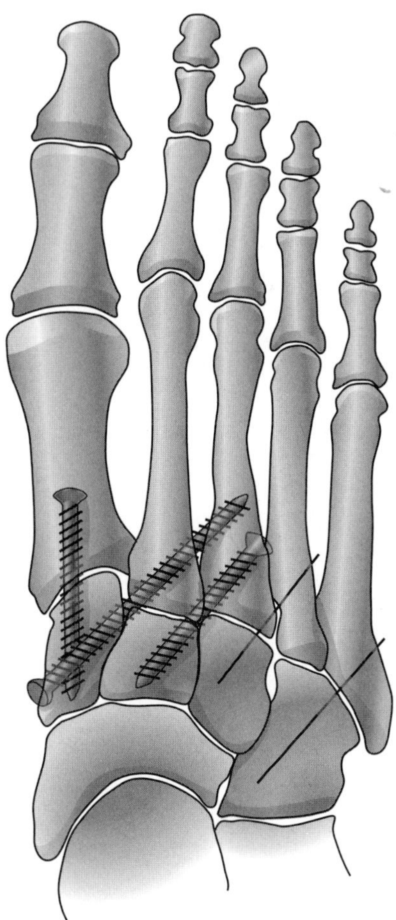

FIGURE 10-57 ■ Fixation of tarsometatarsal joint dislocations. (Redrawn from McClain, E.I., Gruen, G.S., Hansen, S.T.: Fracture-dislocation of the tarsometatarsal joint: Open reduction and internal fixation with screw fixation. In Heckman, J.D. (ed.) Perspectives in Orthopaedic Surgery. New York, Thíeme, 1991, pp. 35–44.)

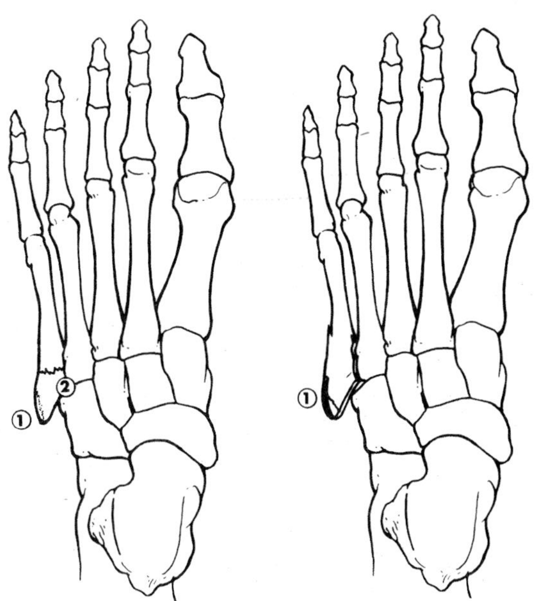

FIGURE 10-58 ■ Jones versus pseudo-Jones fractures. (From Connolly, J.F., ed.: Depalma's The Management of Fractures and Dislocations, an Atlas, 3rd ed. Philadelphia, WB Saunders, 1981, pp. 2065–2066; reprinted by permission.)

2. Treatment
   a. Nonoperative Treatment
      (1) NWB SLC for 6–8 weeks
      (2) 12% require late surgery
   b. Operative Treatment
      (1) Athletes
      (2) Percutaneous screw fixation
      (3) Faster healing and return of function
3. Complications
   a. Nonunion—Treat with screw fixation/bone graft

K. **Fifth Metatarsal Fractures**—Pseudo-Jones fracture
1. Evaluation/Classification (see Fig. 10-58)
   a. Avulsion fracture base of fifth metatarsal (peroneus brevis tendon)
2. Treatment
   a. Cast/healing shoe for 2–3 weeks
   b. WBAT

L. **Metatarsophalangeal Joint Dislocation**
1. Evaluation/Classification
   a. First MTP most common
   b. Dorsal
2. Treatment
   a. Closed reduction
   b. Cast/healing shoe
   c. WBAT

M. **Phalangeal Fractures**
1. Treatment
   a. Nonoperative Treatment
      (1) Indicated for almost all phalangeal fractures
      (2) Buddy-taping
      (3) WBAT
   b. Operative Treatment
      (1) Indications—Intra-articular fractures of great toe; open fractures

SECTION 3

Pediatric Trauma

I. Introduction—Fractures and dislocations in children are often unique; several features of the injuries are not found in adults (Tables 10-9 through 10-20). Children's bones are more ductile than adult bones and bowing is thus unique to children. The terms *greenstick* and *torus* imply a partial fracture with some part of the bone intact. The periosteum in children is much thicker and often remains intact on the concave (compression) side, allowing for less displacement and better reduction of fractures. Children's fractures heal more quickly and with less immobilization than adults' fractures. Contractures are also less likely. However, because bones are actively growing in pediatric fractures, malunion and growth plate injuries are an important concern. Remodeling is more thorough, thus displacement and angulation that would not be acceptable in an adult are often so in children. The exception to this rule is intra-articular fractures, in which the same axioms apply.

II. Child Abuse

A. Introduction—Unfortunately, child abuse does occur and one must always be alert for the "battered child." All states now require physicians to report suspected child abuse. Suspicions should be raised when seeing fractures in children less than 3 years old (most common age group) with multiple healing bruises, skin marks, burn, unreasonable histories, signs of neglect, and so on.

B. Fracture Locations—The most common locations of fractures in children of abuse are the humerus, tibia, and femur, in that order. Skeletal surveys are appropriate, if suspicions are high, in children with delayed development, and in some metaphyseal and spiral fractures. Diaphyseal fractures are also common with abuse (four times as common as metaphyseal fractures). Skeletal surveys are not as helpful in children over 5 years old. Instead, a bone scan may be done as an alternative or an adjunctive study. Nonorthopaedic injuries found in abuse include head injuries, burns, and blunt abdominal visceral injuries.

C. Treatment—In addition to normal fracture care, early involvement of social workers and pediatricians is essential. If the abuse is missed, there is a greater than 1:3 chance of further abuse and a 5-10% chance of death in affected children.

III. Physeal Fractures

A. Introduction—Fracture of the physis, or growth plate, is more likely than injury to attached ligaments, thus assume there is a fracture of the physis until proved otherwise.

B. Characteristics—Although physeal fractures are classically thought to be through the zone of provisional calcification (within the zone of hypertrophy) of the growth plate, the fracture can be through many different layers. The blood supply of the epiphysis is tenuous, and injuries can disrupt small physeal vessels supplying the growth center. This can lead to many complications associated with these injuries (e.g., limb length discrepancies, malunion, bony bars). The most common physeal injuries occur in the distal radius, followed by the distal tibia.

C. Classification—The Salter-Harris (SH) classification modified by Rang is the gold standard for physeal injuries (Fig. 10-59, Table 10-9).

D. Treatment

1. Gentle reduction should be attempted initially for SH I and II fractures, sometimes utilizing conscious sedation protocols. With reduction and immobilization, these fractures will do well without a significant amount of growth arrest (except in the distal femur). SH III and IV fractures are intra-articular by definition and usually require ORIF. Follow-up radiographs are required for all physeal injuries. Remodeling is also common with pediatric fractures (up to 20 degrees). This depends on location and age of the patient. Tables 10-9 through 10-20 detail the tolerances for each fracture during childhood. Harris-Park growth arrest lines (transverse radiodense lines) may be the only evidence of a physeal injury on follow-up radiographs.

E. Partial Growth Arrest

1. Physeal bars or bridges result from growth plate injuries that arrest a part of the physis and leave the uninjured physis to grow normally. This results in angular growth and deformity. Physeal bridge resection with interposition of fat graft or artificial material is reserved for patients with >2 cm of growth remaining, and <50% physeal involvement. Smaller, peripheral bars in young patients have the highest success rate. MRI and CT scans can help define location and amount of physeal closure. Arrest involving >50% of the physis should be treated with ipsilateral completion of the arrest and contralateral epiphysiodesis or ipsilateral limb lengthening.

Table 10-9. SALTER-HARRIS CLASSIFICATION OF PHYSEAL INJURIES

TYPE	DESCRIPTION	PROGNOSIS
I	Transverse fractures through physis	Excellent
II	Fractures through the physis with metaphyseal fragment	Excellent
III	Fractures through physis and epiphysis	Good, but with potential for intra-articular deformity; may require ORIF
IV	Fractures through epiphysis, physis, and metaphysis	Good, but unstable fragment requires ORIF
V	Crush injury to the physis	Poor with growth arrest
VI	Injury to perichondrial ring	Good, may cause angular deformities

ORIF, open reduction and internal fixation.

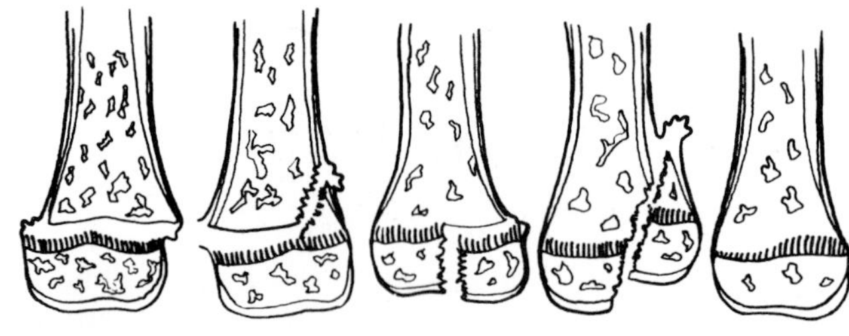

FIGURE 10-59 ■ Salter-Harris classification of injuries to the physis. (From Bora, F.W.: The Pediatric Upper Extremity. Philadelphia, WB Saunders, 1986, p. 154.)

Table 10-10. PEDIATRIC WRIST AND HAND TRAUMA

INJURY	EPONYM	CLASSIFICATION	TREATMENT	COMPLICATIONS
Phalanx fractures (Fig. 10-60)	(Watch for mallet equivalent)	Based on phalanx and SH classification	Closed reduction for most; ORIF if condylar; SH III/IV, >25 degrees if <10 yo, >10 degrees if >10 yo; dynamic traction for pilon equivalents	Residual deformities, tendon imbalance, nail deformities.
MC fractures (Fig. 10-61)		Based on location	Reduce; ORIF if irreducible	Avascular necrosis of metacarpal head
Thumb MC fractures (Fig. 10-62)	D = Bennett equivalent	A: Metaphyseal; B: SH II (medial); C: SH II (lateral); D: SH III	Closed reduction except for D, which requires ORIF	
IP dislocation			Closed reduction and splint; open reduction if irreducible, incongruous on x-ray study, or redisplaces with movement	
MCP dislocation			Attempt closed reduction; open reduction if irreducible	
CMC dislocation			Reduce with finger traps; CRPP with Kirschner wire to carpus and adjacent MC	
Distal radius		SH fractures I–V	CRPP types III & IV	Deformity, loss of reduction
	Torus	Tension side intact	SAC for 3 wk	Infection (open fracture), Volkmann's contracture
	Greenstick	Tension side with plastic deformation	Reduce if angulation >10 degrees	Growth arrest, malunion refracture, TFCC
	Complete	Both cortices disrupted	Reduce and place in LAC	Tears, carpal tunnel syndrome

SH, Salter-Harris; *ORIF*, open reduction and internal fixation; *yo*, year old; *MC*, metacarpal; *MCP*, metacarpophalangeal joint; *CMC*, carpometacarpal; *CRPP*, closed reduction/percutaneous pinning; *TFCC*, triangular fibrocartilage complex; *LAC*, long arm cast.

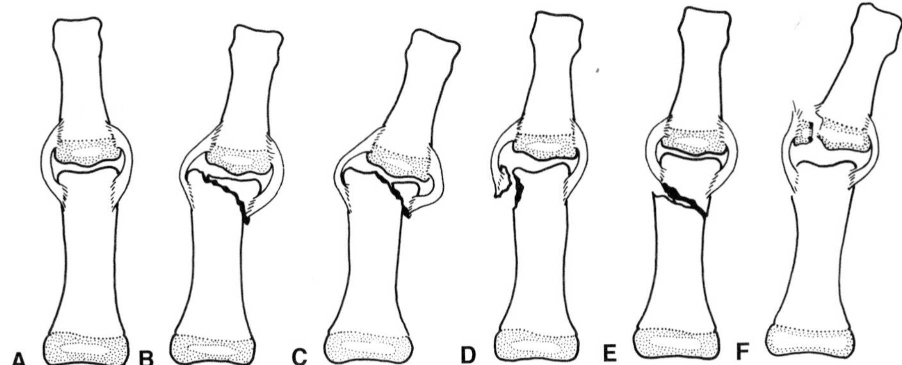

FIGURE 10-60 ■ Pediatric finger interphalangeal fractures. *A,* Normal; *B,* Unicondylar; *C,* Partial condylar; *D,* Lateral avulsion; *E,* Bicondylar; *F,* SH III. (From Ogden, J.A.: Skeletal Injury in the Child, 2nd ed. Philadelphia, WB Saunders, 1990, p. 530.)

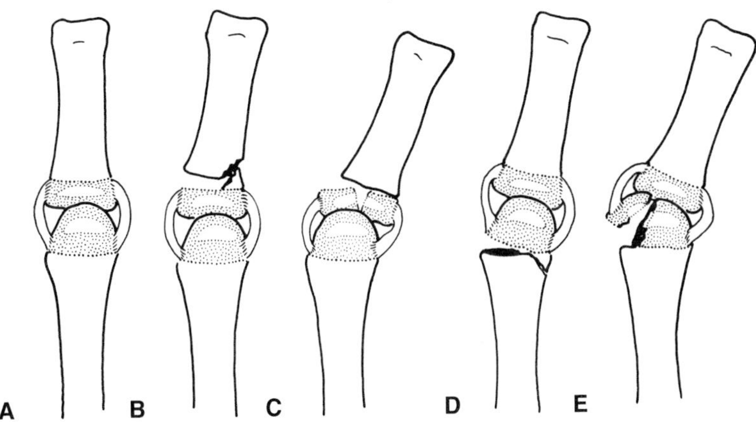

FIGURE 10-61 ■ Pediatric metacarpophalangeal (MCP) fractures. *A,* Normal; *B,* SH II proximal phalanx; *C,* SH III proximal phalanx; *D,* SH II metacarpal; *E,* SH III metacarpal. (From Ogden, J.A.: Skeletal Injury in the Child, 2nd ed. Philadelphia, WB Saunders, 1990, p. 530.)

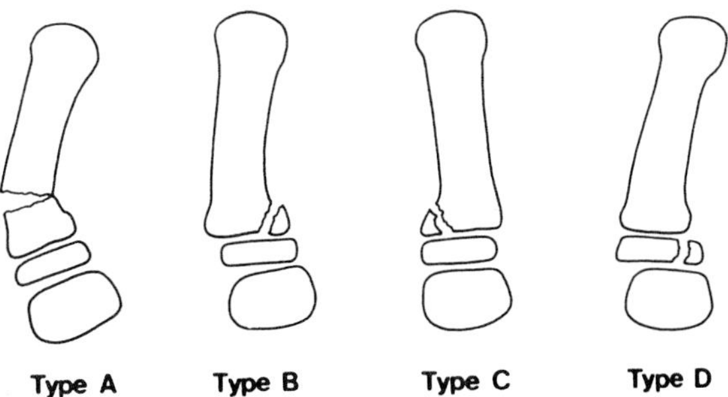

FIGURE 10-62 ■ Classification of pediatric thumb metacarpal fractures. *A,* Metaphyseal; *B,* SH II medial; *C,* SH II lateral; *D,* SH III. (From O'Brien, E.T.: Fractures of the hand and wrist region. In Rockwood, C.A., Jr., Wilkins, K.E., and King, R.E., eds.: Fractures in Children, 2nd ed. Philadelphia, JB Lippincott, 1984, p. 257.)

Table 10-11. PEDIATRIC RADIAL AND ULNAR SHAFT TRAUMA

INJURY	EPONYM	CLASSIFICATION	TREATMENT	COMPLICATIONS
Radius & ulna	Both bone	Greenstick compression complete	Correct rotation with pronation/supination with <10 degrees angulation: LAC 3–4 wk if <10 yo; bayonet opposition okay if growth remains	Refracture, limb ischemia, malunion (especially in <10 yo with inadequate reduction), nerve injury, synostosis
Plastic deformation		Based on bones involved (ulna >radius)	Reduction with pressure as a fulcrum, the most deformed bone first. Must reduce >20 degrees in 4 years; less in older children	Persistence of deformity
Ulna fx and radial head dislocation (Fig. 10-63)	Monteggia	I: Ulna angulation & radial head ant. (extension)	Reduce (traction flexion) LAC 100 degrees flexion supination	Late diagnosis (reconstruct annular ligament), decreased ROM
		II: Ulna angulation & radial head post. (flexion)	Reduce (traction extension), LAC in some extension	Missed wrist injury, nonunion, persistent radial head dislocation
		III: ulna ant. angulation, radial head lat. (adduction)	Reduce (extension), LAC 90 degrees flexion supination	Periarticular ossification
		IV: Ulna and proximal {1/3} radius fracture (both angulated ant.)	Reduce (supinate); may require ORIF	
Radial head dislocation (ant.)	Monteggia equivalent		Supination & pressure on radial head LAC 100 degrees of flexion supination	Synostosis, PIN injury, loss of reduction
Ulna fx and radial neck fx	Check for Monteggia equivalent		Reduce (traction pressure on radial head varus stress) LAC at 90 degrees	
Ulna fx & proximal radius fx	Check for Monteggia equivalent		Reduce (traction supination) LAC 90 degrees supination	
Radius fx & distal radioulnar dislocation	Galeazzi		Reduce (traction supination if ulna dorsal; pronation if ulna volar); ORIF if >12 yo or reduction fails	Malunion, nerve injury (AIN), RU subluxation, loss of radial bow

yo, year old; *fx*, fracture; *LAC*, long arm cast; *ROM*, range of motion; *PIN*, posterior interosseous nerve; *AIN*, anterior interosseous nerve; *RU*, radioulnar.

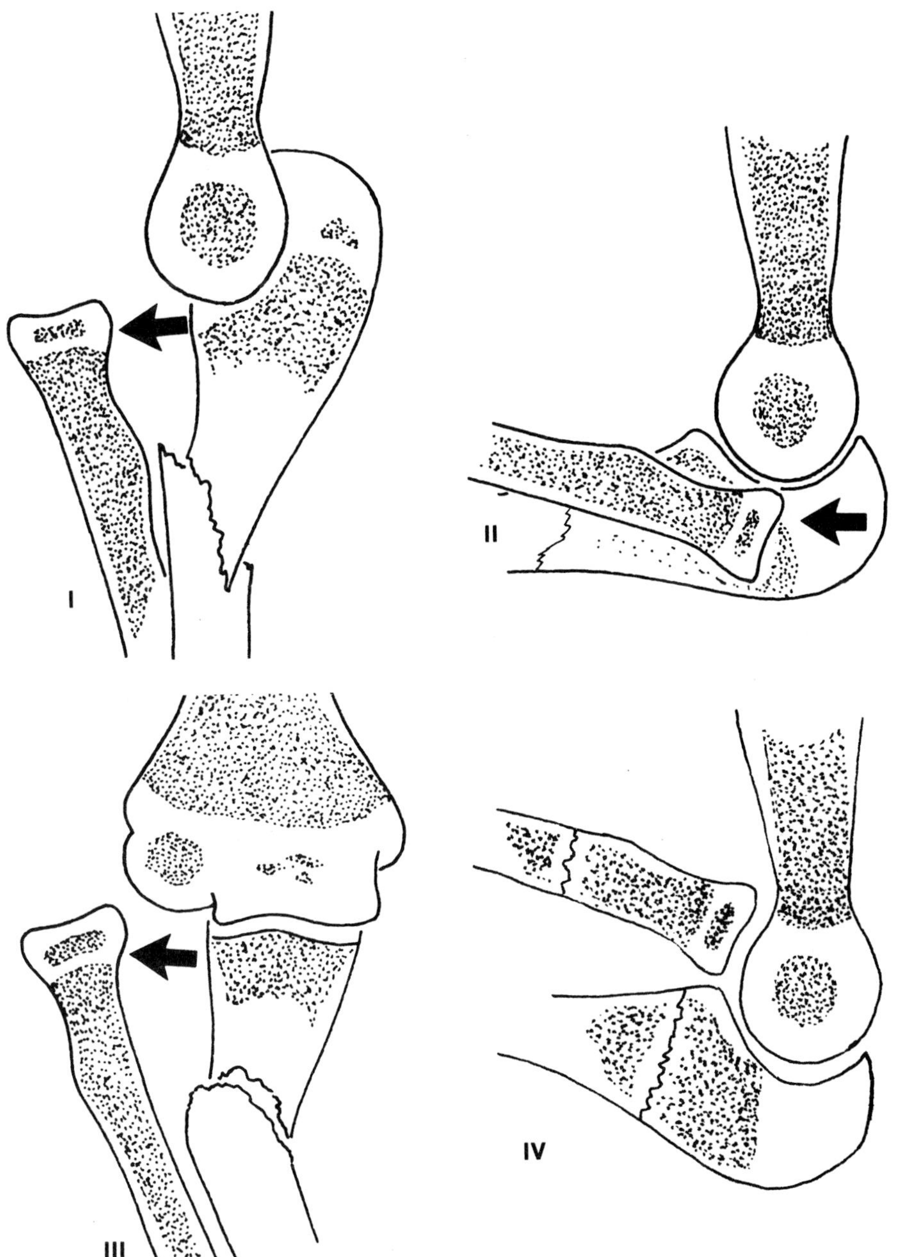

FIGURE 10-63 ■ Pediatric Monteggia fractures. *I,* Anterior; *II,* Posterior; *III,* Lateral; *IV,* BB fracture. (*I–III* from Ogden, J.A.: Skeletal Injury in the Child, 2nd ed. Philadelphia, WB Saunders, 1990, p. 480–481.)

Table 10-12. PEDIATRIC ELBOW TRAUMA

INJURY	EPONYM	CLASSIFICATION	TREATMENT	COMPLICATIONS
Supracondylar (6–8 yo) (Fig. 10-64)		I: Extension (98%), undisplaced	Immobilize 3 wk	Nerve injury (AIN & radial), vascular injury (1%); decreased ROM; if pulse present but then lost, explore; if no pulse but pink hand, watch; if no pulse and cold, explore
		II: displaced (posterior cortex intact)	Reduce; cast vs. CRPP (must re-create Baumann's angle) (Fig. 10-65)	HO, cubitus varus (5–10%), ipsilateral fxs
		III: displaced	Reduce; CRPP vs. open pinning	
		Flexion (distal fragment ant.)	Reduce in extension; CRPP vs. casting in extension	Nerve injury (ulnar), malunion-decreased extension
Lateral condyle (6 yo) (Fig. 10-66)		Milch I: SH IV, II: SH II into trochlea	Minimally displaced (<2 mm), splint; displaced, ORIF with pins or cannulated screws	Overgrowth/spur "fish tail deformity," nonunion, cubitus valgus, AVN, ulnar nerve palsy
Medial condyle (9–14 yo)		Nondisplaced: <10mm displacement; displaced: >10 mm displacement	Minimally displaced, splint; displaced, ORIF	Cubitus varus, AVN
Entire distal humeral physis (<7 yo) (Fig. 10-67)		A: infant (SH I); B: 7mo–3 yo (SH I); C: 3–7 yo (SH II)	Closed reduction, LAC; displaced, CRPP	Child abuse, common late dx, cubitus varus
Medial epicondylar apophysis (11 yo) (Fig. 10-68)		I: Acute injuries		Highly associated with elbow dislocation (50%), valgus instability, loss of extension
		A: Undisplaced	Immobilize 1 wk	
		B: Minimally displaced	Immobilize 1 wk	
		C: Significantly displaced (may be dislocated)	ORIF for valgus instability, otherwise early ROM	
		D: Entrapment of fragment in joint	Manipulative extraction ORIF (especially with ulnar nerve entrapment)	
		E: Fracture through epicondylar apophysis	Immobilization vs. ORIF	
	Little League elbow	II: Chronic tension stress injury	Change in throwing activities	
T condylar fx		Based on fracture	ORIF	Decreased ROM
Radial head/neck (>4 yo) (Fig. 10-69)		A: SH I or II physeal fracture; B: SH IV fracture; C: transmetaphyseal fracture; D: with elbow dislocation; E: with elbow dislocation	Immobilize if <60 degrees pronation/supination; ORIF if markedly displaced or >60 degrees primarily	Decreased ROM, radial head overgrowth, neck notching, AVN synostosis, nonunion
Proximal olecranon physis (rare)		I: Physeal-metaphyseal border (younger children) II: Physis with large metaphyseal fragment (older children)	ORIF if significantly displaced	Watch for osteogenesis imperfecta, epiphyseal overgrowth spurs
Olecranon metaphysis		A: Flexion	If undisplaced (<3 mm), immobilize 3 wk; ORIF if defect	Rare: delay/nonunion
		B: Extension	Reduction in extension	
		C: Shear	Immobilize in hyperflexion	ORIF if periosteal tear
Elbow dislocation (11–20 yo)		Based on direction of dislocation	Reduction and cast for <2 wk	Watch for associated fractures and nerve injuries (ulnar > median), HO, recurrent dislocation
Radial head subluxation (15 mo–3 yo)	Nursemaid's elbow	Stretching of annular ligaments	Reduce (supination flexion)	Unreduced subluxations, recurrence, irreducible (rare)

yo, year old; *CRPP*, closed reduction/percutaneous pinning; *HO*, heterotopic ossification; *AVN*, avascular necrosis; *SH*, Salter-Harris; *LAC*, long arm cast; *dx*, diagnosis; *ORIF*, open reduction and internal fixation; *ROM*, range of motion.

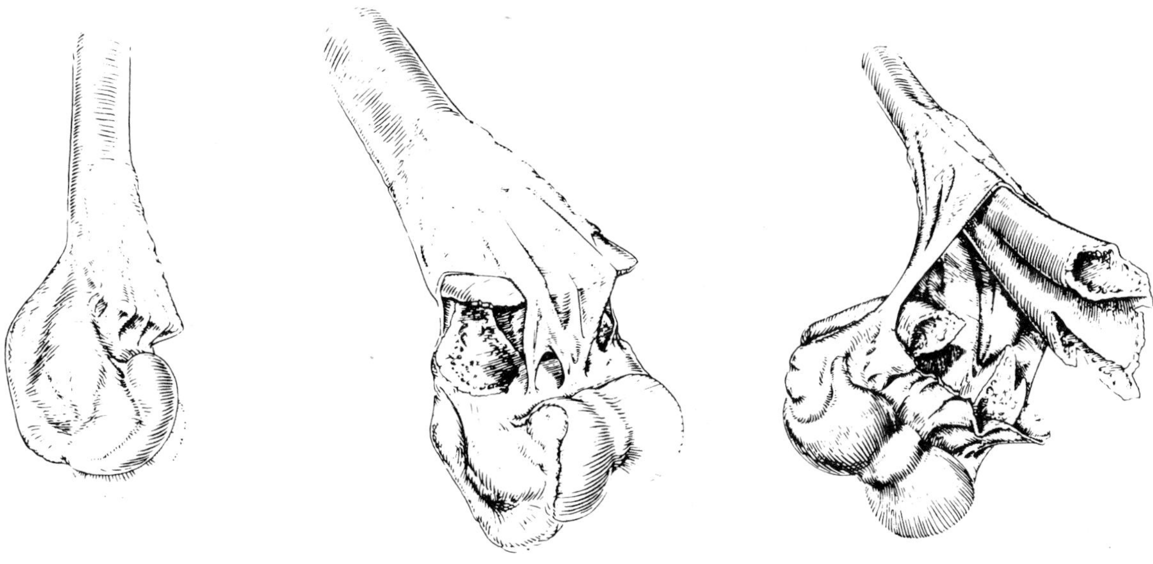

FIGURE 10-64 ■ Supracondylar fractures. (From Abraham, E., et al,: Experimental hyperextension supracondylar fractures in monkeys. Clin. Orthop. 171:313, 314, 1982.)

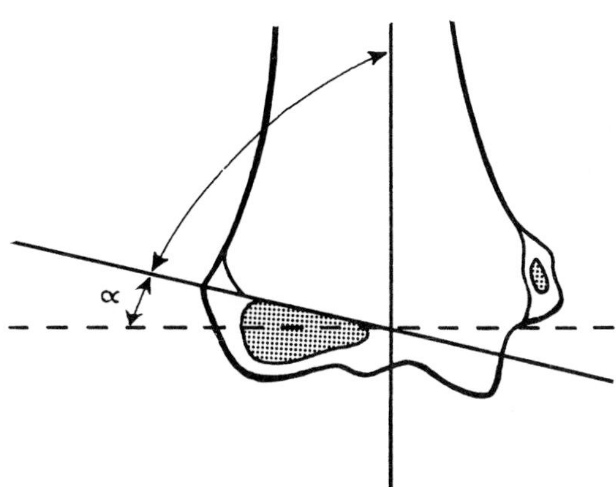

FIGURE 10-65 ■ Baumann's angle is created by the intersection of a line drawn down the proximal margin of the capitellare ossification center and a line drawn perpendicular to the long axis of the humeral shaft. (From Herring, J.A.: Tachdjian's Pediatric Orthopaedics, 3rd ed. Philadelphia, WB Saunders, 2002, p. 2145.)

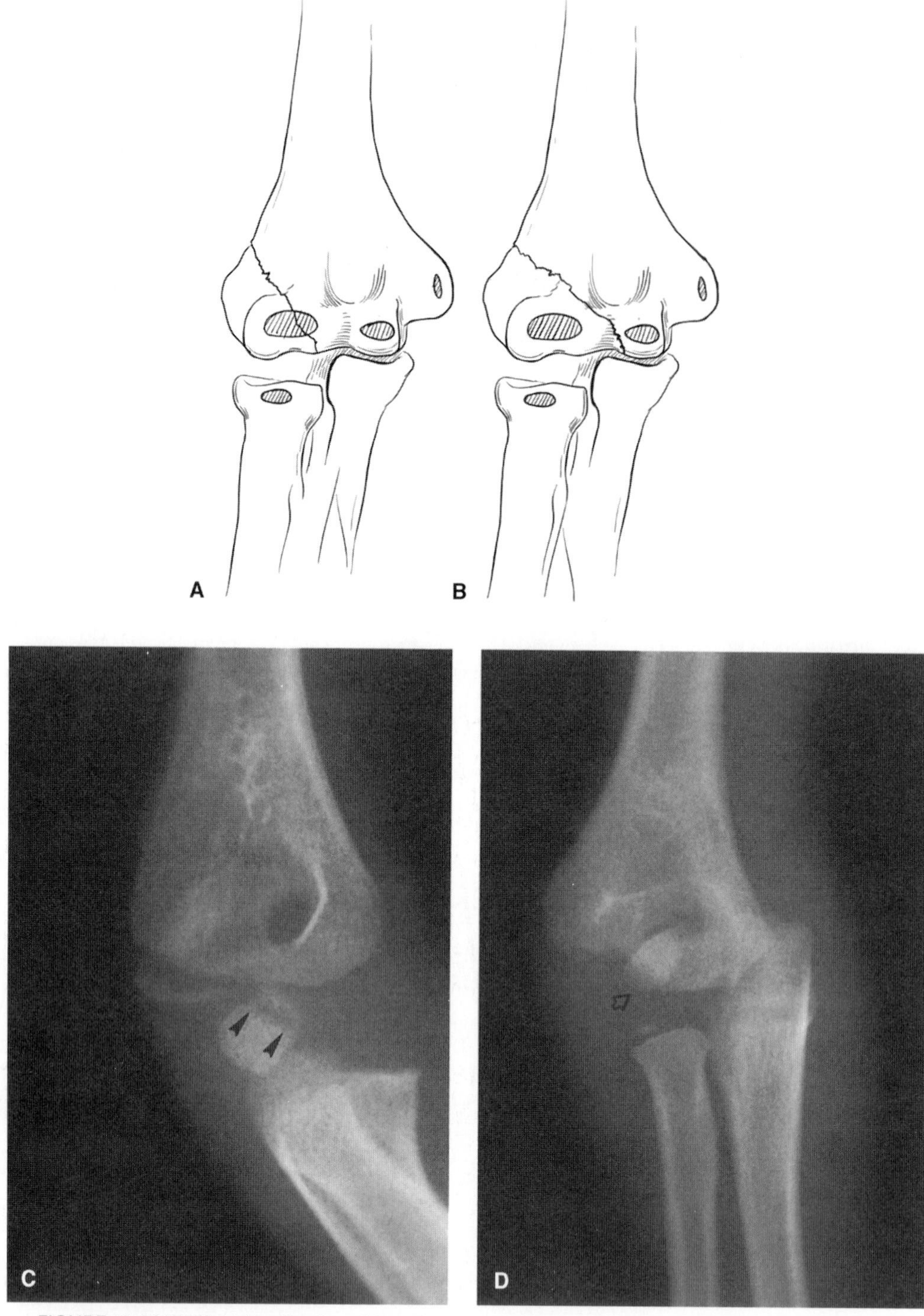

FIGURE 10-66 ■ Milch classification of lateral condyle fractures. *A,* Type I—the fracture extends through the secondary ossification center of the capitellum. *B,* Type II—the fracture crosses the epiphysis and enters the joint medial to trochlear groove. (From Herring, J.A.: Tachdjian's Pediatric Orthopaedics, 3rd ed. Philadelphia, WB Saunders, 2002, p. 2179.)

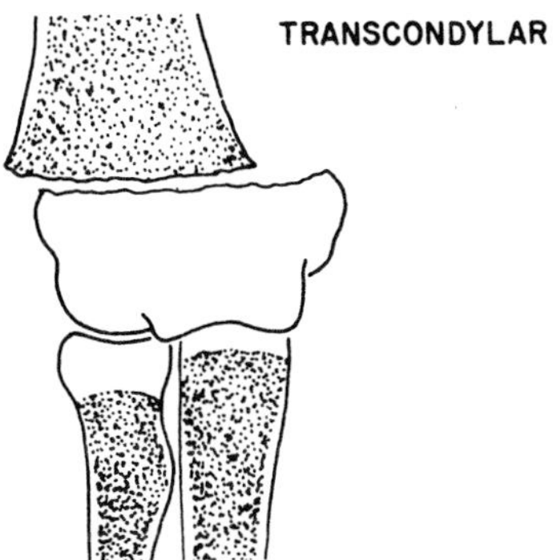

FIGURE 10-67 ■ Total condylar fracture. (From Ogden, J.A.: Skeletal Injury in the Child, 2nd ed. Philadelphia, WB Saunders, 1990, p. 388.)

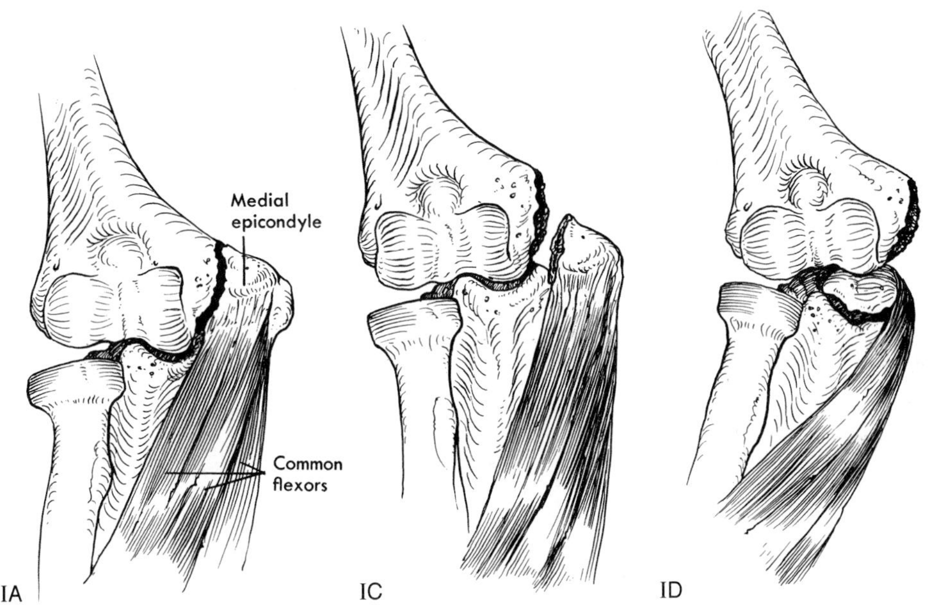

FIGURE 10-68 ■ Medial epicondyle fractures. *IA,* Undisplaced; *IC,* Displaced; *ID,* Entrapped. (From Tachdjian, M.O.: Pediatric Orthopaedics, 2nd ed. Philadelphia, WB Saunders, 1990, p. 3122.)

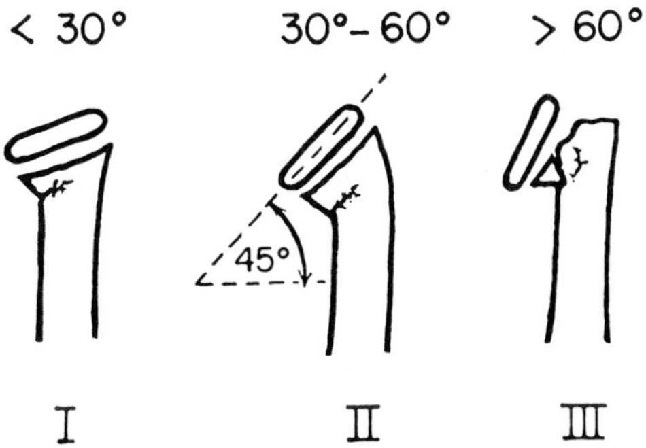

FIGURE 10-69 ■ Radial head fractures. (From Tachdjian, M.O.: Pediatric Orthopaedics, 2nd ed. Philadelphia, WB Saunders, 1990, p. 3140.)

Table 10-13. PEDIATRIC SHOULDER TRAUMA

INJURY	EPONYM	CLASSIFICATION	TREATMENT	COMPLICATIONS
Humeral shaft		Neonate	Small splint or splint to side	Compartment syndrome, radial nerve palsy, rotational deformity
		<3 yo	Collar and cuff (okay if <12 yo) growth disturbance (<15 mm not noticeable)	
		3–12 yo	Figure of eight brace	
		>12 yo	Figure of eight brace	
Proximal humeral physis		SH (I most common in <5 yo)	Sling if minimally displaced, gentle manipulation for displaced fractures; PCP vs. ORIF for <50% opposition, >45 degrees angulation	
Proximal humeral metaphysis (common)		Based on location	Sling	
Midshaft clavicle		≤2 yo	Supportive sling if symptomatic	Rare: malunion or nonunion neurovascular compromise
		>2 yo	Figure eight vs. sling	
Medial clavicle		Usually SH I or II physeal separations	Sling for 1 wk	
Lateral clavicle		I: Nondisplaced; intact AC & CC ligaments IIA: Clavicle displaced superiorly; fx medial to CC ligament IIB: Clavicle displaced superiorly; conoid ligament tear	Sling vs. figure eight; may use ORIF type II	
AC joint (Fig. 10-70)		Same as adult	Same as adult	Watch for coracoid fracture
SC joint		Ant. & post.	Same as adult	
Clavicle dislocation (rare)			Open reduction with repair of periosteal tube	
Scapula fractures		Based on location	Same as adult	
Glenohumeral dislocation		Traumatic vs. nontraumatic	Initial immobilization followed by rehabilitation; reconstruction for recurrent instability	Recent research shows >60% chance of redislocation when patient is <21 yo

yo, year old; *SH*, Salter-Harris; *PCP*, percutaneous pin fixation; *AC*, acromioclavicular; *CC*, coracoclavicular; *SC*, sternoclavicular.

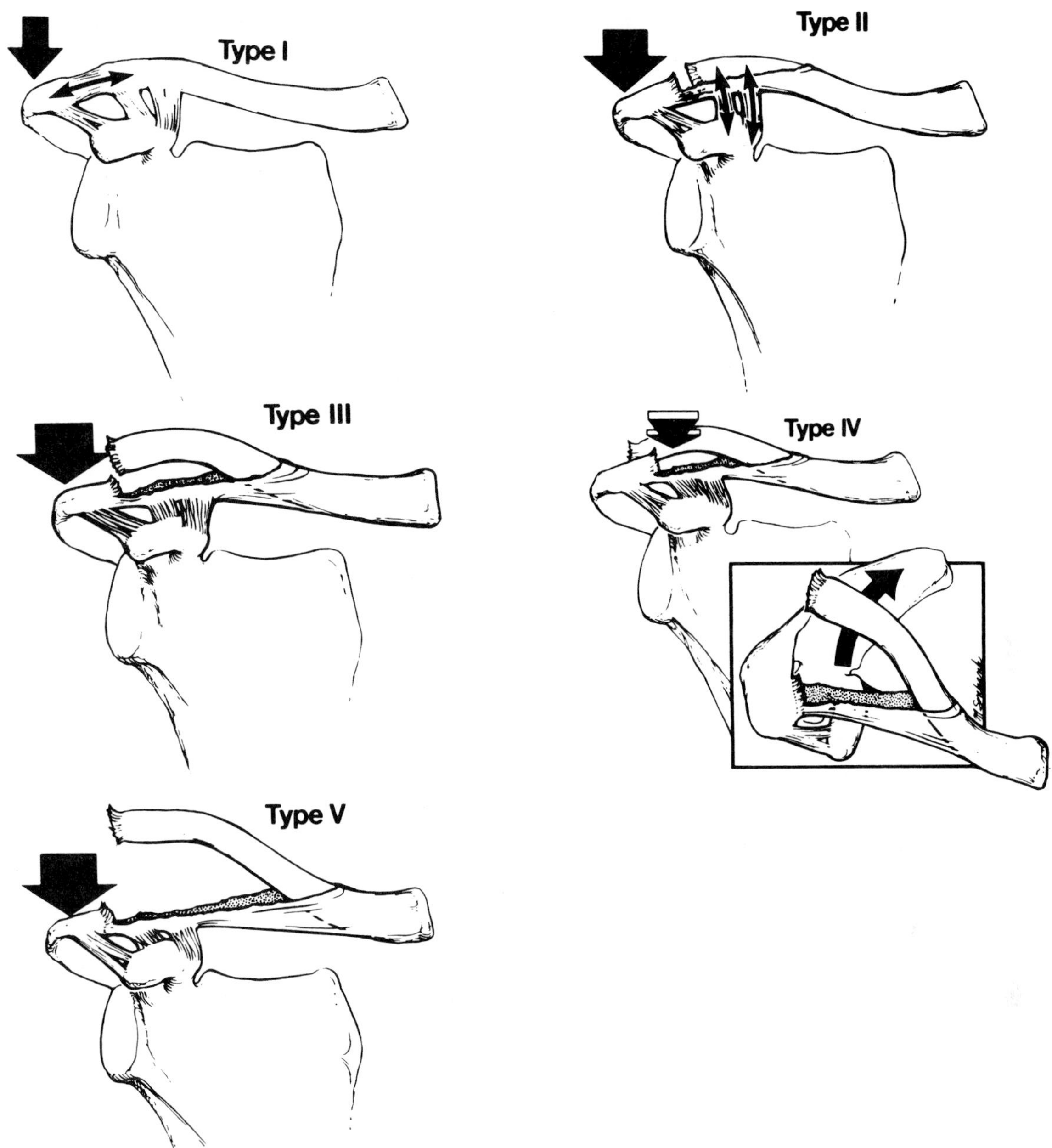

FIGURE 10-70 ■ Classification of pediatric acromioclavicular (AC) injuries. (From Rockwood, C.A., Jr., Wilkins, K.E., and King, R.E., eds.: Fractures in Children, 2nd ed. Philadelphia, JB Lippincott, 1984, p. 636.)

Table 10-14. PEDIATRIC SPINE TRAUMA

INJURY	EPONYM	CLASSIFICATION	TREATMENT	COMPLICATIONS
Occiput–C1 dissociations			Reduced with traction; craniovertebral fusion later	Often fatal
C1–C2 dissociations		Traumatic ligament disruption	Reduce in extension; immobilize with halo for 8–12 wk	Vertebral artery is a risk with surgery
	Grisel's syndrome	Ligament laxity from local inflammation	Traction immobilize for 6–8 wk	
	Rotatory subluxation	I: Without C1 shift; II: <5 mm C1 ant. shift; III: >5 mm C1 ant. shift; IV: post. shift	I: Soft collar; II, III, & IV: Traction & immobilization 6 wk, C1–C2 fusion if recurrence/neurologic injury	
		Odontoid-physeal or os odontoindeum	Reduce (hyperextension). Immobilize in halo for 12 wk	Less nonunion for type II vs. adults
C2–C3 dislocation		True vs. pseudo (more likely)		
Cervical facet dislocation			Same as adults	
Thoracic and lumbar fxs		Same as adults	Same as adults	
Spondylosis		Stress fx of pars (likely at L5–S1)	Acute: immobilize in brace; otherwise surgical treatment; fusion for refractory cases	
Spinal cord injury without radiographic abnormality (SCIWORA)		Spinal cord injury without radiographic abnormality	Evaluation with MRI and supportive treatment	Scoliosis (especially <8 yo)

MRI, magnetic resonance imaging; *yo*, year old.

Table 10-15. PEDIATRIC PELVIC TRAUMA

INJURY	EPONYM	CLASSIFICATION	TREATMENT	COMPLICATIONS
Pelvic Fractures				
		Key and Cornwell's		In general, less than adults
		I: Ring intact (Figs. 10-71and 72)		
		Avulsions (ASIS AIIS IT)	BR flexed hip for 2 wk; guarded WB for 4 wk	Loss of reduction, delayed union,
		Pubis/ischium	BR 3–7 days; limited WB for 4 wk	DJD, malunion, organ injury
	Duverney	Iliac wing	BR with leg abducted; progress to WB	Sacral nerve injury
		Sacrum/coccyx	BR 3–6 wk, if severe (sacral)	
		II: Single break in ring (Fig. 10-73)		
		Ipsilateral ramii	BR 2–4 wk; non-WB	
		Symphysis pubis	BR with sling or spica	
		SI joint (rare)	BR with progressive WB	
		III: Double break in ring (see Fig. 10-73)		
	Straddle	Bilateral pubic ramii	BR with flexed hip 2–4 wk	Often unstable with associated injuries
	Malgaigne	Ant. & post. ring with migration	Skeletal traction; external fixator for 3–6 wk	
		IV: Acetabular fractures		
		Small fragment with dislocation	BR with progress to ambulation	
		Linear: Nondisplaced	Treat associated pelvic fracture	
		Linear: Hip unstable	Skeletal traction; ORIF if incongruous	
		Central	Lateral traction for reduction; ORIF if severe	HO, especially with ORIF

BR, bed rest; *ASIS*, anterior superior iliac spine; *AIIS*, anterior inferior iliac spine; *IT*, ischial tuberosity.

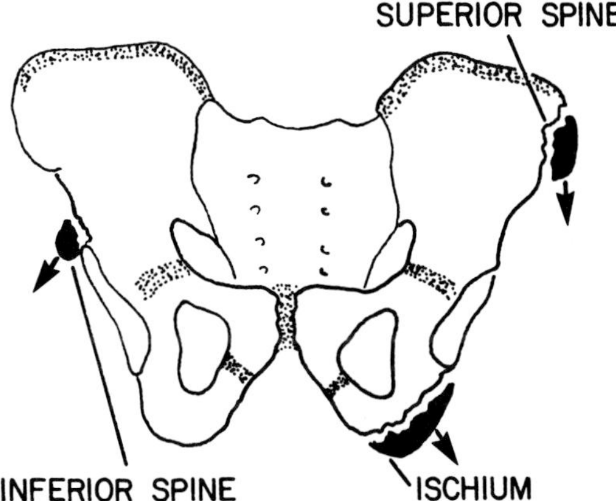

FIGURE 10-71 ■ Avulsion fractures of the pelvis. *Superior spine,* Sartorius avulsion; *Inferior spine,* Rectus avulsion; *Ischium,* Hamstring avulsion. (From Ogden, J.A.: Skeletal Injury in the Child, 2nd ed. Philadelphia, WB Saunders, 1990, p. 635.)

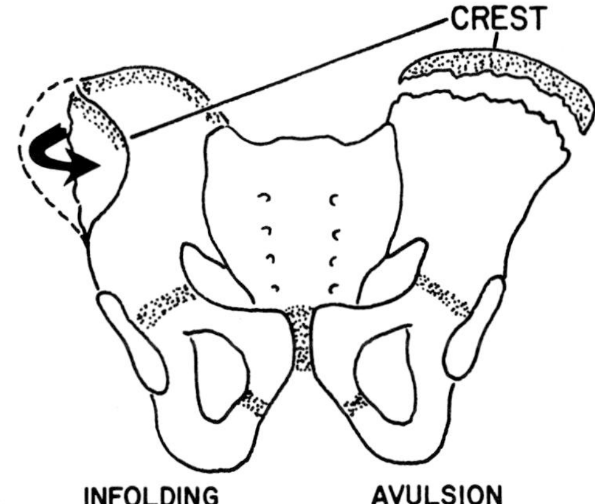

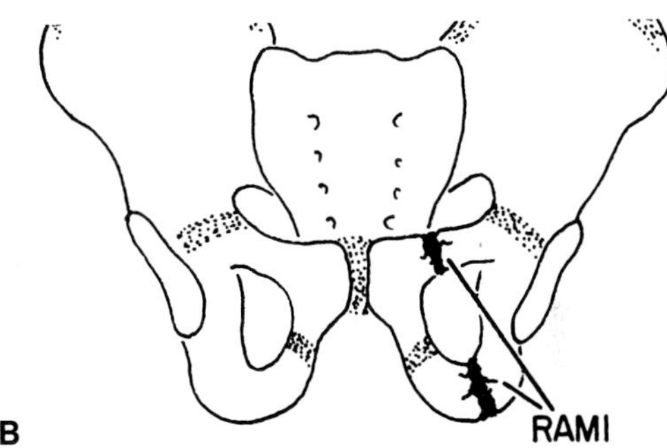

FIGURE 10-72 ■ Stable pelvic fractures. (From Ogden, J.A.: Skeletal Injury in the Child, 2nd ed. Philadelphia, WB Saunders, 1990, p. 634.)

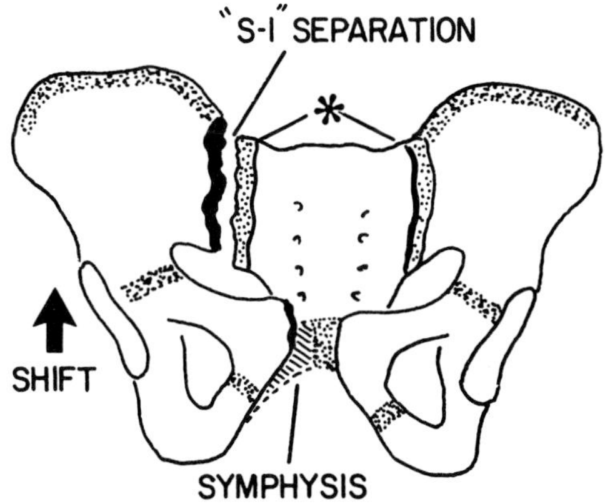

FIGURE 10-73 ■ Unstable pelvic fractures. (From Ogden, J.A.: Skeletal Injury in the Child, 2nd ed. Philadelphia, WB Saunders, 1990, p. 388.)

Table 10-16. PEDIATRIC HIP TRAUMA

INJURY	EPONYM	CLASSIFICATION	TREATMENT	COMPLICATIONS
Hip fractures (Fig. 10-74)				
		Delbet		
		IA: Transepiphyseal with dislocation	Closed reduction or ORIF with pin	AVN close to 100%
		IB: Transepiphyseal without dislocation	CRPP with spica	AVN in up to 60%
		II: Transcervical	CRPP with spica	Coxa vara (25%): Treat with subtrochanteric valgus osteotomy
		IIIA: Cervical trochanteric (displaced)	CRPP with spica	Nonunion (6%)
		IIIB: Cervical trochanteric (nondisplaced)	Spica cast in abduction	Growth arrest
		IV: Intertrochanteric	Spica cast: ORIF if unstable	May cross physis if it creates greater fracture stability
Femoral neck stress fx				
		Devas		
		Superior transverse	CRPP (otherwise displaces)	Displacement causes more problems: Varus deformities
		Inferior (compressive)	NWB	
Traumatic dislocation		Post. or ant.	Closed reduction: Open if incongruous joint	AVN (10%) recurrent dislocation HO DJD

AVN, avascular necrosis; *CRPP*, closed reduction/percutaneous pinning; *fx*, fracture; *NWB*, non-weight-bearing; *HO*, heterotopic ossification; *DJD*, degenerative joint disease.

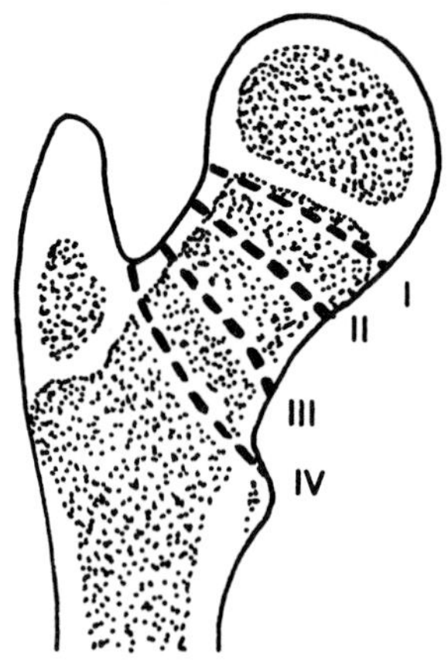

FIGURE 10-74 ■ Femoral neck fractures in children. *I*, Transepiphyseal; *II*, Transcervical; *III*, Cervical-trochanteric; *IV*, Intertrochanteric. (From Ogden, J.A.: Skeletal Injury in the Child, 2nd ed. Philadelphia, WB Saunders, 1990, p. 689.)

Table 10-17. PEDIATRIC FEMORAL SHAFT TRAUMA

INJURY	EPONYM	CLASSIFICATION	TREATMENT	COMPLICATIONS
Femur fracture (to include subtrochanteric fractures)		≤6 yo	Spica cast: May need period of traction if >2 cm short followed by spica casting	LLD: Angular deformity (avoid >10 degrees frontal and >30 degrees sagittal malalignment
		6–13 yo	Current trend to use flexible titanium nails with possible additional immobilization but may also use ex-fix (higher refracture rate) plate (need to remove and causes large scar formation) or traction (rare)	Rotational deformity >10 degrees); expect 0.9 centimeter overgrowth in <10 yo.
		≥14 yo (skeletally mature)	IM nail	AVN reported with IM nails in children with growth remaining

yo, year old; *LLD*, leg length discrepancy; *ex-fix*, external fixation; *IM*, intramedullary; *AVN*, avascular necrosis.

Table 10-18. PEDIATRIC KNEE TRAUMA

INJURY	EPONYM	CLASSIFICATION	TREATMENT	COMPLICATIONS
Distal femoral epiphysis (Figs. 10-75–10-77)	"Wagon wheel"	SH I–IV (II most common)	Closed reduction: LLC; CRPP in SH III or IV; open if soft tissue interposition or displaced III & IV	Popliteal artery or peroneal nerve injury, recurrent displacement; growth plate injuries because of undulating physis
Proximal tibial epiphysis		SH I–IV (II most common)	Nondisplaced: LLC in 30° of flexion; displaced: CRPP	**Popliteal artery injury**, growth plate injury
Floating knee		Letts		
		A: Both fractures diaphyseal	ORIF in one; closed reduction in the other	Infection, nonunion, malunion, injuries
		B: One fracture diaphyseal & one metaphyseal	ORIF diaphyseal & closed reduction of metaphyseal	
		C: One fracture diaphyseal & one epiphyseal	CRPP epiphyseal fx & ORIF diaphyseal	
		D: One fracture open & one closed	Débride/ex-fix open & closed reduction of closed fx	
		E: Both fx open	Débride/ex-fix both	
Tibial tubercle avulsion (14–16 yo in jumping sport) (Fig. 10-78)		Odgen		
		1: Small distal piece fractured	If minimally displaced with extension then cast; otherwise ORIF	Genu recurvatum, decreased ROM, laxity
		2: Fx at junction of primary and secondary oss centers		
		3: Fx through one epiphysis (SH III)		
Tibial spine (most common hemarthrosis in preadolescent) (Fig. 10-79)		Meyers & McKeever		
		I: Incomplete/ nondisplaced	Attempt closed reduction in extension for all; if remains displaced then may use arthroscope and ACL guide to fix with suture	Meniscal entrapment
		II: Hinged (posterior rim intact)		
		III: Completely displaced		
Patella		Undisplaced	Aspiration and cast vs. brace in 5° of flexion	Patella alta, extensor lag, infection
		Displaced (>2 mm)	ORIF with tension band	
	Sleeve fx (Fig. 10-80)	Avulsion of the distal pole & articular cartilage	ORIF with tension band	
Femorotibial dislocations		Same as adult	Same as adult: Arteriogram	Popliteal artery injury
Patella dislocations			Closed-reduction cast for 3 wk; consider fixing MPFL; open if fragment	Predisposition: Down's syndrome arthrogryposis

SH, Salter-Harris; *LLC*, long leg cast; *CRPP*, closed reduction/percutaneous pinning; *ORIF*, open reduction and internal fixation; *fx*, fracture; *ex-fix*, external fixation; *ACL*, anterior cruciate ligament; *MPFL*, medial patellofemoral ligament.

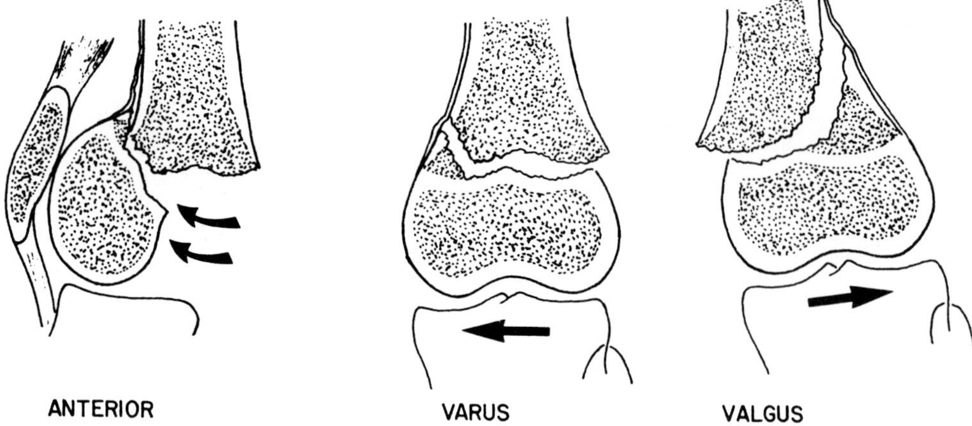

FIGURE 10-75 ■ Distal femoral physeal fractures. (From Ogden, J.A.: Skeletal Injury in the Child, 2nd ed. Philadelphia, WB Saunders, 1990, p. 725.)

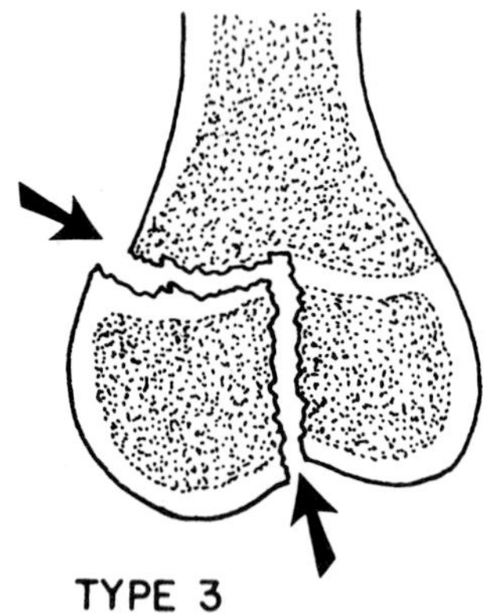

FIGURE 10-76 ■ Distal femoral Salter-Harris III fracture. (From Ogden, J.A.: Skeletal Injury in the Child, 2nd ed. Philadelphia, WB Saunders, 1990, p. 727.)

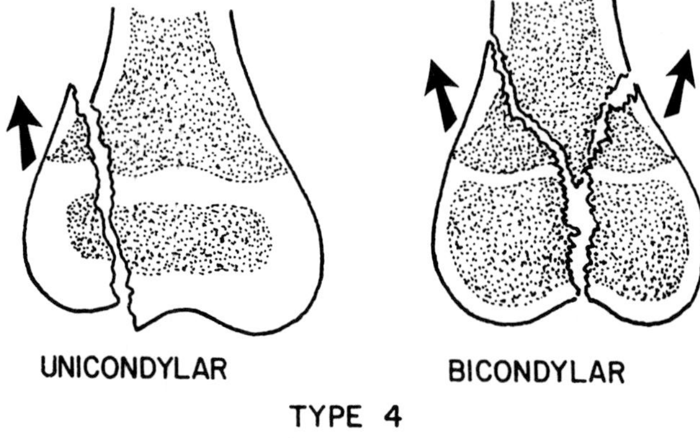

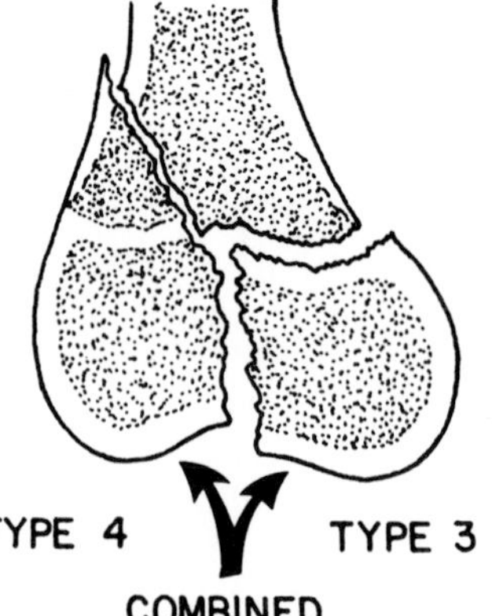

FIGURE 10-77 ■ Salter-Harris III and IV fractures of the distal femur. (From Ogden, J.A.: Skeletal Injury in the Child, 2nd ed. Philadelphia, WB Saunders, 1990, p. 689.)

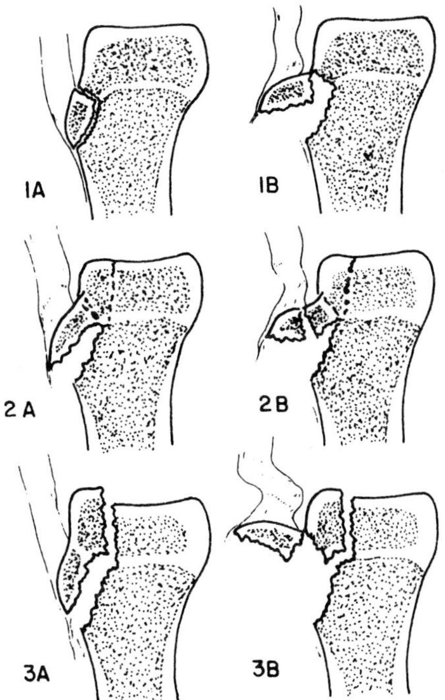

FIGURE 10-78 ■ Fractures of the tibial tubercle. (From Ogden, J.A.: Skeletal Injury in the Child, 2nd ed. Philadelphia, WB Saunders, 1990, p. 808.)

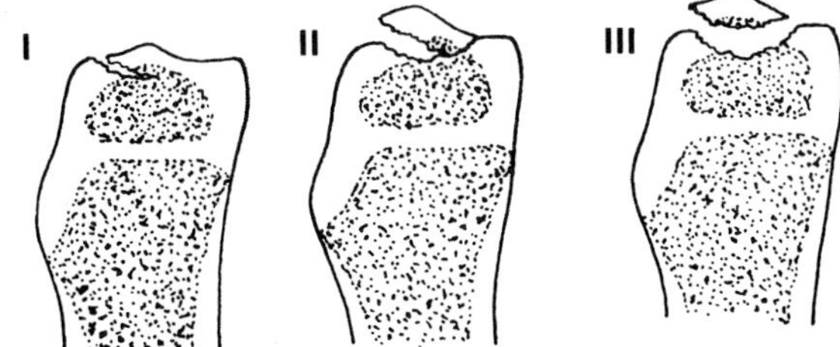

FIGURE 10-79 ■ Tibial spine fractures. (From Ogden, J.A.: Skeletal Injury in the Child, 2nd ed. Philadelphia, WB Saunders, 1990, p. 689.)

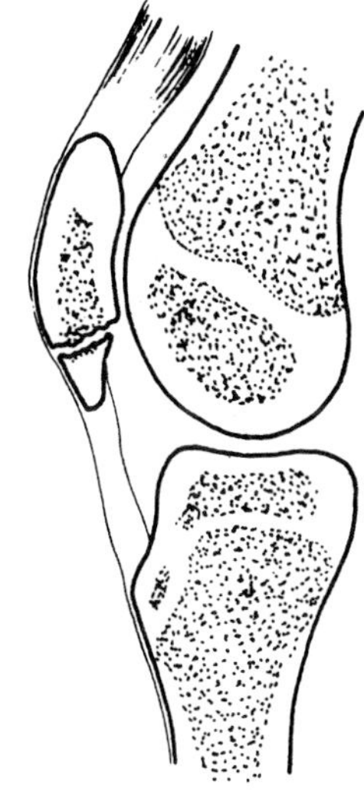

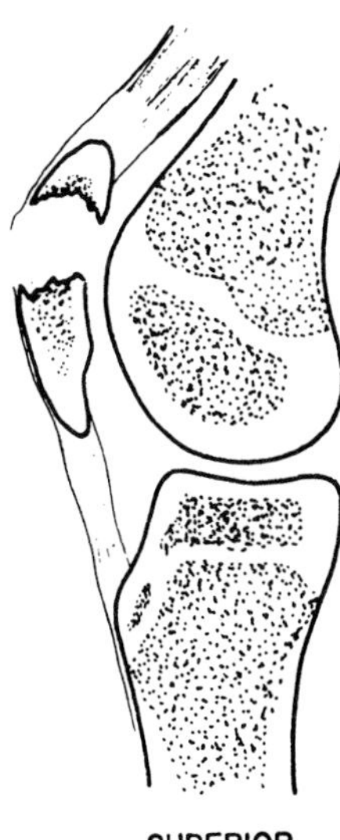

FIGURE 10-80 ■ Patellar sleeve fractures. (From Ogden, J.A.: Skeletal Injury in the Child, 2nd ed. Philadelphia, WB Saunders, 1990, p. 762.)

Table 10-19. PEDIATRIC TIBIAL SHAFT TRAUMA

INJURY	EPONYM	CLASSIFICATION	TREATMENT	COMPLICATIONS
Tibia-fibula	Greenstick	Incomplete	LLC in slight flexion for 6–8 wk unless >10 degrees AP or >5 degrees V/V then must do manipulation	Angular deformity (valgus)
		Complete	Closed reduction and cast	LLD (may see overgrowth with <10 yo), malrotation, vascular injury
Tibial spiral	Toddler's	Spiral tibia fx in <6 yo	LLC 3–4 wk	
Bike spoke injury		Soft tissue disruption	Admit and observe	Compartment syndrome, need for soft tissue coverage
Proximal tibial metaphysis (Fig. 10-81)	Cozen's	Greenstick in 3–6 yo (complete in older children)	LLC in varus for 6 wk	Genu valgum arterial injury, physeal injury

LLC, long leg cast; *AP*, anteroposterior; *V/V*, varus or valgus; *yo*, year old; *fx*, fracture.

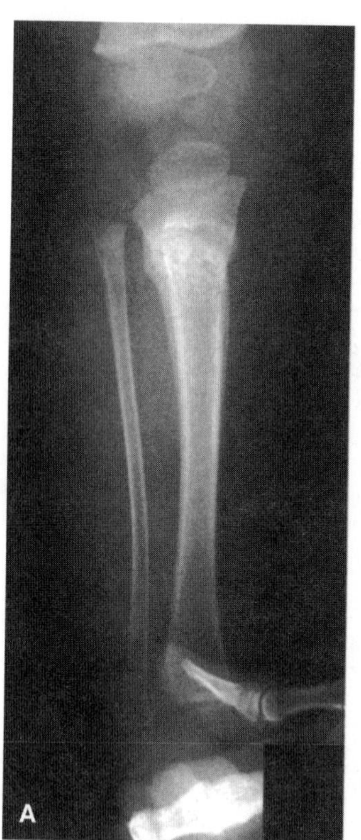

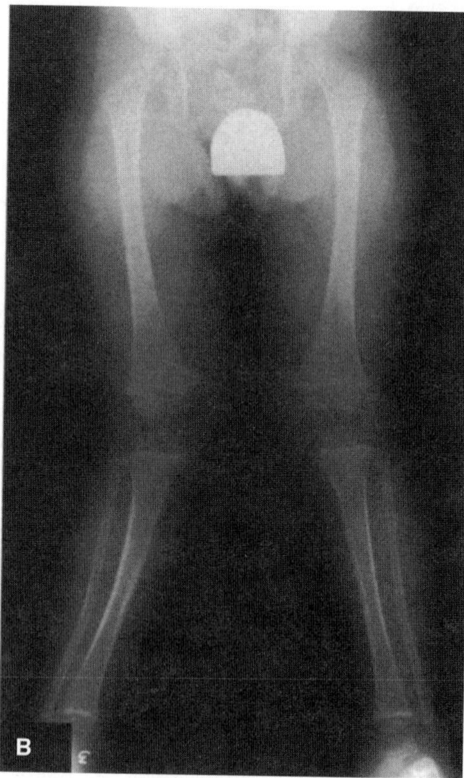

FIGURE 10-81 ■ Valgus deformity following a proximal metaphyseal tibial fracture in a 3-year-old boy. *A,* Radiograph showing healing at 4 weeks. *B,* One year later there was obvious valgus deformity on the injured leg. (From Herring, J.A.: Tachdjian's Pediatric Orthopaedics, 3rd ed. Philadelphia, WB Saunders, 2002, p. 2374.)

Table 10-20. PEDIATRIC ANKLE AND FOOT TRAUMA

INJURY	EPONYM	CLASSIFICATION	TREATMENT	COMPLICATIONS
Ankle fractures		Salter-Harris (SH) and Dias-Tachdjian (Fig. 10-82)	If SH I or II injury then treat with SLWC; if SH III or IV then with CRPP after reduction vs. ORIF if not acceptable	Angular deformity, bony bridge (poor prognosis with distal tibia) LLD, DJD, Rotational deformity, AVN
	Juvenile Tillaux (Fig. 10-83)	SH III of lateral tibial physis (because medial is closed in this age group)	May use LLC if <2 mm displacement; if greater, treat with ORIF and visualization of joint line	
	Wagstaff	SH III of distal fibular physis	Closed reduction and cast; open if required	
	Triplane (Fig. 10-84)	Complex SH IV with components in all three planes	ORIF if >2 mm articular step-off (fixation achieved parallel to physis in metaphysis and epiphysis	Must use CT to delineate fracture
Talus		Same as adult	Closed reduction and cast unless >5 mm or 5° of displacement	AVN
Calcaneus	Essex-Lopresti	Same as adult	Same as adult	
Tarsometatarsal		Fx of base of second metatarsal and cuboid fracture	Closed reduction vs. CRPP if unstable	
Base of the fifth metatarsal	Same as adult	Same as adult	Same as adult	Nonunion

SLWC, short-leg walking cast; *CRPP*, closed reduction/percutaneous pinning; *ORIF*, open reduction and internal fixation; *LLD*, leg length discrepancy; *DJD*, degenerative joint disease; *AVN*, avascular necrosis; *LLC*, long leg cast; *CT*, computed tomography; *fx*, fracture.

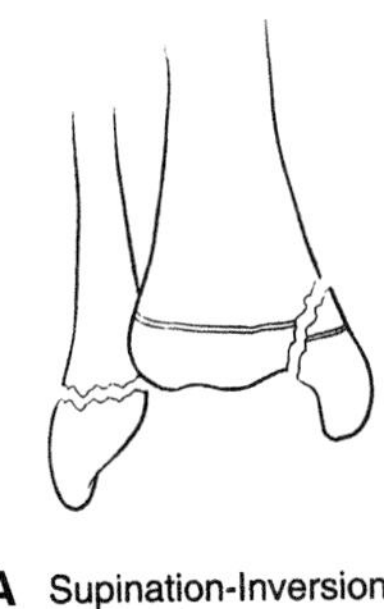

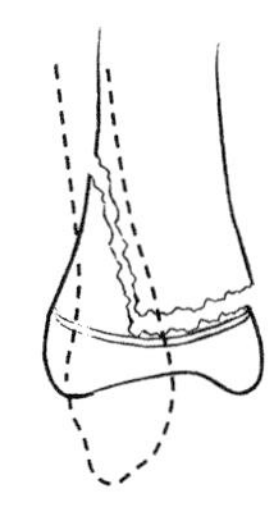

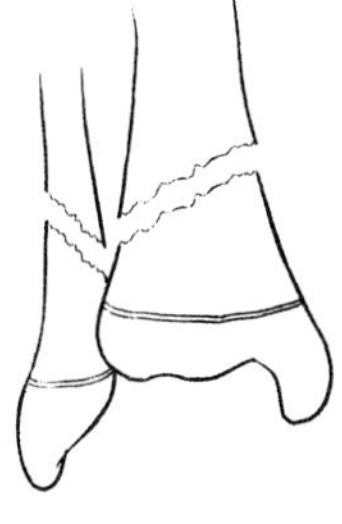

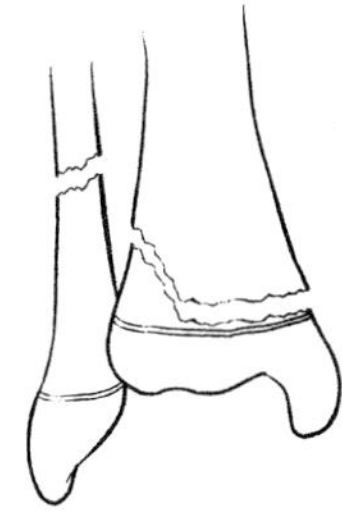

FIGURE 10-82 ■ The Dias-Tachdjian modification of the Lauge-Hansen classification of ankle fractures in children (*A-D*). (From Herring, J.A.: Tachdjian's Pediatric Orthopaedics, 3rd ed. Philadelphia, WB Saunders, 2002, p. 2393,)

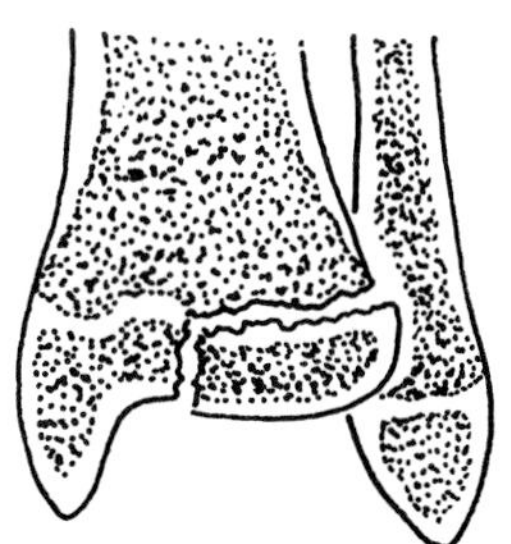

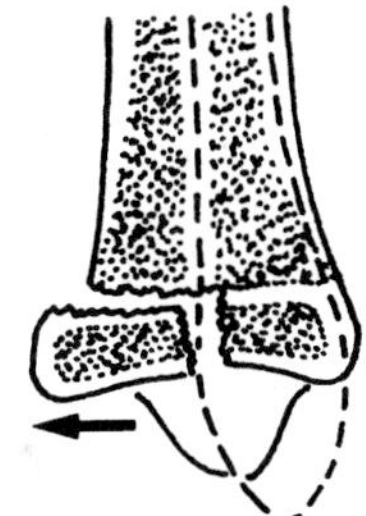

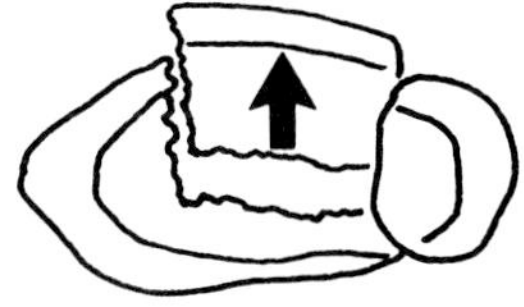

TYPE 3 - FRACTURE OF TILLAUX

FIGURE 10-83 ■ Juvenile Tillaux fracture. (From Ogden, J.A.: Skeletal Injury in the Child, 2nd ed. Philadelphia, WB Saunders, 1990, p. 838.)

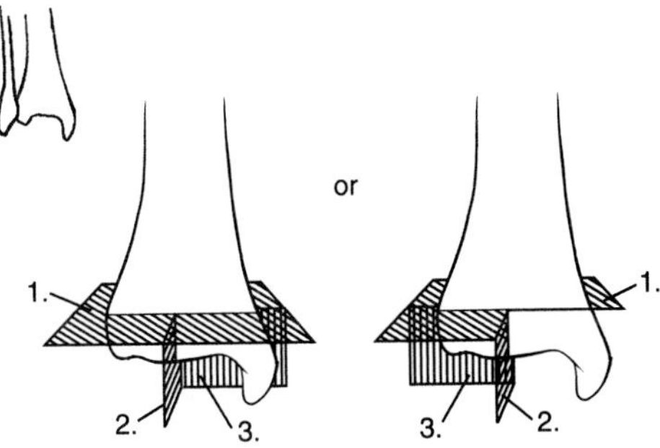

FIGURE 10-84 ■ The triplane fracture pattern. Note the fracture pattern in three planes: *1,* Axial plane; *2,* Sagittal plane; *3,* Frontal plane. (From Herring, J.A.: Tachdjian's Pediatric Orthopaedics, 3rd ed. Philadelphia, WB Saunders, 2002, p. 2410.)

SECTION 4

Spine

TABLE 10-21 SPINE TRAUMA

LEVEL	INJURY TYPE	CLASSIFICATION	COMMON NAME	MECHANISM OF INJURY	RISK OF NEUROLOGIC INJURY
Occipitocervical dislocation					
	Type I	Traynelis et al.	(anterior)	anterior translation	very high
	Type II		(distraction)	pure distraction	very high
	Type III		(posterior)	posterior translation	very high
Occipital condyle fracture		Anderson-Montesano			
	Type I		Impacted condyle fx	compression of skull	low
	Type II		occipital condyle and basilar skull fx	compression of skull	low
	Type III		avulsion fx of alar ligament	distraction of skull	moderate to high
C1 ring fracture					
	posterior arch fracture		lamina fracture	hyperextension	low
	two and three part fracture		lateral mass fracture	lateral compression	low
	four part fracture		Jefferson fracture	axial compression	low
C2 fracture					
	Traumatic spondylolisthesis	Levine	hangmans Fx		
	Type I or Ia		Ia called atypical hangmans	hyperextension	low
	Type II or IIa			hyperextension with secondary flexion	low to moderate
	Type III		bilateral facet dislocation	hyperextension with secondary flexion/distraction	high
	Odontoid Fracture	Anderson-D'Alonzo			
	Type I		avulsion fx	hyperextension of distraction	low
	Type II		fx at junction of odontoid and body	multiple mechanims	moderate
	Type III		fx into C2 body	multiple mechanims	moderate
	C2 Body fracture			similar to subaxial cervical spine	low
Transverse ligament disrution			C1-2 instability	severe flexion	mod to high
C1-2 Rotatory Subluxation		Fielding-Hawkins			
	Type I		rotatory fixation	rotational trauma	low
	Type II		rotatory fixation with 3-5 mm of anterior displacement	rotational trauma	moderate
	Type III		rotatory fixation with >5 mm anterior displacement	rotational trauma	moderate
	Type IV		rotatory fixation with posterior displacement	rotational trauma	moderate to high
Subaxial cervical spine		Allen-Ferguson		mechanims implied by name	depends on stage of injury
	Compressive flexion			compression and flexion	low to high
	Distractive flexion			distraction and flexion	low to high
	Axial compression			axial compression	low to high
	Compressive extension			compression and extension	low to high
	Distractive extension			distraction and extension	low to high
	Lateral flexion			lateral bending	low to moderate
			Compression	flexion	low
			Burst	axial compression	moderate to high
			Flexion teardrop	compression and flexion	high
			Facet dislocation	flexion and distraction	high
			Posterior element fracture (e.g. spinous process)	extension (sometimes flexion or rotation)	low
Thoracolumbar spine	Compression	Denis		flexion and axial loading	
	Burst			axial loading	
	stable				
	unstable				
	Seatbelt injury		Chance Fx(bony injury)	distraction and flexion	
	Fracture-dislocation			rotation and shear	

TREATMENT	INDICATION FOR SURGERY	IMPORTANT POINTS
occipitocervical fusion	surgery indicated	very unstable, rarely survive injury
occipitocervical fusion	surgery indicated	very unstable, rarely survive injury
occipitocervical fusion	surgery indicated	very unstable, rarely survive injury
collar	usually not required	alar ligament and tectoral membrane usually intact
collar	usually not required	alar ligament and tectoral membrane usually intact
collar, halo or surgery depending on stability	more than 1 mm of displacement	potential for ligament disruption
immobilization	not indicated	hyperextension
immobilization	not indicated	
immobilization, sometimes traction	optional for widely displaced lateral masses	>7 mm of offset of lateral mass indicated transverse ligament rupture
collar		prove stable with supervised flexion-extension radiographs
Immobilization, avoid traction with IIa	osteosythesis optional	type II use traction, type IIa avoid traction
Surgical reduction of facet dislocation and C2-3 fusion	surgery required to reduce facets	open reduction of facets required
collar	none	watch for associated occipitocervical instability
halo vs. internal fixation	unstable fracture or nonunion	high rate of nonunion
halo vs. internal fixation	unstable fracture or nonunion	lower rate of nonunion
immobilization	rare	usually stable
C1-2 fusion	ADI >3-5 mm	often associated with dizziness, syncope, respiratory problems and blurred vision
immobilization/traction/surgery	indicated for chronic cases with fixed deformity and spasm or instability	many causes, infection and trauma most common
immobilization/traction/surgery	indicated for chronic cases with fixed deformity and spasm or instability	
immobilization/traction/surgery	indicated for chronic cases with fixed deformity and spasm or instability	
immobilization/traction/surgery	indicated for chronic cases with fixed deformity and spasm or instability	
depends on stage of injury	instability of neurologic deficit with cord compression	
	instability of neurologic deficit with cord compression	
	instability of neurologic deficit with cord compression	
	instability of neurologic deficit with cord compression	
	instability of neurologic deficit with cord compression	
	instability of neurologic deficit with cord compression	
collar		watch for signs of posterior ligament disruption
halo vs. anterior decompression/fusion	cord compression	anterior decompression especially indicated with incomplete cord injury
halo vs. anterior decompression/fusion	cord compression	very unstable
reduction of facet, fusion	bilateral facet dislocation	possible disc herniation, consider MRI before reduction
collar	floating lateral mass	most are stable
bracing	greater than 50% anterior colapse or spinous process widening	osteoporotic compression fracture require work-up and treatment of underlying condition
bracing	progressive deformity or neurologic compromise	watch for any sign of posterior ligament rupture
surgery	>30degrees kyphosis, incomplete cord injury with cord compression	cord decompression required if neurologic deficit present
surgery for posterior ligament ruptures, bracing for post	>17% kypphosis with bony injury, posterior ligament injury	high rate of associated intra-abdominal injuries
surgical aligment, fusion, instrumentation	all require surgery	long segmental posterior construct

Selected Bibliography

INTRODUCTION

Bosse, M.J., et al.: An analysis of outcomes of reconstruction or amputation after leg-threatening injuries. N. Engl. J. Med. 347(24):1924–1931, 2002.

PHYSEAL INJURY (PEDIATRIC)

Ogden, J.A.: The evaluation and treatment of partial physeal arrest. J. Bone Joint Surg. [Am.] 69(8):1297–1302, 1987.

Salter, R.B., Harris, W.R.: Injuries involving the epiphyseal plate. J. Bone Joint Surg. [Am.] 45:587–622, 1963.

WRIST AND HAND (PEDIATRIC)

Campbell R.M., Jr.: Operative treatment of fractures and dislocations of the hand and wrist region in children. Orthop. Clin. North Am. 21(2):217–243, 1990.

Dicke, T.E., Nunley, J.A.: Distal forearm fractures in children. Complications and surgical indications. Orthop. Clin. North Am. 24(2):333–340, 1993.

Light, T.R.: Carpal injuries in children. Hand Clin. 16(4):513–522, 2000.

Noonan, K. J., Price, C.T.: Forearm and distal radius fractures in children. J. Am. Acad. Orthop. Surg. 6(3):146–156, 1998.

Torre, B.A.: Epiphyseal injuries in the small joints of the hand. Hand Clin. 4(1):113–121, 1988.

RADIAL AND ULNAR SHAFT (PEDIATRIC)

Flynn, J.M.: Pediatric forearm fractures: decision making, surgical techniques, and complications. AAOS Instr. Course Lect. 51:355–360, 2002.

Goodwin, R.C., Kuivila, T.E.: Pediatric elbow and forearm fractures requiring surgical treatment. Hand Clin. 18(1):135–148, 2002.

Ring, D., Jupiter, J.B., Waters, P.M.: Monteggia fractures in children and adults. J. Am. Acad. Orthop. Surg. 6(4):215–224, 1998.

Ring, D., et al.: Pediatric floating elbow. J. Pediatr. Orthop. 21(4):456–59, 2001.

ELBOW (PEDIATRIC)

Bast, S.C., Hoffer, M.M., Aval, S.: Nonoperative treatment for minimally and nondisplaced lateral humeral condyle fractures in children. J. Pediatr. Orthop. 18(4):448–450, 1998.

Dias, J.J., et al.: Management of severely displaced medial epicondyle fractures. J. Orthop. Trauma. 1(1):59–62, 1987.

Finnbogason, T., et al.: Nondisplaced and minimally displaced fractures of the lateral humeral condyle in children: a prospective radiographic investigation of fracture stability. J. Pediatr. Orthop. 15(4):422–425, 1995.

Lins, R.E., Simovitch, R.W., Waters, P.M.: Pediatric elbow trauma. Orthop. Clin. North Am. 30(1):119–132, 1999.

Shimada, K., et al.: Osteosynthesis for the treatment of non-union of the lateral humeral condyle in children. J. Bone Joint Surg. [Am.] 79(2):234–240, 1997.

Skaggs, D.L., et al.: Operative treatment of supracondylar fractures of the humerus in children. The consequences of pin placement. J. Bone Joint Surg. [Am.] 83-A(5):735–740, 2001.

Sponseller, P.D.: Problem elbow fractures in children. Hand Clin. 10(3):495–505, 1994.

SPINE (PEDIATRIC)

Akbarnia, B.A.: Pediatric spine fractures. Orthop. Clin. North Am. 30(3):521–536, 1999.

Bosch, P.P., Vogt, M.T., Ward, W.T.: Pediatric spinal cord injury without radiographic abnormality (SCIWORA): the absence of occult instability and lack of indication for bracing. Spine 27(24):2788–2800, 2002.

Sun, P.P., et al.: Spectrum of occipitoatlantoaxial injury in young children. J. Neurosurg. 93(Suppl. 1):28–39, 2000.

PELVIS (PEDIATRIC)

Grisoni, N., et al.: Pelvic fractures in a pediatric level I trauma center. J. Orthop. Trauma. 16(7):458–463, 2002.

Tolo, V.T.: Orthopaedic treatment of fractures of the long bones and pelvis in children who have multiple injuries. AAOS Instr. Course Lect. 49:415–423, 2000.

HIP (PEDIATRIC)

Bagatur, A.E., Zorer G.: Complications associated with surgically treated hip fractures in children. J. Pediatr. Orthop., Part B. 11(3):219–228, 2002.

Canale, S.T.: Fractures of the hip in children and adolescents. Orthop. Clin. North Am. 21(2):341–352, 1990.

Davison, B.L., Weinstein, S.L.: Hip fractures in children: a long-term follow-up study. J. Pediatr. Orthop. 12(3):355–358, 1992.

Hughes, L.O., Beaty, J.H.: Fractures of the head and neck of the femur in children. J. Bone Joint Surg. [Am.] 76(2):283–292, 1994.

Spiegel, P.G., Mast, J.W.: Internal and external fixation of fractures in children. Orthop. Clin. North Am. 11(3):405–421, 1980.

Thompson, G.H., Bachner, E.J., Ballock, R.T.: Salter-Harris type II fractures of the capital femoralepiphysis. J. Orthop. Trauma. 14(7):510–514, 2000.

FEMUR (PEDIATRIC)

Buckley, S.L.: Current trends in the treatment of femoral shaft fractures in children and adolescents. Clin. Orthop. 338:60–73, 1997.

Sponseller, P.D.: Surgical management of pediatric femoral fractures. AAOS Instr. Course Lect. 51:361–365, 2002.

KNEE (PEDIATRIC)

Beaty, J.H., Kumar A.: Fractures about the knee in children. J. Bone Joint Surg. [Am.] 76(12):1870–1880, 1994.

Davies, E.M., McLaren M.I.: Type III tibial spine avulsions treated with arthroscopic Acutrak screw reattachment. Clin. Orthop. 388:205–208, 2001.

Hallam, P.J., et al.: An alternative to fixation of displaced fractures of the anterior intercondylar eminence in children. J. Bone Joint Surg. [Br.] 84(4):579–582, 2002.

Qidwai, S.A.: Intramedullary Kirschner wiring for tibia fractures in children. J. Pediatr. Orthop. 21(3):294–297, 2001.

Roberts, J.M.: Operative treatment of fractures about the knee. Orthop. Clin. North Am. 21(2):365–379, 1990.

Zionts, L.E.: Fractures around the knee in children. J. Am. Acad. Orthop. Surg. 10(5):345–355, 2002.

TIBIA (PEDIATRIC)

D'Souza, L.G., et al.: The bicycle spoke injury: an avoidable accident? Foot Ankle Int. 17(3):170–173, 1996.

Letts, M., Vincent, N., Gouw, G.: The "floating knee" in children. J. Bone Joint Surg. [Br.] 68(3):442–446, 1986.

Muller, I., et al.: Results of proximal metaphyseal fractures in children. Arch. Orthop. Trauma Surg. 122(6):331–333, 2002.

Yue, J.J., et al.: The floating knee in the pediatric patient. Nonoperative versus operative stabilization. Clin. Orthop. (376):124–136, 2000.

FOOT AND ANKLE (PEDIATRIC)

Buoncristiani, A.M., Manos, R.E., Mills, W.J.: Plantar-flexion tarsometatarsal joint injuries in children. J. Pediatr. Orthop. 21(3):324–327, 2001.

Crawford, A.H.: Ankle fractures in children. AAOS Instr. Course Lect. 44:317–324, 1995.

Kling, T.F., Jr.: Operative treatment of ankle fractures in children. Orthop. Clin. North Am. 21(2):381–392, 1990.

Trott, A.W.: Fractures of the foot in children. Orthop. Clin. North Am. 7(3):677–686, 1976.

PELVIS AND HIP

Bosse, M.J., Poka, A., Reinert, C.M., et al.: Heterotopic ossification as a complication of acetabular fracture: Prophylaxis with low-dose irradiation. J. Bone Joint Surg. [Am.] 70:1231–1237, 1988.

Bucholz, R.W.: The pathologic anatomy of Malgaigne fracture-dislocations of the pelvis. J. Bone Joint Surg. [Am.] 63:400–404, 1981.

Dalal, S.A., Burgess, A.R., Siegal, J.H., et al.: Pelvic fracture and multiple trauma. Classification by mechanism is key to pattern of organ injury, resuscitative requirements and outcome. J. Trauma 29:981–1000, 1989.

Denis, F., Davis, S., and Comfort, T.: Sacral fractures: An important problem: Retrospective analysis of 236 cases. Clin. Orthop. 227:67-81, 1988.

Dreinhofer, K.E., Schwarzkopf, S.R., Haas, N.P., et al.: Isolated dislocation of the hip: Long term results in 50 patients. J. Bone Joint Surg. [Br.] 76:6-12, 1994.

Epstein, H.C.: Traumatic Dislocation of the Hip. Baltimore, Williams & Wilkins, 1980.

Epstein, H.C., Wiss, D.A., and Cozen, L.: Posterior fracture dislocation of the hip with fractures of the femoral head. Clin. Orthop. 201:9-17, 1985.

Fassler, P.R., Swiontkowski, M.F., Kilrow, A.W., and Routt, M.L.: Injury of the sciatic nerve associated with acetabular fracture. J. Bone Joint Surg. [Am.] 75:1157-1166, 1993.

Hanson P.B., Milne, J.C., and Chapman, M.W.: Open fractures of the pelvis—review of 43 cases. J. Bone Joint Surg. [Br.] 73:325-329, 1991.

Horwitz, S.M.: The management of pathological hip fractures. Op. Tech. Orthop. 4:122-129, 1994.

Judet, R., Judet, J., and Letournel, E.: Fractures of the acetabulum: Classification and surgical approaches for open reduction. J. Bone Joint Surg. [Am.] 46:1615-1646, 1964.

Juliano, P.J., Bosse, M.J., and Edwards, K.J.: The superior gluteal artery and complex acetabular procedures: A cadaveric angiographic study. J. Bone Joint Surg. [Am.] 76:244-248, 1994.

Koval, K.J., and Zuckerman, J.D.: Current concepts review: Functional recovery after fracture of the hip. J. Bone Joint Surg. [Am.] 76:751-758, 1994.

Koval, K.J., and Zuckerman, J.D.: Hip fractures: I. Evaluation and treatment of femoral neck fractures. II. Hip fractures: Evaluation and treatment of intertrochanteric fractures. J. Am. Acad. Orthop. Surg. I:2:141-149, 1994; II: 2:150-156, 1994.

Kyle, R.F.: Fractures of the proximal part of the femur. J. Bone Joint Surg. [Am.] 76:924-950, 1994.

Kyle, R.F., Wright, T.M., and Burstein, A.H.: Biomechanical analysis of the sliding characteristics of compression hip screw. J. Bone Joint Surg. [Am.] 62:1308-1314, 1980.

Lange, R.H., and Hansen, S.T., Jr.: Pelvic ring disruptions with symphysis pubis diastasis: Indications, technique, and limitations of anterior internal fixation. Clin. Orthop. 201:130-137, 1985.

Latenser, B.A., Gentilello, L.M., Tarver, A.A., et al.: Improved outcome with early fixation of skeletally unstable pelvic fractures. J. Trauma 31:28-31, 1991.

Letournel, E., and Judet, R.: Fractures of the Acetabulum. Elson, R. A., transl., ed. New York, Springer-Verlag, 1981.

Lu-Yao, G.L., Keller, R.B., Littenberg, B., and Wennberg, J.E.: Outcomes after displaced fractures of the femoral neck—meta analysis of 106 published reports. J. Bone Joint Surg. [Am.] 76:15-25, 1994.

Matta, J., Anderson, L., Epstein, H., and Henricks, P.: Fractures of the acetabulum: A retrospective analysis. Clin. Orthop. 205:230-240, 1986.

Matta, J.M., and Saucedo, T.: Internal fixation of pelvic ring fractures. Clin. Orthop. 242:83-97, 1989.

Matta, J.M., Mehne, D.K., and Roffi, R.: Fractures of the acetabulum: Early results of a prospective study. Clin Orthop. 205:241-250, 1986.

McMurtry, R., Walton, D., Dickinson, D., et al.: Pelvic disruption in the polytraumatized patient: A management protocol. Clin. Orthop. 151:22-30, 1980.

Mears, D.C., and Rubash, H.: Pelvic and acetabular fractures. Thorofare, NJ, Slack, 1986.

Mears, D.C., Capito, C.P., and Deleeuw, H.: Posterior pelvic disruptions managed by the use of the double cobra plate. Instr. Course Lect. 37:143-150, 1988.

Naam, N.H., Brown, W.M., Hurd, R., et al.: Major pelvic fractures. Arch. Surg. 118:610-616 1983.

Riemer, B.L., Butterfield, S.L., Ray, R.L., and Daffner, R.H.: Clandestine femoral neck fractures with ipsilateral diaphyseal fractures. J. Orthop. Trauma 7:443-449, 1993.

Rizzo, P.F., Gould, E.S., Lyden, J.P., et al.: Diagnosis of occult fractures about the hip: Magnetic resonance imaging compared with bone-scanning. J. Bone Joint Surg [Am.] 75:395-401, 1993.

Routt, M.L.C., Jr., and Swiontkowski, M.F.: Operative treatment of complex acetabular fractures: Combined anterior and posterior exposures during the same procedure. J. Bone Joint Surg. [Am.] 72:897, 1990.

Stahaeli, J.W., Frassica, F.J., and Sim, F.H.: Prosthetic replacement of the femoral head for fracture of the femoral neck in patients who have Pakinson disease. J. Bone Joint Surg. [Am.] 70:565-568, 1988.

Swiontkowski, M.F.: Current concepts review: Intracapsular fractures of the hip. J. Bone Joint Surg. [Am.] 76:129-138, 1994.

Tile, M.: Fractures of the Pelvis and Acetabulum. Baltimore, Williams & Wilkins, 1984.

Tile, M.: Pelvic ring fractures: Should they be fixed? J. Bone Joint Surg. [Br.] 70:1-12, 1988.

Young, J.W.R., and Burgess A.R.: Radiographic Management of Pelvic Ring Fractures: Systematic Radiographic Diagnosis. Baltimore: Urban & Schwarzenberg, 1987.

THIGH AND LEG

Arneson, T.J., Melton, L.J., III, Lewallen, D.G., et al.: Epidemiology of diaphyseal and distal femoral fractures in Rochester, Minnesota, 1965-1984. Clin. Orthop. 234:188-194, 1988.

Behrens, F., and Searls, K.: External fixation of the tibia: Basic concepts and prospective evaluation. J. Bone Joint Surg. [Br.] 68:246-254, 1986.

Blair, B., Koval, K.J., Kummer, F., et al.: Basicervical fractures of the proximal femur: A biomechanical study of 3 internal fixation techniques. Clin. Orthop. 306:256-263, 1994.

Bonar, S.K., and Marsh, J.L.: Unilateral external fixation for severe pilon fractures. Foot Ankle 14:57-64, 1993.

Bone, L., and Bucholz, R: The management of fractures in the patient with multiple trauma. J. Bone Joint Surg. [Am.] 68:945-949, 1986.

Bone, L.B., Cassman, S., Stegemann, P., and France, J.: Prospective study of union rate of open tibial fractures treated with locked unreamed intramedullary nails. J. Orthop. Trauma 8:45-49, 1994.

Bone, L.B., Johnson, K.D., Weigelt, J., et al.: Early versus delayed stabilization of femoral fractures: A prospective randomized study. J. Bone Joint Surg. [Am.] 71:336, 1989.

Boynton, M.D., and Schmeling, G.J.: Nonreamed intramedullary nailing of open tibial fractures. J. Am. Acad. Orthop. Surg. 2:107-114, 1994.

Brumback, R.J., Ellison, T.S., Molligan, H., et al.: Pudendal nerve palsy complicating intramedullary nailing of the femur. J. Bone Joint Surg. [Am.] 74:1450-1455, 1992.

Brumback, R.J., Reilly, J.P., Poka, A., et al.: Intramedullary nailing of femoral shaft fractures. J. Bone Joint Surg. [Am.] 70:1441-1462, 1988.

Caudle, R.J., and Stern, P.J.: Severe open fractures of the tibia. J. Bone Joint Surg. [Am.] 69:801-807, 1987.

Cierny, G., III, Byrd, H.S., and Jones, R.E.: Primary versus delayed soft tissue coverage for severe open tibial fractures: A comparison of results. Clin. Orthop. 178:54-63, 1983.

Delamarter, R.B., Hohl, M.E., Jr.: Ligament injuries associated with tibial plateau fractures. Clin. Orthop. 250:226-233, 1990.

DeLee, J.C., and Stiehl, J.B.: Open tibia fracture with compartment syndrome. Clin. Orthop. 160:175-184, 1981.

Den Hartog, B.D., Bartal, E., and Dooke, F.: Treatment of the unstable intertrochanteric fracture: Effect of the placement of the screw, its angle of insertion, and osteotomy. J. Bone Joint Surg. [Am.] 73:726-733, 1991.

Desjardins, A.L., Roy, A., Paiement, G., et al.: Unstable intertrochanteric fracture of the femur: A prospective randomised study comparing anatomical reduction and medial displacement osteotomy. J. Bone Joint Surg. [Br.] 75:445-447, 1993.

Gustilo, R.B., Mendoza, R.M., and Williams, D.N.: Problems in the management of type III (severe) open fractures: A new classification of type III open fractures. J. Trauma 24:742-746, 1984.

Gustilo, R.B., Merkow, R.L., and Templeman, D.: Current concepts review: The management of open fractures. J. Bone Joint Surg. [Am.] 72:299, 1990.

Hack, D.J., and Johnson, E.E.: The use of the unreamed nail and tibial fractures with concomitant preoperative or intraoperative elevated compartment pressure or compartment syndrome. J. Orthop. Trauma 8:203-211, 1994.

Hansen, S.T., and Winquist, R.A.: Closed intramedullary nailing of the femur: Kuntscher technique with reaming. Clin. Orthop. 138:56-61, 1979.

Holbrook, J.L., Swiontkowski, M.F., and Sanders, R.: Treatment of open fractures of the tibial shaft: Ender nailing versus external fixation: A randomized, prospective comparison. J. Bone Joint Surg. [Am.] 71:1231, 1989.

Hume, E., and Catalano, J.B., Ipsilateral neck and shaft fractures of the femur. Op. Tech. Orthop. 4:111–115, 1994.
Lachiewicz, P.F., and Funcik, T.: Factors influencing the results of open reduction and internal fixation of tibial plateau fractures. Clin. Orthop. 259:210–215, 1990.
Lhowe, D.W., and Hansen, S.T.: Immediate nailing of open fractures of the femoral shaft. J. Bone Joint Surg. [Am.] 70:812–820, 1988.
Mast, J.W., Spiegel, F.G., and Pappas, J.N.: Fractures of the tibial pilon. Clin. Orthop. 230:68–82, 1988.
Mawhinney, I.N., Maginn, P., and McCoy, G.F.: Tibial compartment syndromes after tibial nailing. J. Orthrop. Trauma 8:212–214, 1994.
Nowotarski, P., and Brumback, R.J.: Immediate interlocking nailing of fractures of the femur caused by low to mid velocity gunshots. J. Orthop. Trauma. 8:134–141, 1994.
Pritchett, J.W.: Supracondylar fractures of the femur. Clin. Orthop. 184:173–177, 1984.
Richards, R.R., Waddell, J.P., Sullivan, T.R., et al.: Infra-isthmal fractures of the femur: A review of 82 cases. J. Trauma 24:735–741, 1984.
Rhimer, B.L., Butterfield, S.L., Ray, R.L., et al.: Clandestine femoral neck fractures with ipsilateral diaphyseal fractures. J Orthop. Trauma 7:443–449, 1993.
Schatzker, J., and Lambert, D.C.: Supracondylar fractures of the femur. Clin. Orthop. 138:77–83, 1979.
Suedkamp, N.P., Barbey, N., Vueskens, A., et al.: The incidence of osteitis in open fractures: An analysis of 948 open fractures (a review of the Hanover experience). J. Orthop. Trauma 7:473–482, 1993.
Swiontkowski, M.F., Hansen, S.T., Jr., and Kellam, J: Ipsilateral fractures of the femoral neck and shaft: A treatment protocol. J. Bone Joint Surg. [Am.] 66:260–268, 1984.
Talucci, R.C., Manning, J., Lampard, S., et al.: Early intramedullary nailing of femoral shaft fractures: A cause of fat embolism syndrome. Am. J. Surg. 146:107–110, 1983.
Tornetta, P., Bergman, M., Watnik, N., et al.: Treatment of grade III B open tibial fractures—a prospective randomized comparison of external fixation in non-reamed locked nailing. J. Bone Joint Surg. [Br.] 76:13–19, 1994.
Webb, L.X., Winquist, R.A., and Hansen, S.T.: Intramedullary nailing and reaming for delayed union or nonunion of the femoral shaft: A report of 105 consecutive cases. Clin. Orthop. 212:133–141, 1986.
Whittle, A.P., Russell, T.A., Taylor, J.C., and Lavelle, D.G.: Treatment of open fractures of the tibial shaft with the use of interlocking nailing without reaming. J. Bone Joint Surg. [Am.] 74:1162–1171, 1992.
Winquist, R.A., Hansen, S.T., Jr., and Clawson, D.K.: Closed intramedullary nailing of femoral fractures: A report of five hundred and twenty cases. J. Bone. Joint Surg. 66A:529–539, 1984.
Wiss, D.A., and Brien, W.W.: Subtrochanteric fractures of the femur: Results of treatment by interlocking nailing. Clin. Orthop. 283:231–236, 1992.
Zickel, R.E.: Subtrochanteric femoral fractures. Orthop. Clin. North Am. 11:555–568, 1980.

KNEE

Benirschke, S.K., Agnew, S.G., Mayo, K.A., et al.: Immediate internal fixation of open, complex tibial plateau fractures: Treatment by standard protocol. J. Orthop. Trauma 6:76–86, 1992.
Carpenter, J.E., Kasman, R., and Matthews, L.S.: Fractures of the patella. J. Bone Joint Surg. [Am.] 75:1550–1561, 1993.
Fernandez, D.L.: Anterior approach to the knee with osteotomy of the tibial tubercle for bicondylar tibial fractures. J. Bone Joint Surg. [Am.] 70:208–219, 1988.
Georgiadis, G.M.: Combined anterior and posterior approaches for complex tibial plateau fractures. J. Bone Joint Surg. [Br.] 76:285–289, 1994.
Haas, S.B., and Callaway, H.: Disruptions of the extensor mechanism. Orthop. Clin. North Am. 23:687–695, 1992.
Iannacone, W.M., Bennett, F.S., DeLong, W.G., et al.: Initial experience with the treatment of supracondylar femoral fractures using the supracondylar intramedullary nail: A preliminary report. J. Orthop. Trauma 8:322–327, 1994.
Jensen, D.B., Rude, C., Duus, B., and Bjerg-Nielsen, A.: Tibial plateau fractures; A comparison of conservative and surgical treatment. J. Bone Joint Surg. [Br.] 72:49–52, 1990.
Koval, K., Sanders, R., Borrelli, J., et al.: Indirect reduction and percutaneous screw fixation of displaced tibial plateau fractures. J. Orthop. Trauma 6:340–346, 1992.
Moore, T.M.: Fracture-dislocation of the knee. Clin. Orthop. 156:128–140, 1981.
Saltzman, C.L., Goulet, J.A., McClellan, R.T., et al.: Results of treatment of displaced patellar fractures by partial patellectomy. J. Bone Joint Surg. [Am.] 72:1279, 1990.
Sanders, R.: Patella fractures and extensor mechanism injuries. In Browner, B.D., Jupiter, J.B., Levine, A.M., et al. (eds.): Skeletal Trauma: Fractures, Dislocations, Ligamentous Injuries, vol. 2. Philadelphia, WB Saunders, 1992, pp. 1685–1716.
Schatzker, J., McBroom, R., and Bruce, D.: The tibial plateau fracture: The Toronto experience, 1968–1975. Clin. Orthop. 138:94–104, 1979.
Siliski, J.M., Mahring, M., and Hofer, H.P.: Supracondylar-intercondylar fractures of the femur: Treatment by internal fixation. J. Bone Joint Surg. [Am.] 71:95–104, 1989.
Weber, M.J., Janecki, C.J., McLeod, P., et al.: Efficacy of various forms of fixation of transverse fractures of the patella. J. Bone Joint Surg. [Am.] 62:215–220, 1980.

ANKLE AND FOOT

Canale, S.T., and Kelly, F.B.: Fractures of the neck of the talus. J. Bone Joint Surg. [Am.] 60:143–156, 1978.
DeCoster, T.A., and Miller, R.A.: Management of traumatic foot wounds. J. Am. Acad. Orthop. Surg. 2:226–230, 1994.
DeLee, J.C., and Curtis, R.: Subtalar dislocation of the foot. J. Bone Joint Surg. [Am.] 64:433–437, 1982.
Faciszewski, T., Burks, R.T., and Manaster, B.J.: Subtle injuries of the Lisfranc joint. J. Bone Joint Surg. [Am.] 72:1519, 1990.
Giachino, A.A., and Uhthoff, H.K.: Current concepts review: Intraarticular fractures of the calcaneus. J. Bone Joint Surg. [Am.] 71:784–787, 1989.
Goossens, M., and De Stoop, N.: Lisfranc's fracture-dislocations: Etiology, radiology, and results of treatment: A review of 20 cases. Clin. Orthop. 176:154–162, 1983.
Harper, M.C., and Hardin, G.: Posterior malleolar fractures of the ankle associated with external rotation-abduction injuries: Results with and without internal fixation. J. Bone Joint Surg. [Am.] 70:1348–1356, 1988.
Lindsay, W.R.N., and Dewar, R.P.: Fractures of the Os Calcis. Am. J. Surg. 95:555–576, 1958.
Macey, L.R., Benirschke, S.K., Sangeorzan, B.J., and Hansen, S.T.: Acute calcaneal fractures: Treatment, options, and results. J. Am. Acad. Orthop. Surg. 2:36–43, 1994.
Marti, R.K., Raaymakers, E.L., and Nolte, P.A.: Malunited ankle fractures—the late results of reconstruction. J. Bone Joint Surg. [Br.] 72:709–713, 1990.
McReynolds, I.S.: The Case for Operative Treatment of Fractures of the OS Calcis. Philadelphia, WB Saunders, 1982.
Ovadia, D.N., and Beals, R.K.: Fractures of the tibial plafond. J. Bone Joint Surg. [Am.] 68:543–551, 1986.
Sangeorzan, B.J., Benirschke, S.K., Mosca, V., et al.: Displaced intraarticular fractures of the tarsal navicular. J. Bone Joint Surg. [Am.] 71:1504, 1989.
Segal, D.: Displaced Ankle Fractures Treated Surgically and Postoperative Management. St. Louis, CV Mosby, 1979.
Stephenson, J.R.: Treatment of displaced intra-articular fractures of the calcaneus using medial and lateral approaches, internal fixation, and early motion. J. Bone Joint Surg. [Am.] 69:115–130, 1987.
Swanson, T.V., Bray, T.J., and Holmes, G.B.: Fractures of the talar neck: A mechanical study of fixation. J. Bone Joint Surg. [Am.] 74:544–551, 1992.

SHOULDER

Flatow, E.L., Pollock, R.G., and Bigliani, L.U.: Operative treatment of two part, displaced surgical neck fractures of the proximal humerus. Op. Tech. Orthop. 4:2–8, 1994.
Goss, T.P.: Current concepts review: Fractures of the glenoid cavity. J. Bone Joint Surg. [Am.] 74:299–305, 1992.
Goss, T.P.: Double disruptions of the superior shoulder suspensory complex. J. Orthop. Trauma 7:99–106, 1993.
Green, A., and Norris, T.R.: Humeral head replacement for four part fractures and fracture dislocations. Op. Tech. Orthop. 4:13–20, 1994.
Herscovici, D., Jr., Fiennes, A.G., Allgower, M., et al.: The floating shoulder-ipsilateral, clavical and scapular neck fractures. J. Bone Joint Surg. [Br.] 74:362–366, 1992.
Jaberg, H., Warner, J.P., and Jakob, R.P.: Percutaneous stabilization of unstable fractures of the humerus. J. Bone Joint Surg. [Am.] 74:508–515, 1992.
Klassen, J.F., and Cofield, R.H.: Surgical management of scapular fractures, Op. Tech. Orthop. 4:58–63, 1994.

Schlegel, T.F., and Hawkins, R.J.: Displaced proximal humeral fractures: Evaluation and treatment. J. Am. Acad. Orthop. Surg. 2:54-66, 1994.

Schlegel, T.F., and Hawkins R.J.: Hemiarthroplasty for the treatment of proximal humeral fractures. Op. Tech. Orthop. 4:21-25, 1994.

Schlegel, T.F., and Hawkins, R.J.: Internal fixation of three part proximal humeral fractures. Op. Tech. Orthop. 4:9-12, 1994.

Sidor, M.L., Zuckerman, J.D., Lyon, T., and Koval, K: The Neer classification system for proximal humeral fractures—an assessment of interobserver reliability and intraobserver reproducibility. J. Bone Joint Surg. [Am.] 75:1745-1750, 1993.

Siebenrock, K.A., and Gerber, C.: The reproducibility of classification of fractures of the proximal end of the humerus. J. Bone Joint Surg. [Am.] 75:1751-1755, 1993.

Stableforth, P.G.: Open reduction and internal fixation of displaced four part segment fractures of the proximal humerus. Op. Tech. Orthop. 4:26-30, 1994.

Tanner, M.W., and Cofield, R.H.: Prosthetic arthroplasty for fractures and fracture-dislocations of the proximal humerus. Clin. Orthop. 179:116-128, 1983.

Wilkins, R.M., and Johnston, R.M.: Ununited fractures of the clavicle. J. Bone Joint Surg. [Am.] 65:773-778, 1983.

Zdrovkovic, D., and Damholt, V.V.: Comminuted and severely displaced fractures of the scapula. Acta Orthop. Scand. 45:60-65, 1974.

HUMERUS

Amillo, S., Barrios, R.H., Martinez-Peric, R., and Losada, J.I.: Surgical treatment of the redial nerve lesions, associated with fractures of the humerus. J. Orthop. Trauma 7:211-215, 1993.

Horne, G.: Supracondylar fractures of the humerus in adults. J. Trauma 20:71-74, 1980.

Jupiter, J.B., Barnes, K.A., Goodman, L.J., and Saldana, A.E.: Multiplane fractures of the distal humerus. J. Orthop. Trauma 7:216-220, 1993.

Jupiter, J.B., Neff, U., Holzach, P., et al.: Intercondylar fractures of the humerus: An operative approach. J. Bone Joint Surg. [Am.] 67:226-239, 1985.

Pollock, F.H., Drake, D., Bovill, E.G., et al.: Treatment of radial neuropathy associated with fractures of the humerus. J. Bone Joint Surg. [Am.] 63:239-243, 1981.

Prietto, C.A.: Supracondylar fractures of the humerus. J. Bone Joint Surg. [Am.] 61:425-428, 1979.

ELBOW

Broberg, M.A., and Morrey, B.F.: Results of delayed excision of the radial head after fracture. J. Bone Joint Surg. [Am.] 68:669-674, 1986.

Jupiter, J.B.: Internal fixation for fractures about the elbow. Op. Tech. Orthop. 4:31-48, 1994.

Mehlhoff, T.L., Noble, P.C., Bennett, J.B., and Tullos, H.S.: Simple dislocation of the elbow in the adult: Results after closed treatment. J. Bone Joint Surg. [Am.] 70:244, 1988.

O'Driscoll, S.W.: Prosthetic elbow replacement for distal humeral fractures and nonunions. Op. Tech. Orthop. 4:54-57, 1994.

O'Driscoll, S.W.: Technique for unstable olecranon fracture—subluxations. Op. Tech. Orthop. 4:49-53, 1994.

Regan, W., and Morrey, B.: Fractures of the coronoid process of the ulna. J. Bone Joint Surg. [Am.] 71:1348, 1989.

Silberstein, M.J., Brodeur, A.E., and Graviss, E.R.: Some vagaries of the lateral epicondyle. J. Bone Joint Surg. [Am.] 64:444-448, 1992.

FOREARM

Chapman, M.W., Gordon, J.E., and Zissimos, A.G.: Compression-plate fixation of acute fractures of the diaphyses of the radius and ulna. J. Bone Joint Surg. [Am.] 71:159, 1989.

DeLuca, P.A., Linsey, R.W., and Ruwe, P.A.: Refracture of bones in the forearm after removal of compression plates. J. Bone Joint Surg. [Am.] 70:1372-1376, 1988.

Gelberman, R.H., Garfin, S.R., Hergenroeder, P.T., et al.: Compartment syndromes of the forearm: Diagnosis and treatment. Clin. Orthop. 161:252-261, 1981.

Grace, T.G., and Eversmann, W.W.: Forearm fractures. J. Bone Joint Surg. [Am.] 62:433-438, 1980.

Moed, B.R., Kellam, J.F., Foster, R.J., et al.: Immediate internal fixation of open fractures of the diaphysis of the forearm. J. Bone Joint Surg. [Am.] 68:1008-1017, 1986.

Vince, K.G., and Miller, J.E.: Cross union complicating fracture of the forearm: I. Adults. J. Bone Joint Surg. [Am.] 69:640-653, 1987.

HAND AND WRIST

Bednar, J.M., and Osterman, A.L.: Carpal instability: Evaluation and treatment. J. Am. Acad. Orthop. Surg. 1:11-17, 1993.

Bradway, J.K., Amadio, P.C., and Cooney, W.P.: Open reduction and internal fixation of displaced, comminuted intra-articular fractures of the distal end of the radius. J. Bone Joint Surg. [Am.] 71:839, 1989.

Herbert, T.J., and Fisher, W.E.: Management of the fractured scaphoid using a new bone screw. J. Bone Joint Surg. [Br.] 66:114-123, 1984.

Herndon, J.H., ed.: Scaphoid Fractures and Complications. Monograph Series. Rosemont, IL, American Academy of Orthopaedic Surgeons, 1994.

Jupiter, J.B.: Current concepts review: Fractures of the distal end of the radius. J. Bone Joint Surg. [Am.] 73:461-469, 1991.

Jupiter, J.B., and Lipton, H.: The operative treatment of intraarticular fractures of the distal radius. Clin. Orthop. 292:48-61, 1993.

Jupiter, J.B., and Masen, M.: Reconstruction of post-traumatic deformity of the distal radius and ulna. Hand Clin. 4:377-390, 1988.

Letournel, E.: The treatment of acetabular fractures through the ilioinguinal approach. Clin. Orthop. 292:62-76, 1993.

Melone, C.P., Jr.: Open treatment for displaced articular fractures of the distal radius. Clin. Orthop. 202:103-111, 1986.

Stickland, J.W., and Steichen, J.B., eds.: Difficult Problems in Hand Surgery. St. Louis, CV Mosby, 1982.

Taleisnik, J.: Current concepts review: Carpal instability. J. Bone Joint Surg. [Am.] 70:1262-1268, 1988.

SPINE

Anderson LD, D'Alonzo RT: Fractures of the odontoid process of the axis. J Bone Joint Surg Am. 1974 Dec;56(8):1663-74

Anderson PA, Montesano PX: Morphology and treatment of occipital condyle fractures. Spine. 1988 Jul;13(7):731-6.

Traynelis VC, Marano GD, Dunker RO, Kaufman HH: Traumatic atlanto-occipital dislocation. Case report. J Neurosurg. 1986 Dec;65(6): 863-70.

Jefferson G: Fractures of the altas vertebrae. Br J Surg 7:407, 1920.

Spence KF, Decker S, Sell KW: Bursting atlantal fracture associated with rupture of the transverse ligament. J Bone Joint Surg Am 52:543-49, 1970.

Anderson LD, D'Alonzo RT: Fractures of the odontoid process of the axis. J Bone Joint Surg Am 56:1663, 1974.

Fielding JW, Hawkins RJ: Atlanto-axial rotatory fixation. (Fixed rotatory subluxation of the atlanto-axial joint). J Bone Joint Surg Am. 1977 Jan;59(1):37-44.

Dickman CA, Mamourian A, Sonntag VK, Drayer BP: Magnetic resonance imaging of the transverse atlantal ligament for the evaluation of atlantoaxial instability. J Neurosurg. 1991 Aug;75(2):221-7

Effendi B, Roy D, Cornish B, Dussault RG, Laurin CA: Fractures of the ring of the axis. A classification based on the analysis of 131 cases. J Bone Joint Surg Br. 1981;63-B(3):319-27.

Levine AM, Edwards CC: The management of traumatic spondylolisthesis of the axis. J Bone Joint Surg Am. 1985 Feb;67(2):217-26.

Allen BL Jr, Ferguson RL, Lehmann TR, O'Brien RP: A mechanistic classification of closed, indirect fractures and dislocations of the lower cervical spine. Spine. 1982 Jan-Feb;7(1):1-27.

Babcock JL: Cervical spine injuries. Diagnosis and classification. Arch Surg. 1976 Jun;111(6):646-51.

Denis F: Spinal instability as defined by the three-column spine concept in acute spinal trauma. Clin Orthop. 1984 Oct;(189):65-76.

Magerl F, Aebi M, Gertzbein SD, Harms J, Nazarian S: A comprehensive classification of thoracic and lumbar injuries. Eur Spine J. 1994;3(4):184-201.

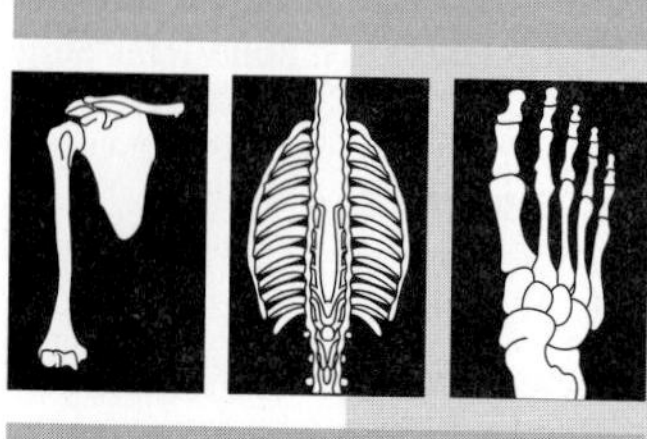

11 Anatomy

FRANKLIN D. SHULER

I. Introduction

A. **Osteology**—The human skeleton has 206 bones: 80 bones in the axial skeleton and 126 bones in the appendicular skeleton. Ossification, the formation of bone, can be intramembranous (without a cartilage model; as in the skull) or enchondral (with a cartilage model; most bones). Enchondral growth begins in the diaphyses of long bones at a primary ossification center, most of which are present at birth (Table 11-1). Secondary ossification centers usually develop in the periphery of bones and are important for growth and the treatment of childhood fractures.Anatomic landmarks of the skeleton and their related structures are listed in Table 11-2.

B. **Arthrology**—Joints are commonly classified into three types based on their freedom of movement: (1) synarthroses, (2) amphiarthroses, and (3) diarthroses. Although **synarthroses,** such as the sutures in the skull, may have motion during early childhood, they usually have no motion at maturity and simply serve to join two bony elements. **Amphiarthrodial** joints, such as the symphysis pubis, have hyaline cartilage and intervening discs. Limited motion is possible. In true **diarthrodial** joints, motion is enhanced and is characterized by hyaline cartilage, synovial membranes, capsules, and ligaments. Diarthrodial joints are further classified based on degrees of freedom of motion and their shape. Uniaxial joints (ginglymus [i.e., hinge] and trochoid [i.e., pivot]) allow movement in one plane. Biaxial joints (e.g., condyloid, ellipsoid, saddle joints) allow movement in two planes. Polyaxial joints (spheroidal [ball and socket]) allow movement in any direction. Finally, plane (gliding) joints allow only slight sliding of one joint surface over another.

C. **Myology**—Several arrangements of fibers allow classification of muscles into the following categories: parallel (e.g., rhomboids), fusiform (e.g., biceps brachii), oblique (with tendinous interdigitation—further subclassified as pennate, bipennate, multipennate), triangular (e.g., pectoralis minor), and spiral (e.g., latissimus dorsi).

D. **Nerves**—Most peripheral nerves originate from the ventral rami of spinal nerves and are distributed via several plexii (cervical, brachial, lumbosacral). The mnemonic **SAME** can be used to help understand function of nerves: **S**ensory = **A**fferent, **M**otor = **E**fferent. Efferent, or motor, fibers carry impulses from the central nervous system to muscles; afferent, or sensory, fibers carry information toward the central nervous system. The autonomic nervous system controls visceral structures and consists of the parasympathetic (craniosacral) and sympathetic (thoracolumbar) divisions. Preganglionic neurons of parasympathetic nerves arise in the nuclei of cranial nerves (CN) III, VII, IX, and X and in the S2, S3, and S4 segments of the spinal cord; they synapse in peripheral ganglia. Preganglionic neurons in the sympathetic system are located in the spinal cord (T1–L3) and synapse in chain ganglia adjacent to the spine and collateral ganglia along major abdominal blood vessels.

E. **Vessels**—Consist of arteries, veins, and lymphatics. Of primary concern to the orthopaedist is avoiding major injury to these structures. Their courses and relationships are important and are highlighted in this chapter.

F. **Standard Surgical Approaches Summary Tables**—Table 11-3 Upper extremity; Table 11-4 Lower extremity.

G. **Ossification**—Summary provided in Table 11-1.

II. Shoulder

A. **Osteology**—The shoulder girdle is composed of the scapula and clavicle, and serves to attach the upper limb to the trunk. The shoulder (glenohumeral) joint is the attachment of the upper humerus (see the following discussion on the arm) to the shoulder girdle.

Table 11-1. SUMMARY OF OSSIFICATION PATTERNS

BONE	OSSIFICATION CENTER	AGE AT APPEARANCE	AGE AT FUSION
Scapula	Body (primary)	8 weeks (fetal)	
	Coracoid (tip)	1 year	
	Coracoid	15 years	
	Acromion	15 years	
	Acromion	16 years	
	Inferior angle	16 years	
	Medial border	16 years	
Clavicle	**Medial (primary)**	**5 weeks (fetal)**	
	Lateral (primary)	**5 weeks (fetal)**	**25 years**
	Sternal	19 years	
Humerus	Body (primary)	8 weeks (fetal)	Blends at 6 years and unites at 20 years
	Head	1 year	
	Greater tuberosity	3 years	
	Lesser tuberosity	5 years	
	Capitulum	2 years	Blends and unites with body at 16–18 years
	Medial epicondyles	5 years	
	Trochlea	9 years	
	Lateral epicondyles	13 years	
Ulna	Body (primary)	8 weeks (fetal)	
	Distal ulna	5 years	20 years
	Olecranon	10 years	16 years
Radius	Body (primary)	8 weeks (fetal)	
	Distal radius	2 years	17–20 years
	Proximal radius	5 years	15–18 years
Pelvis	Ilium (primary)	2 months	15 years
	Ischium (primary)	4 months	15 years
	Pubis (primary)	6 months	15 years
	Acetabulum	12 years	15 years
Tibia	Body (primary)	7 weeks (fetal)	
	Proximal (secondary)	birth	20 years
	Distal (secondary)	2 years	18 years
Fibula	Body (primary)	8 weeks (fetal)	
	Proximal (secondary)	3 years	25 years
	Distal (secondary)	2 years	20 years

Table 11-2. SKELETAL GROOVES, NOTCHES, AND POINTS

REGION	GROOVE OR NOTCH	IMPORTANT RELATED STRUCTURES
Hand	Hook of Hamate	Ulnar nerve
	Trapezial groove	FCR tendon
Wrist	Distal ulna	ECU
	Radial styloid	EPL
Elbow	Medical supracondylar process	Median nerve, brachial artery
Shoulder	Scapular notch	Suprascapular nerve
	Supraglenoid tubercle	Long head biceps brachii
	Infraglenoid tubercle	Long head triceps brachii
Hip	ASIS	Sartorius
	AIIS	Dir. head of rectus femoris
	Ischial spine	Coccygeus, levator ani
	Lesser sciatic foramen	Pudendal nerve
	Piriformis fossa	Obturator externus
	Tip of greater trochanter	Piriformis
	Quadrate tubercle	Quadratus femoris
	Lesser trochanter	Psoas minor
Knee	Hunter's canal	Femoral → popliteal artery
	Adductor tubercle	Adductor magnus
	Gerdy's tubercle	IT band
	Fibular neck	Common peroneal nerve
Foot	Henry's knot	FDL-FHL intersection
	Sustentaculum tali	Spring ligament (FHL inferior)
	Base of fifth metatarsal	Peroneus brevis/plantar aponeurosis
	Tuberosity of navicular	Tibialis posterior
	Cuboid groove	Peroneus longus
	Sinus tarsi	Ligamentum cervis tali and EDB

FCR, Flexor carpi radialis; ECU, extensor carpi ulnaris; EPL, extensor pollicis longus; ASIS, anterior superior iliac spine; AIIS, anterior inferior iliac spine; IT, iliotibial; FDL, flexor digitorum longus; FHL, flexor hallucis longus; EDB, extensor digitorum brevis.

Table 11-3. SUMMARY OF POPULAR ORTHOPAEDIC SURGICAL APPROACHES: UPPER EXTREMITY

REGION	APPROACH	EPONYM	MUSCULAR INTERVAL 1 (NERVE)	MUSCULAR INTERVAL 2 (NERVE)	DANGERS
Shoulder	Anterior	Henry	Deltoid (axillary)	PEC. Major (med./lat. pectoral)	MC N/cephalic V
	Lateral		Deltoid (splitting (axillary)	Deltoid (splitting) (axillary)	Axillary N
	Posterior		Infraspinatus (susprascapular)	Teres minor (axillary)	Ax. N/post. cir. hum. A
Prox. humerus	Anterolateral		Deltoid/Pec. major (axillary/ med./lat. pectoral)	Radial and axillary N/ant cir. hum. A	
Distal humerus	Anterolateral		Triceps/branchialis (radial/musculocutaneous)	Brachioradialis (radial)	Radial N
	Lateral		Lat. triceps/branchioradialis (radial)	Radial N	
Humerus	Posterior		Long triceps (radial)	Radial N/brachial A	
Elbow	Anterolateral	Henry	Brachialis/pron. teres (musculocut./median)	Brachioradialis (radial)	Lat. ABC N/ radial N
	Posterolateral	Kocher	Anconeus (radial)	Ext. carpi ulnaris (PIN)	PIN (diss. to ann. lig.)
	Medial		Brachialis (musculocutaneous)	Triceps/pron. teres (radial/median)	Ulnar N
Forearm	Anterior	Henry	Brachioradialis (radial)	Pronator teres/FCR (median)	PIN
	Dorsal	Thompson	ECRB (radial)	EDC/EPL (PIN)	PIN
	Ulnar		ECU (PIN)	FCU (ulnar)	Ulnar N and A
Wrist	Dorsal		Third compartment (PIN)	Fourth compartment (PIN)	
Scaphoid	Volar	Russe	FCR or through sheath (median)	Radial A	Radial A
	Dorsolateral	Matti	First compartment (PIN)	Third compartment (PIN)	Sup. rad. N/radial A

N, Nerve; A, artery; V, vein; PIN, posterior interosseous nerve; MC, musculocutaneous; ABC, antebrachial cutaneous; ECRB, extensor carpi radialis brevis; EDC, extensor digitorum communis; FCU, flexor carpi ulnaris.

1. **Scapula**—Spans the second through seventh ribs and serves as an attachment for 17 muscles and four ligaments. The scapular glenoid is retroverted approximately 5 degrees. Key anatomic processes are the scapular spine, coracoid, and acromion. Attachments to the coracoid include the coracoacromial ligament, coracoclavicular ligaments (conoid and trapezoid [lateral]), cojoined tendon (coracobrachialis and short head of biceps), and pectoralis minor. Make the distinction between the suprascapular notch and the spinoglenoid notch. The **suprascapular notch** has the superior transverse scapular ligament separating the suprascapular artery (superior) from the suprascapular nerve (inferior). The **spinoglenoid notch** has both the artery and nerve inferior to the inferior transverse scapular ligament. Long-term nerve compression at the spinoglenoid notch (i.e., ganglion [think labral pathology]) results in infraspinatus atrophy.
2. **Clavicle**—Acts as a fulcrum for lateral movement of the arm. It has a double curvature (sternal-ventral, acromial-dorsal) and serves as an attachment for the upper extremity. The clavicle is the **first bone in the body to ossify (5 weeks fetal) and the last to fuse (*medial* epiphysis at 25 years of age).** Fracture of the clavicle is the most common musculoskeletal birth injury.

B. **Arthrology**—The shoulder area has one major (glenohumeral) and several minor (sternoclavicular, acromioclavicular, scapulothoracic) articulations. Additionally, numerous ligaments are associated with each articulation.

1. **Glenohumeral Joint** (Fig. 11-1)—Spheroidal (ball-and-socket) joint. The articular surface of the glenoid is thickest at the periphery. This joint has the greatest range of motion of any joint, but motion is at the expense of stability. There are static and dynamic restraints of shoulder motion. **Static restraints** include articular anatomy, glenoid labrum, negative pressure, capsule, and ligaments. **Dynamic restraints** include the rotator cuff, biceps tendon and scapulothoracic motion. Important shoulder-stabilizing structures are summarized in the chart below.

GLENOHUMERAL STABILIZERS

STRUCTURE	FUNCTION
Coracohumeral ligament	Primary restraint to inferior translation of the adducted arm and to ER
Glenoid labrum	Increases surface area, static stabilizer
SGHL	Primary restraint to ER in adducted or slightly abducted arm
	Primary restraint to inferior translation in the adducted arm
MGHL (absent up to 30%)	Primary stabilizer to anterior translation with the arm abducted to 45 degrees
IGHLC	**Primary stabilizer for anterior and inferior instability in abduction**

ER, external rotation; SGHL, superior glenohumeral ligament; MGHL, middle glenohumeral ligament; IGHLC, inferior glenohumeral ligament complex.

Table 11-4. SUMMARY OF POPULAR ORTHOPAEDIC SURGICAL APPROACHES: LOWER EXTREMITY

REGION	APPROACH	EPONYM	MUSCULAR INTERVAL 1 (NERVE)	MUSCULAR INTERVAL 2 (NERVE)	DANGERS
Iliac crest	Posterior		Gluteus maximus (inferior gluteal)	Latissimus dorsi (thoracodorsal)	Clunial N, SGA, Sciatic N
	Anterior		TFL/glut. Med. & min. (superior gluteal)	Ext. abd. oblique (segmental)	ASIS/LFCN
Hip	Anterior	Smith-Peterson	Sartorius/rectus fem. (femoral)	TFL/gluteus medius (sup. gluteal)	LFCN, Fem. N, Asc. br. LFCA
	Anterolateral	Watson-Jones	Tensor fasciae latae (sup. gluteal)	Gluteus medius (sup. gluteal)	Fem. NAV/Profunda A
	Lateral	Hardinge's	Splits glut. med. (sup. gluteal)	Splits vastus lat. (femoral)	Femoral NVA/LFCA (transverse br.)
	Posterior	Moore-Southern	Splits glut. max. (inf. gluteal)	N/A	Sciatic, inf. glut. A
	Medial	Ludloff	Add. longus/add. brevis (ant. div. obt.)	Gracilis/add. magnus (obt./tibial)	Ant. div. obt. N/MFCA
Thigh	Lateral		Vastus lateralis (femoral)	Vastus lateralis (femoral)	Perf. br. profundus
	Posterolateral		Vastus lateralis (femoral)	Hamstrings (sciatic)	Perf. br. profundus
	Anteromedial		Rectus femoris (femoral)	Vastus medialis (femoral)	Med. sup. geniculate A
Distal femur	Posterior		Biceps femoris (sciatic)	Vastus lateralis (femoral)	Sciatic N/PFCN
Knee	Med. parapatellar		Vastus medialis (femoral)	Rectus femoris (femoral)	Infrapatellar br. saphenous N
	Medical		Vastus medialis (femoral)	Sartorius (femoral)	Infrapatellar br. saphenous N
	Lateral		Iliotibial band (sup. gluteal)	Biceps femoris (sciatic)	Peroneal N/popliteus ten.
	Posterior		Semimem/lat. gastroc. (tibial)	Biceps/lat. gastroc. (tib.)/(tib.)	Med. sural cut. N/tib. N/peroneal N
	Lateral		Vastus lateralis (femoral)	Biceps femoris (sciatic)	Peroneal N/lat. sup. gen. A
Tibia	Posterolateral		GS, soleus, FHL (tibial)	Peroneus brevis/longus (sup. peroneal)	Lesser saph. V/post. tib. A
	Anterior		Tibialis anterior (peroneal)	Periosteum	Long saph. V
Ankle	Anterior		EHL (deep peroneal)	EDL (deep peroneal)	S and D peroneal N/ant. tib. A
Med. malleolus	Posterior		Tibialis posterior	FDL	Saphenous N and V
Ankle	Posterolateral		Peroneus brevis (sup. peroneal)	FHL (tibial)	Sural N/sm saph. V
Distal fibula	Lateral		Peroneus tertius (deep peroneal)	Peroneus brevis (sup. peroneal)	Sural N
Foot	Anterolateral		Peroneal muscles (sup. peroneal)	EDC and per. tertius (deep peroneal)	Deep per. N/ant. tib. A
	Posteromedial		TP or FDL	FDL or FHL	Post. tib. A/tib N

A, Artery; V, vein; N, nerve; S, superficial; D, decreased; LFCA, lateral femoral circumflex artery; MFCA, medial femoral circumflex artery; SGA, superior gluteal artery; PFCN, posterior femoral cutaneous nerve; LFCN, lateral femoral cutaneous nerve; EDL, extensor digitorum longus; EHL, extensor hallucis longus; TP, tibialis posterior.

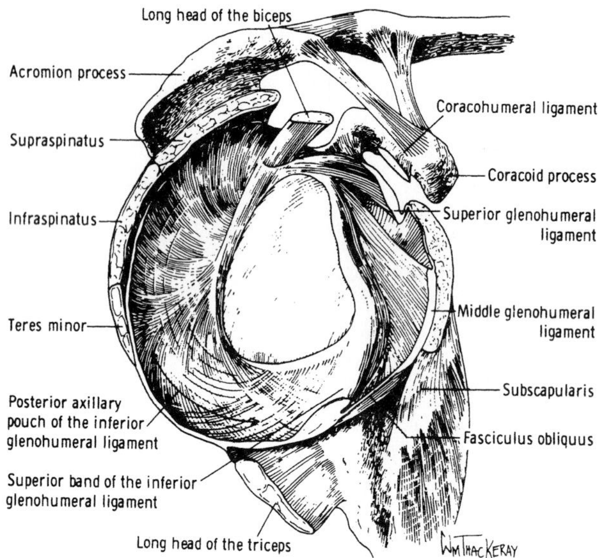

FIGURE 11-1 ■ Glenohumeral ligaments and rotator cuff muscles. The **rotator interval** is between the anterior border of the supraspinatus and the superior border of the subscapularis. This interval helps limit flexion and external rotation of the shoulder. Within the rotator interval is the **SGHL**: primary restraint to inferior translation in the adducted shoulder and primary restraint to external rotation in adducted or slightly abducted arm. The **MGHL**, absent in up to 30% of shoulders, is a primary stabilizer to anterior translation with the arm slightly abducted (45 degrees). **The IGHLC is the primary stabilizer for anterior and inferior instability in abduction**. (From Turkel, S.J., Panio, M.W., Marshall, J.L., et al.: Stabilizing mechanisms preventing anterior dislocation of the glenohumeral joint. J. Bone Joint Surg. [Am.] 63:1209, 1981.)

2. **Sternoclavicular Joint**—Double gliding joint with an articular disc. Its ligaments include the capsule, anterior and posterior sternoclavicular ligaments, an interclavicular ligament, and a costoclavicular ligament. The sternoclavicular joint rotates 30 degrees with shoulder motion.
3. **Acromioclavicular Joint**—Plane/gliding joint that also possesses a fibrocartilagenous disc. Its ligaments (Fig. 11-2) include the capsule, acromioclavicular ligament, and coracoclavicular ligament (with trapezoid [anterolateral] and conoid [posteromedial and stronger] component ligaments). The acromioclavicular ligaments prevent anteroposterior displacement of the distal clavicle. **The coracoclavicular ligament prevents superior displacement of the distal clavicle.** When the arm is maximally elevated, about 5–8 degrees of rotation occurs at the acromioclavicular joint although the clavicle rotates approximately 40–50 degrees.
4. **Scapulothoracic Joint**—Although not a true joint, this attachment allows scapular movement against the posterior rib cage. It is fixed primarily by the scapular muscular attachments. Glenohumeral motion as compared with scapulothoracic motion is a 2 : 1 ratio.
5. **Intrinsic Ligaments of the Scapula**—Include the superior transverse scapular ligament (which separates the suprascapular nerve [inferior] and vessels [superior] at the suprascapular notch), the inferior transverse scapular ligament (spinoglenoid notch), and the **coracoacromial ligament** (which is a frequent cause of impingement). The coracoacromial ligament is important in superior-anterior restraint in rotator cuff deficiencies and **should be preserved when débriding painful massive rotator cuff tears** that cannot be surgically repaired. The **acromial branch of the thoracoacromial artery** runs on the medial aspect of the coracoacromial ligament.

C. **Muscles of the Shoulder** (Fig. 11-3)—Five muscles help connect the upper limb to the vertebral column (trapezius, latissimus, both rhomboids, and the levator scapulae). Four muscles connect the upper limb to the thoracic wall (both pectoralis muscles, subclavius, and serratus anterior). Finally, six muscles act on the shoulder joint itself (deltoid, teres major, and the four rotator cuff

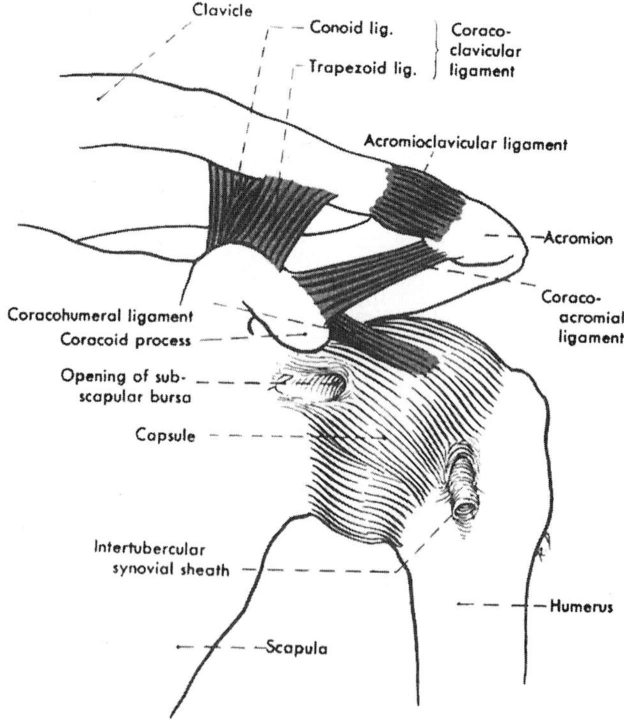

FIGURE 11-2 ■ Ligaments about the shoulder. The **acromioclavicular ligaments** (superior, inferior, anterior, and posterior) prevent anterior-posterior translation of the distal clavicle. The superior ligament is most important and is reinforced by fibers from the trapezius and deltoid muscles. The **coracoclavicular ligaments** (conoid [posteromedial] and trapezoid [anterolateral]) prevent superior translation of the distal clavicle. The **coracoacromial (CA) ligament** should be preserved in massive rotator cuff defects because it provides superior restraint to the humeral head. Bleeding encountered during release of the CA ligament is from the acromial branch of the thoracoacromial artery (second part of axillary artery [Figure 11-6]). (From Jenkins, D.B.: Hollinshead's Functional Anatomy of the Limbs and Back, 6th ed., Philadelphia, WB Saunders, 1991, p. 71.)

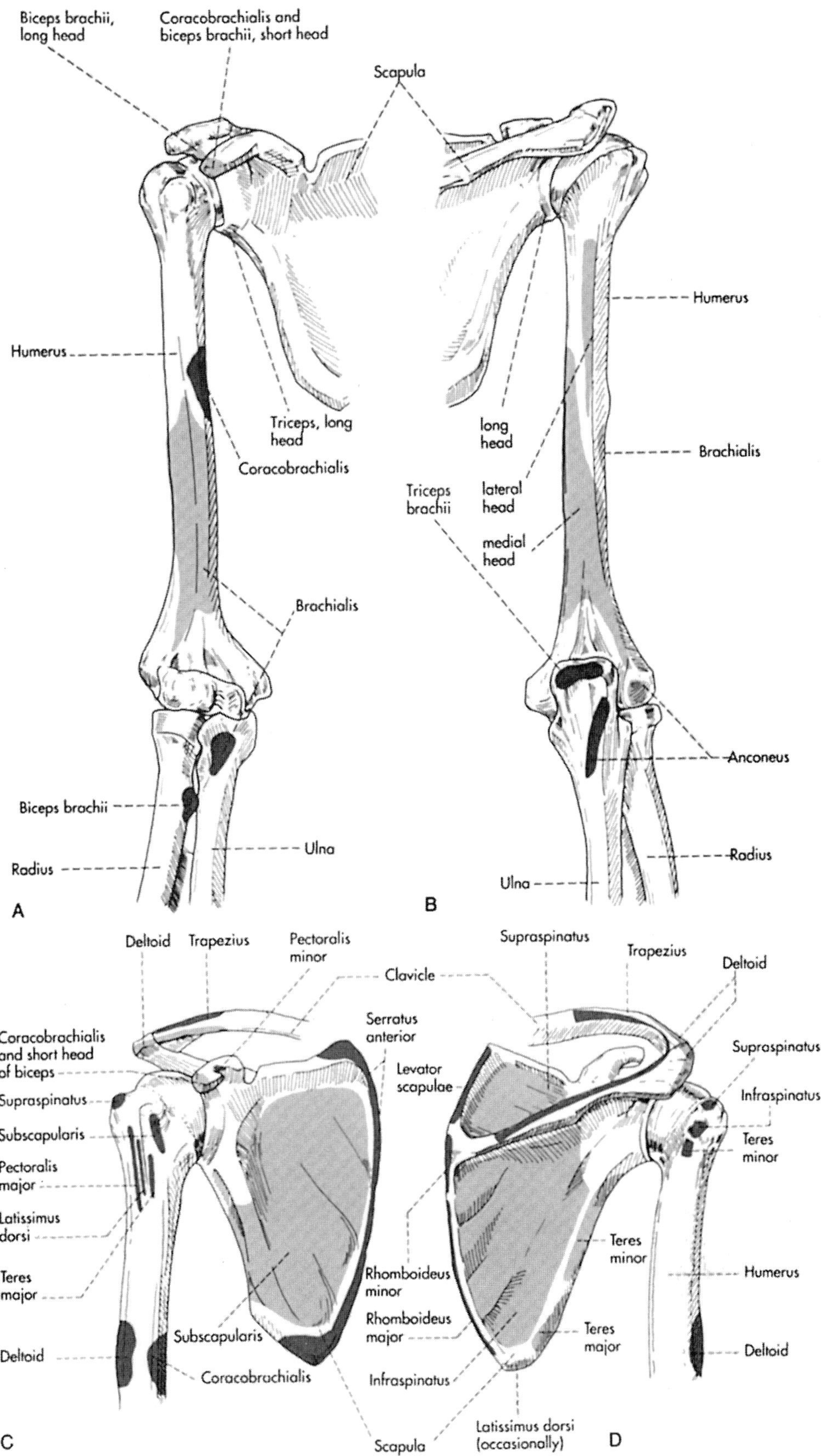

FIGURE 11-3 ■ Origins and insertions of muscles about the shoulder girdle. (From Jenkins, D.B.: Hollinshead's Functional Anatomy of the Limbs and Back, 6th ed., Fig. 5-3. Philadelphia, WB Saunders, 1991.)

Table 11-5. MUSCLES OF THE SHOULDER

MUSCLE	ORIGIN	INSERTION	ACTION	INNERVATION
Trapezius	Spin. proc. C7–T12	Clavicle, scapula (AC, SP)	Rotate scapula	CN XI
Lat. dorsii	Spin. proc. T6–S5, ilium	Humerus (ITG)	Ex., add., IR humerus	Thoracodorsal
Rhomboid maj.	Spin. proc. T2–T5	Scapula (med. border)	Adduct scapula	Dorsal scapular
Rhomboid min.	Spin. proc. C7–T1	Scapula (med. spine)	Adduct scapula	Dorsal scapular
Lev. scapulae	T. proc. C1–C4	Scapula (sup. med.)	Elevate, rotate scapula	C3, C4
Pectoralis maj.	Sternum, ribs, clavicle	Humerus (L-ITG)	Add., IR arm	M and L PN
Pectoralis min.	Ribs 3–5	Scapula (coracoid)	Protract scapula	MPN
Subclavius	Rib 1	Inf. clavicle	Depress clavicle	U trunk
Serratus ant.	Ribs 1–9	Scapula (vent. med.)	Prevent winging	Long thoracic
Deltoid	Lateral clavicle, scapula	Humerus (deltoid tub.)	Abduct arm (2)	Axillary
Teres major	Inf. scapula	Humerus (M-ITG)	Add., IR, ext.	L subscapular
Subscapularis	Ventral scapula	Humerus (LT)	IR arm, ant. stability	U and L subscapular
Supraspinatus	Sup. scapula	Humerus (GT)	Abd. (1), ER arm stability	Suprascapular
Infraspinatus	Dorsal scapula	Humerus (GT)	Stability, ER arm	Suprascapular
Teres minor	Scapula (dorsolateral)	Humerus (GT)	Stability, ER arm	Axillary

ITG, Intertubercular groove; AC, acromion; SP, spinous process; LT, lesser tuberosity; GT, greater tuberosity.

muscles [supraspinatus, infraspinatus, teres minor, subscapularis]). The rotator cuff muscles serve to depress and stabilize the humeral head against the glenoid. The **greater tuberosity** of the humerus serves as an attachment for three rotator cuff muscles: *supraspinatus, infraspinatus,* and the *teres minor.* The **lesser tuberosity** of the humerus serves as the attachment site for the *subscapularis* muscle (shoulder internal rotator).

The shoulder internal rotators (pectoralis major, latissimus dorsi, and subscapularis) are stronger than the external rotators (teres minor and infraspinatus), which is why posterior shoulder dislocations happen more commonly with electrical shock and seizures. Table 11-5 presents specifics on these muscles. The shoulder has been described as having four supporting layers (Fig. 11-4)

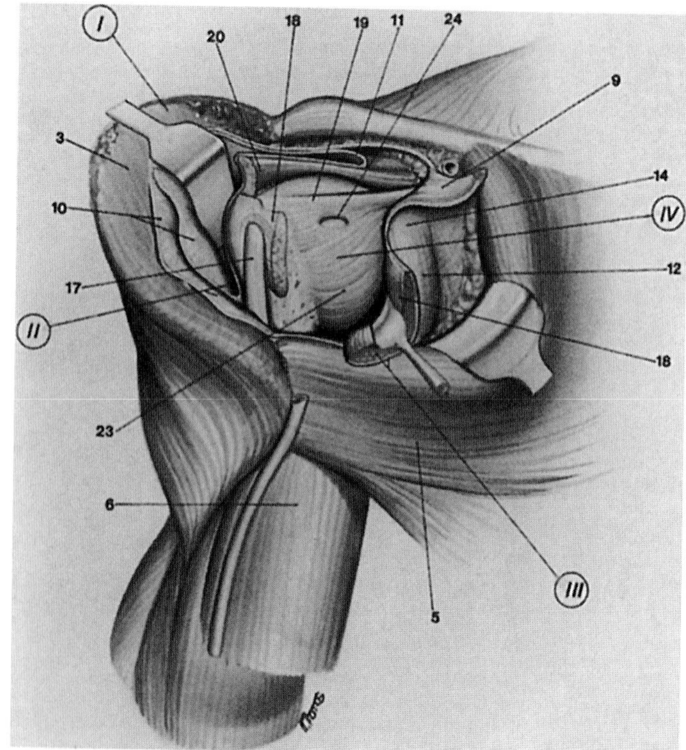

FIGURE 11-4 ■ Anterior aspect of the right shoulder depicting the four layers *(circled roman numerals).* The lateral retractor is placed deep to layer II, demonstrating the ease of dissection in the plane of the bursa around the lateral aspect of the proximal humerus. The subscapularis and supraspinatus (layer III) have been reflected, disclosing layer IV (capsule and coracohumeral ligament). The usual shape and position of the defect in the rotator interval (if present) is depicted; it is variable. *3* = deltoid; **5 = pectoralis major**; *6* = biceps; *9* = coracoacromial ligament; *10* = fasciae (II); *11* = deep layer of subdeltoid bursa; *12* = conjoined tendon; *14* = tip of coracoid process; *17* = biceps long head; *18* = deep layer subdeltoid bursa and subscapularis; *19* = coracohumeral ligament; *20* = supraspinatus under deep bursa layer; *23* = joint capsule; *24* = hiatus in capsule. (From Cooper, D.E., O'Brien, S.J., and Warren, R.F.: Supporting layers of glenohumeral joint. Clin. Orthop. 289:151, 1993.)

SHOULDER-SUPPORTING LAYERS

LAYER	STRUCTURE
I	Deltoid Pectoralis major
II	Clavipectoral fascia Cojoined tendon, short head biceps, and coracobrachialis
III	Deep layer of subdeltoid bursa Rotator cuff muscles (SITS—supraspinatus, infraspinatus, teres minor, subscapularis)
IV	Glenohumeral joint capsule Coracohumeral ligament

BRACHIAL PLEXUS CORD TERMINATIONS

CORD	TERMINATION
Lateral	**Musculocutaneous nerve** Lateral pectoral nerve
Posterior	**Radial and axillary nerve** Upper and lower subscapular nerve Thoracodorsal nerve
Medial	**Ulnar nerve** Medial pectoral nerve Medial brachial cutaneous nerve Medial antebrachial cutaneous nerve
Medial and lateral	**Median nerve**

D. **Nerves**—The **brachial plexus** (Fig. 11-5) is formed from the **ventral primary rami of C5–T1** and lies under the clavicle **between the scalenus anterior and scalenus medius**. Dorsal rami of C5-T1 innervate dorsal neck musculature and skin. The brachial plexus is organized into five components: ***r*oots, *t*runks, *d*ivisions, *c*ords, and *b*ranches** (remember the mnemonic *R*on *T*aylor *d*rinks *c*old *b*eer). There are five roots (C5-T1, although C4 and T2 can have small contributions), three trunks (upper, middle, lower), six divisions (two from each trunk), three cords named because of anatomic relationship to the axillary artery (posterior, lateral, medial), and multiple branches. The termination of each cord is worth mentioning.

Note that there are ***four preclavicular branches*** **(from roots and upper trunk): dorsal scapular nerve, long thoracic nerve, suprascapular nerve,** and **nerve to subclavius. Preganglionic (proximal to the dorsal root ganglion) brachial plexus lesions would be expected to produce scapular winging** (because of paralysis of the preclavicular long thoracic nerve) and Horner's syndrome (injury to brachial plexus at C8-T1—involving the inferior/stellate ganglion). Postganglionic brachial plexus injuries should therefore not have Horner's syndrome, winged scapula, diaphragmatic paralysis, or rhomboid paralysis. Additional review of obstetric brachial plexus palsies is shown in the following chart.

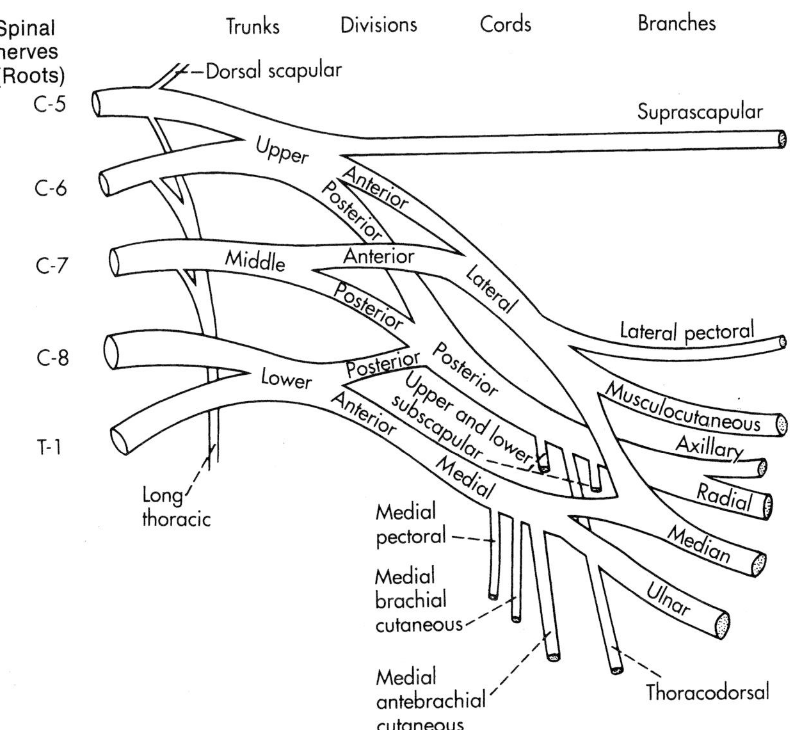

FIGURE 11-5 ■ **Brachial plexus**. Remember the four preclavicular/supraclavicular branches: long thoracic nerve (serratus anterior muscle), dorsal scapular nerve (rhomboids muscle), suprascapular nerve (supraspinatus and infraspinatus muscle) and the nerve to the subclavius (not shown). (From Jenkins, D.B.: Hollinshead's Functional Anatomy of the Limbs and Back, 6th ed., Fig. 5-7. Philadelphia, WB Saunders, 1991.)

BRACHIAL PLEXUS PALSY SUMMARY

PALSY	ROOTS	DEFICIT	PROGNOSIS
Erb-Duchenne	C5,C6	Deltoid, rotator cuff, elbow flexors, wrist and hand extensors "Waiter's tip"	Best
Klumpke	C8, T1	Wrist flexors, intrinsics, Horner's syndrome	Poor
Total plexus	C5–T1	Flaccid arm	Worst

ROTATOR CUFF MUSCLE INNERVATION—ALL C5,C6

MUSCLE	INNERVATION
External rotators	
Supraspinatus	Suprascapular nerve (C5,C6)
Infraspinatus	Suprascapular nerve (C5,C6)
Teres minor	Axillary nerve (C5,C6)
Internal rotator	
Subscapularis	Upper (C5) and lower subscapular nerve (C5,C6)

Understand the difference between scapular-trapezius winging and serratus anterior scapular winging. Injury to the spinal accessory nerve causes **scapular-trapezius winging,** resulting in shoulder depression with scapular *translation laterally* and the *inferior angle rotated laterally* because of the unopposed pull of the serratus anterior. Injury to the long thoracic nerve causes **serratus anterior scapular winging,** resulting in superior elevation with scapular *translation medially* and the *inferior angle rotated medially.* Innervation of all rotator cuff muscles is derived from C5,C6 of the brachial plexus.

E. **Vessels** (Fig. 11-6)—The subclavian artery arises either directly from the aorta (left subclavian) or from the brachiocephalic trunk (right subclavian). It then emerges between the scalenus anterior and medius muscles and becomes the axillary artery at the outer border of the first rib. **The axillary artery is divided into three portions based on its relationship to the pectoralis minor** (the first is medial to it, the second is under it, and the third is lateral to it). Each part of the artery has as many branches as the number of that portion (e.g., the second part

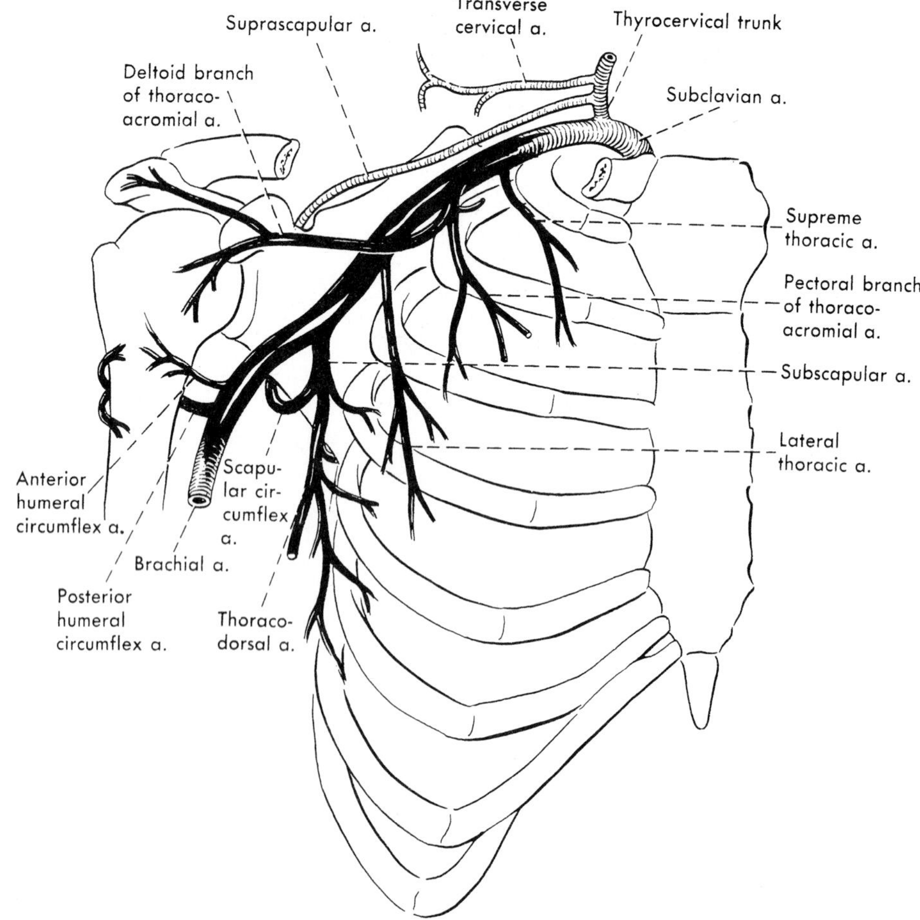

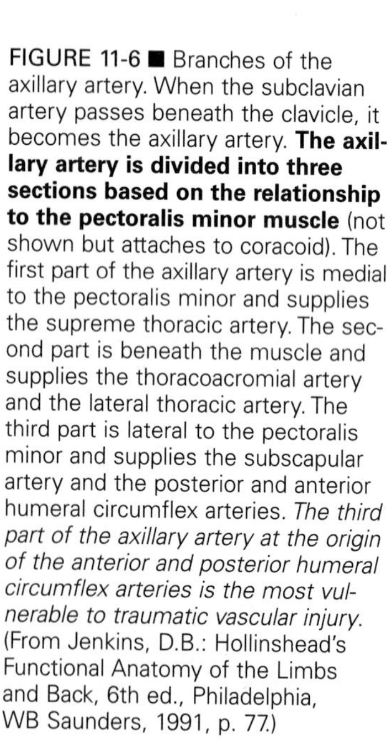
FIGURE 11-6 ■ Branches of the axillary artery. When the subclavian artery passes beneath the clavicle, it becomes the axillary artery. **The axillary artery is divided into three sections based on the relationship to the pectoralis minor muscle** (not shown but attaches to coracoid). The first part of the axillary artery is medial to the pectoralis minor and supplies the supreme thoracic artery. The second part is beneath the muscle and supplies the thoracoacromial artery and the lateral thoracic artery. The third part is lateral to the pectoralis minor and supplies the subscapular artery and the posterior and anterior humeral circumflex arteries. *The third part of the axillary artery at the origin of the anterior and posterior humeral circumflex arteries is the most vulnerable to traumatic vascular injury.* (From Jenkins, D.B.: Hollinshead's Functional Anatomy of the Limbs and Back, 6th ed., Philadelphia, WB Saunders, 1991, p. 77.)

AXILLARY ARTERY BRANCHES

PART	BRANCH	COURSE
1	Supreme thoracic	Medial to serratus anterior and pectorals
2	Thoracoacromial	Four branches (deltoid, acromial, pectoralis, clavicular)
	Lateral thoracic	Descends to serratus anterior
3	Subscapular	Two branches (thoracodorsal and circumflex scapular **[triangular space]**)
	Anterior humeral circumflex	Blood supply to humeral head—arcuate artery lateral to bicipital groove
	Posterior humeral circumflex	Branch in the **quadrangular space** accompanying the axillary nerve

has two branches). *The third part of the axillary artery at the origin of the anterior and posterior humeral circumflex arteries is most vulnerable to traumatic vascular injury.*

F. **Surgical Approaches to the Shoulder (Table 11-3)**—Include the anterior approach (reconstructions and arthroplasties), lateral approach (acromioplasty and cuff repair), and posterior approach (posterior reconstruction). A summary chart is shown in the next column.

1. **Anterior Approach (Henry)** (Fig. 11-7)—Explores the interval between the **deltoid (axillary nerve) and the pectoralis major (medial and lateral pectoral nerve).** The cephalic vein is dissected and retracted laterally with the deltoid, and the underlying subscapularis is exposed. The subscapularis is then divided (preserving the most inferior

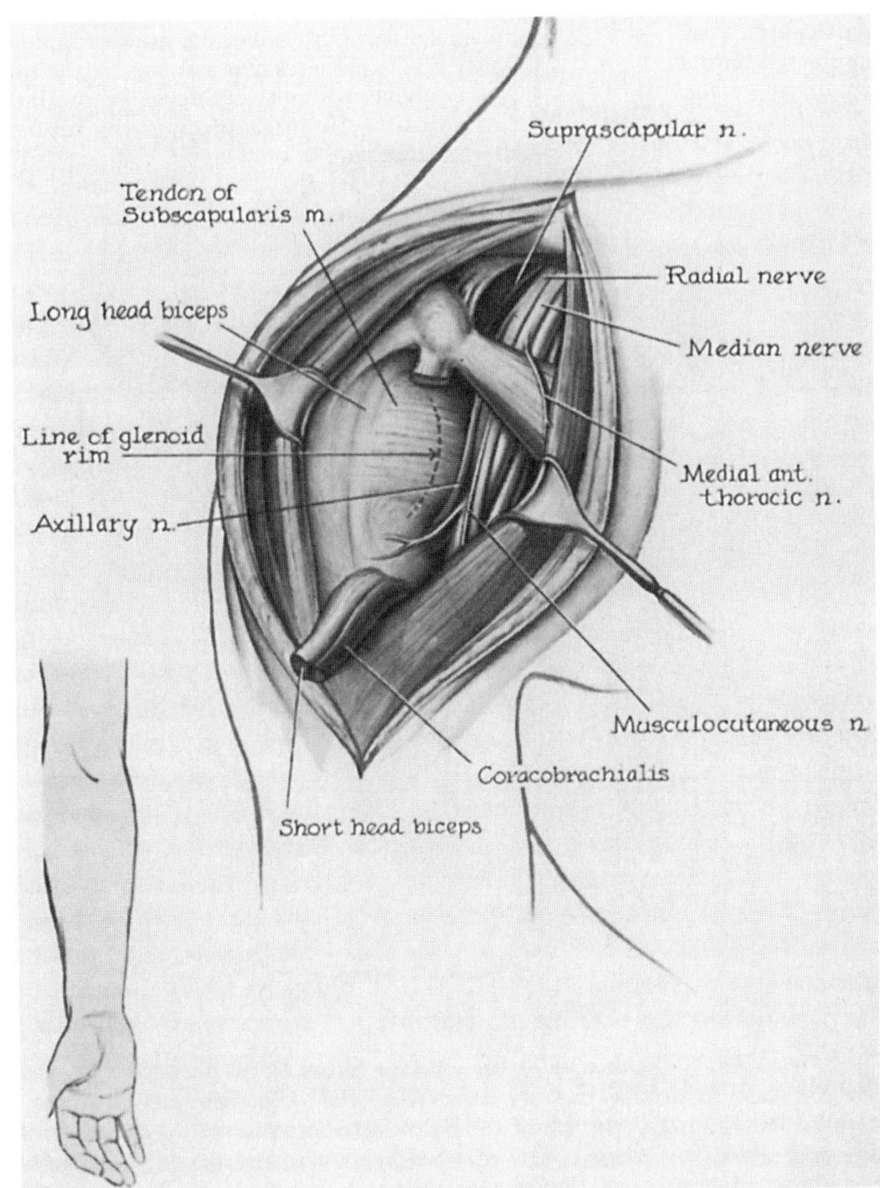

FIGURE 11-7 ■ Anterior approach (Henry) to the shoulder. The interval between the **deltoid (axillary nerve)** and the **pectoralis major (medial and lateral pectoral nerve)** is explored. Avoid excessive medial retraction (see medial retractor) on the coracobrachialis or dissection medial to this muscle to prevent injury to the **musculocutaneous nerve**. Avoid the **axillary nerve**, which is inferior to the shoulder capsule. Positioning the arm in adduction and external rotation helps displace the axillary nerve from the surgical field. (From Kaplan, E.B.: Surgical Approaches to the Neck, Cervical Spine, and Upper Extremity. Philadelphia, WB Saunders, 1966, p. 57.)

fibers to protect the axillary nerve), and the shoulder capsule is encountered. Division of the subscapularis does not lead to denervation because innervation enters medially. There is a leash of three vessels (one artery and the superior and inferior venae comitantes) that mark the lower border of the subscapularis. Protect the **musculocutaneous nerve** (lateral cord brachial plexus) by avoiding vigorous retraction of the cojoined tendon and avoiding dissection medial to the coracobrachialis. This nerve usually penetrates the biceps/coracobrachialis 5–8 cm below the coracoid, but it enters these muscles proximal to this 5-cm "safe zone" almost 30% of the time. Palsy of the musculocutaneous nerve would affect the coracobrachialis, biceps brachii and the brachialis muscles, and sensation in the *lateral antebrachial cutaneous nerve* (termination of the musculocutaneous nerve). The **axillary nerve** (posterior cord brachial plexus), which is **just inferior to the shoulder capsule**, must be protected during procedures in this area. *Adduction and external rotation of the arm will help displace the axillary nerve from the surgical field.*

2. **Lateral Approach**—Involves splitting the deltoid muscle or subperiosteal dissection of the muscle from the acromion. The **deltoid should not be split more than 5 cm below the acromion** to avoid injury to the **axillary nerve** (posterior cord brachial plexus exiting from quadrangular space). If dissection extends >5 cm inferior, denervation of the deltoid can occur in a location anterior to the muscle split because of the posterior innervation of the muscle. The supraspinatus tendon is exposed and allows for repairs of the rotator cuff.
3. **Posterior Approach** (Fig. 11-8)—Uses the internervous plane between the **infraspinatus (suprascapular nerve)** and **teres minor (axillary nerve)**. This plane can be approached by detaching the deltoid from the scapular spine or by splitting the deltoid (Rockwood's). After this interval is found, the posterior capsule lies immediately below it. The axillary nerve and the posterior circumflex humeral artery both run in the **quadrangular space** below the teres minor, so it is important to stay above this muscle. **Excessive medial retraction of the infraspinatus can injure the suprascapular nerve.**

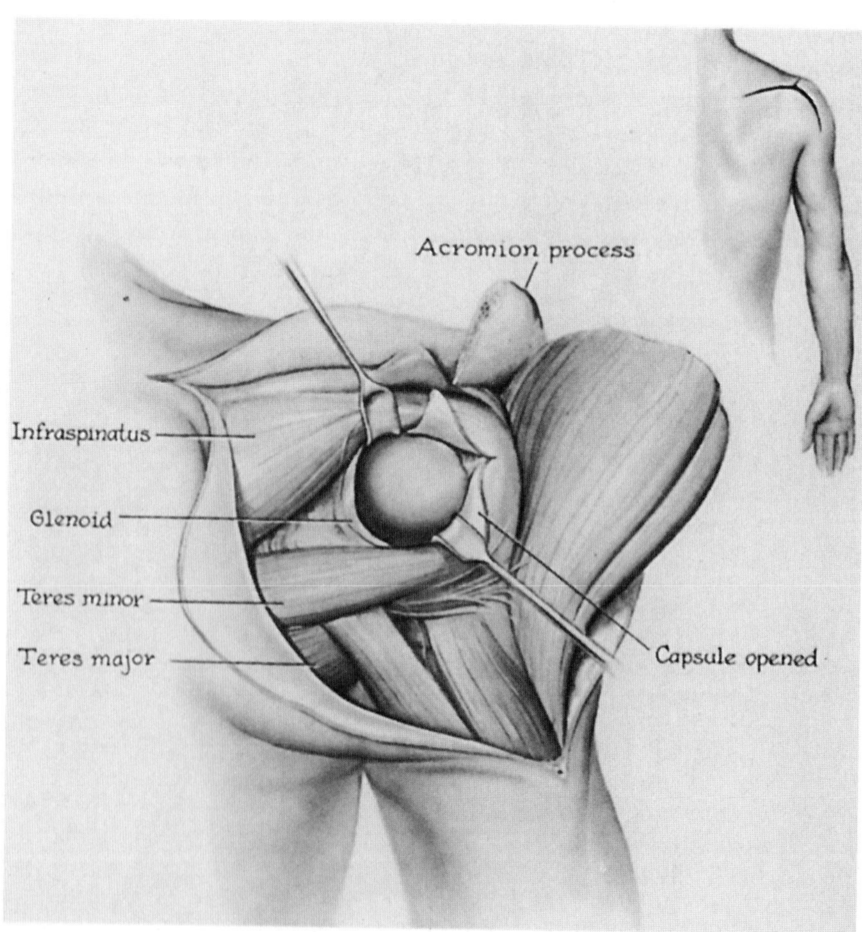

FIGURE 11-8 ■ Posterior approach to the shoulder. The interval between the **infraspinatus (suprascapular nerve)** and **teres minor (axillary nerve)** is explored. **Do not dissect below the teres minor**. Dissections below the teres minor risk injury to the structures in the **quadrangular space: posterior humeral circumflex artery and the axillary nerve**. The axillary nerve divides into the deep (deltoid) and superficial branches (teres minor and cutaneous branch [Hilton's law]) within the quadrangular space. Also **avoid excessive retraction of the infraspinatus** to avoid suprascapular nerve palsy. (From Kaplan, E.B.: Surgical Approaches to the Neck, Cervical Spine, and Upper Extremity. Philadelphia, WB Saunders, 1966, p. 61.)

SHOULDER SURGICAL APPROACHES

APPROACH	INTERVAL	RISKS
Anterior (Henry)	Deltoid (axillary nerve) and pectoralis major (medial and lateral pectoral nerve)	Axillary nerve limits inferior exposure (place arm in adduction and ER) Musculocutaneous nerve—avoid vigorous retraction and medial dissection to the cojoined tendon/ coracobrachialis
Lateral	Deltoid splitting (axillary nerve)	Avoid deltoid split >5 cm below acromion to avoid damaging axillary nerve
Posterior	Infraspinatus (suprascapular nerve) and teres minor (axillary nerve)	Dissection inferior to the teres minor risks **quadrangular space** structures: axillary nerve and posterior humeral circumflex artery Avoid excessive medial retraction on infraspinatus, which can injure suprascapular nerve

G. **Arthroscopy**—Portals for arthroscopy (discussed in Chapter 3, Sports Medicine) include the anterior superior (musculocutaneous nerve at risk with portals medial), the anterior inferior (must be above the subscapularis and lateral to the conjoined tendon), and the posterior (inferior portals may risk the axillary nerve).

III. Arm

A. **Osteology**—The humerus is the only bone of the arm and the largest and longest bone of the upper extremity. It is composed of a shaft and two articular extremities. The hemispheric head, directed superiorly, medially, and slightly dorsally, articulates with the much smaller scapular glenoid cavity. The *anatomic neck,* directly below the head, serves as an attachment for the shoulder capsule. The *surgical neck* is lower and is more often involved in fractures. The **greater tuberosity**, lateral to the head, serves as the attachment for the *supraspinatus, infraspinatus, and teres minor* muscles (anterior to posterior, respectively). The **lesser tuberosity**, located anteriorly, has only one muscular insertion: the last rotator cuff muscle, the *subscapularis.* The bicipital groove (for the tendon of the long head of the biceps) is situated between the two tuberosities. The shaft of the humerus has a posterior spiral groove adjacent to the deltoid tuberosity. This groove is approximately 13 cm above the articular surface of the trochlea. Distally, the humerus flares into medial and lateral epicondyles and forms half of the elbow joint with a medial spool-shaped trochlea (articulates with the olecranon of the ulna) and a globular capitellum (which opposes the radial head). The normal articular alignment of the distal humerus has a 7 degree valgus tilt (carrying angle). Additionally, the **humeral head is retroverted approximately 30 degrees** relative to the transepicondylar axis of the humerus with the **scapular glenoid approximately 5 degrees retroverted**.

B. **Arthrology**—The humerus articulates with the scapula on its upper end, forming the glenohumeral joint (discussed earlier), and with the radius and ulna on its lower end, forming the elbow joint. The elbow is composed of a compound ginglymus (hinge) joint (the humeroulnar articulation) and a trochoid (pivot) joint (the humeroradial articulation). The axis of rotation for the elbow is centered through the trochlea and capitellum and passes through a point anteroinferior on the medial epicondyle.

ELBOW JOINT ARTICULATIONS

ARTICULATION	COMPONENTS
Humeroulnar	Trochlea and trochlear notch
Humeroradial	Capitulum and radial head
Proximal radioulnar	Radial notch and radial head

The elbow joint has capsuloligamentous tissues that are a key source of testable material (Fig. 11-9). The elbow capsule allows maximal distension at approximately 70–80 degrees of flexion, which is why patients with effusions hold their arms in this most comfortable position. Also, the anterior capsule attaches at a point approximately 6 mm distal to the tip of the

ELBOW LIGAMENTS

LIGAMENT	COMPONENTS	COMMENTS
Medial collateral (MCL)	**Anterior bundle MCL (ulnar collateral)**; Posterior bundle; Transverse bundle (Cooper's ligament)	Anterior bundle (strongest of all elbow ligaments): anterior band taut from 60 degree flexion to full extension, posterior band taut from 60–120 degree flexion
Lateral collateral	**LUCL**; Annular ligament; Quadrate (annular ligament to radial neck) and oblique cord	Deficiency of LUCL results in posterolateral rotator instability

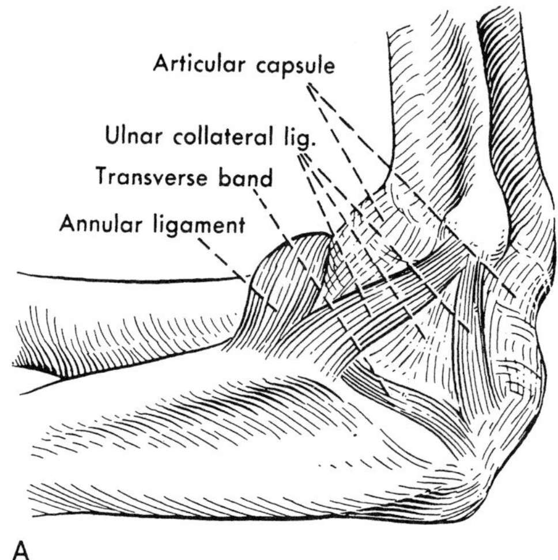

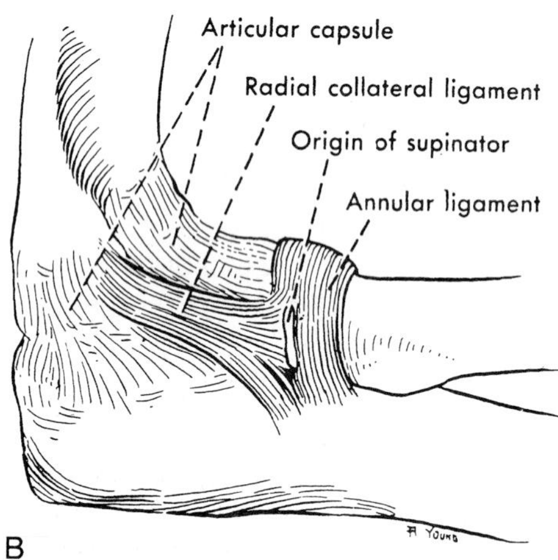

FIGURE 11-9 ■ Elbow ligaments. *A,* Medial view. The most important portion of the medial collateral ligament is the anterior bundle or ulnar collateral ligament. *B,* Lateral view. The most important portion of the lateral collateral ligament complex is the lateral ulnar collateral ligament (LUCL) or radial collateral ligament. Deficiency of the LUCL results in posterolateral rotatory instability. (From Jenkins, D.B.: Hollinshead's Functional Anatomy of the Limbs and Back, 6th ed., Philadelphia, WB Saunders, 1991, p. 108.)

coronoid. Because of this, the coronoid tip is an intra-articular structure that is visualized during elbow arthroscopy. Other testable coronoid attachments include the anterior bundle of the medial collateral ligament (18 mm distal to the coronoid tip) and brachialis (11 mm distal to the coronoid tip). The **medial collateral ligament** (anterior bundle, posterior bundle and transverse bundle) arises from the anteroinferior portion of the medial humeral epicondyle and provides stability to valgus stress. The **anterior bundle is most important in helping resist valgus forces**. Remember that *valgus stability with the arm in* ***pronation*** suggests an *intact anterior bundle of the medial collateral ligament.* The lateral collateral ligament or radial collateral ligament (annular, radial, and ulnar parts) originates on the lateral humeral epicondyle near the axis of elbow rotation. The **lateral ulnar collateral ligament** (LUCL) is an essential elbow stabilizer and runs from the lateral epicondyle to the ulna crista supinatoris (supinator crest). **Deficiency of the LUCL manifests as posterolateral rotatory instability of the elbow.**

C. **Muscles of the Arm**—There are four muscles of the arm (Table 11-6). The triceps muscle helps form borders for two important spaces (Fig. 11-10). The **triangular space** is bordered by the teres minor (superiorly), teres major (inferiorly), and long head of the triceps (laterally); it contains the **circumflex scapular vessels**. The **quadrangular (quadrilateral) space** is also bordered by the teres minor (superiorly) and the teres major (inferiorly), with the long head of the triceps forming its medial border and the humerus forming the lateral border. The quadrangular space transmits the **posterior humeral circumflex vessels and the axillary nerve**. The **triangular interval** is immediately inferior to the quadrangular space and is bordered by the teres major (superiorly), long head of the triceps (medially), and lateral head of the triceps or the humerus (laterally). Through this interval the **profunda brachii artery** and **radial nerve** can be seen.

Table 11-6. MUSCLES OF THE ARM

MUSCLE	ORIGIN	INSERTION	ACTION	INNERVATION
Coracobrachialis	Coracoid	Mid. humerus medial	Flexion, adduction	Musculocutaneous
Biceps	Coracoid (SH) Supraglenoid (LH)	Radial tuberosity	Supination, flexion	Musculocutaneous
Brachialis	Ant. humerus	Ulnar tuberosity (ant.)	Flexes forearm	Musculocut., radial
Triceps	Infraglenoid (LH) Post. humerus (lat H) Post. humerus (MH)	Olecranon	Extends forearm	Radial

SH, Short head; LH, long head; lat H, lateral head; MH, medial head.

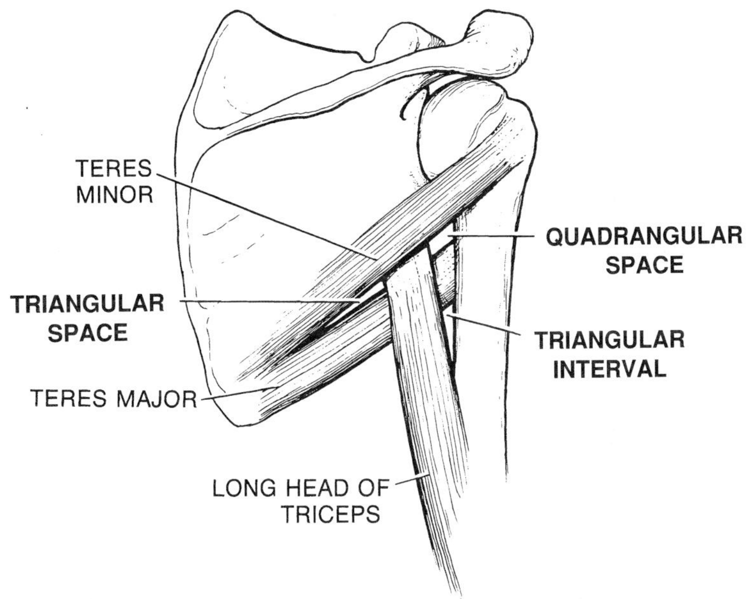

FIGURE 11-10 ■ Borders of key spaces and intervals from posterior. **Quadrangular space** (axillary nerve and posterior humeral circumflex artery), **triangular space** (circumflex scapular vessels), and **triangular interval** (radial nerve and profunda brachii artery). (From Kaplan, E.B.: Surgical Approaches to the Neck, Cervical Spine, and Upper Extremity. Philadelphia, WB Saunders, 1966, p. 53.)

SHOULDER SPACES AND INTERVALS

SPACE	BORDERS	NERVE	VESSEL
Quadrangular (quadrilateral) space	Superior—lower border teres minor; Lateral—surgical neck of humerus; Medial—long head of triceps; Inferior—upper border of teres major	Axillary nerve	Posterior humeral circumflex a
Triangular space	Superior—lower border of teres minor; Lateral—long head of triceps; Medial—teres major		Circumflex scapular a
Triangular interval	Superior—lower border teres major; Lateral—shaft of humerus; Medial—long head of triceps	Radial nerve	Profunda brachii a

Muscles controlling elbow motion include the flexors (biceps, brachialis, and brachioradialis) and the extensors (triceps). **Tennis elbow** (lateral epicondylitis) primarily involves the extensor carpi radialis brevis **(ECRB)**.

D. **Nerves**—Four major nerves traverse the arm, two giving off branches to arm musculature and two that innervate distal musculature (Fig. 11-11). Most of the cutaneous innervation of the arm arises directly from the brachial plexus.

1. **Musculocutaneous Nerve (Lateral Cord)**—Pierces the coracobrachialis 5–8 cm distal to the coracoid and then branches to supply this muscle, the biceps, and the brachialis. It also gives off a branch to the elbow joint before it becomes the **lateral antebrachial cutaneous nerve** of the forearm, which is located *lateral to the cephalic vein.*
2. **Radial Nerve (Posterior Cord)**—Spirals around the humerus (medial to lateral) in the spiral groove at a distance of approximately 13 cm from the trochlea. It emerges on the lateral side of the arm after piercing the lateral intermuscular septum approximately 7.5 cm above the trochlea between the brachialis and brachioradialis anterior to the lateral epicondyle (where it supplies the anconeus muscle).
3. **Median Nerve (Medial and Lateral Cords)**—Accompanies the brachial artery along the arm, crossing it during its course (lateral to medial). It supplies some branches to the elbow joint but has no branches in the arm itself.
4. **Ulnar Nerve (Medial Cord)**—Medial to the brachial artery in the arm and then runs behind the medial epicondyle of the humerus, where it is quite superficial. It also has branches to the elbow but not arm branches.
5. **Cutaneous Nerves**—The supraclavicular nerve (C3, C4) supplies the upper shoulder. The axillary nerve supplies the shoulder joint

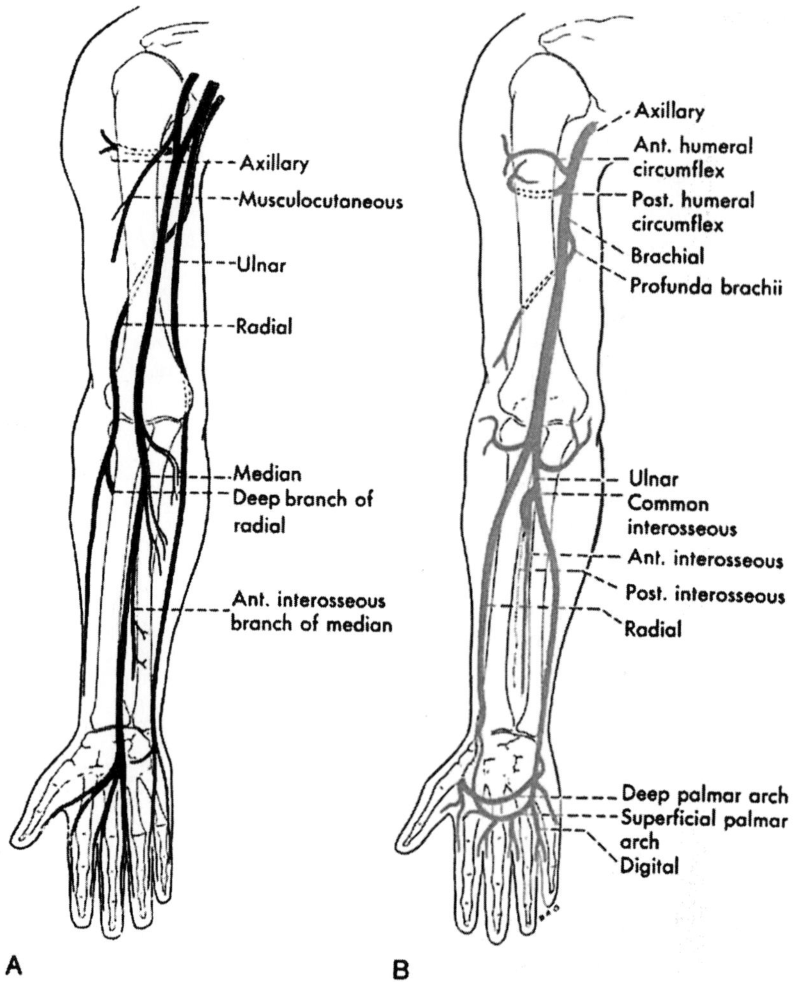

FIGURE 11-11 ■ Nerves and vessels of the upper extremity. *A,* Principal nerves. *B,* Chief arteries. (From Jenkins, D.B.: Hollinshead's Functional Anatomy of the Limbs and Back, 6th ed. Philadelphia, WB Saunders, 1991, p. 62.)

and the overlying skin (in accordance with Hilton's law). The medial, lateral, and dorsal brachial cutaneous nerves supply the balance of the cutaneous innervation of the arm. The lateral antebrachial cutaneous nerve is the termination of the musculocutaneous nerve (see Fig. 11-40 for dematome summary).

E. **Vessels**—The brachial artery originates at the lower border of the tendon of the teres major and continues to the elbow, where it bifurcates into the radial and ulnar arteries (see Fig. 11-11). Lying medial in the arm, the brachial artery curves laterally to enter the cubital fossa (formed by the distal humerus proximally, the brachioradialis laterally, and the pronator teres medially). Its principal branches include the deep brachial (also known as the profunda, this artery accompanies the radial nerve posteriorly in the triangular interval), the superior and inferior ulnar collaterals, and nutrient and muscular branches. The supratrochlear artery is the least flexible branch; these collateral vessels can bind up the brachial artery with distal humerus fractures.

F. **Surgical Approaches to the Arm**—A summary chart is provided on the following page.
   1. **Anterolateral Approach to the Humerus** (Fig. 11-12)—Depends on the internervous plane between the **deltoid (axillary nerve)** and the **pectoralis major (medial and lateral pectoral nerves) proximally** and between the fibers of the **brachialis (radial nerve and musculocutaneous nerve) distally**. The radial and axillary nerves are at risk mainly because of forceful retraction.The anterior circumflex humeral vessels may need to be ligated with a proximal approach.
   2. **Posterior Approach to the Humerus** (Fig. 11-13)—Uses the interval between the lateral and long heads of the triceps superficially and a **muscle-splitting approach for**

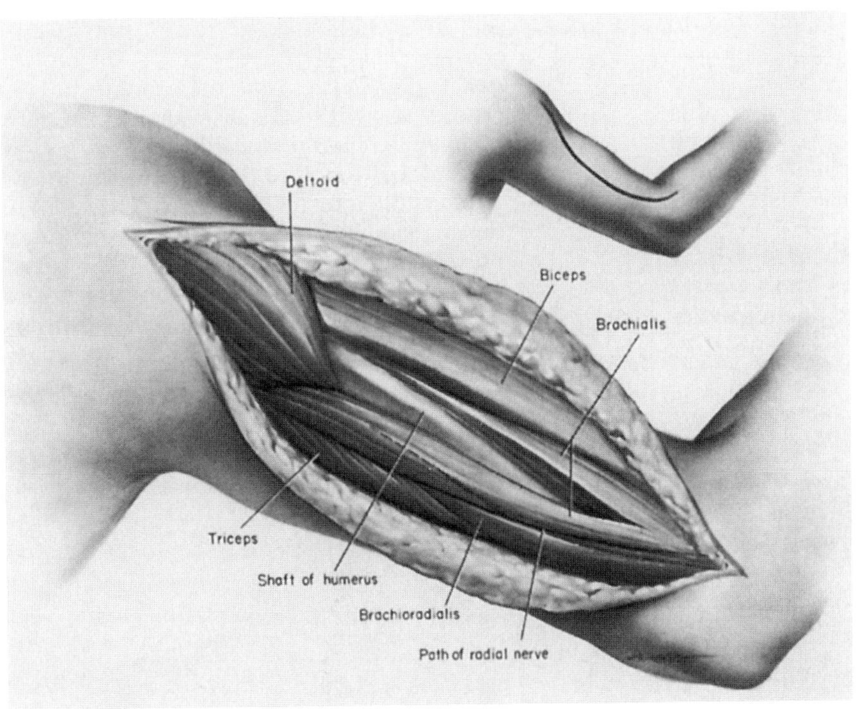

FIGURE 11-12 ■ Lateral approach to the arm. (From Kaplan, E.B.: Surgical Approaches to the Neck, Cervical Spine, and Upper Extremity. Philadelphia, WB Saunders, 1966, p. 74.)

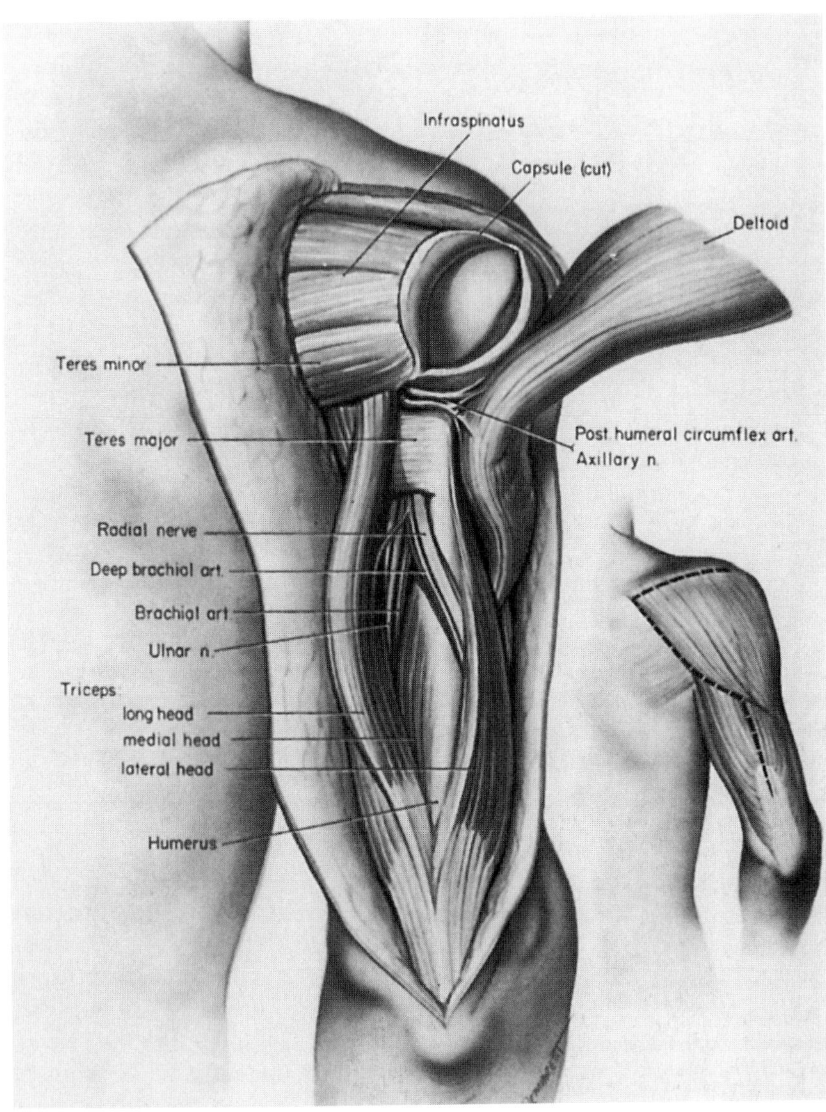

FIGURE 11-13 ■ Posterior approach to the arm. The medial, or deep head, of the triceps is split in this approach. (From Kaplan, E.B.: Surgical Approaches to the Neck, Cervical Spine, and Upper Extremity. Philadelphia, WB Saunders, 1966, p. 73.)

the medial (deep) head. The radial nerve (which limits proximal extension of this approach) and deep brachial artery must be identified and protected. The ulnar nerve is jeopardized unless subperiosteal dissection of the humerus is meticulous.

3. **Anterolateral Approach to the Distal Humerus** (Fig. 11-14)—Uses the interval between the **brachialis (musculocutaneous and radial nerves)** and the **brachioradialis (radial nerve).** The radial nerve again must be identified and protected.
4. **Lateral Approach to the Distal Humerus**—Exploits the interval between the triceps and the brachioradialis by elevating a portion of the common extensor origin from the lateral epicondyle. Proximal extension jeopardizes the radial nerve.

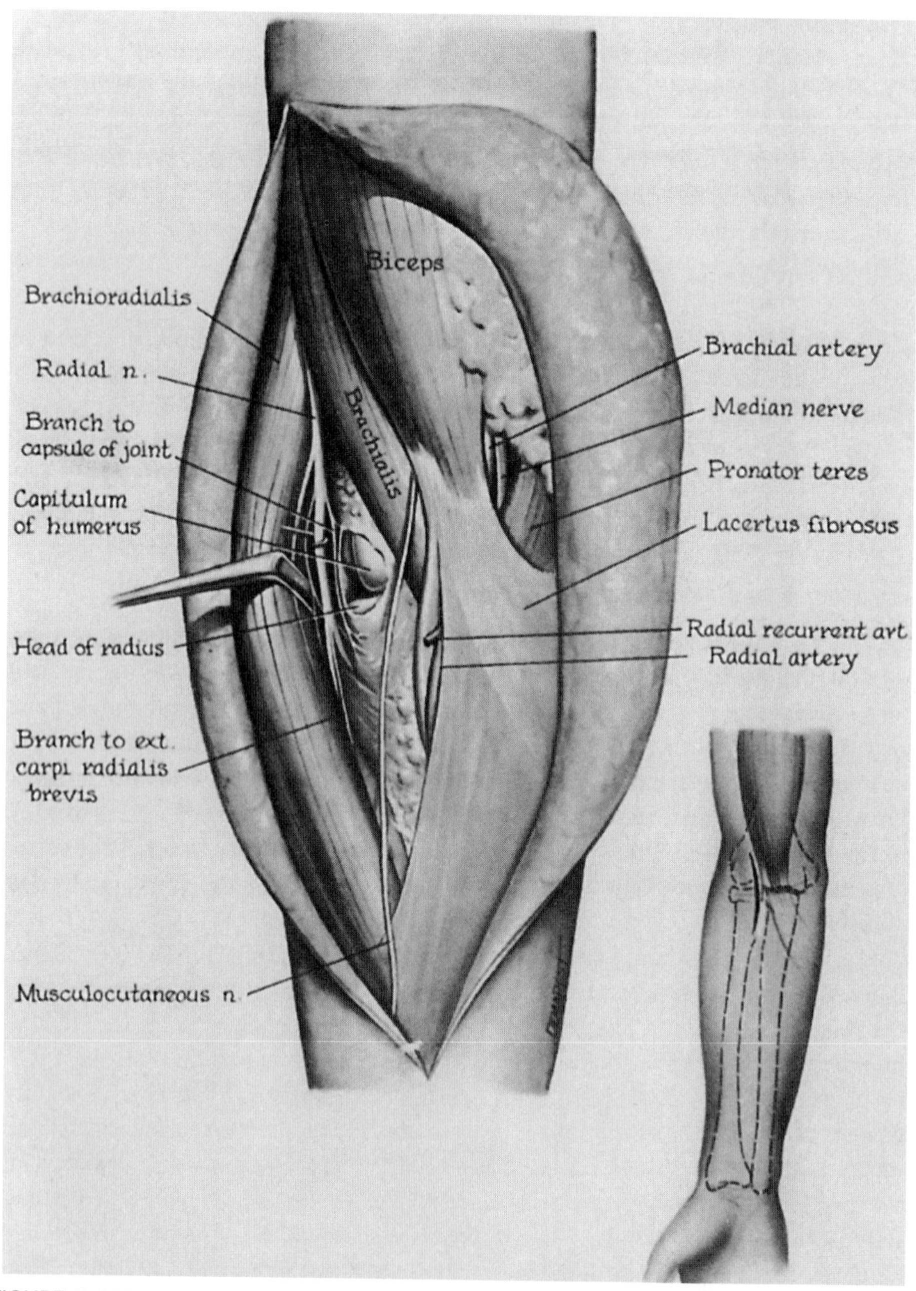

FIGURE 11-14 ■ Anterior elbow anatomy. For the lateral distal humerus exposure, the interval between the brachioradialis (radial nerve) and the brachialis (radial and musculocutaneous nerve) is explored protecting the radial nerve. (From Kaplan, E.B.: Surgical Approaches to the Neck, Cervical Spine, and Upper Extremity. Philadelphia, WB Saunders, 1966, p. 77.)

HUMERAL SURGICAL APPROACHES

APPROACH	INTERVAL	RISKS
Anterolateral—proximal	Proximal: Deltoid (axillary nerve) and pectoralis major (medial and lateral pectoral nerve) Distal: Brachialis (radial and musculocutaneous nerve)	Radial nerve Axillary nerve Anterior humeral circumflex artery
Posterior	Triceps (radial nerve): lateral and long heads	Radial nerve Deep brachial artery
Anterolateral—distal	Brachialis (musculocutaneous and radial nerve) and brachioradialis (radial nerve)	Radial nerve
Lateral	Triceps (radial nerve) and brachioradialis (radial nerve)	Radial nerve with proximal extension

G. **Surgical Approaches to the Elbow**—Standard approaches are discussed below and a summary chart is provided.

1. **Posterior Approach to the Elbow** (Fig. 11-15)—Detachment of the extensor mechanism of the elbow gives excellent exposure for many elbow fractures. The olecranon osteotomy (best done with a chevron cut 2 cm distal to the tip) should be predrilled and the ulnar nerve protected. An alternative approach splits the triceps and leaves the olecranon intact.
2. **Medial Approach to the Elbow**—Exploits the interval between **the brachialis (musculocutaneous nerve)** and the **triceps (radial nerve) proximally** and the **brachialis and pronator teres (median nerve) distally.** The ulnar and medial antebrachial cutaneous nerves are in the field and must be protected.

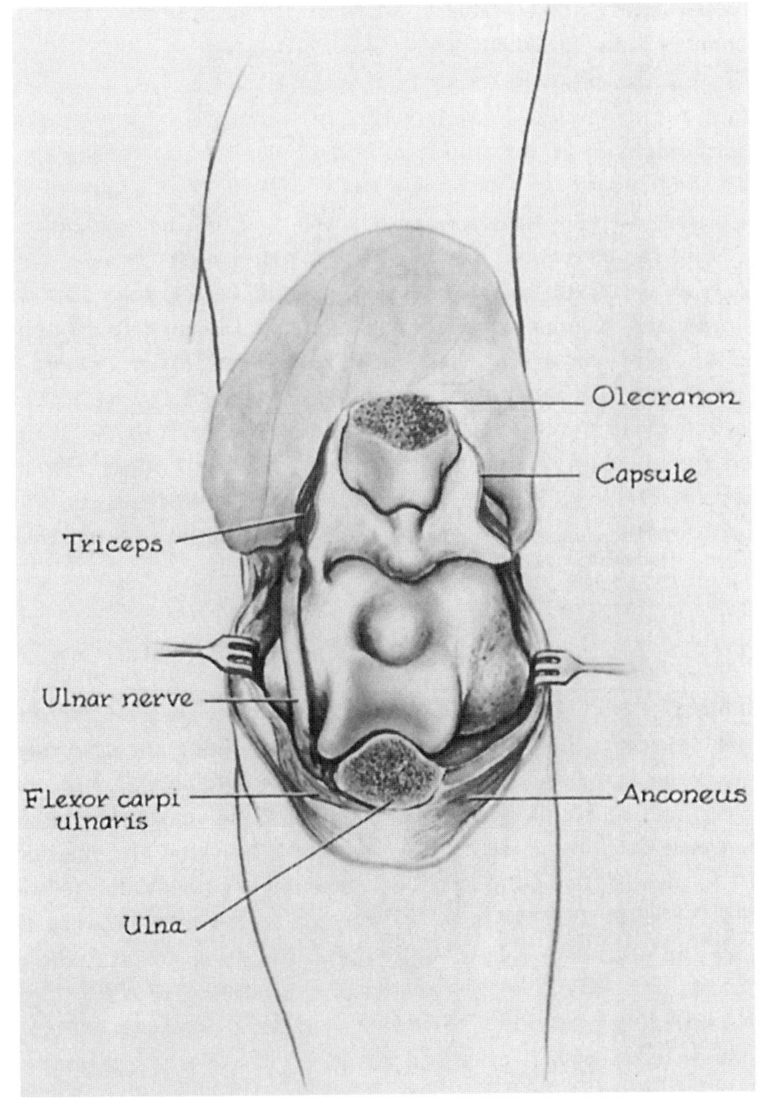

FIGURE 11-15 ■ Posterior approach to the elbow. An olecranon osteotomy is shown. (From Kaplan, E.B.: Surgical Approaches to the Neck, Cervical Spine, and Upper Extremity. Philadelphia, WB Saunders, 1966, p. 82.)

3. **Anterolateral Approach to the Elbow (Henry's)**—An extension of the same approach to the distal humerus, this approach is a brachialis (musculocutaneous nerve) splitting approach proximally and is between the pronator teres (median nerve) and the brachioradialis distally. The lateral antebrachial cutaneous nerve must be protected superficially and the radial nerve (and its branches) deep (supinate the forearm). Additionally, the brachial artery (which lies under the biceps aponeurosis) must be carefully protected. Branches of the radial recurrent artery must be ligated with this approach.
4. **(Postero) Lateral (Kocher's) Approach to the Elbow** (Fig. 11-16)—Uses the interval between the **anconeus (radial nerve)** and the main extensor origin **(extensor carpi ulnaris [ECU] [posterior interosseous nerve—PIN]). Pronation of the arm moves the PIN anteriorly and radially**, and the radial head is approached through the proximal supinator fibers. Extending this approach distal to the annular ligament increases the risk to the PIN.

ELBOW SURGICAL APPROACHES

APPROACH	INTERVAL	RISKS
Posterior	Detach triceps or olecranon osteotomy	Ulnar nerve Olecranon nonunion
Medial	Proximally: Brachialis (musculocutaneous nerve) and triceps (radial nerve) Distally: Brachialis and pronator teres (median nerve)	Ulnar nerve Medial antebrachial cutaneous n.
Anterolateral (**Henry's**)	Proximally: Brachialis (musculocutaneous nerve) splitting Distally: Pronator teres (median nerve) and brachioradialis (radial nerve)	Lateral antebrachial cutaneous nerve Radial nerve Ligation of radial recurrent artery Protect brachial artery **SUPINATE FOREARM**
Posterolateral (**Kocher's**)	Anconeus (radial nerve) and ECU (PIN of radial nerve)	PIN (pronation moves PIN anteriorly and radially) **PRONATE FOREARM**

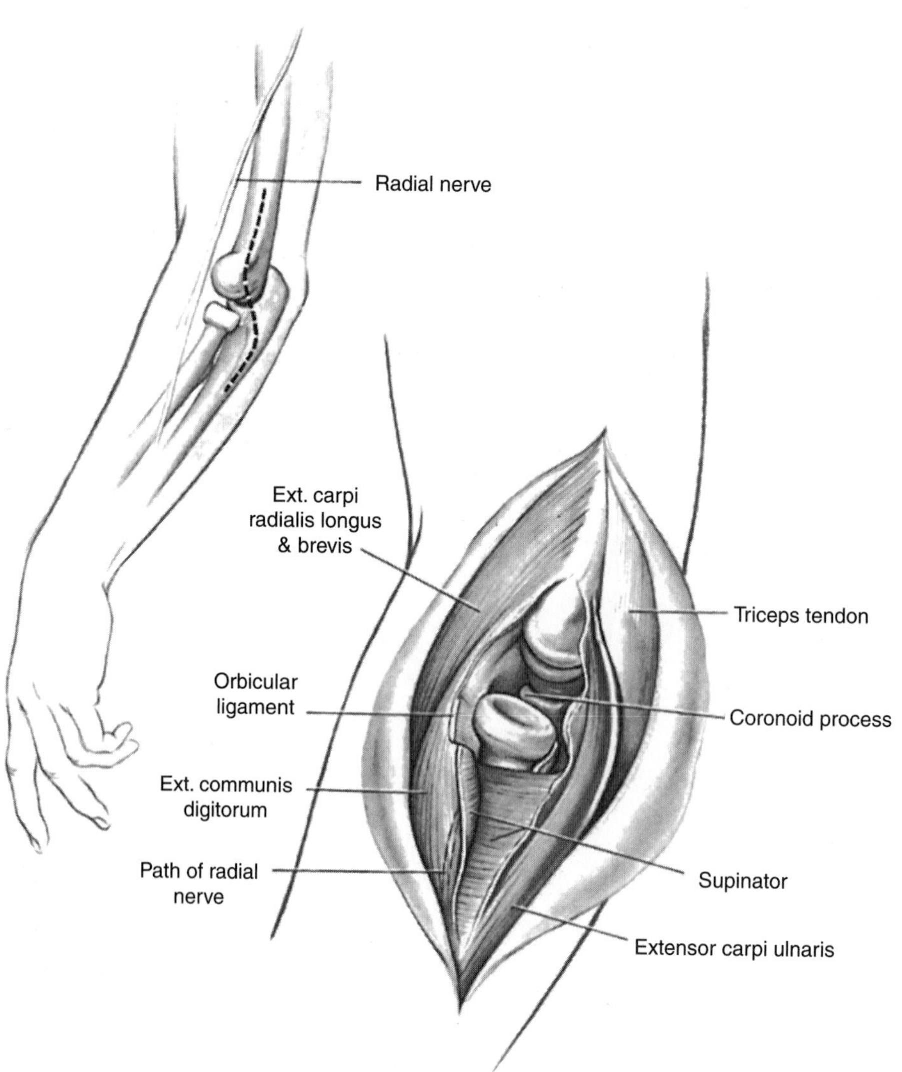

FIGURE 11-16 ■ Lateral approach to the elbow. This approach explores the interval between the anconeus (radial nerve) and the ECU (PIN). Arm **pronation** helps move the PIN away from the surgical field. (From Kaplan, E.B.: Surgical Approaches to the Neck, Cervical Spine, and Upper Extremity. Philadelphia, WB Saunders, 1966, p. 83.)

H. **Arthroscopy**—Portals for elbow arthroscopy include the anterolateral portal (radial nerve risk), the anteromedial portal (risks the medial antebrachial cutaneous and median nerves), and posterolateral portals.

IV. Forearm

A. **Osteology**—The forearm includes two long bones—the ulna and radius, which articulate with the humerus (principally the ulna) and the carpi (principally the radius).

1. **Ulna**—Proximally, the ulna is composed of two curved processes, the olecranon and the coronoid processes, with an intervening trochlear notch. Distally, the ulna tapers and ends in a lateral head and a medial styloid process.
2. **Radius**—The proximal radius is composed of a head with a central fovea, a neck, and a proximal medial radial tuberosity (for insertion of the biceps tendon). The radius has a gradual bend (convex laterally) and gradually increases in size distally. Restoration of the radial bow is important in fixation of radial shaft fractures. The distal extremity of the radius is composed of the carpal articular surface, an ulnar notch, a dorsal tubercle (Lister's tubercle, which is at the level of the scapholunate joint), and a lateral styloid process.

B. **Arthrology**—The radius and ulna articulate proximally at the elbow joint (discussed earlier) and distally at the wrist. The wrist consists primarily of the radiocarpal joint but also includes the distal radioulnar articulation (most stable in supination) with its triangular fibrocartilage complex.

1. **Radiocarpal Joint**—An ellipsoid joint involving the distal radius and the scaphoid, lunate, and triquetrum. This joint is usually located at the level of the proximal wrist flexion crease. Covered by a loose capsule, the wrist relies heavily on ligaments, especially volar ligaments, for stability. They include the volar and dorsal radiocarpal ligaments and the ulnar and radial collateral ligaments.
2. **Triangular Fibrocartilage Complex (TFCC)** (Fig. 11-17)—Originates from the most ulnar portion of the radius and extends into the caput ulna and the ulnar wrist to the base of the fifth metacarpal. It includes the following components:

COMPONENTS OF THE TFCC

COMPONENT	ORIGIN	INSERTION
Dorsal and volar radioulnar ligament	Ulnar radius	Caput ulna
Articular disc	Radius/ulna	Triquetrum
Prestyloid recess	Disc	Meniscus homologue
Meniscus homologue	Ulna/disc	Triquetrum/UCL
Ulnar collateral ligament (UCL)	Ulna	Fifth metacarpal

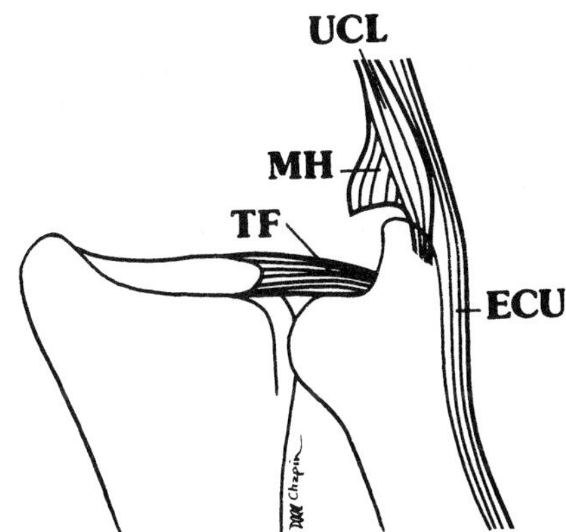

FIGURE 11-17 ■ Triangular fibrocartilage complex (TFCC). UCL, ulnar collateral ligament; MH, meniscal homologue; TF, transverse fibers (radioulnar ligament); ECU, extensor carpi ulnaris. (From Weissman, B.N., and Sledge, C.B.: Orthopedic Radiology. Philadelphia, WB Saunders, 1986, p. 115.)

C. **Muscles of the Forearm** (Fig. 11-18)—Arrangement based on both location and function into volar flexors (superficial and deep) and dorsal extensors (superficial and deep) (Table 11-7).

D. **Nerves**—The nerves of the upper arm continue into the forearm (Fig. 11-19).

1. **Radial Nerve**—Anterior to the lateral epicondyle, the **radial nerve runs between the brachialis and brachioradialis** and divides into anterior and deep (PIN) branches. The PIN splits the supinator and supplies all of the extensor muscles (except the mobile wad [brachioradialis, extensor carpi radialis brevis—ECRB—extensor carpi radialis longus—ECRL]). Compression of the PIN can occur at six places (see page 613, Summary of Compressive Neuropathies of the Forearm.). The superficial branch of the radial nerve passes to the dorsal radial surface of the hand in the distal third of the forearm by passing between the brachioradialis and ECRL.

RADIAL NERVE INNERVATION

NERVE	INNERVATION
Radial nerve (posterior cord)	Triceps, brachioradialis, ECRL, ECRB
PIN	Supinator, ECU, ED, EDM, AbdPL, EPL, EPB, EIP

2. **Median Nerve**—Lies medial to the brachial artery at the elbow, superficial to the brachialis muscle. In the forearm the **median nerve splits** the two heads of the **pronator teres** and then **runs between the flexor digitorum superficialis (FDS) and flexor**

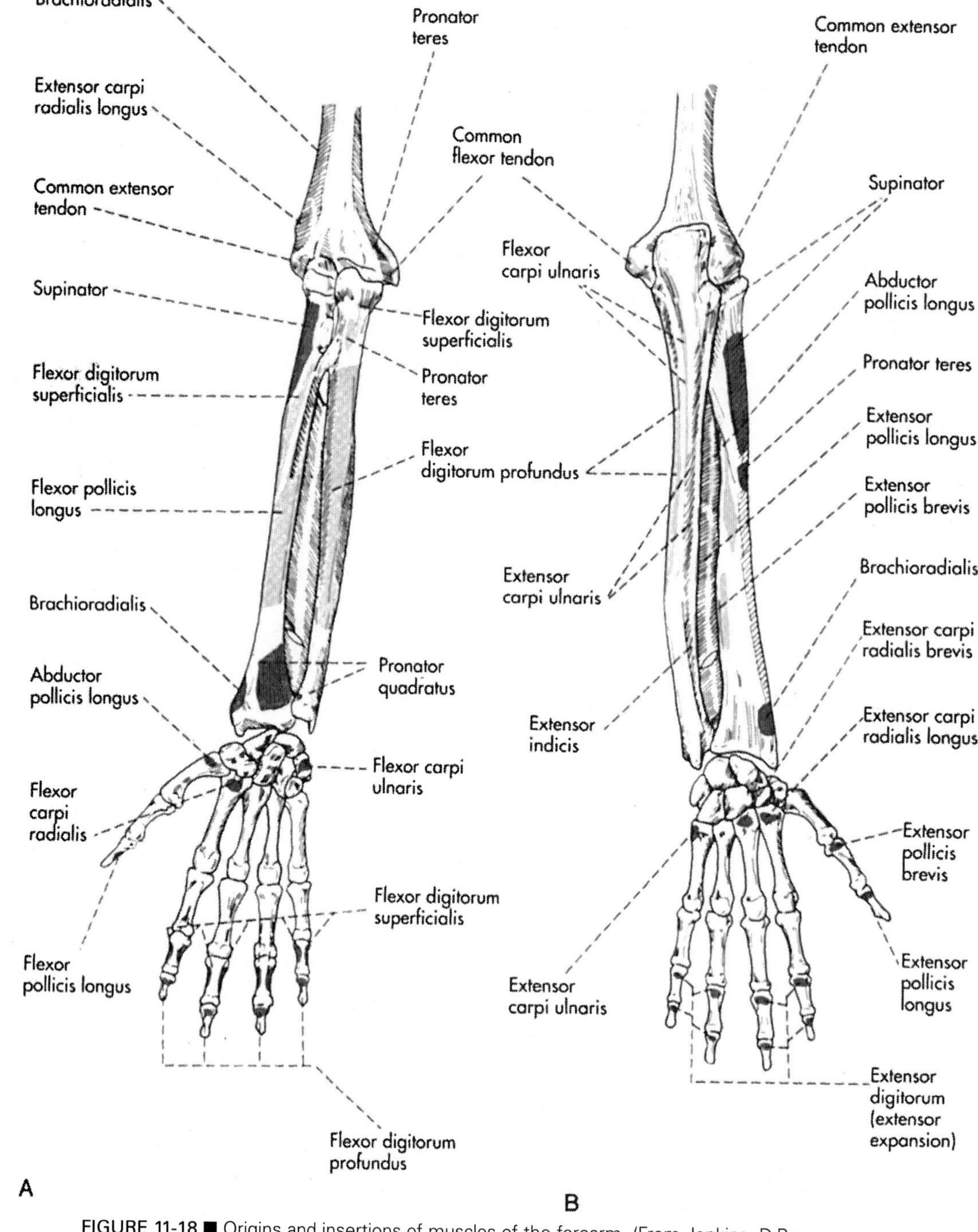

FIGURE 11-18 ■ Origins and insertions of muscles of the forearm. (From Jenkins, D.B.: Hollinshead's Functional Anatomy of the Limbs and Back, 6th ed., Fig. 8-4. Philadelphia, WB Saunders, 1991.)

digitorum profundus (FDP), becoming more superficial at the flexor retinaculum, where it continues into the hand. It has branches to all the superficial flexor muscles of the forearm except the flexor carpi ulnaris (FCU). Its anterior interosseous branch, which runs between the flexor pollicis longus (FPL) and FDP, supplies all the deep flexors except the ulnar half of the FDP.

MEDIAN NERVE INNERVATION

NERVE	INNERVATION
Median nerve (medial and lateral cord)	PT, FCR, PL, FDS, AbdPB, FPB supinator head, OP, 1st & 2nd lumbrical
AIN (anterior interosseous nerve)	FDP (I & II), FPL, PQ

Table 11-7. MUSCLES OF THE FOREARM

MUSCLE	ORIGIN	INSERTION	ACTION	INNERVATION
Superficial Flexors				
Pronator teres (PT)	Med. epicondyle and coronoid	Mid. lat. radius	Pronate, flex forearm	Median
Flexor carpi radialis (FCR)	Med epicondyle	2nd and 3rd Metacarpal bases	Flex wrist	Median
Palmaris longus (PL)	Med. epicondyle	Palmar aponeurosis	Flex wrist	Median
Flexor carpi ulnaris (FCU)	Med. epicondyle and post. ulna	Pisiform	Flex wrist	**Ulnar**
Flexor digitorum superficialis (FDS)	Med. epicondyle and ant. radius	Base of middle phalanges	Flex PIP	Median
Deep Flexors				
Flexor digitorum profundus (FDP)	Ant. and med ulna	Base of distal phalanges	Flex DIP	**Median-ant. interosseous/and ulnar**
Flexor pollicis longus (FPL)	Ant. and lat. radius	Base of distal phalanges	Flex IP, thumb	Median-ant. interosseous
Pronator quadratus (PQ)	Distal ulna	Volar radius	Pronate hand	Median-ant. interosseous
Superficial Extensors				
Brachioradialis (BR)	Lat. supracondylar humerus	Lat. distal radius	Flex forearm	Radial
Ext. carpi radialis longus (ECRL)	Lat. supracondylar humerus	2nd Metacarpal base	Extend wrist	Radial
Ext. carpi radialis brevis (ECRB)	Lat. epicondyle of humerus	3rd Metacarpal base	Extend wrist	Radial
Anconeus	Lat. epicondyle of humerus	Proximal dorsal ulna	Extend forearm	Radial
Extensor digitorum (ED)	Lat. epicondyle of humerus	Extensor aponeurosis	Extend digits	Radial-post. interosseous
Extensor digiti minimi	Common extensor tendon	Small finger extensor carpi ulnaris	Extend small finger	Radial-post. interosseous
Ext. carpi ulnaris (ECU)	Lat. epicondyle of humerus	5th Metacarpal base	Extent/adduct hand	Radial-post. interosseous
Deep Extensors				
Supinator	Lat. epicondyle of humerus, ulna	Dorsolateral radius	Supinate forearm	Radial-post. interosseous
Abductor pollicis longus (APL or AbdPL)	Dorsal ulna/radius	1st Metacarpal base	Abduct thumb, extend	Radial-post. interosseous
Extensor pollicis brevis (EPB)	Dorsal radius	Thumb proximal phalanx base	Extend thumb MCP	Radial-post. interosseous
Extensor pollicis longus (EPL)	Dorsolateral ulna	Thumb dorsal phalanx base	Extend thumb IP	Radial-post. interosseous
Extensor indicis proprius (EIP)	Dorsolateral ulna	Index finger extensor apparatus (ulnarly)	Extend index finger	Radial-post. interosseous

PIP, Proximal interphalangeal joint; DIP, distal interphalangeal joint; MCP, metacarpophalangeal joint.

3. **Ulnar Nerve**—Enters the forearm between the two heads of the FCU, which it supplies, and then **runs between the FCU and FDP** (and **innervates the ulnar half of this muscle**). It lies more superficial at the wrist and enters the hand through Guyon's canal.

ULNAR NERVE INNERVATION

NERVE	INNERVATION
Ulnar nerve (medial cord)	FCU, FDP (III & IV), PB, AbdDM, ODM, FDM 3rd & 4th lumbrical, interossei, AddP, deep head FPB

4. **Summary of Important Forearm Neuroanatomic Relationships**

FOREARM NEUROANATOMIC RELATIONSHIPS

NERVE	RELATIONSHIP
Radial nerve	Between brachialis and brachioradialis
PIN	Splits supinator
Superficial radial	Between brachioradialis and ECRL
Median nerve	Medial to brachial artery at elbow
AIN	Splits pronator teres and runs between FDS and FDP
	Between FPL and FDP
Ulnar nerve	Between FCU and FDP

5. **Cutaneous Nerves**—The forearm has the **lateral antebrachial cutaneous nerve** (the continuation of the musculocutaneous nerve **that passes lateral to the cephalic vein** after emerging laterally from between the

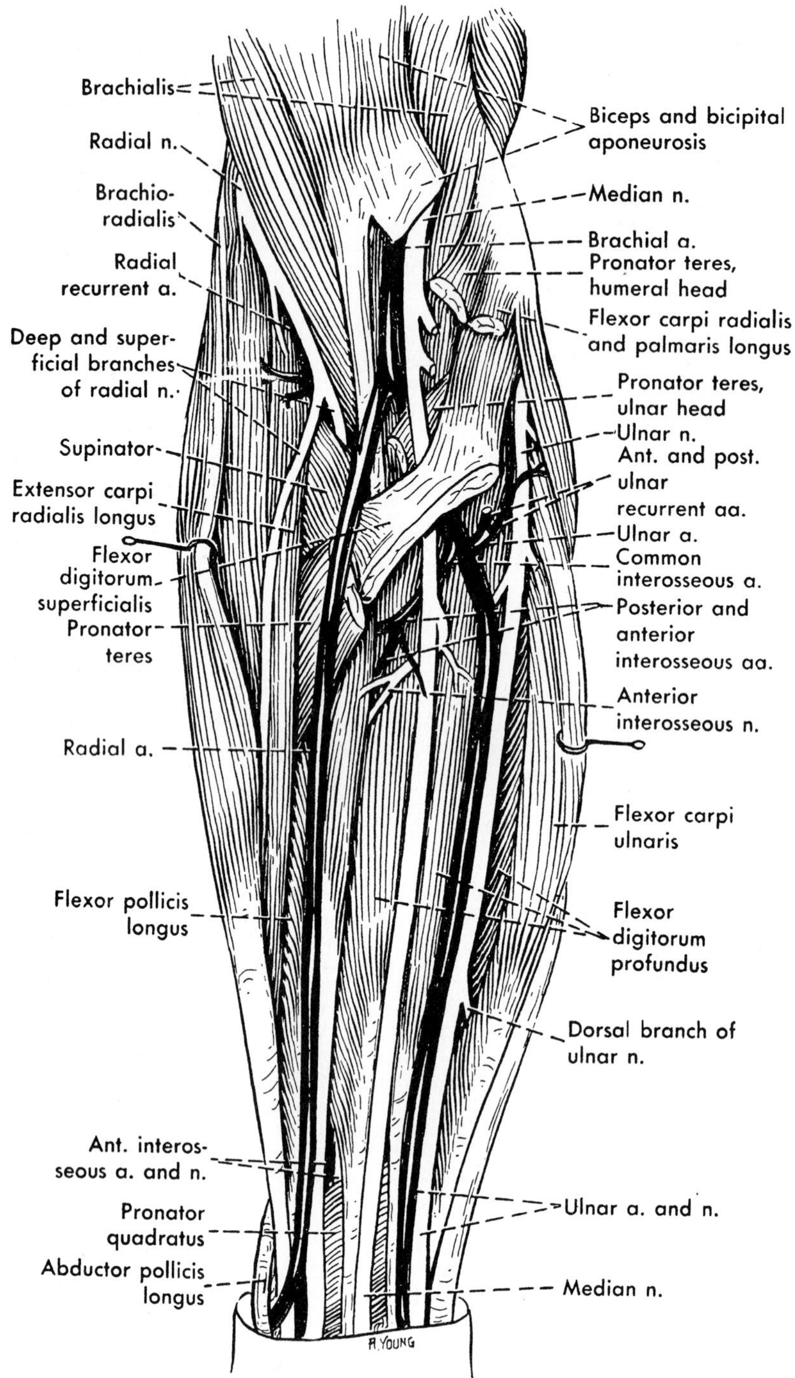

FIGURE 11-19 ■ Arteries *(black)* and nerves *(white)* of the forearm. (From Jenkins, D.B.: Hollinshead's Functional Anatomy of the Limbs and Back, 6th ed. Philadelphia, WB Saunders, 1991, p. 131.)

biceps and brachialis at the elbow), the medial antebrachial cutaneous nerve (a branch from the medial cord of the brachial plexus), and the posterior antebrachial cutaneous nerve (a branch of the radial nerve given off in the arm) (see Fig. 11-40).

6. **Summary of Compressive Neuropathies of the Forearm**

An example of key testable material on compressive neuropathies would be which muscle is last to return following PIN palsy release. Since the PIN innervates in order the supinator, ECU, ED, EDM, AbdPL, EPL, EPB, and EIP, the last muscle to return to function, the extensor indices proprius (EIP), is the most distally innervated muscle.

NERVE COMPRESSION SYNDROMES OF THE ARM/FOREARM

SYNDROME	NERVE INVOLVED	SITE(S) OF COMPRESSION
Pronator	Median nerve	Supercondylar process of humerus and ligament of Struthers Lacertus fibrosis (bicepital aponeurosis) Pronator teres Arch of FDS
AIN	AIN of median nerve	Deep head of PT FDS Aberrant vessels Accessory muscles (i.e., Gantzer's)
Cubital tunnel	Ulnar nerve	Arcade of Struthers Medial intermuscular septum Medial epicondyle Cubital tunnel Proximal edge of FCU (Osborne's fascia) Deep flexor pronator aponeurosis
PIN Radial tunnel	PIN of radial nerve	**F**ibrous bands **R**ecurrent leash of Henry **E**CRB **A**rcade of Frohse (proximal edge of superficial head of supinator) **S**upinator distal margin
Superficial radial nerve	Superficial radial nerve	Between the Brachioradialis (BR) and ECRL

E. **Vessels** (see Fig. 11-19)—At the elbow the brachial artery enters the cubital fossa (bordered by the two epicondyles, the brachioradialis, and the pronator teres and overlying the brachialis and supinator). It then divides at the level of the radial neck into the radial and ulnar arteries.

1. **Radial Artery**—Runs initially on the pronator teres, deep to the brachioradialis, and continues to the wrist between this muscle and the flexor carpi radialis (FCR). Forearm branches include the radial recurrent (see earlier discussion) and muscular branches.
2. **Ulnar Artery**—The larger of the two branches, it is covered by the superficial flexors proximally (between the FDS and FDP). Distally, the artery lies on the FDP, between the tendons of the FCU and FDS. Forearm branches include the anterior and posterior ulnar recurrent (discussed earlier), the common interosseous (with anterior and posterior branches), and several muscular and nutrient arteries.

FOREARM VASCULAR ANATOMIC RELATIONSHIPS

ARTERY	RELATIONSHIP
Radial	On pronator teres deep to brachioradialis Enters wrist between BR and FCR
Ulnar	Proximally between FDS and FDP Distally lies on FDP between FCU and FDS

F. **Surgical Approaches to the Forearm**

1. **Anterior Approach (Henry's)** (Fig. 11-20)—Utilizes the interval between the **brachioradialis (radial nerve)** and the **pronator teres (or FCR distally) (median nerve).** Proximally it is necessary to isolate and ligate the **leash of Henry** (radial artery branches) and subperiosteally to strip the supinator from its insertion. It is essential to protect the superficial branch of the radial nerve (retract laterally) and the brachioradialis. Distally, it is necessary to dissect off the FPL and pronator quadratus. Supination of the forearm displaces the PIN ulnarly.
2. **Dorsal (Posterior) Approach (Thompson)** (Fig. 11-21)—Uses the interval between the **extensor carpi radialis brevis (radial nerve) and extensor digitorum communis (or extensor pollicis longus distally) (PIN).** The PIN must be identified and protected when using this surgical approach. **Excessive retraction of the supinator can injure the posterior interosseous nerve.**
3. **Exposure of the Ulna**—Via the interval between the **extensor carpi ulnaris (PIN) and the FCU (ulnar nerve).**

FOREARM SURGICAL APPROACHES

APPROACH	INTERVAL	RISKS
Anterior (Henry's)	Brachioradialis (radial nerve) and pronator teres (median nerve) Distally: FCR (median nerve)	Ligate leash of Henry (radial artery branches) Superficial branch radial nerve
Dorsal posterior (Thompson's)	ECRB (radial nerve) and EDC (PIN) Distally: EPL	PIN. Avoid excessive retraction of supinator
Ulna	ECU (PIN) and FCU (ulnar nerve)	

4. **Cross-Sectional Diagrams of Middle and Distal Forearm** (Figs. 11-22 and 11-23, Table 11-8).

V. Wrist and Hand (See Chapter 6, Hand and Microsurgery)

A. **Osteology**

1. **Carpal Bones**—Each carpal bone has six surfaces, with proximal, distal, medial, and lateral surfaces for articulation and palmar and dorsal surfaces for ligamentous insertion. **Ossification begins at the capitate** (usually present at 1 year of age) and **proceeds in a counterclockwise direction.** Therefore the hamate is the second carpus to ossify (1–2 years), followed by the triquetrum (3 years), lunate (4–5 years), scaphoid (5 years), trapezium (6 years), and trapezoid (7 years). The pisiform, which is a large sesamoid bone, is the last to

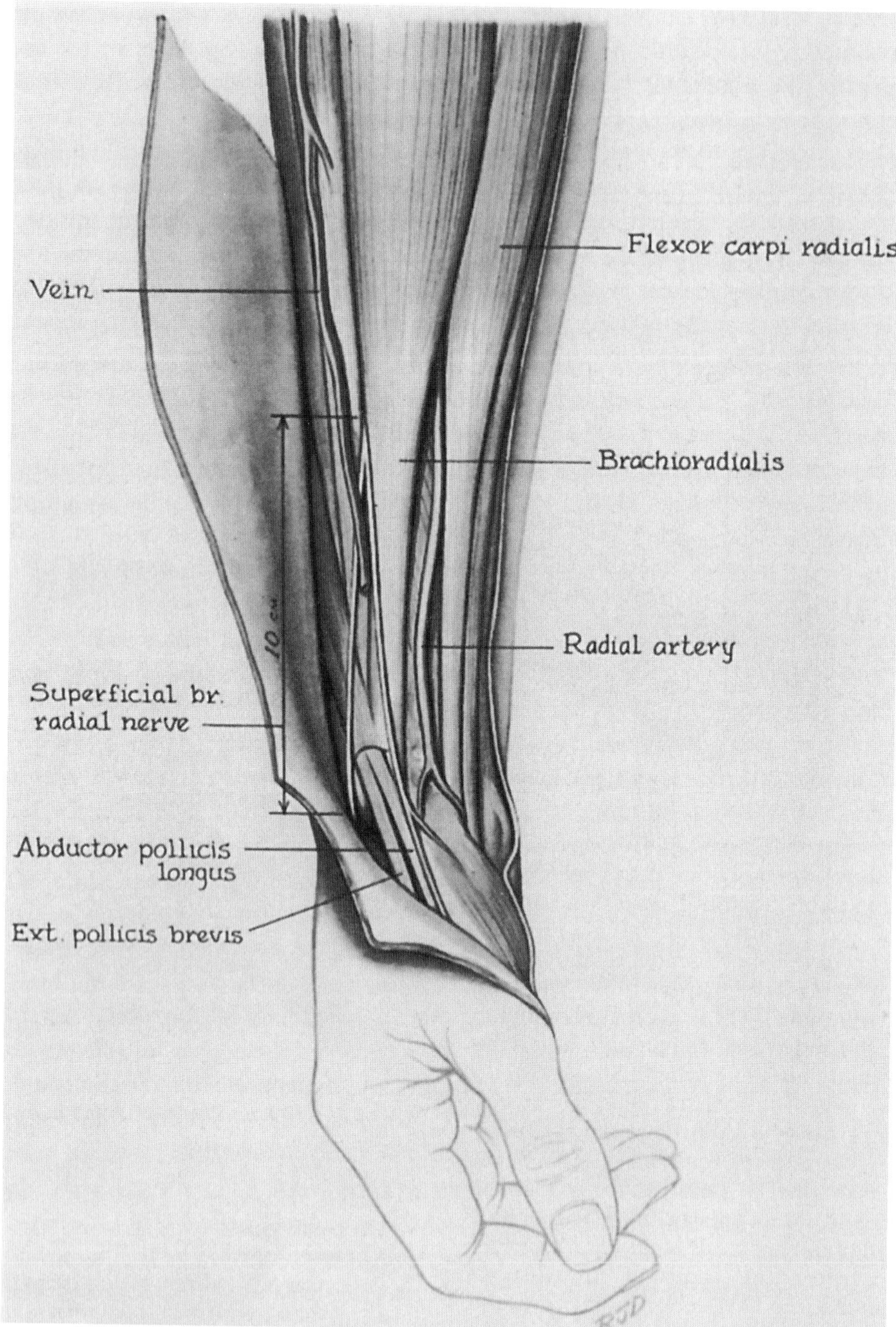

FIGURE 11-20 ■ Anterior (Henry's) approach to the forearm. The interval between the brachioradialis (radial nerve) and the PT or FCR (median nerve) is explored. Protect the superficial radial nerve that lies underneath the brachioradialis. (From Kaplan, E.B.: Surgical Approaches to the Neck, Cervical Spine, and Upper Extremity. Philadelphia, WB Saunders, 1966, p. 92.)

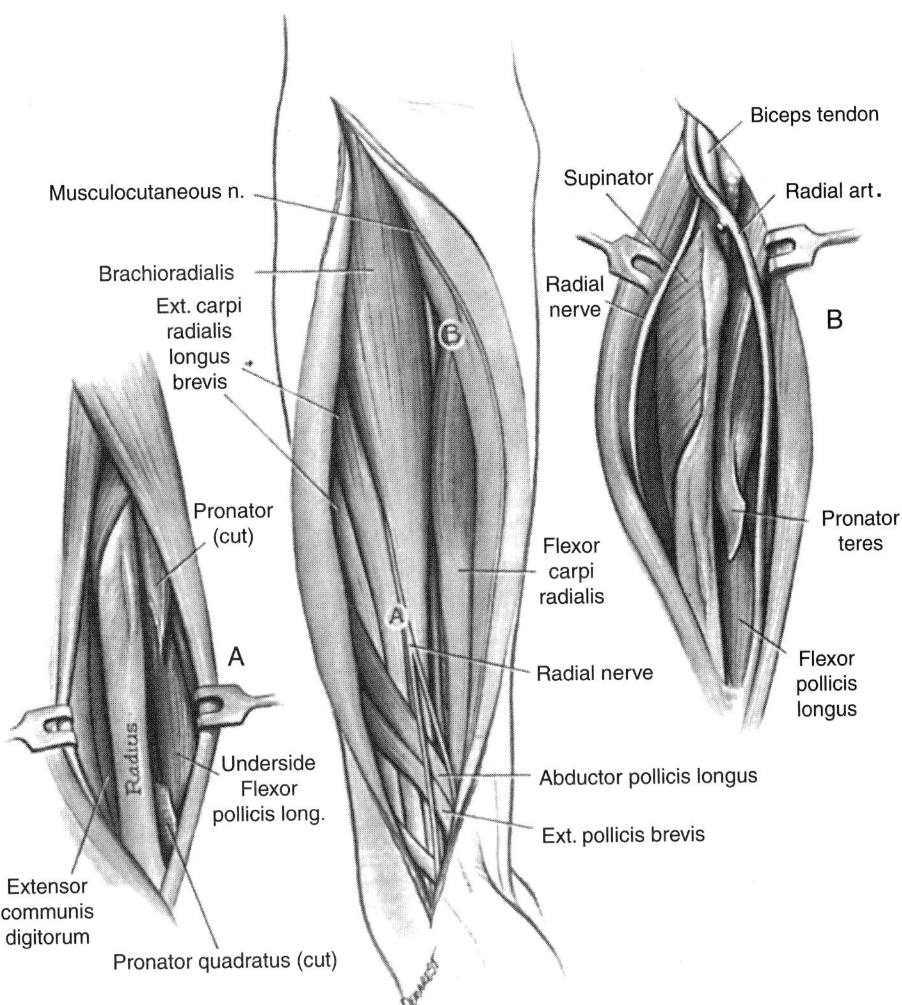

FIGURE 11-21 ■ Dorsal (Thompson) approach to the forearm. The interval between the ECRB (radial nerve) and the EDC (PIN) is explored. (From Kaplan, E.B.: Surgical Approaches to the Neck, Cervical Spine, and Upper Extremity. Philadelphia, WB Saunders, 1966, p. 90.)

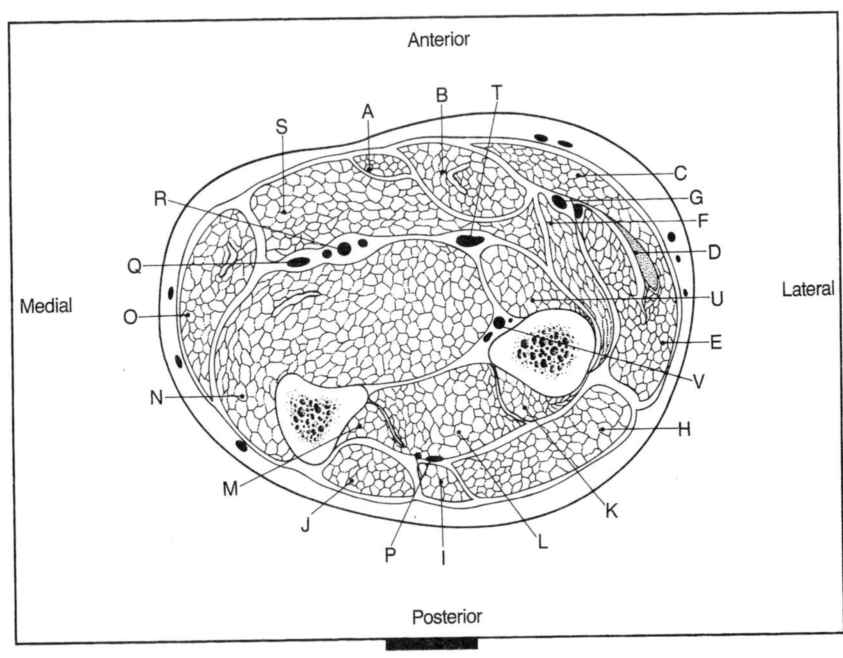

FIGURE 11-22 ■ Cross-section of the mid-forearm. Practice labeling the diagram. See Table 11-8 for key. (From Callaghan, J.J., ed.: Anatomy Self-Assessment Examination, Fig. 39. Park Ridge, Ill, American Academy of Orthopaedic Surgeons, 1991.)

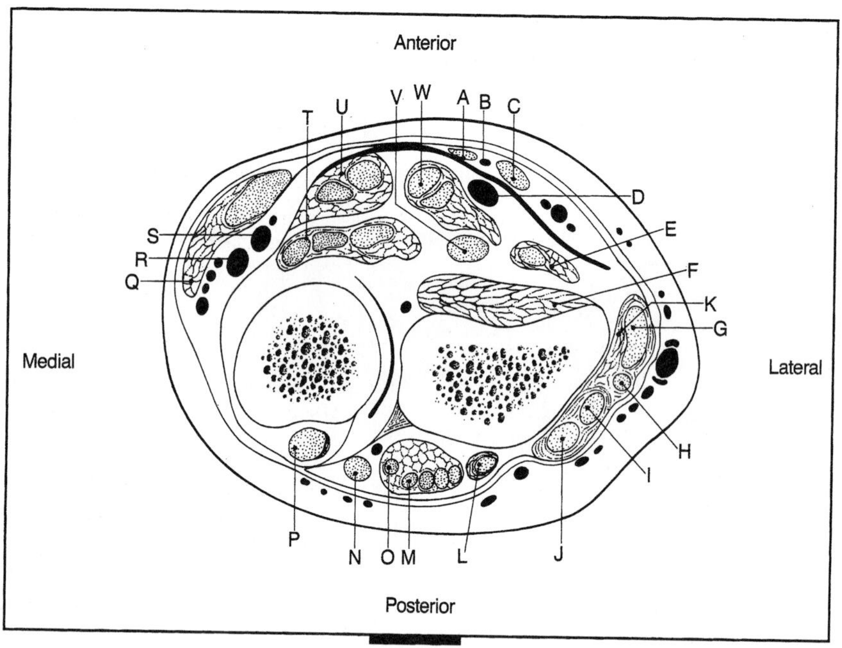

FIGURE 11-23 ■ Cross-section of the distal forearm proximal to the distal radioulnar joint. Practice labeling the diagram. See Table 11-8 for key. (From Callaghan, J.J., ed.: Anatomy Self-Assessment Examination, Fig. 38. Park Ridge, Ill, American Society of Orthopaedic Surgeons, 1991.)

Table 11-8. CROSS-SECTIONAL ANATOMY FIGURE KEY

FIGURE 11-22: MID-FOREARM	FIGURE 11-23: DISTAL FOREARM	FIGURE 11-56: PROXIMAL THIGH
A—Palmaris longus M	A—Palmaris longus M	A—Sartorius M
B—Flexor carpi radialis M	B—Palmar branch median N	B—Rectus femoris M
C—Brachioradialis M	C—Flexor carpi radialis M	C—Vastus medialis M
D—Extensor carpi radialis longus M	D—Median N	D—Vastus intermedius M
E—Extensor carpi radialis brevis M	E—Flexor pollicus longus M	E—Vastus lateralis M
F—Pronator teres M	F—Pronator quadratis M	F—Short head biceps femoris M
G—Superficial branch radial N	G—Abductor pollicus longus M	G—Sciatic N
H—Extensor digitorum M	H—Extensor pollicus brevis M	H—Long head biceps femoris M
I—Extensor digiti minimi M	I—Extensor carpi radialis longus M	I—Semitendinosus M
J—Extensor carpi ulnaris M	J—Extensor carpi radialis brevis M	J—Semimembranosus M
K—Abductor pollicus longus M	K—tendon of Brachioradialis M	K—Adductor magnus M
L—Extensor pollicus brevis M	L—Extensor pollicis longus M	L—Gracilis M
M—Extensor pollicus longus	M—Extensor digitorum M	M—Adductor brevis M
M—also Extensor indicis M	N—Extensor digiti minimi M	N—Adductor longus M
N—Flexor digitorum profundus M	O—Extensor indicis M	O—Femoral A and V
O—Flexor carpi ulnaris M	P—Extensor carpi ulnaris M	P—Deep femoral A and V
P—Posterior interosseous N and A	Q—Flexor carpi ulnaris M	
Q—Ulnar N	R—Ulnar N	
R—Ulnar A	S—Ulnar A	
S—Flexor digitorum superficialis M	T—Flexor digitorum profundus M	
T—Median N	U—Flexor digitorum superficialis M	
U—Flexor pollicus longus M	V—Flexor digitorum profundus M	
V—Anterior interosseous A and N	W—Flexor digitorum superficialis M	

M, Muscle; N, nerve; V, vein; A, artery.

ossify (9 years). Several key features are important to recognize in the individual carpal bones.

CARPAL BONE FEATURES

BONE	IMPORTANT FEATURES	NO. ARTICULATIONS
Scaphoid	Tubercle (TCL [transverse carpal lig.], APB) distal vascular supply	5
Lunate	Lunar shape	5
Triquetrum	Pyramid shape	3
Pisiform	Spheroidal (TCL, FCR)	1
Trapezium	FCR groove, tubercle (opponens, APB, FPB, TCL)	4
Trapezoid	Wedge shape	4
Capitate	Largest bone, central location	7
Hamate	Hook (TCL)	5

2. **Metacarpals**—Have two ossification centers: one for the body (primary center of ossification), which ossifies at 8 weeks of fetal life (like most long bones), and one at the neck, which usually appears before age 3. *The first metacarpal is a primordial phalanx and has its secondary ossification center located at the base (like the phalanges)*. Several characteristics allow identification of the individual metacarpals.

METACARPAL FEATURES

METACARPAL	DISTINCTIVE FEATURES
I (thumb)	Short, stout, base is saddle shaped
II (index)	Longest, largest base, medial at base
III (middle)	Styloid process
IV (ring)	Small quadrilateral base, narrow shaft
V (small)	Tubercle at base (ECU)

3. **Phalanges**—The 14 phalanges (three for each finger and two for the thumb) are similar. They all have secondary ossification centers at their bases that appear at ages 3 (proximal), 4 (middle), and 5 (distal). The bases of the proximal phalanges are oval and concave, with smaller heads ending in two condyles. The middle phalanges have two concave facets at their bases and pulley-shaped heads. The distal phalanges are smaller and have palmar ungual tuberosities distally.

B. **Arthrology**

1. **Radiocarpal (Wrist) Joint**—Ellipsoid joint made up of the distal radius, scaphoid, lunate, triquetrum, and the ligamentous structures listed in the chart in the next column.

   The palmar/volar radiocarpal ligament is the strongest supporting structure, although it has a weak area on the radial side (the space of Poirier) that lends less support to the scaphoid, lunate, and trapezoid.

RADIOCARPAL WRIST LIGAMENTS

STRUCTURE	ATTACHMENTS	DISTINCTIVE FEATURES
Articular capsule	Surrounds joint	Reinforced by volar and dorsal RCL
Volar radiocarpal ligament (RCL)	Radius, ulna, scaphoid, lunate, triquetrum, capitate	Oblique ulnar, strong
Dorsal radiocarpal ligament	Radius, scaphoid, lunate, triquetrum	Oblique radial, weak
Ulnar collateral ligament	Ulna, triquetrum, pisiform, TCL	Fan-shaped, two fascicles
Radial collateral ligament	Radius, scaphoid, trapezium, TCL	Radial artery adjacent

2. **Intercarpal Joints**
   a. **Proximal Row**—Scaphoid, lunate, and triquetral are gliding joints. Two dorsal intercarpal ligaments connect the scaphoid and lunate and the lunate and triquetral bones. Two palmar intercarpal ligaments connect the scaphoid and lunate and the lunate and triquetral bones. The dorsal intercarpal ligaments are stronger. Interosseous ligaments are narrow bundles connecting the lunate and scaphoid and the lunate and triquetral bones (Fig. 11-24).
   b. **Pisiform Articulation**—The pisotriquetral joint has a thin articular capsule. The ulnar collateral and palmar radiocarpal ligaments also connect the pisiform proximally. The pisohamate ligament and pisometacarpal ligaments help extend the pull of the FCU.
   c. **Distal Row**—Trapezium, trapezoid, capitate, and hamate gliding joints. The dorsal intercarpal ligaments connect the trapezium with the trapezoid, the trapezoid with the capitate, and the capitate with the hamate. The palmar ligaments do the same. The interosseous ligaments are much thicker in the distal row, connecting the capitate and hamate (strongest), the capitate and trapezoid, and the trapezium and trapezoid (weakest).
   d. **Midcarpal Joint**—Transverse articulations between the proximal and distal rows are reinforced by palmar and dorsal intercarpal ligaments and carpal collateral ligaments (radial is stronger).
3. **Carpometacarpal (CMC) Joints**
   a. **Thumb CMC Joint**—A highly mobile saddle joint. It is supported by a capsule and radial, palmar, and dorsal CMC ligaments.
   b. **Finger CMC Joints**—Gliding joints with capsules, dorsal CMC ligaments (strongest), palmar CMC ligaments, and interosseous CMC ligaments.
4. **Metacarpophalangeal Joints**—Ellipsoid joints covered by palmar (volar plate), collateral, and deep transverse metacarpal ligaments.

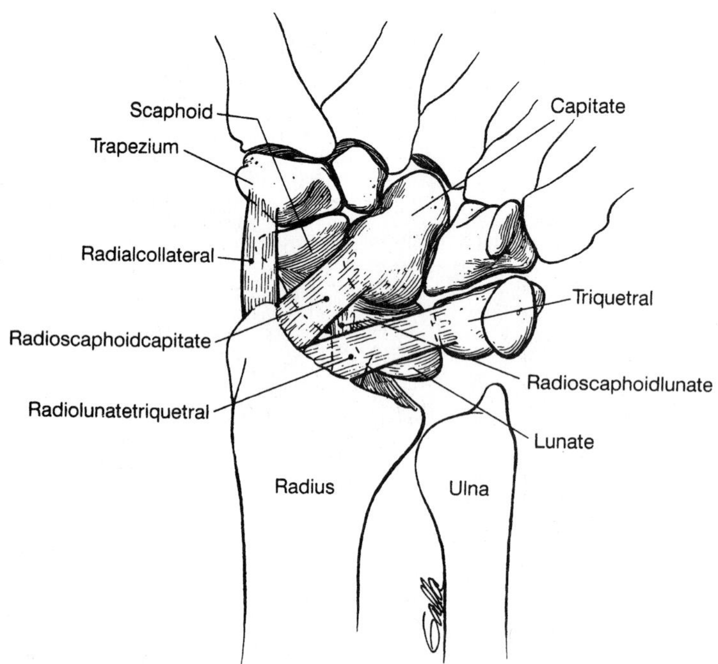

FIGURE 11-24 ■ Extrinsic radiocarpal ligaments. (From Mooney, J.F., Siegel, D.B., and Koman, L.A.: Ligamentous injuries of the wrists in athletes. Clin. Sports Med., 11:1291–1139, 1992.)

5. **Interphalangeal Joints**—Hinge joints with capsules and obliquely oriented collateral ligaments.
6. **Other Important Structures**
   a. **Extensor Retinaculum**—Covers the dorsum of the wrist and contains six synovial sheaths (Figs. 11-25, 11-26). Orientation of the extensor tendons at the wrist is key testable material. The first dorsal compartment contains the abductor pollicis longus (APL) and the extensor pollicis brevis (EPB). The **EPB tendon is ulnar to the APL tendon** (frequently the APL has multiple tendon slips—address during release for de Quervain's tenosynovitis). In the second dorsal compartment the **ECRL tendon is radial**

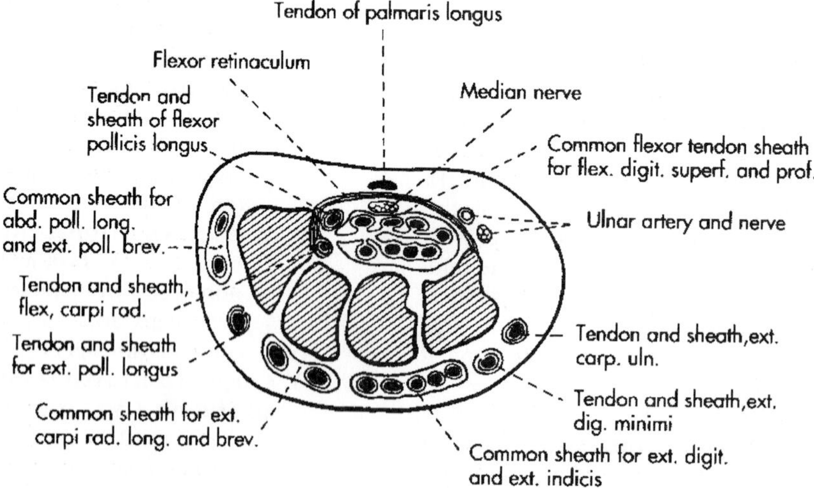

FIGURE 11-25 ■ Components of the carpal tunnel. The roof of the carpal tunnel is the flexor retinaculum composed of the deep forearm fascia, transverse carpal ligament (TCL), and the distal aponeurosis between the thenar and hypothenar muscle. The carpal tunnel contains the median nerve and nine tendons (FPL, four FDS and four FDP). Please note that the FCR passes under the TCL and is not considered a tendon within the carpal tunnel. The FPL is located volar to the FCR, which is the most dorsal radial tendon passing under the flexor retinaculum. (From Jenkins, D.B.: Hollinshead's Functional Anatomy of the Limbs and Back, 6th ed. Philadelphia, WB Saunders, 1991, p. 162.)

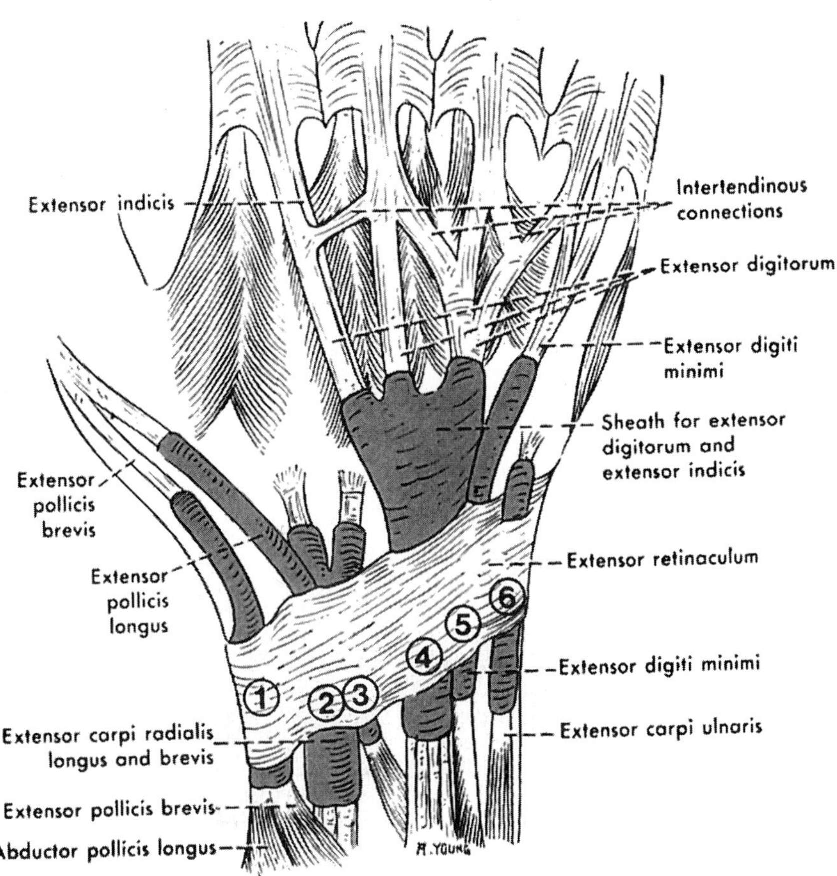

FIGURE 11-26 ■ Extensor compartments of the wrist *(1–6)*. See summary chart in text. (From Jenkins, D.B.: Hollinshead's Functional Anatomy of the Limbs and Back, 6th ed. Philadelphia, WB Saunders, 1991, p. 174.)

to the ECRB tendon. Thus the EPL tendon is ulnar to the ECRB tendon at wrist level. The anatomic snuffbox is bordered by tendons of the first and third dorsal wrist compartments with the EPB tendon serving as the radial snuffbox border and the EPL tendon as the ulnar border. Please note that the posterior interosseous nerve is contained within the floor of the fourth dorsal wrist compartment.

DORSAL WRIST COMPARTMENTS

COMPARTMENT	CONTENTS	PATHOLOGIC CONDITION
1	APL, EPB	De Quervain's tenosynovitis
2	ECRL, ECRB	Extensor tendonitis (intersection syndrome)
3	EPL	Rupture at Lister's tubercle (after wrist fractures), Drummer's wrist
4	EDC, EIP	Extensor tenosynovitis
5	EDM	Rupture (RA—Vaughn-Jackson syndrome)
6	ECU	Snapping at ulnar styloid

b. **Transverse Carpal Ligament ([TCL]; Flexor Retinaculum)**—The TCL is actually one component of the flexor retinaculum that serves as the roof of the carpal tunnel (see Fig. 11-25). The flexor retinaculum is attached medially to the pisiform and the hook of the hamate and laterally to the tuberosity of the scaphoid and the ridge of the trapezium. The **carpal tunnel** decreases in volume with wrist flexion. This tunnel **contains the median nerve and nine tendons (FPL, 4 FDS and 4 FDP).** *In the tunnel the FDS tendons of the long and ring finger are volar to the tendons of the index and small fingers.* The flexor retinaculum also forms the floor of Guyon's canal, which is bordered as well by the hook of the hamate and the pisiform and is covered by the volar carpal ligament. Entrapment of the ulnar nerve in this canal is possible (Fig. 11-27).

c. **Triangular Fibrocartilage Complex—** Formed by the triangular fibrocartilage, ulnocarpal ligaments (volar ulnolunate and ulnotriquetral ligaments), and a meniscal homologue. Injuries to this structure are a common cause of ulnar wrist pain (see Fig. 11-17).

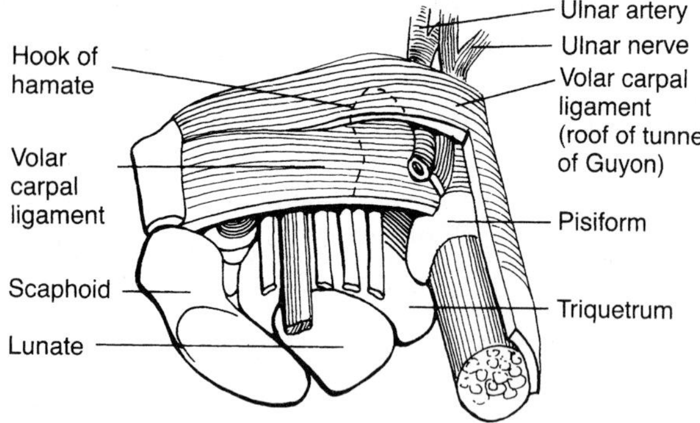

FIGURE 11-27 ■ The carpal tunnel is formed by the transverse carpal ligament volarly and the carpal bones on the floor and sides. Guyon's canal is formed by the volar carpal ligament (roof), the hamate (lateral wall), and the pisiform (medial wall). (From DeLee, J.C., and Drez, D., Jr.: Orthopaedic Sports Medicine: Principles and Practice, vol. 1. Philadelphia, WB Saunders, 1994, p. 932.)

d. **Intrinsic Apparatus**—Complex arrangement of structures that surround the digits (Fig. 11-28). The following structures are important:

INTRINSIC APPARATUS

STRUCTURE	ATTACHMENTS	SIGNIFICANCE
Sagittal bands	Covers MCP	Allows MCP extension
Transverse (sagittal) fibers	Volar plate	Allows MCP flexion (interossei)
Lateral bands	Covers PIP	Allows PIP extension (lumbricals)
Oblique retinacular ligament (Landsmeer's ligament)	A4 pulley, terminal tendon	Allows DIP extension (passive)

e. **Flexor Sheath** (Fig. 11-29)—Covers the flexor tendons in the finger, protecting and nourishing the tendons (vincula). Also forms five pulleys (A1–A5) with three intervening

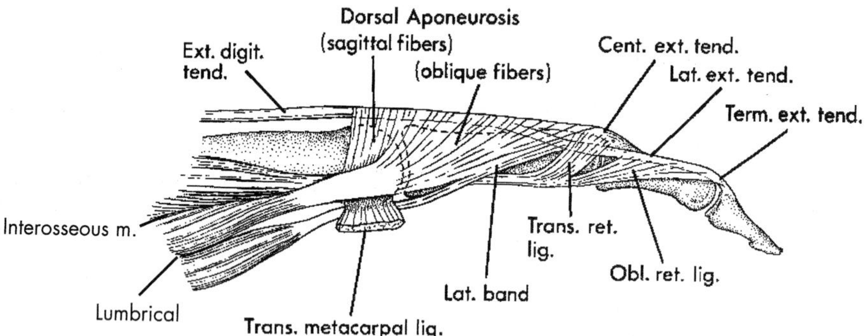

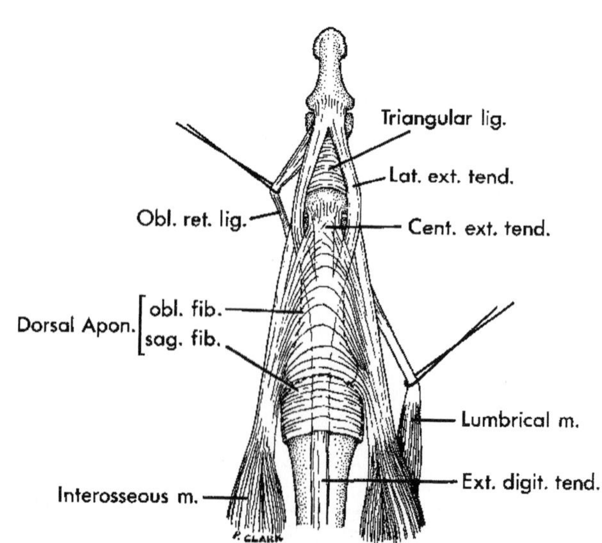

FIGURE 11-28 ■ Dorsal extensor apparatus. (Adapted from Bora, F.W.: The Pediatric Upper Extremity. Philadelphia, WB Saunders, 1986, p. 93.)

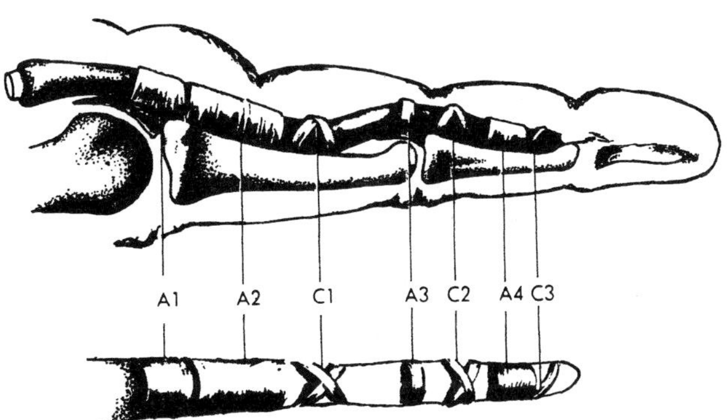

FIGURE 11-29 ■ Flexor pulleys. A1 pulley is the source of trigger digits. (From Tubiana, R.: The Hand, vol. 3. Philadelphia, WB Saunders, 1985, p. 173.)

cruciate attachments (C1–C3). The **A2 pulley,** overlying the proximal **phalanx, is the most important** one, **followed by A4,** which covers the middle phalanx. **The A1 pulley is involved in trigger digits.**

C. **Muscles** (Table 11-9) **Origins and Insertions** (Fig. 11-30)

D. **Nerves** (Fig. 11-31)

1. **Median Nerve**—Enters the wrist just under the transverse carpal ligament between the FDS and the FCR. The palmar cutaneous branch, which arises proximal to the transverse carpal ligament between the palmaris longus and FCR, supplies the thenar skin. The deep (muscular) branch runs radially and supplies thenar muscles. Digital nerves supply the lumbricals and the volar aspect of the radial 3½ digits.

MEDIAN NERVE INNERVATION

NERVE	INNERVATION TO HAND IS BOLD PRINT
Median nerve (medial and lateral cord)	PT, FCR, PL, FDS, **AbdPB, FPB supinator head, OP, 1st & 2nd lumbrical**

2. **Ulnar Nerve**—Enters the wrist through Guyon's canal and divides into a superficial branch (palmaris brevis and skin) and a deep branch. The deep branch travels with the deep palmar arch and passes between the abductor digiti minimi and flexor digiti minimi brevis giving off motor branches to the deep musculature (three hypothenar muscles, two ulnar lumbricals, all interossei and the adductor pollicis) and terminating in digital nerves for the ulnar 1½ digits. The dorsal cutaneous branch swings dorsally at the wrist and can be injured with either arthroscopic portal placement or surgical incisions.

ULNAR NERVE INNERVATION

NERVE	INNERVATION TO HAND IS BOLD PRINT
Ulnar nerve (medial cord)	FCU, FDP (III & IV), PB, **AbdDM, ODM, FDM, 3rd & 4th lumbrical, interossei, AddP, deep head FPB**

Table 11-9. MUSCLES OF THE HAND AND WRIST

MUSCLE	ORIGIN	INSERTION	ACTION	INNERVATION
Thenar Muscles				
Abductor pollicis brevis (APB or AbdPB)	Scaphoid, trapezoid	Base of proximal phalanx, radial side	Abduct thumb	Median
Opponens pollicis	Trapezium	Thumb metacarpal	Abduct, flex, med. rotation	Median
Flexor pollicis brevis (FPB)	Trapezium, capitate	Base of proximal phalanx, radial side	Flex MCP	Median, ulnar
Adductor pollicis (AddP)	Capitate, 2nd/3rd metacarpals	Base of proximal phalanx, ulnar side	Adduct thump	Ulnar
Hypothenar Muscles				
Palmaris brevis (PB)	TCL, palmar aponeurosis	Ulnar palm	Retract skin	Ulnar
Abductor digiti minimi (ADM or AbdDM)	Pisiform	Base of proximal phalanx, ulnar side	Abduct small finger	Ulnar
Flexor digiti minimi brevis (FDMB)	Hamate, TCL	Base of proximal phalanx, ulnar side	Flex MCP	Ulnar
Opponens digiti minimi (ODM)	Hamate, TCL	Small finger metacarpal	Abduct, flex, lat. ratation	Ulnar
Intrinsic Muscles				
Lumbricals	Flexor digitorum profundus (FDP)	Lateral bands (radial)	Extend PIP	Median, ulnar
Dorsal interosseous (DIO)	Adjacent metacarpals	Proximal phalanx base/ extensor apparatus	Abduct, flex, MCP	Ulnar
Volar interosseous (VIO)	Adjacent metacarpals	Proximal phalanx base/ extensor apparatus	Abduct, flex MCP	Ulnar

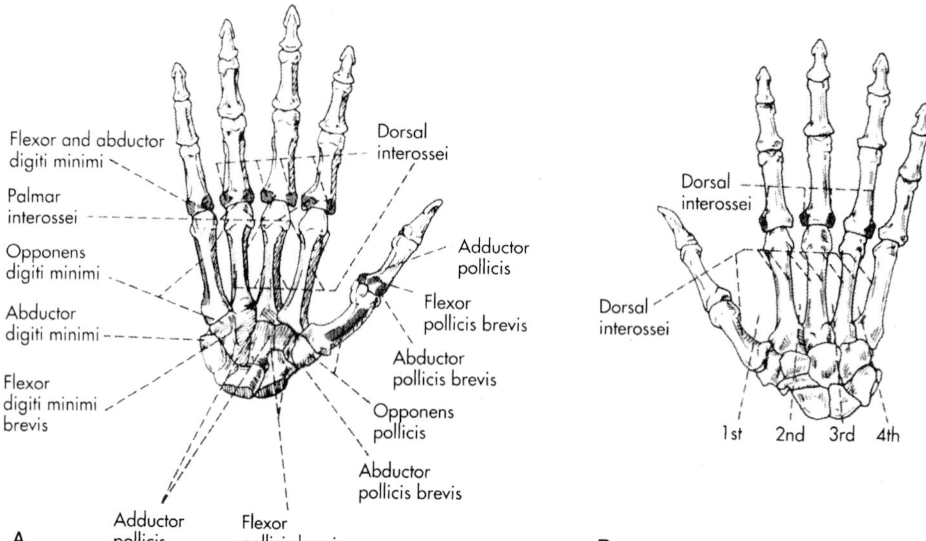

FIGURE 11-30 ■ Origins and insertions of muscles of the wrist and hand. (From Jenkins, D.B.: Hollinshead's Functional Anatomy of the Limbs and Back, 6th ed., Philadelphia, WB Saunders, 1991, Fig. 11-9.)

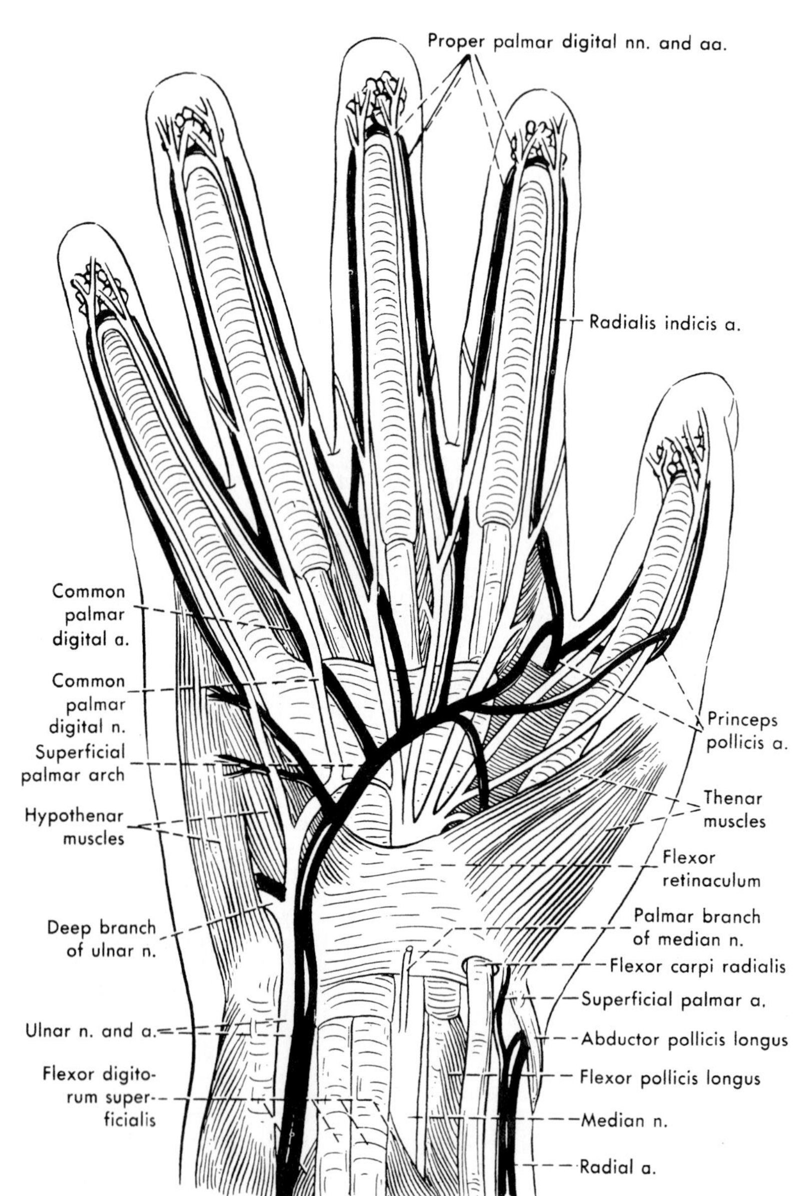

FIGURE 11-31 ■ Nerves and vessels of the hand. (From Jenkins, D.B.: Hollinshead's Functional Anatomy of the Limbs and Back, 6th ed., Fig. 11-11. Philadelphia, WB Saunders, 1991.)

3. **Sensation to the Thumb**—Composed of five branches: lateral antebrachial cutaneous nerve, superficial and dorsal digital branches of the radial nerve, and digital and palmar branches of the median nerve.

E. **Vessels** (see Fig. 11-31)

1. **Radial Artery**—At the wrist the radial artery reaches the dorsum of the carpus by passing between the FCR and the abductor pollicis longus and extensor pollicis brevis tendons (snuffbox). Before this, it gives off a superficial palmar branch that communicates with the superficial arch (ulnar artery). In the hand it forms the *deep palmar arch.* **The dorsal carpal branch of the radial artery enters the scaphoid dorsally and distally.**
2. **Ulnar Artery**—At the wrist, the ulnar artery lies on the TCL, gives off a deep palmar branch (which anastomoses with the deep arch), and then forms the *superficial palmar arch,* which is *distal to the deep arch.*
3. **Digital Arteries**—Arise from the superficial palmar arch and **run dorsal to the nerves.**

F. **Surgical Approaches**

1. **Dorsal Approach to the Wrist** (Fig. 11-32)—Through the third and fourth extensor

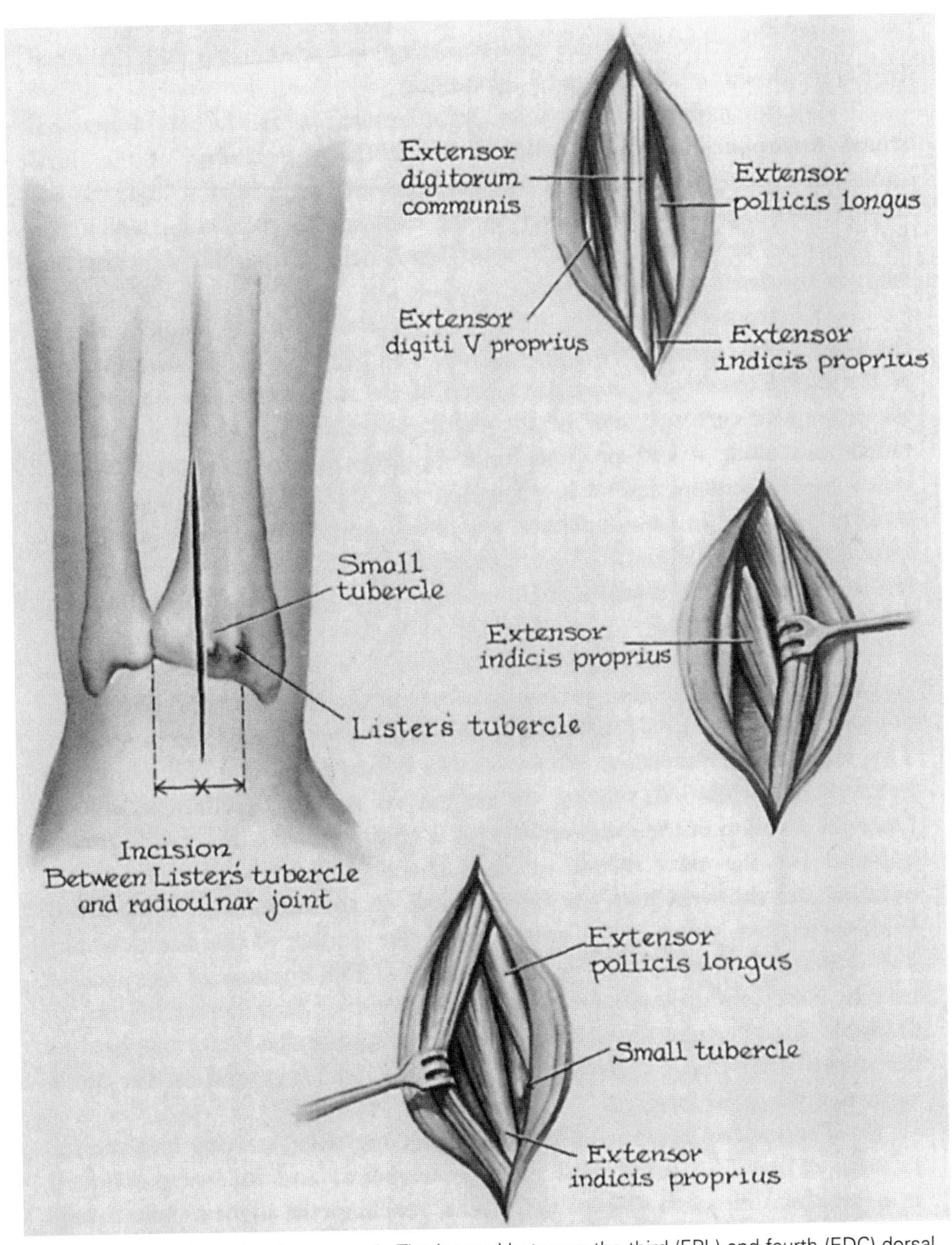

FIGURE 11-32 ■ Dorsal wrist approach. The interval between the third (EPL) and fourth (EDC) dorsal wrist compartments is explored. (From Kaplan, E.B.: Surgical Approaches to the Neck, Cervical Spine, and Upper Extremity. Philadelphia, WB Saunders, 1966, p. 112.)

compartments (extensor pollicis longus and EDC). Protecting and retracting these tendons allows access to the distal radius and the dorsal radiocarpal joint.

2. **Volar Approach to the Wrist**—Used most commonly for carpal tunnel release, the incision is usually made in line with the fourth ray to avoid the palmar cutaneous branch of the median nerve. Careful dissection through the transverse carpal ligament is necessary to avoid injury to the median nerve or its motor branch. The median nerve and flexor tendons can be retracted to allow access to the distal radius and carpus. See Fig. 11-33 for relevant anatomy.
3. **Volar Approach to the Scaphoid (Russé)** (Fig. 11-34)—Uses the interval between the FCR and the radial artery. An approach through the radial aspect of the FCR sheath is often easier and protects the radial artery.
4. **Dorsolateral Approach to the Scaphoid** (Fig. 11-35)—Utilizes an incision within the anatomic snuffbox (first and third dorsal wrist compartment), protecting the superficial radial nerve and radial artery (deep).
5. **Volar Approach to the Flexor Tendons (Bunnell's)**—Zigzag incisions across the flexor creases help to expose the flexor sheaths. The digital sheaths should be avoided.
6. **Midlateral Approach to the Digits**—Good for stabilization of fractures and neurovascular exposure, this approach uses a laterally placed incision at the dorsal extent of the interphalangeal (IP) creases. Exposure of the digital neurovascular bundle is carried out volar to the incision.

WRIST SURGICAL APPROACHES

APPROACH	INTERVAL	RISKS
Dorsal wrist	Third (EPL) and fourth (EDC) compartments	Transection of the PIN innervation to the wrist capsule can be performed
Volar wrist	FCR	Palmar cutaneous branch median nerve
Volar scaphoid	FCR and radial artery	Radial artery
Dorsolateral scaphoid	First and third compartments	Superficial radial nerve and radial artery

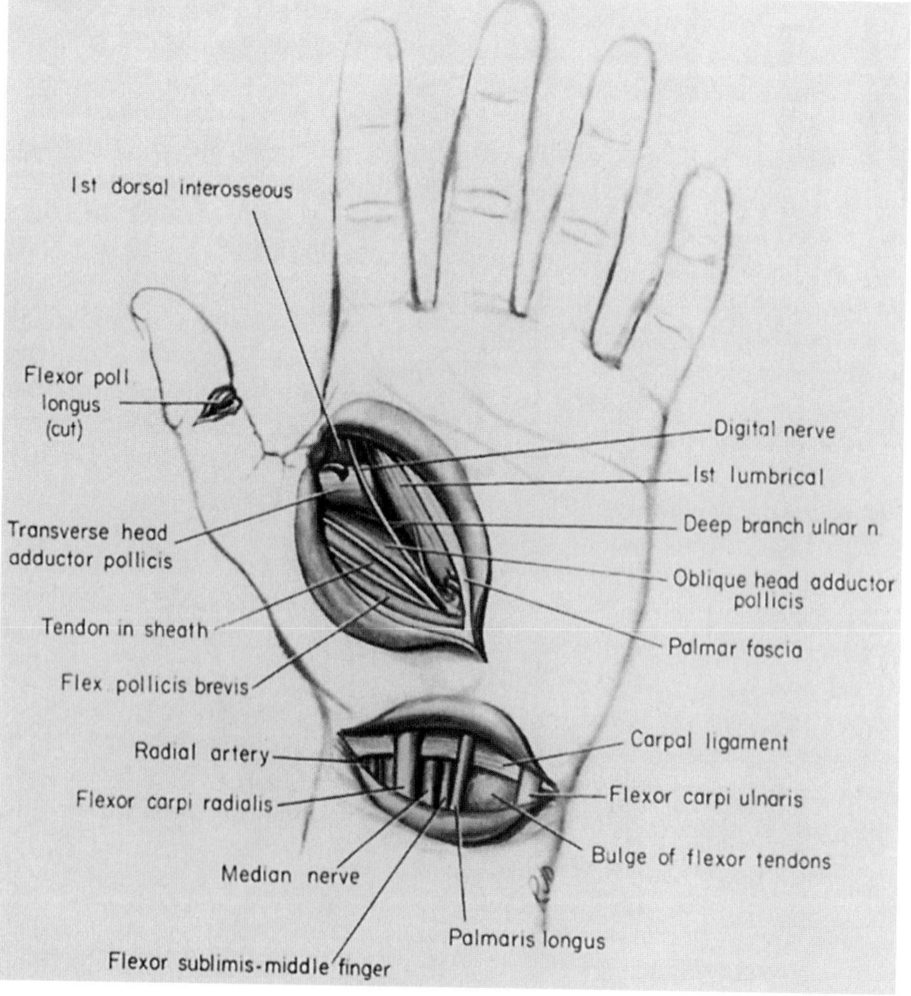

FIGURE 11-33 ■ Relevant anatomy of the carpal tunnel and thenar muscles. (From Kaplan, E.B.: Surgical Approaches to the Neck, Cervical Spine, and Upper Extremity. Philadelphia, WB Saunders, 1966, p. 97.)

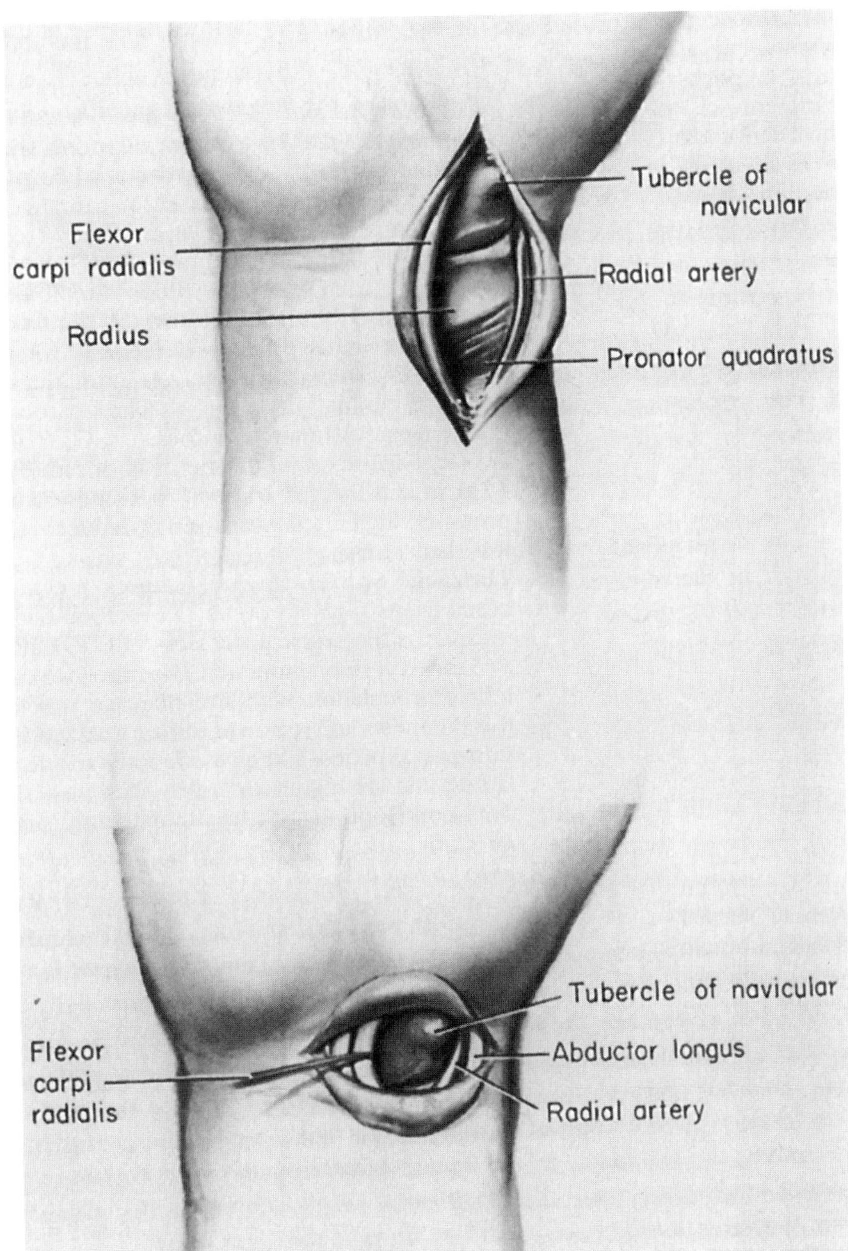

FIGURE 11-34 ■ Russé's approach to the scaphoid. The interval between the FCR and radial artery is used. (From Kaplan, E.B.: Surgical Approaches to the Neck, Cervical Spine, and Upper Extremity. Philadelphia, WB Saunders, 1966, p. 101.)

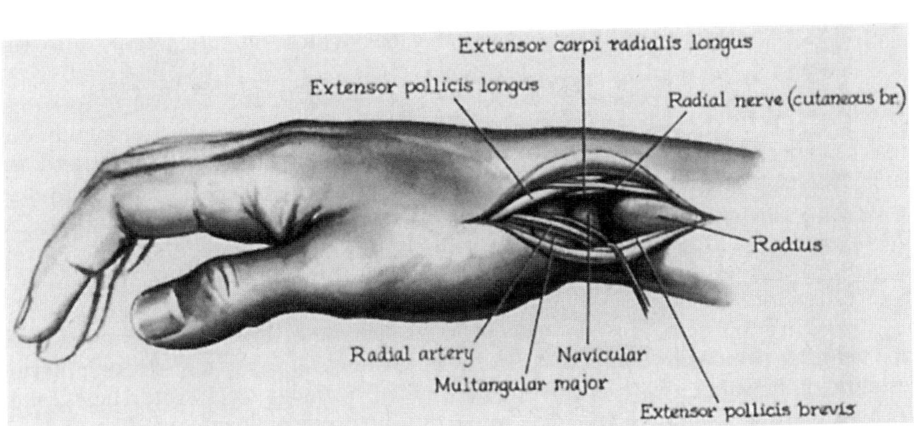

FIGURE 11-35 ■ Dorsal approaches to the scaphoid. The interval between the first and third dorsal wrist compartments is explored. (From Kaplan, E.B.: Surgical Approaches to the Neck, Cervical Spine, and Upper Extremity. Philadelphia, WB Saunders, 1966, p. 107.)

G. **Arthroscopy**—Portals used for wrist arthroscopy are based on the dorsal compartments. The 1-2 portal (risks the radial artery), 6-R and 6-U portals (radial and ulnar to the sixth compartment—risks the ulnar nerve and artery) are the most dangerous. The commonly used 3-4 and 4-5 portals are safer.

H. Summary of Upper-Extremity Innervation

SUMMARY OF UPPER-EXTREMITY INNERVATION

NERVE	INNERVATION
Musculocutaneous nerve (lateral cord)	Coracobrachialis, biceps, brachialis
Axillary nerve (posterior cord)	Deltoid, teres minor
Radial nerve (posterior cord)	Triceps, brachioradialis, ECRL, ECRB
PIN	Supinator, ECU, ED, EDM, AbdPL, EPL, EPB, EI
Median nerve (medial and lateral cord)	PT, FCR, PL, FDS, AbdPB, FPB supinator head, OP, 1st & 2nd lumbrical
AIN	FDP (I & II), FPL, PQ
Ulnar nerve (medial cord)	FCU, FDP (III & IV), PB, AbdDM, ODM, FDM, 3rd & 4th lumbrical, interossei, AddP, deep head FPB

VI. Spine

A. Osteology

1. **Introduction**—The spine contains 33 vertebrae: 7 cervical, 12 thoracic, 5 lumbar, 5 fused sacral, and 4 fused coccygeal vertebrae. Normal curves include cervical lordosis, thoracic kyphosis, lumbar lordosis, and sacral kyphosis. The vertebral bodies generally increase in width craniocaudally, with the exception of T1–T3. Locations of important topographic landmarks are bold in the following chart.

SPINE VERTEBRAL BODIES

TOPOGRAPHIC LANDMARK	SPINAL LEVEL
Mandible	C2-3
Hyoid cartilage	**C3**
Thyroid cartilage	C4-5
Cricoid cartilage	**C6**
Vertebra prominens	C7
Scapular spine	T3
Distal tip of scapula	T7
Iliac crest	L4-5

2. **Cervical Spine**— The atlas (C1) has no vertebral body and no spinous process. C1 has two concave superior facets that articulate with the occipital condyles. *The highest percentage of neck flexion and extension occur at the occiput-C1 articulation (50% of total).* The axis (C2) develops from five ossification centers with an initial cartilaginous junction between the dens and vertebral body (subdental synchondrosis) that fuses at 7 years of age. The base of the dens narrows because of the transverse ligament. The *atlantoaxial articulation is responsible for the majority of neck rotation with 50% of total rotation occurring at the C1-C2 articulation.* The **atlantoaxial joint is a diarthrodial joint**, which explains why pannus in RA can affect this articulation and result in instability (see Chapter 7, Spine). Vertebrae C2–C7 have foramina in each transverse process and bifid spinous processes (except for C7 nonbifid posterior spinous process—vertebral prominens). The vertebral artery travels in the transverse foramina of C6–C1. The carotid (Chassaignac's) tubercle is found at C6. **The cervical spine canal diameter is normally 17 mm** and the cervical cord becomes compromised when the diameter is reduced to less than 13 mm.
3. **Thoracic Spine**—Unique features include costal facets (present on all 12 vertebral bodies and the transverse processes of T1–T9) and a rounded vertebral foramen. The thoracic vertebrae articulation with the rib cage makes this the most rigid region of the axial skeleton.
4. **Lumbar Spine**—These vertebrae are the largest and are higher anteriorly than posteriorly contributing to the lumbar lordosis. *Lumbar lordosis ranges from 55-60 degrees with apex at L3 with most of the lordosis because of the intervertebral disc spaces.* The majority of **lumbar lordosis (66%) occurs from L4 to sacrum**. Lumbar vertebrae contain short laminae and pedicles. They also have mammillary processes (separate ossification centers) that project posteriorly from the superior articular facet. Do not forget that **spondylolysis** is a **defect in the pars interarticularis** and the *most common cause of back pain in children and adolescents.*
5. **Sacrum**—Fusion of five spinal elements. The sacral promontory is the anterosuperior portion that projects into the pelvis. There are usually four pairs of pelvic sacral foramina located both anteriorly and posteriorly that transmit respective ventral and dorsal branches of the upper four sacral nerves. There is also a sacral canal, which opens caudally into the sacral hiatus.
6. **Coccyx**—Fusion of the lowest four spinal elements; it attaches dorsally to the gluteus maximus, the external anal sphincter, and the coccygeal muscles.

B. **Spinal Ligaments**—Include the anterior and posterior longitudinal ligaments, ligamentum flavum and the supraspinous, interspinous, and intertransverse ligaments.

1. **General Arrangement**—The vertebral bodies are bound together by the strong anterior longitudinal ligament (**ALL**) and the weaker posterior longitudinal ligament (**PLL**). The ALL

is usually thickest at the center of the vertebral body and thins at the periphery. Separate fibers extend from one to five levels. The ALL resists hyperextension. The PLL extends from the occiput (tectorial membrane) to the posterior sacrum. It is separated from the center of the vertebral body by a space that allows passage of the dorsal branches of the spinal artery and veins. The PLL is hourglass-shaped, with the wider (yet thinner) sections located over the discs. Ruptured discs tend to occur lateral to these expansions. Ligamentous capsules overlying the zygapophyseal joints and the intertransverse ligaments contribute little to interspinous stability. The **ligamentum flavum** is a strong, yellow, elastic ligament connecting the laminae. It runs from the anterior surface of the superior lamina to the posterior surface of the inferior lamina and is constantly in tension. Hypertrophy of the ligamentum flavum is said to contribute to nerve root compression. The **supraspinous** and **interspinous** ligaments lie dorsal to and between the spinous processes, respectively. The supraspinous ligament begins at C7 and is in continuity with the ligamentum nuchae (which runs from C7 to the occiput).

2. **Spine Stability (Denis)** —The three-column system is summarized in the following chart.

DENIS SPINE COLUMNS

COLUMN	COMPOSITION
Anterior	ALL, anterior two-thirds of annulus and vertebral body
Middle	Posterior third of body and annulus, PLL
Posterior	Pedicles, facets and facet capsules, spinous processes, posterior ligaments including interspinous and supraspinous ligaments, ligamentum flavum

3. **Specialized Ligaments**
   a. **Atlanto-Occipital Joint**—Consists of two articular capsules (anterior and posterior) and the **tectorial membrane** (a cephalad extension of the PLL). It is further stabilized by the ligamentous attachments to the dens.
   b. **Atlantoaxial Joint**—The **transverse** ligament is the major stabilizer of the median atlantoaxial joint. This articulation is further stabilized by the apical ligament (longitudinal), which together with the transverse ligament composes the **cruciate** ligament. Additionally, a pair of **alar,** or **"check," ligaments** run obliquely from the tip of the dens to the occiput (Fig. 11-36). Do not forget that *an atlantodens interval of >7-10 mm or a posterior space of <13 mm is a relative contraindication to elective orthopaedic surgery* and the spine should be stabilized first. Common measurements in C1-C2 disorders are covered in Chapter 7 (Fig. 7-2).

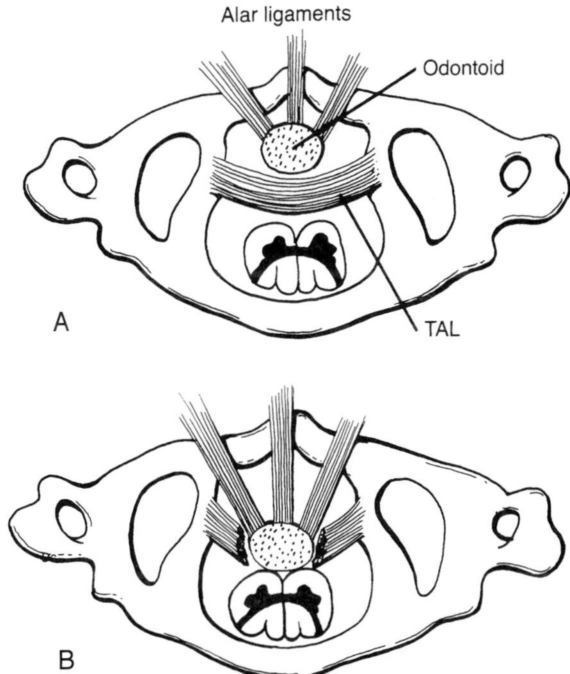

FIGURE 11-36 ■ The atlantoaxial complex as seen from above *(A)*. The disruption of the transverse ligament (TAL) with intact alar ligaments results in C1–C2 instability without cord compression *(B)*. (From DeLee, J.C., and Drez, D., Jr.: Orthopaedic Sports Medicine, Principles and Practices, vol. 1. Philadelphia, WB Saunders, 1994, p. 432; *B* redrawn from Hensinger, R.N.: Congenital anomalies of the atlantoaxial joint. The Cervical Spine Research Society Editorial Committee. The Cervical Spine, 2nd ed. Philadelphia, J.B. Lippincott, 1989, p. 242.)

   c. **Iliolumbar Ligament**—This stout ligament connects the transverse process of L5 with the ilium. Tension on this ligament in patients with unstable vertical shear pelvic fractures can lead to avulsion fractures of the transverse process.

4. **Facet (Apophyseal) Joints**—The orientation of the facets of the spine dictates the plane of motion at each relative level. The facet orientation varies with spinal level and is summarized in the chart below.

ORIENTATION OF SPINE FACETS

SPINE REGION	SAGITTAL FACET ORIENTATION	CORONAL FACET ORIENTATION
Cervical	35 degrees at C2 increasing to 55 degrees at C7	Neutral, 0 degrees
Thoracic	60 degrees at T1 increasing to 70 degrees at T12	20 degrees posterior
Lumbar	137 degrees at L1 decreasing to 118 degrees at L5	45 degrees anterior

In the cervical spine the superior articular facet is anterior and inferior to the inferior articular process of the vertebra above. Nerve roots exit near the superior articulating process. In the lumbar spine the superior articular facet is anterior and lateral to the inferior articular facet.

5. **Intervertebral Discs**—The intervertebral discs are fibrocartilaginous, with an obliquely oriented **annulus fibrosus** composed of **type I collagen** and a softer central **nucleus pulposus** made of **type II collagen.** The nucleus pulposus has a high polysaccharide content and is approximately 88% water. Aging results in the loss of water and conversion to fibrocartilage. The discs account for 25% of the total spinal columnar height. They are attached to the vertebral bodies by hyaline cartilage, which is responsible for the vertical growth of the column. **Intradiscal pressure is position dependent:** pressure is **lowest when lying supine** and highest when sitting and flexed forward with weights in hands.

C. **Spinal Musculature**

1. **Neck**—The neck is divided, for functional purposes, into the anterior and posterior regions.
   a. **Anterior**—The anterior neck muscles include the superficial platysma muscle (CN VII innervated), stylohyoid and digastric muscles (CN XII innervated) above the hyoid, and "strap" muscles below the hyoid. Important strap muscles include the sternohyoid and omohyoid in the superficial layer and the thyrohyoid and sternohyoid in the deep layer; all are innervated by the ansa cervicalis (C1-C3). Laterally, the sternocleidomastoid (CN XI and ansa) runs obliquely across the neck, rotating the head to the contralateral side. The **anterior triangle** (borders: sternocleidomastoid, midline of the neck, and the lower border of the mandible) is the largest area. Three smaller triangles include the submandibular, carotid (bordered by the posterior aspect of the digastric and the omohyoid, and used for the anterior approach to C5), and posterior (bordered by the trapezius, sternocleidomastoid, and clavicle).
   b. **Posterior**—The posterior neck muscles form the borders of the **suboccipital triangle.** The superior and inferior heads of the obliquus capitis muscle and the rectus capitis posterior major muscle forms this triangle. The vertebral artery and the first cervical nerve are within this triangle, and the greater occipital nerve (C2) is superficial.
   c. **Frequently Tested Relationships**—Contents of carotid sheath: internal carotid artery, common carotid artery, internal jugular vein and CN X (vagus).

SPINAL MUSCLE RELATIONSHIPS

MUSCLE	RELATIONSHIP
Longus capitus	Anterior to longus colli Posterior to sympathetic chain
Longus colli	Anterior to vertebral artery Posterior to longus capitus

2. **Back**—The back is blanketed by the trapezius (superiorly) and the latissimus dorsi (inferiorly). The rhomboids and levator scapulae are deep to this layer. The deep muscles of the back are arranged into two groups: erector spinae and transversospinalis group. The erector spinae run from the transverse and spinous processes of the inferior vertebrae to the spinous processes of the superior vertebrae. They stabilize and extend the back. All of the deep back musculature is innervated by dorsal primary rami of spinal nerves.

D. **Nerves**

1. **Spinal Cord**—The cord extends from the brain stem to the inferior border of L1, where it terminates as the conus medullaris. It is enclosed within the bony spinal canal with variable amounts of space (greatest in the upper cervical spine). The cord also varies in diameter (widest at the origin of plexi). In cross-section, the cord has both geographic and functional boundaries (Fig. 11-37). It is

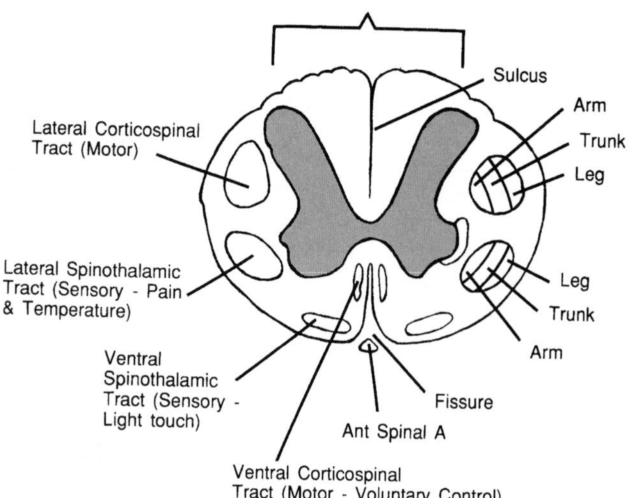

FIGURE 11-37 ■ Cross-section of the spinal cord illustrating functions of the ascending and descending tracts. **Ascending tracts (sensory)**; dorsal columns, lateral spinothalamic, ventral or anterior spinothalamic. **Descending (motor)**: lateral corticospinal and ventral or anterior corticospinal.

divided in the midline anteriorly by a fissure and posteriorly by the sulcus. Functions of the ascending (sensory) and descending (motor) tracts are summarized in the following chart.

SPINAL CORD TRACTS

	TRACTS	FUNCTION
Ascending (sensory)	Dorsal columns	Deep touch, proprioception, vibratory
	Lateral spinothalamic	Pain and temperature
	Anterior spinothalamic	Light touch
Descending (motor)	Lateral corticospinal	Voluntary motor
	Anterior corticospinal	Voluntary motor

The posterior funiculi **(dorsal columns)** are located dorsally and receive ascending fibers, which deliver deep touch, proprioception, and vibratory sensation. The **lateral spinothalamic tract** transmits pain and temperature. (It is the site for chordotomy for intractable pain.) Descending in the **lateral corticospinal tract** are fibers that transmit instructions for voluntary muscle contraction. Sacral structures are most peripheral in the lateral corticospinal tracts with cervical structures more medial. (This is why central cord syndrome affects the upper extremities more than the lower extremities—see following chart). The **ventral (anterior) spinothalamic tract** transmits light touch sensation, and the **ventral (anterior) corticospinal tract** delivers cortical messages of voluntary contraction. Deficits associated with incomplete spinal cord injury patterns are predicted by the anatomy of the ascending and descending tracts. Do not forget that **prognosis with incomplete spinal cord injury** is *unaffected by the bulbocavernosis reflex.* A summary is provided in the following chart.

INCOMPLETE SPINAL CORD INJURY PATTERNS

INJURY PATTERN	FUNCTIONAL DEFICIT	RECOVERY
Central **(most common)**	UE>LE, usually quadriplegic with sacral sparing. Flaccid paralysis of UE and spastic paralysis of LE	75%
Anterior	Complete motor deficit	10% **(worst prognosis)**
Posterior	Loss of deep pressure, deep pain and proprioception	
Brown-Séquard	Unilateral cord injury with ipsilateral motor deficit and contralateral pain and temperature deficit (two levels below injury)	>90% recovery

UE, Upper extremity; LE, lower extremity.

The **spinal cord tapers at L1 (conus medullaris)**, and a small filum terminale continues with surrounding nerve roots contained within a common dural sac (cauda equina) to its termination in the coccyx. Spinal cord injury at this level may permanently interrupt the bulbocavernosis reflex.

2. **Nerve Roots** (Fig. 11-38)—Thirty-one pairs of spinal nerves: 8 cervical, 12 thoracic, 5 lumbar,

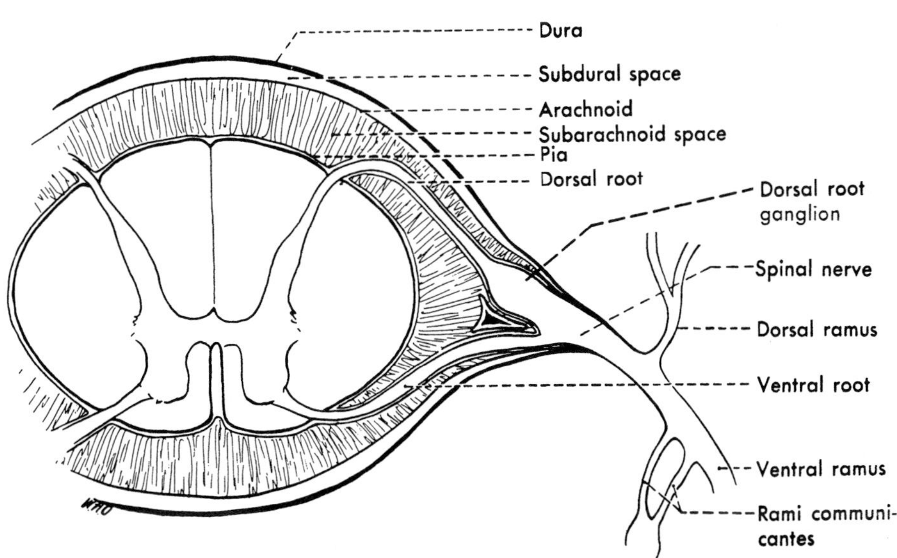

FIGURE 11-38 ■ Spinal nerves. Please note that the facet joints are innervated by the medial branch of the dorsal primary ramus and sinuvertebral nerve. (From Jenkins, D.B.: Hollinshead's Functional Anatomy of the Limbs and Back, 6th ed. Philadelphia, WB Saunders, 1991, p. 205.)

5 sacral, and 1 coccygeal. Within the subarachnoid space the dorsal root (and ganglia) and ventral roots converge to form the spinal nerve. The nerve becomes "extradural" as it approaches the intervertebral foramen (dura becomes epineurium) at all levels above L1. Below this level the nerves are contained within the cauda equina. After exiting the foramen the spinal nerve delivers dorsal primary rami, which supply the muscles and skin of the neck and back regions. Innervation of structures within the spinal canal including periosteum, meninges, vascular structures, and articular connective tissue is from the **sinuvertebral nerve**. The ventral rami supply the anteromedial trunk and the limbs. With the exception of the thoracic nerves, ventral rami are grouped in plexuses before delivering sensorimotor functions to a general region. In the **cervical spine the numbered nerve exits at a level *above* the pedicle of corresponding vertebral level (e.g., C2 exits at C1–C2)**. In the lumbar spine the nerve root traverses the respective disc space above the named vertebral body and exits the respective foramen under the pedicle (Fig. 11-39). Herniated discs usually impinge on the traversing nerve root and the facet joint. For example, a disc herniation at L4-L5 would cause compression of the traversing L5 nerve root resulting in a positive tension sign (straight-leg raise) and diminished strength in the hip abductors, EHL, and pain and numbness in the lateral leg to the dorsum of the foot (see Fig. 11-40). A far lateral L4-L5 disc herniation would compress the exiting L4 nerve root, resulting in a positive tension sign (femoral nerve stretch test) and L4 compromise. Do not forget that the L5 nerve root is relatively fixed to the anterior sacral ala and can be damaged by sacral fractures and errant anteriorly placed iliosacral screws.

3. Quick Summary of Key Testable Neurologic Levels

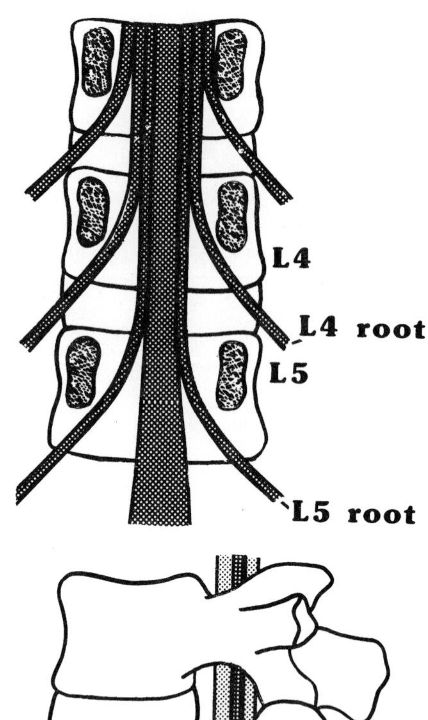

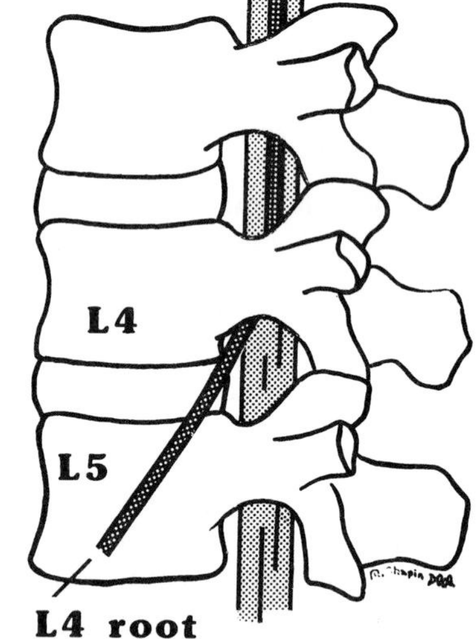

FIGURE 11-39 ■ Lumbar spine nerve root locations in relation to vertebral landmarks. Central disc herniation between L4–L5 would compress the traversing root and therefore affect L5. A far lateral disc herniation between L4–L5 would affect the exiting root L4. In the cervical spine the numbered nerve exists at a level above the pedicle of the corresponding vertebral level. (From Weissman, B.N., and Sledge, C.B.: Orthopedic Radiology. Philadelphia, WB Saunders, 1986, p. 283.)

KEY TESTABLE NEUROLOGIC LEVELS

NEUROLOGIC LEVEL	REPRESENTATIVE MOTOR	REFLEX
C5	Deltoid	Biceps
C6	Wrist extension	Brachioradialis
C7	Wrist flexion	Triceps
C8	Finger flexion	
T1	Interossei	
L4	Tibialis anterior	Patellar
L5	Toe extensors	
S1	Peroneal	Achilles

A summary of findings of nerve root compression is highlighted in Chapter 7 (Table 7-2 [cervical] and Table 7-4 [lumbar]). Dermatomes are key testable items shown in Fig. 11-40.

4. **Sympathetic Chain**—The cervical sympathetic chain lies **posterior** and medial **to the carotid sheath**. It is *anterior to the longus capitus muscle.* The cervical sympathetic chain has three ganglia: superior, middle, and inferior. **Disruption of the inferior ganglia can lead to Horner's syndrome.** There are 3 ganglia in the cervical region, 11 in the thoracic region, 4 in the lumbar region, and 4 in the sacral region.

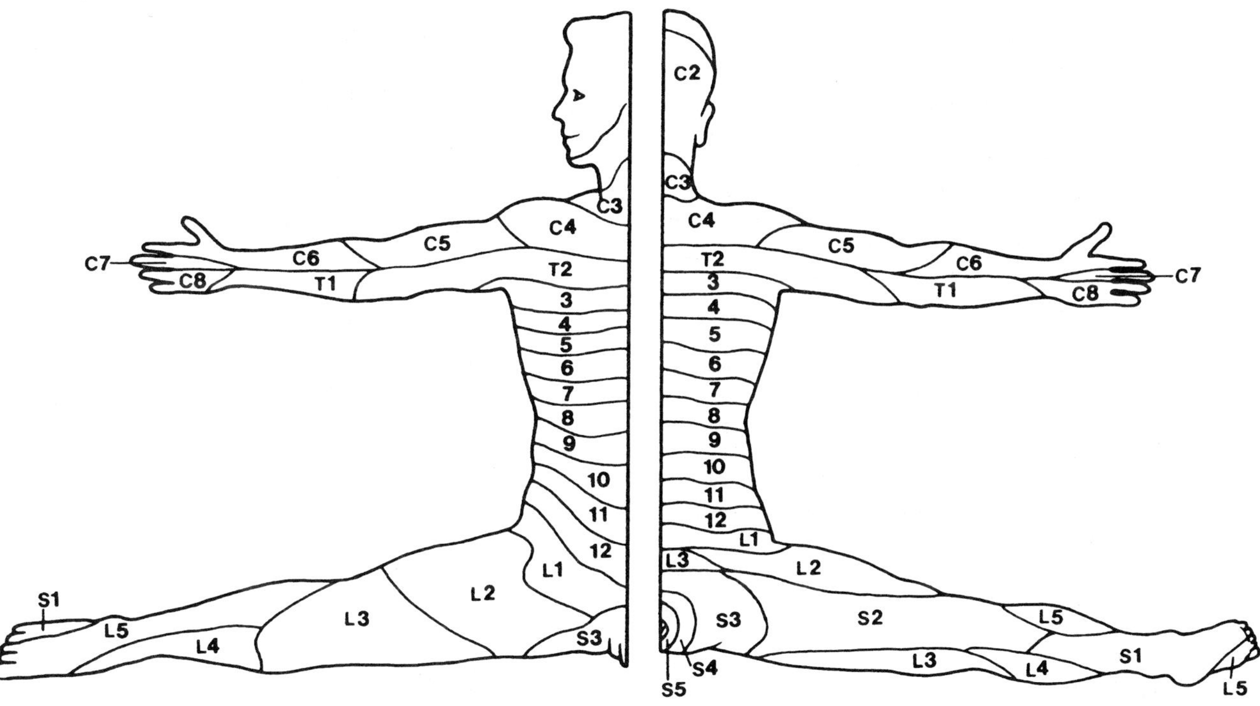

FIGURE 11-40 ■ Dermatomal patterns.

CERVICAL SYMPATHETIC GANGLIA

GANGLIA	LOCATION	OTHER
Superior	C2–C3	Largest
Middle	C6	Variable
Inferior	C7–T1	Stellate

E. **Vascular Supply to the Spine**

Spinal blood supply is usually derived from the segmental arteries located at vertebral midbodies via the **aorta (which lies on the left side of the vertebral column with the inferior vena cava and azygos vein on the right)**. The primary supply to the dura and posterior elements is from the dorsal branches. The ventral branches supply the vertebral bodies via ascending and descending branches, which are delivered underneath the PLL in four separate ostia. **The vertebral artery** (a branch of the subclavian) ascends through the transverse foramina of C1-C6 (anterior to and not through C7), **posterior to the longus colli muscle**, then posterior to the lateral masses, along the cephalad surface of the posterior arch of C1 (atlas), passes ventromedially around the spinal cord and through the foramen magnum before uniting at the midline basilar artery. *The distance from the spinous process of C1 laterally to the vertebral artery is 2 cm* (safe distance for dissections would therefore be less than 2 cm). The artery of **Adamkiewicz** (great anterior medullary artery) enters through the **left** intervertebral foramen in the lower thoracic spine from **T8 to T12**. It supplies the interior two-thirds of the anterior cord. Arterial supply to the spinal cord is from anterior and posterior spinal arteries and segmental branches of the vertebral artery and dorsal arteries, which travel via the dorsal and ventral rootlets to the respective dorsal and anterolateral portions of the cord. The venous drainage of the vertebral bodies is primarily via the central sinusoid located on the dorsum of each vertebral body.

F. **Surgical Approaches to the Spine**

1. **Anterior Approach to the Cervical Spine**—A transverse incision is based on the desired level (e.g., for C5 one should enter the carotid triangle). The platysma is retracted with the skin. The pretracheal fascia is exposed to explore the interval between the **carotid sheath (contains the internal and common carotid arteries, the internal jugular vein, and the vagus nerve [CN X])** and the trachea. The prevertebral fascia is sharply incised and the longus colli muscle gently retracted (protecting the recurrent laryngeal nerve [a branch of the vagus nerve

that lies outside the sheath]) to expose the vertebral body. Increased risk of injury to the **recurrent laryngeal nerve** occurs with right-sided approaches (paralysis is identified by a hoarse, scratchy voice from unilateral vocal cord paralysis visualized with direct laryngoscopy). The recurrent laryngeal nerve arises from the vagus at the level of the subclavian artery on the right with the left arising at the level of the aortic arch. Lower left-sided anterior cervical approaches risk injury to the **thoracic duct** that is *posterior to the carotid sheath.* By dissecting the longus muscles subperiosteally, one also protects the stellate ganglion (avoiding Horner's syndrome). The anterior surface of the vertebral body is exposed.

2. **Posterior Approach to the Cervical Spine**—After a midline approach through the ligamentum nuchae, the superficial layer (trapezius) and intermediate layer (splenius, semispinalis, longissimus capitis) are reflected laterally, and the vertebrae are exposed. The vertebral artery is especially vulnerable as it leaves the foramen transversarium and travels above and medially to pierce the atlanto-occipital membrane at its lateral angle. The greater occipital nerve (C2) and the third occipital nerve (C3) should also be protected in the suboccipital region. Access to the spinal canal is via laminectomy or facetectomy (Fig. 11-41).
3. **Anterior (Transthoracic) Approach to the Thoracic Spine**—A transverse incision is made approximately two ribs above the level of interest. Dissection over the top of the rib is carried out to avoid injuring the intercostal neurovascular bundle (which lies on the inferior internal surface of the rib). The rib is further dissected and removed from the field. **The right-sided approach is favored to avoid the aorta, segmental arteries, artery of Adamkiewicz, and thoracic duct (in the upper thoracic spine on the left side of the esophagus and behind the carotid sheath).** The esophagus, aorta, vena cava, and pleura of the lungs should be identified and protected.
4. **Posterior Approach to the Thoracolumbar Spine**—A straight midline incision is made over the spinous processes and carried down through the thoracolumbar fascia. The plane between the two segmentally innervated erector spinae muscles is used. Paraspinal musculature is subperiosteally dissected from the attached spinous processes, exposing the posterior elements. Structures at risk include the posterior primary rami (near facet joints) and segmental vessels (anterior to the plane connecting the transverse processes). Partial laminectomy allows greater exposure of the cord and discs. Pedicle screw placement is at the junction of the lateral border of the superior facet and the middle of the transverse process. These screws should be angled 15 degrees medially and in line with the slope of the vertebra, as seen on lateral radiographs.
5. **Anterior Approach to the Lumbar Spine (Transperitoneal)**—Longitudinal incision from below the umbilicus to just above the pubic symphysis. Split the rectus abdominis muscles and incise the peritoneum. Protect and retract bladder distally and bowel cephalad and incise the posterior peritoneum longitudinally over the sacral promontory. The aorta bifurcation is revealed and the middle sacral artery is ligated. Expose the L5–S1 disc space. Injury to the lumbar plexus, particularly the **superior hypogastric plexus of the sympathetic plexus that lies over the L5 vertebral body**, can cause **sexual dysfunction and retrograde ejaculation**. Do not forget that ejaculation is a predominantly sympathetic nervous system function and erection is a predominantly parasympathetic nervous system function.
6. **Anterolateral Approach to the Lumbar Spine (Retroperitoneal)**—Provides access from L1 to sacrum. An oblique incision is centered over the 12th rib to the lateral border of the rectus abdominis muscle. The external oblique, internal oblique, and transversus abdominis muscles are incised in line with the skin incision. Elevate the retroperitoneal fat revealing the psoas major muscle and **genitofemoral nerve**. Ligate the segmental lumbar vessels and mobilize the aorta and vena cava to expose the desired vertebral level. Protect the **sympathetic chain** (medial to the psoas and lateral to the vertebral body) and **ureters** (between peritoneum and psoas fascia).

FIGURE 11-41 ■ Surgical procedures on the cervical spine. (From Rothman, R.H., and Simeon, F.A.: The Spine, 2nd ed. Philadelphia, WB Saunders, 1982, p. 484.)

SPINE SURGICAL APPROACHES

APPROACH	INTERVAL	RISKS
Anterior cervical	Carotid sheath and the trachea	Recurrent laryngeal nerve Sympathetic ganglion
Posterior cervical	Midline approach between paracervical muscle	Vertebral artery
Anterior thoracic	Transverse between ribs two levels above surgical site	Dissect over top of rib to avoid intercostal neurovascular bundle
Posterior thoracolumbar	Midline approach over spinous processes	Posterior primary rami and segmental vessels. Protect nerve root
Anterior lumbar (transperitoneal)	Between segmentally innervated rectus abdominis	Presacral plexus of parasympathetic nerve

7. **Anatomy Important to Placement of Halo Pins**—Optimal position for placement of anterolateral halo pins is approximately 1 cm superior to the orbital rim in the outer two-thirds of the orbit below the equator of the skull (Fig. Unn 11-1). This position will then place the temporal fossa and temporalis muscle lateral and the supraorbital nerve, supratrochlear nerve, and frontal sinus medially. The supraorbital nerve is lateral to the supratrochlear nerve that overlies the frontal sinus. The most commonly injured *cranial nerve* with halo traction is the abducens (CN VI), which is identified by a loss of lateral gaze.

VII. Pelvis and Hip

A. **Osteology**—The pelvic girdle is composed of two innominate (coxal) bones that articulate with the sacrum. Each innominate bone is composed of three united bones: ilium, ischium, and pubis. The ilium has two important anterior prominences: the anterior superior (ASIS) and anterior inferior (AIIS) iliac spines. The anterior superior iliac spine is palpable at the lateral edge of the inguinal ligament. It is the origin for the sartorius muscle and the transverse and internal abdominal muscles. The anteroinferior iliac spine is less prominent and provides the origin of the direct head of the rectus femoris and the iliofemoral ligament (Y ligament of Bigelow). The ilium also has a posterior superior iliac spine that is usually located 4–5 cm lateral to the S2 spinous process. The greater sciatic notch is located posterior and superior to the acetabulum. The iliopectineal eminence is a raised region anteriorly that represents the union of the ilium and pubis. The iliopsoas muscle traverses a groove between this eminence and the anteroinferior iliac spine. The acetabulum is anteverted (15 degrees) and obliquely oriented (45 degrees caudally). The posterosuperior articular surface is thickened to accommodate weight-bearing. The inferior surface is deficient and contains the acetabular, or cotyloid, notch bound by the transverse acetabular ligament. The proximal femur is composed of the femoral head, neck, and greater and lesser trochanters. The femoral neck is anteverted approximately 14 degrees in relation to the femoral condyles. The femoral neck shaft angle averages 127 degrees. Hip trabecular architecture is illustrated in Fig. 11-42.

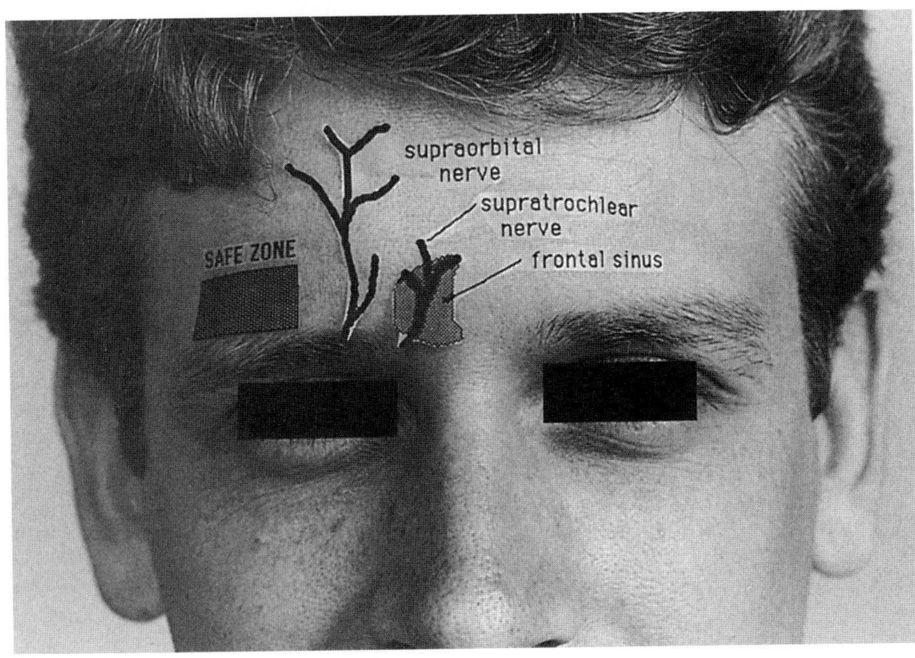

FIGURE UNN11-1 ■ Safe placement of halo pins.

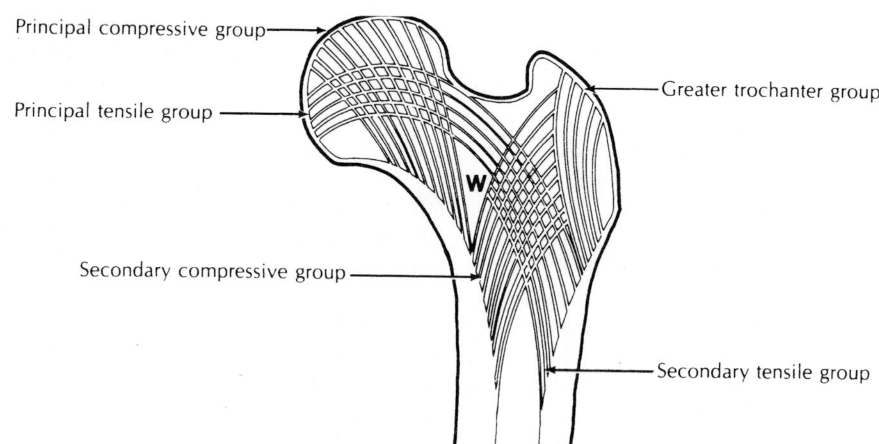

FIGURE 11-42 ■ Hip trabeculae. Trabecular patterns help determine the presence of osteopenia (Singh index). If all trabecular groups are visualized, a Singh grade VI is established (normal). Also, the difference between Garden type III and IV displaced femoral neck fractures is determined by the alignment of trabecular patterns of the femoral head and acetabulum. Alignment occurs in type IV because the femoral head assumes a normal position in the acetabulum. (From DeLee, J.C.: Fractures and dislocations of the hip. In Rockwood, C.A., Jr., Green, D.P., and Buchholz, R.W., eds.: Fractures in Adults, 3rd ed. Philadelphia, J.B. Lippincott, 1991, p. 1488.)

B. **Arthrology**

1. **Hip**—The hip joint is a spheroidal, or ball-and-socket, type of diarthrodial joint. Its stability is based primarily on the bony architecture. The acetabulum is deepened by the fibrocartilaginous labrum. The joint capsule extends anteriorly across the femoral neck to the trochanteric crest; however, posteriorly it extends only partially across the femoral neck leaving the basicervical and intertrochanteric crest regions extracapsular (Fig. 11-43). A series of three ligaments compose the capsule anteriorly. The *iliofemoral,* or Y ligament of Bigelow is the strongest ligament in the body and attaches the anteroinferior iliac spine to the intertrochanteric line in an inverted Y fashion. The remaining anterior ligaments, the *ischiofemoral* and *pubofemoral* ligaments, are weaker but lend additional stability. Inside the joint the **ligament of teres** arises from the apex of the cotyloid notch and attaches to the fovea of the femoral head. It transmits an arterial branch of the posterior division of the **obturator artery** to the femoral head (less significant in adults). Blood supply to the femoral head changes with age and key points are highlighted in the following chart. This chart helps explain why the standard antegrade femoral nailing start point is undesirable for pediatric femur fractures. Using the piriformis start point would damage the posterosuperior retinacular vessels, causing avascular necrosis of the femoral head. Additionally, in adults, one avoids completely transecting the quadratus femoris muscle in the posterior acetabular approach to avoid damage to the main blood supply to the femoral head-medial femoral circumflex artery.

AGE-DEPENDENT CHANGES TO FEMORAL HEAD BLOOD SUPPLY

AGE	BLOOD SUPPLY
Birth to 4 years	Primary medial and lateral circumflex arteries (from deep femoral artery) Ligamentum teres with obturator artery posterior division
4 years to adult	Negligible lateral circumflex artery Minimal ligamentum teres *Posterosuperior* and posteroinferior retinacular from medial femoral circumflex artery
Adult	Medial femoral circumflex to lateral epiphyseal artery

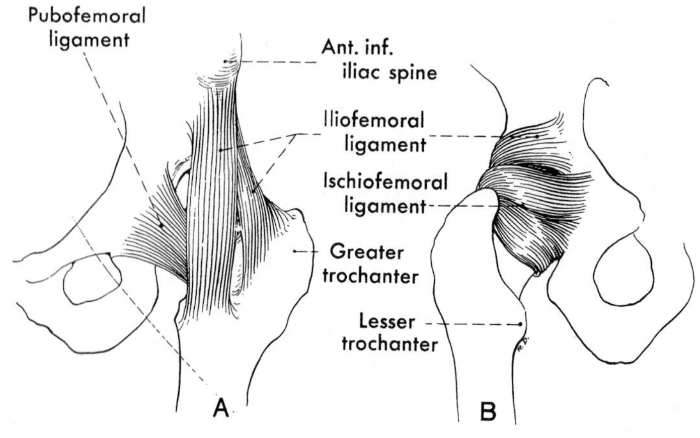

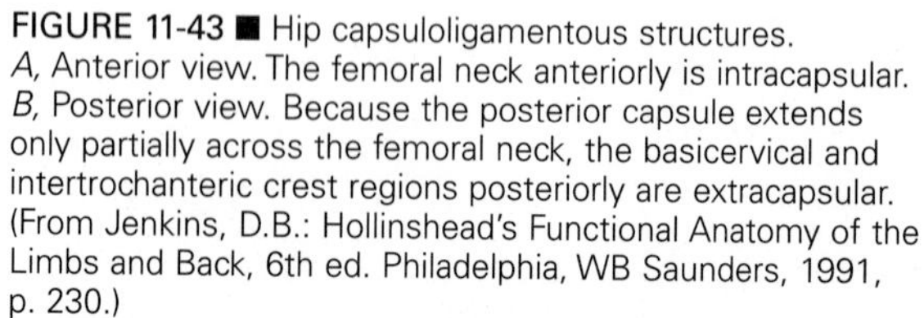
FIGURE 11-43 ■ Hip capsuloligamentous structures. *A,* Anterior view. The femoral neck anteriorly is intracapsular. *B,* Posterior view. Because the posterior capsule extends only partially across the femoral neck, the basicervical and intertrochanteric crest regions posteriorly are extracapsular. (From Jenkins, D.B.: Hollinshead's Functional Anatomy of the Limbs and Back, 6th ed. Philadelphia, WB Saunders, 1991, p. 230.)

2. **Sacroiliac (SI) Joint**—A true diarthrodial gliding joint supported by three groups of ligaments: posterior SI ligaments, anterior SI ligaments, and interosseous ligaments.
3. **Symphysis Pubis**—Connects the two hemipelvi anteriorly and is united with a fibrocartilaginous disc and supported by the superior pubic ligament and the arcuate pubic ligament.
4. Other ligaments include the sacrospinous and sacrotuberous ligaments, which outline the boundaries for the greater and lesser sciatic foramina. The **sacrospinous ligament** (anterior sacrum ischial spine) is the inferior border of the greater sciatic foramen and the superior border of the lesser sciatic foramen. The lesser sciatic foramen is bordered inferiorly by the **sacrotuberous ligament** (anterior sacrum ischial tuberosity). The piriformis, sciatic nerve, and other important structures exit the greater sciatic foramen. The short external rotators of the hip exit the lesser sciatic foramen.

C. **Muscles of the Pelvis and Hip** (Table 11-10; Fig. 11-44)—The following chart lists key neurologic levels controlling functions of the lower extremities.

SUMMARY OF IMPORTANT LOWER-EXTREMITY NEUROLOGY

JOINT	FUNCTION	NEUROLOGIC LEVEL
Hip	Flexion	T12, L1–L3
	Extension	S1
	Adduction	L2–L4
	Abduction	L5
Knee	Flexion	L5, S1
	Extension	L2–L4
Ankle	Dorsiflexion	L4, L5
	Plantarflexion	S1, S2
	Inversion	L4
	Eversion	S1

Principal hip **flexor** muscles are the iliopsoas, rectus femoris, and sartorius. Hip **extensor** muscles are the gluteus maximus and hamstrings (semitendinosus, semimembranosus, and long head of biceps femoris). Hip **abduction** primarily results from the actions of the gluteus medius and minimus. The tensor fascia lata also helps with abduction in a flexed hip. Hip **adduction** primarily results from the actions of the adductor brevis, longus and magnus, pectineus, and gracilis. Hip **external rotation** results from the action of the obturator internus, obturator

Table 11-10. MUSCLES OF THE PELVIS AND HIP

MUSCLE	ORIGIN	INSERTION	NERVE	SEGMENT
Flexors				
Iliacus	Iliac fossa	Lesser trochanter	Femoral	L2-4 (P)
Psoas	Transverse processes of L1-L5	Lesser trochanter	Femoral	L2-4 (P)
Pectineus	Pectineal line of pubis	Pectineal line of femur	Femoral	L2-4 (P)
Rectus femoris	AIIS, acetabular rim	Patella → tibial tubercle	Femoral	L2-4 (P)
Sartorius	ASIS	Proximal medial tibia	Femoral	L2-4 (P)
Adductors				
Post. adductor magnus	Inferior pubic ramus/ischial tuberosity	Linea aspera/adductor tubercle	Obturator (P) and Sciatic (tibial)	L2-4 (A)
Adductor brevis	Inferior pubic ramus	Linea aspera/pectineal line	Obturator (P)	L2-4 (A)
Adductor longus	Anterior pubic ramus	Linea aspera	Obturator (A)	L2-4 (A)
Gracilis	Inf. symphysis/pubic arch	Proximal medial tibia	Obturator (A)	L2-4 (A)
External Rotators				
Gluteus maximus	Ilium post to post gluteal line	Iliotibial band/gluteal sling (femur)	Inf. gluteal	L5-S2 (P)
Piriformis	Ant. sacrum/sciatic notch	Proximal greater trochanter	Piriformis	S12 (P)
Obturator externus	Ischiopubic rami/obturator membrane	Trochlear fossa	Obturator	L2-4 (A)
Obturator internus	Ischiopubic rami/obturator membrane	Medial greater trochanter (MGT)	Obturator internus	L5-S2 (A)
Superior gemellus	Outer ischial spine	MGT	Obturator internus	L5-S2 (A)
Inferior gemellus	Ischial tuberosity	MGT	Obturator femoris	L4-S1 (A)
Quadratus femoris	Ischial tuberosity	Quadrate line of femur	Obturator femoris	L4-S1 (A)
Abductors				
Gluteus medius	Ilium between post, and ant. gluteal lines	Greater trochanter	Superior gluteal	L4-S1 (P)
Gluteus minimus	Ilium between ant. and inf. gluteal lines	Ant. border of greater trochanter	Superior gluteal	L4-S1 (P)
Tensor fasciae latae (TFL) [tensor fascia femoris (TFF)]	Anterior iliac crest	Iliotibial band	Superior gluteal	L4-S1 (P)

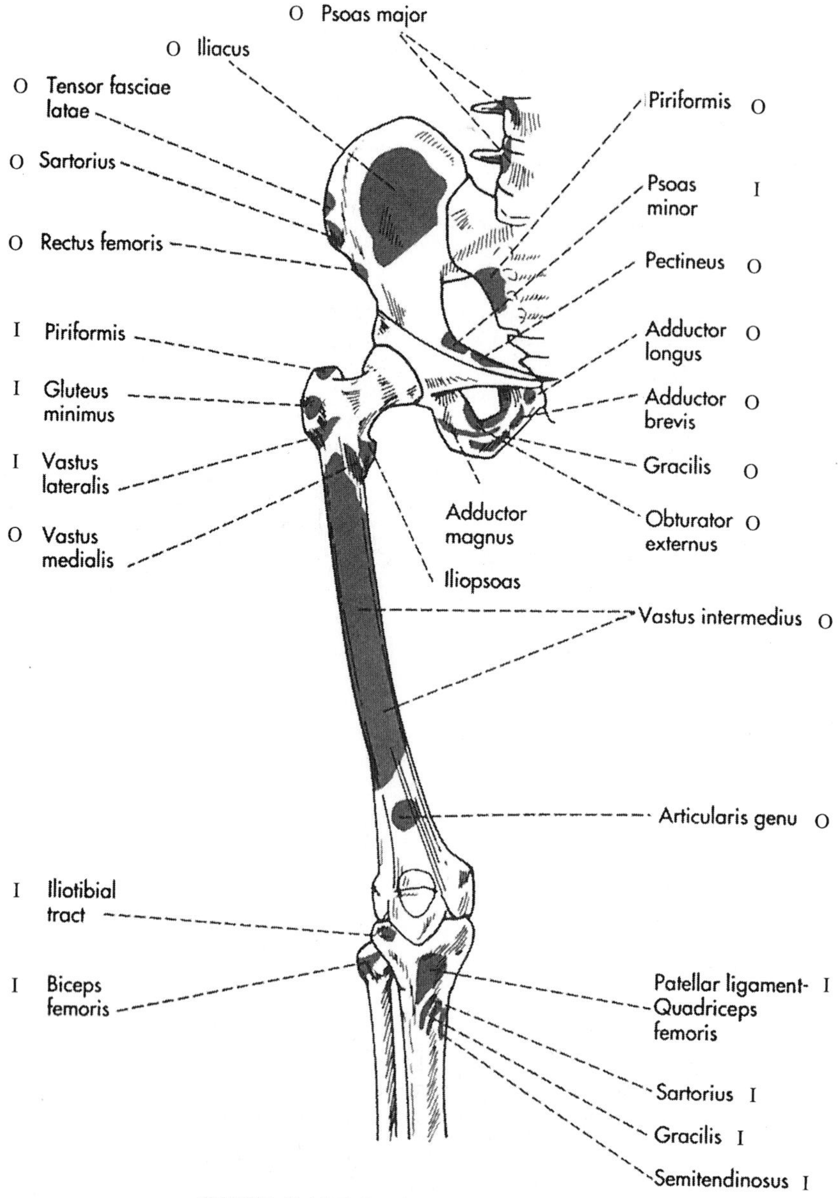

FIGURE 11-44 ■ *See legend on opposite page*

externus, superior and inferior gemellus, quadratus femoris, and the piriformis. Hip **internal rotation** is provided by secondary actions of the anterior fibers of the gluteus medius and minimus, tensor fascia lata, semimembranosus, semitendinosus, pectineus, and posterior part of the adductor magnus.

D. **Nerves**

1. **Lumbosacral Plexus** (Fig. 11-45)—The lumbosacral plexus is composed of **ventral rami from T12–S3** and lies **posterior to the psoas muscle**. The sciatic nerve (L4-S3) has an anterior preaxial tibial nerve division and a postaxial peroneal nerve division. The spatial orientation of the sciatic nerve also places the peroneal division more lateral than the tibial division. This orientation makes it more vulnerable to injury at the time of surgery. For example, the most common neural injury at the time of primary total hip arthroplasty is the peroneal division of the sciatic nerve. Bonus questions: (1) What is the only muscle innervated by the peroneal division of the sciatic nerve above the level of the fibular neck? (Short head of the biceps femoris.) (2) The peroneal division of the sciatic nerve runs on the deep surface of what muscle? (Long head of the biceps femoris.)

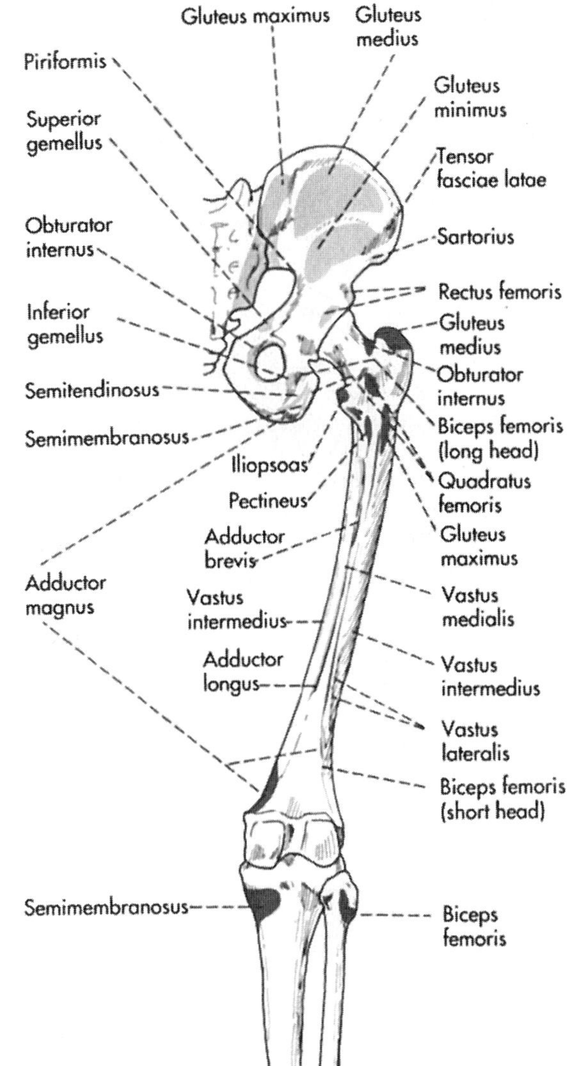

FIGURE 11-44 ■ Origins and insertions of muscles of the hip and leg. O, origin; I, insertion. Origins = light areas; insertions = dark areas. (Adapted from Jenkins, D.B.: Hollinshead's Functional Anatomy of the Limbs and Back, 6th ed., Figs. 16-7, 17-3. Philadelphia, WB Saunders, 1991.)

LUMBOSACRAL PLEXUS DIVISIONS

NERVES	LEVEL	INNERVATION
Anterior Division Tibial	L4–S3	Semimembranosus/semitendinosus/biceps (long head)/adductor magnus/sup. gemellus/soleus/plantaris/popliteus/tibialis posterior/flexor digitorum longus/flexor hallucis longus
Quadratus femoris	L4–S1	Quadratus femoris/inf. gemellus
Obturator internus	L5–S2	Obturatorius internus/sup. gemellus
Pudendal	S2–S4	Sensory: perineal Motor: bulbocavernosus/urethra/urogenital diaphragm
Coccygeus	S4	Coccygeus
Levator ani	S3–S4	Levator ani
Posterior Division		
Peroneal	L4–S2	Biceps (short head)/tibialis anterior/extensor digitorum longus/peroneus tertius/extensor hallucis longus Peroneus longus and brevis/extensor hallucis brevis/extensor digitorum brevis
Sup. gluteal	L4–S1	Gluteus medius and minimus/TFL
Inf. gluteal	L5–S2	Gluteus maximus
Piriformis	S2	Piriformis
Post. femoral cutaneous (PFCN)	S1–S3	Sensory: posterior thigh

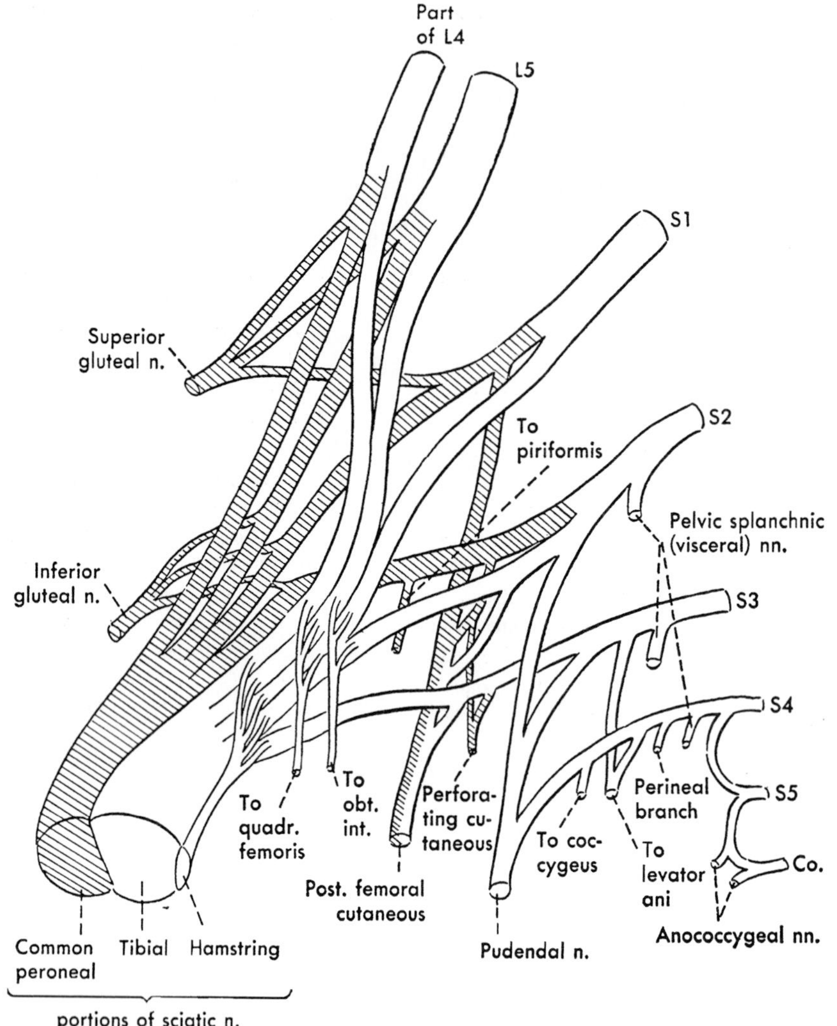

FIGURE 11-45 ■ Sacral plexus. Anterior division *(unshaded)* and posterior division *(shaded)*. (From Jenkins, D.B.: Hollinshead's Functional Anatomy of the Limbs and Back, 6th ed. Philadelphia, WB Saunders, 1991, p. 256.)

2. **Anatomic Spatial Relationships**—The lumbar plexus is found on the anterior surface of the quadratus lumborum under (and within) the substance of the psoas major muscle. The genitofemoral nerve pierces the psoas and then lies on the anteromedial surface of the psoas. The femoral nerve lies between the iliacus and the psoas. The lateral femoral cutaneous nerve lies on the surface of the iliacus muscle and exits the pelvis under the lateral attachment of the inguinal ligament. Virtually all important nerves about the hip leave the pelvis by way of the sciatic foramen. The major reference point for the greater sciatic nerve and related structures in the hip is the piriformis muscle ("key" to the sciatic foramen). The **superior gluteal nerve and artery lie above the piriformis**, and virtually everything else leaves below the muscle (remember POP'S IQ [lateral to medial nerves]: *p*udendal, *o*bturator internus, *p*ostfemoral cutaneous, *s*ciatic, *i*nferior gluteal, *q*uadratus femoris). Two nerves leave the greater sciatic foramen and re-enter the pelvis via the lesser foramen (pudendal and nerve to obturator internus). Anteriorly, the great nerves and vessels enter the thigh (and into the **femoral triangle**) under the inguinal ligament (Fig. 11-46). The borders of this triangle include the sartorius laterally, the pectineus medially, and the inguinal ligament superiorly. Within the triangle, from lateral to medial, are the femoral *n*erve, *a*rtery, and *v*ein *a*nd the *l*ymphatic vessels (remember

NAVAL). The **floor of the femoral triangle** (again, lateral to medial) is made up of the **iliacus**, psoas, pectineus, and the adductor longus. The femoral nerve descends between the iliacus and psoas and delivers numerous branches to muscle, overlying skin, and the hip joint (in accordance with Hilton's law). A spontaneous **iliacus hematoma may irritate the femoral nerve,** owing to its proximity. Also, do not forget that hip pain can also present from Pott's disease (tuberculous spondylitis) of the spine because of the attachment of the iliopsoas to the lumbar spine. At the apex of the triangle the saphenous nerve branches off and travels under the sartorius muscle. The obturator nerve exits the pelvis via the obturator canal. It splits into anterior and posterior divisions within the canal. The anterior division proceeds anteriorly to the obturator externus and posteriorly to the pectineus, supplying the adductor longus and brevis and the gracilis; it then delivers cutaneous branches to the medial thigh. The posterior division supplies the obturator externus, adductor brevis, and upper part of the adductor magnus, and it delivers other branches to the knee joint. Referred pain from the hip to the knee can be from the continuation of the obturator nerve anterior that can provide sensation to the medial side of the knee. **Retractors placed behind the transverse acetabular ligament can injure the obturator nerve and artery.**

E. **Vessels** (Fig. 11-47)—The aorta branches into the common iliac arteries anterior to the L4 vertebral body. The common iliac vessels, in turn, divide into the internal (or *hypogastric*; medial) and external (lateral) iliacs at the S1 level. Important **internal iliac artery** branches include the **obturator** (the posterior branch **supplies the transverse acetabular ligament), superior gluteal** (can be injured in the sciatic notch), **inferior gluteal** (supplies the gluteus maximus and the short external rotators), and **internal pudendal** (reenters the pelvis through the lesser sciatic notch) (Fig. 11-48). **Anteroinferior screws and acetabular retractors jeopardize the obturator artery and vein.** The **external iliac artery** continues

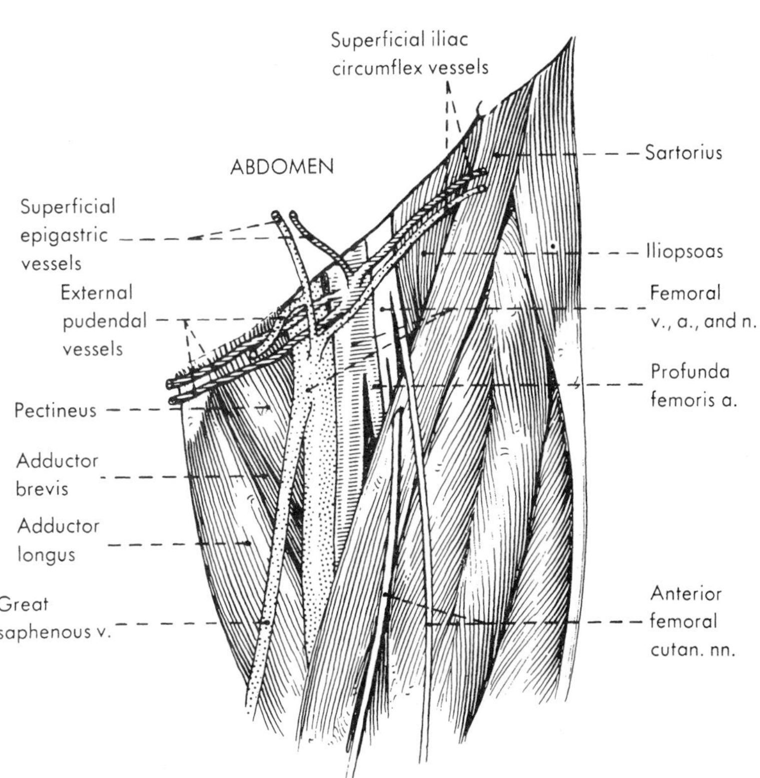

FIGURE 11-46 ■ Femoral triangle. The order of structures of the femoral canal from lateral to medial: iliopsoas/iliacus, femoral nerve, femoral artery, femoral vein, pectineus. (From Jenkins, D.B.: Hollinshead's Functional Anatomy of the Limbs and Back, 6th ed. Philadelphia, WB Saunders, 1991, p. 243.)

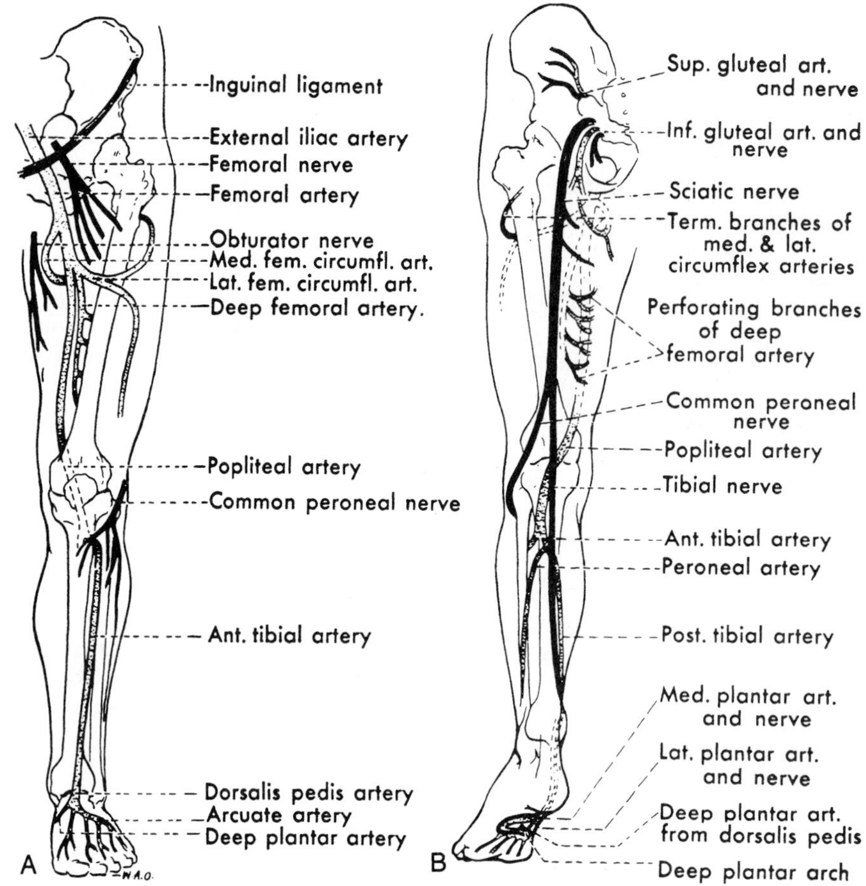

FIGURE 11-47 ■ Nerves and vessels of the lower extremity. *A*, Anterior view. *B*, Posterior view. (From Jenkins, D.B.: Hollinshead's Functional Anatomy of the Limbs and Back, 6th ed. Philadelphia, WB Saunders, 1991, p. 221.)

under the inguinal ligament to become the femoral artery. It **can be injured by anterosuperior quadrant acetabular screw placement** during total hip arthroplasty. A summary of key issues for acetabular screw placement is shown in the following chart.

ACETABULAR SCREW PLACEMENT ZONES

ACETABULAR ZONE	STRUCTURES AT RISK
Posterior superior	Safe zone
Posterior inferior	Safe zone
Anterior superior	External iliac artery and vein
Anterior inferior	Anterior inferior obturator nerve, obturator artery and vein

The femoral artery enters the femoral triangle and delivers the profunda femoris, which supplies the anteromedial portion of the thigh and the perforators, which pierce the lateral intermuscular septum to supply the vastus lateralis muscle. The profunda has two other important branches: the medial and lateral femoral circumflex arteries. The lateral femoral circumflex travels obliquely and deep to the sartorius and rectus femoris. It delivers an ascending branch (at risk during anterolateral approaches) that proceeds to the greater trochanteric region and a descending branch that travels laterally under the rectus femoris. The **medial femoral circumflex**, which supplies most of the blood to the **femoral head**, runs between the pectineus and the iliopsoas, then in the interval between the obturator externus and adductor brevis muscles, and in the **interval between the adductor magnus and brevis**. It proceeds distally anterior to the quadratus femoris on its cranial edge just distal to the obturator externus. The cruciate anastomosis is the confluence of the ascending branch of the first perforating artery, the descending branch of the inferior gluteal artery, and the transverse branches of the medial and lateral femoral circumflex arteries. It lies at the inferior margin of the quadratus femoris muscle. The superficial femoral artery continues on the medial side of the thigh (between the vastus medialis and

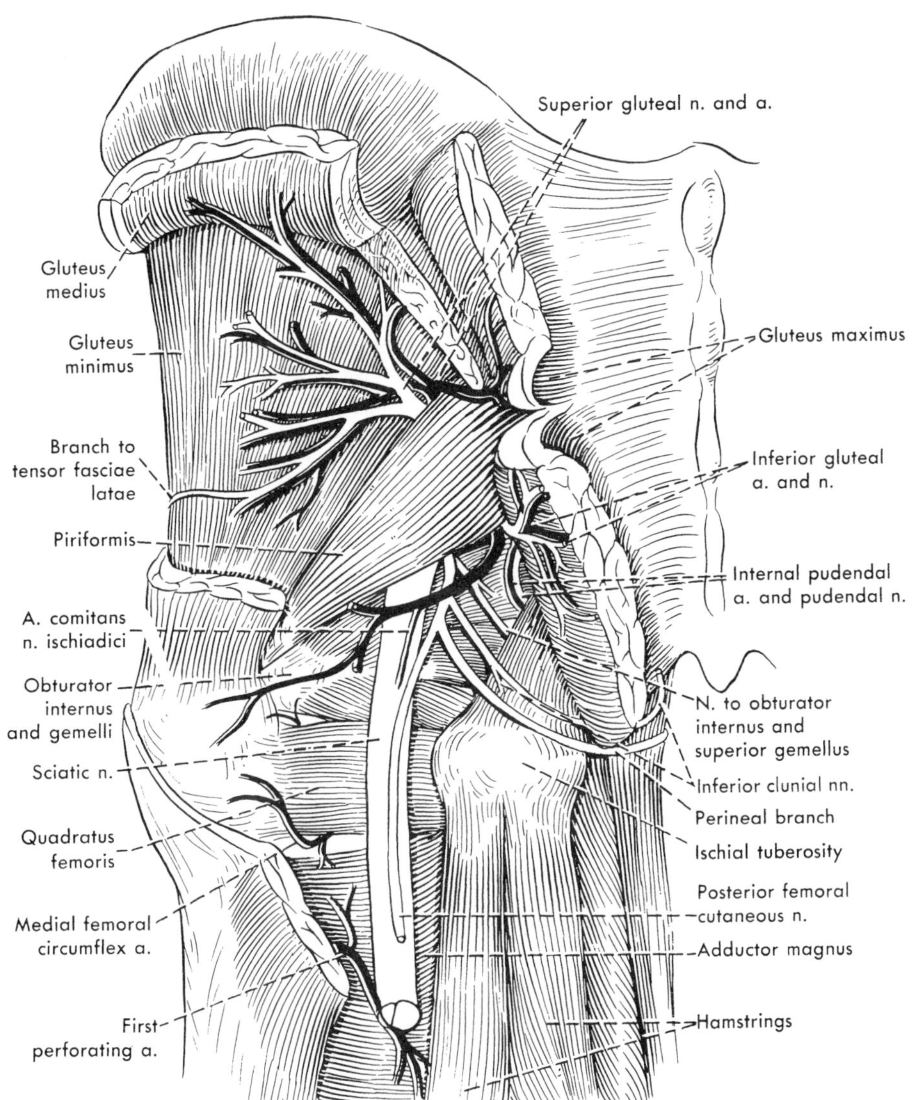

FIGURE 11-48 ■ Posterior hip anatomy. Note relationship of structures to the piriformis muscle. (From Jenkins, D.B.: Hollinshead's Functional Anatomy of the Limbs and Back, 6th ed., Philadelphia, WB Saunders, 1991, p. 260.)

adductor longus) toward the adductor (Hunter's) canal. In the posteromedial thigh it becomes the popliteal artery in the popliteal fossa.

F. **Approaches to the Pelvis and Hip**

1. **Posterior Approach to the Iliac Crest**—A curvilinear incision is made just inferior to the crest, beginning at the posterior superior iliac spine. After identifying the iliac crest, the gluteus maximus fibers are subperiosteally dissected from the outer table. Risks of this approach include to the greater sciatic notch (superior gluteal artery and sciatic nerve) and the **cluneal nerves (8 cm anterolateral to the posterior superior iliac spine)**.
2. **Anterior Approach to the Iliac Crest**—An oblique incision is made lateral to the anterior superior iliac spine, and the crest is exposed through the interval between the external oblique and the gluteus medius. Risks are to the greater sciatic notch, the inguinal ligament, and the lateral femoral cutaneous nerve.
3. **Anterior (Smith-Peterson) Approach to the Hip** (Fig. 11-49)—Takes advantage of the internervous plane between the **sartorius (femoral nerve)** and the **tensor fascia lata (superior gluteal nerve)**. It is useful for hemiarthroplasty and open reduction of the congenitally dislocated hip. Retract the lateral femoral cutaneous nerve anteriorly and ligate the **ascending branch of lateral femoral circumflex artery (which lies superficial to the rectus)**. For deeper dissection, approach the interval between the gluteus medius and rectus femoris. Detach the origin of both heads of the rectus femoris. **Reflection of the conjoined rectus tendon too distally can risk injury to the descending branch of the lateral femoral circumflex artery.** Retract the

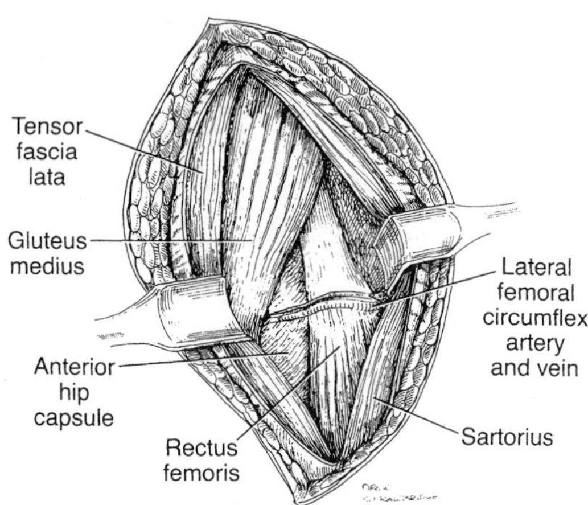

FIGURE 11-49 ■ Anterior (Smith-Peterson) approach to the hip. The interval between the sartorius/rectus femoris (femoral nerve) and the TFL/gluteus medius (superior gluteal nerve) is explored. The ascending branch of the lateral femoral circumflex artery is ligated. (From Steinberg, M.E.: The Hip and Its Disorders. Philadelphia, WB Saunders, 1991, p. 92.)

rectus medially and the gluteus medius laterally. Dissect any attachments of the iliopsoas to the inferior capsule and perform a capsulotomy. Dangers are to the **lateral femoral cutaneous nerve**, which is located anterior or medial to the sartorius about 6–8 cm below the anterior superior iliac spine. The superficial circumflex artery penetrates the fascia lata just anterior to the lateral femoral cutaneous nerve. The femoral nerve and vessels can sometimes be injured with aggressive medial retraction of the sartorius.

4. **Anterolateral (Watson-Jones) Approach to the Hip** (Fig. 11-50)—This approach can be used for total hip arthroplasty, as popularized by Watson-Jones. There is no true internervous plane, but it utilizes the **intermuscular plane between the tensor fascia femoris and gluteus medius**. After the incision and superficial dissection, the fascia lata is split to expose the vastus lateralis. Detach the anterior third of the gluteus medius from the greater trochanter and the entire gluteus minimus. Dissect the reflected head of the rectus femoris (and capsular attachment of the iliopsoas if necessary) and retract medially. Perform a capsulotomy. Dangers of this approach include damage to the femoral nerve by excessive medial retraction, denervation of the tensor fascia femoris if the intermuscular interval is exploited too superiorly (the superior gluteal nerve lies about 5 cm above the acetabular rim), and injury to the descending branch of the **lateral femoral circumflex artery** with anterior and inferior dissection.
5. **Lateral (Hardinge's) Approach to the Hip** (Fig. 11-51)—Useful for total hip arthroplasty, bipolar hemiarthroplasty, and revision work. This approach utilizes an incision that **splits both the gluteus medius and the vastus lateralis** in tandem. Incise the skin and the fascia lata to expose the gluteus medius and the vastus. Incise the gluteus medius from the greater trochanter, leaving a cuff of tissue and the posterior one-half to two-thirds attached. Extend this incision to split the gluteus medius proximally. Distally, split the vastus along its anterior one-fourth down to the femoral shaft. Detach the gluteus minimus from its insertion. The hip capsule is exposed for further dissection. Dangers include injury to the femoral nerve and possible denervation of the gluteus medius **(superior gluteal nerve), if the split is too proximal (more than 5 cm proximal to the greater trochanter)**.
6. **Posterior (Moore or Southern) Approach to the Hip** (Fig. 11-52)—The internervous

FIGURE 11-50 ■ Anterolateral (Watson-Jones) approach to the hip. The interval between the TFL (superior gluteal nerve) and the gluteus medius (superior gluteal nerve) is explored. (From Steinberg, M.E.: The Hip and Its Disorders. Philadelphia, WB Saunders, 1991, p. 93.)

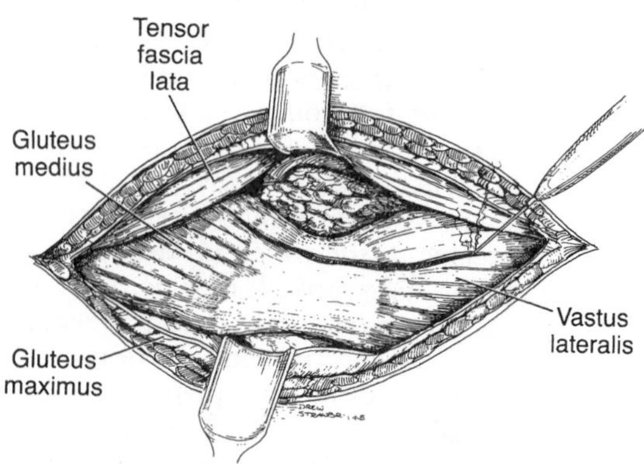

FIGURE 11-51 ■ Lateral (Hardinge's) approach to the hip. The interval between the gluteus medius (superior gluteal nerve) and the vastus lateralis (femoral nerve) is explored. (From Steinberg, M.E.: The Hip and Its Disorders. Philadelphia, WB Saunders, 1991, p. 95.)

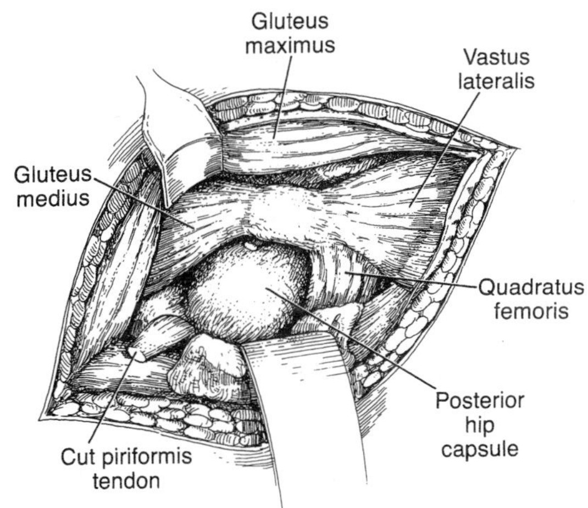

FIGURE 11-52 ■ Posterior (Moore or Southern) approach to the hip. The interval between the gluteus maximus (inferior gluteal nerve) and the gluteus medius/TFL (superior gluteal nerve) is explored. (From Steinberg, M.E.: The Hip and Its Disorders. Philadelphia, WB Saunders, 1991, p. 98.)

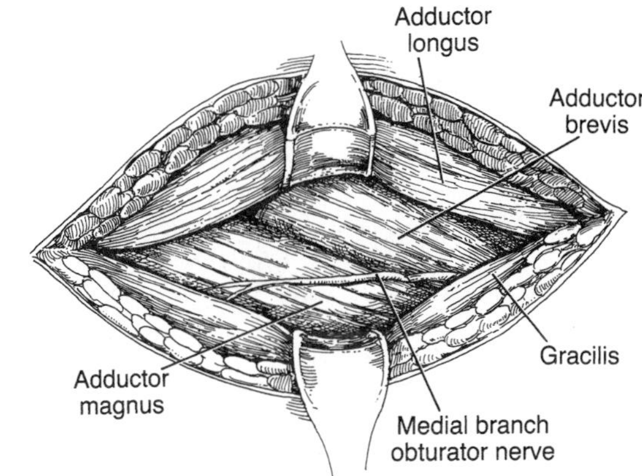

FIGURE 11-53 ■ Medial (Ludloff) approach to the hip. The interval between the adductor longus (obturator nerve) and the gracilis (obturator nerve) is explored. (From Steinberg, M.E.: The Hip and Its Disorders. Philadelphia, WB Saunders, 1991, p. 99.)

plane in one version is between the **gluteus maximus (inferior gluteal nerve)** and the **gluteus medius and the tensor fascia lata (superior gluteal nerve)**. Most surgeons, however, approach the hip by splitting the fibers of the gluteus maximus. Incise the skin and the fascia lata along the posterior border of the femur, and then split the fibers of the gluteus maximus bluntly. Next, expose the short external rotators close to their insertion into the greater trochanter. Reflect them laterally to protect the sciatic nerve and expose the posterior hip capsule. A portion of the quadratus femoris may be taken down with the short external rotators, but one must be aware of the significant bleeding that can come from the inferior portion of this muscle (ascending branches of medial femoral circumflex artery). Dangers include sciatic neurapraxia if the sciatic nerve is not properly protected by the short external rotators. Additional trouble may be encountered if the inferior gluteal artery is damaged during the splitting of the gluteus maximus.

7. **Medial (Ludloff) Approach to the Hip** (Fig. 11-53)—Used occasionally for pediatric adductor releases and open reductions, this approach uses the interval between the adductor longus and gracilis. Deep, the interval is between the adductor brevis and magnus. Structures at risk include the anterior division of the **obturator nerve and medial femoral circumflex artery** (between the adductor brevis and the adductor magnus/pectineus). **The deep external pudendal artery (anterior to the pectineus near the adductor longus origin) is also at risk proximally.**
8. **Acetabular Approaches**—Used primarily for open reduction and internal fixation (ORIF) of pelvic fractures, these approaches are basically extensions of incisions for exposure of the hip (discussed earlier). The Kocher-Langenbeck incision is a posterolateral approach that provides access to the posterior column/acetabulum (Fig. 11-54). The ilioinguinal incision relies on mobilization of the rectus abdominis and iliacus, exposing the anterior column. Three windows are available with this approach. The first window gives access to the internal iliac fossa and the anterior sacroiliac joint. The second window (between the iliopectineal fascia and the external iliac vessels) gives access to the pelvic brim and part of the superior pubic ramus. The third window (below the vessels and the spermatic cord) provides access to the quadrilateral plate and retropubic space (Fig. 11-55). The extended iliofemoral incision allows access to both

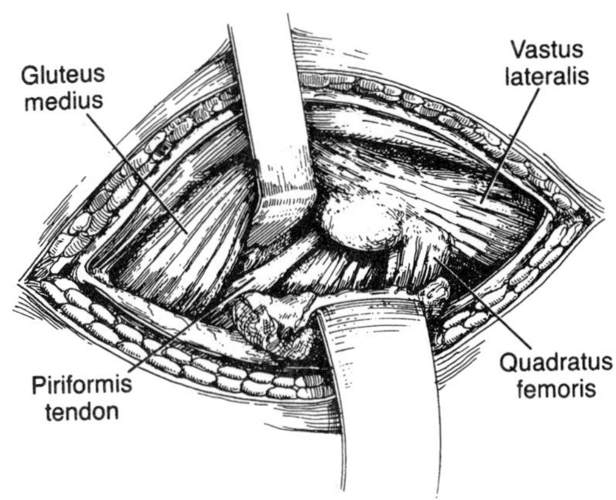

FIGURE 11-54 ■ Posterolateral approach to the hip. (From Steinberg, M.E.: The Hip and Its Disorders. Philadelphia, WB Saunders, 1991, p. 96.)

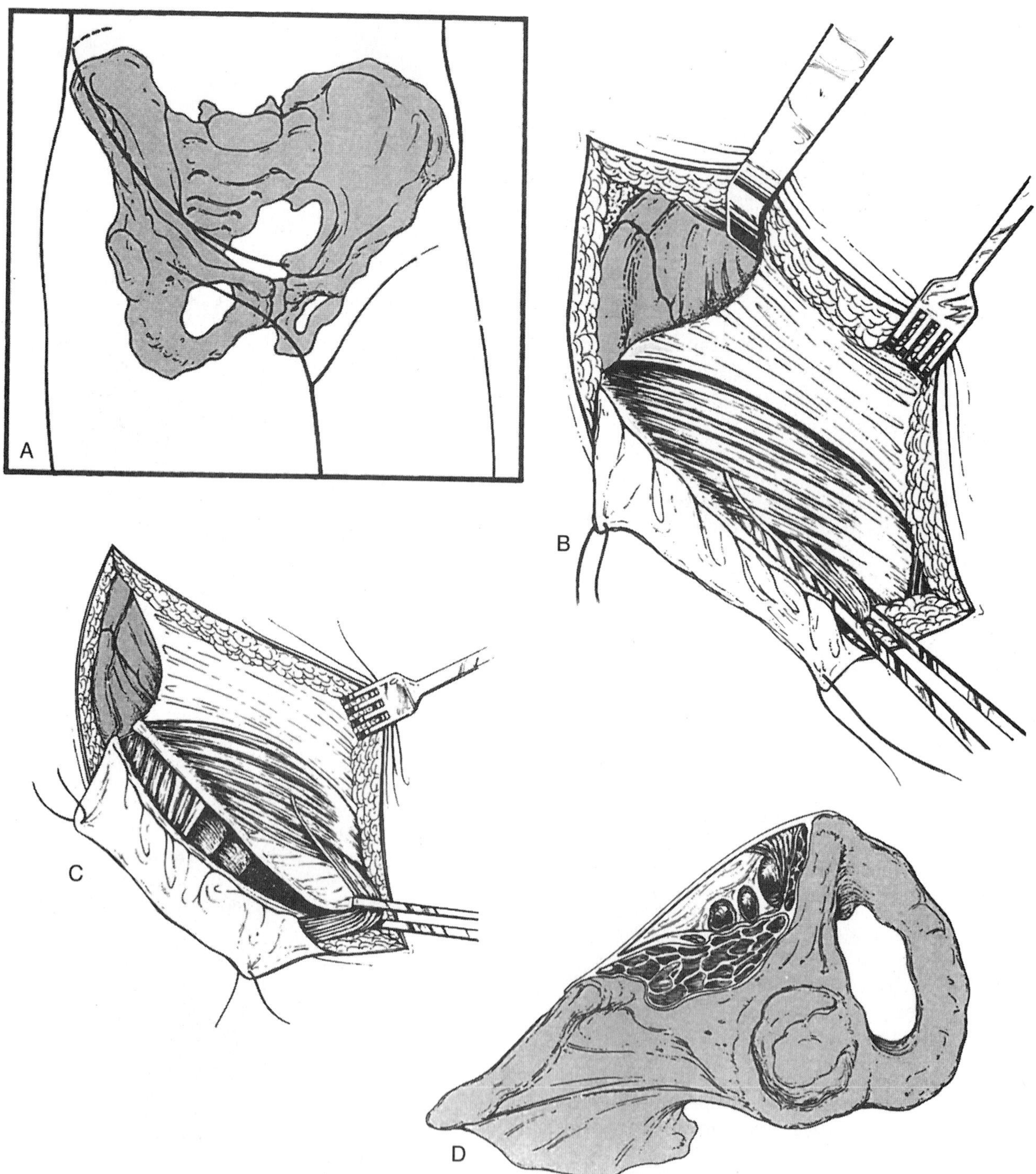

FIGURE 11-55 ■ The ilioinguinal approach. *A,* The skin incision. *B,* The internal iliac fossa has been exposed, and the inguinal canal has been unroofed by distal reflection of the external oblique aponeurosis. *C,* An incision along the inguinal ligament detaches the abdominal muscles and transversalis fascia, giving access to the psoas sheath, the iliopectineal fascia, the external aspect of the femoral vessels, and the retropubic space of Retzius. *D,* An oblique section through the lacuna musculorum and lacuna vascularum at the level of the inguinal ligament.

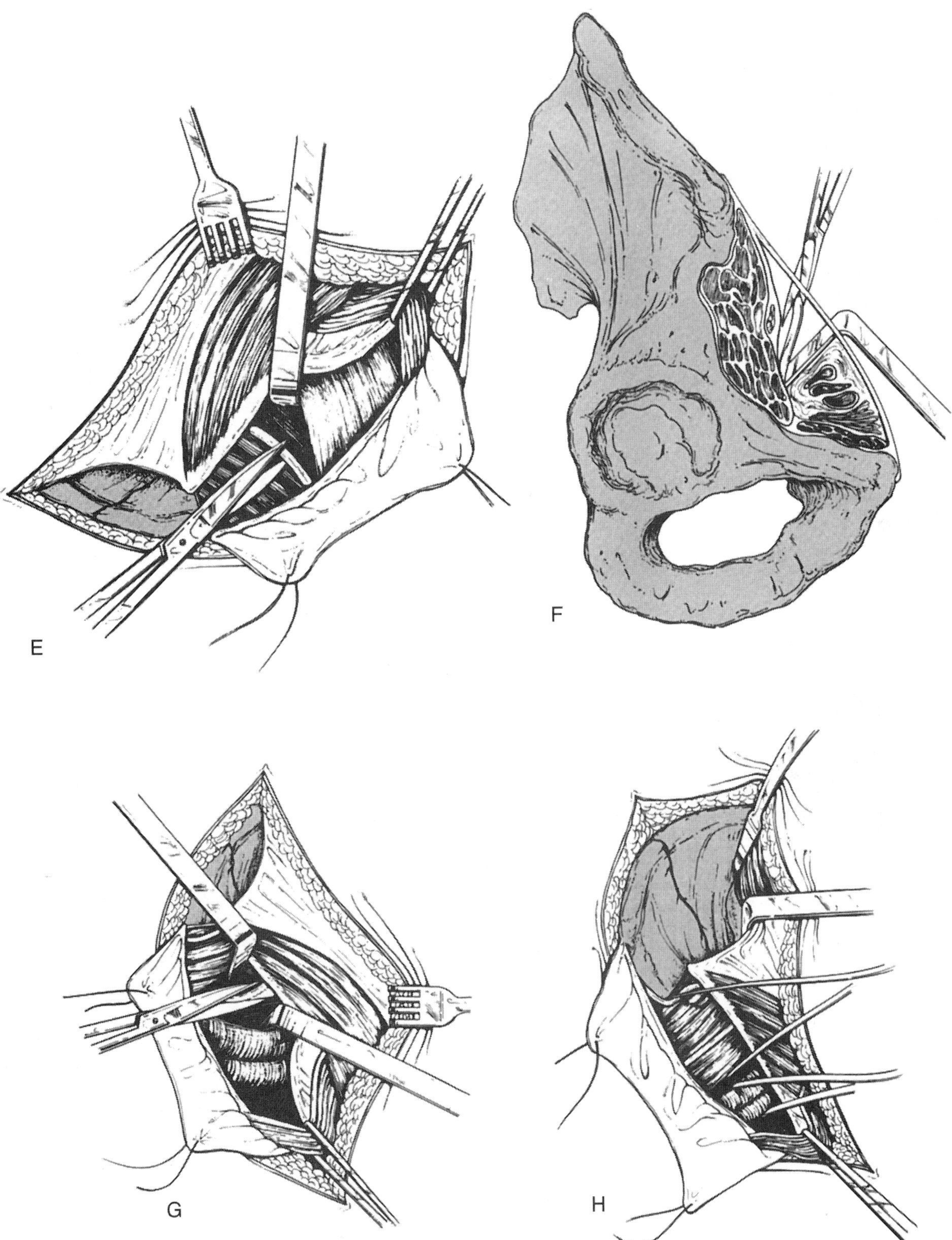

FIGURE 11-55—cont'd ■ *E,* Division of the iliopectineal fascia to the pectineal eminence. *F,* An oblique section that demonstrates division of the iliopectineal fascia. *G,* Proximal division of the iliopectineal fascia from the pelvic brim to allow access to the true pelvis. *H,* The first window of the ilioinguinal approach, which gives access to the internal iliac fossa, the anterior sacroiliac joint, and upper portion of the anterior column.

Illustration continued on following page

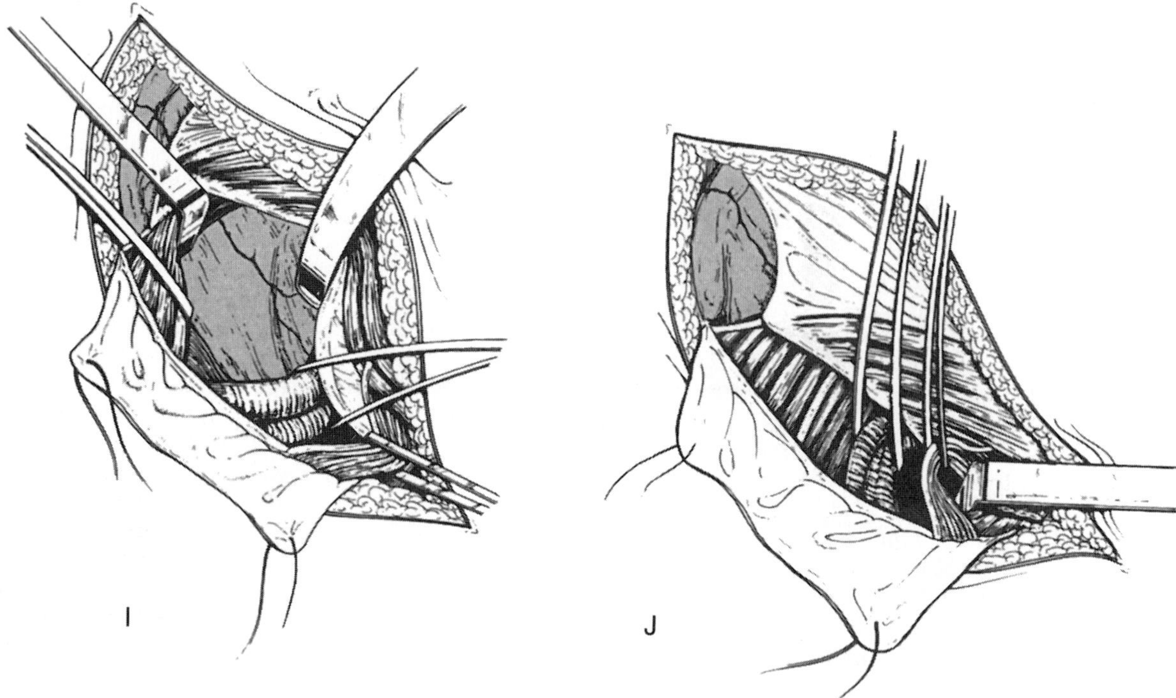

FIGURE 11-55—cont'd ■ *I*, The second window of the ilioinguinal approach, giving access to the pelvic brim from the anterior sacroiliac joint to the lateral extremity of the superior pubic ramus. The quadrilateral surface and posterior column are accessible beyond the pelvic brim. *J*, Access to the symphysis pubis and retropubic space of Retzius, medial to the spermatic cord and femoral vessels. (From Browner B.D., Jupiter J.B., Levine, A.M., and Trafton, P.G.: Skeletal Trauma: Fractures, Dislocations, Ligamentous Injuries, Fig. 32-5*A–J*. Philadelphia, WB Saunders, 1992, pp. 907–909.)

columns by reflecting the gluteal muscles and tensor posteriorly and dividing the obturator internus and piriformis.

HIP SURGICAL APPROACHES

APPROACH	INTERVAL	RISKS
Anterior (Smith-Peterson)	Sartorius/rectus femoris (femoral nerve) and tensor fascia lata/gluteus medius (superior gluteal nerve)	Lateral femoral cutaneous nerve (6–8 cm below ASIS anterior or medial to sartorius) Ligation of ascending branch of lateral femoral circumflex artery (lies superficial to rectus femoris muscle)
Anterolateral (Watson-Jones)	Between TFL (supinator gluteal nerve) and gluteus branch of medius (supinator gluteal nerve)	Femoral nerve because of excessive medial retraction Injury to descending lateral femoral circumflex artery
Lateral (Hardinge's)	Gluteus medius (supinator gluteal nerve) and vastus lateralis (femoral nerve)	Femoral nerve, artery, vein Lateral femoral circumflex artery
Posterior (Moore-Southern)	Gluteus maximus (inferior gluteal nerve) gluteus medius/TFL (supinator gluteal nerve)	Sciatic nerve and inferior gluteal artery during the gluteus maximus muscle split. If quadratus femoris transected, ligation of medial femoral circumflex artery
Medial (Ludloff)	Adductor longus and adductor brevis (obturator nerve) and gracilis/adductor magnus (obturator/tibial nerve)	Anterior division of obturator nerve Medial femoral circumflex artery Deep external pudendal artery

G. **Arthroscopy**—Hip arthroscopy portals include the anterolateral and posterolateral portals (adjacent to the superior border of the greater trochanter) and the anterior portal (femoral nerve and lateral femoral cutaneous nerve risk).

VIII. Thigh

A. Osteology of the Femur

1. **Introduction**—The femur is the largest bone of the body. The neck-shaft angle averages approximately 127 degrees, although it begins at 141 degrees in the fetus. The anteversion varies from 1 to 40 degrees but averages 14 degrees. The femur has an

Table 11-11. MUSCLES OF THE ANTERIOR THIGH

MUSCLE	ORIGIN	INSERTION	INNERVATION
Vastus lateralis	Iliotibial line/greater trochanter/lateral linea aspera	Lateral patella	Femoral
Vastus medialis	Iliotibial line/medial linea aspera/supracondylar line	Medial patella	Femoral
Vastus intermedius	Proximal anterior femoral shaft	Patella	Femoral

anterior bow. There are two femoral condyles; the medial condyle is larger. The more prominent medial epicondyle supports the adductor tubercle.

2. **Ossification**—Important areas of femoral ossification include the head and the distal femur. The femoral head is usually not present at birth but appears as one large physis that includes both trochanters at about 11 months and fuses at 18 years. Slipped capital femoral epiphysis occurs through the femoral head epiphysis (zone of hypertrophy). The distal femoral physis appears at birth and fuses at 19 years. Do not forget about knee stress examinations for the evaluation of distal femoral physeal fractures in pediatric patients.

B. **Muscles of the Thigh**
   1. **Anterior Thigh** (Table 11-11)—See Table 11-8 for rectus femoris, sartorius.
   2. **Medial Thigh**—See adductors in Table 11-10.
   3. **Posterior Thigh** (Table 11-12)
   4. **Cross-Sectional Diagram** (Fig. 11-56)

C. **Nerves and Vessels** (see also the preceding discussion on the pelvis and hip and the following discussion on the knee and leg)—The **sciatic nerve** (L4–S3) emerges from its foramen anterior to the piriformis muscle (through the piriformis in 2% of people) and lies posterior to the other short external rotators. It descends below the gluteus maximus and proceeds posteriorly to the adductor magnus and between the long head of the biceps and the semimembranosus. Before it emerges from the popliteal fossa, it divides into the common peroneal nerve and the tibial nerve. The **peroneal division** has one innervation in the thigh—**short head of biceps femoris.** The common peroneal nerve diverges laterally and traverses the lateral knee region under cover of the biceps femoris. The tibial nerve emerges into the popliteal fossa lateral, proceeds posteriorly to the vessel, and then descends between the heads of the gastrocnemius. The **femoral nerve** (L2–4) is the largest branch of the lumbar plexus and supplies the thigh muscles in the following chart. The *largest branch of the femoral nerve is the saphenous nerve.* The infrapatellar branch of the saphenous nerve supplies the skin of the medial side of the front of the knee and patellar ligament and can be damaged during total knee replacement surgery. The **lateral femoral cutaneous nerve** (L2-3) supplies skin and fascia on the anterolateral thigh surface from the greater trochanter to the knee. It can be damaged with acetabular approaches that dissect around its course underneath the lateral end of the inguinal ligament. The **obturator nerve** (L2–4) can be damaged during various hip and acetabular approaches (screw placement in anteroinferior quadrant), resulting in sensation decrease in the medial thigh and loss of hip adductor function. The obturator nerve has two branches after it passes through the obturator foramen: the anterior branch (adductor longus, adductor brevis, gracilis) and the posterior branch (obturator externus, adductor magnus, adductor brevis [variable]). Please note that **the anterior branch of the obturator nerve can provide sensation to the medial side of the knee and can be a source of referred pain from hip pathology**.

Table 11-12. MUSCLES OF THE POSTERIOR THIGH

MUSCLE	ORIGIN	INSERTION	INNERVATION
Biceps (long head)	Medial ischial tuberosity	Fibular head/lateral tibia	Tibial
Biceps (short head)	Lat. linea aspera/lat. intermuscular septum	Lateral tibial condyle	Peroneal
Semitendinosus	Distal med. ischial tuberosity	Anterior tibial crest	Tibial
Semimembranosus	Proximal lat. ischial tuberosity	Oblique popliteal ligament Posterior capsule Posterior/medial tibia Popliteus Medial meniscus	Tibial

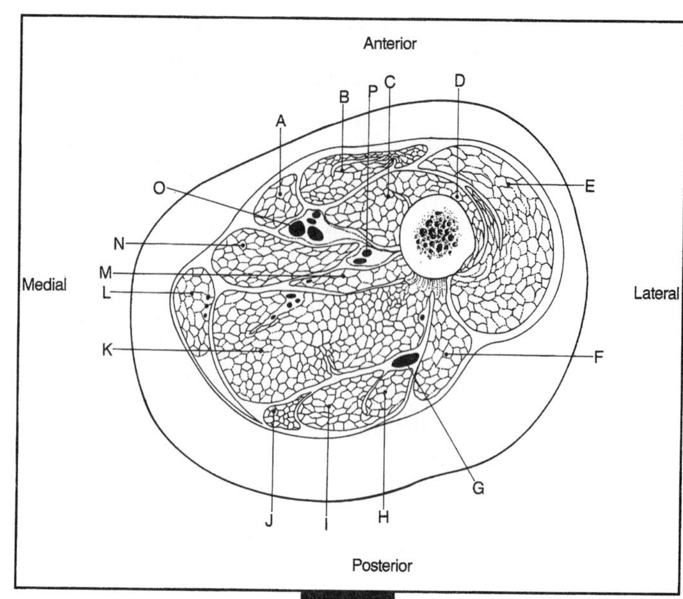

FIGURE 11-56 ■ Cross-section of the proximal thigh. Practice labeling the diagram. See Table 11-8 for key. (From Callaghan, J.J., ed.: Anatomy Self-Assessment Examination, Fig. 53. Park Ridge, Ill, American Academy of Orthopaedic Surgeons, 1991.)

Always evaluate clinically and radiographically a joint above and below a patient's complaint. A summary of innervation patterns in the thigh is shown in the following chart.

THIGH MUSCLE INNERVATION

NERVE IN THIGH	COMPONENTS	INNERVATION
Femoral	L2–4	Iliacus, psoas major (lower part), sartorius, pectineus, quadriceps, articularis genus muscles
Obturator	L2–4	Obturator externus, hip adductors (brevis, longus, magnus), gracilis
Sciatic	L4–S3	**Peroneal division—short head biceps femoris**
		Tibial division—hamstrings (semitendinosus, semimembranosus), part of adductor magnus, long head biceps femoris

The *external iliac artery* becomes the **femoral artery** after traversing the inguinal ligament arriving into the femoral triangle. The femoral artery branches to become the deep femoral artery and the superficial femoral artery. The **deep femoral artery** gives rise to the medial and lateral femoral circumflex arteries. The **medial femoral circumflex artery is the major blood supply to the femoral head in the adult** and lies anterior to the quadratus femoris muscle. After supplying the profundus (described earlier), the superficial femoral artery descends under cover of the sartorius muscle and proceeds between the adductor group and the vastus medialis into the adductor canal. At the level above the medial femoral condyle, the artery supplies a descending geniculate branch, then passes through a defect in the adductor magnus (adductor hiatus) and emerges in the popliteal fossa. The vein is usually posterior to the artery. The **obturator artery** is a branch of the ***internal iliac artery*** and its posterior branch supplies the ligamentum teres acetabular artery. This arterial supply is an important blood supply to the femoral head from birth to 4 years old. The internal iliac artery also supplies the superior and inferior gluteal arteries.

THIGH VESSELS AT RISK DURING SURGICAL APPROACHES

APPROACH	VASCULAR STRUCTURE AT RISK
Anterior hip (Smith-Peterson)	Ascending branch of lateral femoral circumflex artery (superficial to rectus femoris muscle)
Anterolateral hip (Watson-Jones)	Descending branch of lateral femoral circumflex artery
Medial hip (Ludloff)	Medial femoral circumflex artery and deep external pudendal artery (at risk during percutaneous tenotomy of adductor longus)
Lateral and posterolateral thigh	Perforators from profunda femoris artery
Anteromedial distal femur	Medial superior geniculate artery

D. **Approaches to the Thigh**

1. **Lateral Approach to the Thigh**—The lateral approach is used for ORIF of intertrochanteric and femoral neck fractures. This approach can be extended for access to

shaft and supracondylar fractures. There is no true internervous plane. Split the fascia lata in line with the femoral shaft. Include part of the tensor fascia femoris, if necessary. Then bluntly dissect the vastus lateralis in line with its fibers or dissect the fibers of the intermuscular septum. Identify and coagulate the various perforators from the profunda femoris.

2. **Posterolateral Approach to the Thigh**—This approach may be used for exposure of the entire length of the femur through an internervous plane. It exploits the interval between the **vastus lateralis (femoral nerve) and the hamstrings (sciatic nerve)**. Incise the fascia under the iliotibial band and retract the vastus superiorly. Continue anteriorly to the lateral intermuscular septum with blunt dissection until the periosteum over the linea aspera is reached. The danger of this dissection lies in the series of perforating vessels from the profundus that pierce the lateral intermuscular septum to reach the vastus. If approached without care, these vessels can retract and bleed underneath the septum.
3. **Anteromedial Approach to the Distal Femur**—This approach may be used for ORIF of distal femoral and femoral shaft fractures. Explore the interval between the **rectus femoris and vastus medialis (femoral nerve)** and extend to a point medial to the patella. Retract the rectus laterally. Explore the interval to reveal the vastus intermedius. It may be necessary to open the knee joint. If so, incise the medial patellar retinaculum and split a portion of the quadriceps tendon just lateral to the medial border. After identifying the vastus intermedius, split it along its fibers to expose the femur. Dangers include injury to the medial superior geniculate artery and the infrapatellar branch of the saphenous nerve, because both cross the site of exposure. Additionally, one must leave an adequate cuff of tissue for a strong patellar retinacular repair or risk lateral subluxation of the patella.
4. **Posterior Approach to the Thigh**—This rare approach may be used for exploration of the sciatic nerve. It makes use of the internervous interval between the **biceps femoris (sciatic nerve) and the vastus lateralis (femoral nerve)**. Identify and protect the posterior femoral cutaneous nerve (between the biceps and the semitendinosus). Next, explore the interval between the biceps and the lateral intermuscular septum. Detach the origin of the short head of the biceps from the linea aspera. This maneuver allows exposure of the femur at the midshaft level. In the lower thigh retract the long head of the biceps laterally to expose the sciatic nerve. It lies on the surface of the adductor magnus and may be retracted laterally to expose this portion of the femur.

THIGH SURGICAL APPROACHES

APPROACH	INTERVAL	RISKS
Lateral	Vastus lateralis (femoral nerve)	Perforators from the profunda femoris artery
Posterolateral	Vastus lateralis (femoral nerve) and hamstrings (sciatic nerve)	Perforators from the profunda femoris artery
Anteromedial (distal)	Rectus femoris (femoral nerve) and vastus medialis (femoral nerve)	Medial superior geniculate artery, infrapatellar branch of saphenous nerve
Posterior	Biceps femoris (sciatic nerve) and vastus lateralis (femoral nerve)	Posterior femoral cutaneous nerve (between biceps and semitendinosus) and sciatic nerve

IX. Knee and Leg

A. Osteology

1. **Patella**—The patella is the largest sesamoid bone. It serves three functions: it is a fulcrum for the quadriceps; it protects the knee joint; and it enhances lubrication and nutrition of the knee. An accessory or "bipartite" patella may represent failure of fusion of the superolateral corner of the patella and is commonly confused with patellar fractures.
2. **Tibia**—The tibia articulates with the distal femur with proximal medial (oval and concave) and lateral (circular and convex) facets. Gerdy's tubercle lies on the lateral side of the proximal tibia and is the insertion of the iliotibial tract. The tibial shaft is triangular in cross-section and tapers to its thinnest point at the junction of the middle and distal thirds and then again widens to form the tibial plafond. Distally, the tibia forms an inferior quadrilateral surface for articulation with the talus and the pyramid-shaped medial malleolus. Laterally, the fibular notch forms an articulation with the fibula.
3. **Fibula**—The styloid process of the head serves as the attachment for the fibular collateral ligament and the biceps tendon. Lying just below the head, the neck of the fibula is grooved by the common peroneal nerve. The expanded distal fibula is known as the lateral malleolus and extends beyond the distal margin of the medial malleolus. Together with the inferior distal surface of the tibia, these structures make up the ankle mortise.

B. Arthrology

1. **Knee**—The knee is a compound joint consisting of two condyloid joints and one sellar joint (patellofemoral articulation). The knee is enclosed in a **capsule** that has posteromedial

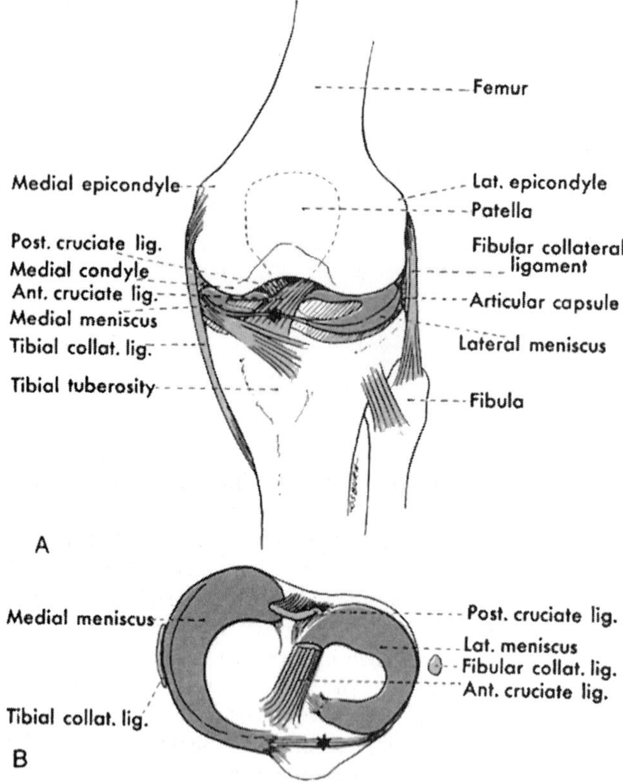

FIGURE 11-57 ■ Ligaments of the knee. (From Jenkins, D.B.: Hollinshead's Functional Anatomy of the Limbs and Back, 6th ed., Fig. 16-1. Philadelphia, WB Saunders, 1991.)

and posterolateral recesses, which **extend 15 mm distal to the subchondral surface of the tibial plateau** (be careful to avoid intra-articular pin placement). The medial and lateral femoral condyles articulate with the corresponding tibial facets. Intervening menisci serve to deepen the concavity of the facets, help protect the articular surface, and assist in rotation of the knee (Fig. 11-57).

The **peripheral third of the menisci are vascular** (and can be repaired); the inner two-thirds are nourished by synovial fluid. The medial meniscus tears three times more often than the more mobile lateral meniscus. Protect the saphenous nerve during medial meniscus repairs. The lateral meniscus is associated with meniscal cysts, discoid menisci, and is the most common site of tears in acute ACL injuries. Protect the peroneal nerve during repairs on the lateral meniscus. Stability of the knee is enhanced by a complex arrangement of ligaments (Table 11-13; Fig. 11-58). The cruciate ligaments are crucial to anteroposterior stability, and the collateral ligaments provide varus/valgus stability. Each cruciate ligament is made up of two portions, or bundles. The ACL and PCL anterior bundles are tight in flexion. *The PCL has an anterolateral bundle and the ACL has an anteromedial bundle.* Remember **PAL**: **P**CL has **a**nterol**a**teral. Thus the **anterior cruciate ligament** is composed of an **anteromedial** portion that is **tight in flexion** and a **posterolateral** portion that is **tight in extension**. The **posterior cruciate ligament** has an **anterolateral** portion that is **tight in flexion** and a **posteromedial** portion that is **tight in extension**. The PCL lies between the ligament of Humphrey (anterior) and Wrisberg's ligament (posterior). The posterolateral corner (PLC) comprises the arcuate ligament, popliteus, posterolateral capsule, lateral collateral (LCL), popliteofibular ligament, and lateral head of gastrocnemius. Injuries to the PCL and PLC provide key testable material. Isolated injuries to the PCL cause greatest instability at 90 degrees of knee flexion. Combined PCL and PLC injuries result in increasing instability as the knee is flexed from 30–90 degrees. Isolated PLC injuries result in increasing

Table 11-13. LIGAMENTS OF THE KNEE

LIGAMENT	ORIGIN	INSERTION	FUNCTION
Retinacular	Vastus medialis and lateralis	Tibial condyles	Forms anterior capsule
Posterior fibers	Femoral condyles	Tibial condyles	Forms posterior capsule
Oblique popliteal	Semimembranosus tendon	Lateral femoral condyle/posterior capsule	Strengthens capsule
Deep medial collateral (MCL)	Medial epicondyle	Medial meniscus	Holds med. meniscus to femur
Superficial MCL	Medial epicondyle	Medial condyle of tibia	Resists valgus force
Arcuate	Lat. femoral condyle, over popliteus	Post. tibia/fibular head	Posterior support
Lateral collateral (LCL)	Lateral epicondyle	Lateral fibular head	Resists varus force
Anterior cruciate (ACL)	Anterior intercondylar tibia	Posteromed. lat. femoral condyle	Limits hyperextension/sliding
Posterior cruciate (PCL)	Posterior sulcus tibia	Anteromed. femoral condyle	Prevents hyperflexion/sliding
Coronary	Meniscus	Tibial periphery	Meniscal attachment
Wrisberg	Posterolateral meniscus	Med. femoral condyle (behind PCL)	Stabilizes lat. meniscus
Humphrey	Posterolateral meniscus	Med. femoral condyle (in front)	Stabilizes lat. meniscus
Transverse meniscal	Anterolateral meniscus	Anteromedial meniscus	Stabilizes menisci

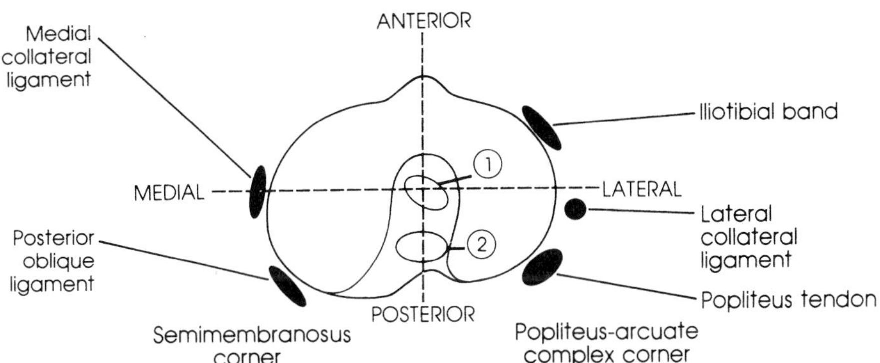

FIGURE 11-58 ■ Ligaments of the knee. *1,* Anterior cruciate ligament; *2,* posterior cruciate ligament. (From Magee, D.J.: Orthopedic Physical Assessment. Philadelphia, WB Saunders, 1987, p. 285.)

instability most notable at 30 degrees with instability decreasing as the knee is flexed to 90 degrees. In addition, several muscles and tendons traverse the knee, giving it dynamic stability. Please note that the hamstring tendons used for autograft ACL reconstruction are the gracilis and semitendinosus.

2. **Superior Tibiofibular Joint**—A plane or gliding joint that is strengthened by the anterior and posterior ligaments of the head of the fibula.

C. **Muscles of the Leg**—Commonly divided into groups based on compartments (anterior, lateral, superficial posterior, and deep posterior) (Table 11-14). The **posterior compartments are supplied by the tibial nerve** and contain preaxial muscles.The **anterior and lateral compartments are supplied by the common peroneal nerve** (anterior-deep, lateral-superficial) and contain postaxial muscles. Origins and insertions are noted in Figure 11-59. The popliteal fossa is bordered by the gastrocnemius muscles, semimembranosus, and biceps. The plantaris muscle makes up the floor of the fossa. Four compartment releases of the leg are key testable material and are summarized in the chart on the next page. Please note that the saphenous nerve (termination of the femoral nerve) is subcutaneous.

Table 11-14. MUSCLES OF THE LEG

MUSCLE	ORIGIN	INSERTION	ACTION	INNERVATION
Anterior Compartment				
Tibialis anterior	Lateral tibia	Med. cuneiform, 1st metatarsal	Dorsiflex, invert foot	Deep peroneal (L4)
Extensor hallucis longus (EHL)	Mid. fibula	Great toe distal phalanx	Dorsiflex, extend toe	Deep peroneal (L5)
Extensor digitorum longus (EDL)	Tibial condyle/fibula	Toe middle and distal phalanges	Dorsiflex, extend toes	Deep peroneal (L5)
Peroneus tertius	Fibula and EDL tendon	5th metatarsal	Evert, plantar flex, abduct foot	Deep peroneal (S1)
Lateral Compartment				
Peroneus longus	Proximal fibula	Med. cuneiform, 1st metatarsal	Evert, plantar flex, abduct foot	Superficial peroneal (S1)
Peroneus brevis	Distal fibula	Tuberosity of 5th metatarsal	Evert foot	Superficial peroneal (S1)
Superficial Posterior Compartment				
Gastrocnemius	Post. med. and lat. femoral condyles	Calcaneus	Plantar flex foot	Tibial (S1)
Soleus	Fibula/tibia	Calcaneus	Plantar flex foot	Tibial (S1)
Plantaris	Lat. femoral condyle	Calcaneus	Plantar flex foot	Tibial (S1)
Deep Posterior Compartment				
Popliteus	Lat. femoral condyle, fibular head	Proximal tibia	Flex, IR knee	Tibial (L5,S1)
Flexor hallucis longus (FHL)	Fibula	Great toe distal phalanx	Plantar flex great toe	Tibial (S1)
Flexor digitorum longus (FDL)	Tibia	2nd-5th toe distal phalanges	Plantar flex toes, foot	Tibial (S1,S2)
Tibialis posterior	Tibia, fibula, interosseous membrane	Navicular, med. cuneiform	Invert/plantar flex foot	Tibial (L4,L5)

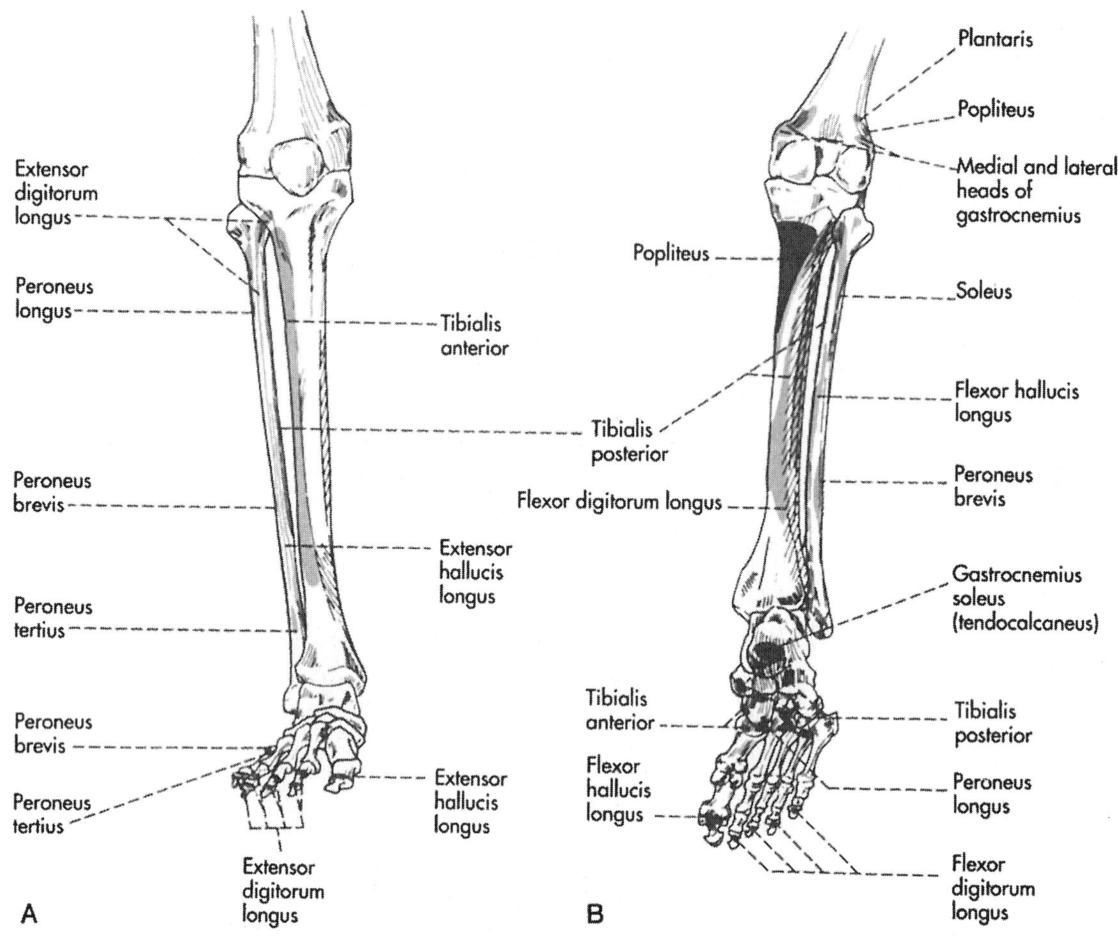

FIGURE 11-59 ■ Origins and insertions of leg and foot muscles. (From Jenkins, D.B.: Hollinshead's Functional Anatomy of the Limbs and Back, 6th ed., Fig. 19-3. Philadelphia, WB Saunders, 1991.)

COMPARTMENT RELEASES OF LEG

COMPARTMENT	MUSCLES	NEUROVASCULAR STRUCTURES RELEASED
Anterior	TA, EHL, EDL, PT	Deep peroneal nerve and anterior tibial artery
Lateral	PL, PB	Superficial peroneal nerve
Superficial posterior	GSC, plantaris	Sural nerve
Deep posterior	Popliteus, FHL, FDL, TP	Posterior tibial artery and vein, tibial nerve, peroneal a. and vein

D. **Nerves** (Fig. 11-60)

1. **Tibial Nerve (L4–S3)**—Continues in the thigh, deep to the long head of the biceps, and enters the popliteal fossa. It then crosses over the popliteus muscle and splits the two heads of the gastrocnemius, passing deep to the soleus on its course to the posterior aspect of the medial malleolus. It terminates as the medial and lateral plantar nerves. Muscular branches supply the posterior leg along its course (**superficial and deep posterior compartments**).

TIBIAL NERVE INNERVATION

NERVE	INNERVATION DISTAL TO KNEE
Tibial nerve	Gastrocnemius, soleus, tibialis posterior, FDL, FHL, medial and lateral plantar nerve

2. **Common Peroneal Nerve (L4–S2)**—The smaller terminal division of the sciatic, this nerve runs laterally in the popliteal fossa in the interval between the medial border of the biceps and the lateral head of the gastrocnemius. Then it winds around the neck of the fibula, deep to the peroneus longus, where it divides into superficial and deep branches. **This nerve can be injured with traction and with lateral meniscal repair.**
   a. **Superficial Peroneal Nerve**—Runs along the border between the lateral and anterior compartments in the leg, supplying muscular branches to the peroneus longus and brevis (**lateral compartment**). It terminates in two cutaneous branches (medial dorsal and intermediate dorsal cutaneous nerve)

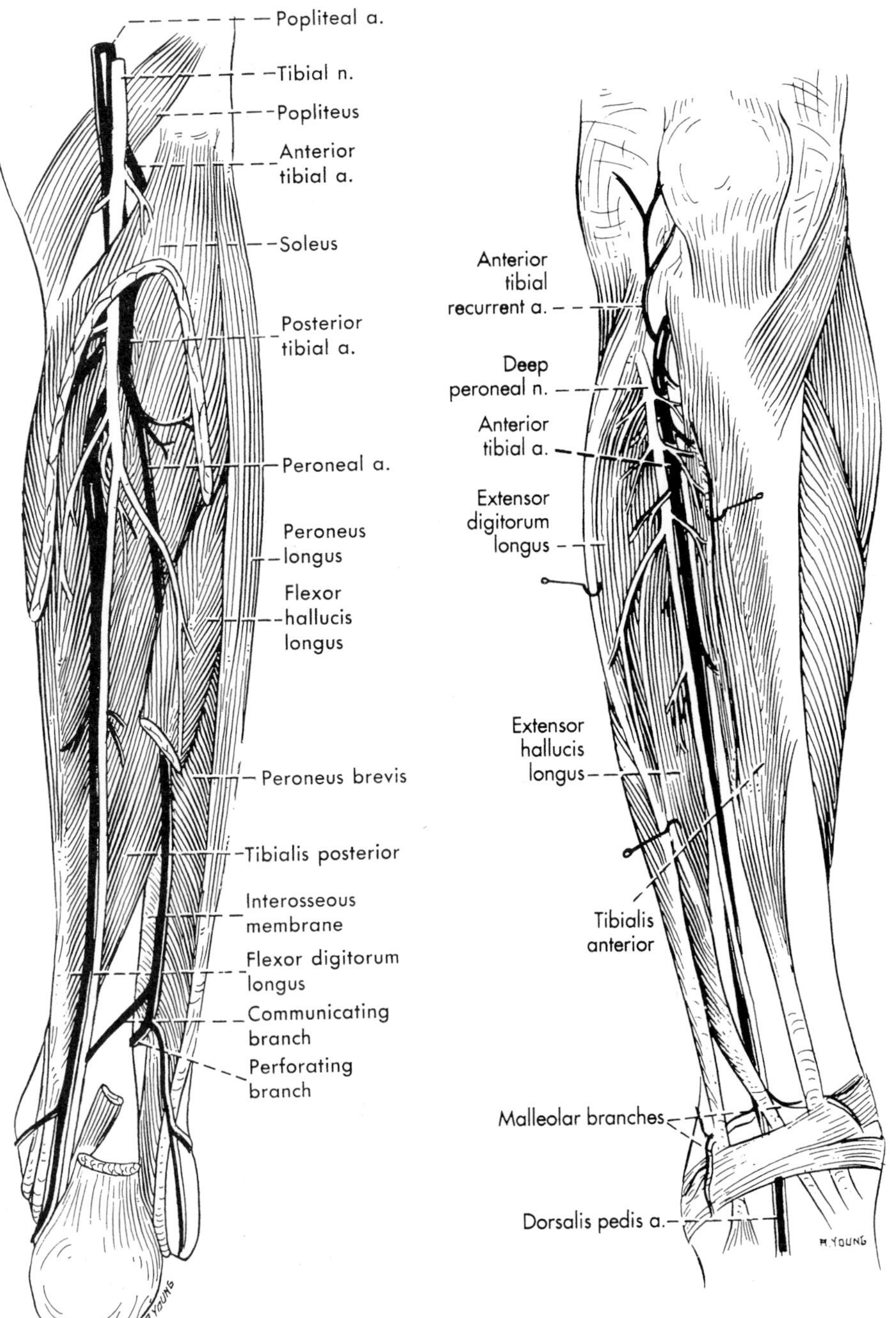

FIGURE 11-60 ■ Nerves and vessels of the leg. *Left,* Posterior. *Right,* Anterior. (From Jenkins, D.B.: Hollinshead's Functional Anatomy of the Limbs and Back, 6th ed. Philadelphia, WB Saunders, 1991, pp. 292, 296.)

supplying the dorsal foot. Please note that the superficial peroneal nerve supplies dorsal medial sensation to the great toe.

SUPERFICIAL PERONEAL NERVE INNERVATION

NERVE	INNERVATION
Superficial peroneal nerve	Peroneus longus and brevis

b. **Deep Peroneal Nerve**—Sometimes known as the anterior tibial nerve, this nerve runs along the anterior surface of the interosseous membrane, supplying the musculature of the **anterior compartment** (TA, EHL, EDL, PT). The first web space sensation is provided by the deep peroneal nerve.

DEEP PERONEAL NERVE INNERVATION

NERVE	INNERVATION
Deep peroneal nerve	Tibialis anterior, EDL, EHL, PT, EDB

3. **Cutaneous Nerves** (see Fig. 11-40)—Important cutaneous nerves include the saphenous nerve (L3-4) and the sural nerve (S1-2). The saphenous nerve is the continuation of the femoral nerve of the thigh, and it becomes subcutaneous on the medial aspect of the knee between the sartorius and gracilis (where it is sometimes injured during procedures about the knee, e.g., meniscal repair). The saphenous nerve supplies sensation to the medial aspect of the leg and foot. The sural nerve, which is often used for nerve grafting and can cause painful neuromas when inadvertently cut, is formed by cutaneous branches of both the tibial (medial sural cutaneous) and common peroneal (lateral sural cutaneous) nerves. It lies on the lateral aspect of the leg and foot.

E. **Vessels** (see Fig. 11-60)—Branches of the popliteal artery, the continuation of the femoral artery, supply the leg. The artery enters the popliteal fossa between the biceps and semimembranosus and descends underneath the tibial nerve and terminates between the medial and lateral heads of the gastrocnemius, dividing into the anterior and posterior tibial arteries. Several genicular branches are given off in the popliteal fossa, including the medial and lateral geniculates (which supply the menisci) and the **middle geniculate (which supplies the cruciate ligaments)**. The superior lateral geniculate can be injured during lateral release procedures. The descending geniculate artery (a branch of the femoral artery proximal to Hunter's canal) supplies the vastus medialis at the anterior border of the intermuscular septum. The **inferior geniculate artery** passes between the popliteal tendon and fibular collateral ligament in the posterolateral corner of the knee.

1. **Anterior Tibial Artery**—The first branch of the popliteal artery, this vessel passes between the two heads of the tibialis posterior and the interosseous membrane to lie on the anterior surface of that membrane between the tibialis anterior and extensor hallucis longus until it terminates as the dorsalis pedis artery.
2. **Posterior Tibial Artery**—Continues in the deep posterior compartment of the leg, coursing obliquely to pass behind the medial malleolus, where it terminates by dividing into medial and lateral plantar arteries. Its main branch, the **peroneal artery**, is given off 2.5 cm distal to the popliteal fossa and continues in the deep posterior compartment, lateral to its parent artery, between the tibialis posterior and flexor hallucis longus (FHL), eventually terminating in calcaneal branches.

F. **Surgical Approaches to the Knee and Leg**

1. **Medial Parapatellar Approach to the Knee**—Used most commonly for total knee arthroplasty, this approach utilizes a midline incision and a medial parapatellar capsular incision. The infrapatellar branch of the saphenous nerve is sometimes cut with incisions that stray too far medially, leading to a painful neuroma.
2. **Medial Approach to the Knee** (Fig. 11-61)—Used for repair of the medial collateral ligament (MCL) and capsule, this approach is in the interval between the sartorius and medial patellar retinaculum. The saphenous nerve and vein must be identified and protected. Three layers are commonly recognized (from superficial to deep): (1) pes anserinus tendons, (2) superficial MCL, and (3) deep MCL and capsule.
3. **Lateral Approach to the Knee** (Fig. 11-62)—Used primarily for exploring and repairing damaged ligaments, this approach utilizes the plane between the **iliotibial band (superior gluteal nerve) and the biceps (sciatic nerve)**. The common peroneal nerve, located near the posterior border of the biceps, must be isolated and retracted. The popliteus tendon is also at risk and should be identified. **The lateral inferior geniculate artery is posterior to the lateral collateral ligament between the lateral head of the gastrocnemius and the posterolateral capsule; it must also be identified and coagulated. The superior lateral geniculate artery is located between the femur and vastus lateralis.**
4. **Posterior Approach to the Knee**—Occasionally required to address posterior capsular pathology, this approach uses an S-shaped incision, beginning laterally and ending medially (distally). The popliteal fossa is exposed using the small saphenous vein and medial sural cutaneous nerves as landmarks. The two heads of the gastrocnemius can be detached if greater exposure is necessary. An alternative approach is to mobilize the medial head of the gastrocnemius (lateral to the semimembranosus) and retract it laterally, using its muscle belly to protect the neurovascular structures.
5. **Anterior Approach to the Tibia**—May be used for ORIF of fractures and bone grafting; it relies on subperiosteal elevation of the tibialis anterior.
6. **Posterolateral Approach to the Tibia**—Used typically for bone grafting of tibial nonunions, this approach utilizes the internervous plane between the **soleus and the FHL (tibial nerve) and the peroneal muscles (superficial peroneal nerve)**. The FHL is detached from its origin on the fibula, and the tibialis posterior is detached from its origin along the interosseous membrane to reach the tibia. Neurovascular structures in the posterior compartment (including the peroneal artery)

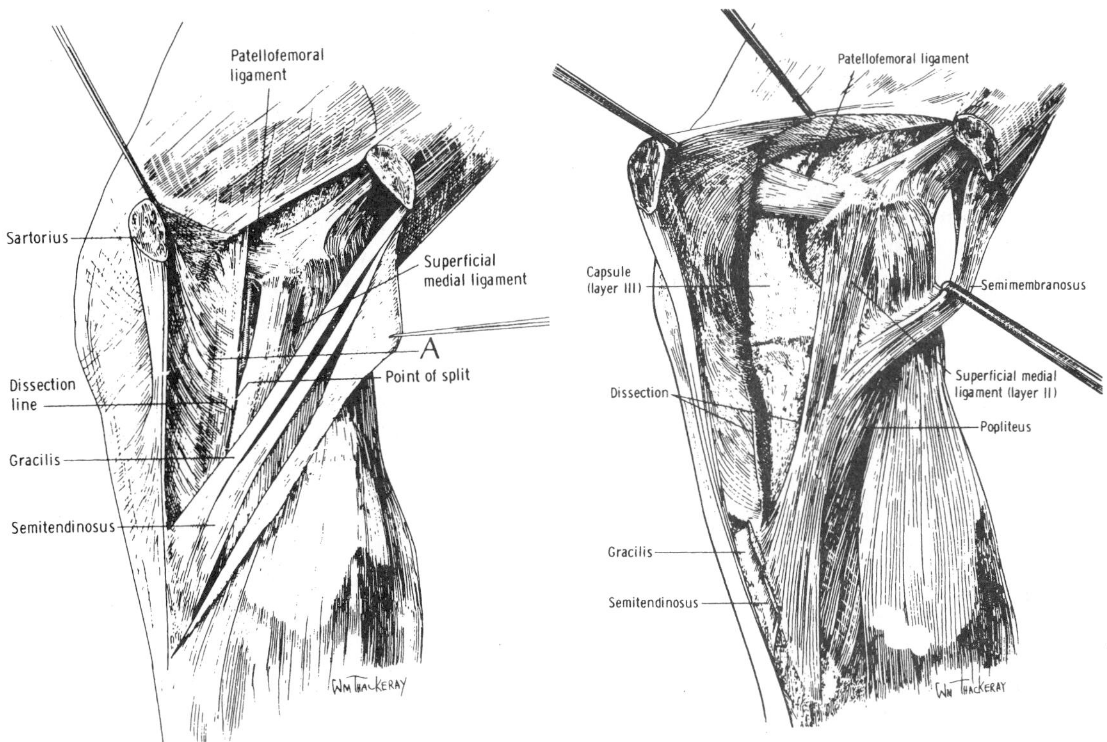

FIGURE 11-61 ■ Medial structures of the knee. (Warren, L.F., and Marshall, J.L.: The supporting structures and layers of the medial side of the knee. J. Bone Joint Surg. [Am.] 61:58, 1979.)

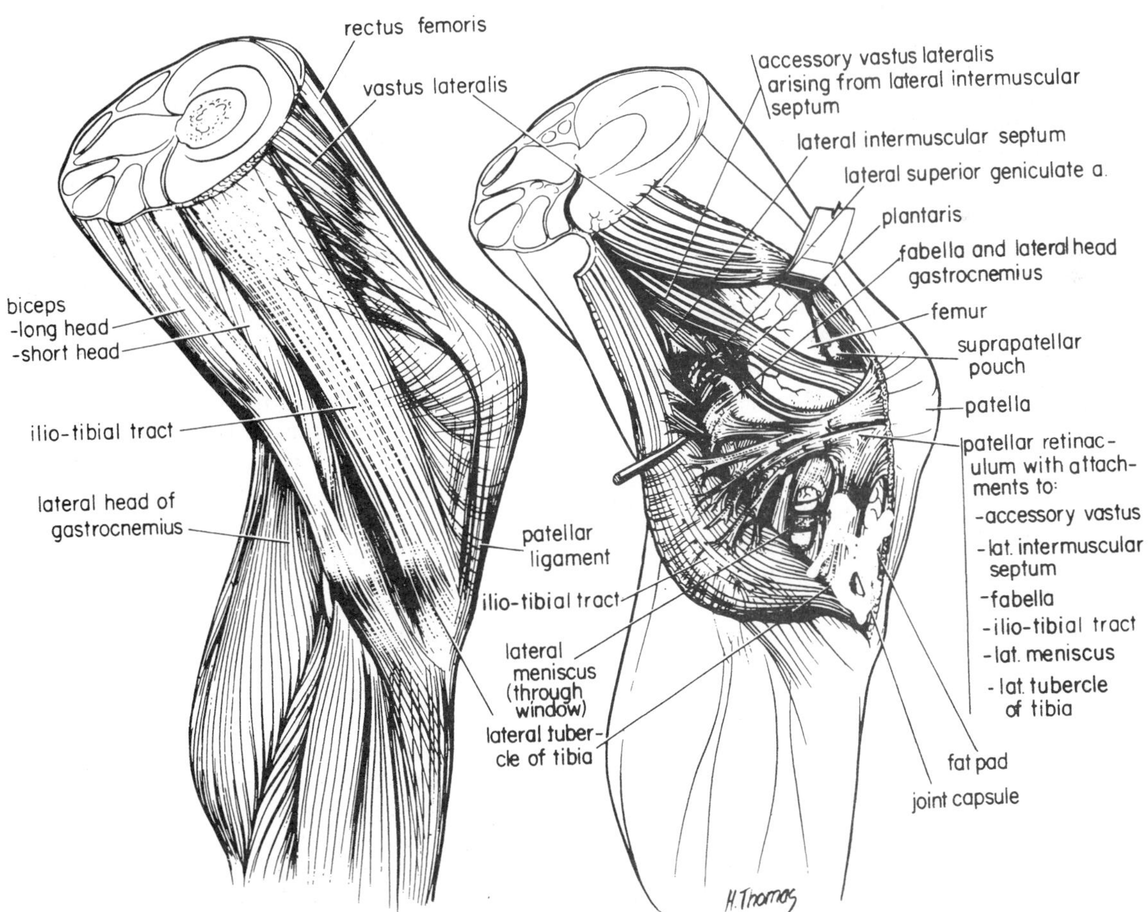

FIGURE 11-62 ■ Lateral structures of the knee. (From Seebacher, J.R., Inglis, A.E., Marshall, J.L., and Warren R.F.: The structure of the posterolateral aspect of the knee. J. Bone Joint Surg. [Am.] 64:533, 1982.)

are protected by the muscle bellies of the FHL and tibialis posterior.

7. **Approach to the Fibula**—Through the same interval as the posterolateral approach to the tibia, but stays more anterior and relies on isolation and protection of the common peroneal nerve in the proximal dissection.

KNEE AND LEG SURGICAL APPROACHES

APPROACH	INTERVAL	RISKS
Medial parapatellar knee	Through quadriceps tendon	Infrapatellar branch saphenous nerve
Medial knee	Sartorius and medial patellar retinaculum	Saphenous nerve and vein
Lateral knee	Iliotibial band (supinator gluteal nerve) and biceps femoris (sciatic nerve)	Common peroneal nerve Popliteus tendon Lateral inferior geniculate artery
Anterior tibia	Elevation of TA	
Posterolateral tibia	Soleus and FHL (tibial nerve) and peroneals (supinator peroneal nerve)	Peroneal artery

G. **Arthroscopy**—Arthroscopic portals for knee arthroscopy commonly include the inferomedial and inferolateral portals and a proximal (medial or lateral) portal. Posterior portals can place certain neurovascular structures at risk (lateral—common peroneal nerve; medial—saphenous nerve and vein).

X. Ankle and Foot

A. **Osteology**—The 26 bones of the foot include 7 tarsal bones, 5 metatarsals, and 14 phalanges. The foot is divided into the hindfoot (talus and calcaneus), midfoot (navicular, cuboid, and three cuneiforms), and forefoot (metatarsals and phalanges).

1. **Tarsus**—Includes the talus, calcaneus, cuboid, navicular, and three cuneiforms.
   a. **Talus**—Articulates with the tibia and fibula in the ankle mortise and with the calcaneus and navicular distally. It is made up of a body that is wider anteriorly with three articular surfaces (the trochlea [including surfaces for the malleoli articulations], and the posterior and middle calcaneal facets) and a posterior process (for the posterior talofibular ligament). The neck of the talus connects with the head, which in turn articulates with the navicular distally and the calcaneus inferiorly. The talus has no muscular attachments but has a groove posteriorly for the tendon of the flexor hallucis longus. Additionally, two-thirds of the talus is covered with cartilage. The **primary blood supply to the talar body is from the artery of the tarsal canal** (posterior tibial artery). The other blood supplies include the superior neck vessels (anterior tibial artery) and the artery of the tarsal sinus (dorsalis pedis).
   b. **Calcaneus**—Largest and strongest bone in the foot. It has three surfaces that articulate with the talus: a large posterior facet, an anterior facet, and a middle facet. Distally, there is an articular surface that receives the cuboid bone. The **sustentaculum tali** is an overhanging horizontal eminence on the anteromedial surface of the calcaneus. The sustentaculum tali supports the middle articular surface above it has an *inferior groove for the FHL tendon.*
   c. **Cuboid**—Lies on the lateral aspect of the foot, is grooved on the plantar surface by the peroneus longus, and has four facets for articulation with the calcaneus, the lateral cuneiform, and the fourth and fifth metatarsals.
   d. **Navicular**—The most medial tarsal bone; lies between the talus and the cuneiforms. Proximally, the surface is oval and concave for its articulation with the head of the talus. Distally, the navicular has three articular surfaces, one for each of the cuneiforms. The medial plantar projection serves as the insertion for the posterior tibial tendon.
   e. **Cuneiforms**—Medial, intermediate, and lateral, these three bones articulate with the navicular and posterior cuboid (lateral cuneiform) and the first three metatarsals. The intermediate cuneiform does not extend as far distally as the medial cuneiform, allowing the second metatarsal to "key" into place.
2. **Metatarsals**—Five bones, numbered from medial to lateral, span the distance between the tarsals and the phalanges. In general, their shape and function are similar to those of the metacarpals of the hand. The first metatarsal has a plantar cristae that articulates with the fibular and tibial sesamoids contained within the flexor hallucis brevis tendon.
3. **Phalanges**—Also similar to the hand. The great toe has two phalanges, and the remaining digits have three.
4. **Ossification**—Each tarsus has a single ossification center, except the calcaneus, which has a second center posteriorly. The calcaneus, talus, and usually the cuboid are present at birth. The lateral cuneiform appears during the first year, the medial cuneiform during the second year, and the intermediate cuneiform and navicular during the third year. The posterior center for the calcaneus usually appears at the eighth year. The second through fifth metatarsals have two ossification centers: a primary center in the shaft and a secondary

center for the head that appears at age 5–8. The phalanges and first metatarsal have secondary centers at their bases that appear during the third or fourth year proximally and the sixth to seventh year distally.

B. **Arthrology**

1. **Inferior Tibiofibular Joint**—Formed by the medial distal fibula and the notched lateral distal tibia, this joint is supported by four ligaments: anterior and posterior inferior tibiofibular ligaments, transverse tibiofibular ligament and an interosseous ligament. The **anteroinferior tibiofibular ligament** is an oblique band that connects the bones anteriorly. Avulsion of this ligament may result in a **Tillaux fracture**.
2. **Ankle Joint** (Fig. 11-63)—A ginglymus, or hinge, joint is formed by the malleoli and the talus. The medial collateral (deltoid) ligament comprises two layers: (1) superficial—tibionavicular and tibiocalcaneal, (2) deep—anterior and posterior tibiotalar. The lateral fibular ligaments are the anterior talofibular ligament (ATFL), calcaneofibular ligament (CFL) and posterior talofibular ligament (PTFL). **The ATFL is the weakest and is intracapsular** (intracapsular thickening). Position of the ankle is critical when testing the lateral ligament complex: plantar flexion tightens the ATFL and inversion with neutral flexion tightens the CFL.

ANKLE JOINT LIGAMENTS

LIGAMENT	ORIGIN	INSERTION
Capsule	Tibia	Talus
Deltoid		
Tibionavicular	Med. malleolus	Navicular tuberosity
Tibiocalcaneal	Med. malleolus	Sustentaculum tali
Posterior tibiotalar	Med. malleolus	Inner side of talus
Anterior tibiotalar	Med. malleolus	Medial surface of talus
ATFL	Lateral malleolus	Transversely to talus anteriorly
PTFL	Lateral malleolus	Transversely to talus posteriorly
CFL (calcaneofibular)	Lateral malleolus	Obliquely posteriorly to calcaneus

3. **Subtalar Joint**—Talar plantar facets articulate with the calcaneus. Stability is derived from four ligaments: the medial, lateral, and interosseous talocalcaneal and cervical ligaments.
4. **Intertarsal Joints** (Fig. 11-64)—Relatively self-explanatory, but there are several ligamentous structures that deserve notice (Table 11-15).
5. **Other Joints**—Tarsometatarsal joints are gliding joints supported by dorsal, plantar, and interosseous ligaments. The base of the first metatarsal is not ligamentously connected to

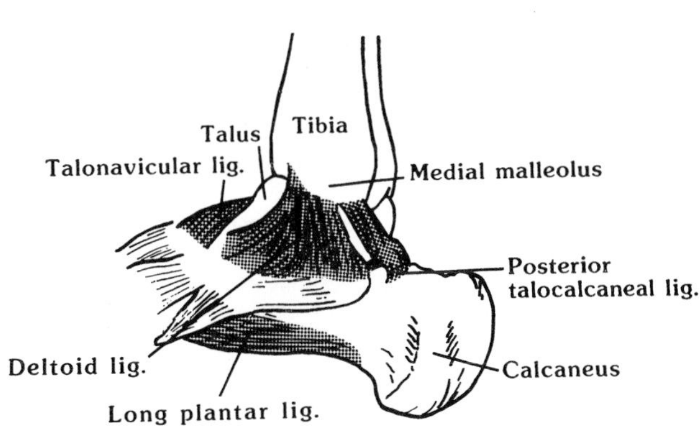

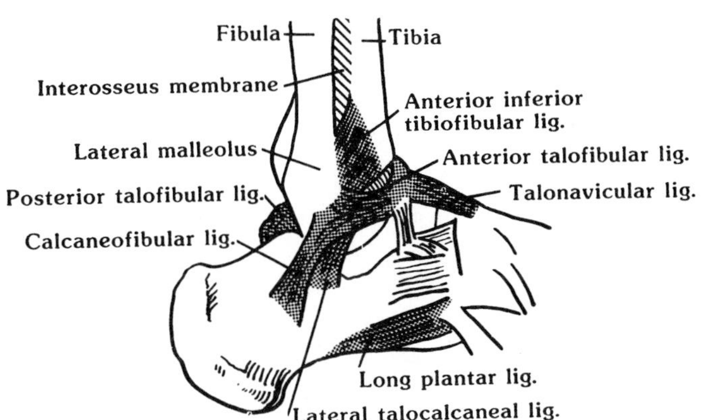

FIGURE 11-63 ■ Ankle ligaments. *Top,* Medial. *Bottom,* Lateral. (From Weissman, B.N., and Sledge, C.B.: Orthopedic Radiology. Philadelphia, WB Saunders, 1986, pp. 593, 594.)

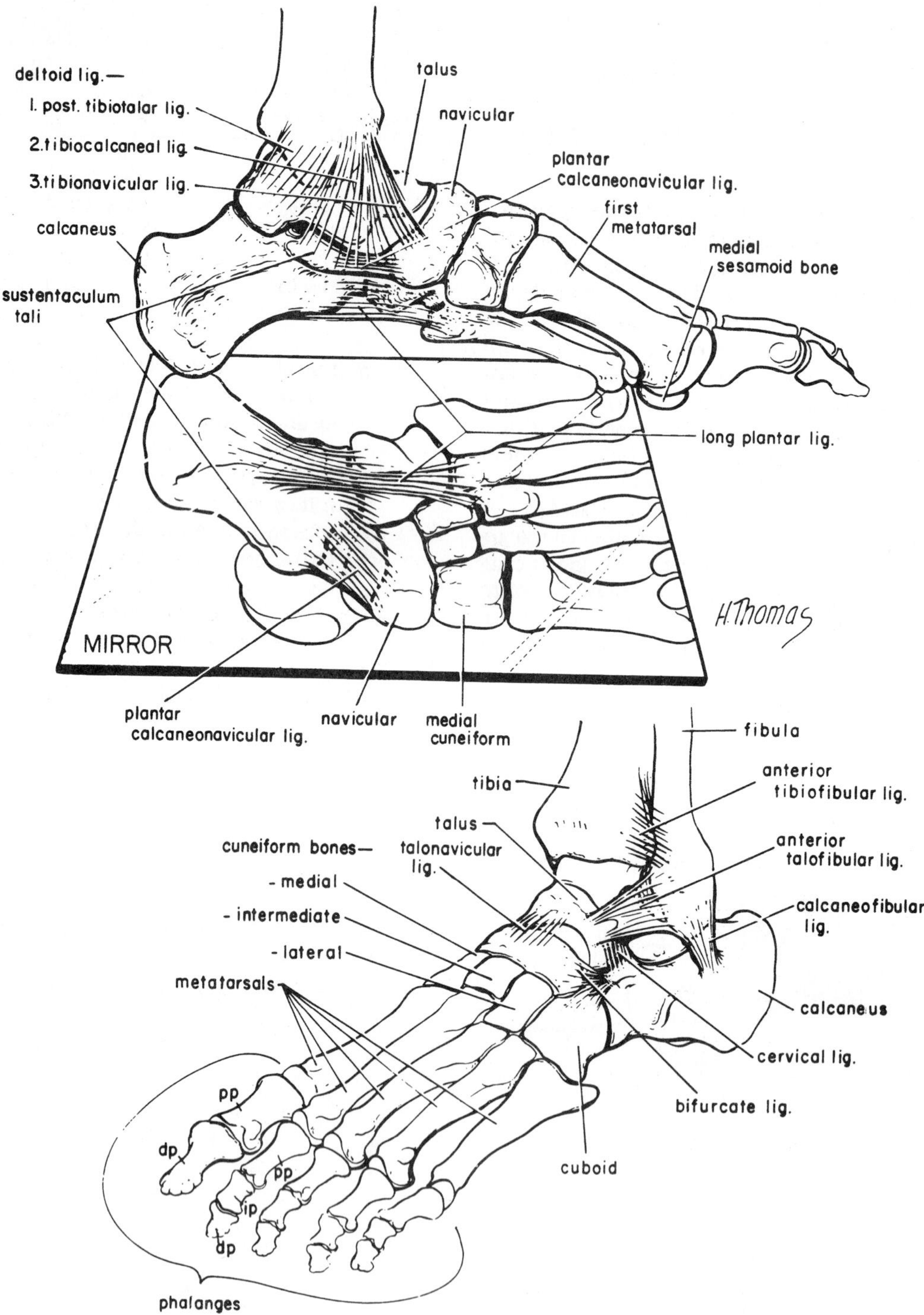

FIGURE 11-64 ■ Ligaments of the foot. (From Jahss, M.H.: Disorders of the Foot. Philadelphia, WB Saunders, 1982, p. 14.)

Table 11-15. LIGAMENTS OF THE INTERTARSAL JOINTS

LIGAMENT	COMMON NAME	ORIGIN	INSERTION
Interosseous talocalcaneal	Cervical	Talus	Calcaneus
Calcaneocuboid/calcaneonavicular	Bifurcate	Calcaneus	Cuboid and navicular
Calcaneocuboid-metatarsal	Long plantar	Calcaneus	Cuboid and 1st-5th metatarsals
Plantar calcaneocuboid	Short plantar	Calcaneus	Cuboid
Plantar calcaneonavicular	Spring	Sustentaculum tali	Navicular
Tarsometatarsal	Lisfranc	Med. cuneiform	2nd metatarsal base

the second metatarsal. The **Lisfranc ligament** connects the medial (shortest) cuneiform to the second (longest) metatarsal. In about 20% of patients it exists as a plantar and dorsal structure. The deep transverse metatarsal ligaments interconnect the metatarsal heads. The digital nerve courses plantar under the **transverse metatarsal ligament** and is the spot where interdigital neuritis (**Morton's neuroma**—usually second or third interdigital space) occurs. Additionally, the transverse metatarsal ligament attaches the second metatarsal head to the fibular sesamoid. This ligament holds the hallucal sesamoids in place and gives the appearance of sesamoid subluxation when the first metatarsal moves medially in hallux valgus. Plantar and collateral ligaments support the metatarsophalangeal joints. The primary stabilizing structure of the metatarsophalangeal joint is the plantar plate. IP joints are supported mainly by their capsules.

C. **Muscles**—Origins and insertions of muscles are shown in Figure 11-65, and tendons about the foot and ankle are shown in Figure 11-67. A total of 13 tendons cross the ankle joint: **Posterior**—Achilles; **Lateral**—Peroneals with longus (superficial) and brevis (deep); **Anterior** (from lateral to medial)—Peroneus tertius, EDL, EHL, TA; and **Medial** *(Tom, Dick, and Harry)—t*ibialis posterior, F*D*L, F*H*L. Key testable material comes from understanding what muscles are active during the different periods of the gait cycle (Chapter 9, Rehabilitation; Gait, Amputations, Prosthetics, Orthotics). Please note that the Achilles tendon's maximum anteroposterior dimension on magnetic resonance imaging is 8 mm. The arrangement of muscles and tendons in the foot is best considered in layers (Table 11-16). On the plantar

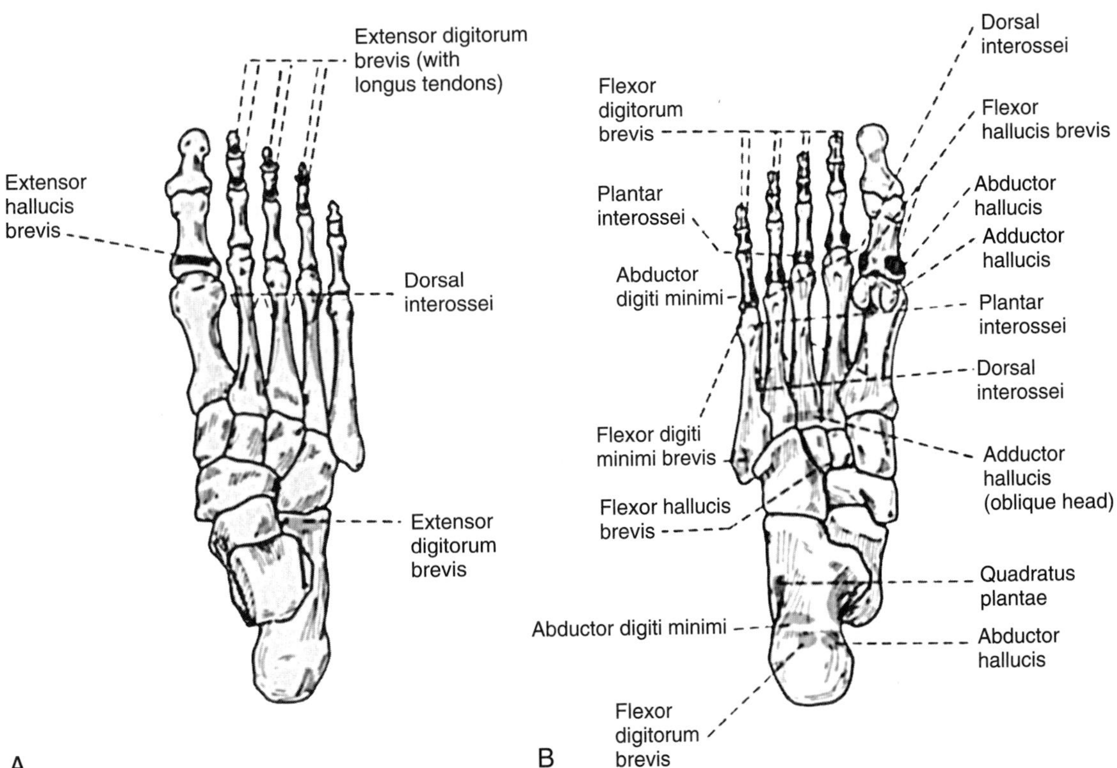

FIGURE 11-65 ■ Origins and insertions of muscles of the foot. *A*, Dorsal view. *B*, Plantar view. (From Jenkins, D.B.: Hollinshead's Functional Anatomy of the Limbs and Back, 6th ed., Fig. 20-7. Philadelphia, WB Saunders, 1991.)

Table 11-16. MUSCLES OF THE ANKLE AND FOOT

MUSCLE	ORIGIN	INSERTION	ACTION	INNERVATION
Dorsal Layer				
Extensor digitorum brevis (EDB)	Superolateral calcaneus	Base of proximal phalanges	Extend	Deep peroneal
First Plantar Layer				
Abductor hallucis	Calcaneal tuberosity	Base of great toe proximal phalanx	Abduct great toe	Med. plantar
Flexor digitorum brevis (FDB)	Calcaneal tuberosity	Distal phalanges of 2nd-5th toes	Flex toes	Med. plantar
Abductor digiti minimi	Calcaneal tuberosity	Base of 5th toe	Abduct small toe	Lat. plantar
Second Plantar Layer				
Quadratus plantae	Med. and lat. calcaneus	FDL tendon	Helps flex distal phalanges	Lat. plantar
Lumbricals	FDL tendon	EDL tendon	Flex MTP, extend IP	Med. and lat. plantar
FDL and FHL	Tibia/fibula	Distal phalanges of digits	Flex toes/invert foot	Tibial
Third Plantar Layer				
Flexor hallucis brevis (FHB)	Cuboid/lat. cuneiform	Proximal phalanx of great toe	Flex great toe	Med. plantar
Adductor hallucis	Oblique: 2nd-4th metatarsals	Proximal phalanx of great toe lat.	Adduct great toe	Lat. plantar
Flexor digiti minimi brevis (FDMB)	Base of 5th metatarsal head	Proximal phalanx of small toe	Flex small toe	Lat. plantar
Fourth Plantar Layer				
Dorsal interosseous	Metatarsal	Dorsal extensors	Abduct	Lat. plantar
Plantar interosseous	3rd-5th Metatarsals	Proximal phalanges medially	Adduct toes	Lat. plantar
(Peroneus longus and tibialis posterior)	Fibula/tibia	Med. cuneiform/navicular	Evert/invert foot	Superficial peroneal/tibial

Note: For abduction and adduction in the foot, the second toe serves as the reference.

surface intrinsic muscles dominate the first and third layers, and extrinsic tendons are more important in the second and fourth layers. There is **one dorsal intrinsic muscle of the foot—EDB** (lateral terminal branch of **the deep peroneal nerve**). Plantar **heel spurs** originate in the **flexor digitorum brevis** (medial plantar nerve innervation). Tendons are arranged about the toe, as shown in Figure 11-66. Lumbricals are located plantar to the transverse metatarsal ligament and interossei tendons are dorsal.

D. **Nerves** (see Fig. 11-47)—Nerves of the ankle and foot are branches of proximal nerves discussed earlier. A summary of muscle/nerve function is shown in the following chart.

FOOT NEUROMUSCULAR INTERACTIONS

FOOT FUNCTION	MUSCLE	INNERVATION
Inversion	Tibialis anterior	Deep peroneal nerve (L4)
	Tibialis posterior	Tibial nerve (S1)
Dorsiflexion	Tibialis anterior, EDL, EHL	Deep peroneal n.: TA (L4), EDL, and EHL (L5)
Eversion	Peroneus longus and brevis	Superficial peroneal nerve (S1)
Plantar flexion	Gastrocsoleus, FDL, FHL, tibialis posterior (also hindfoot inverter)	Tibial nerve (S1)

Please note: the posterior tibial tendon is the initiator of hindfoot inversion during gait (Chapter 9). This explains why a person cannot single-stance toe rise with posterior tibial tendon deficiency and a normal Achilles tendon.

1. **Tibial Nerve—The tibial nerve supplies all intrinsic foot muscles except the EDB (deep peroneal nerve).** The tibial nerve splits into two branches under the flexor retinaculum: medial and lateral plantar nerves. Both of these nerves run in the second layer of the foot. The medial plantar nerve runs deep to the abductor hallucis, and the lateral plantar nerve runs obliquely under the cover of the quadratus plantae. The most proximal branch of the lateral plantar nerve is the nerve to the abductor digit quinti (Baxter's nerve). **The distribution of the sensory and motor branches of the plantar nerves is similar to that in the hand.** The medial plantar nerve (like the median nerve of the hand) supplies plantar sensation to the medial 3½ digits and motor to only a few plantar muscles (flexor hallucis brevis, abductor hallucis, flexor digitorum brevis, and first lumbrical). The lateral plantar nerve (like the ulnar nerve in the hand) supplies plantar sensation to the lateral 1½ digits and the remaining intrinsic muscles of the foot. The third web space digital nerve consists of branches from both the medial and lateral plantar nerves.

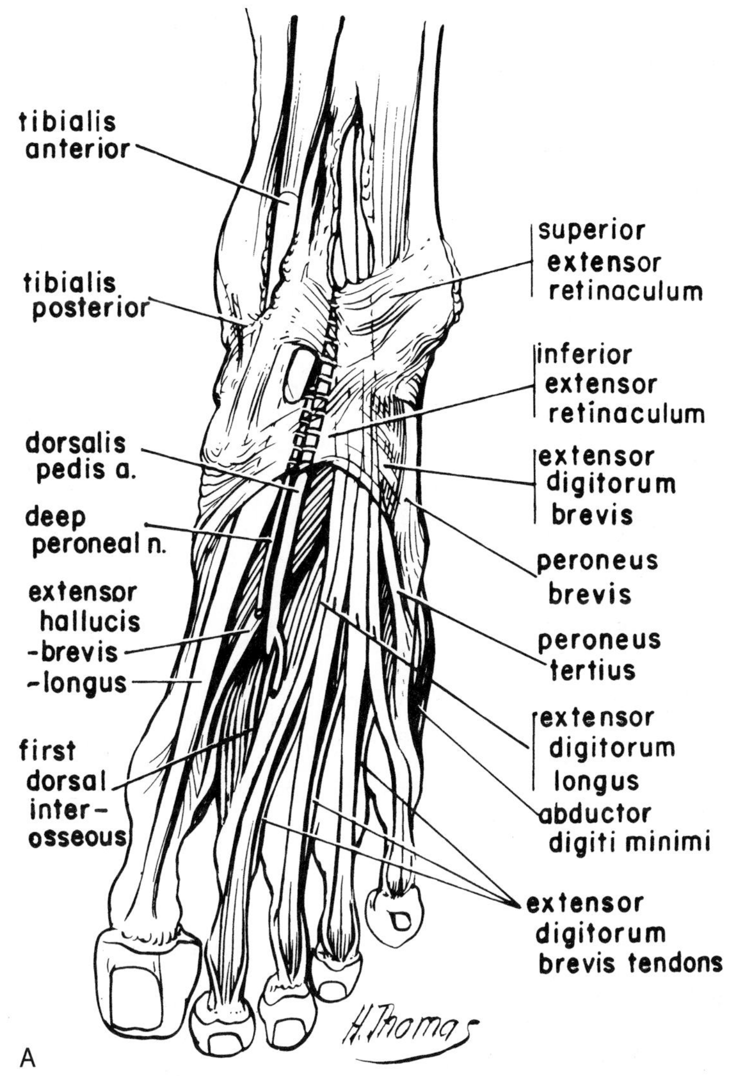
tibialis anterior
superior extensor retinaculum
tibialis posterior
inferior extensor retinaculum
dorsalis pedis a.
extensor digitorum brevis
deep peroneal n.
peroneus brevis
extensor hallucis
-brevis
-longus
peroneus tertius
extensor digitorum longus
first dorsal inter-osseous
abductor digiti minimi
extensor digitorum brevis tendons
H. Thomas
A

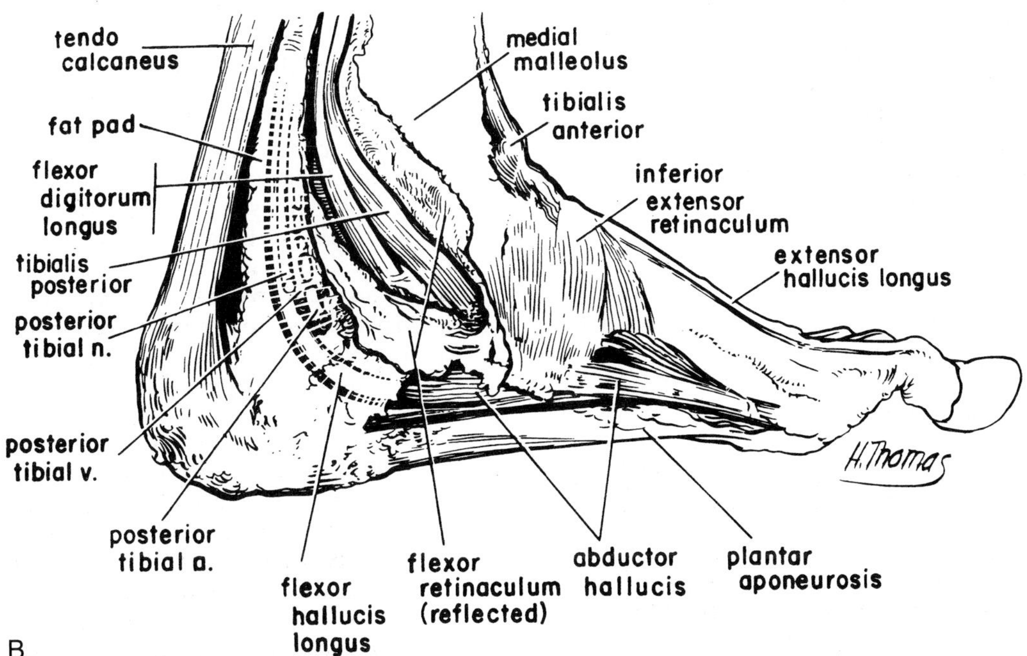
tendo calcaneus
medial malleolus
tibialis anterior
fat pad
flexor digitorum longus
inferior extensor retinaculum
tibialis posterior
extensor hallucis longus
posterior tibial n.
posterior tibial v.
H. Thomas
posterior tibial a.
flexor hallucis longus
flexor retinaculum (reflected)
abductor hallucis
plantar aponeurosis
B

FIGURE 11-66 ■ *See legend on following page*

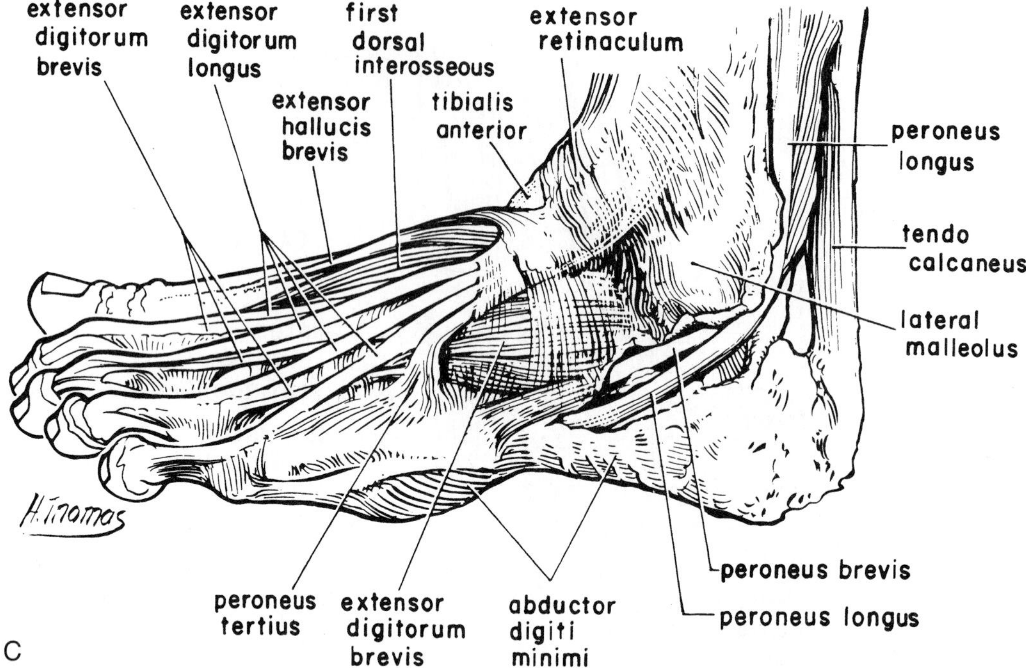

FIGURE 11-66 ■ Cross-section of the toe at the metatarsal base. **Lumbricals are plantar** to the transverse metatarsal ligament and **interossei are dorsal** to this ligament. The interossei and lumbricals (except the first lumbrical [medial plantar nerve]) are innervated by the lateral plantar nerve (From Jahss, M.H.: Disorders of the Foot. Philadelphia, WB Saunders, 1982, p. 623.)

MEDIAL AND LATERAL PLANTAR NERVE INNERVATION

NERVE	INNERVATION
Medial plantar nerve	FHB, abductor hallucis, FDB, 1st lumbrical
Lateral plantar nerve	QP, ADM, FDM, adductor hallucis, interossei, 2nd–4th lumbricals

2. **Common Peroneal Nerve**—Splits into superficial and deep branches in the leg and has terminal branches in the foot as well. The lateral terminal branch of the deep peroneal nerve ends in the proximal dorsal foot by supplying the extensor digitorum brevis (EDB) muscle. The medial terminal branch of the deep peroneal nerve supplies sensation to the first web space. The **medial and intermediate dorsal cutaneous nerves of the superficial peroneal nerve supply the bulk of the remaining sensation to the dorsal foot**. The dorsal intermediate branch is at risk during placement of the anterolateral ankle arthroscopic portal discussed below. All sensation of the foot is supplied by the sciatic nerve except the medial ankle and foot (saphenous nerve [termination of femoral nerve]). Please note that the **dorsal medial cutaneous nerve (branch of the superficial peroneal nerve)** crosses the EHL from lateral to medial and **supplies sensation to the dorsomedial aspect of the great toe**.

E. **Vessels**—Like the nerves that run with them, there are two main arteries that supply the ankle and foot.
   1. **Dorsalis Pedis Artery**—Continuation of the anterior tibial artery of the leg, it provides the blood supply to the dorsum of the foot via its lateral tarsal, medial tarsal, arcuate, and first dorsal metatarsal branches. Its largest branch, the deep plantar artery, runs between the first and second metatarsals and contributes to the plantar arch (see Fig. 11-67*A*).
   2. **Posterior Tibial Artery**—Divides into medial and lateral plantar branches under the abductor hallucis muscle. The larger lateral branch receives the deep plantar artery and forms the plantar arch in the fourth layer of the plantar foot.

F. **Important Neurovascular Relationships**—May be seen in a coronal section (Fig. 11-68).

G. **Surgical Approaches**
   1. **Anterior Approach to the Ankle**—Used primarily for ankle fusion, this approach uses the interval between the **extensor hallucis longus and extensor digitorum longus (both deep peroneal nerve)**. Before incising the extensor retinaculum, care must be taken to protect the superficial peroneal nerve. The deep peroneal nerve and anterior tibial artery, which lie directly in this interval, must be retracted medially with the extensor hallucis longus.

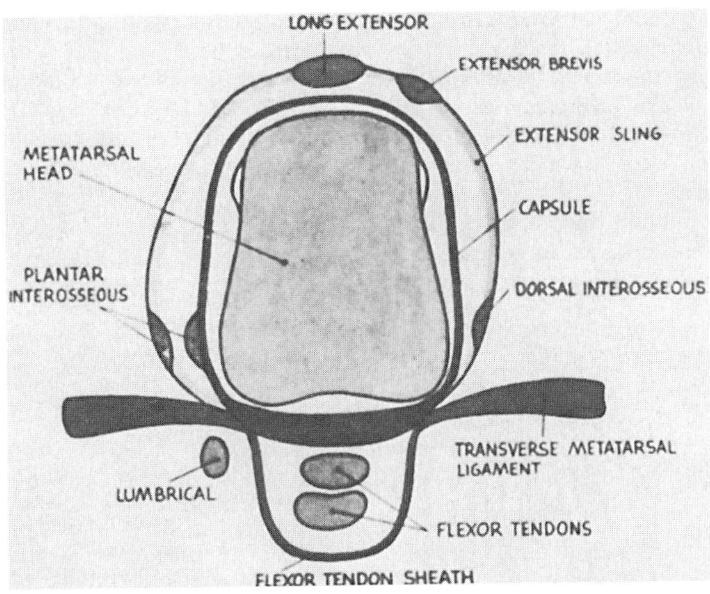

FIGURE 11-67 ■ Muscles and tendons of the foot. *A,* Dorsal view. *B,* Medial view. *C,* Lateral view. (From Jahss, M.H.: Disorders of the Foot. Philadelphia, WB Saunders, 1982, pp. 18–20.)

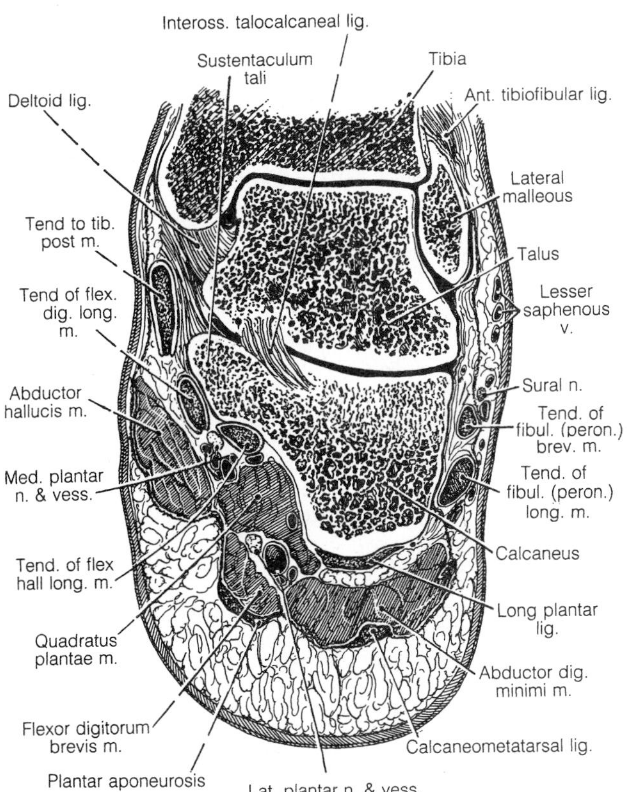

FIGURE 11-68 ■ Vertical section of the ankle. Note the FHL groove under the sustentaculum tali of the calcaneus. (From Essentials of Human Anatomy, 9th ed., by Russell T. Woodburne and William E. Burkel. Copyright 1957, 1994 by Oxford University Press, Inc. Used by permission of Oxford University Press, Inc.)

2. **Approach to the Medial Malleolus**—This approach is commonly used for ORIF of ankle fractures. It is superficial and can be approached anteriorly or posteriorly. The anterior approach jeopardizes the saphenous nerve and the long saphenous vein; the posterior approach places the structures running behind the medial malleolus (posterior tibial artery; FDL; posterior tibial artery, vein, and nerve; and FHL) at risk. A posteromedial approach, behind the medial malleolus, can be made through the tendon sheath of the posterior tibialis.
3. **Posteromedial Approach to the Ankle/Foot**—Used for clubfoot release in children, this approach begins medial to the Achilles tendon and curves distally along the medial border of the foot. Care must be taken to protect the posterior tibial nerve/artery and their branches. The posterior tibialis tendon is a landmark for the location of the subluxated navicular in the clubfoot.
4. **Lateral Approach to the Ankle**—Used for ORIF of distal fibula fractures, this approach is subcutaneous. The sural nerve (posterolateral) and the superficial peroneal nerve (anterior) must be avoided.
5. **Lateral Approach to the Hindfoot**—Used for triple arthrodesis, this approach uses the internervous plane between the **peroneus tertius (deep peroneal nerve) and peroneal tendons (superficial peroneal nerve).** The fat pad covering the sinus tarsi is removed, and the EDB is reflected from its origin to expose the joints. The lateral branch of the deep peroneal nerve (which supplies the EDB) must be protected with this approach.

Deep penetration with an instrument from this approach can injure the FHL.

6. **Anterolateral Approach to the Midfoot**—Requires release of the EDB. The risk of this approach, commonly used for excision of a calcaneonavicular bar, is to the calcaneal navicular (Spring) ligament.
7. Approach to the midfoot and digits is direct and is not discussed in detail. In general, care must be taken to protect digital nerves/arteries.

FOOT AND ANKLE SURGICAL APPROACHES

APPROACH	INTERVAL	RISKS
Anterior ankle	EHL (deep peroneal nerve) EDL (deep peroneal nerve)	Superficial and deep peroneal nerve, Anterior tibial artery
Anterior medial malleolus ankle		Saphenous nerve and vein
Distal fibula		Sural nerve (posterolateral) and superficial peroneal nerve (anterior with variable position)
Lateral hindfoot	Peroneus tertius (deep peroneal nerve) and peroneal tendons (supinator. peroneal nerve)	Lateral branch of deep peroneal nerve
Anterolateral midfoot	Release EDB	Calcaneal navicular ligament

H. **Arthroscopy**—Portals used in ankle arthroscopy can put important structures at risk. The anterolateral portal can jeopardize the dorsal intermediate cutaneous branch of the superficial peroneal nerve. The anteromedial portal can damage the greater saphenous vein. Anterior central portals are no longer recommended because of risk to the dorsalis pedis artery. Posteromedial portals can injure the posterior tibial artery (and are not recommended), and the posterior lateral portal can injure the sural nerve.

ANKLE ARTHROSCOPY PORTALS

PORTAL	LOCATION	RISKS
Anterolateral	Medial to lateral malleolus, lateral to peroneus tertius	Dorsal intermediate cutaneous branch of superficial peroneal nerve
Anteromedial	Medial to TA tendon, lateral to medial malleolus	Saphenous nerve and saphenous vein
Posterolateral	Medial to peroneal tendons, lateral to Achilles tendon	Sural nerve and small saphenous vein
Anterocentral	Medial to EDC, lateral to EHL	Deep peroneal nerve and anterior tibial artery

I. Summary of Lower-Extremity Innervation

SUMMARY OF LOWER EXTREMITY INNERVATION

NERVE	INNERVATION
Femoral nerve	Iliacus, psoas, quadriceps femoris (rectus femoris and the vastus lateralis, intermedius, and medialis)
Obturator nerve	Adductor brevis, longus, and magnus (along with tibial nerve), gracilis
Superior gluteal nerve	Gluteus medius, gluteus minimus, tensor fascia lata
Inferior gluteal nerve	Gluteus maximus
Sciatic nerve	Semitendinosus, semimembranosus, biceps femoris (long head [tibial division] and short head [peroneal division]), adductor magnus (with obturator nerve)
Tibial nerve	Gastrocnemius, soleus, tibialis posterior, FDL, FHL, medial and lateral plantar nerve
Deep peroneal nerve	Tibialis anterior, EDL, EHL, PT, EDB
Superficial peroneal nerve	Peroneus longus and brevis

XI. Summary

A. Important anatomic landmarks are summarized in Table 11-1.

B. **Surgical Approaches**—Key internervous intervals are summarized in Tables 11-2 and 11-3.

Selected Bibliography

Arnoczky, S.P., and Warren, R.F.: Microvasculature of the human meniscus. Am. J. Sports Med. 10(2):909–905, 1982.

Bohlman, H.H.: The Neck. In D'Ambrosia, R., ed.: Musculoskeletal Disorders. Philadelphia, J.B. Lippincott, 1977.

Bora, F.W.: The Pediatric Upper Extremity. Philadelphia, WB Saunders, 1986.

Browner, B.D., Jupiter, J.B., Levine, A.M., et al.: Skeletal Trauma. Philadelphia, WB Saunders, 1992.

Callaghan, J.J., ed.: Anatomy Self-Assessment Examination. Park Ridge, Ill, American Academy of Orthopaedic Surgeons, 1991.

Callaghan, J.J., ed.: Anatomy Self-Assessment Examination. Park Ridge, Ill, American Academy of Orthopaedic Surgeons, 1996.

Cervical Spine Research Education Committee: The Cervical Spine, 2nd ed. Philadelphia, J.B. Lippincott, 1989.

Chapman, M.W., ed.: Operative Orthopaedics. Philadelphia, J.B. Lippincott, 1988.

Chapman, M.W., ed.: Gray's Anatomy, 30th American ed. Philadelphia, Lea & Febiger, 1985.

Cohen, M.S., and Bruno R.J.: The collateral ligaments of the elbow. Clin. Orthop. 383:123–130, 2001.

Cooper, D.E., O'Brien, S.J., and Warren, R.F.: Supporting layers of the glenohumeral joint. Clin. Orthop. 289:1441–1455, 1993.

Corley, F.G., ed.: Shoulder and Elbow Self-Assessment Examination. Park Ridge, Ill, American Academy of Orthopaedic Surgeons, 1996.

Corley, F.G., ed.: Shoulder and Elbow Self-Assessment Examination. Park Ridge, Ill, American Academy of Orthopaedic Surgeons, 1999.

Crock, H.V.: An atlas of the arterial supply of the head and neck of the femur in man. Clin. Orthop. 152:17, 1980.

DeCoster, T.A., ed.: Anatomy Self-Assessment Examination. Park Ridge, Ill, American Academy of Orthopaedic Surgeons, 1999.

DeCoster, T.A., ed.: Anatomy Self-Assessment Examination. Park Ridge, Ill, American Academy of Orthopaedic Surgeons, 2002.

DeLee, J.C., and Drez, D., Jr.: Orthopaedic Sports Medicine: Principles and Practice. Philadelphia, WB Saunders, 1994.

Doyle, J.R.: Anatomy of the finger flexor tendon sheath and pulley system. J. Hand Surg. [Am.] 13:4734-4784, 1988.

Girgis, F.G., Marshall, J.L., and Monajem, A.R.S.: The cruciate ligaments of the knee joint: Anatomical, functional, and experimental analysis. Clin. Orthop. 106:216-231, 1975.

Green, D.P., Hotchkiss, R.N., and Pederson, W.C.: Green's Operative Hand Surgery, 4th ed., New York, Churchill Livingstone, 1999.

Harding, K.: The direct lateral approach to the hip. J. Bone Joint Surg. [Br.] 64:171-179, 1982.

Henry, A.K.: Extensive Exposure, 2nd ed. New York, Churchill Livingstone, 1973.

Hollinshead, W.H.: Anatomy for Surgeons, vol. 3, 2nd ed. New York, Harper & Row, 1969.

Hoppenfield, S., and DeBoer, P.: Orthopaedics: The Anatomic Approach. Philadelphia, J.B. Lippincott, 1984.

Hoppenfeld, S.: Orthopaedic Neurology: A Diagnostic Guide to Neurological Levels. Philadelphia, Lippincott-Raven, 1997.

Jahss, M.H.: Disorders of the Foot. Philadelphia, WB Saunders, 1987.

Jenkins, D.B.: Hollinshead's Functional Anatomy of the Limbs and Back, 6th ed. Philadelphia, WB Saunders, 1991.

Kaplan, E.B.: Surgical Approaches to the Neck, Cervical Spine, and Upper Extremity. Philadelphia, WB Saunders, 1966.

Ludloff, K.: The open reduction of the congenital hip dislocation by an anterior incision. Am. J. Orthop. Surg. 10:438, 1913.

Magee, D.J.: Orthopaedic Physical Assessment. Philadelphia, WB Saunders, 1987.

Mooney, J.F., Siegel, D.B., and Koman, L.A.: Ligamentous injuries of the wrist in athletes. Clin. Sports Med. 11(1):129-139, 1992.

Morrey, B.F., and An, K.N.: Articular and ligamentous contributions to the stability of the elbow joint. J. Sports Med. 11:315-319, 1983.

Morrey, B.F., and An, K.N.: Functional anatomy of the ligaments of the elbow. Clin. Orthop. 210:84-90, 1985.

Myerson, M.S., ed.: Foot and Ankle Self-Assessment Examination. Park Ridge, Ill, American Academy of Orthopaedic Surgeons, 1997.

Myerson, M.S., ed.: Foot and Ankle Self-Assessment Examination. Park Ridge, Ill, American Academy of Orthopaedic Surgeons, 2000.

Netter, F.H.: The CIBA Collection of Medical Illustrations, vol. 8: Musculoskeletal System, Part I. Summit, NJ, Ciba-Geigy, 1987.

Orthopaedic Knowledge Update Home Study Syllabus I, II, and III. Chicago, American Academy of Orthopaedic Surgeons, 1984, 1987, 1990.

Place, H.M., ed.: Adult Spine Self-Assessment Examination. Park Ridge, Ill, American Academy of Orthopaedic Surgeons, 1997.

Place, H.M., ed.: Adult Spine Self-Assessment Examination. Park Ridge, Ill, American Academy of Orthopaedic Surgeons, 2000.

Rockwood, C.A., Jr., and Green, D.P., eds.: Fractures in Adults, 3rd ed. Philadelphia, J.B. Lippincott, 1991.

Rothman, R.H., and Simeon, F.A.: The Spine, 2nd ed. Philadelphia, WB Saunders, 1982.

Ruge, D., and Wiltse, L.L., eds.: Spinal Disorders: Diagnosis and Treatment. Philadelphia, Lea & Febiger, 1977.

Sarrafian, S.K.: Anatomy of the Foot and Ankle. Philadelphia, J.B. Lippincott, 1983.

Seebacher, J.R., Inglis, A.E., Marshall, J.L., et al.: The structure of the posterolateral aspect of the knee. J. Bone Joint Surg. [Am.] 64:536-541, 1982.

Steinberg, M.E.: The Hip and Its Disorders. Philadelphia, WB Saunders, 1991.

Tubiana, R.: The Hand. Philadelphia, WB Saunders, 1985.

Turkel, S.J., Panio, M.W., Marshall, J.L., and Girgis, F.G.: Stabilizing mechanisms preventing anterior dislocation of the gleno-humeral joint. J. Bone Joint Surg. [Am.] 63: 1208-1217, 1981.

Verbiest, H.A.: Lateral approach to the cervical spine: Technique and indications. J. Neurosurg. 28:191-203, 1968.

Warren, I.F., and Marshall, J.L.: The supporting structures and layers on the medial side of the knee. J. Bone Joint Surg. [Am.] 61:56-62, 1979.

Watkins, R.G.: Surgical Approaches to the Spine. New York, Springer-Verlag, 1983.

Weissman, B.N., and Sledge, C.B.: Orthopedic Radiology. Philadelphia, WB Saunders, 1986.

Wilson, F.C., and Dirschl, D.R.: Orthopaedics: PreTest and Self-Assessment and Review. New York, McGraw-Hill, 1996.

Woodburne, R.T., and Burkel, W.E.: Essentials of Human Anatomy, 9th ed. New York, Oxford University Press, 1994.

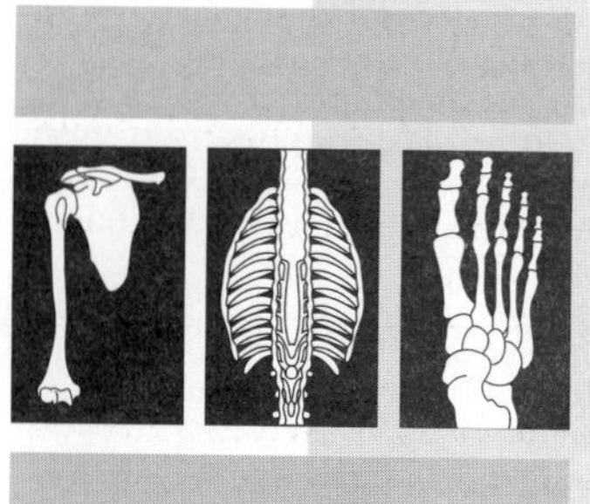

12 Principles of Practice and Statistics

DAMIAN M. RISPOLI
KERRY G. JEPSEN
KEVIN D. PLANCHER

SECTION 1

Principles of Practice

I. Impairment, Disability, Handicap

A. Impairments

1. Impairments are conditions that interfere with an individual's activities of daily living. Impairments are **the loss of use or derangement of any body part, system, or function**. It is determined by the physician based on the objective results of a physical examination. An impaired individual is not necessarily disabled. For example, a surgeon who loses a hand will be disabled in terms of the ability to operate; the surgeon may be fully capable of being the chief of a hospital medical staff and may not be at all disabled with respect to that occupation.
2. Permanent Impairment—Impairment that has become static or well stabilized with or without medical treatment and is not likely to remit despite maximal medical treatment.

B. Disability

1. Disability is an alteration of an individual's capacity to meet personal, social, or occupational demands or statutory or regulatory requirements because of impairment. Disability may be thought of as the gap between what a person can do and what the person needs or wants to do. To meet the definition of disability, an individual's impairment or combination of impairments must be of such severity that he or she is not only unable to do the work previously done, but also cannot perform any other kind of substantial gainful work, considering the individual's age, education, and work experience.
2. Permanent Disability—Disability that has become static or well established and is not likely to change despite continuing use of medical or rehabilitative measures.
3. **Provisions of the Americans with Disabilities Act (ADA)**—Effective July 22, 1992, for private-sector organizations that employ 25 or more employees.
   a. Accommodation refers to modifications of a job or workplace that enables a disabled employee to meet the same job demands and conditions required of any other employee in the same or similar job.
   b. Under the ADA, identification of an individual as having a disability does not depend on the results of a medical examination.
   c. An individual may be identified as having a disability if there is a record of an impairment that has substantially limited one or more major life activities.
4. **Morbidity Associated with Disability**
   a. Feelings of displacement, depression, and suicide increase as disabilities protract.
   b. There is a higher incidence of drug and alcohol abuse, family disruption, and divorce among disabled workers.
   c. Return to employment must be the goal of treatment.

C. Handicap

1. A handicap is related to, but different from, the concepts of disability and impairment. Under federal law an individual is handicapped if he or she has an impairment that substantially limits one or more of life's activities, has a record

of such impairment, or is regarded as having such impairment. This definition is so broad that almost any person may be considered to be handicapped.

II. Informed Consent—A legal doctrine that requires a physician to obtain consent for treatment to be rendered, an operation to be performed, and many diagnostic procedures.

Informed consent is a process and not simply a form or document. It represents an exchange of information between the surgeon and the patient (or legal representative) that ultimately culminates in the selection of and agreement to undergo a specific form of treatment. Without proper consent the surgeon may be guilty of an assault, battery, or trespass against the patient. Most litigation results from unexpected consequences of a procedure. Properly informed patients will be aware of and have decided to accept both the benefits and risks. Consent must be obtained by the attending surgeon.

The **attending physician should explain in layperson's terms the following**:

- The patient's diagnosis and the nature of the condition or illness necessitating intervention
- The nature and purpose of the proposed treatment/procedural plan
- The risk and complications of the treatment or procedure.
- All options or alternatives (including no treatment), with their associated risks/complications
- The probability of success. **No** guarantee of success should be expressed or implied

A. Decision-Making Capacity
   1. A patient must be able to understand the clinical circumstances and the indications for a procedure.
   2. A patient must be able to understand the alternative approaches to the procedure.
   3. A patient must be able to weigh the alternative approaches and be able and willing to express in an understandable fashion his or her choices.

B. The level of capacity required of a patient is related to the risks of a procedure and the risk-benefit ratio.
   1. In circumstances when a patient lacks the ability for decision making, informed consent may be obtained by a legal guardian, or in situations deemed medically necessary, by a physician.
   2. Special informed-consent rules apply to emergencies and minors.
      a. A medical emergency is an unconscious or incapacitated person with a life- or limb-threatening condition requiring immediate medical attention. Treatment can proceed without informed consent. Ensure that a description of the patient's medical condition at the time of the emergency is documented in the record, specifically addressing the reason for the emergent condition and why treatment needed to be rendered.
      b. Consent rules for minors vary greatly from state to state. The surgeon must be aware of those rules that apply locally. Generally, consent for treatment of minors is obtained from the parent or guardian for all but emergency conditions.

C. Informed consent may be documented in the following three basic ways:
   - A long form (i.e., detailed form that includes all the specific details of elements noted in previous discussion)
   - A short form (may not contain all the specific details, simply states that the risks/benefits have been explained)
   - A detailed note in the patient's record. A short or long form is usually combined with the note, creating so-called **double consent**

D. Standards of Disclosure—The degree of disclosure varies among the states, and the courts have developed two standards that may be applied.
   1. **Professional or Reasonable Physician Standard.** Used by most states. Based on what is customary practice in a specific medical community for surgeons to divulge to the patients.
   2. **Patient Viewpoint Standard.** This is based on the level of information a reasonable person would want to know in a similar circumstance. The courts have showed some preference for this standard in recent years.

III. Elements of Malpractice

A. Malpractice is defined as negligence by a health-care provider that results in injury to a patient. A malpractice suit is a civil action filed by a patient alleging that a physician's negligence resulted in an injury for which the patient desires compensation. The requirement of the law is proof by a preponderance of the evidence.
   1. Negligence is the result of failure to exercise the degree of diligence and care that a reasonable and prudent person would exercise under the same or similar conditions.
   2. Medical negligence comprises four elements: **duty, breach of duty, causation,** and **damages**.
      a. Duty begins when the surgeon offers to treat the patient, and the patient accepts that offer. The duty of the physician is to provide care equal to the same standard of care ordinarily executed by surgeons in the same medical specialty.
         (1) Standard of care is not uniform and is established by local expert opinion.
         (2) **Residents and fellows are held to the same standard of care as board-certified orthopaedists.**
      b. **Breach of duty** occurs when action or failure to act deviates from the standard of care. This may be an act of commission (doing what one should not have) or omission (failing to do what one should have).

c. **Causation** is present when it is demonstrated that failure to meet the standard of care was the direct cause of the patient's injuries.
d. **Damages** are monies awarded as compensation for injuries sustained as the result of medical negligence.
   (1) **Special damages** are actual expenses, such as medical/rehabilitative expenses and lost wages.
   (2) **General damages,** or noneconomic losses, are awards for pain and suffering, disfigurement, and so on.
   (3) **Punitive/exemplary damages** serve as a penalty for blatant disregard or incompetence. These are seldom awarded in medical malpractice cases.
   (4) **Ad damnum clause** is the portion of a plaintiff's complaint that specifies the amount of money sought for damages in a suit. Some states do not allow this clause to be included as part of a lawsuit.

3. The **comparative negligence doctrine** awards damages based on the percentage of responsibility for the result by each party.
4. **Contributory negligence** bars recovery of damages if there was negligence on the part of the plaintiff.
5. **Modified comparative fault** bars recovery of damages if the plaintiff's percentage of negligence exceeds 50%.

B. Bad Faith Action—The filing of a claim and pursuit of action regardless of the lack of reasonable grounds for filing the claim. In these circumstances the physician may countersue for damages.

C. Expert Testimony
1. The American Academy of Orthopaedic Surgeons' (AAOS) guidelines for expert testimony are that a physician must have:
   a. A current, valid, and unrestricted license to practice medicine in the applicable state
   b. Satisfactorily completed the educational requirements of the American Board of Orthopaedic Surgery or a recognized specialty board
   c. **Experience, education, or demonstrated competence in the subject of the case**
   d. Familiarity with clinical practice and applicable standard of care in orthopaedic surgery at the time of the incident
   e. Full awareness of all the pertinent facts and history of the case at the time of the incident
2. Expert testimony is used to determine the standard of care and whether a breach of conduct has occurred.
3. An orthopaedic treating physician has an ethical and legal responsibility to provide accurate and truthful testimony at a patient's request.
4. The expert should ensure the testimony is nonpartisan, scientifically correct, and clinically accurate. The expert should testify only to the facts and be prepared to provide documentation for the basis of testimony (personal experience, clinical references, currently accepted orthopaedic opinion).
5. It is unethical to accept compensation based on the outcome of the litigation; however, reasonable compensation commensurate with time and expertise is acceptable.

D. Res ipsa loquitor
1. Certain cases do not require expert testimony.
2. This is the legal doctrine of ***res ipsa loquitor*** ("the thing speaks for itself"). Examples of this are wrong-site surgery, surgical equipment inadvertently left in the patient, and failure of a physician to attend to a persistently complaining patient in distress.

E. Statute of Limitations—A plaintiff must file a malpractice suit within the statute of limitations.
1. Commonly, the **statute of limitations is 2 years**. However, this varies by state.
2. The statute of limitations for **minors** may also vary by state; it is generally **2 years from the time of the incident or until the individual's 18th birthday**.

F. Discovery
1. Discovery is the process by which both parties find out about each other's cases and is a period of information gathering.
2. Discovery is formed by several techniques of fact gathering.
   a. **Interrogatories**—Written questions answered in writing under oath.
   b. **Deposition**—Pretrial oral testimony given under oath.
   c. **Production Request**—Producing documents regarding a claim.
   d. **Request for Admission**—Admitting or denying factual statements under oath.

IV. Medical Records

A. Medical records represent the best defense in a malpractice lawsuit.
1. Medical records must be maintained for 7 years after the last date of treatment.
2. Medical records are confidential and cannot be reproduced or discussed with parties not involved in treating the patient without the patient's written approval.

B. Accurate and complete medical records protect both the patient and physician from errors and misinterpretations. Records should be:
1. Well documented, detailing the history, observations, reasons for treatment provided, and patient noncompliance
2. Legible and clear
3. Accurate and properly identify the patient
4. A logical sequence of the events and factors affecting treatment decisions

5. An outline of the treatment plan, including risks, benefits, and alternatives
6. Free from editorial comments or casual criticism of the patient or other health-care providers

C. Medical records should never be altered.
1. All corrections should be made by amendments. Amendments should accurately reflect the reason for correction and be placed following the last entry.
2. An errant entry should be lined through so that it remains legible. The reason for the correction, date, time, and physician's initials must be included.
3. Removing or obscuring an entry shatters credibility and is indefensible.
4. Attempts to supplement or clarify entries after notification of a lawsuit constitutes tampering.

D. On notification of a lawsuit, the medical records should be secured, inventoried, and copied. Copies of the medical record must be made available to the patient or the attorney in a reasonable amount of time. **The medical record must not be withheld as ransom for outstanding bills.**

V. Physician-Patient Relationship ("The Central Focus")

The *Code of Medical Ethics and Professionalism for Orthopaedic Surgeons states the following:*

"The physician-patient relationship has a contractual basis and is based on confidentiality, trust, and honesty. Both the patient and the orthopaedic surgeon are free to enter or discontinue the relationship within any existing constraints of a contract with a third party. An orthopaedic surgeon has an obligation to render care only for those conditions that he or she is competent to treat. The orthopaedist shall not decline to accept patients solely on the basis of race, color, gender, sexual orientation, religion, or national origin or on any basis that would constitute illegal discrimination." (Section IB)

A. The physician-patient relationship is a consensual relationship.
1. The relationship is established by a telephone call, a visit, or by the choice of a consultant from a provider list.
2. Rights and Responsibilities Related to the Relationship
   a. The patient has a right to courteous, confidential, and prompt treatment.
   b. The patient has the responsibility to be compliant with the treatment plan.
   c. Physicians have the responsibility to request appropriate consultation and to relinquish responsibility when the care of the patient reaches outside their scope of practice.
   d. Physicians must read their managed care contract before committing to the relationship. They must understand their legal responsibilities before executing an agreement to be supervising physicians for an allied health-care company.

B. Communication
1. Physicians who use empathy in their day-to-day interactions with patients increase the perception that they are caring and enhance their day-to-day enjoyment of medical practice.
2. Effective communication enhances patient compliance, increases quality of outcome, and is an excellent risk-management tool.
3. Time constraints make patient-focused communications skills very important. Key tools for effective communication are:
   a. Displaying empathy and respect
   b. Attentive listening
   c. Obtaining an accurate history of symptoms
   d. Explaining relevant facts, addressing concerns and fears, and honestly answering questions
   e. Empowering the patient or guardian by involving them in the medical-decision process
   f. Demonstrating cultural/ethnic sensitivity
4. Office staff interactions with the patient may have a direct effect on the physician-patient relationship.
   a. Having established policies and procedures to guide the patient through the system will foster a positive relationship.
   b. As an employer, hire wisely, supervise diligently, and weigh carefully the needs of your practice and your patients when hiring employees.

C. The Difficult Patient
1. Each patient's needs should be identified and focused on by the physician rather than responded to generally.
   a. Characterization of patients in terms such as "loser," "addict," "druggie," "troll," or "gomer" is stereotyping. Such terms divert the physician's attention from the issue that must be tackled with each individual.
   b. It is helpful to attempt to understand difficult patients by exploring the individual circumstances from the patient's perspective.
   c. Try to evaluate goals for care in terms that the patient would both agree with and understand.
   d. The physician may need to modify the aim. This may include the need at times to reformulate the focus from cure to incremental improvement or palliation.
2. Ending the Physician-Patient Relationship
   a. Physicians must always provide emergent treatment to patients.
   b. For patients with whom an insolvable conflict occurs, or for patients who can no longer pay for service, the physician may sever the physician-patient relationship so long as an alternative source of care can be identified.
   c. This is best accomplished in writing and should provide the patient with ample time to establish care with the new provider.

d. Medical records should be forwarded to the accepting physician, including a medical history and a summary of treatments rendered. Date of shipping and receipt of records should be documented.

D. Abandonment
  1. Wrongful termination of the physician-patient relationship consists of four basic elements.
     a. There must be an established physician-patient relationship.
     b. The patient must have a reasonable expectation that care will be provided.
     c. The patient must have a medical need that requires medical attention, the absence of which will result in harm or injury.
     d. Causation must be established. The failure to provide care must produce injury or harm.
  2. Abandonment may take many forms.
     a. It may be alleged that the patient's follow-up is inadequate to recognize common complications.
     b. Failure to provide an appointment to an established patient even if the patient has not paid previous bills, has missed other appointments, has been noncompliant, or has sought interim care from another provider.
     c. Premature discharge from an inpatient setting.
     d. If illness, personal conflict, or vacation prevents the physician from attending to patient care, immediate notice must be issued to allow the patient the opportunity to seek care elsewhere.
     e. If a patient does not appear for important follow-up appointments, a certified letter should be sent instructing the patient to follow-up.

E. Medical Referrals
  1. A medical referral aims to obtain services that the referring physician is unable to render to the patient.
     a. Selection of a consultant should be based primarily on the consultant's ability to handle the patient's clinical care.
     b. Choice of a consultant involves not only consideration of technical skill but also the elements of the physician-patient relationship, insurance type accepted by the consultant, and perhaps even factors such as gender or ethnicity.
     c. Under no circumstances should consideration be influenced by factors such as kickbacks.
     d. Monetary compensation in exchange for referrals is illegal.
     e. It is also unacceptable for the primary care physician to choose a consultant incapable of providing the necessary care just because that consultant was picked by a health plan.
     f. It is the physician's responsibilities to ensure that health plans to which they subscribe permit adequate access to qualified specialists. If not, the physicians must lobby for referral outside their panel.

VI. Malpractice Insurance

A. There are two basic types of malpractice insurance: occurrence and claims made.
  1. **Occurrence coverage** covers the insured for all claims resulting from action during the period of employment covered by the policy, regardless of when the claim is filed. It continues to cover the physician for occurrences during a specific period even after the physician has ceased working at that particular job/location.
  2. **Claims-made coverage** covers the insured during a particular period of employment covered by the policy. Claims filed after the expiration of the policy (usually when the physician leaves a particular job/employer) are not covered even if the events occurred during the period of coverage.
     a. **Tail coverage** is a separate policy that covers the physician for all claims made for actions occurring during the period of coverage; this essentially makes an occurrence policy.
     b. **Prior acts coverage** protects the insured from claims resulting from events for which claims have yet to be filed.
     c. **Locum tenens coverage** is coverage that is extended to a physician temporarily replacing the policyholder.
     d. **Slot coverage** covers duties encountered while practicing in a specific position through which several physicians may rotate.

B. Policies may have specific restrictions or exclusions.
  1. Some policies cover only direct patient care.
  2. Activities such as peer review, quality assurance, and utilization review may be covered by the insurance policy or by a health-care contract.
  3. **Nearly all resident/fellow policies have an exclusion for moonlighting.** The resident or fellow must ensure that either the institution where they are moonlighting provides coverage or they should purchase professional liability insurance on their own behalf.
  4. **Hold Harmless Clause**—This contractual statement attempts to shift liability from the employer to the physician. Insurance carriers do not generally cover this contractual obligation.

E. **Surcharging or Experience Rating**—Insurance plans may assess points against a physician based on the number of claims filed and dollar amounts awarded on behalf of the insured.

F. **The Good Samaritan Act**—This act grants immunity for good faith acts performed by persons at the scene of an emergency. Immunity is not given if the act constitutes gross, willful, or wanton neglect. This does not extend to care given in expectation of payment by persons who routinely render care in an emergency room or by the patient's admitting, attending, or treating physician.

G. The AAOS recommends that a resident or fellow make a point of obtaining evidence of insurance for each year of residency and saving this evidence in personal files.

VII. Special Liability Status of Residents and Fellows—The status of residents and fellows as licensed physicians who are functioning as employees while in a training/educational program creates a special relationship between them and their patients and supervisors.

A. Failure to inform a patient of residency/fellow status may result in claims of fraud, deceit, misrepresentation, assault, battery, and lack of informed consent.

B. Residents and fellows are responsible for their own actions. In addition, their supervisors may also be held accountable for the actions of their residents and fellows. This is known as **vicarious liability**.

C. **Respondeat Superior**—An agency relationship is established from the fact that the resident has been authorized to act for or represent the supervising physician. As an agent for the supervisor, all acts of the relationship are considered to be under the direction of the supervisor. This term means, "Let the master answer." This doctrine is also known as "borrowed servant" or the "captain of the ship." This relationship is independent of the specific employer of the trainee.

D. **Residents and fellows are held to the same standard of care as a fully trained practicing orthopaedist, regardless of their level of training.** Residents should not attempt to perform procedures that are beyond their level of training. Appropriate consultation with their supervisor is imperative in any situation. Lack of appropriate consultation puts the resident at risk of acting independent of the supervisor.

The AAOS recommends that residents and fellows permanently retain documentation regarding the resolution of any adverse decision in which they may be named. Adverse decisions will be reported to the National Practitioner Data Bank, and this information made available to all health-care facilities, as will any pending litigation. Documentation regarding the individual cases and information on the resolution of adverse decisions will be necessary when the individual seeks privileges at any health-care facility.

VIII. HIV Testing and Treatment of the HIV-Infected Patient.

A. Some states mandate that explicit informed consent is required for HIV testing.

B. The AAOS has adopted a policy that HIV testing of hospitalized patients be performed in the same unrestricted manner as any other lab test at the order of the attending physician, without specific consent.

C. The AAOS advocates state and federal legislation consistent with the aforementioned policy.

D. HIV testing may have substantial social and economic consequences for the individual who tests positive.

E. Performing Procedures on Patients Who Are HIV-Infected

1. Avoiding procedures would diminish a patient's access to necessary medical care and in almost all cases is ethically unacceptable.
2. The physician has a fiduciary responsibility to act in the best interest of his or her patient, but this does not include actions that place the physician at substantial risk.
3. It has been shown that many physicians overestimate their risk of HIV transmission from a patient.
4. To decide whether a particular surgical procedure places an undue risk on the surgeon and the operative team, the surgeon must attempt to accurately gauge the actual risk associated with the patient.

VIII. Industry and the Orthopaedic Surgeon

Medicine and industry work together in improving the treatment of patients. This relationship is even more pronounced in orthopaedics because of the required implants, materials, and techniques. Ethical conduct demands that the educational support of the orthopaedist by industry is not excessive, does not profit the company directly, and has the purpose of improving patient care through education. The *Code of Medical Ethics and Professionalism For Orthopaedic Surgeons* states:

"The practice of medicine inherently presents potential conflicts of interest. When a conflict of interest arises, it must be resolved in the best interest of the patient. The orthopaedic surgeon should exercise all reasonable alternatives to ensure that the most appropriate care is provided to the patient. If the conflict of interest cannot be resolved, the orthopaedic surgeon should notify the patient of his or her intention to withdraw from the relationship."

A. Guidelines

1. Gifts or financial support from the industry should primarily benefit the patient and in no way should influence treatment decisions.
2. Gifts with "strings" attached should not be accepted.

3. Social functions not associated with an educational element should not be offered to or accepted by orthopaedic surgeons.
4. Cash gifts should be neither offered nor accepted.
5. Continuing medical education (CME) subsidies that support educational programs (CME credits provided) are acceptable when they improve patient care. **Educational subsidies should not be applied to personal expenses (travel, lodging) for attendees.** Any subsidy should be paid directly to the conference sponsor.
6. Faculty at CME courses may accept reasonable honoraria and reimbursement for travel, lodging, and meal expenses.
7. Educational events not tied to CME credits are acceptable at the discretion of the orthopaedic surgeon. Potential for conflict of interest exists in these circumstances and the surgeon must use sound ethical judgment when evaluating and considering such offers.
8. Genuine consultants may accept reasonable honoraria and reimbursement for travel, lodging, and meal expenses.
9. Scholarships to allow residents or fellows to attend CME courses are permitted. Selection for those attending must be made by the residents or fellows program director.

B. Loyalties and Conflicts of Interest
1. The physician's role is to use his or her expertise to select the best possible orthopaedic hardware, medication, or treatment for a particular patient's needs. Decisions should be based on:
   a. Clinical trials in the published medical literature
   b. The clinician's expertise
   c. The clinician's perspective of the patient's preference
   d. Monetary issues, which should enter into the decision process in the realm of cost effectiveness
      (1) Monetary considerations may include limitations of the patient's resources or needs.
      (2) There is no role in this decision for consideration of factors that benefit the physician. This is particularly true for financial compensation.
2. Compensation may potentially affect a physician's decision making concerning the choice of particular hardware, medication, or treatment. **In this circumstance the physician must disclose to the patient that he or she receives this financial compensation.**
3. In circumstances in which a physician has developed a novel therapeutic modality that is clearly superior to anything else available, the clinician might state to the patient, "I participated in development of this product and receive compensation for its use. Based on published clinical trials and in my opinion, it is the best product for your use."
4. Any financial relationship or ownership in a durable medical goods provider, imaging center, surgery center, or other health care facility must be disclosed to the patient if not immediately obvious.

C. Advertising
1. Federal and state antitrust laws protect truthful advertising.
2. Truthful advertising must not contain any overtly false claim nor imply a false claim that would affect a reasonably prudent person. It should include only claims that can be substantiated by the physician and not omit any fact that would influence a reasonably prudent person.
3. Claims should be representative of expected results for the average patient.
4. Care should be exercised when using terms such as "safe and effective," because the layperson equates these terms with no risk and a guarantee of a good result.
5. Advertising of physicians' qualifications should reflect the amount of formal training and degree of expertise and competence.

D. Royalties
1. Similar to financial interests, any items of money, including royalties received from a manufacturer, must be disclosed to the patient.
2. It is unethical to receive any payment (excluding royalties) from the manufacturer for the use of its product.
3. It is unethical for the physician to agree to exclusively use a product for which the physician receives royalties.

E. Patents—The nature of medical practice builds on innovations and ideas, and to claim exclusive rights to a procedure denies all former individual contributions.The additional fallout from such patents would limit medical education, increase the cost of delivered services, and jeopardize the quality of patient care. The AAOS states that procedure patents are unethical.

F. Second Opinions—Definition of specific relationships between physicians and their responsibilities to their colleagues and patients can avoid inappropriate actions. Clear and direct communication between parties involved can eliminate most problems.
1. **Consultation** implies that the treating physician retains care for the patient but is requesting additional diagnostic or treatment expertise from the consultant. **It is unethical for the consulting physician to solicit care of a patient** or to make slanderous accusations about the referring physician.

2. **Referral** implies the treating physician desires to share care of the patient for a specific service. This request may be temporary or permanent and should be made clear at the outset by the physicians involved.
3. **Transfer** by the treating physician implies complete transfer of care to the accepting physician. All transfers must be made with the consent of the patient.
4. Second opinions secured by third-party payers before authorizing procedures are usually governed by contractual agreements. The physician must be aware of provisions in the contract regarding assumption of care.

IX. Research—Clinical and basic research provides a tremendous opportunity for improvement of the diagnosis and treatment of orthopaedic disease.

A. Ethical research is conducted when the primary goal is to improve methods of detection or treatment of illness. It should be designed to produce useful, reproducible information and should not be redundant or serve to further individuals or institutions financially or professionally.

B. Results should be reported honestly, accurately, and in a timely fashion. Misrepresentation or falsifying data is unethical.

C. Withholding critical information to protect financial interest may create an ethical conflict and jeopardize patient care.

D. Sponsorship by industry has represented a potential conflict of interest or bias; however, significant developments have been made possible by their involvement, and this form of cooperative effort is gaining acceptance. Specific ethical problems arise with this type of research funding.
1. Financial interests of the researcher through stock holdings, stock options, or profit-sharing agreements with the funding corporation may introduce bias or jeopardize objectivity in reporting results.
2. It is unethical once a researcher is involved in a project funded by a corporation to buy or sell the corporation's stock until the project is complete or results are made a matter of public record.
3. All areas of corporate involvement, including resources, materials, and sponsorship, must be disclosed as part of reporting results.
4. Researchers may be retained as consultants or lecturers but compensation must be commensurate with his or her actual efforts.

E. **Human research subjects must provide voluntary informed consent before participating** in any research protocol. Their medical care must not be contingent on their participation, and they must be allowed to withdraw from the study at any time without penalty. Each subject must be able to demonstrate understanding of the information and the ability to make a responsible decision. The decision must be voluntary and not the result of undue pressure or influence. A voluntary informed consent must include the following:
1. An explanation of the proposed procedure
2. Likely effects and risks of the procedure
3. An explanation of possible side effects in language easily understood by the patient
4. Methods and conditions of participation

F. Animal Use in Research
1. The AAOS states the humane use of animals in research is justified to enhance the quality of life of both humans and animals.
2. The use of animals is only ethical when no suitable alternatives are available.
3. Protocols should be designed to minimize the number of animals used. The animals must be utilized in a manner that avoids abuse and maintains all appropriate animal care standards.
4. Animal Care and Use Committee approval is mandatory as is following all applicable regulations and standards.

G. Responsibilities of the Principal Investigator (PI) and Coauthors
1. The PI remains responsible for all aspects of the research project, even when duties have been delegated to others.
2. The PI is also responsible for accurately representing efforts of individuals or agencies involved in the research and citing contributions from other researchers or publications.
3. **Coauthors must have made a significant contribution to the design of, collection of data for, and forming of the research project.**
4. Each coauthor should sign an affidavit stating that he or she has reviewed the manuscript and agrees with all results and conclusions presented therein before publication.
5. Resident research should be conducted under the supervision of an attending surgeon. However, the attending surgeon must contribute to the work in actual fact or in a consultative capacity.

H. Scientific Publications—Scientific publications create information that affects other research and direct care of patients. If error in scientific method, or failure to replicate results is found, the PI is responsible for accurately reporting this.

I. World Medical Association Declaration of Helsinki (October 2000)
1. Written by the World Medical Association to provide ethical guidance for medical research.
2. Based on the duty of a physician to "promote and safeguard the health of the people."

X. The Impaired Physician

A. A surgeon (resident, fellow, or attending) who discovers chemical impairment, dependence, or incompetence in a colleague or supervisor has the responsibility to ensure the problem is identified and treated.

B. Mechanisms exist for the proper identification and treatment of the impaired physician.

C. Misconduct can be reported to state and local agencies. One must be sure to act in good faith with reasonable evidence when reporting such incidences.

D. If a patient is at risk for immediate harm or injury by an impaired physician, one should assert authority and relieve the physician of the patient care and then address the problem with the senior hospital staff as soon as possible.

XI. Sexual Misconduct—Sexual misconduct in a physician's relationships with patients, co-workers, staff, or colleagues cannot be tolerated. Sexual relationships between individuals while maintaining a professional supervisor/trainee relationship, even if consensual, create the potential for sexual exploitation and the loss of objectivity. Supervisors may need to be reassigned or responsibilities may need to be modified to avoid potential conflict.

A. Sexual harassment can be characterized as
   1. Quid Pro Quo—Harassment is directly linked to employment or advancement.
   2. Hostile Environment Harassment—Verbal or physical conduct (gestures, innuendo, humor, pictures, etc.) of a sexual nature or a general hostility due to gender that promotes a hostile environment in the workplace. Actual sexual advances are not necessary to create a hostile work environment.

B. The adopted standard for offensive behavior is the "reasonable woman" test. If a reasonable woman would have found the behavior objectionable, then harassment may have occurred.

C. Individuals in medical training programs are considered employees of the school that is training them. This status allows them to pursue harassment claims under the Civil Rights Act.

D. Sexual Misconduct with Patients
   1. This is simply a form of sexual exploitation.
   2. Such misconduct is unethical and may represent malpractice or even criminal acts of assault. Courts have maintained that a patient is unable to give meaningful consent to sexual or romantic advances.
   3. Physicians are encouraged to report instances of sexual misconduct by their colleagues.
   4. Many states have laws prohibiting physicians from pursuing relationships with current or former patients.
      a. These laws protect the patient from exploitation.
      b. They help the physician to maintain objectivity in diagnosis and treatment.

E. The physician-patient relationship must be terminated before pursuing any romantic interest. Even then, it may still be unethical if the physician exploits certain confidences, trust, or emotions learned while serving as the patient's physician. The Academy recommends consultation with a colleague before initiating a relationship with a former patient.

XII. Violence—Each year intentional violence claims 20,000 lives, is responsible for more than 300,000 hospitalizations, and causes millions of injuries. It is estimated that 1.4 million children in the United States suffer some form of maltreatment each year. As many as 2000 children die each year from abuse.

The U.S. Child Abuse Prevention and Treatment Act of 1974 requires orthopaedic surgeons to report all suspected cases of child abuse to local authorities. Failure to report suspected child abuse might result in state disciplinary actions.

A. Child protective services and social workers should be alerted and the events and home circumstances should be investigated.

B. These statutes provide immunity for physicians when reporting such cases provided they act in good faith, even if the information is protected by the physician-patient privilege.

C. Elderly abuse has been estimated to affect 2 million older Americans each year. A 1989 Congressional study indicated that 1 of every 25 Americans over age 65 suffers some serious form of abuse, neglect, or exploitation. Many states have provided legislation to protect physicians who report elderly abuse from liability.

D. Reporting of spousal abuse is not protected. A physician may encourage a patient to pursue such measures. If the physician believes that an individual is truly incapable of self-protection, then a court order may be obtained to permit reporting.

XIII. Managed Care—Health maintenance organizations (HMOs) have become increasingly prevalent. A large number of persons with health insurance are enrolled in HMOs. This shift has necessitated physician groups to contract with HMOs. HMOs are shifting to create direct access to certain specialties. Orthopaedics is a specialty that lends itself to direct contracting with managed care groups. To re-establish both economic control and clinical autonomy, many physicians are forming alliances to compete for and negotiate contracts with HMOs. The following ethical considerations are from the AAOS: *Opinions on Ethics and Professionalism: The Orthopaedic Surgeon in the Managed Care Setting.*

A. Prior to joining a managed care organization (MCO) the surgeon should be fully aware of the utilization guidelines and reimbursement policies to ensure the patient's welfare remains at the forefront.

B. The obligation to ensure the patient's welfare remains in this setting.

C. All interactions should be conducted in a professional manner to ensure that the psychologic and physical welfare of the patient is preserved.

D. Cost is an ethical consideration in determining appropriate treatment plans.
E. The surgeon has the ethical responsibility to practice within the scope of their training and experience.
F. Once engaged in care the surgeon has the responsibility to continue to provide appropriate care within the limits established by the MCO.
G. According to sound ethical principle, the surgeon should report any unethical conduct by the members or administration of the MCO.
H. The surgeon also has the ethical responsibility to be an educator of musculoskeletal care within the MCO.

XIV. Physician Statements by the AAOS

A. Regarding the scope of orthopaedic practice and the managed care arrangement:
   1. The AAOS opposes any arrangement in which orthopaedic surgeons are excluded from the provision of musculoskeletal care.
   2. The AAOS approves immediate performance and interpretation of diagnostic imaging and studies.
   3. The AAOS opposes any policy that prohibits orthopaedists from performing x-ray studies. Orthopaedists are entitled to adequate compensation for their interpretation of diagnostic imaging studies.
B. Regarding second opinions, both the patient and the orthopaedist are free to enter or discontinue the relationship with any existing contract with a third party.
C. **Regarding Discovery of Wrong-Site Surgery**
   1. If after the surgical procedure it is determined that the surgery was performed at the wrong site, as soon as reasonably possible the surgeon should discuss the mistake with the patient and, if appropriate, with the patient's family and recommend an immediate plan to rectify the mistake unless there is a medical reason not to proceed.

SECTION 2

Statistics

I. Introduction to Statistics—As a consumer of medical research, the orthopaedic surgeon needs to have a firm grasp of statistical concepts. The ability to discern superior from inferior research allows the surgeon to make sound clinical decisions and enhance surgical outcomes. An ability to understand statistics allows a surgeon to generalize with confidence about a given population based on the study of a small subset of that population. It enables critical evaluation of large chunks of data by reducing them to understandable indices.

A. Basic Terminology

1. **Basic Terminology in Design**

a. **Hypothesis**—A supposition or unproved theory.

(1) The research hypothesis is the theory believed to be true.

(2) The null hypothesis is the opposite of the research hypothesis.

b. **Theory**—A hypothesis with proof; a grouping of relationships based on scientific proof.

c. **Natural Law**—A collection of proven theories; an event or occurrence that has been proved to occur in a specific manner in a given set of circumstances.

d. **Population**—A collection of all possible measurements that could be used to address a hypothesis.

e. **Sample**—A subset of the population.

(1) Samples should be random; that is, all members of the population should have an equal chance of being selected to ensure the sample is representative of the population as a whole. Non-random samples introduce bias into the study.

f. **Bias**—A flaw in impartiality that alters the manner in which measurement, analysis, or assessment is recorded, conducted, or interpreted. Ways to minimize the introduction of bias into a study include randomization, masking (formerly referred to as blinding), and meticulous attention to the study protocol.

(1) Selection bias is introduced by a non-random selection of a sample from a given population.

(2) Observational or informational bias occurs when a measurement/outcome is affected by the characteristics of the study group itself.

g. **Confounding Factors**—Variables that can interfere with the researcher's ability to draw statistically valid conclusions. Matching (see following definition) is a strategy to minimize the effect of confounding factors. Always try to minimize bias and confounding factors to increase the strength of a study.

h. **Efficacy**—A term important in outcomes research that refers to a treatment working under ideal conditions.

i. **Effectiveness**—Another term important in outcomes research that refers to how a treatment works in real-world conditions.

j. **Inclusion/Exclusion Criteria**—Criteria determined during experimental design that define the study population.

k. **Randomization**—Minimizes confounding variables to equalize them in all small groups.

l. **Accuracy**—This tests the issue of data differentiation. The ideal test is always accurate.

m. **Precision**—The ability to repeat measurements accurately.

n. **Matching**—Matching controls decreases confounding variables. For example, all people with the same age are put together in a study.

o. **Instrument**—A measurement tool.

2. **Basic Terminology in Assessment**

Once a study has been evaluated or designed using the preceding principles, then the manner in which the data are subsequently collected or interpreted must be designed or assessed. This leads to the principle of accuracy: specifically, the ability to correctly identify data collected or evaluated by a study. The concept of precision is slightly different; it is the ability to arrive at the same data point with repeated testing. Other critical concepts in assessment of tests are sensitivity, specificity, positive predictive value, and negative predictive value.

a. **Sensitivity**—The ability of a test to detect that which is truly positive.

Sensitivity

$$= \frac{\text{All positive test results}}{\text{All specimens with condition present}} \times 100$$

b. **Specificity**—The ability to detect that which is truly negative.

Specificity

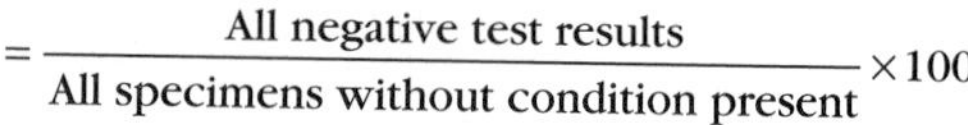

$$= \frac{\text{All negative test results}}{\text{All specimens without condition present}} \times 100$$

c. Positive predictive value—The chance that a condition is present if identified by a positive test.

Positive Predictive Value

$$= \frac{\text{All positive test results with condition present}}{\text{All positive test results}} \times 100$$

d. Negative predictive value—The opposite of positive predictive value, the chance that a condition is not present as identified by a negative test result.

Negative Predictive Value

$$= \frac{\text{All negative test results without condition present}}{\text{All negative test results}} \times 100$$

When dealing with a clinical condition, it is important to remember that these concepts are intimately intertwined. As the sensitivity of a test increases, the negative predictive value increases, a desirable trait for a screening test for an uncommon condition. If a condition is common, then a test with higher specificity and subsequently a higher positive predictive value is more desirable.

B. Statistical Power/Power Analysis—Accepting or rejecting the null hypothesis is the basic thrust of all scientific studies. The research hypothesis becomes that which the scientist theorizes to be true. The null hypothesis is the antithesis; it is that which the scientist hopes to statistically reject. The scientist may be correct or incorrect.

1. **Type I and Alpha Errors—Rejecting a true null hypothesis/false positive**—In this case the scientist's research hypothesis was erroneously accepted as positive; hence a false-positive result. The probability of committing a type I error is the P-value. Alpha is the frequency of occurrence of a type I error. **Protect against alpha error with significance levels.**
2. **Type II and Beta Errors—Accepting a false null hypothesis/false negative**—The scientist has erroneously accepted a negative null hypothesis; hence a false-negative result. Beta signifies the frequency of a type II error occurring. Protect against beta error with statistical power. Alpha and beta are inversely related.
3. Power—Power is the likelihood that a statistically significant difference would be found between two groups given that a difference truly did exist. Increasing sample size and improving experimental design can maximize power. Sample size is the number of subjects in a study population. A **power analysis** is a statistical process experimenters use to determine the sample size that allows them to make statistically valid conclusions based on a study design. A simple estimate of sample size can be determined using the rule of three: if a condition has an occurrence of 1 in 10, then the researcher needs a population three times this number (30) for a statistically significant study.

Probability mathematics allows one to quantify uncertainty and randomness. There are many different statistical tests that can be used to arrive at a probability statement, or P-value, for a given study design. The P-value is defined as the probability that the null hypothesis is true; thus it is the probability of the researcher committing a type I error. The stated P-value in a study alerts the reader of the magnitude of chance that the study arrived at the conclusion serendipitously. This sets the criteria of rejecting the null hypothesis and is known as significance level. It is imperative to note that the chance of making a conclusion by chance alone increases in a multiple-comparison study, and the P-value should be adjusted downward.

C. Hypothesis Testing—P-values less than 0.05 are generally accepted as statistically significant. A P-value less than a given number assigns statistical significance to a finding. This, however, does not immediately assign clinical significance to a finding. This is where the idea of confidence intervals assists critical evaluation of a study. Based on a normal distribution, the 95% confidence interval means all values falling within $\pm \approx 2$ standard deviations (SDs) from the mean. A confidence interval is the range of values that includes the true value within a given probability (usually 95%).

D. Statistical Tests

1. Discrete data is also known as noncontinuous, categorical, or qualitative. This type of data is defined by its ability to be placed into specific categories. It is statistically evaluated using P-values, the chi-square test, and Fisher's exact test. The chi-square test concerns the frequency with which an observation occurs and is used to evaluate discrete data to generate a P-value. Fisher's exact test generates a more conservative estimate of the P-value and is used when the study numbers are small.
2. Continuous data vary over a continuous range. Continuous data are evaluated using these statistical measures: central tendency, variation, and distribution of the data. Tests for continuous data include the one-sample t-test, the independent two-sample t-test, the paired t-test, and the analysis of variance (ANOVA) test. T-tests were developed by W.S. Gosset, writing under the pseudonym of Student, and may be referred to as the Student's t-tests.
   a. One-Sample T-Test—Compares the sample mean value to a known mean of a standard variable. This test calculates a t-value that is used to obtain a P-value from a statistics chart.
   b. Two-Sample T-Test—Compares the mean values with two independent groups. The paired t-test allows comparison between two dependent samples.
   c. ANOVA—Simply an extension of the t-test and allows determination of a statistically

significant difference in the mean values when more than two independent groups are being compared. It relies on two sources of variation: between group and within group.

d. These statistical tests represent only the most basic of statistical procedures; the careful investigator will enlist the aid of a trained statistician to assist in data analysis.

E. The Normal Distribution—This is a key concept to understand. Normal is a statistical concept; it is not related to an anatomic condition or disease state. Some refer to the normal distribution as Gaussian distribution to avoid such confusion (Fig. 12-1). The normal distribution is a theoretic probability distribution determined by two quantities, the mean and SD. The mean is the numeric sum of all the values divided by the number of values. The SD is simply the square root of the variance, where variance is the mean of the squared deviations about the mean of the data. Changing the mean shifts the entire curve along the x-axis (abscissa), whereas changing the SD changes the width of the curve along the x-axis. The normal distribution is unimodal, bell-shaped, and symmetric at a horizontal line equal to the mean value. Virtually all observations in a normal distribution occur within mean ± 3 SD, 95% within mean ± 2 SD, and two-thirds within mean ± 1 SD. The mean is a measure of central tendency.

F. Terms
1. Median—The middlemost observation.
2. Mode—The most frequently occurring observation.
3. Standard Deviation—A measure of spread or variation.
4. Range—The highest minus lowest value.
5. Mean Deviation—The average value of all deviation from the mean.
6. Variance—The average of the squares of each observation's deviation from the mean.
7. Standard Error of the Mean—When comparing different samples with different means, the standard error of the mean must be used, which is the SD of the distribution of sample means.

G. Correlation analysis and regression analysis refer to methods by which two variables are shown to be related.
1. Correlation analysis gives a value that allows assessing the extent to which two sets of data or variables are related.
2. Regression analysis uses a mathematical equation to calculate approximate values of a variable from known values of another variable.

H. Validity and Reliability
1. Reliability refers to the ability to repeat a study's measurements and get the same results.
   a. Intra-observer and inter-observer error can affect reliability and must be adequately accounted for and controlled within the experimental design.
2. Validity refers to the extent to which an experimental value represents a true value.
   a. The study of biologic systems introduces biologic variability into an investigation.
   b. The ANOVA test distinguishes biologic variability from measurement error and provides a reliability coefficient/interclass correlation coefficient.

II. Types of Statistical Studies

A. Descriptive—Descriptive studies take available data and arrange and present them to highlight or demonstrate differences or significant findings. These studies cannot show cause-and-effect relationships, but they are highly useful in showing

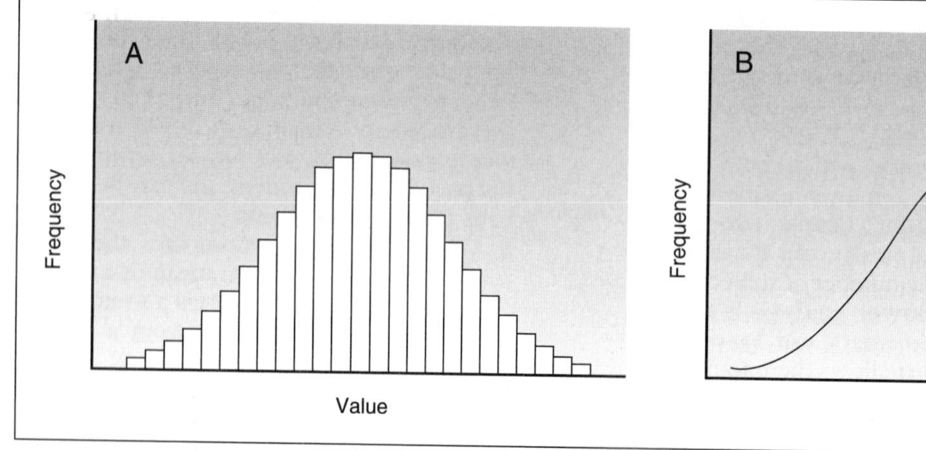

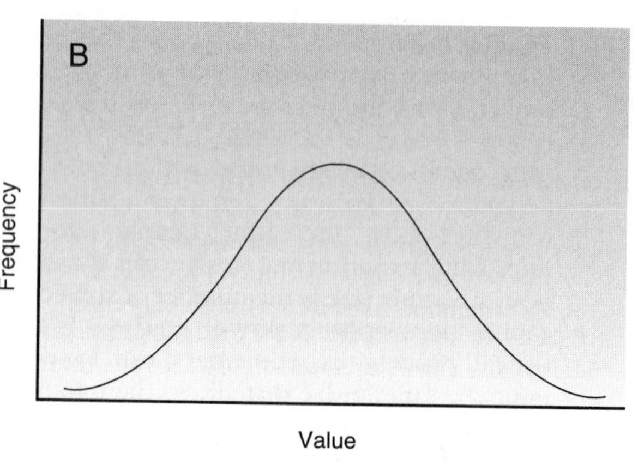

FIGURE 12-1 ■ Normal (Gaussian) distribution. *A*, Probability distribution of actual data, plotted as a histogram with very narrow ranges. *B*, The simplified way this idea is represented in textbooks, articles, and tests. (From Jekel, J.F., Elmore, J.G., and Katz, D.L.: Epidemiology, Biostatistics, and Preventive Medicine. Philadelphia, WB Saunders, 1996.)

associations or generating a research hypothesis that may be studied further.

1. Case Reports and Case Series—A case report is a presentation/description of a disease or condition that occurred in one patient. Case series present information from multiple patients with a similar disease or condition. These generate speculative associations, which can be further tested by analytic studies.
2. Correlational Studies—Studies that use very large sample sizes to identify associations between a disease or injury and another studied variable. Correlational studies are best used to generate a research hypothesis and a worthy study, but no conclusions can be drawn from them.
3. Cross-Sectional Studies—This type of study evaluates a group at one point in time. Often described as a "snapshot" of a population or sample. Causal links between diagnosis and variables are found, but no conclusions are drawn.

B. Analytic—Analytic studies are designed to compare exposures to risk factors with disease states. They allow hypothesis testing and statistical analysis. The two major types of analytic studies are cohort and experimental. Cohort studies are those in which the researcher does not influence or alter the conditions of the group being studied. The researcher is an observer who records occurrences as they happen. In experimental studies, the researcher is actively involved in controlling and altering the conditions of the group as a part of the experimental design or protocol.

1. **Case Control**—Subjects in the study group are chosen based on the presence of an injury or the presence of a disease. The group is then analyzed to identify associated, clinically relevant information. Case-control studies by definition begin with a population and its disease and cannot be evaluated prospectively to determine exposure.
2. **Prospective Cohort Study**—A study in which a group of disease-free subjects is followed over time to identify onset of disease or injury. This type of study identifies incidence. Cohort studies are useful for establishing relative risk.
3. **Meta-Analysis**—The combining of several smaller cohort studies into one larger cohort to examine treatment and outcome variables.
4. Survival Analysis—A type of cohort study where outcome is plotted over time.
5. Outcomes Research—A branch of clinical epidemiology that makes a scientific measurement of the effect of a condition on the life of a patient. The data are reported in a way that allows comparison with the work of other investigators. The rising cost of health care, varying regional practice patterns, and poor methods of clinical research in the past have spawned the recent interest in outcomes research.
6. Interventional Study—Also known as a clinical trial and involves the testing of an intervention. The gold standard of studies is the randomized, blind clinical trial. This type of study is usually designed to minimize the impact of bias and confounding factors.

III. Epidemiology

A. Epidemiology is the study of the frequency and cause of disease in human populations. The terminology of this field permeates the medical literature and therefore an understanding of these terms is critical in the evaluation and design of experiments. Concepts such as prevalence and incidence measure the frequency of disease within a given population. Measures of disease association, such as relative risk and the odds ratio, allow definition of the relationship between exposure to a risk factor and the disease or condition studied.

1. Prevalence—The total number of affected individuals at a single point in time divided by the total number of individuals at risk for the disease or condition in a population.
2. Incidence—The number of new cases of the disease or condition that arise during a specified time interval.
3. Cumulative Incidence—The incidence (new cases that develop over time) divided by the total number of individuals at risk for the disease or condition in a population. (It does not account for varying time periods.)
4. Incidence Rate—The number of new cases in a specified time interval divided by the population at risk but without disease. It gives a far better estimation of the significance of exposure.
5. Relative Risk—The incidence in the exposed group divided by the incidence in the unexposed group. Relative risk can be approximated retrospectively by calculating the odds ratio. As the relative risk approaches 1, the incidence rates of both groups reach equality. Above 1, a positive correlation between the risk and the condition being studied exists. Below 1, the exposure is exerting a protective effect on the population being exposed.
6. Odds Ratio—The odds of exposure in those with the condition/disease compared with the odds in those without disease.

Selected Bibliography

American Academy of Orthopaedic Surgeons: Advisory Statement: Orthopaedic Medical Testimony. February 2001.

American Academy of Orthopaedic Surgeons: Advisory Statement: The Importance of Good Communication in the Physician-Patient Relationship. 2002.

American Academy of Orthopaedic Surgeons: Code of Medical Ethics and Professionalism for Orthopaedic Surgeons. October 1988, revised May 2002.

American Academy of Orthopaedic Surgeons: Opinions on Ethics and Professionalism: Advertising by Orthopaedic Surgeons. May 2002.

American Academy of Orthopaedic Surgeons: Opinions on Ethics and Professionalism: Ethics in Health Research in Orthopaedic Surgery. May 2002.

American Academy of Orthopaedic Surgeons: Opinions on Ethics and Professionalism: Gifts and the Orthopaedic Surgeon's Responsibility with Industry. May 2002.

American Academy of Orthopaedic Surgeons: Opinions on Ethics and Professionalism: Medical and Surgical Procedure Patents. May 2002.

American Academy of Orthopaedic Surgeons: Opinions on Ethics and Professionalism: Reporting of Suspected Abuse or Neglect of Children, Disabled Adults, or the Elderly. May 2002.

American Academy of Orthopaedic Surgeons: Opinions on Ethics and Professionalism: Sexual Harassment and Exploitation. May 2002.

American Academy of Orthopaedic Surgeons: Opinions on Ethics and Professionalism: Sexual Misconduct in the Physician-Patient Relationship. May 2002.

American Academy of Orthopaedic Surgeons: Opinions on Ethics and Professionalism: Second or Additional Medical Opinions in Orthopaedic Surgery. May 2002.

American Academy of Orthopaedic Surgeons: Opinions on Ethics and Professionalism: The Orthopaedic Surgeon in the Managed Care Setting. May 2002.

American Academy of Orthopaedic Surgeons: Principles of Medical Ethics and Professionalism in Orthopaedic Surgery. December 1995.

Brickmeyer, N.J., and Weinstein, J.N.: Clinical epidemiology. In Beaty, J.H., ed.: Orthopaedic Knowledge Update 6. Am. Acad. Orthop. Surg. 89–95, 1999.

Colton, T.: Statistics in Medicine. Boston, Little Brown & Co., 1974.

Committee on Professional Liability: Guide to the Ethical Practice of Orthopaedic Surgery, 3rd ed. Rosemont, IL, AAOS, 1998.

Committee on Professional Liability: Managing Orthopaedic Malpractice Risk. Rosemont, IL, AAOS, 1996.

Committee on Professional Liability: Medical Malpractice: A Primer for Orthopaedic Residents and Fellows. Rosemont, IL, AAOS, 1993.

Dawson-Saunders, B., and Trapp, R.G., eds.: Basic and Clinical Biostatistics. Norwalk, Conn, Appleton & Lange, 1990.

Elam, K., Taylor, V., Ciol, M.A., et al.: Impact of a workers' compensation practice guideline on lumbar spine fusion in Washington state. Med. Care 35:417–424, 1997.

Ellrodt, G., Cook, D.J., Lee, J., et al.: Evidence-based disease management. J.A.M.A. 278:1687–1692, 1997.

Ellwood, P.M.: Shattuck lecture: Outcomes management, a technique of patient experience. N. Engl. J. Med. 318:1549–1556, 1988.

Epstein, A.M.: The outcomes movement: Will it get us where we want to go? N. Engl. J. Med. 323:266–270, 1990.

Feinstein, A.R., ed.: Clinical Epidemiology: The Architecture of Clinical Research. Philadelphia, WB Saunders, 1985.

Ficarra, B.: Medicolegal Examination, Evaluation, and Report. Florida, CRC Press Inc., 1987.

Fletcher, R.H., Fletcher, S.W., and Wagner, E.H., eds.: Clinical Epidemiology: The Essentials, 2nd ed. Baltimore, Williams & Wilkins, 1988.

Gartland, J.J.: Orthopaedic clinical research: Deficiencies in experimental design and determinations of outcome. J. Bone Joint Surg. [Am.] 70:1357–1364, 1988.

Gottlieb, S., and Einhorn, T.: Beyond HMOs: Understanding the next wave of changes in health-care organization. J. Am. Assoc. Orthop. Surg. 6:75–83, 1998.

Greenfield, M.V., Kuhn, J.E., and Wojyts, E.M.: Current concepts: A statistical primer. Am. J. Surg. Med. 24:3–6; 25:1–6; 26:1–3.

Hennekens, C.H., Buring, J.E., and Mayrent, S.L., eds.: Epidemiology in Medicine. Boston, Little Brown & Co., 1987.

Hinkle, D.E., Jurs, S.G., and Wiersma, W.: Applied Statistics for the Behavioral Sciences. Boston, Houghton-Mifflin, 1979.

Hulley, S.R., and Cumings, S.R., eds.: Designing Clinical Research. Baltimore, Williams & Wilkins, 1988.

Ingelfinger, J.A., Mosteller, F., Thibodeau, L.A., et al., eds.: Biostatistics in Clinical Medicine, 3rd ed. New York, McGraw-Hill, 1994.

Kelsey, J.L., ed.: Epidemiology of Musculoskeletal Disorders. New York, Oxford University Press, 1982.

Kreder, H.J., Wright, J.G., and McLeod, R.: Outcome studies in surgical research. Surgery 121:223–225, 1997.

Laupacis, A., Sekar, N., and Stiell, G.: Clinical prediction rules: A review and suggested modifications of methodological standards. J.A.M.A. 277:488–494, 1997.

Lieber, R.L.: Experimental design and statistical analysis. In Simon, S.R., ed.: Orthopaedic Basic Science. Chicago, AAOS, 1994.

Martin, D.P., Engelberg, R., Agel, J., et al.: Development of a musculoskeletal extremity health status instrument: The Musculoskeletal Function Assessment Instrument. J. Orthop. Res. 14:173–181, 1996.

Mozena, J.P., Emerick, C.E., and Black, S.C., eds.: Clinical Guideline Development: An Algorithm Approach. Gaithersburg, Md, Aspen Publishers, 1996.

National Health Lawyers Association: Colloquium report on legal issues related to clinical practice issues. Washington, DC, 1995.

Petitti, D.B., ed.: Meta-Analysis, Decision Analysis, and Cost-Effectiveness Analysis: Methods for Quantitative Synthesis in Medicine. New York, Oxford University Press, 1994.

Rosenberg, A.G.: Practice guidelines. In Beaty, J.H., ed.: Orthopaedic Knowledge Update 6. Am. Acad. Orthop. Surg. 97–102, 1999.

Schootman, M., Powell, J.W., and Albright, J.P.: Statistics in sports injury research. In DeLee, J.C., and Drez, D., Jr.: Orthopaedics Sports Medicine: Principles of Practice. Philadelphia, WB Saunders, 1994.

Szabo, R.M.: Statistical analysis as related to hand surgery. J. Hand Surg. 22A:376–384, 1997.

Szklo, M.: Design and conduct of epidemiological studies. Prev. Med. 16:142–149, 1987.

Whimster, W.F.: Biomedical Research. New York, Springer-Verlag, 1997.

Winslade, W.J.: The Texas Medical Jurisprudence Examination: A Self-Study Guide. Texas: University of Texas Medical Branch, 1997.

World Medical Association Declaration of Helsinki, Ethical Principles for Medical Research Involving Human Subjects. 52nd WMA General Assembly, Edinburgh, Scotland, October 2000.

Wright, J.G.: Outcomes Assessment. In Beaty, J.H., ed.: Orthopaedic Knowledge Update 6. Am. Acad. Orthop. Surg. 103–106, 1999.

Wright, J.G., McLeod, R.S., and Lossing, A.: Measurement in surgical clinical research. Surgery 119:241–244, 1996.

Index

Page numbers followed by f indicate figures; t, tables; b, boxes.

B

C

D

E

F

I

J

K

L

M

N

O

P

Q

R

S

T

U

V

W

X

Y